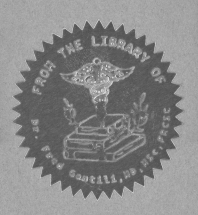

OUTPATIENT SURGERY

EDITED BY

GEORGE J. HILL, II, M.D.

Professor of Surgery
Washington University School of Medicine
St. Louis

formerly
Associate Professor of Surgery
University of Colorado School of Medicine
Denver

W. B. SAUNDERS COMPANY · PHILADELPHIA · LONDON · TORONTO

W. B. Saunders Company: West Washington Square
Philadelphia, Pa.   19105

12 Dyott Street
London, WC1A 1DB

833 Oxford Street
Toronto, Ontario M8Z 5T9, Canada

Outpatient Surgery   ISBN 0-7216-4675-1

Print No: 9   8   7   6   5   4   3   2

To Lanie,
for infinite patience

Contributors

M. DENNIS BARTON, M.D. Assistant Professor of Anesthesiology, University of Colorado School of Medicine. Attending Anesthesiologist, University of Colorado Medical Center, Veterans Administration Hospital, Denver General Hospital, Denver, Colorado.

WATSON A. BOWES, JR., M.D. Associate Professor of Obstetrics and Gynecology, University of Colorado Medical Center, Denver, Colorado. Consultant, Fort Carson Army Hospital, Fort Carson, Colorado.

PAUL W. BROWN, M.D. Professor of Orthopaedic Surgery, Chief, Division of Hand Surgery, Department of Orthopaedics and Rehabilitation, University of Miami School of Medicine. Chief of Hand Surgery, Jackson Memorial Hospital; Consultant in Hand Surgery, Veterans Administration Hospital, Miami, Florida.

JOHN D. BURRINGTON, M.D., F.R.C.S.(C), F.A.A.P. Associate Professor of Surgery, University of Colorado Medical Center. Surgeon-in-Chief, Children's Hospital; Consultant in Pediatric Surgery, Fitzsimons Army General Hospital, Denver, Colorado.

JAMES R. CERASOLI, M.D. Assistant Professor of Ophthalmology, University of Colorado School of Medicine. Chief, Ophthalmology, Denver General Hospital, Consultant, Denver Veterans Administration Hospital, Denver, Colorado.

THOMAS K. CRAIGMILE, M.D. Associate Clinical Professor of Neurological Surgery, University of Colorado School of Medicine Attending Neurosurgeon, Colorado General Hospital, Veterans Administration Hospital, St. Joseph Hospital, Presbyterian Hospital, St. Luke's Hospital, General Rose Memorial Hospital, Denver, Colorado.

ALFRED J. DE FALCO, M.D. Associate Clinical Professor of Surgery, University of Colorado School of Medicine, Attending Staff, Children's Hospital, Lutheran Hospital, St. Anthony Hospital, Colorado General Hospital; Consultant, Fitzsimons Army General Hospital, Denver, Colorado.

WILLIAM DROEGEMUELLER, M.D. Associate Professor of Obstetrics and Gynecology, University of Colorado Medical Center, Denver, Colorado.

BEN EISEMAN, M.D. Professor of Surgery, University of Colorado School of Medicine. Director of Surgery, Denver General Hospital, Denver, Colorado.

GERALD M. ENGLISH, M.D. Assistant Clinical Professor of Otolaryngology, University of Colorado School of Medicine. Chief of Otolaryngology, Porter Swedish Hospital. Attending Staff, General Rose Memorial Hospital, Denver Veterans Administration Hospital, Denver Children's Hospital, St. Luke's Hospital, Denver General Hospital, St. Anthony Hospital, Denver, Colorado.

JOHN Q. GALLAGHER, M.D. Assistant Clinical Professor of Surgery, University of Colorado School of Medicine. Attending Surgeon, University of Colorado Medical Center, Presbyterian Medical Center, St. Joseph Hospital, Denver, Colorado.

LELAND G. HAWKINS, M.D. Associate Professor of Surgery, University of Colorado School of Medicine. Chief, Division of Orthopedic Surgery, Denver General Hospital, Denver, Colorado.

GEORGE J. HILL, II, M.D. Professor of Surgery, Washington University School of Medicine. Chief, Washington University Surgical Service, St. Louis City Hospital; Assistant Attending Surgeon, Barnes Hospital; Staff Surgeon, St. Louis Veterans Administration Hospital, St. Louis, Missouri.

ROBERT R. LARSEN, M.D. Clinical Instructor in Surgery, Denver General Hospital, Denver, Colorado.

MELVIN M. NEWMAN, M.D. Associate Professor of Surgery, University of Colorado School of Medicine. Attending Staff, Colorado General Hospital, Denver, Colorado.

LAWRENCE W. NORTON, M.D. Associate Professor of Surgery, University of Colorado School of Medicine. Assistant Director of Surgery, Denver General Hospital; Attending Surgeon, Colorado General Hospital; Staff, St. Joseph Hospital, Presbyterian Hospital, General Rose Memorial Hospital, Denver, Colorado.

J. CUTHBERT OWENS, M.D. Professor of Surgery, University of Colorado School of Medicine, Denver, Colorado.

BRUCE C. PATON, M.R.C.P.(Ed.), F.R.C.S.(Ed.) Professor of Surgery, University of Colorado School of Medicine. Attending Staff, Colorado General Hospital, Denver General Hospital, Denver Veterans Administration Hospital; Consultant, Fitzsimons Army General Hospital, Denver, Colorado.

ISRAEL PENN, M.D., F.R.C.S.(Eng.), F.R.C.S.(C.) Associate Professor of Surgery, University of Colorado School of Medicine. Chief of Surgery, Veterans Administration Hospital; Attending Surgeon, Colorado General Hospital, General Rose Memorial Hospital, Children's Hospital, Denver, Colorado.

NORMAN E. PETERSON, M.D. Assistant Professor of Urology, University of Colorado School of Medicine. Chief, Division of Urology, Denver General Hospital. Consultant in Urology, Veterans Administration Hospital, Denver, Colorado.

ERICK R. RATZER, M.D. Assistant Clinical Professor of Surgery, University of Colorado School of Medicine. Attending Surgeon, Colorado General Hospital, Veterans Administration Hospital; Staff, Presbyterian Hospital, St. Joseph Hospital, General Rose Memorial Hospital, Denver General Hospital; Director, Bonfils Tumor Clinic, University of Colorado Medical Center, Denver, Colorado.

SHELDON ROGER, M.D. Clinical Instructor in Surgery, University of Colorado School of Medicine. Attending Staff, General Rose Memorial Hospital, Mercy

Hospital, Presbyterian Hospital, Children's Hospital, Veterans Administration Hospital, Denver, Colorado.

WILLIAM ROBERT ROSS, D.P.M. Chief, Podiatry Clinic, Denver General Hospital, Denver, Colorado.

ROBERT B. RUTHERFORD, M.D. Associate Professor of Surgery, Univeristy of Colorado School of Medicine. Director of Emergency Services, University of Colorado Medical Center, Denver, Colorado.

JOHN EDWARD LAWSON SALES, M.A., M. Chir., F.R.C.S. Senior Surgical Registrar, St. Bartholomew's Hospital; Clinical Assistant, St. Mark's Hospital, London, England.

R. C. A. WEATHERLEY-WHITE, M.A., M.D. Assistant Clinical Professor of Surgery (Plastic). University of Colorado School of Medicine. Chief, Plastic Surgery Section, Denver General Hospital; Attending Plastic Surgeon, St. Joseph Hospital, Children's Hospital, Denver, Colorado.

DAVID S. WOLF, D.P.M. Volunteer Faculty, University of Colorado Medical Center, Denver, Colorado. Staff Podiatrist, La Junta Medical Center, La Junta, Colorado.

Foreword

In 1966, George J. Hill, II, M.D. joined the faculty of the University of Colorado with an appointment of Instructor in the Department of Surgery. Although he was originally from the Midwest, his professional associations for the preceding decade had been on the East Coast, mostly at Harvard. In the ensuing seven years from 1966 to 1973, Dr. Hill rose on the academic ladder at the University of Colorado to the rank of Associate Professor of Surgery. The combination of his early and later associations made him an eloquent spokesman for outpatient surgery as it has been and is practiced in widely separated parts of the country. This breadth of view, as well as his special talents as a writer, editor, and organizer, made him an ideal choice to undertake the difficult task of producing a worthy successor to the historically important *Christopher's Textbook of Minor Surgery*. The job was completed just before Dr. Hill moved in January, 1973, to St. Louis, with the appointment of Professor of Surgery at Washington University and Chief of Surgery, St. Louis City Hospital.

The contributors to this volume were recruited exclusively from the faculty of the University of Colorado. Their position in the administrative framework of the Medical School at the time they prepared their chapters is of interest. Eleven of the authors held full-time appointments at the Colorado General or the Veterans Administration Hospitals. Five had full-time appointments at the Denver General Hospital. An additional ten were private practitioners who were donating their time with either token financial remuneration or none at all. The magnitude of input from the volunteer faculty provides some insight into the community support that Colorado surgeons have provided for their state university.

A group versatile enough to provide excellent coverage of so many topics of ambulatory care cannot be developed overnight, and this is particularly true when most of the input is from a single department. For the last twenty years, the Department of Surgery at the University of Colorado has grown and differentiated under the wise stewardship of two exceptional Chairmen, Dr. Henry Swan, II, from 1950 to 1961, and Dr. William R. Waddell, from 1961 to 1972. Both attracted talented staff members by fostering daring and imaginative innovations in surgery. But, at the same time, they encouraged and insisted upon the highest professional performance in less dramatic activities. This premium on quality as expressed by Dr. George Hill and his collaborators has quite naturally extended to the outpatient clinics that provide the setting for the text that follows.

THOMAS E. STARZL, M.D., PH.D.

Professor and Chairman
Department of Surgery
University of Colorado School of Medicine

Preface

The weary, frightened faces crowded together in the waiting rooms of large hospitals and busy offices are a constant reminder that our methods are imperfect and we must labor to improve them. This book was prepared to assist in the delivery of more effective, efficient care to all who appear at the doors of our medical facilities — to help surgeons and their assistants select, treat and release those patients who can be managed in the context of the Outpatient Department. Anyone who has heard the commotion, smelled the fear and anger, and seen the turmoil of the Outpatient Department will appreciate the need for better service in this area. It is to this end the authors have worked to prepare a guide for outpatient surgery.

GEORGE J. HILL
St. Louis, Missouri   63110

Acknowledgments

The editor is indebted to many of his colleagues for the opportunity to write and to assemble this information. The impetus to initiate the project came from Mr. John Dusseau, Vice-President of W. B. Saunders Company, and from Dr. Ben Eiseman, Professor of Surgery and Chief of Surgery at Denver General Hospital.

Many physicians, surgeons, students and laymen have contributed ideas and assistance toward the completion of this book. It is possible to mention only a few of these men and women here, and it is my hope that many others will recognize their contributions within the text. It is particularly fitting to thank the patients and their families who suffered during the trials and errors of the authors during their years as students and resident surgeons.

I particularly appreciate the time spent by my teachers and preceptors at the Peter Bent Brigham Hospital, and give special thanks for the many hours which Dr. John Brooks spent in the Surgical Outpatient Department with the house staff. Dr. Francis Moore, Dr. Robert Gross, Dr. Dwight Harken, Dr. Richard Wilson, Dr. Joseph Murray, Dr. Richard Warren and Dr. John Shillito all gave unselfishly of their time, demonstrating and assisting in outpatient or office practice. Among my fellow residents, Dr. Judson Randolph, Dr. Menelaos Aliapoulios and Dr. C. E. Zimmerman showed exceptional skill in the difficult challenge of outpatient surgery.

My past experiences as an observer and outpatient surgeon in areas outside of university hospitals have played a large role in the formulation of this book. The doctors and ranchers of Wheatland County, Montana, are responsible for these experiences—especially Mr. and Mrs. Wilbur "Pete" White, and Mr. and Mrs. Robert T. Stevens. The physicians and citizens of Carroll County, New Hampshire, have played a similar role in demonstrating the needs and opportunities in outpatient work—in particular, Mr. and Mrs. James Simonds, and the Rev. and Mrs. David Works.

I am pleased to acknowledge the comments and suggestions made by the staff of the U. S. Naval Dispensary, Kodiak, Alaska, and the staff and directors of the Hospital de Apartado, Antioquia, Colombia, South America, particularly Mr. and Mrs. David Parry. I continue to draw on the memories and medical challenges presented by my fellow members of the Harvard Mountaineering Club in expeditions and weekend climbs.

This book was prepared by a long-distance cooperative effort between the authors, in Denver, and our invaluable artist, Mrs. Dorothy Irwin, in Toronto, and the staff of W. B. Saunders Company, in Philadelphia, which included Mr. John Hanley, Mr. Herb Powell and Miss Lorraine Battista. Various parts of the text were read and valuable comments were offered by Dr. Jurgen Kogler, Dr. Theodore Eickhoff, Dr. Jack Chang, Dr. E. H. Fralick, and Dr. Kent Kirkland. The text was faithfully typed and collated by Miss Nancy Matthews, and by my secretary, Mrs. Kathy Krall.

Of the many other students and faculty who helped directly or indirectly with this work, I wish to give thanks especially to Dr. William R. Waddell, to the summer student Fellows supported by the United States Public Health Service, to Miss Priscilla Parkin, and to my students in Surgery 520, "Clinical Applications of the Basic Sciences."

This work was supported in part by a Junior Faculty Fellowship of The American Cancer Society, by donations to the Cancer Chemotherapy Account and by United States Public Health Service grants CA12204, CA8086, and FR00051.

Finally, I wish to acknowledge the continuous enthusiasm registered by my children, David, Sarah and Helena, and the almost unbelievable patience and help given by my wife.

Contents

Introduction

C'est par l'etude de La Petite Chirurgie que le chirurgien commence son apprentissage.

— MAISONNET

I think that there ought to be a book in the hands of the pupil to direct him in his studies . . . in which the lessons he has detailed to him at length by his teachers may be found more shortly expressed . . . to which, as a surgeon, he can turn for the detail of what is necessary to be done in preparing for an operation . . .

Every surgeon . . . ought to bring his judgment maturely to bear on all the points of the case; the objects to be attained; the dangers to be expected; the resources which he ought to have in readiness against probable mischance . . .

By anticipating he may avoid embarrassment, maintain his self-possession undisturbed, and save himself from the distraction of consultation and whispering.

SIR CHARLES BELL (1774–1842), *Professor of Surgery, University of Edinburgh ("Bell's palsy")*

This book was written to help young surgeons, interns and medical students in their work outside of the regular inpatient hospital wards. The major theme is the diagnosis and treatment of surgical patients in the Outpatient Clinic, Emergency Room and overnight ward.

We wish to encourage outpatient care whenever it can be done safely, for the economic burden is thereby reduced, the anxiety of the patient alleviated, and the danger of hospital-acquired sepsis is in part relieved.

Outpatient care is frequently delegated to junior house staff with relatively little supervision. A large patient load is thrust upon the young surgeon, and he has responsibility to make prompt and accurate decisions. The patient desires economy, speed, accuracy and sympathy. Since many outpatient procedures must be done under local anesthesia, awareness of the patient's pain and anxiety is essential for success.

Mixed in with routine or relatively minor problems, sudden emergencies may appear which require an entirely different magnitude of treatment. Usually these patients will soon be transferred to inpatient status, but responsibility for them is initially that of the outpatient surgeon. Guidelines for management of major surgical emergencies are therefore included as an integral part of this text.

Relatively minor complaints may be the hallmark of a serious impending crisis. The outpatient surgeon must be alert to these possibilities.

We have included descriptions of conditions and operations which can be treated by utilizing an overnight period of observation, because many hospitals have a small overnight ward adjacent to the outpatient-emergency facility under the control of the outpatient surgical team.[11] Patients may therefore be operated upon in the main operating room or undergo major diagnostic procedures such as angiography as part of their stay in the Outpatient Department, since they can be placed in a regular hospital bed to recover for up to 24 hours.[13] Many patients can be handled in this way only if they can return either to a good home or to an ambulatory care facility staffed with competent personnel. Procedures such as herniorrhaphy, saphenous vein surgery, lung biopsy, and cervical cone biopsy appear in this context.

All of the procedures described in this book have been performed as described by the authors. These are procedures which can technically be performed in an Outpatient Clinic and a well-outfitted Emergency Room which is equipped for brief major operations, and in which convalesence is speedy enough to permit release from the hospital within 24 hours. Nevertheless, we recommend that good judgment be used in selecting patients for outpatient surgery. It must be remembered that the patient should always be hospitalized if there is any question regarding the advisability of performing the procedure in the office or outpatient department, or as an overnight admission to the hospital.

Outpatient Surgery incorporates many of the ideas developed for American physicians by Frederick Christopher in Minor Surgery (1930), based on the previous textbooks by Wharton, Foote, Maisonnet and Hertzler, and the immensely popular Manual of Minor Surgery by Heath which appeared in 20 editions. Christopher's textbook was a classic which was published in six editions over an 18-year period, and which was carried on in two additional editions by Drs. Alton Ochsner and Michael DeBakey. Members of the Department of Surgery at the University of Colorado began to work together on a description of their work in this field in 1967. The first publication of this team effort was the volume of Surgical Clinics of North America entitled Improved Techniques in Everyday Surgery (1969), edited by Dr. Ben Eiseman. Outpatient Surgery is a textbook which was designed to carry forward the work which was begun by Drs. Christopher, Ochsner, DeBakey and Eiseman.

The topics presented here cover subjects which comprise most of the entire field of surgery, which we define as the healing art which utilizes physical procedures such as incision, repair and other manipulations. Thus the specialties of gynecology and obstetrics, anesthesi-

ology, podiatry, transplantation and oncology are represented, as well as the conventional categories of general surgery, trauma, cardiovascular and thoracic surgery, otolaryngology, urology, plastic surgery, pediatric surgery, orthopedics and proctology. Special chapters are presented regarding surgical considerations in areas far removed from teaching hospitals, such as developing countries and expeditions into remote areas. The latter topics are covered in this text because of the interest which many young surgeons have shown in extending their service into these very special outpatient situations. We also wish to acknowledge the fact that the procedures used in the outpatient department of American university hospitals are not necessarily the procedures which will or should be used in developing countries[8] or remote areas.

The authors have described the conditions and treatments which constitute the majority of their own outpatient practice. In some instances, the work is primarily diagnostic, whereas in other clinics it consists in large part of minor and major operations. In every case, each author has presented his personal experience as a guide for the young men and women who plan to work in the outpatient specialty clinics and offices.

The long-term follow-up of all patients will be emphasized, since the results of inpatient care must be measured by the surgeon in his office or outpatient clinic over an extended period of time.[2]

It is our hope that this text may serve as a useful reference for office practice as well as for the hospital Outpatient Department. The degree to which this will be possible will obviously vary greatly with the facilities, assistance, training and skill of the physician who uses this book.

References

1. Bell, C.: A System of Operative Surgery Founded on the Basis of Anatomy. 1st

American ed. Hartford, Goodwin, 1816 (pp. iv–v).

2. Brook, R. H., Appel, F. A., Avery, C., Orman, M., and Stevenson, R. L.: Effectiveness of inpatient follow-up care. New Eng. J. Med., *285*:1509–1514, 1972.

3. Christopher, F.: Minor Surgery. 1st–6th eds. Philadelphia, W. B. Saunders Co., 1930–1948.

4. Eiseman, B. (ed.): Improved Techniques in Everyday Surgery. Surg. Clin. N. Amer., *49*(6):1199–1553, 1969.

5. Foote, E. M.: A Textbook of Minor Surgery. 1st–5th eds. New York, Appleton Century Crofts, 1908–1924.

6. Heath, C.: A Manual of Minor Surgery and Bandaging for the Use of House Surgeons, Dressers and Junior Practitioners. 1st–20th eds. Philadelphia, Blakiston and F. A. Davis Co., 1861–1930. Late editions by G. Williams.

7. Hertzler, A. E., and Chesky, V. E.: Minor Surgery. St. Louis, C. V. Mosby Co., 1927.

8. Ingelfinger, F. J.: Western medicine in tropical islands. New Eng. J. Med., *285*:1535–1536, 1972.

9. Maisonnet, P. J. F. R.: Petite Chirurgie. 1st–4th eds. Paris, G. Doin & Cie, 1928–1942.

10. Ochsner, A., and DeBakey, M. E. (eds.): Christopher's Minor Surgery. 7th–8th eds. Philadelphia, W. B. Saunders Co., 1955–1959.

11. Ruckley, C. V., MacLean, Mary, Smith, A. M., and Falconer, C. W. A.: Team approach to early discharge and outpatient surgery. Lancet, *1*:177–180, 1971.

12. Wharton, H. R.: Minor Surgery and Bandaging. 1st–6th eds. Philadelphia, Lea Bros., 1891–1905.

13. Zimmerman, C. E.: Techniques of Patient Care; A Manual of Bedside Procedures for Students, Interns and Residents. Boston, Little, Brown and Co., 1970.

1

Organization – Design, Function and Operation of Outpatient Clinics and Emergency Rooms

By ROBERT B. RUTHERFORD, M.D.

CURRENT PROBLEMS IN EMERGENCY AND OUTPATIENT CARE

The patterns of utilization of both the Emergency Department and Outpatient Clinics of U.S. hospitals have changed greatly in the last decade. To date, most of the changes have been unintentionally brought about by changing patient or "consumer" practices. Indeed, a significant proportion of the operational problems currently plaguing our Emergency Rooms and other Outpatient facilities can be traced to the hospital's failure to appreciate or adequately adjust to changes in the public's attitude and approach to obtaining medical care.

Thus, most of the current changes represent stop-gap measures and quantitative adjustments rather than basic or qualitative changes in the system of health care delivery. However, with increasing awareness of the problems and the need for change among physicians and hospital administrators, with continuing public pressure and with federal and state governments and other "third parties" playing an increasing role as the patient's advocate in establishing standards and exerting controls governing the provision and cost of health care, most substantive if not radical changes can be anticipated in the coming decade. Whether or not the final product or system will embody any of the relatively new concepts such as the health maintenance organization, the Surgi-Center, the convenience clinic or the neighborhood health center, or the newly emerging health professionals such as the full-time "emergency physician," nurse-practitioner, physician's associate or emergency medical technician remains to be seen.

Most existing emergency rooms were originally designed, equipped, staffed and organized to deal with the acutely ill and injured. Outpatient clinics, on the other hand, have generally been geared toward new or unsolved problems of a nonemergent nature, but with the emphasis on outpatient diagnostic evaluation as a basis for definitive therapeutic decisions, whether or not the latter involves admission or operation. In the past, any outpatient treatment or long-term follow-up of these problems was usually left to the patient's primary physician, the same physician who cared for his acute self-limited illnesses and other "minor" medical problems and provided for regular physical check-ups and the long-term care of chronic illnesses.

However, increasing medical specialization and the decreasing number and availability of general practitioners and other physicians providing primary medical care, increasing population growth and motility (the latter disrupting and discouraging the re-establishment of stable doctor-patient relationships), increasing expectations on the part of the patient and his physician (particularly in terms of the more complex diagnostic equipment and therapeutic facilities offered by the hospital as opposed to the physician's office), and the increasing influence of third party medical payment plans have all contributed to increased utilization of hospital emergency and outpatient clinic facilities by the public.

Most hospitals' outpatient clinics, particularly in the larger institutions, have not really attempted to accommodate this demand. To the contrary, many of them have followed, if not led, the way to increasing specialization by em-

phasizing secondary or tertiary rather than primary medical care, so that in major hospitals today, the patient usually finds himself in a menage of clinics with labels such as cleft palate, cancer chemotherapy, renal hypertension, audiology, epilepsy, glaucoma, hand, orthoptics, peripheral vascular, speech, adolescent psychiatry, collagen vascular, pediatric allergy, and so on. Attempts to have even a simple complaint such as persistent headaches evaluated and treated in such a setting frequently result in multiple visits to different specialty clinics interspersed with long delays, an unfortunate and too common situation which has been labeled "outpatient ping pong." Even if the cause of the patient's complaint is fairly evident, the decision as to which clinic he should be sent to is not always clear to someone unfamiliar with the hospital's ground rules.

While these particular problems are more likely to be encountered in the major medical centers, the patient is likely to be confronted with a loosely coordinated menage of specialty clinics in any sizable hospital, each with its limited hours of operation, restrictive admission policies, and long waiting times. The cost, let alone the time consumed (particularly for the working patient) in seeking medical care in the traditionally organized outpatient clinic, may be prohibitive. On the other hand, there stands the Emergency Room, completely equipped, staffed in all specialties, and open to the public night and day. The inevitable and predictable result, given these factors, has been called the "Emergency Room population explosion." The patient census of many hospital emergency departments has doubled and in some cases tripled in the last decade, and the rate of increase is accelerating. Thus, whereas the inpatient admissions increased by 8 per cent per capita in this country in the 60's and outpatient visits increased by 18 per cent, Emergency Room visits increased by 79 per cent; and whereas the rate of increase in outpatient census was four times greater than that of the inpatient between 1952 and 1962, in the next decade it was approximately eight times greater.

However, the problem is greater than statistics alone would indicate because those same Emergency Rooms that were designed, equipped and staffed to deal with emergent or at least urgent medical problems now find themselves obliged to provide services formerly rendered by office visits or house calls made by physicians practicing in the community. Currently, this type of patient constitutes approximately two-thirds of the national Emergency Room census. Such patients indirectly interfere with the effective delivery of care to the true or serious emergencies, although in general, once the acutely ill or injured person has reached a major medical facility, emergency medical care is excellent and continues to improve. Treatment priorities often dictate that the patients with relatively minor or nonurgent problems must wait the *longest* time for the *least* treatment. Pressure on the emergency department staff to keep up with this flood of patients not only is responsible for treatment errors (mainly those of omission) but often leads to hurried impersonal care which, when combined with long waiting times, creates a degree of friction between the patients and the Emergency Room staff which is a source of most of the unpleasant incidents which erupt there.

The practice of treating nonemergent problems in an emergency department results in "episodic, expensive and ineffective" medical care. Patients pay double for this "convenience," since they are charged both a physician's fee for service and a facilities fee which is necessarily high because of expensive equipment, drugs and other supplies kept on hand for the management of all kinds of emergencies. Furthermore, there is a tendency for the attending physician to order more laboratory and x-ray studies on these patients than he would if he were the patient's regular physician, and there is usually little follow-up care

and a great deal of repetition by each of the several physicians who may treat these patients over the course of a year of episodic walk-in medical care. Thus, while it may be referred to as "supermarket medicine," the use of an Emergency Room to obtain nonemergent medical care provides only the convenience of availability and not the speed, efficiency and inexpensive features one expects at the neighborhood supermarket.

It is clear, then, that major changes are needed in our system (if it may be called that) of delivering ambulatory or outpatient care. To be successful, not only must whatever changes evolve lead to better, more comprehensive medical care at a reasonable cost, but they will have to do so in a way that is convenient, logical and attractive enough to gain public acceptance. Too much of the current public "abuse" of emergency care facilities has been blamed on lack of patient education. While this may be a problem, it must be appreciated that the public will not use outpatient facilities in the intended way if they do not satisfy the patient's needs and expectations, regardless of how well they are indoctrinated and how well the facilities are conceived and organized from the point of view of the hospital and its medical staff.

DESIGN OF EMERGENCY AND OUTPATIENT CARE FACILITIES

General Approach

The planning and building of an outpatient or emergency care facility involves several rather distinct phases:

1. *The program planning phase.* This includes determining the need for the facility and its role in the delivery of health care in the community at large and within the hospital complex itself. It must determine the intended scope of capabilities and the medical and surgi-

cal services it will offer, estimating the cost of the facility and its financial feasibility in terms of the availability of construction funds. A master plan and schematic drawings must be completed.

2. *The physical planning phase*, in which final architectural drawings are completed and construction documents are drawn up.

3. *The actual construction phase*.

4. *The "moving-in" phase*, in which painting, decorations and internal furnishings are completed and movable equipment is installed.

Bids for architectural and construction firms are let out between each of the first three phases respectively, and the whole process usually requires three to five years from start to finish. Although it is recognized that the major input from the medical staff must go into the initial phase, the importance of involving the architects as early as possible is not generally appreciated. It is advantageous to involve them during the conceptual period, long before the formal architectural work actually begins. One cannot expect an architect to come up with a good functional design if he has not received adequate input from the hospital staff.

The individual characteristics of each hospital and its staff, the community in which it is located and the patient population which it serves vary so widely that no single design concept will prove universally satisfactory. Therefore one should beware of pre-packaged or "off the shelf" plans. Nothing less than a custom-tailored job will do, and nowhere is the advice that architectural "design must be based on function" more applicable. Careful prospective study of precisely the same variables offers the best prospect for success in planning for a new, expanded or renovated emergency or outpatient facility.

But before focusing on the actual design or internal features of the new facility, there is a series of basic preliminary steps which must be taken. One must first establish the need for the new facility as well as the availability of construction funds before going very far. The next step is to establish clearly the type of care to be offered in this new facility. In doing this, differences must be resolved between the type of care the hospital can provide and the type of care the community needs and seeks. Considerations must be based on the desires and capabilities of the medical staff and the type of care offered by other facilities in the same area. The importance of these points and the need to have them settled at the outset cannot be overemphasized. It may seem that most hospitals let community needs determine the type of care they give and the manner in which it will be provided. However, this is rarely the sole determinant and sometimes not even the major one. Administratively, most hospitals exercise a number of constraints over outpatient as well as inpatient admissions. These constraints are frequently present even if they are not formally set forth in the form of eligibility rules pertaining to residency, financial status, service-connected disability, and so forth. A subtler but equally powerful influence is the attitude of the medical staff toward patient care. For example, the faculty of a university hospital might feel that it should attempt to function as a referral center for problems of special interest or complexity and not provide community health care in its broadest sense. Such an attitude would not be readily apparent to patients from the community presenting themselves for care at that hospital nor would it influence their choice. Those responsible for organizing outpatient and emergency care in such institutions will find themselves caught in the middle in this situation.

The situation in community hospitals presents other difficulties. Established practitioners on the staffs of these hospitals understandably wish to center (and schedule) their own outpatient care activities in their offices. They may rarely use the hospital's outpatient clinics and may view the Emergency Room as a convenient place in which to meet their private patients to handle off-hour emergencies or to perform special procedures for which their offices are not adequately equipped. Many of these hospitals are encountering increasing difficulties in providing adequate coverage for their Emergency Rooms and Outpatient Clinics from their own "volunteer" staff.

Obviously these two different situations require entirely different approaches in the organization and planning of outpatient operations. It should be clear that the guiding philosophies behind each institution's outpatient activities need to be formally clarified at the highest administrative level and approval of the medical staff must be gained before proceeding very far with the actual design phase.

Similarly, the patient population to be served by this outpatient facility should be analyzed and sufficient demographic data obtained to identify not only the present patient population but also changing trends that will affect its future make-up. Finally, one must investigate all other existing or planned outpatient facilities in the community or region. More than one metropolitan medical center has found its outpatient facilities overwhelmed as one or more neighboring hospitals have joined in the flight to the suburbs. Nor is it a unique situation for two neighboring hospitals to launch independent expansion programs almost simultaneously for their outpatient and emergency care facilities. This lack of inter-hospital cooperation, communication and coordination is responsible for the emergence of regional medical planning programs.

The contemporary movement toward *categorization* of emergency medical facilities is a first step in regional medical planning. Standards have been drawn up by the A.M.A. Commission on Emergency Medical Services for four distinct levels of capability in providing emergency medical services. Professional staffing, facilities and equipment, supporting diagnostic services and intensive care units, and communications capabilities are evaluated in four categories: I (Comprehensive); II (Major); III(General); and IV (Basic Emergency Medical Services). It is anticipated that these guidelines will be adopted and categorization will be accomplished with the voluntary cooperation of the hospitals by survey questionnaire and site visit. It is felt that each hospital should be allowed to achieve as high a category as it wishes. Each will be expected to function effectively at its chosen level of capability, participating in the regional planning for the delivery of emergency medical services. This movement recognizes that not all hospitals have the capability or desire to handle any and all emergencies, but that all should at least have an effective capability for resuscitation and referral. It is based on the assumption that a more efficient system of delivering emergency medical care should result from establishing the specific capabilities and desires of each hospital. Obviously these standards must be kept in mind in building a new or enlarged facility, since the standard guidelines will probably serve as a major basis for successful application for federal funds to support such a building program.

Other preliminary considerations include the determination of basic space needs, the choice between expansion and renovation versus rebuilding, and the selection of the optimum building site. Space needs are difficult to estimate without the help of an experienced architect. There are no universally accepted factors for converting the patient load of an outpatient or emergency department to square footage. Large facilities tend to be more efficient than small ones in minimizing poorly utilized or dead space. Similarly, busy clinics, which have staggered appointment systems and a minimum of special examination or treatment rooms, will require less space for a given patient load. In general, a surgical clinic will handle patients at almost twice the rate of a medical clinic. The average time spent by a surgeon with each patient is 20 minutes, and the complete cycle, allowing time for tidying the room and changing the "linen," for the patient to dress and undress, and for the doctor to complete the patient's medical record usually takes at least one-half hour. Complicated new cases may take twice as long, and simple follow-up visits half this time. However, one should not extend this observation too strictly in planning space. For example, two patients an hour, eight hours a day, per hundred square feet of examining room would *under*estimate the overall space needed by a factor of as much as 10. Appearances to the contrary, even a busy clinic rarely achieves more than a 50 per cent utilization rate and even the most efficient design will require at least 50 per cent of the space for waiting room, corridors, administrative and other nonpatient care areas. Thus in practice, the space needs for an outpatient clinic may run as high as 25 to 50 square feet per patient per day.

One might think that an Emergency Room, open 24 rather than 8 hours daily, would utilize more space more efficiently. However the E.R. must be designed to handle peak loads which may last for only a few hours a day and its spacious and well-equipped trauma-resuscitation area may be in use only 10 per cent of the time. Because of such essential but poorly utilized areas, the smaller emergency departments are usually more inefficient in space utilization. There is no linear conversion factor, but a convenient figure to work from is 10,000 gross square feet for a daily patient load of 100 patients. This may seem high, but one must remember that there are few emergency departments in this country that are big enough to handle the clinical demands placed on them.

The choice between expansion and renovation as opposed to rebuilding is usually not difficult. The availability of construction funds, space in which to expand, and the suitability of the external relationships of the present structure will ordinarily make the choice obvious. It should go without saying that the hospital's various outpatient components should be spatially related to each other in a functional manner and, to a lesser degree, to essential administrative and supporting services. Inappropriate "external" relationships may seriously detract from an otherwise well-conceived Emergency Room plan.

As far as the "internal" design is concerned, it is usually advisable to begin with a rough plan based on patient flow and services performed, and then adjust the size of each area to meet expected peak demands. At this point the architect can complete the details after consultation with the personnel who will be involved in the daily operation of each area. Architects can only produce a satisfactory design if provided with proper and specific information such as magnitude and type of patient load, anticipated maximum patient input rates, nature and frequency of services and procedures performed, special diagnostic or therapeutic equipment, and so forth.

The simplest outpatient facility will consist of a common receiving area for all outpatients, served by a number of basic examining rooms and one large multi-purpose treatment area for special procedures and resuscitation. It should be located close to the hospital's x-ray and laboratory facilities. In larger hospitals, emergency and nonurgent outpatient care should be provided in separate (though preferably adjacent) areas. In most hospitals, a significant proportion of the outpatient traffic is of an unscheduled but nonemergent nature, so there should be a screening clinic located immediately adjacent to the outpatient clinic's main entrance.

Some of the above concepts can be better appreciated from the consideration of Figure 1–1, a schematic representation of the layout of a nonexistent outpatient facility. The oversimplified arrangement depicted here does not indicate the vertical or horizontal access to important inpatient areas and supporting services, such as the operating room and blood bank. Important details of internal design are also deliberately

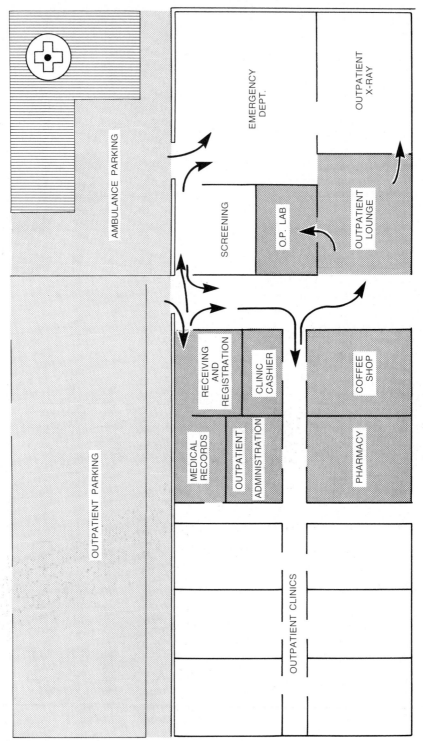

Figure 1–1   A moderate-sized outpatient facility.

omitted. This figure is not intended to recommend a specific plan but to illustrate the considerations involved in arriving at a functionally satisfactory layout. Note, for example, that the Emergency Department parking area is separate from that for general outpatient use. Each parking area should have well-marked, separate access ways to facilitate traffic control. The concept of separate but adjacent entrances is carried from the parking lot into the hospital so that the acutely ill and injured enter directly into the Emergency Department, whereas the ambulatory ill enter through the main outpatient entrance. The main outpatient entrance is flanked by a receiving and registration area on one side and a screening or triage clinic on the other. With this arrangement, the patient can receive proper directions as soon as he enters the outpatient area. He can be registered and his records sent for at the same station. The administrative core area is completed by the clinic cashier and outpatient administrative offices. After registration, the unscheduled patient is seen in the screening clinic and either referred to the Emergency Department or the appropriate Outpatient Clinic, or given simple treatment on the spot. The diagnostic laboratory and the x-ray unit are positioned to serve both the Emergency Department and the Outpatient Clinics. There is a general waiting area located on the outpatient side of the diagnostic facilities and this, in turn, is conveniently located across from a coffee shop or refreshment stand. Adjacent to it, at the exit from the Outpatient Clinic areas, is the pharmacy.

Emergency Department Design

Many of the considerations mentioned above in regard to the overall design of an ambulatory care complex apply individually to the design of an Emergency Department. Again, design should be based on function. However, few Emergency Rooms function identically, so before proceeding with the actual design of a new, expanded or renovated Emergency Department, responsible members of the hospital staff must decide a number of practical questions pertaining to E.R. function.

For example:

Will the Emergency Department function as such in a strict sense, or will it also serve as an ambulance-admitting area or walk-in ambulatory care facility?

Will the surgical and orthopedic treatment areas be used for elective procedures?

Will there be an emergency observation ward or will all patients be admitted to one of the inpatient services?

Will lacerations be sutured, casts applied and abscesses drained in special treatment areas, or in examining cubicles using portable equipment and sterile supplies?

Will patients with major trauma receive resuscitation and definitive diagnostic and therapeutic procedures in the Emergency Department or will they be transferred immediately to either the operating room or intensive care areas?

Will pediatric, medical, surgical, obstetric and gynecological, and psychiatric problems all be seen in a common suite of examining rooms, or will separate, but adjacent facilities be required?

Will patient registration and financial arrangements be handled in the Emergency Department or elsewhere?

Will the Emergency Department serve as the outpatient complex's "front door," or will there be a separate receiving and screening clinic?

Will the Emergency Room serve as a focus for any of the institution's special treatment programs (e.g., alcoholism, drug addiction, hemophilia, asthma)?

Will clinical research be conducted in the Emergency Room?

Will regular educational programs be conducted in the Emergency Room for physicians, medical students, nurses, emergency medical technicians or other allied health personnel?

Will basic diagnostic tests be performed in the Emergency Room, or will all specimens be sent to the main laboratory?

The answers to these and other basic questions about the functional requirements of the Emergency Department will place one in a better position to estimate the basic space requirements as discussed above, keeping in mind future growth, the need to plan for peak loading conditions and the fact that few emergency rooms in this country, including a surprising number less than five years old, are adequate for their current daily operations. Before turning to the details of internal design, the facilities and services whose external relationships are important to the Emergency Department should be carefully considered: blood bank, x-ray department (if there is no x-ray unit in the Emergency Department), diagnostic laboratory, operating room, central receiving and admissions, screening clinic (if separate), other outpatient clinics, medical records, patient parking areas, pharmacy, central supply, and the hospital's "front door." The spatial relationship of the Emergency Department to these other departments may be of great importance.

Attention must also be given to the following aspects of internal design: the need for controlled, orderly patient flow; separate access to the Emergency Department for ambulance and ambulatory patients, and for Emergency Department personnel; adequate waiting areas for patients *and* the friends and relatives who accompany them; special and multipurpose treatment areas; lavatories; dressing rooms; lounges and sleeping quarters for physicians; nurses' lounges and conference rooms for in-service teaching programs; an area for extended observation and treatment (emergency observation ward); areas for storage and supplies; areas for clean and dirty linens; and areas for x-ray and laboratory procedures.

As the details of the Emergency Department layout unfold, compromises will be needed. For example, maximum visibility of the patients by Emergency Department staff is desirable, but on the other hand, there is a need to provide an adequate degree of privacy for special diagnostic or therapeutic procedures. Similarly, in this era of specialization, there is a tendency to develop special areas which are specifically designed and equipped for the management of certain emergencies. If this trend is followed to its inevitable conclusion, the result might be a trauma receiving area, cardiac emergency area, laceration area, poison or overdose area, dirty or incision and drainage area, orthopedic area or cast room, eye, ear, nose and throat examining rooms, gyn or "pelvic" rooms, and minor surgery areas. Only in the largest of emergency departments can this degree of specialization be economically justified. In most medium-sized emergency departments, it is usually preferable to combine all of the special emergency equipment in one spacious trauma-resuscitation area. This equipment includes EKG monitoring, oscilloscope, defibrillator, respirator, Ambu bags, laryngoscopes, endotracheal tubes, emergency drugs, special procedure trays, and catheterization equipment. To avoid unnecessary duplication, the multipurpose examining rooms should be equipped so that they can be used not only for examination but for minor treatments by bringing in portable equipment or special trays of instruments. A selection of equipment includes cast cart, IV cart, incision and drainage tray, and suture tray. For this approach to be successful, the individual examining rooms must be larger than usual and must have good lighting, oxygen, suction and multiple electric outlets. They should be at least 9 by 12 feet in size, preferably 10 by 14 feet, and should be equipped with a good stretcher or mobile cart rather than a fixed examining table.

The following is a series of arbitrary recommendations regarding Emergency Room design and—indirectly—function. Of necessity, they reflect personal opinion and are not intended to represent the final solution. Since they are based on personal experience in specific emergency departments, they might be better appreciated by referring to Figure 1–2, a suggested layout for a

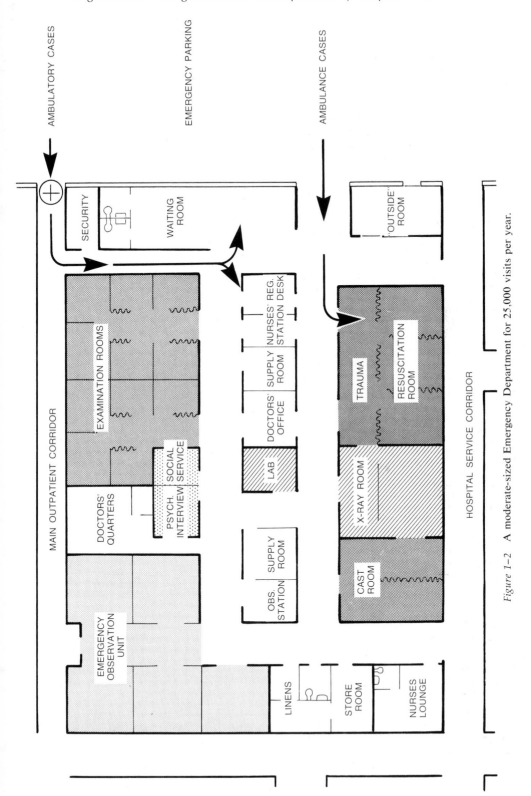

Figure 1–2 A moderate-sized Emergency Department for 25,000 visits per year.

moderate-sized Emergency Department which might comfortably accommodate about 25,000 visits a year. This plan is actually a stylized version of the layout of the Emergency Department at the Colorado General Hospital, with some of the undesirable features excluded and other desirable features included to give a more functional design.

The Emergency Room entrance and parking area should be clearly marked and well lit, with the signs visible from a distance of 75 to 100 yards. Signs indicating the direction of the Emergency Room entrance should also be posted at other main hospital entrances and at major intersections leading to the hospital. The Emergency Room entrance should be partly covered for protection from the elements and there should be room for at least two ambulances to pass and park easily. No extended parking privileges should be allowed at the ambulance entrance itself. If adjacent emergency parking is provided, it should be identifiably separate from ambulance parking and approximately 12 parking spaces should be provided per 20,000 annual visits. Such emergency parking should be closely supervised or it will soon cease to serve the needs of the Emergency Department's patients. The ambulance unloading area should be visible from the front desk within the Emergency Room through clear glass windows or doors. The entrance doors themselves should be double-width as should all the main coridors of the Emergency Department, easily accommodating a stretcher with people walking on both sides. There should be a double set of these doors which open automatically as well as manually in case of power failure. This ambulance entrance should provide direct access to the Emergency Department's receiving area. Thus the seriously ill and injured patients can pass directly into the trauma resuscitation area without going through the main waiting room. There should be a security station near this entrance as well as a "parking space" for additional stretchers and wheel-

chairs (2 per 4000 annual visits). Also near this entrance, there should be an "outside room" with direct and separate access from both outside and inside the Emergency Department. This room can serve as a decontamination station for patients contaminated with radionuclides, riot control gases and other noxious substances which would be undesirable if directly introduced into the internal environment of the Emergency Department. It can also be used for holding patients who are dead on arrival pending their transfer to the morgue or the medical examiner's office. In addition, it may be appropriate to have an area with drop curtains, shower and hose immediately outside this room for large-scale decontamination procedures.

Clearly separate from the ambulance entrance there should be an ambulatory entrance which allows patients to enter the Emergency Department waiting area from both the outside parking lot and a main hospital corridor. The waiting area of the Emergency Department should be large, with at least twice the number of seats as the average number of patients seen per hour. Waiting rooms are usually made too small because of the idealistic philosophy that patients shouldn't have to wait. However, the time and magnitude of peak patient input loads are unpredictable and allowance must also be made for friends and relatives accompanying the patient. The waiting area should be well furnished with television or background music, current reading material, beverage and candy vending machines, adjacent rest rooms and telephones. The reception desk should be open. It should face the Emergency Department entrances and the main waiting area. It is important to avoid having patients and their relatives or friends milling around the reception desk. Ordinarily, each new arriving patient, after stating his problem, should be given a number and asked to take a seat until registration can be completed. On the other hand, if the patient obviously is an emergency requiring immediate evaluation and treatment on admission, he should be ushered promptly into a treatment room. The registration desk should be backed by a nurses' station from which the nurses can clearly see both registering and waiting patients, and which will allow the nurses to be easily consulted by the clerks regarding problem patients. During overload periods, when there is a backup of waiting patients, nurses should make an attempt to go out into the waiting room and at least briefly interview each waiting patient to assess the urgency of their problem and advise them as to the anticipated waiting time they will encounter. An operations control board placed across from the doctor and nurses' office in the patient examining area has been found to be extremely helpful. The name and time of admission of each patient to an examining room as well as their presenting problem is listed and initialed by the nurse at the time of admission. The physician initials the next column to indicate that he has accepted that patient. After examination and treatment, he lists the diagnostic studies and consultations ordered as well as any other items necessary for final disposition. A glance at this board as well as the adjacent boxes of charts of patients not as yet admitted enables the Emergency Department personnel to assess its operational status and decide on appropriate action.

The supply room should be centrally located to minimize unnecessary movement. There should be a separate doctor's station where records can be completed, telephone calls received, consultations made and diagnostic studies reviewed. A small diagnostic laboratory should be provided, in which white counts, hematocrits and urinalysis can be done, and smears stained or cultured, even though most of the studies may be done in the main laboratory. Both the general examining rooms and special treatment areas should be readily accessible and within hearing—if not visible—from the doctors' or nurses' station. Ideally, an x-ray unit should be located inside or immediately adjacent to the Emergency Depart-

ment, preferably between the orthopedic room and the trauma resuscitation area. The x-ray unit should have a multipurpose capability, but most important, it should have a rapid developer. The other features shown in Figure 1–2 are self-explanatory. More will be said of the emergency observation ward subsequently. This design (Figure 1–2) is adequate for a moderate-sized Emergency Room in the true sense of the word. A larger Emergency Room requires considerably more functional specialization, particularly when there is an admixture of nonurgent or ambulatory care problems. Figure 1–3 illustrates the basic layout of an Emergency Department designed to receive 100,000 or more emergency and nonemergent visits annually. It represents a preliminary plan for an expanded emergency and ambulatory care facility to be built at the Colorado General Hospital. It shows a degree of functional separation into specialty areas appropriate only in the largest of emergency departments. The present Emergency Room occupies the upper left hand section of this plan.

Outpatient Clinic Design

The basic purpose of an outpatient clinic is to provide a convenient place for outpatient—physician contact. In its simplest form, an outpatient clinic combines in a single unit: a waiting area, reception desk, nurses' and doctors' stations, and a series of examining or treatment rooms. As in the case of the Emergency Department, the need for compromise between the desirable features of specialization and the economical features of multi-usage is encountered. In the smaller hospital, one often finds a combination of general purpose and specialty examination and treatment rooms combined in a single outpatient clinic. In larger hospitals, one usually encounters a series of specialty clinics. A few of these, such as an ophthalmology or otolaryngology clinic, may require very specialized and fixed examination and treatment facilities. Among the others, the assignment of one or two

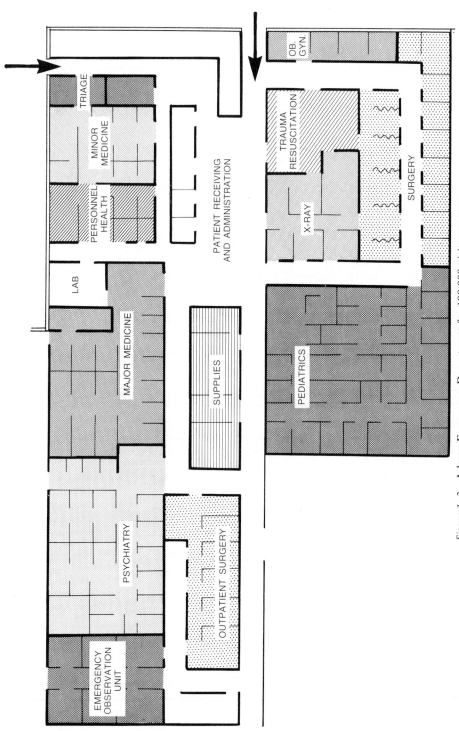

Figure 1–3   A large Emergency Department for 100,000 visits per year.

rooms as special treatment areas will allow multiples of a basic clinic design to be used in overlapping fashion by wide varieties of specialties. With minor adjustments, these special treatment rooms can be used for applying casts, for cystoscopy, for sigmoidoscopy or for surgical dressing changes. Similarly, the judicious use of treatment carts (such as dressing carts or cast carts) will allow the same basic clinic to be used for hematology or dermatology in the morning and orthopedics or urology in the afternoon.

Regardless of the basic clinic layout in terms of waiting room, reception desk, nurses' and doctors' stations and special equipment and supply rooms, the most important part of the design of any out-patient clinic area is the individual examination and treatment room. Figure 1–4 shows three variations on the same

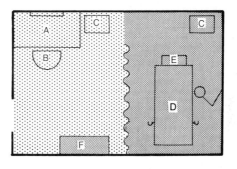

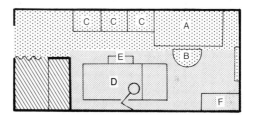

Figure 1–4   Examples of treatment rooms
A — Physician's desk
B — Physician's chair
C — Chairs for patients and relatives, friends or interpretors
D — Examining table
E — Foot stool
F — Supply cabinet

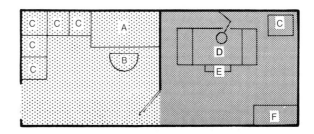

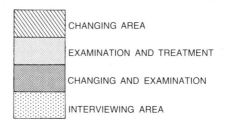

CHANGING AREA

EXAMINATION AND TREATMENT

CHANGING AND EXAMINATION

INTERVIEWING AREA

theme, each differing slightly in size and elaborateness. Each provides for a patient interview, undressing and dressing, and examination and treatment (with portable treatment carts) within the same unit. This arrangement allows the doctor and patient (with a relative or interpreter if necessary) to go quickly through the steps of interview, undressing, and examination. If necessary, treatment can be given with a minimum of interruption, embarrassment or scene changing. The size of these rooms will vary between 9 by 12 and 10 by 14 feet. In most surgical clinics, these rooms will include a modified dressing cart and a wash basin.

EMERGENCY OBSERVATION UNIT

The emergency observation unit is a controversial feature of many large Emergency Departments, and is more typical of a university, city or county hospital than of a private community hospital. The large Emergency Departments usually receive a higher proportion of "disposition cases." They are staffed by physicians on full-time duty and have more specialized, independent inpatient services. Observation units are sometimes denigrated on the theoretical grounds that if a patient needs more than a few hours of observation or treatment, he ought to be admitted. However, most large metropolitan hospitals find these units invaluable from a practical point of view. The situation is analogous to waiting rooms in Emergency Departments: ideally there should not be a need for a large waiting room, but it is a practical necessity in most Emergency Departments.

There are several valid reasons for the existence of these observation units. Their real *raison d'etre* is to allow for continued, frequent observation of patients by the same physician over the course of several hours, but less than a day. The assumption is that the majority of these patients will be discharged from the hospital within 24 hours. Subsequent developments in some patients will clarify a need for continued hospitalization which was not apparent on admission. A typical example of this use of an observation unit is the patient with acute abdominal pain who may be developing "a surgical abdomen." Other examples are patients with a history of a significant blow to the head or frank concussion with no neurologic signs or residual symptoms, and patients with an acute psychiatric crisis, drug overdose, or suicidal gesture, in whom immediate admission to a psychiatric hospital would be a threat or stigma. Patients who have been involved in a serious automobile accident, but appear on initial evaluation to have escaped serious injury should be observed for several hours before discharge from the hospital. All of these patients deserve repeated evaluation or extended observation by the same physician. If these physicians are on full-time duty in a busy Emergency Department, their patients cannot readily be observed if they are scattered around the inpatient wards of the hospital. On the one hand, these patients do not need the degree of nursing care provided in an intensive care unit, but on the other hand, they need more observation than is usually provided overnight on a regular ward. These observation problems should be confined in one area, under the eye of a single nurse and conveniently close to the doctors who are responsible for their care. This plan not only is convenient and economical but promotes good patient care.

The real controversy usually arises because of the use of these observation units for other purposes, such as a buffer against "undesirable," untimely and unrewarding admissions, on inpatient services. These units are often used as overnight or weekend holding areas for other disposition cases, until they can be sent to a more "appropriate" medical facility. Examples are short-term admission areas for more complicated diagnostic procedures (arteriography, liver or spleen biopsy) and the short-term treatment of selected "surgical infections," which would benefit from a brief period of intensive antibiotic and topical therapy following drainage or débridement in the Emergency Department. The observation units are used as areas for the treatment of selected hematologic problems by the administration of whole blood, packed cells or other blood components, and for short-term observation of "completed" abortions. Other uses are short-term treatment of recurrent "medical" problems with established diagnosis for which prompt resolution under treatment can be reasonably expected (e.g., asthmatic crises, epileptic seizures, complications of ethanol intoxication, and so on). Therapeutic crises in cancer chemotherapy patients are sometimes managed in observation units to avoid unnecessary hospitalization. Depending on the particular circumstances which pertain in a given hospital, the above indications for admission to an emergency observation unit may be considered acceptable. Unless acceptable exceptions to the traditional indications for admission to the emergency observation unit are specifically set down in the Emergency Department's written procedures, there is a tendency for this unit to be used for the management of such conditions as acute pancreatitis, acute cholecystitis, spontaneous pneumothorax, acute pelvic inflammatory disease and other medical and surgical problems which usually cannot be controlled within 24 hours. However, as long as the use of emergency observation beds is carefully supervised, they can be one of the best areas of bed utilization in a modern medical center. The minimum essentials of design for this unit should include a central nursing station with good visibility of multiple semi-open patient cubicles, drug and linen supply areas and adequate toilet facilities. One or two of the units may be specially modified for the protective custody of psychiatric problems or patients under surveillance by a law enforcement agency. One observation bed per 100 inpatient beds usually suffices.

EQUIPMENT, SUPPLIES AND DRUGS

The Emergency Room

It goes without saying that even the best trained professional staff can not deliver emergency medical care without appropriate equipment, supplies and drugs. A discussion of specific choices is beyond the scope of this chapter. The following are offered as check lists and should not be considered complete or all-inclusive, since they were taken from the inventory of a single emergency department.

1. Equipment, Minor
alcohol lamp
bandage scissors
blood agar plates
blood sampling sets
blood sampling equipment
　(vacutainers, syringes, tubes)
catheters (intravenous, urinary, nasogastric,
　pediatric peritoneal dialysis, assorted
　thoracostomy, central venous)
counter pressure device (G-suit)
culture tubes, swabs
drains
esophageal balloon (Sengstaken)
flashlights, bulbs, batteries
hot water bottles
ice bags
incubator
instrument stands
ophthalmoscope
otoscope
selected special and extra instruments
　(in sterile pan)
selected suture material
soaking basins and tubs
sterile dressings
thermometers
tracheostomy tubes, multiple sizes
Thioglycolate broth tubes
2. Equipment, Major
arm boards
cardiopulmonary resuscitation cart
defibrillator—monitor
irrigation stands
Kelly pads
operating or "laceration" tables
operating lights
　(overhead movable and portable)
orthopedic cart
portable oxygen tank
　(in addition to wall oxygen)

portable suction machine
  (in addition to wall suction)
refrigerator
splints (Thomas, universal, hand and other
  selected splints)
sphygmomanometers (wall mounted and
  portable)
trauma cart
trauma (x-ray) stretchers
ventilatory support equipment
  (oropharyngeal airways, padded tongue
  blades, laryngoscopes, endotracheal and
  nasotracheal tubes, McGill forceps, ambu
  bags, mechanical ventilator)
  3. Special Procedure Sets
burn dressing—major
central venous pressure catheterization tray
cutdown tray
D and C tray, lumbar puncture
ENT tray (including nasal packing)
gastric lavage tray, paracentesis
Kirschner wire set
minor dressing pack
minor pelvic tray
sigmoidoscopy tray
suture tray
suture tray with "plastic" instruments
thoracotomy tray (with vascular clamps)
tracheostomy tray
tube thoracostomy tray

Comment. The cardiopulmonary resuscitation cart includes all the equipment, drugs and supplies which might be needed in the event of a cardiopulmonary arrest. This would ordinarily be kept in the trauma-resuscitation area, particularly if one section of this is specifically set aside for the management of cardiac and respiratory crises. In the same area, a defibrillator and electrocardiogram or cardiac monitor is kept. However, cardiac or respiratory arrests do not always occur where they are supposed to, so it is important that all this equipment be easily portable. On the other hand, except in the event of multiple injuries or minor disasters, most of the major trauma will be managed in the area designated for this purpose. It is wise to have a "trauma" cart separate from the cardiopulmonary resuscitation cart, on which is placed all the items that might ordinarily be requested by the physician or the nurse during the first

ten minutes of arrival of a major trauma victim. These items should include, for example, lactated Ringer's solution, Plasmanate, infusion sets, venous pressure sets, Intracaths, Foley catheters, nasogastric tubes, blood sampling syringes and tubes, multiple syringes and needles. The trauma cart or carts should also hold tourniquets, sterile gloves, oxygen nasal cannula and mask, organic iodide prep, antibiotic ointment, adhesive tape, sterile lubrication jelly, suction catheters, three-way stop cocks, alcohol sponges, large and small gauze dressings, arm boards, sand bags, lidocaine, epinephrine, calcium chloride and sodium bicarbonate. Since victims of serious multiple injuries are usually cared for by a team of physicians and nurses, we have found it appropriate to divide the materials between four smaller carts. The one placed near the patient's head includes all the equipment needed for airway control and the insertion of nasogastric tubes. A second one at the patient's side has all the equipment necessary for insertion of a central venous pressure catheter. A third cart on the patient's other side has equipment for insertion of a peripheral intravenous catheter plus that needed for performing abdominal paracentesis. The fourth cart has everything needed for insertion of an indwelling urinary catheter. This allows each of the attending physicians to perform those procedures quickly which are almost routinely applied to serious trauma victims, without having to struggle to reach a common "crash" cart or bother the nurse. The nurse is in turn free either to monitor the vital signs or to respond to special requests.

Although most orthopedic treatment can best be carried out in a specific area equipped with sinks having plaster traps, x-ray view boxes, splints, slings, traction equipment and so on, it is usually expedient, for simpler procedures, to take a plaster cart to the patient rather than to have the patient wait until this "cast room" is cleared of more complicated cases. This is just one example of the need for flexibility rather than commitment to one fixed procedure.

4. *Drugs.* The following is a list of drugs maintained in our Emergency Department. Depending on the convenience and availability of the hospital pharmacy or one nearby, it may be necessary for the Emergency Department to stock single days' supplies of important or commonly used drugs such as antibiotics, in addition to those listed here. In addition, the Emergency Room must stock crutches, canes, Ace bandages and other take-home supplies for the patients, if they are not readily available elsewhere in the hospital on a 24-hour basis.

DRUGS STOCKED IN THE EMERGENCY DEPARTMENT

acetylsalicylic compound
albumin, normal human serum
aminophylline
ammonia, aromatic spirits
amphetamine sulfate
antivenin, coral snake
antivenin, polyvalent snake
antivenin, spider bite
apomorphine hydrochloride
atropine sulfate
bacitracin ointment
benedryl
benzalkonium chloride solution
caffeine and sodium benzoate
calamine lotion
calcium chloride
calcium gluconate
chloral hydrate
chlordiazepoxide hydrochloride
chlorpromazine
codeine
codeine terpin hydrate, dehydrocodeine cough mixture
cortisone acetate
dextran
diazepam
digitoxin
digoxin
dehydroergotamine
Dilantin
diphenhydramine hydrochloride
edathamil calcium–disodium
ephedrine sulfate
ephedrine sulfate, NF
epinephrine
ergonovine maleate
ethyl chloride spray
fibrinogen, human
fluorescein sodium
glucose
globulin, immune serum
glycerine suppositories
glyceryl trinitrate
heparin, sodium
hexachlorophene solution
hydrocortisone acetate

hydrocortisone sodium sulfate
hydrogen peroxide solution
hyperimmune globulin, tetanus
insulin
iodine and organic iodide solutions
isoproterenol
isopropyl alcohol
kaolin with pectin mixture
levarterenol bitartrate
lidocaine hydrochloride
magnesium sulfate
meperidine hydrochloride
meprobamate
methylene blue
morphine sulfate
nalorphine hydrochloride
neomycin sulfate ointment
neostigmine bromide
neostigmine methylsulfate
naloxone hydrochloride
norepinephrine
oxytocin
papaverine hydrochloride
paraldehyde
Peruvian balsam
phenobarbital
phenol
phenylephrine hydrochloride
physostigmine
phytonadione
plasma protein fraction, human
potassium permanganate tablets
procainamide hydrochloride
procaine hydrochloride
promethazine hydrochloride, NF
protamine sulfate
quinidine sulfate
silver nitrate applicators
sodium amytal
sodium bicarbonate
talc
tetanus antitoxin, bovine
tetanus toxoid
tetracaine hydrochloride
tincture of benzoin
zinc chloride

5. Furniture. Each examining room should have a desk and two chairs and be stocked with changes of linen, examining gowns and commonly used supplies: cotton swabs, gloves, lubricants, adhesive tape, simple dressings, medical record forms, prescription pads, requisition forms for laboratory and x-ray studies, disposable towels, Kleenex tissues, flashlight, reflex hammer, otoscope and ophthalmoscope, stethoscope, sphygmomanometer, and so on. The ideal patient cart or stretcher should have a radiolucent top which is flexible and adjustable so that the head can be elevated and the knees bent. It should be adjustable in height, have its own IV standard and be equipped with stirrups, safety straps, side rails, and wheel brakes. Few models fit all these specifications.

Outpatient Clinic

A surgical clinic has more complicated supply needs than the usual medical or pediatric clinic, but they are much simpler than those of an Emergency Room. In most surgical clinics, certain rooms will be set aside as surgical dressing rooms. These may even be used for minor surgical procedures such as small superficial biopsies, débridement, incision and drainage, and for changing surgical dressings. Each of these rooms should have a surgical dressing cart and either the room or the cart should be stocked with all the necessary equipment and supplies used in changing dressings, including:

band-aids, assorted
drains: Penrose and "cigarette"
gauze packing (iodoform and plain)
gauze rolls
gauze squares, small, medium and large
gloves, nonsterile (rectal)
gloves, sterile
instruments: mosquito clamps, Crile clamps, Adson forceps, Kelly clamps, needle holder, suture scissors, dissecting scissors, scalpel handle and blades, probes and groove directors
petrolatum gauze
prepping solutions: tincture of iodine, tinc-

ture of Merthiolate, organic iodide preparations, hexachlorophene solutions, benzalkonium solutions, merbromin solution, ether, acetone, 70 % alcohol
tape, adhesive
tape, blastoplast
tape, nonallergenic
topical agents: Vaseline, zinc oxide, bacitracin ointment, Sulfamylon cream, peroxide, balsam of Peru
tube gauze

Both clean and sterile linens should be stocked in this room, particularly packs of sterile towels and drape sheets. If minor surgical procedures are to be done frequently, individual packs for these procedures can be prepared in central supply and kept stocked in this room. It is, of course, of utmost importance that the surgical dressing cart be used with scrupulous technique, using transfer forceps to take sterile dressings and instruments from the cart to a separate sterile field. In addition, a fully equipped surgical dressing cart should be sent daily from central supply to be exchanged for the used one.

It is not necessary to use the special surgical dressing room to see all postoperative patients and patients with simple wounds. Each room should be equipped with the common dressing needs, including gauze dressings, adhesive tape and suture packs, as well as the standard prepping solutions. This overcomes the necessity of moving patients into the surgical dressing room simply to have a few sutures removed. In addition to the simple dressing materials, each room in the surgical clinic should have a desk, stocked with history paper, prescription pads, laboratory, x-ray and consultation request slips, and with the common tools used in physical examination such as a thermometer, sphygmomanometer, flashlight, pin and brush, tuning fork, reflex hammer and stethoscope. A supply of less commonly used drugs and equipment can be stocked in the supply or utility room of each clinic to save time requesting them from the pharmacy or central supply. These might include various suture materials, specimen cups with formalin, additional instruments (biopsy forceps, IV needles, catheters and solutions, sterile rubber cathers and irrigation sets), Ace bandages and Unna's paste boots, and vaginal specula. No matter how remote the possibility may seem, each major clinic area should also be equipped with one emergency cart for cardiopulmonary resuscitation. This cart should be used only for emergencies and its stock must be checked on a regular basis.

EMERGENCY DEPARTMENT STAFFING PATTERNS AND DUTIES

The staffing requirements of an Emergency Department have traditionally been broken down into categories for physicians, nurses and administrators. Unfortunately, this same separatism often carries into the job descriptions of these personnel, and into the lines of authority and responsibility. In the last few years, the clear lines of distinction between the roles of the doctor, the nurse and the clerk have been obscured by the appearance in the Emergency Department of "corpsmen" or emergency medical technicians, physician's associate, patient's ombudsmen, social workers and other allied health personnel. In addition, there has been a steady trend toward expanding and upgrading the roles of both nursing and administrative personnel in the Emergency Department. Thus, inflexibility regarding the roles of the various personnel involved in the Emergency Department is now being relaxed in the cause of efficiency and economy. Efforts are being made to pass many of the routine duties formerly performed by the physician and the nurse onto the nurse and clerk respectively, so that the time and effort of each member of the staff are more efficiently spent performing duties and skills for which they were trained and which, indeed, require the degree of training and skill which they have had. The objective is to allow the physician

to concentrate on those tasks which require his skill and judgment. Nurses, technicians or other allied health personnel carry out more of the routine tasks, such as gathering historical background, recording vital signs and making other simple physical observations, as well as some of the more common manipulative or therapeutic skills (taking EKG's, starting IV's, drawing blood samples, for example). These activities are carried out under the direction and supervision of the physician rather than being performed by him personally. Similarly, expansion of the duties of the clerk in the Emergency Department will free the nurse of paperwork and allow her to concentrate on patient care. These upward shifts will gradually bring about changes in the relationships and ratios between the patient, physician, nurse and allied health personnel. Theoretically, since everyone will be working closer to the upper limits of his ability and skill, there should be a greater degree of job satisfaction, and assuming a commensurate level of responsibility, the entire operation should be more economical and efficient. The basic duties performed in an Emergency Department will not change, but there will be a gradual change in the personnel performing them, with a broadening base of auxiliary personnel. Even if new types of personnel such as emergency medical technicians and physician's associates are not introduced into an Emergency Room and the basic physician-nurse-clerk staffing continues, the duties and responsibilities of each member of the team can be expected to shift upward.

To operate efficiently, the Emergency Department must have direction, and this can best be provided by interested and involved physicians, although it is not always feasible for every Emergency Room to have a full-time physician director. While this may be a goal worth striving for in any large Emergency Department, practical considerations require that some compromise be made in smaller, less active Emergency Departments. Few traditionally trained surgeons have the background or inclination to devote themselves full-time to this effort, although, as will be discussed later, the new breed of "emergency physicians" may eventually do much to solve this dilemma. The Emergency Department is an unpredictably busy, 168-hour-a-week operation which cannot be given full-time direction by any single physician, even if he works long hours. To achieve round-the-clock direction, a responsive system is necessary, with clear lines of authority which are followed in a responsible manner. Formalized, well-disseminated Emergency Department policies are necessary. Standard procedures, lines of authority and delegated responsibility can provide this essential direction whether the director of the Emergency Department is immediately present or not.

If there is a physician-director who devotes a significant proportion of his time to this job, he will ordinarily work closely with the head nurse and/or a unit manager or administrative assistant, seeing that the operational policies of the Emergency Department which they formulate together are carried out on a daily basis. Another common organizational pattern consists of an Emergency Department committee, made up of staff physicians representing different clinical interests, one of whom acts as chairman of the committee. Such a committee may provide overall policy direction, with day-to-day operation of the Emergency Department being left to the head nurse or manager who receives consultation as necessary with the chairman of the committee. Weekly "business" meetings of the Emergency Department committee should be held, with appropriate nursing and administrative representatives. Current Emergency Department operational problems should be discussed and operational statistics should be reviewed, including incidents, deaths and complications, and overnight ward utilization. In most Emergency Departments, the nursing and adminis-

trative staff provide the only permanence to the professional staff, since physician coverage of the Emergency Department tends to be temporary and fragmented.

There are several basic patterns of Emergency Department physician coverage commonly seen today. These are: (1) a rotation of the entire attending staff of the hospital, (2) a rotation of interns and residents supervised by a small group of full-time staff members, (3) coverage provided by a large incorporated group from the hospital's own attending staff (Pontiac Plan), (4) a group of full-time (contract) emergency physicians (Alexandria Plan) and (5) various combinations of the above, including attending staff coverage supplemented by "moonlighting" physicians who regularly work in nearby university training programs or federal health care institutions.

There are advantages and disadvantages to each of these staffing plans. While no one plan will satisfy all Emergency Departments, one or a combination of them will prove more suitable than others for a given hospital. The traditional approach in community hospitals has been a rotation of the entire "volunteer" attending staff, supplemented in some hospitals by house staff in training. The traditional approach in the larger university-affiliated hospitals has been to staff the Emergency Department with a full complement of house staff. The interns serve as primary physicians. Specialty interests are covered by residents of varying degrees of experience, backed by faculty. The overall supervision is provided by one or more members of the full-time faculty. Both of these approaches have failed to stand up under the stresses of the previously described "Emergency Room population explosion."

In the community hospital, the heavier patient load has resulted in a need for greater staff coverage, which in turn has caused increasing conflicts with the private practices of the attending staff. This situation has been aggravated by the increasing difficulties of community hospitals in competing with university-affiliated hospitals for qualified house staff. Furthermore, a larger proportion of the hospital's staff are specialists who find that Emergency Room problems are frequently outside their areas of special interest and clinical competence. As more and more of these "specialists" are excused from Emergency Room duty, a disproportionately greater load falls on the remaining "generalists." Frequently, Emergency Department duty is neither financially nor professionally rewarding, particularly when a significant proportion of the case load is routine, and a large percentage of patients are either indigent or "bad risk" financially. Increasing medical-legal risks are also associated with Emergency Room practice. Hospital staffs have therefore abandoned traditional coverage in favor of other approaches. The Pontiac and Alexandria plans were developed out of the necessity created by these circumstances.

Emergency Department coverage by an incorporated group of the attending staff is typified by the Pontiac Plan (named because of its origin at the Pontiac General Hospital in Pontiac, Michigan in 1961). This increasingly popular plan offers full-time Emergency Department coverage by a relatively large group of staff physicians who still retain their individual practices in the community, but contractually agree to devote varying amounts of time on duty in the hospital's Emergency Department. When the group is large enough, part-time participation is more flexible and therefore can be varied to a degree compatible with the participant's private practice. The participating staff physician retains his usual staff privileges and professional relationships at the hospital while participating in this plan. For this reason, he is more likely to work in harmony with the remainder of the medical staff in the community during the time he is covering the Emergency Department. This arrangement also provides the opportunity for the benefits of corporate practice such as retirement plans, group insurance coverage, and

so on. Coverage by a larger group provides less of the consistency and continuity that a smaller group of full-time emergency physicians might provide. The heaviest contributors to this type of group coverage plan tend to be young physicians trying to get started in practice and older physicians wishing to withdraw from the rigors of an open private practice. There have been problems with some of the former viewing the Emergency Department as a source of new private patients. In addition, some of these groups have experienced difficulties in attracting the participation and cooperation of the more established, successful practitioners in the community. In other groups, the income has been disappointing, partly because of the expensiveness or inefficiency of their billing system and the high proportion of nonpaying patients. Some hospitals have solved these problems by getting the hospital to agree to the use of its billing system and to provide a guaranteed minimum income for services rendered to nonpaying patients.

The other major alternative to traditional Emergency Department coverage at a community hospital is called the Alexandria Plan because of its city of origin (Alexandria, Virginia, 1961). This plan provides full-time coverage by physicians who have no outside practice, although they may serve more than one Emergency Department. These physicians, usually four in number, may form a partnership or corporation. In general an Emergency Department census of 18,000 to 20,000 visits a year is required to sustain a four-man group without the necessity for financial assistance from the hospital. As the Emergency Department census increases, an additional physician is usually added for every 7000 to 10,000 patient visits a year. The advantage of coverage by a group of full-time contract physicians is that the clinical activities are performed by a few physicians who are accustomed to the clinical problems presenting to an Emergency Room and can see large numbers of patients efficiently. These physicians have no admission privileges and provide no follow-up care. Therefore there is no concern about patient "stealing." Staff physicians may resent the fact that emergency physicians command relatively large incomes considering their negligible investment in setting up a practice, limited hours of work and minimal on-going patient care responsibilities. This resentment is usually offset by appreciation for relief from Emergency Room on-call responsibilities. A more lasting concern is whether this approach may perpetuate a system that provides ambulatory care on an episodic basis in Emergency Rooms. This practice has been shown to be expensive and ineffective. There may also be grounds for challenging the validity of "emergency medicine" as a specialty and a long-term solution to this aspect of health care delivery, even though it appears to be a *fait accompli* and certainly provides an attractive immediate solution to many of our current Emergency Department staffing problems. There is also a potential conflict between the role of the emergency physician, as viewed by himself—the compleat specialist in emergency medical problems—and the practical role which he is usually asked to fill: namely, someone to initiate resuscitation of the seriously ill or injured until the appropriate specialists can be summoned and to handle the increasing burden of general practice or minor medical problems which have fallen upon most Emergency Rooms today.

The problems of who should train the emergency physician and what his education should consist of are also still unsettled. Currently, two-year residencies in emergency medicine have been established in a few university hospitals. In the vast majority of university medical centers the emphasis remains in favor of the establishment of trauma or emergency medical care centers restricted to "true" emergencies, with the less urgent ambulatory care problems being handled in other outpatient facilities. Only the future will answer whether either of these approaches will survive and flourish, or whether some other approach—such as a modification of those used in certain European countries—will supervene.

In the university or university-affiliated hospital, there has usually been an increase in trauma, and patients with emergency problems are turning to larger, better-equipped Emergency Departments. Nevertheless, the disproportionate part of the increase in patient census has still come from nonemergent, general medical problems. Most of the trainees in university and university-affiliated hospitals are there for specialty training. Understandably, they and the heads of their departments or divisions resist their devoting an increasingly large proportion of their training period to this type of "service." Thus, there is an increasingly stiffer effort being made by many departments in university hospitals to restore and maintain a more favorable balance between "education" and "service." The other pressures forcing a reconsideration of the role of house staff in Emergency Departments are financial and ethical. Financially, university hospitals are losing the opportunity to collect significant sums in professional fees when most of the patient care is being provided by house staff. Ethically, the problem arises from the steadily increasing percentage of patients presenting to university hospital emergency departments that can no longer be considered indigent by any standards. The proportion of indigent to those who pay directly or are covered by some third-party plan has been completely reversed. In addition, there is the recurring ciritcism that "nowhere else in medicine are the most seriously ill left in the hands of the least experienced." Studies show that the emergency medical care of serious injuries provided by university hospitals is generally better than elsewhere in the community, but the pressure from this criticism persists. Triage systems have been developed in most large Emergency Departments, but they have simply dislocated the problem to other outpatient areas. New approaches will undoubtedly develop, but at the moment an increasing number of university hospitals are abandoning their traditional coverage plan or at least significantly modifying it. Some have resorted to using salaried physicians to handle these "service commitments" either in "walk-in" or "evening" clinics or in the Emergency Room itself. Others are superimposing faculty panels on top of house staff coverage, to provide for better supervision and teaching as well as the collection of fees for service to private patients.

The problems with the nursing and administrative staffing in the Emergency Department are somewhat less complex but by no means simple. Fortunately, a number of "traditional" restraints are being overcome. Nurses are no longer considered simply as physician's aides. They are being allowed to make many routine clinical decisions and to perform procedures such as withdrawing blood samples, starting intravenous therapy, taking electrocardiograms, dressing wounds, and performing other minor manipulative procedures. The parallel development of the emergency medical technicians and physician's associates has served to break down resistance to upgrading the role of the nurse. In many institutions where nursing shortages are experienced, corpsmen returning from the Armed Forces, trained emergency medical technicians, licensed practical nurses and physician's associates are used to fill the professional ranks in the Emergency Department formerly held by nurses.

This effort to unburden the physician and nurse of "nonprofessional" responsibilities has resulted in an additional burden being placed on the nonprofessional administrative staff. Unfortunately, the Emergency Department clerks usually have been gradually saddled with these increasing responsibilities without adequate training or additional help. They are frequently underpaid as well as undertrained for their more important and sensitive duties, which include receiving outside telephone calls regarding emergencies, greeting patients and conducting registration and financial interviews. Rarely are they selected for their ability to maintain their equanimity under pressure or their natural respect for and sincere interest in patient welfare. In their position, between the waiting patient and the physician and nurse, they hold one of the most important public relations positions in the hospital. For just as the Emergency Department is the hospital's "front door," so are these clerks the Emergency Department's front line, in as much as they hold a major responsibility for the impression patients receive of the Emergency Department.

Although staffing patterns are easier to work out for nursing and clerical personnel, it is important to recognize that the traditional pattern of three shifts a day popularized by inpatient nursing services is frequently inappropriate when applied to an Emergency Department. One must recognize peak periods of clinical activity both by hour and by day and in some instances by season. An adequate coverage for nursing and administrative personnel must be developed accordingly. Uneven and overlapping shifts may be required. In a smaller Emergency Room, a head nurse may handle the bulk of the administrative decisions and organizational tasks. In a larger Emergency Department, it is advisable to have both a head nurse and administrative assistant or manager. In addition, there should be an identifiable charge nurse and/or chief clerk for any period of the day when there is more than one nurse or clerk present. Contingency plans for backup personnel in *all* categories of personnel must be provided to meet every situation from natural disasters and civil disturbances to vacations and illnesses. In summary, one cannot overemphasize the importance of selection for proper attitude, careful orientation and training for specific duties, written policies and procedures, clear job descriptions and adequate salaries.

STAFFING OF THE SURGICAL OUTPATIENT CLINIC

Generally this is a simple task. The simplest professional unit consists of a clerk, a nurse and a physician. If multiple surgeons are in attendance at one time, additional nurses will be necessary, particularly if minor surgical procedures are being performed. Personnel providing secretarial support, maintenance and so on are usually pooled or shared with other outpatient and inpatient services. In general, staffing patterns are less of a problem than staffing attitudes. A new ten hour, four day week may help solve the problems of staffing the surgical clinics, most of which are too busy for an eight hour day. The surgical clinic may place demands on nursing personnel that are lacking in other outpatient areas because of the special procedures that are performed there, but even this is rarely a problem. Most of the problems in running a surgical clinic are not due to inadequate numbers or abilities or the auxiliary staff, but of attitudes or organization. The key to a smooth, efficient clinic operation is timing of and preparation for the patient-doctor encounter. When the patient is given an appointment time, he should be asked to arrive 10–15 minutes prior to that time. During this preliminary period, patients should have been welcomed by name by the receptionist, who will log the patient in, prepare or obtain the patient's record, and introduce the patient to the nurse, who after reading (preferably in advance) the patient's record and asking a few pertinent questions, should usher the patient into the examining room. If necessary, specific instructions should be given regarding the patient's dress. The patient should be assisted as necessary in preparing for the arrival of the doctor. The doctor should always strive to arrive on time and move on to the next patient on schedule. One of the best guarantees of accomplishing this is advance preparation of oneself and the clinic personnel. The clinic receptionist or nurse should have been informed of the general nature of the patient's problem at the time of the appointment. The estimated time of the examination should be noted, or treatments as well as any special procedures that might be performed. Preferably the doctor's note should be dictated immediately after the examination or treatment is completed or at the completion of the visit. Most well-organized physicians can dictate a history while the patient undresses and the physical examination while the patient dresses again. In parting, the physician should summarize his instructions to the patient. If feasible, instructions to the patient should be legibly written and handed to the patient along with any prescriptions and the time of the next appointment. Immediate dictation of the record avoids obvious problems caused by reliance on memory and allows legible copies to be available at an early date for the hospital's records and the physician's own files, as well as those of referring physicians.

PATIENT MANAGEMENT AND RECORDS

Emergency Department

The basic principles regarding the management of patients in the Emergency Department are generally accepted. Some of these are covered in the *Standards for Accreditation of Hospitals*. Others have been included for the sake of completeness.

1. All patients presenting for treatment at the Emergency Department must be considered as having an emergent medical problem until proven otherwise.
2. From a practical point of view, the patient's definition of emergency must be favored over the physician's.
3. All patients presenting to the Emer-

gency Department should be seen (however briefly) by a physician, and the physician must bear the ultimate responsibility for that patient's treatment.

4. Within a short time of their arrival at the Emergency Department, all patients should be at least interviewed by a nurse, particularly if significant delays for evaluation and treatment are predictable.

5. The patient should be advised of potential treatment delays to be encountered in the Emergency Department.

6. The request of a patient or his private physician for transfer to another institution for evaluation and treatment should be honored as long as (and only if) the transfer is not expected to prove detrimental to the treatment of the patient.

7. Whenever possible, attempts should be made to contact the patient's private physician regarding treatment in the Emergency Department.

8. Financial consideration should have no bearing upon the emergency medical services provided by a particular Emergency Department.

9. A written record of each patient's Emergency Department visit should be kept and these records should be subject to periodic review.

10. There should be an up-to-date written set of policies and procedures covering every important aspect of Emergency Department operations, including policies regarding the management of specific conditions.

The patient's Emergency Department record should be written on a form specially designed for this purpose. There are almost as many emergency record forms as there are emergency departments. There obviously should be some uniformity here, at least in terms of the minimum essential information. It is the author's opinion that the more cluttered a form is with multiple spaces reserved for specific aspects of the history and physical, the more impractical the form is. Essential information should include patient's name, address, telephone number, means of arrival, name of personal or private physician, and chief complaint. The time of arrival and departure should also be noted. The physician's note should include the time the patient is first seen, vital signs, history and physical, diagnostic impressions, diagnostic studies ordered, treatment administered, patient instructions and final disposition. Preferably the patient's instructions should be written legibly. An additional carbon copy tear-off sheet at the bottom of the record where disposition, treatment and instructions are written along with the next clinic appointment and the doctor's signature serves this purpose nicely. In addition, a carbon copy of the entire record is extremely useful in allowing for medical record audit on a daily basis without the need to hold up the permanent copy. In a teaching institution, a regular audit of the medical records of the Emergency Department is extremely valuable and brings to light a number of aspects of patient care which would otherwise go unnoticed.

Surgical Outpatient Clinic

Surgical clinic patients present only a few special problems. Convalescent care units and physical medicine and rehabilitation services are commonly involved because of the disabilities associated with surgical operations and injuries and the need for special provisions for transportation and social service support. In addition, cooperation with medical records in filling out disability affidavits and insurance forms is necessary. Such problems are not encountered with new patients, but occur in patients returning for follow-up care after surgery. Ordinarily surgical follow-up care is brief, but occasionally it must be extended—for example, in patients with carcinomas, major vascular procedures, or gastric resection. In addition, there are a number of conditions traditionally cared for by surgeons which do not involve surgery, such as stasis ulcers and chronic low back pain, for example.

Surgical clinic records should not differ from those of other clinics except when special examinations are involved. In these instances special forms can be followed. It is helpful to use anatomic stamps to help illustrate the physical examination. New surgical patients can fill out the past history and review of systems with the help of a nurse or receptionist prior to the interview by the surgeon. He is then free to concentrate on the present illness and those aspects of the past history and review of systems brought out by the questionnaire, without having to do a complete detailed history himself. In the case of patients who are followed for certain conditions, such as vascular surgical patients on anticoagulant therapy or cancer chemotherapy patients, it is important that the patient arrive far enough in advance of the appointment with the physician so that the necessary preliminary laboratory work can be completed. Patients should be given staggered clinic appointments, the intervals being determined by the nature of the visit, such as one hour for a complete new patient work-up, a half hour for a specialty consultation and 15 to 20 minutes for a follow-up visit including suture removal. In general, a nurse or auxiliary personnel should be in attendance at the time the procedures are performed. The same can be said for pelvic and rectal examinations. Removal of sutures or dressing changes should not require an assistant or chaperone.

FINANCIAL ASPECTS OF AMBULATORY SURGICAL CARE

The rapidly rising increases in cost of medical care are to a considerable degree related to the high cost of inpatient services. Organized opposition is growing to these rising costs at a national level. It is expected that an emphasis on outpatient care will be a major result.

Already insurance companies are offering incentives for prehospital or outpatient diagnostic work-ups, a change from the days in which insurance companies would not honor any outpatient diagnostic studies. Once the remaining barriers to coverage of outpatient care costs by insurance have been eliminated and incentives rather than penalties have become associated with outpatient as opposed to inpatient care, one can expect a tremendous impetus to the development of this kind of surgical care. All possible surgical procedures will be done on an outpatient basis. An example of what can be expected is seen in the new concept of a SURGICENTER®, a special facility in which simple elective surgery is performed in an environment oriented around anesthesia, surgery, and minimal pre- and postoperative care. The operations include herniorrhaphies, breast biopsies, transurethral resections, vasectomies, varicose vein strippings, cosmetic plastic surgery and other relatively minor surgical procedures requiring a general anesthetic. These procedures are well tolerated physiologically and do not require extended hospital care. They may soon be performed almost exclusively as outpatient procedures in good-risk patients.

It is beyond the scope of this book to study alternative billing systems, facilities, fees and overhead charges, and the advantages of prepaid medical plans versus the usual third-party programs. However, it is important that the physician retain the right to establish his fee. The facilities fee, if included in the bill, should be identified as such or listed separately. The facilities fee should include only those administrative charges, expenses and services which directly affect the care received by the patient. It is also important that the patient be aware of the breakdown of charges, and that the physician receive a copy of each bill sent to the patient. It should personally be consulted before the bill is referred to a collection agency or before a legal suit is undertaken. That is, while it is efficient to have the bills "aged" and sent out on an automatic basis with a certain prearranged sequence regarding the type of bill or notice sent to the patient, the doctor-patient relationship must not be circumvented in this and the doctor must have the final say in any major decision regarding his patient's bill.

2

Anesthesia for Outpatients

By DENNIS BARTON, M.D.

There are many procedures that require anesthesia but do not require overnight hospitalization. This chapter will examine anesthetic techniques and point out methods which have been found useful for outpatients.

With in-hospital charges rapidly approaching one hundred dollars per day, there has been increasing interest in keeping relatively minor surgical problems out of the hospital. Inpatient facilities are hampered by nursing shortages (estimated as 285,000 nurses nationally in 1967),[1] and to some degree by the incidence of nosocomial infections, (9.4 per cent in one hospital's surgery service).[2] Some hospitals have organized a formal outpatient surgery program[3,4] in which patients come to the outpatient facility for a preoperative visit, are examined for their fitness for surgery, undergo the necessary preoperative laboratory examinations, and are then given written instructions to prepare them for the day of surgery. The patients return for their operation, recover from anesthesia in the same facilities used by inpatients, and go home to bed. Of course, there are many patients who arrive at the hospital as emergencies who have not been so well prepared. Emergency surgical patients can frequently be treated and sent home also.

All outpatient surgery—whether elec-

32

tive or emergency—should be done at an inpatient facility. Unexpected complications will arise even in patients who have been carefully selected for fitness for outpatient surgery. The incidence of complications requiring hospitalization is quite low (4.1 per cent in one large series).

There are many patients and procedures not suitable for outpatient anesthesia. The procedure itself may be relatively minor, but the patients may be a poor anesthetic risk because of severe systemic disease. Some patients may have no one to look after them at home. One series[5] found that 5.4 per cent of patients previously selected for outpatient surgery were unable to follow their normal occupation on the day after anesthesia. This incidence alone warrants the precept that no patient should be returned to an isolated home environment. Other patients who may be unable to follow written instruction must also be hospitalized.

Emergency patients with head injuries or stupor resulting from alcohol or drug abuse cannot be sent out but must be kept for observation. Patients undergoing surgical procedures with a high incidence of postoperative blood loss or other complications must also be kept in the hospital: mammoplasty, extensive varicose vein stripping and perhaps tonsillectomy fall into this category.

This chapter will consider regional and general anesthetic techniques. The pharmacology of local anesthetics will be presented first, followed by presentations of useful regional anesthetic techniques. The regional anesthetic techniques in this chapter have wide application to various surgical disciplines. Those techniques peculiar to a particular surgical speciality are found elsewhere in the appropriate chapter. The last section of this chapter will consider pertinent facts relating to drugs for premedication and general anesthetic agents.

Table 2–1 summarizes the pharmacology of the well-known local anesthetic agents. The maximum permitted doses in a typical adult are shown in Table 2–2.

The physician usually desires local anesthetic drugs of rapid onset, low toxicity and prolonged duration. Unfortunately, drugs of rapid onset tend to be of short duration, and one must choose a drug compatible with the length of the proposed procedure. The converse is also true, and longer acting drugs tend to have slower onset times. Some attempts have been made to shorten the onset of action of longer acting drugs by using carbonated salts of the local anesthetic base. Unfortunately, these drugs are not yet available clinically.[7]

One will occasionally encounter allergy to local anesthetic agents. This is usually manifested as a rash, urticaria or even wheezing.[8] One must distinguish between allergy to the anesthetic drug and allergy to the preservative in the drug vial (methylparaben).[9] If a patient has a history of allergy to a drug in the para-aminobenzoic acid-ester series (procaine, chlorprocaine, tetracaine), skin testing may reveal no allergy to other local anesthetics. Anaphylactic shock reaction to minute amounts of local anesthetic drug is extremely rare. Two cases in 55,000 regional blocks are reported by Moore.[6]

Most histories of allergy to local anesthetics are actually histories of inadvertent intravascular injection, especially with epinephrine-containing solutions. Fright at the sight of an injection needle is probably the most common cause of "allergy to local anesthetics." One still encounters cases where the well-publicized dose limits of various anesthetic drugs have been exceeded by physicians somehow ignorant of the deadly potency of local anesthetic agents.

Close verbal contact is kept between the physician and the patient undergoing local block so that early signs of toxicity can be detected. The patient may become nauseated or drowsy, or complain of tinnitus or generalized numbness and tingling. The physician may detect jerky, myoclonic movements. Full blown toxicity can result in coma, grand mal seizures, and cardiac and respiratory arrest.

TABLE 2–1 PHARMACOLOGY OF LOCAL ANESTHETIC AGENTS*

DRUG (TRADE NAME)	SUPPLIED	MAXIMUM PERMITTED DOSE	ONSET OF ACTION	DURATION	TOXICITY
Cocaine Not for injection	As powder made up in 1–4% solution	100 mgm total Some authors use up to 6.6 mgm/kg	Rapid – topical	1 hr	Convulsions, coma, respiratory arrest
Dyclonine (Dyclone) Not for injection	Solution, 0.5% concentration	200 mgm in adult	Rapid – topical	20–30 mins	Very rarely reported
Procaine (Novocaine)	1–2% solution	10–15 mgm/kg	Rapid	30 mins to 1 hr	Tinnitus, nausea, convulsions rare
Chlorprocaine (Nesacaine)	1–2% solution	10–20 mgm/kg	Very rapid	1 hr	Less toxic than Procaine
Tetracaine (Pontocaine)	Made up from Niphinoid crystal as required to 0.05–0.15% solutions (10 mgm crystal/vial)	1.5 mgm/kg (not to exceed 150 mgm)	Slow (15–45 min) (Usually combined with faster-acting agents)	3–6 hrs	Drowsiness→coma Convulsions rare
Tetracaine (Pontocaine) Topical	1–3% solution Also ingredient of Cetacaine (see text)	1.5 mgm/kg (not to exceed 150 mgm)	Moderate speed (*Topical use*) Sometimes combined with other agents (see text)	2 hrs	As above
Lidocaine (Xylocaine)	0.5–2% solution	4 mgm/kg	5–30 minutes	2 hrs	Drowsiness→coma Convulsions also se
(Lignocaine)	2–4% solution	4 mgm/kg	Rapid (*Topical use*)	1 hr	Drowsiness→coma Convulsions also se
Mepivacaine (Carbocaine)	1.0–2.0% solutions	7 mgm/kg (do not exceed 1000 mgm/ 24 hrs)	5–30 minutes	2–3 hrs	Drowsiness→coma Convulsions
Lidocaine with 1:200,000 epinephrine	0.5–2.0% solution	7 mgm/kg	5–30 minutes	2–3 hrs	Drowsiness→coma Convulsions. Do ne use more than 50 c 1:200,000 epinephr solution
Prilocaine (Citanest)	1.0–3.0% solutions	Dose not to exceed 700 mgm in adult	5–30 minutes	2–3 hrs	Drowsiness→coma or convulsions. Methemoglobinemia with overdose (see text)
Bupivacaine (Marcaine)	0.25–0.5% solution	Max. dose 250 mgm in adult	7–30 minutes	4–6 hrs or 25% longer than tetracaine	Tremor, shivering, nausea. Rare convulsions

*1% solutions of drugs listed have 10 mgm drug per 1 cc; 2% solutions have 20 mgm per cc, etc.

The management of such an emergency is treated elsewhere in this book (see Chapter 26). Major blocks should not be attempted unless resuscitative gear is at hand. An intravenous line should be set up in cases where drug doses near the permitted maximum are planned.

Blocks may fail or may need renewal. As a general rule, the maximum permitted dose should never be exceeded at one sitting. Many of the blocks described

TABLE 2–2 Maximum Volume of 1 Per Cent Solution of Local Anesthetics for a 70 Kgm Adult* (10 mg/ml)

Anesthetic	Maximum Volume
Procaine (Novocaine)	70–105 cc
Chlorprocaine (Nesacaine)	70–140 cc
Lidocaine (Xylocaine, Lignocaine)	28 cc
Lidocaine with epinephrine	50 cc
Mepivacaine (Carbocaine)	50 cc
Prilocaine (Citanest)	70 cc

*Calcuations based on maximum doses specified in Table 2–1.

in this chapter will require nearly the maximum permitted dose and should not be renewed until several hours have passed. Less extensive blocks that fail can be attempted several times, provided a drug with a high maximum dose is chosen. Tachyphylaxis to local anesthetic agents is often encountered with repeated injection of a certain drug. The block can be re-established with a different local anesthetic drug.

Topical Anesthesia — Cocaine, Cetacaine, Tetracaine, Dyclonine

Cocaine, dyclonine and Cetacaine are used exclusively as surface analgesics. Lidocaine in viscous form or as a 5 per cent solution, as well as tetracaine are also available as topical agents. Cocaine is the only agent in the series that has vasoconstrictive properties, and this may be the reason why the drug still enjoys popularity. Great care must be exercised in its use — a measured amount of the drug in a 1 to 2 per cent solution is placed in a medicine cup (totaling 50–100 mgm) and this dose is never exceeded. (However, one author has used up to 6.6 mgm per kg cocaine and has never encountered a toxic reaction.)[10] The cocaine is applied with a swab; a spray is inefficient. Overdose with cocaine is manifested by hyperirritability leading to convulsions, coma and respiratory arrest.

Tetracaine (Pontocaine, Amethocaine) can be employed as a topical anesthetic either alone or in combination with other topical anesthetic agents.

If tetracaine alone is chosen, a 1.0 to 2.0 per cent solution is used. The limit of the dose for tetracaine is 1.5 mgm per kg. Overdose usually results in drowsiness, progressing to shallow respirations and coma. Convulsions are rarely encountered.[6] The use of other topical agents with tetracaine gives the physician a faster onset of anesthesia. Cetacaine, a combination of tetracaine with ethylamino and butylamino benzoate, is used frequently at our hospitals. The latter two chemicals are poorly soluble in water, a property which causes these drugs to be absorbed slowly into the body, and they provide only surface anesthesia.

Dyclonine is an excellent topical anesthetic,[11] differing in its structural formula from other anesthetic agents. It is confined to topical use because it is rather irritative to tissue when injected locally. The topical effect lasts around 20 minutes. In dose ranges used clinically (4–20 cc of 0.5 per cent solution) no toxic reactions have been reported; indeed doses of 200–500 mgm IV in man have been without toxic effects.

Local and Regional Drugs

Procaine. Has a wide margin of safety, and up to 15 mgm per kg total of the drug can be used. The onset of action is extremely rapid (seven minutes for nerve blocks), but it cannot be expected to last for more than an hour. Convulsions are reported to occur with overdose, but extremely large and unrealistic doses are necessary to achieve this.

Chlorprocaine. Is said to be even less toxic than procaine.[12] Twenty mgm per kg of this drug have been used without toxic effects. Again the onset of action is extremely rapid, but the drug cannot be used for prolonged surgery. Both procaine and chlorprocaine are de-activated via hydrolysis by the pseudo-cholinesterase system in the blood. This fact may have practical importance, for there are certain rare patients that are hereditarily deficient in this enzyme system.

Tetracaine. Has been mentioned as a topical agent, but it also has a place as an adjuvant with other local anesthetic agents for peripheral nerve block. When used singly, the drug takes 15 to 45 minutes to produce an effect. Its duration is four to six hours. It is useful in a 0.1 to 0.15 per cent solution. The maximum permissible dose appears to be 1.5 mgm per kg, up to 150 mgm total. Tetracaine is also hydrolyzed by the pseudocholinesterase system.

Lidocaine. Offers fairly prolonged anesthesia (one to two hours), with much less delay than tetracaine.[13] The addition of epinephrine 1:200,000 prolongs the action to two to three hours. The volume of 1:200,000 epinephrine solution should not exceed 50 cc to avoid side effects from the epinephrine. The onset of action varies from 5 to 30 minutes. The most common cause of block failure with this drug is impatience. A patient who has been days getting ready for surgery can afford to wait 20 to 30 minutes more for the onset of solid anesthesia.

The maximum doses of lidocaine are listed on the chart. Solutions of 0.5 to 1.0 per cent are used for sensory anesthesia, while 1.5 to 2.0 per cent concentrations are more suitable for motor nerve block, or blocks where a longer duration is required. Minor lacerations can easily be handled with 0.5 per cent solutions. Solutions with epinephrine should never be used on the finger, the toes, or the penis since the resultant ischemia may cause necrosis. Toxicity is usually manifested by drowsiness deepening into coma and cardiorespiratory collapse. Convulsions are rare.

Mepivacaine. Is roughly equivalent to xylocaine with epinephrine in both duration of anesthesia and maximum permitted dose (see Table 2–1). Addition of epinephrine to mepivacaine will prolong the action of the drug only slightly.[13] Mepivacaine accumulates in the body with repeated blocks, and it has been recommended that no more than 1000 mgm of mepivacaine be used in a 24-hour period.[14] Toxicity is manifested by stupor and coma, or rarely by convulsions.

Prilocaine. Was felt to be an advance in local anesthetics because the maximum permitted dose was stated to be 10 mgm per kg. Unfortunately, methemoglobinemia occurs with this drug, owing to the accumulation of a metabolite of prilocaine in the red cells of the patient. Methemoglobinemia is seen as 5 per cent of total hemoglobin at doses of 600 mgm prilocaine.[13] The methemoglobinemia can be reversed with 1–2 mgm per kg IV methylene blue. Nevertheless, the early enthusiasm for the drug has been dimmed by this side effect. As with mepivacaine, the addition of epinephrine will not greatly prolong the action of the drug. Overdose is manifested by tremor, shivering, nausea and vomiting.

Bupivicaine. Has now been released for general use in the United States, and has been widely studied abroad. It has an extremely long duration in peripheral nerve blocks, again with a slow onset of action.[15] Peripheral nerve blocks as long as 24 hours have been reported with this drug, and this may make one hesitate to use it when rapid motor and sensory return is desired.

Regional Anesthetic Techniques

All these techniques will be more satisfactory if premedication with tranquilizers, somnifacients or analgesics is used. For outpatients these drugs are best given IV to allow rapid recovery after the procedure. (See the section on premedication later in this chapter.)

Intravenous Regional Anesthesia. This method was first published by Bier in 1908, but owes its current revival to Holmes, who reintroduced the technique in 1963.[16] The technique is especially useful in emergencies or other procedures where a tourniquet time of an hour or less is foreseen. The technique is illustrated in Figure 2–1. A scalp vein needle is inserted into a vein near the proposed site of operation, and a double cuffed tourniquet is fitted about the upper arm. The hand and arm below the tourniquet are exsanguinated either with an Esmarch bandage, or by gravity drainage in the case of fracture or trauma. The upper (proximal) cuff of the tourniquet is then inflated, and a local anesthetic is injected (see below for dosage) into the scalp vein needle. Analgesia suitable for operation will appear in 10 to 15 minutes in the arm below the tourniquet. (Cuts on fingers that prevent venous spread of the drug may not allow analgesia distal to the cut.) The injected drug spreads through the venous system in the arm and then diffuses through the tissues.[17] Once analgesia is established, the lower (distal) tourniquet is inflated and the upper (proximal) tourniquet is deflated. The inflated tourniquet is now over an analgesic area, and the occurrence of tourniquet pain is reduced. Tourniquet pain can still be a problem with this method, especially if the procedure is prolonged over an hour. Tourniquet time limits analgesia. When the tourniquet is released, sensation is quickly restored. Intravenous bupivacaine evidently allows the physician 20 minutes of analgesia after tourniquet release,[18] and this drug is now available commercially in the United States.

DOSAGE: Three mgm per kg of 0.5 per cent lidocaine is used for intravenous regional analgesia (42 cc in a 70 kgm

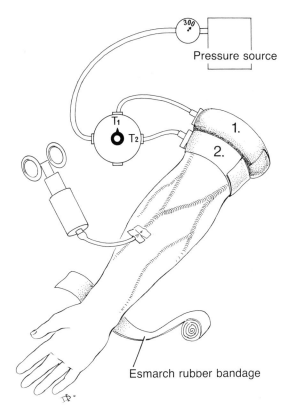

Figure 2–1 Intravenous regional analgesia. A double cuffed tourniquet permits inflation of an occlusive tourniquet over a previously anesthetized area. Such tourniquets are commercially available.

Pressure source

Esmarch rubber bandage

adult). There will be no motor nerve block with this concentration. The physician should not use the drug made up with preservative or with epinephrine. If flaccidity is desired, 1 mgm d-tubocurarine per 40 pounds of body weight can be added to the injection. This small dose will be harmlessly redistributed when the tourniquet is released.

Axillary Block. This block is easily learned, and has been found suitable for emergency and elective surgery of the forearm and hand.[19] The technique is quite useful in children. Needle placement for the block is illustrated in Figure 2–2. The brachial artery is invested with a perivascular fascial sheath. The sheath holds not only the artery but also the median, radial and ulnar nerves.

The patient lies supine, with the arm to be blocked placed so that the hand rests above or near the top of the head. A 23 gauge needle is inserted close to the brachial artery near the lateral border of the pectoralis major muscle. A paresthesia is sought, indicating needle contact with one of the nerves in the perivascular sheath. (The sheath is fairly superficial in the axilla, and the physician will err in going too deep.) The radial nerve lies behind the artery, so the median nerve (above) or the ulnar nerve (below) is usually encountered with the needle. The patient will experience tingling or an electric shock

sensation down the forearm into the hand. The patient should be instructed to say "Now" when the paresthesia is elicited. The entire anesthetic solution can be deposited at the site of the paresthesia. An alternate technique is to deposit half the anesthetic solution at each of two separately elicited paresthesiae, usually the median and ulnar nerves. (See later for dosage.) The anesthetic solution will spread within the perivascular sheath and surround all three nerves. Some patients find this block an unpleasant experience and premedication is required. The physician will also encounter patients who will not experience a paresthesia. In this instance the 23 gauge needle is inserted directly into the brachial artery and its position is checked by aspiration of blood. The needle is then withdrawn to a point just outside the artery where blood can no longer be aspirated. The tip of the needle is presumed to be in the perivascular space, and again the entire amount of anesthetic solution is deposited.

The injection site may not give anesthesia to the musculocutaneous nerve. A sensory branch of this nerve, the lateral antebrachial cutaneous nerve, has a variable distribution in the radial border of the forearm and down into the thenar eminence. The physician will occasionally encounter patients who

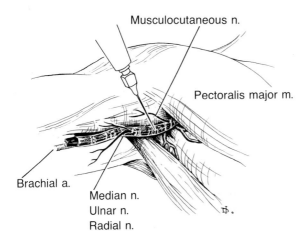

Musculocutaneous n.

Pectoralis major m.

Brachial a.

Median n.
Ulnar n.
Radial n.

Figure 2–2 The axillary block. Note that the musculocutaneous nerve is often missed with this block. The anesthetic solution is held in place by the perivascular sheath that encases both the artery and the nerves.

will experience some sensation if surgical dissection is carried into these areas. The problem is usually solved by local infiltration at the surgical site.

Tourniquet pain is sometimes experienced with this block, owing to tourniquet pressure on the intercostobrachial nerve that innervates a portion of the upper medial aspect of the arm. A line of subcutaneous infiltration of local anesthetic across the axilla above the tourniquet will solve this problem.

DOSAGE: Lidocaine with epinephrine will give around three hours of anesthesia with this block. Dosage of lidocaine with epinephrine 1:200,000 should be limited to 7–8 mgm per kg. A sufficient volume (¼ cc per pound in the adult) to fill the axillary sheath must be used. In children 7–8 mgm per kg of 1 per cent lidocaine with epinephrine will supply sufficient volume. As an example, in a young, fit, 80 kg man, one would use 30 cc of 1.5 per cent lidocaine with epinephrine plus 10 cc of 1.0 per cent lidocaine with epinephrine. This is a volume of 40 cc with a total dosage of 550 mgm. The maximum allowable dose in this man would be 560–640 mgm.

Mepivicaine 1 per cent, also 7–8 mgm per kg can be used. The block can be prolonged to a four to six hour range with the addition of 1 mgm per cc volume tetracaine. In all blocks with near the maximum allowed dose, an IV drip should be placed in the patient. Resuscitation gear should be at hand wherever blocks are done.

Interscalene Block. This block has been developed and promulgated by Dr. Alon P. Winnie.[20] Because of its site of injection it provides immobility at the shoulder joint and anesthesia of the musculocutaneous nerves, features missing with an axillary block. As the intercostobrachial nerve is still intact with the block, subcutaneous axillary infiltration is required if a tourniquet is used on the arm. The approach to the block is different from that used for the classic supraclavicular approach to the brachial plexus. The supraclavicular approach entails a risk of pneumothorax (0.5 to 4 per cent incidence),[6] while the interscalene approach avoids this complication.

The approach to the block is illustrated in Figure 2–3. The anatomy of

Figure 2–3 The interscalene block. The needle is inserted into the interscalene groove at the level of the cricoid cartilage. The needle points inwardly and slightly caudad.

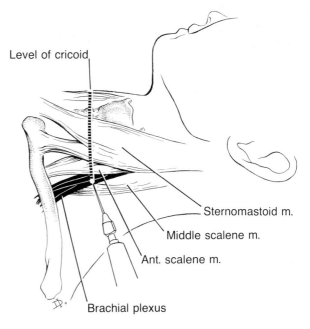

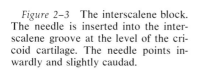

Level of cricoid

Sternomastoid m.

Middle scalene m.

Ant. scalene m.

Brachial plexus

the patient's neck is brought into relief by tilting the head backward and sharply away from the arm to be blocked. The patient is then asked to stretch the arm as if reaching for his knee, and the muscles are brought further into relief by asking the patient to raise his head. Just lateral to the sternocleidomastoid muscle can be felt the anterior scalene muscle. The interscalene groove is palpated lateral to the anterior scalene. A line perpendicular to the interscalene groove is drawn on the skin of the neck from the cricoid cartilage and a 21 gauge needle is inserted at the junction of the interscalene groove with this perpendicular cricoid line. The needle is advanced inwardly and slightly caudad and is kept in an imaginary plane that is perpendicular to the neck at the interscalene groove. Three or four attempts may be needed to elicit a paresthesia, which is mandatory before injection of a drug. The patient will feel the paresthesia down into the hand. No injection is made if the patient has paresthesia in the posterior shoulder, as the block will not succeed. The physician may feel a distinct "pop" as the fibrous tissue investing the brachial plexus is penetrated.

DOSAGE: Adequate volume is necessary for this block. In adults, Winnie suggests the formula $\dfrac{\text{Height (Inches)}}{2} =$ Volume (ml) as a starting point. One to one and a half per cent lidocaine with epinephrine, mepivicaine or prilocaine can be used, provided the maximum allowed dose of these drugs is not exceeded. Low volumes usually result in incomplete block of the ulnar nerve. Larger volumes (40 ml in the adult) will result in block of the supraclavicular nerves as well. Care must be taken not to exceed the maximum allowed mgm per kg dose.

Sciatic-Femoral Block. Sciatic-femoral block was perfected in the United States by the pioneer anesthesiologist Gaston Labat.[21] It is technically more difficult to perform than the other blocks listed in this chapter, but it is included here because of its usefulness in outpatient

and emergency surgery. Surgical incision or manipulation can be performed from 2 cm below the patella. The block will also cover closed manipulation of the knee and the lower portion of the femur. The tourniquet cannot be applied with this block without the additional block of the lateral femoral cutaneous nerve.[6]

The anatomy for the sciatic-femoral block is illustrated in Figures 2–4 and 2–5. The patient lies laterally with the leg to be blocked uppermost and drawn up (Sims' position). A line is drawn from the posterosuperior spine of the ilium to the greater trochanter. The midpoint of the line is located and a perpendicular bisecting line is drawn at this point down the leg. The injection site is 3–5 cm down this bisecting line. A 22 gauge spinal needle is inserted perpendicular to the skin at this point, a depth of 6–8 or even 10 cm being necessary to locate the sciatic nerve. Paresthesia is manifested by tingling or an electric shock sensation down the back of the leg. The patient should be instructed to say "Now" when this paresthesia is obtained.

Bone may be encountered while advancing the needle at this site. This is the rim around the greater sciatic notch. The nerve is usually close to this depth, so the needle need not be advanced much farther.

If no paresthesia is obtained, the needle is redirected either upward or downward in a plane in the body perpendicular to the original bisecting line drawn on the skin surface.

The femoral nerve block is performed with the patient lying supine. The femoral nerve lies lateral at the same depth as the femoral artery. The nerve is best approached from a point 1 cm below the inguinal ligament and just lateral to the artery. The anesthetic solution should be injected in an imaginary triangle. The apex of the triangle is the injection site, while the base is on a plane passing slightly below the femoral artery and nerve (3–3.5 cm). The line of the base is parallel to a line 1 cm below and parallel to the inguinal liga-

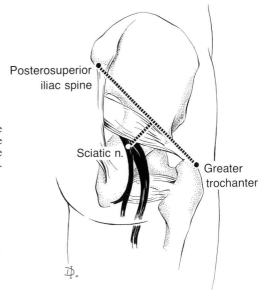

Figure 2–4 Sciatic femoral block. Block of the sciatic nerve. If the needle encounters bone, the operator is at the correct depth, but the needle must be redirected until a paresthesia is elicited.

ment. The injection is carried from the artery laterally at least 1 inch. Usually no paresthesia is elicited.

DOSAGE: Lidocaine (1.0 to 1.25 per cent) with 1:200,000 epinephrine is used. The volume injected at the sciatic nerve varies from 20 to 30 cc. The femoral nerve is injected with 10–15 cc

more fluid. The maximum permitted dose of 7–8 mgm per kg of lidocaine with epinephrine should not be exceeded. In a 70 kg man, this means 30 cc of 1 per cent lidocaine with epinephrine (or 20 cc of 1.5 per cent lidocaine with epinephrine) at the sciatic nerve and 15 cc of 1 percent lidocaine

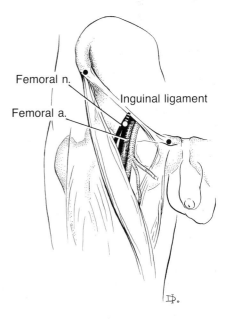

Figure 2–5 Sciatic femoral block. Block of the femoral nerve. No paresthesia is required for this block. The success rate is quite high.

with epinephrine at the femoral nerve. The total dose would then be 450 mgm, while the maximum permitted dose in a 70 kg man is between 490 and 560 mgm.

Anesthesia for Inguinal Hernia.[6,21] Although many surgeons have never used regional anesthesia for this operation, it is a commendable technique. Routine herniorrhaphy is followed by early mobilization and lack of hospitalization. Obviously, complicated hernia

repair should not be attempted on an outpatient basis, but, in experienced hands, the routine herniorrhaphy is of short duration. As will be seen by the description below, the volume of drug injected is fairly large; thus procaine, chlorprocaine or 0.5 per cent xylocaine with epinephrine might be considered the drugs of choice for this surgery. Reference is made in this description to Figure 2–6. Step 1 (Fig. 2–6 *A* and *B*): The operator starts at point X,

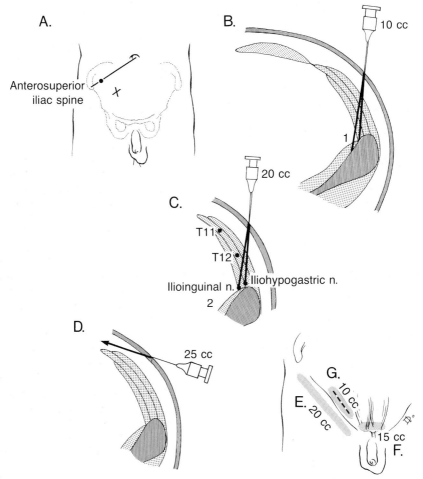

Figure 2–6 Herniorrhaphy. *A.* Point X is roughly 1 inch from the anterior superior iliac spine along the line from this spine to the umbilicus. *B.* Here anesthetic solution is deposited along the inside shelf of the iliac bone. The needle insertion is made at point X. *C.* Muscles lying below the line drawn in *A* are infiltrated in order to block the hypogastric, ilioinguinal and thoracic nerves. *D.* A subcutaneous line of infiltration is carried out on the line drawn in *A*. *E.* Branches of the gluteal and femoral nerves are blocked by a subcutaneous infiltration ½ inch below the inguinal ligament. *F.* Attachments of the rectus abdominis are infiltrated at the pubic bone. *G.* A subcutaneous line of anesthesia is infiltrated where the incision is to be made.

located on the line from the anterior superior iliac spine to the umbilicus. Here 10 cc of anesthetic solution is deposited along the inside shelf of the iliac bone. Step 2 (Fig. 2–6 *C*): The needle is again inserted at point X and a fan-shaped infiltration in the anterior abdominal musculature is made in a plane perpendicular to the line drawn in *A*. Fifteen to twenty cc of solution is used. Multiple redirections are necessary to hit the hypogastric and ilioinguinal nerve as well as thoracic nerves T11 and T12. Step 3 (Fig. 2–6 *D*): Here the needle is directed subcutaneously on the line drawn in Step 1, (Fig. 2–6 *A*). Twenty-five cc of solution is deposited along this line to block thoracic nerves coming down into the operative area. Step 4 (Fig. 2–6 *E*): Subcutaneous infiltration is carried out $1/2$ inch below the inguinal ligament from the anterior superior iliac spine to the groin. This blocks branches of the gluteal and femoral nerves that may go to the operative area. Step 5 (Figs. 2–6 *E*): A deep infection of 15 cc is made along the superior ramus of the pubic bone into the attachment of the rectus abdominis muscle, and into the space between the bladder and pubic bone. Steps 6 and 7 (Fig. 2–6 *E*): Ten cc is injected along the incision line. Tissue in the spermatic cord at the external ring must be blocked when it is exposed, as must the genitofemoral nerve at the internal ring. This should be done by the surgeon after the operation has begun. Attempts at transcutaneous blocking of these structures may result in hematoma formation.

DOSAGE: One hundred cc of either 1 per cent procaine, 1 per cent chlorprocaine or 100 cc of 0.5 per cent xylocaine with 0.25 cc of 1:1000 epinephrine. (Epinephrine concentrations in local anesthetics must not exceed 0.25 cc of 1:1000 total dose.)[6]

Epidural and Subarachnoid Anesthesia.[6,22] These techniques are infrequently used in an outpatient setting for surgery. Spinal anesthesia can be followed by postpuncture headache, a condition caused by the slow leak of cerebrospinal fluid through the puncture hole in the arachnoid membrane. Treatment usually requires bed rest, as the symptoms of this headache are exacerbated by an erect posture. Spinal anesthesia may also result in urinary retention that continues for many hours after sensory nerve block has worn off. This phenomenon is thought to be the result of residual autonomic nerve blockade.[22]

Epidural anesthesia avoids the possibility of postpuncture headache, provided that the epidural needle does not penetrate the arachnoid membrane. This difficulty can occur even in experienced hands, and postpuncture headache may follow. Urinary retention can also follow epidural anesthesia.

Intramuscular and Intravenous Drugs for Outpatient Surgery

In both this section and the section concerning inhalational agents, drugs will be discussed that have actions so powerful and side effects so numerous that administering them should be restricted to those who have clinical training and experience with these drugs. Hopefully this presentation will increase understanding between those wishing to undertake surgery and those anxious to learn about the numerous depressant effects of premedicant and anesthetic drugs.

Premedication. Premedicant or sedative drugs should be kept at a minimum for outpatient surgery. Regional block, however, is more successful with sedation. Thus if sedative drugs are to be administered, they should be of short duration and noncumulative, an ideal difficult to achieve. The drugs are best given in fractional intravenous doses as required.

Antisialagogues. Cholinergic blocking agents are used to prevent excessive salivation. Patient discomfort is increased unnecessarily if these drugs are used with regional block techniques. Atropine (intramuscularly) 0.1 mgm per 15 pounds body weight can be used up to a total dose of 0.4 to 0.5 mgm. Scopolamine is a superior drying agent, and has the effect of amnesia and sedation. Patients will sometimes become delirious with scopolamine, especially in the presence of pain, and therefore the use of it alone in outpatient surgery is not advised.

Narcotics. This group of drugs is useful when preoperative pain is present or postoperative pain is anticipated. The author is best able to gauge the dose by repeated intravenous administration of small doses of narcotics. As a general rule, 2.5 mgm morphine sulfate IV, 20 mgm meperidine (Demerol) IV, or 0.025 mgm fentanyl (Sublimaze) IV give about the same degree of pain relief. The doses can be repeated as required. Ordy et al.[23] found the frequency of nausea the same with all these drugs. Morphine will last somewhat longer than meperidine (one to two hours). Fentanyl, given IV, has a duration of action of only 15 to 30 minutes. Fentanyl has been combined successfully with nitrous oxide analgesia (see below) for outpatient surgery.[54] Overdose with fentanyl, and indeed with all narcotic drugs, is manifested primarily by respiratory depression. Overdose with narcotic drugs can be combatted with a narcotic antagonist levallorphan (Lorfan) 0.5–1.0 mgm IV, nalorphine (Nalline) 5–10 mgm IV, or Naloxone (Narcan) 0.2–0.4 mgm IV. Naloxone has the advantage over other narcotic antagonists in that it has no narcotic depressing properties.

Pentazocine (Talwin) was originally investigated as a narcotic antagonist but is now used as an analgesic. Thirty mgm doses of Talwin can be roughly equated with 10 mgm morphine.[24] The drug was formerly believed to have no addictive effects, but reports of addiction have appeared.[25] The drug also has a "ceiling effect": doses above a certain point—usually 60 mgm—produce no additional analgesia. Nausea and vomiting can be seen with pentazocine.

Most postoperative pain following outpatient surgery can be treated with aspirin or codeine.

Diazepam (Valium). Tranquilizing drugs can also be used in outpatient surgery, but all suffer from the disadvantage that they may cause excessive drowsiness in a patient who is to leave the hospital. As a general rule, phenothiazines are not the drugs of choice in outpatient surgical situations because of their peripheral vasodilating and thus hypotensive properties. Diazepam (Valium)[26] can be given in a 2.5 mgm dose provided it is given slowly into an intravenous drip, as the drug is irritating to the vein. There is more documentation of diazepam as an adjunct in anesthesia than its congener chlordiazepoxide (Librium). Only diazepam has amnestic properties, which is to its advantage. Larger doses cause respiratory depression, especially noticeable when the drug is used with narcotics; diazepam will reduce the emetic effect of narcotics. Although it has no noticeable cardiovascular depressant effects, it does appear to depress patients with alcohol intoxication.

Outpatient dentistry utilizing local analgesia and diazepam has been studied several times.[26] These reports show that diazepam is a valuable adjunct in outpatient surgery, provided that it is not used to produce deep sedation, and the patient is taken home by a responsible party.

Short-Acting Barbiturates. There is no particular use for long-acting barbiturates in outpatient surgery, and the drugs will not be discussed here. Thiopental (Pentothal) and methohexital (Brevital) are mainstays in an outpatient surgical practice. Administration of these drugs may result in respiratory obstruction, hiccoughs, laryngospasm (usually caused by surgical stimulation and too little drug), apnea (caused by overdose), vomiting with consequent aspiration, and cardiovascular depression. Intravenous short-acting barbiturates should not be given to a patient with a full stomach without the prior or subsequent rapid insertion of a cuffed endotracheal tube. The pain of injury will slow gastric motility, and a patient who ate shortly before injury may have food in the stomach *24 hours* after injury. The physician should not use these drugs unless he is prepared to handle the unfortunate consequences that sometimes result.

Thiopental was originally investigated clinically by Lundy at the Mayo Clinic[27] in the early 1930's. The drug is given intravenously in 2.5 per cent concentrations. A test dose of 50 mgm (2 cc) is first administered, followed by gradual injection of the drug to the point where the eyes are fixed and the eyelids no longer contract when the lashes are stroked (wink reflex). The 50 mgm dose will occasionally produce the desired effect in the infirm or demonstrate cardiovascular instability in a hypertensive patient. If hypotension ensues from a test dose, the method should be discontinued. The total dose required will vary from 100 mgm to 1 gm in the adult, and give three to ten minutes of anesthesia.

Once the patient has been anesthetized in this fashion, an operator can perform minor surgical procedures. Thiopental is frequently supplemented with nitrous oxide analgesia (see below) or local anesthetic infiltration. As with all general anesthetics, it is best that one operator handle the thiopental administration, and allow another operator to devote his full attention to the required surgical procedure.

The patient rapidly recovers consciousness from thiopental because of the redistribution of the drug in the body, but drowsiness persists for hours. Longer procedures should not be attempted with thiopental, as the cumulative effects of the drug will produce unnecessary cardiovascular and respiratory depression.[28]

Methohexital (Brevital) is an adequate substitute for thiopental, described first by Gruber et al. in 1956.[29] It is approximately 3.3 times as potent as thiopental.[30] The drug is administered in a 1.0 per cent solution. Many authors feel methohexital has a shorter recovery period.[28, 31] Methohexital is also a respiratory and cardiovascular depressant and should not be used in repetitive doses to prolong anesthesia.[28, 32]

Other Intravenous Agents. Ketamine (Ketalar, Ketaject) marks a new departure in anesthesia and has proved quite useful in outpatient anesthesia work. The drug is not a barbiturate or a narcotic.[33, 34] Miyasaka and Domino[35] have offered evidence that ketamine acts to block or dissociate sensory input from nonspecific thalamic nuclei to the cortex of the brain; ketamine anesthesia is sometimes referred to as a dissociative state. Apnea sometimes appears on induction, but respiration is usually unimpaired. The patient appears to be in a deep sleep, with oropharyngeal reflexes intact. Roving eye movements and random muscle movements herald lightness. Usually the airway is maintained, but the author has encountered patients whose heads must be fully extended or who require a nasopharyngeal airway to keep the airway unobstructed. Preoperative atropine is required to dry secretions in the mouth. The cardiovascular system is stable—indeed, there is an increase in blood pressure. Hypertension is a contraindication for ketamine, and operations that may cause blood or irrigating fluid to enter the mouth or nose are also contraindicated. Laryngospasm may be precipitated by these fluids under ketamine anesthesia, for laryngeal reflexes are not suppressed. The drug is best given IV, and usually 1.0 mgm per pound is sufficient, but the initial dose can be supplemented with 0.5–1.0 mgm per pound doses as required. IM doses of 4–6 mgm per pound can also be used.

There is unfortunately a high incidence of postoperative hallucinations in adults. The incidence will be decreased if the patient is left to recover quietly without external stimulation, but even then the incidence may be unacceptable to many physicians.

The drug has a wide application in pediatric surgery, since children either do not experience or are not bothered by hallucinations. The reason for this difference from the adult experience is not known.

Prolonged procedures are possible

with ketamine alone, using repeat doses of the drug. However, the longer the procedure, the longer the recovery time will be. Single IV doses allow recovery in one or two hours. Adequate postoperative recovery facilities, identical to those used for inpatient surgery, are required.

Propanidid (Epontol). This drug appears to be a useful intravenous agent for outpatient procedures because of its transient action and the rapid recovery that follows its use.[36] The rapid recovery appears to be caused by the drug's metabolism by serum cholinesterase, as well as by drug redistribution. The drug is not available in the United States, but can be obtained elsewhere. Following its administration, first hyperventilation, then hypoventilation or apnea can occur. Administration of larger doses of propanidid can also cause hypotension and its use appears contraindicated in patients with cardiovascular instability. The drug can be considered equipotent to thiopental for induction[30] but with a much faster recovery time. Dose ranges are generally accepted as 5–10 mgm per kg for surgical procedures.

Neurolept-Analgesia. This method of anesthesia is available to the American physician by the use of Innovar, a combination of the ultrashort-acting narcotic fentanyl (Sublimaze) (see earlier discussion), and droperidol (Inapsine), a long-acting tranquilizing agent of the butyrophenone group. Other combinations of drugs, of similar pharmacological properties, are available in other parts of the world. Neurolept-analgesia would appear best reserved for inpatient anesthesia because of the long action (6 to 12 hours) of droperidol.[37]

Agents for Inhalational Analgesia and Anesthesia. The ideal agent for outpatient anesthesia (as yet undiscovered) should offer rapid onset, rapid recovery, no side effects of nausea, vomiting or hallucination, no cardiovascular or respiratory depression, and no need to artificially maintain an airway. Some of the inhalational agents approach this ideal as closely as the drugs previously discussed. Analgesia with inhalational agents may be defined as a state in which peripheral sensation is markedly diminished, but the patient retains consciousness, responds to commands and still maintains his own airway.

Analgesia with methoxyflurane (Penthrane) or trichloroethylene (Trilene) with air or with nitrous oxide and oxygen fulfills many of the requirements for an agent in outpatient anesthesia. The analgesia produced by these agents is usually insufficient to completely mask the pain of surgical procedures. Intelligent patients will tolerate easy dental extractions, sprain and fracture manipulation, joint injections, abscess incision, and other similar procedures, with inhalational analgesia. The greatest clinical experience in this field comes from attempts to control the pain of labor and delivery,[38,39,40] but this clinical experience can be transferred to other areas.[41]

Methoxyflurane (Penthrane) and trichloroethylene analgesia can be self-administered by various commercially available hand-held inhalers (Fig. 2–7). Penthrane is used in a Cyprane or Duke inhaler with the setting in a "full on" position. Both these agents are potent, and general anesthesia can result if too high a concentration is used. This is to the physician's disadvantage, as the patient will lose protective cough and gag reflexes, and possibly aspirate stomach contents. *Inhalational analgesic agents should not be used except by those physicians with the proper facilities and training to handle any consequence of the administration of these drugs.*

General anesthetic agents in common use are summarized in Table 2–3. They all can be used for outpatient surgical work, but some agents seem more suitable than others. These agents can never be given in an emergency unless the airway is fully protected with a cuffed endotracheal tube. Equipotent minimum alveolar concentrations (MAC) are listed to give the reader an idea of the potency of the various agents. The minimum alveolar concentration of an

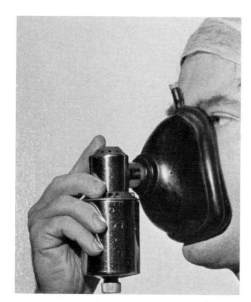

Figure 2–7 A hand-held inhaler. Either trichloroethylene (Trilene) or methoxyflurane (Penthrane) can be used with this device.

anesthetic gas is defined as that concentration required to prevent gross muscular movement in 50 per cent of the subjects in response to a painful stimulus. Values are percentage concentrations at sea level.[42]

Agents that have a low blood gas solubility or low tissue solubility will have a shorter induction and emergence time. The concentration of anesthetic agents in the brain rapidly approaches the concentration of the anesthetic agent in the alveoli when the blood gas solubility is low. When an agent with high blood gas solubility is used, the brain will take longer to receive a sufficient concentration of the agent to induce anesthesia. Emergence time will be delayed by their high blood and tissue solubility. Thus after an ether or methoxyflurane anesthetic, the patient tends to remain somnolent and with diminished postoperative pain for many hours. This may be a distinct advantage with inpatient surgery, but not for the patient who is expected to return home. Agents with a high incidence of postoperative nausea, vomiting, emergence delirium and hallucinations are less acceptable than those agents with a low incidence of these undesirable side effects. These side effects can be controlled with sedatives and antiemetic agents, but such drugs, in turn, will impair the patient when he leaves the hospital.

Explosive agents are becoming less popular as more electrocautery is used and more electrical monitoring equipment is brought into the operating room. Many authorities feel that explosive agents are contraindicated with dental outpatient surgery, as sparks may be produced with drilling or forceps application.

Halothane (Fluothane) is the most widely used inhalational anesthetic in the United States today. It has a low incidence of postoperative nausea and vomiting; it is nonexplosive; and it has a relatively low blood gas solubility. Thus one can predict a brief emergence following short outpatient procedures. Halothane does have a high body fat solubility, and emergence from a longer operation with halothane will be prolonged unless the inspired concentration of the agent is gradually reduced during the case.

Halothane anesthesia can be used in outpatients alone or with atropine premedication only. Lack of heavier preoperative sedation may result in postoperative headache.[3, 43] Also, other preoperative medication will prolong emergence. Even thiopental induction of anesthesia will result in a longer time to complete recovery.[44]

It is highly probable that in rare instances halothane will cause postanesthetic hepatitis.[45] This statement is made against the background of the result of the National Halothane Study, which concludes that halothane is as safe as, if not safer than, other anesthetic agents.[46] Most reported cases of post-halothane hepatitis have a history of prior halothane administration, so that if one forecasts a series of operations for a certain patient, halothane anesthesia should not be used. Halothane is used so widely

TABLE 2–3 Pharmacology of General Anesthetic Agents

Agent (Trade Name)	Supplied	Administered	MAC in O_2	Blood Gas Solubility Coefficient	Flammability	Problems
Di-Ethyl Ether	Copper-lined cans	Open drop or G.M. vaporizer	1.9%	12.1	Flammable and explosive	High incidence nausea and vomiting with emergence
Nitrous Oxide	Gas cylinders	Gas machine	101%	.468	Supports combustion Nonflammable	Inadequate for most procedures
Cyclopropane	Gas cylinders	Gas machine	9.2%	.415	Flammable Highly explosive	High incidence nausea and vomiting, also delirium
Trichlorethylene (Trilene)	Bottles	Gas machine vaporizer Hand-held vaporizer	Est. 1–2%	9.15	Nonflammable within clinical limits of use	Cannot be used with CO_2-absorbing cannister
Halothane (Fluothane)	Bottles	Open drop (rare) G. M. vaporizer	0.76%	2.3	Nonflammable	Emergence shivering, rare incidence hepatitis
Fluroxene (Fluoromar)	Bottles	Gas machine vaporizer	3.4% 0.8% with 77% N20 (48)	1.37	Flammable with conc. > 4%	High incidence nausea and vomiting with emergence
Methoxyflurane (Penthrane)	Bottles	Hand-held vaporizer Gas machine vaporizer	0.16%	13.0	Nonflammable	Rare incidence renal pathology, emergence prolonged

that many patients who have had surgery in the last ten years will have already received the drug. How long should one wait after a halothane anesthetic is administered before giving another? An arbitrary three month period has been recommended.[47] These authors also recommend that until a specific test for viral or halothane hepatitis is developed, the use of halogenated agents in any patient with known liver disease, sepsis, or a recent history of flu-like symptoms should be avoided. A previous halothane administration followed by unexplained postoperative fever or unexplained jaundice is also an indication to avoid further halothane anesthetics. This is but one view, and it remains to be seen if this course of action will decrease the incidence of postoperative halothane hepatitis.

Substitution of methoxyflurane or fluroxene (see Table 2–3) for halothane has been proposed as a solution to this problem. Methoxyflurane is nonexplosive, as is fluroxene in concentrations below 4 per cent. Fluroxene is given in nitrous oxide and oxygen to reduce the potential for explosion.[48] Methoxyflurane, however, has been implicated in the production of postoperative renal toxicity;[49] the mechanism of this reaction has not yet been fully explained. Fluroxene is popular at the author's hospital, but there is limited clinical experience with it in most parts of the country; if it were used as extensively as halothane, it is possible that problems of hepatic toxicity would become apparent. Trichloroethylene (see Table 2–2) with nitrous oxide and oxygen is useful in many outpatient surgical situations. The gas cannot be used with sodalime carbon dioxide absorbing cannisters, as toxic byproducts are formed in the sodalime that are later passed on to other patients.

Endotracheal   General   Anesthesia. Endotracheal intubation is a necessary adjunct for many types of outpatient anesthesia. Adding intubation to an anesthetic will increase the morbidity of the procedure. Mild sore throat is by far the most commonly seen complication. An incidence of 46 per cent has been reported.[50] On the other hand, intubation is necessary for intraoral work, or in patients in whom airway management under anesthesia can present a real problem.

Succinyldicholine (Anectine). Intubation can be facilitated with the use of succinyldicholine, a short-acting muscle relaxant. Its use is mandatory for rapid emergency intubation to gain control of the airway (see Chapter 26). Use of this drug will also increase postanesthetic morbidity, as any dose greater than 10 mgm is associated with varying degrees of muscle ache in patients. The aching, especially in the back of the neck and chest, occurs 18 to 72 hours postoperatively. The incidence can be reduced but not eliminated by small doses of d-tubocurarine IV (3 mgm) preceding succinyldicholine injection.[51] Succinyldicholine administration can also increase intraocular pressure,[52] although here the phenomenon can be blocked by 3 or 6 mgm d-tubocurarine IV. Caution is urged when succinyldicholine is planned for any patient with glaucoma.

Succinyldicholine is metabolized by plasma pseudocholinesterase. Thus apnea following succinyldicholine injection normally lasts only three to five minutes. There are patients who have a hereditary deficiency of this enzyme. The incidence of heterozygous deficiency is about 1 in every 25 patients. Heterozygous patients show a slight prolongation of the drug's action that is not clinically significant. Apnea prolonged up to several hours follows in homozygotes, the incidence being roughly one in every 2500 patients.[53] The deficiency is usually discovered after the injection, as there is no widespread screening procedure for this condition. There is no antidote for succinyldicholine. Apneic patients must be ventilated until the drug wears off.

Despite these drawbacks, succinyldicholine is quite useful in outpatient surgery. The profound but brief relaxation is useful for intubation, reducing fractures and dislocations, or to facilitate abdominal examination under anesthesia. The drug can be given by an intravenous drip or by intermittent injection for periods of muscle relaxation longer than one to three minutes. This drug should be used only by physicians well trained on an anesthesiology service.

Longer-acting muscle relaxants such as d-tubocurarine are infrequently used in outpatient surgery, except with intravenous regional analgesia, or as an adjunct to the use of succinyldicholine in glaucomatous patients.

Summary. This chapter has attempted to cover enough separate anesthetic techniques to allow the reader to intelligently select among them while dealing with outpatient surgical patients. This chapter is not encyclopedic; many useful variations of the techniques described can be found by consulting the appropriate references listed at the end of the chapter.

Anesthetic drugs do not cure disease; their use constitutes a certain risk to every patient who receives them. Intelligent administration of these drugs requires training in a separate branch of medicine, and no physician should attempt these techniques without previous training in anesthesiology.

References

1. 285,00 inactive registered nurses could turn the tide. J.A.M.A., *200*:779–780, 1967.
2. McNamara, M. J., Hill, M. C., Balows, A., and Tucker, E. B.: A study of the bacteriologic patterns of hospital infections. Ann. Intern. Med., *66*:480–488, 1967.
3. Cohen, D. D., and Dillon, J. B.: Anesthesia for outpatient surgery. J.A.M.A., *196*: 1114–1116, 1966.
4. Treloar, E. J.: An out-patient anesthetic service: standards and organization. Can. Anaesth. Soc. J., *14*:596–604, 1967.
5. Fahy, A., and Marshall, M.: Postanesthetic morbidity in out-patients. Br. J. Anaesth., *41*:433–438, 1969.
6. Moore, D. C.: Regional Block: A Handbook for Use in the Clinical Practice of Medicine and Surgery. Springfield: C. C Thomas, 1967.
7. Bromage, P. R.: Improved conduction blockade in surgery and obstetrics: Carbonated local anesthetics. Can. Med. Assoc. J., *97*: 1377–1384, 1967.
8. Adriani, J.: The clinical pharmacology of local anesthetics. Clin. Pharmacol. Ther., *1*:645–673, 1960.
9. Aldrete, J. A., and Johnson, D. A.: Allergy to local anesthetics. J.A.M.A., *207*:356–357, 1969.
10. Proctor, D. F.: Anesthesia for peroral endoscopy and bronchography. Anesthesiology, *29*:1025–1036, 1968.
11. Harris, L. C., Parry, J. C., and Greifenstein, F. E.: Dyclonine – A new local anesthetic agent: Clinical evaluation. Anesthesiology, *17*:648–652, 1956.
12. Foldes, F. F., Molloy, R., McNall, P. G., and Koukal, L. R.: Comparison of toxicity of intravenously given local anesthetic agents in man. J.A.M.A., *172*:1493–1498, 1960.
13. Löfström, B.: Aspects of the pharmacology of local anesthetic agents. Br. J. Anaesth., *42*:194–206, 1970.
14. Moore, D. C., Bridenbaugh, L. D., Bagdi, P. A., and Bridenbaugh, P. O.: Accumulation of mepivacaine hydrochloride during caudal block. Anesthesiology, *29*:585–588, 1968.
15. Moore, D. C., Bridenbaugh, L. D., Bridenbaugh, P. O., and Tucker, G. T.: Bupivacaine hydrochloride: Laboratory and clinical studies. Anesthesiology, *32*:78–83, 1970.
16. Holmes, C. McK.: Intravenous regional analgesia: A useful method of producing analgesia of the limbs. Lancet *1*:245–247, February, 1963.
17. Adams, J. P., Kenmore, P. I., Russell, P. H., and Haas, S. S.: Regional anesthesia in the upper limb. Curr. Pract. Orthop. Surg., *4*:238–261, 1969.
18. Watson, R. L., Brown, P. W., and Reich, M. P.: Venous and arterial bupivacaine concentrations after intravenous regional anesthesia. Anesth. Analg. (Cleveland), *49*: 300–304, 1970.
19. DeJong, R. H.: Axillary block of the brachial plexus. Anesthesiology, *22*:215–225, 1961.
20. Winnie, A. P.: Interscalene brachial plexus block. Anesth. Analg. (Cleveland), *49*: 455–466, 1970.
21. Adriani, J. (ed.): Labat's Regional Anesthesia. Philadelphia: W. B. Saunders Co., 1967.
22. Greene, N. M.: Physiology of Spinal Anesthesia. Baltimore: Williams and Wilkins Co., 1969.
23. Ordy, J. M., Kretchmer, H. E., Gorry, T. H., and Hershberger, T. J.: Comparison of effects of morphine, meperidine, fentanyl, and fentanyl-droperidol. Clin. Pharmacol. Ther., *11*:488–495, 1970.
24. Potter, D. R., and Payne, J. P.: Newer analgesics: With special reference to pentazocine. Br. J. Anaesth., *42*:186–193, 1970.
25. Weber, W. F., and Rome, H. P.: Addiction to pentazocine: Report of two cases. J.A.M.A., *212*:1708, 1970.

26. Dundee, J. W., and Haslett, W. H. K.: The benzodiazepines. A review of their actions and uses relative to anaesthetic practice. Br. J. Anaesth., *42*:217–234, 1970.

27. Lundy, J. S.: Intravenous anesthesia: Preliminary report of the use of two new thiobarbiturates. Proc. Staff Meet. Mayo Clin., *10*:536–543, 1935.

28. Allen, G. D., Kennedy, W. F., Everett, G., and Tolas, A. G.: A comparison of the cardiorespiratory effects of methohexital and thiopental supplementation for outpatient dental anesthesia. Anesth. Analg. (Cleveland), *48*:730–735, 1969.

29. Gruber, C. M., Stoelting, V. K., Hicks, M. L., and Doughty, S.: Clinical experience during anesthesia with a new ultra-short-acting barbiturate. Fed. Proc., *15*:432 (Abstract 1407), 1956.

30. Clarke, R. S. J., Dundee, J. W., Barron, D. W., and McArdle, L.: Clinical studies of induction agents. XXVI: The relative potencies of thiopentone, methohexitone, and propanidid. Br. Anaesth., *40*:593–601, 1968.

31. Thornton, J. A.: Methohexitone and its application to dental anesthesia. Br. J. Anaesth., *42*:255–261, 1970.

32. Wise, C. C., Robinson, J. S., Heath, M. J., and Tomlin, P. J.: Physiological responses to intermittent methohexitone for conservative dentistry. Br. Med. J., *2*:540–543, 1969.

33. Virtue, R. W., Alanis, J. M., Mori, M., Lafarque, R. T., Vogel, J. H. K., and Metcalf, D. R.: An anesthetic agent: 2-orthochlorophenyl, 2-methylamino cyclohexane HC1 (CI-581). Anesthesiology, *28*:823–833, 1967.

34. Corssen, G., Miyasaka, M., and Domino, E. F.: Changing concepts in pain control during surgery: Dissociative anesthesia with CI-581. A progress report. Anesth. Anal. (Cleveland), *47*:746–759, 1968.

35. Miyasaka, M., and Domino, E. F.: Neuronal mechanisms of Ketamine-induced anesthesia. Int. J. Neuropharmacol., *7*:557–573, 1968.

36. Conway, C. M., and Ellis, D. B.: Propanidid. Br. J. Anaesth., *42*:249–254, 1970.

37. Edmonds-Seal, J., and Prys-Roberts, C.: Pharmacology of drugs used in neuroleptanalgesia. Br. J. Anaesth., *42*:207–216, 1970.

38. Smith, B. E., and Moya, F.: Inhalational analgesia with methoxyflurane for vaginal delivery. South. Med. J., *61*:386, 1968.

39. Trichloroethylene. In Bonica, J. J.: Principles and Practice of Obstetric Analgesia and Anesthesia. Philadelphia: F. A. Davis Co., 1967.

40. Hamilton, W. K.: The limited clinical pharmacology of nitrous oxide. Clin. Pharmacol. Ther., *4*:663–672, 1963.

41. Packer, K. J., and Titel, J. H.: Methoxyflurane analgesia for burns dressings: experience with the analgizer. Br. J. Anaesth., *41*: 1080–1085, 1969.

42. Eger, E. I., Brandstater, B., Saidman, L. J., Regan, M. J., Severinghaus, J. W., and Munson, E. S.: Equipotent alveolar concentrations of methoxyflurane, halothane, diethyl ether, fluroxene, cyclopropane, xenon and nitrous oxide in the dog. Anesthesiology, *26*:771–777, 1965.

43. Zohairy, A. F. M.: Postoperative headache after nitrous oxide–oxygen–halothane anesthesia. Br. J. Anaesth., *41*:972–976, 1969.

44. Doenicke, A.: Street fitness after anesthesia in outpatients. Acta Anaesthesiol. Scand. Suppl., *17*:95–97, 1965.

45. Trey, C., Lipworth, L., and Davidson, C. J.: The clinical syndrome of halothane hepatitis. Anesth. Anal. (Cleveland), *48*:1033–1040, 1969.

46. Summary of the national halothane study: Possible association between halothane anesthesia and post-operative hepatic necrosis. J.A.M.A., *197*:775–788, 1966.

47. Lomanto, C., and Howland, W. S.: Problems in diagnosing halothane hepatitis. J.A.M.A., *214*:1257–1261, 1970.

48. Munson, E. S., Saidman, L. J., and Eger, E. I.: Effects of nitrous oxide and morphine on the minimum anesthetic concentration of fluroxene. Anesthesiology, *26*:134–139, 1965.

49. Frascino, J. A., Vanamee, P., and Rosen, P. P.: Renal oxalosis and azotemia after methoxyflurane anesthesia. N. Engl. J. Med., *283*:676–679, 1970.

50. Lewis, R. N., and Swerdlow, M.: Hazards of endotracheal anesthesia. Br. J. Anesth., *36*:504–515, 1964.

51. Hustead, R. F., Atkinson, D. P., and Parmley, R. T.: Succinylcholine-induced muscle pain. Abstracts of Scientific Paper, A.S.A. Meeting 64–65, 1970.

52. Miller, R. D., Way, W. L., and Hickey, R. F.: Inhibition of Succinylcholine-induced increased intraocular pressure by non-depolarizing muscle relaxants. Anesthesiology, *29*:123–126, 1968.

53. Lehmann, H., and Liddell, J.: Human cholinesterase (pseudocholinesterase): genetic variants and their recognition. Br. J. Anaesth., *41*:235–244, 1969.

54. Grell, F. L., Koons, R. A., and Denson, J. S.: Fentanyl in anesthesia: a report of 500 cases. Anesth. Analg. (Cleveland), *49*:523–532, 1970.

3

Trauma

By LAWRENCE W. NORTON, M.D.

INTRODUCTION

The outpatient surgeon must be capable of managing injured patients. The scope of trauma encountered may range from minor injury of an individual to major injuries in mass casualties. While treating the former definitively, the outpatient surgeon initiates for the latter a sequence of treatment involving many hospital services. Common to both functions is his role as first surgeon to receive the injured.

About 50 million persons are injured each year in the United States for a rate of 25 injuries per 100 per year.[1] In 1969, 115,000 died in this country from accidents.[2] The incidence of motor vehicular accidents, accounting for half of these fatalities, is rising at an annual rate of 2 per cent. More than one-third of hospital Emergency Room visits are necessitated by trauma. Most injuries are minor and manageable on an outpatient basis, comprising 15 per cent of all acute conditions necessitating medical care.

Important principles of treatment pertain to all forms of trauma. First, the patient must be promptly attended whether his injury is major or minor. Treatment of minor wounds may be delayed in favor of more pressing problems provided that prompt initial appraisal of the patient is made. Second, care when given must be competent and complete. Complications of injury result from failure to treat as well as incorrect therapy. Third, disposition home or to other care must be prompt, avoiding unnecessary delay.

The outpatient management of trauma will be described in terms of mass casualties from a community disaster, major injuries in an individual patient who will require hospitalization and minor injury in a person who can return home after treatment.

MASS CASUALTIES

Overall Plan and Communications

An active hospital emergency service can seldom receive more than 25 seriously injured patients at one time without immediately expanding staff, supplies and treatment space. A community disaster in which more than this number of casualties are brought to a single hospital should activate a well-rehearsed Disaster Plan. Such a plan assumes that the hospital facility remains intact and that all personnel are capable of reporting for duty. Problems involving radioactivity and toxic gases require separate protocols to protect the hospital staff from contamination. The aim of a Disaster Plan is to give definitive care to all patients within 24 hours of admission. No patient is considered hopelessly injured and the most severely injured are treated first.

The success of an individual hospital's Disaster Plan depends upon community resources for reporting the disaster, triaging victims at the site, transporting patients to local hospitals and maintaining communications among civil authorities, hospital personnel and nonprofessional volunteers. This integration is best accomplished at a municipal or regional level. All agencies to be involved in disaster response should meet under the aegis of a local authority, often the Director of Civil Defense. Police are given responsibility for notifying medical agencies that a disaster has occurred. Word is first given to the hospital which is to supply a field triage team. Such a team consists of at least three doctors and an equal number of clerks or assistants. A communications support person accompanies the team.

The field triage team should be the first medical personnel to reach the disaster scene. Their job is to sort casualties for immediate removal to nearby hospitals. As a doctor assesses the degree of injury, the accompanying clerk tags the patient with information giving number, condition and hospital assignment. The latter is determined arbitrarily by the triage doctor on the basis of known capabilities of local hospitals. Resuscitation is limited to insertion of oral airways in unconscious patients, pressure control of severe external bleeding and splinting of obvious fractures.

As victims are removed from the

disaster site, the communications support person contacts a community radio control center indicating the number of casualties, the proportion severely injured and the number of patients being sent to each local hospital. Central radio control personnel then advise hospitals of similar information and coordinate the assignment of victims among community health facilities if the primary receiving hospitals become overtaxed.

Word of a disaster usually reaches each receiving hospital through a telephone operator. Details of site, type of disaster, estimated number of casualties and the identity and location of the caller are relayed to the designated Director of Disaster Planning who is empowered to activate the Disaster Plan. The Director may be a hospital administrator or chief of a clinical service. Essential personnel in all departments of the hospital are then notified in the order of their importance. The hospital is thereby prepared to receive the injured before existing facilities and personnel are overwhelmed.

Triage

An outpatient surgeon may be designated Triage Officer with responsibility to evaluate arriving casualties, assign priorities of treatment, initiate life-saving procedures and insure rapid disposition for definitive care. The Triage Officer is the key to the success of disaster planning. He should be mature and experienced, for while receiving casualties he must often deal with irrational relatives of patients, demanding newsmen and confused assistants. Unless he maintains rigid authority and awareness of his duties, organization collapses and previous planning becomes valueless.

The first duty of the Triage Officer is to sort casualties in preparation for treatment. He must not neglect this duty by involvement in individual patient care.

Upon activation of the Disaster Plan, he moves to the triage area, usually a large open space with access to emergency vehicle portals, and stations himself at a point from which he can inspect arriving casualties and supervise assistants. Each victim is judged dead-on-arrival (DOA), preoperative or ambulatory. Clerks tag each patient with brief descriptions of number, time of arrival, condition and treatment given. The most seriously injured are selected for priority treatment and identified by special markers such as red ribbons. Ambulatory injured are immediately sent to an Ambulatory Care Area from which they may be hospitalized or treated and discharged. After sorting and tagging, the Triage Officer assigns medical personnel to individual patients as numbers allow to begin emergency treatment. Care in the triage area is limited to maintenance of airway by means of oral airway insertion or endotracheal intubation, ventilation by mouth-to-mouth or resuscitator techniques, control of hemorrhage by pressure dressing, restoration of blood volume by intravenous fluid administration and stabilization of fractures by splinting. A permanently stocked kit containing oral airways, resuscitator bags and masks, laryngoscopes, endotracheal tubes, elastic bandages, splints, intravenous needles and tubing, liter bottles of intravenous crystalloid solution and fresh ampuls of bicarbonate, epinephrine, isoproteranol and morphine should be stored near the triage area. Diagnostic procedures such as thoracentesis or paracentesis are deferred until the patient is admitted to the Preoperative Care Area, although emergency procedures such as pericardiocentesis may be required during triage.

With the opening of a Preoperative Care (Shock) Area, the Triage Officer orders the removal of the most seriously injured (red-tagged) patients from the triage area. It is essential to clear the triage space as rapidly as possible, recognizing strict rules of priority treatment.

Preoperative Care

Critically injured victims are triaged to the Preoperative Care Area whether or not surgery is urgently indicated. Intensive care of the patient begins here and is directed toward reversal of shock and preoperative preparation. Diagnostic procedures including x-ray are now possible and further resuscitative measures such as tube thoracostomy, tracheostomy and mechanical ventilation can be performed.

Ambulatory Care

Outpatient physicians not involved in triage may be assigned to evaluate, treat and arrange disposition of walking wounded. Some of these patients will have no significant injury while others may be emotionally distraught and still others may be ambulatory despite serious injury that requires surgery or plaster immobilization of an extremity. Treatment of lacerations should be as thorough as time and assistance permit with attention to cleaning, débridement, early wound closure, proper dressing, tetanus prophylaxis and follow-up appointment. Sheer numbers may limit individual patient care. In this case closure of wounds by adhesive strips or dressings should replace suture techniques. To all patients with minor injuries, instructions are given to return to the hospital the next day for wound inspection and thorough physical reexamination.

While casualties are being received and treated, the Director of Disaster Planning insures a flow of supplies and personnel to the triage and treatment areas. The security of the hospital and especially the triage area, is maintained by locking all but essential doors and by posting security guards at entrances and exits. Access for hospital personnel and volunteer staff requires identity cards. Control must extend to ambulance areas and nearby streets to maintain open access for emergency vehicles. Relatives, newsmen and curious visitors should be barred from the triage and treatment sites and sequestered in adjacent facilities where information regarding victim identity and condition can be disseminated by hospital administrators.

CS Contamination

Civil disturbances may result in many casualties who are both injured and contaminated with toxic chemicals. Authorities currently use a riot-control agent (orthochlorobenzalmalononitrile) called CS, a symbol derived from the two scientists, B. B. Corson and R. W. Stoughton, who first prepared the substance in 1928. CS is not a gas but a white crystalline powder which is dispersed as an aerosol cloud of finely divided particles. Dispersal is accomplished by blowers, bursting grenades or burning with a fuel.

CS produces immediate irritating effects which persist for five to ten minutes after the victim is removed to fresh air. Severe burning sensation in the eyes, copious tears, coughing, tightness in the chest, rhinorrhea and moist skin stings render the affected individual incapable of effective concerted action. The dose of CS required for severe effects is very small, 10–20 milligrams per cubic meter of air, and this means that even limited exposure results in incapacitation. Despite its irritating effects, CS is remarkably nonlethal. At least 2600 times as much as is irritating is required to produce death in experimental animals. Serious complications in humans are very rare.

Since traumatized persons contaminated with CS may require immediate medical care, attendants and other patients are thus exposed to the agent. Decontamination of the patient is essential to preclude widespread exposure. A decontamination room, preferably outside of the hospital, with water taps or overhead shower and a floor drain should be designated. Hospital personnel wearing gas masks and scrub suits disrobe the patient, wash him thoroughly with soap and water and dress him in clean clothes. After the decontaminated patient has been removed to a treatment area, hospital personnel still wearing gas masks place the patient's clothing in plastic bags or buckets of soapy water. These attendants then remove their own clothing to soak in soapy water, and while still wearing gas masks, take a shower before dressing in fresh clothing. Masks, in turn, are thoroughly washed and dried.

Aqueous solutions of 10 per cent monoethanolamine and 0.3 per cent of a nonionic detergent, such as Triton X–100, dissolve and decontaminate CS on clothes in about two minutes. The decontaminant is then washed off with water. Since large numbers of CS-contaminated patients may be present at one time, it is logistically easier to decontaminate with soap and water than with chemicals.

Radioactive Contamination

Nuclear explosion or industrial contamination with radioactive materials can cause radiation injuries in mass casualties.[3] In the case of explosions, trauma and thermal burns are initially more important problems than radiation injury. Contamination can exist without serious radiation damage. Symptoms are dependent upon total dose of irradiation. In general, if a patient has not vomited within 24 hours after injury, he has not been seriously injured by radiation.

If fallout particles, grossly contaminated with radioactive substances, whether due to military explosion or industrial accident, are not visible during fall or after settling on surfaces, they are likely to have no acute effects. Fallout loses about 90 per cent of its radioactivity within the first seven hours and is virtually inactive after 48 hours. Early fallout carries a high irradiation

dose. As radiation accumulates over several days, however, an increasing dose may result in symptoms. It is important to establish for each victim his distance from the irradiation source and his degree of shielding.

Monitoring for radioactivity should be conducted outside of the triage area. Counters for this purpose are often available from Civil Defense agencies. If counts of radioactivity are high, either on the clothing or the body, decontamination procedures begin before moving the patient inside the hospital. Ambulatory patients should remove all clothing, avoiding contact of outside clothing with unexposed parts of the body. Bathing with soap and water is best accomplished under a shower. Face, hands, fingernails and hair are scrubbed with a brush. Contaminated clothing is placed in tightly covered receptacles until disposed of by trained personnel. Before decontaminated victims are allowed to enter the triage area, they are remonitored for residual radioactivity.

Seriously traumatized and contaminated patients who cannot walk must be undressed and washed. A tub or tank is useful for this purpose. If a tub is unavailable, water may be poured over the skin, concentrating on exposed areas. Open wounds can be sealed with plastic film or tape during bathing. Later they are decontaminated by irrigation with large amounts of water and débridement. Clipping of hair is preferable to shaving, which enhances skin absorption. Alkaline soaps, abrasives and organic solvents also increase skin permeability and penetration of radioactive particles. Wash water used in decontamination is potentially hazardous and should be disposed of without contaminating water supplies. When no water is available for decontamination, wiping or brushing the skin is of some benefit.

Patients who have received heavy radiation exposure (more than 600 rads) will have early nausea, vomiting, malaise, prostration, weakness, fever and diarrhea. With very heavy dosage, collapse and shock may develop within minutes. Hemorrhage, epilation or convulsions are rarely seen after heavy exposure since death supervenes before these signs develop. Since few of these patients survive, only delayed, supportive treatment is justified during a disaster with mass casualties.

The most important treatment category is the medium exposure (200–600 rads) group. These patients will probably constitute the maximum casualty load and provide the best opportunity for effective treatment. Survival in this group is in the range of 50 per cent to 75 per cent, the variation being due to differences in individual response to radiation. Within a few hours of exposure, these patients experience nausea, vomiting and malaise. Recovery thereafter depends upon the severity of hematologic complications which typically occur after a symptom-free period of 7 to 15 days. Initially, patients are supported with antiemetics to control nausea and vomiting. Whole blood or antibiotics are helpful later when bleeding diatheses and infection due to leukopenia have occurred.

Persons receiving under 200 rads of irradiation have had light exposure and rarely die. Transient nausea and vomiting may occur but should disappear within 72 hours. After monitoring and decontamination, these persons may be discharged.

MAJOR TRAUMA

Immediate Reaction of the Outpatient Surgeon and His Team

Initial care of a critically injured patient is the responsibility of the outpatient surgeon. Competent early management is often the key to later recovery. Conversely, initial mistakes cause subsequent morbidity or mortality.

In active hospital emergency rooms a team of doctors, nurses and technicians is available at all times for resuscitation of the severely injured patient. The role of the outpatient surgeon is to command this team by recognizing treatment priorities, assigning individual duties, avoiding confusion and assessing progress. As team leader he should be certain that personnel are trained, rehearsed and ready and that facilities are organized, adequate and available. After the emergency event, he reviews team action to confirm successful management and to correct errors.

The outpatient surgeon who does not have such a team and facilities is responsible for using what he has in the best possible way. He acts alone to preserve the patient's life. Diagnostic and therapeutic measures are limited to the most urgent needs. If help is not imminent and if local facilities are inadequate, the patient must be prepared for referral to a larger treatment center.

Both the team surgeon and the solo outpatient surgeon are confronted by the critically injured patient in terms of immediate life-threatening problems. A detailed accident history is rarely available and time does not permit extensive questioning before treatment begins. When acute needs have been met, medical history relevant to the patient's present condition can be sought.

Examination

In the absence of history and immediate laboratory values, the outpatient surgeon treats the injured patient on the basis of physical findings. Examination is first directed toward respiration and circulation. When these vital functions are assured, overall evaluation of systems may begin. Vital signs are recorded several times within the first quarter hour. If formal records are initially unavailable, state of consciousness and values of blood pressure, pulse and respiration with the time of observation may be written on the linen of the Emergency Room cart.

The state of consciousness must be determined. Pupil size and reaction is recorded. Spinal fluid drainage from the nose or ears, indicating basal skull fracture, should be looked for, though it may easily be missed in the presence of adjacent bleeding wounds. Skull fractures may be palpable. Similarly, injuries of the cervical spine are often associated with deformity and tenderness. The anterior neck is palpated to detect tracheal displacement or injury.

The chest is thoroughly inspected for evidence of paradoxical movement, sucking wounds or abrasions resulting from blunt injury. Auscultation may reveal diminished or absent breath sounds. The quality of heart sounds is rated while auscultating the chest. Fractures may be felt by gently compressing the ribs.

Penetrating abdominal wounds, with or without protruding viscera, are covered with sterile moist dressings while examination is made for abdominal muscle spasm, tenderness and peristalsis. Extremities are rapidly surveyed by requesting active motion in a conscious patient. If the patient cannot comply, extremities are moved passively in a slow, gentle way and are palpated for dislocations or fractures. With thighs in abduction the perineum can be inspected, giving special attention to the perianal area where lacerations related to "blowout" injuries of the pelvis may be seen. The pelvis should be tested for fracture by manual compression of the iliac crests and by pressure on the pubic symphysis.

An important aspect of the examination is palpation of peripheral pulses. Skin color, temperature and muscle activity are affected by major arterial occlusion in the legs.

Priorities and Treatment

The first priority in caring for an injured patient is to assure an open airway and ventilation. Audible or sensible expiration is the most reliable confirmation of an adequate airway and spontaneous breathing. Moving of the chest as respiratory effort does not insure adequate ventilation.

Airway obstruction by the tongue can be relieved by hyperextending the head on the shoulders and advancing the mandible. Foreign bodies obstructing the airway are eliminated by suctioning or cleaning the mouth with a finger. With an open airway, ventilation is possible by means of mouth-to-mouth or mouth-to-nose respiration. These techniques require no apparatus and should be used before attempting endotracheal intubation (see Chapter 26).

Cardiac and pulmonary resuscitation is essentially one activity but adequate ventilation must be achieved before cardiac resuscitation will succeed. The diagnosis of cardiac arrest or inadequate cardiac effort is made when pulsation in a large vessel such as the femoral or carotid artery cannot be felt. Pupillary dilation confirms arrest except in patients with head injury. Electrocardiography is seldom of immediate help unless the equipment is already in place. A normal ECG pattern can exist in the presence of inadequate cardiac output.

Closed cardiac massage begins as soon as the diagnosis of cardiac arrest is made and ventilation is established. Delay of eight to ten minutes is fatal. As the interval is shortened, the chances of complete resuscitation improve. The purpose of massage is to maintain circulation to vital organs until the heart resumes normal pumping. This may require one hour or longer. Successful massage depends upon restoration of blood volume, correction of acidosis and return of myocardial contractile force. The technique of closed massage is described in Chapter 26.

Severe external bleeding can be controlled in most cases by applying finger pressure over the wound. This technique is fast and effective and can be used during cardiorespiratory resuscitation. Later, a pressure dressing replaces the finger. A mound of gauze pads compressed by an elastic bandage makes a satisfactory pressure dressing. The bandage is wrapped tightly enough to tamponade the bleeders but not to occlude intact major vessels. Tourniquet compression of the artery proximal to the wound is very rarely necessary. Tourniquets often increase bleeding by obstructing venous return. They can cause ischemic injury in extremities unless released for several minutes every quarter hour.

Blindly clamping bleeding vessels in a deep wound is unwise. Tissue damage rather than hemostasis usually results. Lacerated major arteries are best controlled by pressure until adequate exposure is possible in the operating room. Ligation of large arteries is seldom justified in the Emergency Room, especially when the risk of subsequent limb ischemia is great. Profuse bleeding is alarming and diverts attention away from more important needs such as restoration of airway and ventilation. Experience and discipline are required to focus on these priorities in the face of dramatic hemorrhage.

After adequate ventilation, effective cardiac function and control of external bleeding have been assured, the outpatient surgeon is responsible for estimating the degree of shock and beginning the restoration of blood volume. Samples of venous blood are drawn for determination of hematocrit and for typing and cross-matching. Arterial blood samples are used for assessing oxygenation and tissue perfusion by means of pO_2, pCO_2 and pH. Vital signs are recorded frequently. A venous channel is urgently required to facilitate and to monitor fluid replacement. Large bore catheters can be placed in peripheral veins such as the basilic vein in the antecubital space. When peripheral veins are collapsed or inaccessible, superior vena cava catheterization or venesection is indicated.

Superior Vena Cava Catheterization

General Discussion

Placement of an indwelling catheter in the superior vena cava for measurement of central venous pressure and administration of fluids is a widely accepted technique in the management of a critically injured patient. Advantages of the technique are (1) rapid procurement of a large caliber intravenous line in a patient with inaccessible peripheral veins, (2) long-term maintenance with relatively few complications, and (3) accurate placement of a catheter tip near the right heart.

Several techniques are available for catheter placement. All are subject to hazards and complications. Common to each venipuncture technique are the risks of perforating the vein with extraluminal catheter placement, arterial puncture, lymphatic duct puncture, brachial plexus injury and air embolism. Catheters positioned by any technique are capable of displacement and thrombus formation. About one-fourth of catheters removed within 72 hours grow micro-organisms when cultured.[4] Pneumothorax, hemothorax, hematoma, mediastinal infiltration, cardiac perforation and subcutaneous emphysema are other reported complications.[5]

Observing certain principles of technique in catheterizing the superior vena cava will minimize the risk of serious complication. The patient should be flat or, preferably, in Trendelenburg position to increase venous filling and to decrease the chance of air embolism. Positioning includes tilting the patient toward the puncture side by placing a pillow or rolled sheet under the opposite shoulder. If the patient holds his breath at the end of expiration or if an assistant firmly presses on the patient's abdomen, filling of subclavian and jugular veins is accentuated.

The skin site for venipuncture is prepared by scrubbing with a surgical soap or an iodophor compound. The area is covered by a sterile drape, and gloves and face mask are mandatory. Local anesthetic is injected to form a skin wheal at the puncture site if the patient is awake.

Subclavian Vein Puncture

The subclavian vein can be cannulated by a supraclavicular or an infraclavicular approach. While the latter is more commonly used, the former entails less risk of pneumothorax.[6]

The infraclavicular subclavian puncture is preferred when the clavicle is higher than the first rib, thereby exposing the subclavian vein to a needle passed below the clavicle. Raising the shoulder toward the head on the side of puncture further exposes the vein. With the patient's head slightly flexed and rotated sharply to the opposite side, the operator places his thumb below the clavicle just lateral to the junction of the middle and lateral thirds. The index finger of the same hand is lodged deeply between the two heads of the ipsilateral sternocleidomastoid muscle just above the clavicle. As the thumb tauts the skin, a 2 inch long 14 gauge needle connected to a 10 ml syringe is inserted through the skin just medial to the thumb (Fig. 3–1 *A*). The barrel of the syringe is depressed to the shoulder to align the needle in a horizontal plane with the subclavian vein. Back pressure is maintained on the plunger of the syringe as the needle is advanced toward the tip of the index finger.

When a free flow of venous blood is obtained, the syringe is carefully removed to avoid displacing the needle. An 8 inch long 16 gauge radiopaque polyethylene or, preferably, silicone catheter is then gently inserted through the needle lumen. After insertion the syringe is attached to the catheter and blood aspirated to insure that the catheter is in a large vein. If flow is not satisfactory, the catheter is withdrawn to a point that yields adequate flow. If this maneuver is unsuccessful, the catheter is replaced.

When backflow of blood is adequate the needle is withdrawn from the skin and either slipped over the end of catheter or retained well away from the skin puncture site. The needle is never advanced over the catheter because this may shear off a portion of tubing within the vein. To retain the catheter and to prevent infection by slight movements

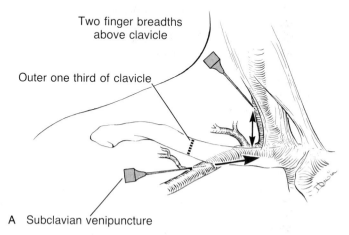

B   Internal jugular venipuncture

Two finger breadths above clavicle

Outer one third of clavicle

A   Subclavian venipuncture

Figure 3–1 Superior Vena Cava Catheterization. A. The infraclavicular approach to the subclavian vein involves percutaneous puncture with a two inch long 14 gauge needle at a site below the clavicle near the junction of the middle and lateral thirds. The needle tip is directed toward the operator's index finger lodged in the suprasternal notch. B. In one technique of internal jugular vein puncture, the needle is inserted lateral to the sternocleidomastoid muscle two finger breadths above the clavicle and advanced toward the suprasternal notch.

in and out of the skin, the catheter is sutured to the skin at the puncture site.

The catheter is connected to infusion tubing and the intravenous bottle lowered to obtain a reflux of blood in the tubing before beginning infusion. Topical antibiotic ointment is applied to the puncture site and a dressing placed which secures the tubing and seals the wound. Chest x-ray is obtained soon afterward to exclude the possibility of pneumothorax or catheter displacement. The dressing is changed and antibiotic ointment reapplied daily. Although catheters have remained in place for several months, removal between three to five days is advised to avoid sepsis.

Supraclavicular subclavian puncture entails less risk of pneumothorax than the infraclavicular approach, especially in patients with emphysema when the subclavian vein, normally overlying the pleural dome, rises to a higher position. Ideal for supraclavicular puncture are patients with a horizontal clavicle and a wide costoclavicular space or obese patients in whom the needle may not reach the subclavian vein when inserted below the clavicle. In this approach the operator stands at the head of the supine patient and presses his index finger, pointing toward the feet, behind the clavicular head of the sternocleidomastoid muscle on the side of the puncture to feel the anterior scalenus tubercle on the first rib. The subclavian artery lies lateral to this tubercle. A needle is inserted in a horizontal plane above and parallel to the anterior scalenus muscle, medial to the subclavian artery. The needle is withdrawn with constant aspiration until a free flow of blood is obtained. The syringe is then lowered toward the shoulder and rotated 180° to place the needle along the axis of the vein with the bevel facing the superior vena cava. Catheter insertion and fixation are performed as described above.

Internal Jugular Vein Puncture

Perhaps the safest technique for placement of a superior vena cava catheter is percutaneous puncture of the internal jugular vein. The incidence of pneumothorax and hemothorax with this technique is negligible. Air embolism, thromboembolism, septicemia and mediastinal infusion of fluid may occur.[7] The internal jugular vein occupies an almost constant anatomic position deep to the sternocleidomastoid muscle and, during a Valsalva maneuver, will be distended to a diameter of at least 2 centimeters in an adult.

With the patient in Trendelenburg position and the head rotated to the opposite side, a needle is introduced at a site along the outer border of the sternocleidomastoid muscle two fingerbreadths above the clavicle. The needle tip is advanced toward the suprasternal notch while suction is maintained. When venous blood returns, a catheter is advanced and secured as described in subclavian puncture (Fig. 3–1 *B*).

An alternative technique for internal jugular puncture is to introduce the needle at the apex of the triangle formed by the dividing sternal and clavicular heads of the sternocleidomastoid and the clavicle. The center of this triangle is directly over the internal jugular vein. The needle is advanced from the apex while maintaining back pressure on the plunger of the syringe, toward the center of the triangle at a 30° angle with the skin. Inadvertent puncture of the carotid artery is seldom dangerous if the needle is withdrawn and direct pressure is applied for several minutes.

Venesection

Percutaneous superior vena cava catheterization has largely replaced venesection as a means of securing a reliable intravenous route in severely traumatized patients. The technique of subclavian or internal jugular puncture is easier and faster than cannulating the saphenous or cephalic veins in the extremities. Nevertheless, the cutdown technique of intravenous infusion occasionally is useful and is essential when superior vena cava catheterization fails and peripheral veins cannot be punctured. It remains a common procedure in pediatric patients in whom percutaneous puncture is technically difficult. Venesection avoids pulmonary or mediastinal complications due to needle puncture or catheter displacement. Problems of thromboembolism and sepsis are not avoided and, in fact, catheters are less well tolerated for prolonged periods in peripheral veins than in larger vessels.

The greater saphenous vein is easily exposed and cannulated at the level of the medial malleolus. Contraindications for venesection at this site are previous excision or thrombosis of the vein, contamination of overlying skin and local injury. Alternate sites are the cephalic vein in the anatomical snuffbox at the wrist, cephalic or basilic veins proximal to the antecubital space and tributaries of the long saphenous vein in the upper thigh. Cannulation of the basilic vein at the antecubital fossa can be performed through a horizontal or longitudinal cutdown incision. Upper extremity routes are preferred for patients with injuries of the liver or vena cava.

The technique of venesection ("cutdown") at the ankle is illustrated in Figure 3–2. A tourniquet is applied about the calf to distend the greater saphenous vein. Skin over the medial aspect of the ankle is prepared with application of an iodophor (organic iodine) paint and draped with sterile towels. The saphenous vein is often visible just anterior to the medial malleolus. One centimeter above and 1 centimeter anterior to the malleolus a 2-centimeter transverse incision is made in the skin over the vein and carried through the scant subcutaneous tissue. By blunt dissection, using the tips of a hemostat, the vein is separated from adjacent tissues, particularly the saphenous nerve, and exposed over a distance of 2 centimeters. Two silk ligatures are passed around the vein. The distal ligature is tied and placed on traction. The untied proximal ligature is retracted upward while a venotomy is made with scissors or pointed scalpel blade midway between ligatures. A polyethylene catheter, 12 or 14 gauge in adults, is beveled slightly at its tip and inserted through the venotomy. As the proximal ligature is relaxed, the tubing is advanced into the vein so that at least 10 centimeters of the catheter lie above the venotomy. The proximal ligature is tied about the vein and tubing in order to secure but not occlude the catheter.

Skin is closed with two or three vertical mattress sutures of silk, one of which is used to encircle the tubing. Antibiotic ointment is applied around the catheter site before a dressing is placed over the wound. Adhesive secures the dressing and further retains the catheter as it lies on the skin of the ankle.

Diagnostic Procedures

Detection of obscure injury, especially after severe blunt trauma, depends upon repeated physical examination of the patient and specific diagnostic procedures performed in the Emergency Room.

X-rays

Head injuries can be studied by skull x-rays, ultra-sound encephalography and carotid arteriography (Chapter 7). Neck pain or tenderness demands that cross-table lateral cervical x-rays be obtained with portable equipment before the patient is moved to avoid spinal cord injury from fractured or dislocated cervical vertebrae. An unconscious, motionless patient should be assumed to have a fractured neck until proved otherwise, especially if found to have a skull fracture. Chest x-ray documents rib fracture, pneumothorax, hemothorax, atelectasis, mediastinal widening or displacement and changes in the cardiac silhouette. X-rays of extremities and the pelvis can, of course, demonstrate fractures or dislocations and peripheral arteriography can show major vessel patency or perforation.

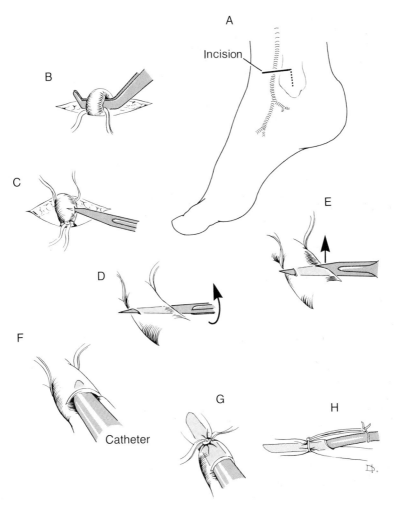

Figure 3–2 Venesection—Greater Saphenous Vein "Cutdown" at Ankle. The technique of greater saphenous venesection at the ankle is illustrated. A. A 2 cm incision is made anterior and cephalad to the medial malleolus. B. The subcutaneous saphenous vein is freed from fascia and the accompanying saphenous vein is freed from fascia and the accompanying saphenous nerve. C. After tying the vein distally and passing a silk ligature proximally, venotomy begins. D. The tip of a #11 scalpel blade is inserted horizontally through the middle of the vein. E. As the blade is rotated vertically the venotomy is completed. F. Polyethylene tubing is advanced proximally through the venotomy and (G) secured with the silk ligature. H. The ligature is passed around the catheter and tied securely to prevent accidental withdrawal.

Abdominal injuries are not often detected by routine x-ray. Free peritoneal air on upright chest x-ray is usually apparent after "blow-out" injuries of the stomach or bowel. Retroperitoneal or subserosal air may be seen in some patients with retroperitoneal rupture of the duodenum or colon. Laceration of organs with bleeding must usually be diagnosed by means other than x-ray, although obliteration of the psoas shadow may be a clue to the presence of retroperitoneal hematoma.

Bladder Catheterization

An indwelling bladder catheter assures precise measurement of urine output which helps in monitoring shock and fluid therapy. Inability to pass a catheter suggests urethral injury and requires percutaneous bladder catheterization or cystostomy. Hematuria is a sign of urinary tract trauma and is an indication for intravenous pyelography (Chapter 19).

Nasogastric Intubation

An 18 F nasogastric tube should be passed in every severely injured patient to reduce gastric content, thereby lessening the risk of aspiration during surgery, and to detect the presence of blood in the stomach. Significant amounts of bright blood returned from the stomach usually indicate gastric or esophageal injury. Stress ulcer bleeding and most types of hemobilia are not seen immediately. Small bowel injuries including duodenal perforation seldom present with blood in the stomach. If gastric perforation is suspected, intermittent suction should be applied to the nasogastric tube. Irrigation is allowed only to maintain tube patency. Sterile saline in small amounts is used for this purpose.

Paracentesis

Paracentesis or peritoneal tap with lavage is a means of detecting injury of abdominal viscera after trauma. It is especially useful in the patient unconscious after blunt trauma in whom physical signs of intraperitoneal injury are often unimpressive. When the tap is positive for blood, laparotomy is usually indicated. When the tap is negative, however, the possibility of intra-abdominal injury cannot be excluded and continued observation with repeated abdominal examination is mandatory.

The four-quadrant needle puncture technique of paracentesis, while simple and rapid, is often falsely negative in cases of slight to moderate hemoperitoneum. It is useful, however, for immediate confirmation of massive intraperitoneal bleeding. A 10 centimeter, 18 or 20 gauge spinal needle attached to a sterile syringe is used to puncture the anterior abdominal wall in the middle of each abdominal quadrant. Skin preparation is limited to single application of tincture of iodine or iodophor antiseptic. Local anesthetic is seldom required. The needle can be felt to perforate the peritoneum by the sudden release of a temporary resistance. Thereafter, the needle is slowly advanced perpendicular to the skin while negative pressure is maintained until blood is obtained or the hub is reached. Very often blood returns as the needle is being withdrawn. Injury to the bowel or other viscera rarely occurs with this technique. Ordinarily the needle tip displaces normal intestine. Perforation of distended or adherent bowel, however, can result in leakage and peritonitis which require laparotomy.[8] Similar peritoneal inflammation has been caused by perforation of an intra-abdominal abscess.[9] Troublesome bleeding from epigastric vessels in the rectus muscle can occur after needle paracentesis. Hematoma is usually prevented by exerting pressure over the puncture site for several minutes.

Peritoneal lavage is currently used in preference to four-quadrant paracentesis. The accuracy of peritoneal lavage in establishing the diagnosis of hemoperitoneum is reported to be as high as 96 per cent. False negatives (3 per cent) were more common than false positives (1 per cent) in a series of 304 patients.[10] The test consists of introducing a catheter into the peritoneal cavity and aspirating for gross blood. If no blood is obtained, the abdominal cavity is irrigated with a balanced salt solution and returning fluid is examined for blood.

The abdomen may be punctured with a trocar, a dialysis catheter or a large bore needle (Fig. 3–3). The latter is preferred because it causes fewer false positive taps due to abdominal wall vessel perforation. A 2 inch 14 gauge needle with a 16 gauge intraluminal catheter, identical to that used for subclavian puncture, is recommended. After painting the skin of the midabdomen with an antiseptic, a skin wheal is raised

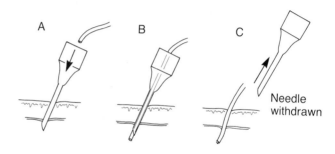

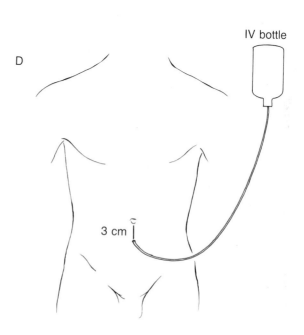

Figure 3–3 Paracentesis and Peritoneal Lavage. A–C. After inserting a two inch 14 gauge needle with stylus through the linea alba 5 cm below the umbilicus, a 16 gauge polyethylene catheter is passed into the abdominal cavity and the needle is withdrawn. D. If gross blood is not obtained, peritoneal lavage is performed by introducing one liter of normal saline solution rapidly into the abdomen and allowing it to freely drain back through the catheter onto a clean, white gauze pad.

with local anesthetic in the midline 5 cm below the umbilicus. The needle is advanced perpendicularly through the abdominal wall to its hub. If aspiration yields gross blood, the procedure is terminated and the patient prepared for laparotomy. If not, the catheter is advanced into the peritoneal cavity and the needle entirely withdrawn. One liter of normal saline solution is introduced rapidly into the abdomen of adults. In children only 500 ml is used. The fluid is then removed by allowing free drainage through the catheter onto a clean white gauze pad. Evidence of even pink-tinged fluid is considered a positive tap.

Examining returned fluid microscopically for erythrocytes and leukocytes has been recommended. Although the exact number of red cells constituting a positive test has not been determined, it appears that 100,000 erythrocytes per cubic millimeter of lavage fluid can be considered significant.[10]

Complications of peritoneal lavage, although unusual, include perforation of bowel, injury of mesentery, transection and loss of the catheter into the abdomen, extra-peritoneal infusion and bleeding from abdominal wall vessels. Peritonitis secondary to lavage has not been reported.

Sinography

Stab wounds of the abdomen may be superficial or they may penetrate the peritoneum. Surgical exploration is usually required in the latter to repair intra-peritoneal injury. Operating on all patients with abdominal stab wounds results in unnecessary exploration rates approaching 50 per cent.[11] To reduce this rate, the outpatient surgeon may wish to determine whether or not the peritoneum has been penetrated by performing stab wound sinography. Shock, peritonitis, a protruding viscus or any other indication for immediate operation obviate the use of sinography. The technique is principally useful to avoid unnecessary exploration when physical findings are inconclusive.

Skin about the stab wound is prepared and draped sterily and wound edges are infiltrated with local anesthetic solution. A 12–18 French rubber catheter is inserted into the wound for a distance of 2 centimeters. The catheter is not pushed more deeply into the wound tract. A purse-string suture of heavy silk is secured in the skin around the catheter to occlude the tract opening. At least 50 cc of meglumine diatrizoate (Renografin 60 per cent) is injected into the catheter by sufficient hand force to evert the skin closed around the tract. The catheter is then clamped and antero-posterior, lateral and oblique roentgenograms of the abdomen promptly taken. Sinography may also be performed under fluoroscopy, following which x-rays are taken (Fig. 3–4).

In penetrating wounds of the peritoneum, contrast medium outlines intra-abdominal structures. In superficial wounds, the medium tends to diffuse along extraperitoneal soft tissue planes. If the chest has been entered, intra-thoracic structures may be outlined.

With multiple stab wounds, each tract should be individually injected and x-rayed to eliminate superimposition of contrast media.

Falsely negative results may occur in as many as 10 per cent of examinations.[12] Insufficient volume of contrast medium

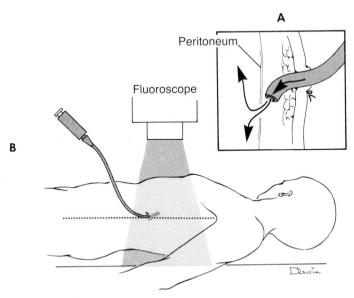

Figure 3–4 Abdominal Sinography. A. A 12–18 French rubber catheter is inserted into a flank stab wound and secured by a purse string suture of heavy silk which occludes the tract opening. Contrast media is injected under some pressure just before anteroposterior, lateral and oblique roentgenograms of the abdomen are taken. B. Contrast media passes into the peritoneal cavity and surrounds visceral structures if the peritoneum has been penetrated.

in multiple stab wounds, or simultaneous chest and abdominal tracts contribute to this error. It is important to perform sinography before diagnostic peritoneal lavage to avoid dilution of radiopaque material within the abdominal cavity.

Complications of sinography include hypersensitivity reactions to the contrast medium and moderate transient pain with injection. The incidence of wound infections, however, is not increased.[12]

MINOR TRAUMA

Most trauma encountered by the outpatient surgeon will consist of minor injuries in patients who return home after treatment.[17,18] Such injuries include contusions, abrasions, lacerations, bites and burns. The essence of treatment in each case is proper wound care. This requires an understanding of tissue injury, inflammation, infection, débridement, repair and healing. Local and constitutional factors influencing these events are discussed elsewhere (Chapters 4 and 6). The practical management of simple wounds, based on knowledge of tissue damage and repair, will be discussed here.

Closed Wounds

Contusions and bruises are nonpenetrating wounds caused by blunt trauma in which subepithelial blood vessels rupture. When blood or pigments disseminate throughout intercellular spaces, without forming a collection of blood, an ecchymosis results. This is identified by an initial blue-black color in subcutaneous tissues which later fades to a brown-green discoloration. If extravasated blood collects in subcutaneous tissue or muscle, a hematoma is formed. Blebs or blisters caused by minor burns or blunt force are another form of closed wound. Because of its thin, easily ruptured wall, however, a bleb is often treated as an open wound.

The important injury in most minor closed wounds is the rupture of capillaries. Other structures are seldom seriously damaged. Inflammatory reaction to the extravasation of blood is generally moderate and, in simple contusions, subsides within a few days. Absorption of blood or serum is rapid unless a hematoma has been formed in large tissue spaces. Then inflammation persists while a capsule of connective tissue encircles the fluid and destroyed cellular elements. Blood in a hematoma ordinarily clots, organizing itself by ingrowing capillaries and connective tissue. Aspiration at this stage is impossible and slow resolution is inevitable.

Treatment of contusions is nonsurgical. Local cold such as an icepack, used early, tends to limit swelling as with any inflammatory process. Later, heat reduces pain and accelerates resolution. Occasionally, a large, early hematoma which is well-defined in subcutaneous tissue and is fluctuant on palpation may require needle aspiration to relieve pain and to hasten healing. The danger here is infecting the evacuated space with micro-organisms introduced with the needle. Aseptic technique in aspirating blood is essential. Overlying skin is painted with tincture of iodine or an iodophor compound. A skin wheal is raised with local anesthetic solution directly over the fluctuant mass. An 18 gauge needle with attached syringe is inserted into the cavity and the syringe advanced and withdrawn or rotated gently until all unclotted blood and serum are aspirated. A sterile gauze dressing is loosely bunched over the site and secured under slight pressure with elastic adhesive to obliterate the empty space and to prevent hematoma recurrence. If drainage is unsatisfactory or if the evacuated space becomes secondarily infected, incision with open drainage is indicated. Rest, elevation, sedation and mild analgesics control pain after such a procedure.

Open Wounds

Certain principles apply to the care of all open wounds regardless of cause, size or location. Inspection must be done aseptically using sterile gloves and a face mask to avoid secondary contamination. No further injury should be caused by unnecessary manipulation during examination, dressing or diagnostic procedures such as x-ray. The whole patient must be evaluated by obtaining an accurate history and performing a physical examination. When multiple injuries have occurred, priority of care is determined so that immediate treatment is given to the most serious problem while no minor injury is neglected.

Abrasions are superficial open injuries in which epithelium of skin or mucous membrane is lost. The wound area may be extensive. Wound depth usually is uneven but no greater than the level of accessory skin structures in the dermis. If all epithelial elements are lost, the lesion is termed "wound with loss of substance." Since nerve endings are exposed, abrasions are painful and may limit the mobility of underlying joints.

Blood, serum and inflammatory cells exuding from abrasions dry to form a crust or scab. Beneath the crust new exudate is formed by inflammation. This either escapes from beneath the crust edge or dries to thicken the eschar. Eventually, mesodermal elements grow from midwound sites and epithelium grows from wound margins to cover the surface. The scab thins and separates to expose an epithelized surface within about ten days.

Dirt and other foreign material may be incorporated into the eschar or imbedded in dermal layers. If inorganic particles remain, a "tattoo" effect is evident after healing. It is important to remove all dirt particles imbedded in abrasions within the limits of pain and new tissue damage. Vigorous washing or scrubbing with sterile water or saline may be required to remove this debris.

The addition of surgical soap is irritating and of little help in freeing particles. Mild antiseptics, such as hexachlorophene, however, may reduce the number of bacteria in the wound. Stronger antiseptics are not indicated as they cause pain and compound tissue injury. It is unlikely that even potent antiseptics kill all contaminating micro-organisms in abrasions since solutions cannot reach deeper tissue spaces.

Since scabs serve to protect abrasions from further trauma and bacterial invasion, they should be preserved during healing. External dressing is optional and dependent upon susceptibility to further trauma. When infection is developing beneath an eschar, however, the scab must be removed and the wound treated openly with nonadherent dressings, saline irrigation and wound support. Infected abrasions may become full-thickness defects if dermal remnants are destroyed. Dressings then involve "wet-to-dry" fine mesh gauze applications as discussed in burns (Chapter 8) and lacerations.

Puncture Wounds

Long, sharp objects may penetrate visceral cavities or injure deep structures in the head, neck and extremities. Evaluation and treatment of such injuries generally require hospitalization. The most frequent puncture injury treated by the outpatient surgeon is nail wound of the foot. Because of the potential for clostridial infection in deep, virtually closed wounds of this type, treatment of nail punctures should be aggressive.

Skin surrounding the puncture site of a nail wound is excised to allow wound irrigation and drainage. After infiltration of skin edges with local anesthetic solution, approximately 3 millimeters of skin is debrided with scissors or knife around the wound margin. Saline irrigation of deeper tissue planes is facilitated by using a syringe and large bore needle. The wound is not closed but dressed lightly for protection if on a weight-bearing surface. Antibiotics in addition to tetanus prophylaxis are indicated.

Lesser puncture wounds caused by needles, wooden splinters or glass may require no treatment except administration of tetanus toxoid. Imbedded foreign bodies need not be removed unless symptomatic, unsightly, infected or the cause of undue patient alarm. Wooden splinters usually produce more pain than metal objects. Often they can be pulled out by grasping a protruding end. A common circumstance is a splinter under the finger nail. Removing a V-shape segment of the nail edge, with the apex overlying the end of the splinter, allows the operator to grasp the splinter. With gentleness the procedure can be carried out painlessly. If necessary, digital nerve block can be used for anesthesia.

While metal objects are readily identified in tissue by x-ray examination, wood and many glass foreign bodies are not. Glass containing lead may be faintly radiopaque. Retained glass is difficult to find in deep wounds regardless of x-ray demonstration. It is rarely identified visually and more often is recognized by a grating sensation when touched by an instrument.

All foreign bodies associated with draining wounds must be removed. If extensive search in deeper tissue spaces is planned or if mechanical aids such as magnets are needed, the procedure is better done in a well-equipped operating room than in an outpatient clinic. It is distressing for both patient and surgeon to hunt unsuccessfully for a possible foreign body under inadequate conditions of light, anesthesia, asepsis and assistance.

An imbedded fish hook is a unique form of puncture wound. The barb must be forced through a wound of exit so that it can be cut off with a wire shears. The remainder of the hook is then withdrawn through the site of entry. An alternative approach for removing a fish hook is described in Chapter 28.

Simple stab wounds and gunshot wounds which do not penetrate the neck, thoracic or peritoneal cavities and do not involve deep structures such as vessels, nerves, tendons or bones can usually be treated on an outpatient basis.

Stab wound tracts seldom require excision or débridement. The cardinal point in care is to keep open the wound of entry allowing free drainage of the wound tract until complete healing has occurred. An effective means of accomplishing this is to excise from $1/2$ to 1 centimeter of full-thickness skin circumferentially at the site of entrance. If the depth of the wound is more than 2 to 3 centimeters, packing with iodine-impregnated gauze keeps skin edges separated and prevents a closed space infection. Packing is replaced during each wound dressing until the deep portion of the tract is healed as determined by gently probing with a sterile applicator stick. At the time of dressing, saline or dilute hydrogen peroxide is used to irrigate the wound tract. If infection develops deeply, the tract must be opened widely or excised to allow adequate drainage.

Superficial gunshot wounds present a greater problem. The degree of tissue damage sustained is related to the tissue velocity of the missile. Entry and exit wound size cannot be related to tissue injury along the bullet tract. Missiles fired from low velocity weapons, such as the .22 caliber rifle, cause relatively little tissue damage. In superficial wounds of this type, entry and exit wounds should be debrided but the tract need not be explored unless heavily contaminated with clothing or other foreign material.

High velocity missile tracts are associated with considerable tissue necrosis. Wounds caused by such missiles should be opened along the entire tract and obviously nonviable tissue debrided. It is unwise to close such wounds primarily. They may be packed loosely, dressed and allowed to heal secondarily. The most common outpatient surgical errors in managing gunshot wounds are failing to recognize injury of deep structures and incompletely debriding high velocity missile wound tracts. If any question exists concerning the adequacy of outpatient débridement, the patient should be hospitalized.

Occasionally the outpatient surgeon will be asked to remove a subcutaneous bullet or missile fragment. It is important that he mark the removed bullet in such a way as to be able to identify it later in court. All bullets removed from patients must be given to police authorities, and gunshot wounds should be reported to the police.

Lacerations

Open wounds caused by objects which incise or tear full-thickness skin are termed lacerations. If deeper tissue damage is slight, as in injury caused by a sharp knife, the lesion is called an "incised wound." Most lacerations are irregular although skin edges remain well-defined. The tendency to gape is due to gravity, contraction of underlying muscle and retraction of tissue fibers lying perpendicular to the laceration. The mechanism of wound healing in lacerations is discussed in Chapter 8.

Minor lacerations are easily managed in the Emergency Room, office and clinic so long as facilities allow adequate anesthesia, débridement and suturing. When deep structures such as nerves, vessels, tendons or bone are involved, repair is best accomplished in the operating room. Since all accidental open wounds are considered contaminated with microorganisms, the surgeon must decide whether or not to attempt primary closure. Wounds of the body and extremities over six hours old are likely to be infected in the sense that contaminating bacteria have invaded tissue. Such wounds are better treated open — anticipating healing by secondary intention. An exception to this principle is wounds of the head and neck which, because of abundant blood supply, can be closed primarily within 12 hours of injury without undue risk of infection. Extensive débridement which removes dead tissue as well as bacteria imbedded in adjacent viable tissue can, of course, transform a potentially infected wound into a relatively clean, moderately contaminated lesion.

Infiltration of anesthetic solution into wound edges is usually sufficient to permit cleansing, débridement and suture repair. Nerve block techniques (Chapter 2) are sometimes more effective and avoid excessive wound manipulation. Minor lacerations are gently irrigated with sterile saline or washed with surgical soap before infiltration of anesthetic solution. More thorough cleansing follows anesthesia. Under aseptic conditions using sterile gloves, mask and wound drapes, lidocaine 1 per cent or 0.5 per cent is injected subcutaneously by means of a 22 or 25 gauge needle around the circumference of the wound. Edges are not grasped with forceps until anesthesia is obtained. The proper plane of injection is the corium which contains nerve endings. Injection of subcutaneous fat is unnecessary.

The most important factor in managing lacerations is adequate débridement. Surface dirt and foreign matter can be removed by vigorous irrigation with saline solution. Several liters may be required in large, heavily contaminated wounds. Surgical soap should not be used in deeper lacerations where muscle, tendon, nerves and blood vessels might be chemically irritated. Soap is useful, however, for cleansing surrounding skin. Iodophor antiseptic solutions usually are applied to skin edges only, although their use in the wound is increasingly common.

Dead or ischemic tissue should be sharply debrided. Devitalized fat or muscle is especially apt to cause wound infection. In sharply incised wounds, the skin border may require no débridement, whereas in avulsion or crush injuries large areas of skin may need excision. Débridement of skin edges is easily accomplished with forceps and scalpel or scissors, and excision is extended to normal-appearing, normal-bleeding tissue.

Bleeders seldom require ties or ligatures, but if they do, an absorbable suture material is used.

It is essential to persist in irrigation and débridement until all devitalized and contaminated tissue is removed. Singleton[13] has shown that the incidence of wound infection is inversely related to the amount of débridement done at the time of injury. The technique of débridement is further described in Chapter 8.

Bites

Animal and Human Bites

These bites produce a combination of puncture and laceration wounds. Common sites of injury are the ankle, forearm and hand. Because of the penetrating nature of the injury, infection with anaerobic micro-organisms is a prime concern. Débridement and drainage prevent deep infection which compounds injury in an otherwise simple lesion. The treatment of teeth injuries is described in Chapters 4, 8 and 13.

Insect Bites

While insect bites are potentially dangerous in terms of hypersensitivity reactions, they seldom result in lesions requiring surgical treatment. A notable exception is the bite of the brown recluse spider which can cause severe local reaction with tissue loss.[14]

The brown recluse spider (*Loxosceles reclusa*) thrives in dark corners of outbuildings, attics and storehouses. It is prevalent in southern and southwestern United States but ranges from the midwest to the Gulf of Mexico and from the Rocky Mountains to the Atlantic coast. The spider's body, 10 to 15 millimeters long, is brown in color with a darker, violin-shaped marking on the back which extends caudally from three pairs of eyes.

The bite is often inconspicuous. Two to eight hours later, however, the area becomes painful. Transient erythema develops at the site followed by formation of a bleb. On the third or fourth day the center of the lesion turns dark red or violet in color and, within another day or two, sloughs to form an ulcer often several centimeters in diameter. Surrounding tissue becomes gangrenous in some cases and underlying joints may be destroyed. Healing is slow as the ulcer remains indolent for several weeks.

Systemic reaction to the bite of the brown recluse spider varies from transient fever, malaise, nausea, vomiting and joint pain to hemolytic anemia and thrombocytopenia which have caused death in children. A petechial skin eruption may occur within 48 hours. Crampy abdominal pain is rarely severe. Edema, jaundice, convulsions and phlebitis have been reported.

Treatment of the brown recluse spider bite varies with the degree of local and systemic reaction. Steroids combined with antihistamines and antibiotics are indicated in severe reactions. Steroid therapy is maintained, with decreasing dosage, for ten days. Local wound care is challenging because of the chronic, therapy-resistant nature of the ulcer. Infection is less a problem than necrosis.

Initial wound care should include cold compresses to reduce local pain and swelling. If an extremity is involved, some degree of immobilization such as elevation is helpful. Dressings prevent inadvertent, painful trauma to the wound site.

Established ulcers heal slowly over several weeks. Skin grafting may accelerate wound closure. If gangrene surrounds the ulcer, excision of all diseased tissue is recommended. This is especially true when the ulcer overlies a finger joint and the danger of secondary osteomyelitis with joint destruction exists. Amputation of fingers has been required in some of these cases.

Suture Repair

Principles

The technique of suturing, as used by the outpatient surgeon in closing wounds, is intended to provide precise coaptation of skin edges and obliteration

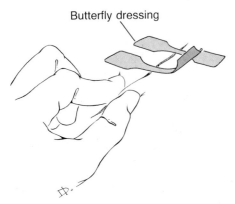

Butterfly dressing

Figure 3–5 "Butterfly" Adhesive Wound Closure. Simple, rapid closure of clean, superficial lacerations can be accomplished without sutures by applying "butterfly" adhesive strips to coapt skin edges.

of subcutaneous spaces. Suturing is a skill resulting from both instruction and experience and it requires that no further tissue damage follow its use. All elements of the procedure must be kept sterile to guard against infection. To minimize trauma, the smallest possible diameter of suture consistent with adequate strength is used. The suture must be easily manipulated, easily tied and, once tied, securely knotted. Occasionally superficial lacerations may be closed securely without sutures, using the "butterfly" adhesive strip shown in Figure 3–5. The butterfly strip can also be used to support a wound following suture removal.

Types of Sutures

There are two types of suture material, absorbable and nonabsorbable. Absorbable sutures are made of animal tissue and are proteolytically dissolved by the host. Plain catgut, made from the submucosa of sheep small intestine, dissolves in human tissue within a week. Impregnating catgut with chromic oxide (chromic catgut) extends resistance to proteolysis for 10 to 40 days, depending upon the degree of impregnation. Polyglycolic acid suture has greater tensile strength than catgut, handles more easily, but is absorbed between 7 and 30 days. The absorbable suture materials are used for closing of subcutaneous

tissues and for ligation of small blood vessels. Their disadvantages are the stimulation of greater local tissue reaction than nonabsorbable materials and the absorption of water which, by causing swelling, loosens knots. Since they are readily absorbed, these substances do not cause chronically draining suture sinuses as do silk sutures.

Silk is the most commonly used nonabsorbable suture material. It consists of the protein fibroin extruded by the silkworm. Its advantages are good tensile strength, little tissue reaction, pliability and secure knots. Cotton shares many of these advantages. Other nonabsorbable materials are monofilamentous synthetic polymers, such as Dacron or nylon, and stainless steel. These substances elicit less trauma reaction than silk but involve either more difficult tying or less knot security. Nonabsorbable sutures are useful for skin closure and for ligation of larger blood vessels.

The size of suture selected for any purpose is determined by its diameter and knot-pull tensile strength. The material used need not be stronger than the tissue it will hold together. Thus catgut used in subcutaneous tissues can be size 3–0. Silk or synthetic suture for approximating the skin is usually size 4–0. Sutures used on the face are often smaller than this and those suitable for injuries of the eye are not larger than size 6–0.

Individually wrapped, sterile sutures are now available in plastic envelopes which open easily by cutting or tearing off the end of the envelope. Material for ties, either absorbable or nonabsorbable, can be unraveled and stored in or under a towel with only the tip of each piece protruding. Thus, each length can be readily grasped. Spools of tie material are not needed in the outpatient repair of most lacerations.

Both absorbable and nonabsorbable suture materials are usually swaged into suitable needles. This arrangement minimizes tissue trauma and the surgeon's effort. Having separate suture material and needle requires that the surgeon place the suture in the needle and hold it there. To do this rapidly the empty needle is best held in the needle holder as it will later be used, the middle of the curve squarely placed about 2 millimeters from the tip of the instrument. While the needle is immobilized in the needle holder, the suture is advanced through the eye for at least one-quarter of its length. It is unnecessary to lock the ends through the holder tips. French-eye needles, which allow the use of heavy sutures on relatively small needles, are threaded by first passing the suture around the tip of the holder and then with tension slipping the material through the notch in the needle eye. Tapered or "round" point needles are used to suture subcutaneous structures. Cutting edge needles which more easily puncture tissue are used to suture skin.

Placement of Sutures

Most minor lacerations require only closure of the skin. If a significant subcutaneous defect exists, the surgeon should suspect injury to deeper structures. When this cannot be confirmed, the subcutaneous tissues are approximated by absorbable sutures placed in Scarpa's fascia. Few sutures are needed to accomplish this closure in most wounds. Since tissue apposition without necrosis from tight sutures is the goal, skin is closed with simple interrupted nonabsorbable sutures. The depth of the suture bite in terms of distance from the skin edge should equal the distance between bites (Fig. 3–6).

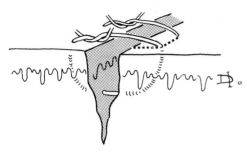

Figure 3–6 Simple Interrupted Suture. In simple interrupted suture technique, the distance from the skin edge should equal the distance apart to avoid tissue ischemia. Bites are taken well through the full thickness of skin.

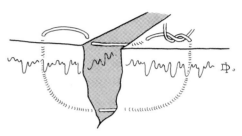

Figure 3–7 Vertical Mattress Suture. The vertical mattress suture which includes bites at the skin edges coapts layers precisely to enhance appearance and healing.

The skin edge can be manipulated by the use of fine-tooth tissue forceps placed on subcuticular structures. This avoids pressure necrosis of epithelial edges. If coaptation of edges is difficult, especially in the center of the wound, vertical mattress sutures can be used (Fig. 3–7).

Arterial bleeders in the depths of a lacerated wound can be securely controlled by means of a suture ligature, as illustrated in Figure 3–8. The ligature is useful when the vessel cannot be grasped with a hemostat. An alternate technique is to pass the needle through the vessel wall and to tie the suture on both sides.

Knot-tying

The outpatient surgeon ties knots to achieve wound hemostasis and closure. Since sutures usually are placed superficially in nonvital tissues, techniques of knot-tying receive little attention. Actually it is just as essential to tie surgical knots well in repairing a laceration as it is in performing other surgery, since the complications of poorly tied knots may be significant. Complications of poor knot-tying include the release of bleeders, skin necrosis and wound separation.

Tension ties are to be avoided but occasionally are needed to approximate wound edges. Simple overhand knots will loosen by the time the rest of the knot is completed unless strands are kept taut throughout.

Two-hand Knot (Fig. 3–9). This is

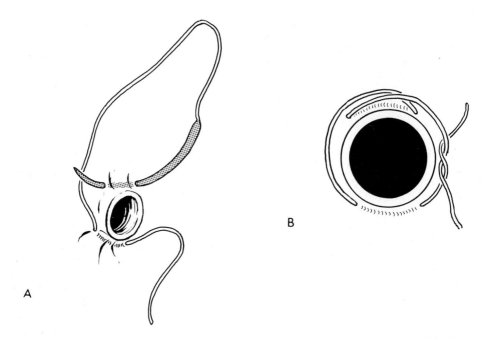

Figure 3–8   Suture Ligature for Retracted Blood Vessel. Arterial bleeders which retract into the wound and cannot be clamped and tied adequately are controlled by means of a suture ligature, usually of fine silk, which circumferentially compresses the vessel.

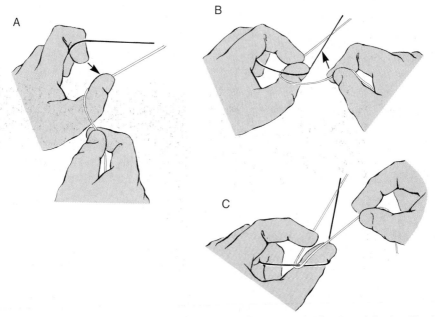

*Figure 3–9   The *two-hand knot* is illustrated. Suture ends are uncrossed as Step A begins. Hands must cross at the end of the first loop tie (Step F) *(opposite page)* to produce a flat knot. Hands are not crossed at the end of the second loop tie (Step J) *(opposite page).*

Illustration continued on opposite page.

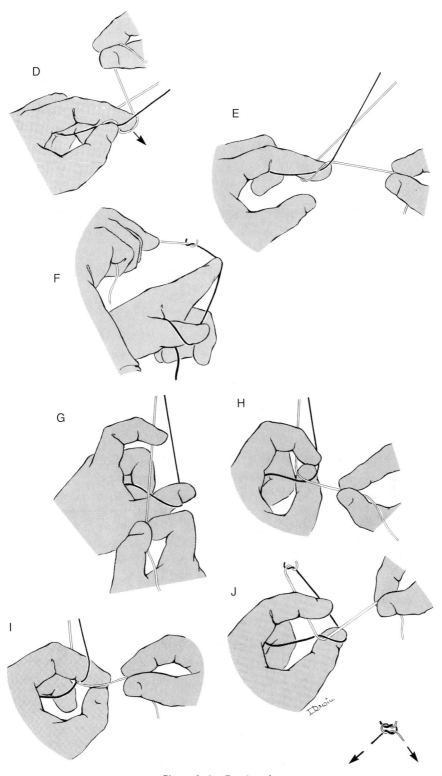

Figure 3–9 Continued.

the most reliable way to tie a square knot. Although slower than the one-hand technique, it insures a more dependable knot, especially under tension. For this reason many surgeons prefer the two-hand tie. It is important to lay the first half of the knot "flat." Unless strands have been crossed initially, this requires crossing the hands between the first and second halves. Two-hand knots tied without crossing the hands at the end of either the first or second half do not lie flat and may become untied.

One-hand Knot (Fig. 3–10).   This tie

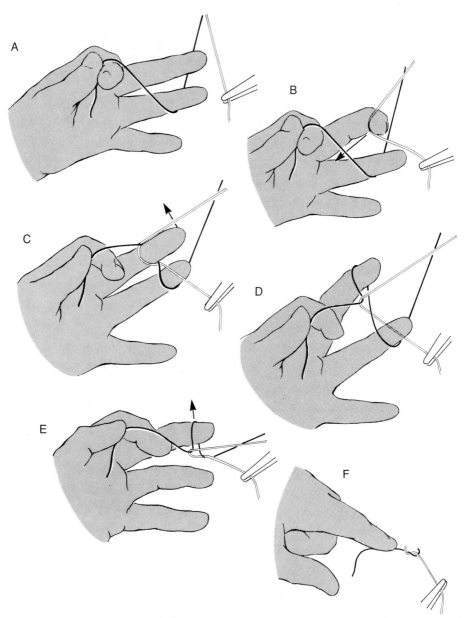

Figure 3–10   The *one-hand knot* is illustrated with one end of the suture grasped by an instrument. In Step A the light colored suture end is crossed over the dark colored suture before beginning the tie. Hands are uncrossed at the end of the first loop tie (Step F) but must be crossed after the second loop tie to produce a flat square knot.

Illustration continued on opposite page.

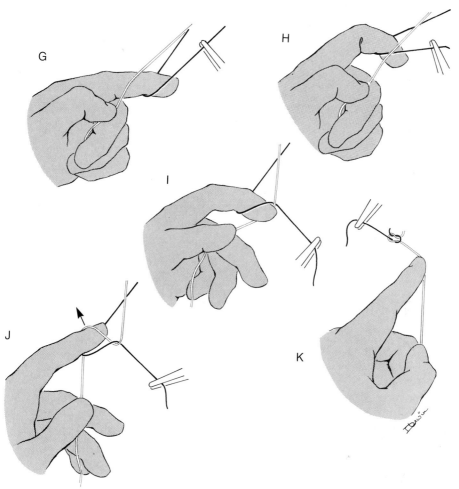

Figure 3–10 Continued.

is executed rapidly and allows the surgeon to retain a needle holder in the opposite hand along with one strand of suture. Again, hands must cross to lay the knot flat and to insure stability.

Instrument Tie (**Fig. 3–11**). Another technique of tying a surgical knot while retaining a needle holder is the instrument tie. Here the instrument acts as a hand in forming loops. The tie is useful only when tension is not required. It is of value when one end of the suture is short and cannot be held.

Wound Dressing

Dressings primarily are used to protect wounds from trauma and contamination. In some instances, they contribute to healing by controlling bleeding, obliterating dead space, supporting structures or relieving pain by immobilizing the wound area. Clean wounds treated early and closed primarily seldom require a protective dressing more than 24 hours. Wound infection rates in dressed and undressed surgical wounds are not significantly different. Open, draining or otherwise complicated wounds, however, benefit from dressings which protect regenerating epithelium, debride developing granulation tissue and absorb exuded fluid.

Surgical dressing is less formalized today than previously. Newer materials allow less bulky dressing and are easily

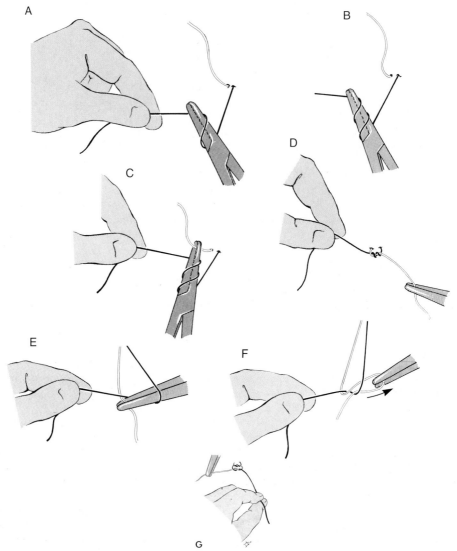

Figure 3–11 The *instrument tie* begins with either single or double (illustrated) looping of the long end of the suture about the needle holder. The first loop is laid flat without crossing hands. Hands must be crossed after the second loop tie (Step G) to produce a flat square knot.

applied and reliably secured. Nevertheless, dressing techniques are important. Certain principles will be discussed here while specific techniques are illustrated in chapters appropriate to the body region.

Closed Wound Dressing

Most closed wounds, such as contusion and hematoma, require no dressing.

Recently sutured lacerations may be protected by covering with wide-mesh gauze secured by adhesive. Squares of gauze, individually wrapped and sterile, are readily available to the outpatient surgeon. After suture repair, the skin is gently washed with sterile water or saline. Sterile gauze pads, two to three layers thick, are placed over the wound when the skin is dry. Antiseptic paint on the suture line is not required. Two or three strips of adhesive secure the gauze without preventing ventilation through the dressing.

Shaving skin hair and applying tincture of benzoin increases the adhesiveness of tape strips. Cloth-backed adhesive, while strong and moderately waterproof, occasionally causes skin irritation which may result in blisters. It is frequently painful to remove from hairy parts of the skin. Tape backed by a nonwoven viscose rayon largely avoids these disadvantages while remaining strongly adherent. It is easily cross-torn by the hands or by a dispenser and is considerably lighter than conventional adhesive. If occlusive or waterproof dressings are required, tape backed with polyethylene plastic may be used. This material contains no sensitizing ingredients and is transparent. Its elasticity makes tearing difficult. Commercially prepared adhesive strips with central gauze squares (e.g., Bandaid) are ideal for protecting small wounds.

Another method of protecting sutured wounds or holding dressings in place is the use of collodion or plastic aerosol sprays. No additional benefit has been shown to result from combining the spray with an antibiotic. When the spray dries, a tough, thick, clear film protects the wound and allows continuing observation. Wounds of the face and neck where dressing is difficult are well-treated with this technique.

Open Wound Dressing

Open wounds exude serum which dries to form a surface eschar. Porous dressings such as gauze become incorporated into the eschar and are sealed to the wound. This can be both helpful and harmful in terms of wound healing. Removing adherent gauze from infected granulations removes tissue debris, thereby debriding the wound. Delicate, new epithelium growing across the wound, on the other hand, may be lost by dressing with adherent gauze. Non-porous materials lack debriding benefits but protect regenerating epithelium. The type of open wound thus dictates the type of dressing needed.

Adherent, porous dressings are ideal for granulating wounds which are heavily contaminated or infected. Fine mesh gauze is used because only small tufts of granulations become fixed in mesh pores and are debrided by dressing removal. The resulting surface is cleaner and more even. Soaking facilitates dressing change and débridement. When a healthy granulating surface is obtained and re-epithelization is likely, nonporous dressings may be used.

Initially clean, superficial open wounds, such as abrasions, are dressed with a nonadherent material such as Telfa. This is a cellophane-like substance with many fine perforations too small to allow tissue ingrowth but large enough to permit circulation of air. Wax or petrolatum-impregnated gauze is another nonadherent dressing. Its disadvantage is skin maceration due to lack of ventilation and drying. Both adherent and nonadherent dressings are backed with gauze and secured by adhesive, plastic spray or bandaging.

Draining wounds present a special problem. Sufficient gauze should cover the wound to absorb all drainage and to keep the skin dry. Dressings of open wounds should be inspected daily and changed if saturated with drainage. Larger amounts of absorbent gauze may be needed to avoid rapid resaturation. Change of dressing is an aseptic procedure requiring sterile gloves, instruments and face mask.

Dressings impregnated with antibacterial agents are helpful in treating minor burns and superficial wounds. In general, however, topical antibiotics are of limited value and may in some cases interfere with tissue regeneration. Deep lacerations which cannot be closed primarily are packed loosely with sterile gauze to keep skin edges apart until secondary healing obliterates the open base.

Pressure Dressing

In order to tamponade superficial wound bleeders or to obliterate tissue spaces, flat or fluffed gauze is heaped over the wound site and maintained under pressure by circumferential bandaging or noncircumferential elastic adhesive. The latter is particularly useful in applying local pressure. Since this type of bandage tends to unroll at the ends or sides, it is surrounded by narrower strips of adhesive plaster.

Bandaging

Bandage materials, once limited to gauze, muslin or flannel, now include a variety of elastic cottons and adhesives. The former is commonly available in rolls 2 to 6 inches wide. Elastic cotton can be rapidly, snugly and neatly applied regardless of previous experience. The elastic qualities of the bandage allow it to conform closely to body contours. While a moderate degree of pressure can be exerted by circular wrapping, occlusion of major arteries is quite unlikely. The material is washable, allowing reuse. This is of some advantage to the outpatient who may be responsible for changing his dressing.

Elastic cotton (Kerlix) is well-suited for use on extremities where circular bandaging is required to stabilize dressings. Figure 3–12 illustrates the appli-

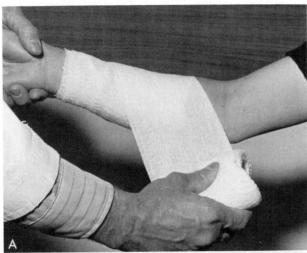

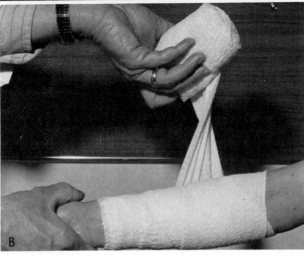

Figure 3–12   Forearm Bandage Technique. A. Elastic cotton is ideal material for bandaging an extremity. To secure a forearm dressing, three inch bandage is wrapped twice around the arm distally and advanced proximally with circular, overlapping turns. B. Snugness of the bandage is increased by rotating the bandage roll 180° after each circular turn to effect a reverse spiral.

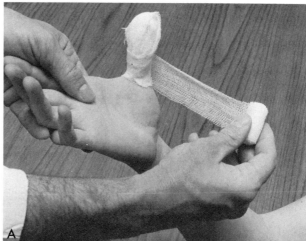

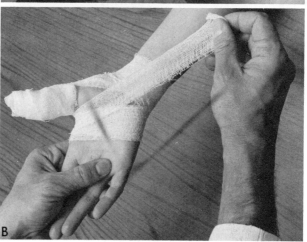

Figure 3–13   Stump Dressing Technique. A. Bandaging a finger with elastic cotton narrowed to one inch in width begins by passing the bandage lengthwise over the digit to effect coverage and locking it in place by circular turns. B. The bandage is secured by passing the roll about the palm and wrist and taping the end.

cation of such a dressing on the forearm. After covering the wound with gauze squares, sterile elastic cotton bandage, 3 inches wide, is wrapped twice around the arm distal to the wound to fix the bandage. The material is unrolled by advancing proximally with circular, overlapping turns. The end of the bandage is secured to the material by adhesive. This dressing may be made more snug by rotating the roll 180 degrees after each circular turn to effect a reverse spiral.

In bandaging any distal area such as an amputation stump or finger, elastic cotton is again useful. Strips of the bandage are rolled lengthwise over the stump and locked in place by circular turns

(Fig. 3–13). Elastic cotton bandaging of joints allows mobility while maintaining dressings in place. When elastic materials are unavailable, a figure-of-eight bandage of gauze or muslin may be used to bandage joints. The technique is shown in Figure 3–14. Several turns are taken distal to the joint to anchor the bandage. The material is then unrolled obliquely across the joint and anchored above by a complete turn. Again the bandage is brought obliquely across the joint space and anchored below by a complete turn. The process is repeated until dressings are securely covered.

The use of elastic adhesive bandages as part of pressure dressings has been described. These materials are also of

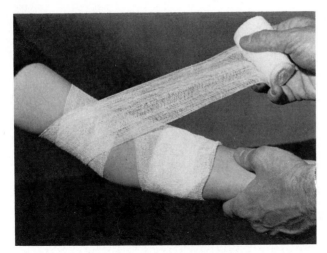

Figure 3–14 Figure of Eight Bandage Technique. To bandage joints, elastic cotton is anchored proximally by taking several turns and then unrolled obliquely across the joint and anchored below by a complete turn. The process is repeated until dressings are securely covered.

value in fixing dressings to the chest, abdomen or pelvis. Elastic adhesive allows the chest to expand and contract without dislodging the bandage, and it can be maintained in areas where other bandages fail to hold. Because of a tendency to unroll at both ends and sides, elastic adhesive should be bordered by ordinary adhesive plaster.

The primary purpose of bandaging is to secure and protect underlying wound dressings. The appearance of the bandage is important, however, in that patients may judge the excellence of their treatment by the neatness of their bandage. While aesthetic considerations are not crucial, they contribute to the technique of bandaging. A trim bandage usually indicates that care has been taken to avoid wrinkles which might create undue pressure and loose turns which might shorten the effective life of the dressing.

References

1. Blanken, G. E.: Current estimates, vital and health statistics HEW, *10*:1–63, 1971.
2. National Safety Council: Accident Facts. Chicago, 1970.
3. Radiation Injury. In McCarroll and P. Skudder (eds.): The Treatment of Mass Civilian Casualties in a National Emergency. Washington, Medical Education for National Defense, 1967.
4. Glover, J. L., O'Byrne, S. A., and Jolly, L.: Infusion catheter sepsis: An increasing threat. Ann. Surg., *173*:148–151, 1971.
5. Smith, B. E., Modell, J. H., Gaub, M. L., and Moya, F.: Complications of subclavian vein catheterization. Arch. Surg., *90*: 228–229, 1965.
6. Yoffa, D.: Supraclavicular subclavian venepuncture and catheterization. Lancet, *2*: 614–617, 1964.
7. Jernigan, W. R., Gardner, W. C., Mahr, M. M., and Milburn, J. L.: Use of the internal jugular vein for placement of central venous catheter. Surg. Gynecol. Obstet., *130*:520–524, 1970.
8. Root, H. D., Hauser, C. W., McKinley, C. R., LaFave, J. W., and Mendiola, Jr., R. P.: Diagnostic peritoneal lavage. Surgery, *57*: 633–637, 1965.
9. Hickman, T. C.: Abdominal paracentesis. Surg. Clin. North Amer., *49*:1409–1412, 1969.
10. Perry, J. F., McMeules, J. E., and Root, H. D.: Diagnostic peritoneal lavage in blunt abdominal trauma. Surg. Gynecol. Obstet., *131*:742–744, 1970.
11. Cornell, W. P., Ebert, P. A., Greenfield, L. F., and Zuidema, G. D.: A new non-operative technique for the diagnosis of penetrating injuries to the abdomen. J. Trauma, *7*:307–314, 1967.
12. Trimble, C.: Stab wound sinography. Surg. Clin. North Amer., *49*:1217–1221, 1969.
13. Singleton, A. O., Jr., David, D., and Julian, J.: The prevention of wound infection following contamination with colon organisms. Surg. Gynecol. Obstet., *108*:389–392, 1959.

14. Frazier, C. A.: Insect Allergy: Allergic and Toxic Reactions to Insects and Other Arthropods. St. Louis: Warren H. Green, Inc., 1969.

15. Ballinger, W. F., II, Rutherford, R. B., and Zuidema, G. D. (eds.): The Management of Trauma. Philadelphia: W. B. Saunders Co., 1968.

16. U. S. Department of Defense. Emergency War Surgery. U. S. Armed Forces Issue of NATO Handbook prepared for use by the Medical Services of NATO nations. Washington: Government Printing Office, 1958.

17. Nealon, T. F.: Fundamental Skills in Surgery. Philadelphia: W. B. Saunders Co., 1971.

18. Red Cross. U. S. American National Red Cross First Aid Textbook. Garden City, N. Y., Doubleday, 1957.

4

Infections

By GEORGE J. HILL, II, M.D.

"If thou examinest a man having a diseased wound in his breast: while the two lips of that wound are ruddy, and that man continues to be feverish, his flesh cannot receive a bandage. I will make cool applications for drawing out the inflammation, applications for drying up the wound, and poultices."

Anon., 3000 B.C.
in Breastead, J. H. (ed.)
The Edwin Smith Surgical Papyrus
Chicago, U. Chicago Press, 1930
Case 41. pp. 371–391

INTRODUCTION

The outpatient surgeon must be concerned with prevention, recognition and treatment of infection. Prevention of contamination is the goal of preparation for elective surgery in clean cases, and reduction in the risk of infection is the goal of preparation for surgery in contaminated cases. Optimum preparation and prophylaxis cannot completely eliminate the risk of infection, so the subtle early signs of infection must be recognized by surgeons and patients in order that effective treatment may begin as soon as possible.[22] Treatment of surgical infections generally consists of either drainage or antibiotics or both. The type of therapy is guided by the location and severity of the infection.

The most difficult challenge for the outpatient surgeon with respect to management of infection is the establishment of adequate follow-up to insure that infections will be recognized promptly. The busy surgeon must find time to instruct his patients or their families on the possible signs and symptoms of sepsis. He should make every effort to see his own patients in follow-up, since the signs of sepsis in clean cases may be easily overlooked, and since the evidence for adequate therapy in infected cases is best obtained by the sequential observations of one physician.

In order to reduce the risk of infection, the outpatient surgeon should utilize optimum management of the wound through the following principles: an aseptic (sterile) environment, mechanical cleanliness of the skin and deep tissues, atraumatic handling of tissues, débridement of devitalized tissue, minimal residual foreign body in the wound, satisfactory hemostasis, elimination of dead space, and careful postoperative observation of the healing wound. These principles pertain to both elective surgery and the repair of traumatic injury — and to the surgery of clean cases as well as to contaminated cases.[23]

Antibiotics are particularly important in the treatment of severe infection in hospitalized patients.[15] On the other hand, infections in outpatients are generally less severe and more superficial than those observed in inpatients. Thus, guidelines for the use of antibiotics in outpatients are somewhat different from those for inpatients. In general, local treatment with moist heat or drainage is sufficient treatment for most infections in outpatients. The use of antibiotics entails the risk of drug reaction (particularly anaphylaxis and blood dyscrasias),

the emergence of resistant strains of bacteria, and additional cost to the patient. When antibiotic treatment is utilized it should be remembered that each hospital and each community has a pattern of resistance to bacteria which may be different from others. In general, bacteria from outpatients are less resistant to antibiotics than bacteria from inpatients.[8] At the University of Colorado Medical Center, we do not commonly use topical antibiotics, except as described below in the section on *Chemotherapy* (neomycin, polymyxin B, bacitracin and nitrofurazone).

PREVENTION

The Environment

The optimum environment for surgery is an operating room fully equipped with the bacteriologic controls available in the surgical suite used for inpatient operations. The main operating room suite has the advantages of minimum personnel traffic and thorough cleansing of the walls, floors and other surfaces between operations. The operations performed in the Outpatient Department may be relatively less complicated than those performed on inpatients, but the morbidity and expense of an infection may nullify the advantages gained by operating in the Outpatient Clinic.[21] The operating rooms in the main surgical suite, obstetrical rooms and in the Outpatient Clinic of Colorado General Hospital are cleansed with a spray down–vacuum pickup technique. The germicide-detergent combination used is a quaternary ammonium compound and non-ionic detergent (Airkem "A-33 Dry"). Rodac plate tests of Airkem "A-33 Dry" showed that it had the best bactericidal activity of any disinfectant studied by the Hospital Epidemiology Committee.

The ideal environment is difficult to achieve and maintain in the major surgical suite, and it is vastly more difficult to achieve high standards of asepsis in the Outpatient Clinic. A rapid turnover of patients, unexpected emergencies, less assistance available, and a relatively high incidence of contaminated wounds and abscesses are factors which reduce the opportunity to maintain rigid control of environmental contamination in outpatient operations. Although compromises become necessary, the surgeon should always endeavor to maintain as wide a field of sterility about his patient as possible. Accidental contamination is almost inevitable when the sterile field contracts simply to the wound itself, a small drape and sterile gloves.

Every effort should be made to maintain an optimum environment for elective procedures in clean cases, such as biopsy, paracentesis or other similar operations. Although theoretically the operating room should be thoroughly cleansed after each patient has been treated, practical considerations often dictate otherwise. Application of plaster, colonic irrigations and drainages of abscesses are inherently more likely to leave residual contamination in the operating room than procedures such as a biopsy or suture of a laceration. Patients with major traumatic injuries are often attended by police, clergy, family or bystanders. Clothing and debris are widely scattered, contaminating even the most ideal environment. Taking these factors into consideration, it may be best to establish one or two major trauma-receiving rooms near the clinic entrance, another room for "dirty" cases, including application of plaster, and one or more operating rooms further from the entrance, for elective outpatient surgery and closure of small lacerations.[1]

The cases in the rooms used for resuscitation are expected to be at greater risk of infection than those in the inner rooms used predominantly for elective surgery. The use of antibiotics should be considered for patients who have a high risk of sepsis.

The outpatient surgeon should scrub his hands and arms for ten minutes[6] with an iodophor detergent (e.g., G.S.I., Betadine or E–Z Prep with Iodophor) or a phenolic-based germicide (e.g., pHisoHex). He should be fully clothed in cap, mask, gown and gloves. It is important for the outpatient surgeon to maintain short, clean fingernails, neat hair on face and scalp, and sleeves which do not reach below the elbows. It is then possible to don gloves and begin work immediately on patients who are brought to the clinic with multiple lacerations and deep visceral penetration. Equipment should be sterilized in the hospital's central sterile supply area, or else it should be prepackaged, sterilized, disposable equipment. The risk of hepatitis or sepsis from inadequate sterilization makes the small countertop steam sterilizer obsolete, except in remote and poverty-stricken areas.

Preparation and Draping for Surgery

Preparation of the patient's skin should be performed as thoroughly as that of the surgeon's hands and arms. Hair is shaved from the operative area immediately prior to surgery. Skin preparations should be performed in a centrifugal fashion, except for badly contaminated wounds which will be excised, or for abscesses prior to drainage. The latter types of wounds are com-

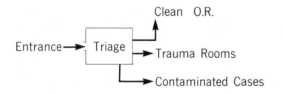

Figure 4–1 Organization of clinic facilities to reduce contamination: receiving rooms for trauma near entrance, and inner rooms for "dirty" and "clean" cases.

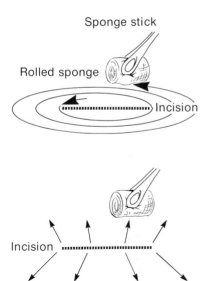

Figure 4–2 Skin preparation: Two acceptable techniques of centrifugal scrubbing and application of disinfectant.

monly prepared by centripetal application of the sterilizing agent.

In most cases the prep is best performed by a ten minute scrub with an iodophor or phenolic-based germicidal soap. The experience in Vietnam with a shorter period of preparation using iodides (iodophors) was satisfactory enough to warrant use of this method in traumatized patients who require immediate surgery. Further experience will be required to determine if skin preparation for elective operations can be safely achieved by preparation with a single application of iodophor. Skin preparation can also be performed effectively by tincture of iodine, which is removed by alcohol after it has dried. This preparation requires only a minute or two, but has the risk of iodine allergy or dermatitis if the iodine is not scrupulously removed by the alcohol rinse.

Zephiran (benzalkonium chloride) is a quaternary ammonium disinfectant which may be used for skin preparation. Zephiran is particularly useful for preparation of the face, since it is relatively nonirritating to the mucosa and eyes in aqueous solution. Lacerations and incisions on the face can be sutured with maximum cosmetic effect if the face is prepared with Zephiran and draped to allow full exposure of the entire face. Tinted tincture of Zephiran is a useful preparation for the torso and extremities, and the orange color outlines the field of preparation nicely. The best method for use of Zephiran is the use of alternate sponges of Zephiran and 70 per cent ethyl alcohol for a ten minute scrub of the skin. Although Zephiran and alcohol are compatible, it should be emphasized that the quaternary ammonium disinfectants are neutralized by anionic compounds such as soap and synthetic soap substitutes.

Sterile towels and other drapes should be applied as in a major operation. The most commonly used barrier around an outpatient wound is a towel with a small hole in its center. While this is adequate for scalp, trunk and thigh, it is inadequate for many other procedures. It tends to slip, revealing underlying nonsterile areas, or—on the face—obscuring the natural lines of symmetry. A larger sterile field can be obtained with towels affixed by clips or sutures through wheals of skin infiltrated with local anesthetic. An alternative method, especially useful on the extremities, is a circumferential prep and drape.

Management of the Wound

Infection is clearly a significant hazard in wounds which are roughly handled and inadequately debrided. In traumatic injuries the wound itself and the deep tissues immediately next to the wound should be searched for foreign bodies by inspecting and gently palpating with the finger and an instrument. Frequently a metallic click on a forceps or a hemostat is a clue to the presence of a foreign body. X-ray of a wound will often reveal opaque foreign bodies which would otherwise be overlooked. The history of the wounding agent will be a guide to the possible presence of foreign bodies and the depth to which foreign bodies may have penetrated. Sharp débridement of the wound edges with a scalpel provides ideal débridement of devitalized tissue and facilitates removal of impacted foreign bodies. However, débridement of the skin is neither necessary nor recommended on the face except when it is utterly destroyed. On the other hand, deep tissues should ordinarily be removed if their viability is in question in order to minimize the danger of anaerobic infection. Occasionally when vital structures are involved, final débridement of deep tissues may be deferred to the second or third day, provided the wound is left open to prevent the proliferation of anaerobic organisms.

Satisfactory hemostasis should be achieved with sutures of minimum but adequate size. Larger suture materials simply add foreign bodies to the wound and increase the likelihood of sepsis. Catgut is commonly used in potentially infected wounds, but silk, cotton or synthetic suture materials are also satisfactory and may be advantageous since closure can be performed with finer material. In any case, serious effort should be made to ligate only the blood vessels, and not a mass of tissue surrounding the blood vessels. If blind ligatures are required to control hemorrhage, the ligatures should be tied as gently as possible, in order to avoid strangulation of tissue. A useful technique for hemostasis in difficult cases is the placement of deep sutures which extend through the skin, and which may be completely removed seven to ten days later. Elimination of dead space should be achieved with sutures rather than drains. If loss of tissue from biopsy or trauma precludes reapproximation of the wound edges, it is better to pack the wound loosely with gauze for subsequent grafting or delayed closure, rather than to draw the wound edges together under great tension. Wounds with dead spaces have a high incidence of infection.

The true incidence of wound infections in outpatient operations is unknown. Infection rates in major operations range from 0.1 per cent to 37 per cent,[10,14,20] with variability resulting from the type of operation (herniorrhaphy,

colon resection, and so on) and the presence or absence of preexisting infection ("clean" vs. "contaminated"). Other important factors are airborne contamination, transfer of bacteria from hospital personnel,[4] endogenous sources of bacteria, and the accuracy of reporting of infections.

Elective major operations in uninfected patients have a wound infection rate of 1 to 3 per cent in university hospitals in the U.S.[20,21] However, it is apparent that the outpatient surgeon must judge his own work carefully. He should accept no existing standard as a guide for an "acceptable" rate of infections, but seek in every way to improve his own record from year to year.

Specific precautions should be taken in cases which entail a high risk of infection, such as a heavy bacterial contamination. The duration of time from injury until repair should also be taken into consideration. As a general rule, wounds which have been untreated for more than six hours should be considered heavily contaminated. Contaminated wounds may be excised and closed primarily but the risk of infection is obviously greater than in clean wounds. Primary closure of contaminated wounds is ordinarily not advisable. However, if severe functional impairment would result unless the wound is closed, débridement and closure of the deep tissues are in order. The skin and subcutaneous tissue can be left open. These cases ordinarily should be treated with antibiotics, and observation in the hospital for one to two days following injury is advisable.

Allergic Reactions

Epinephrine 1:1000 should be available in 1.0 ml ampoules, along with needles and syringes, whenever immunizations with biological products or injections of antibiotics are given to patients. Before vaccines or serum products are administered, the patient should be asked about a history of allergy, specifically "hives," erythematous reactions, fevers or other untoward reactions to biological products. Skin and conjunctival tests should be performed when indicated, as described in the manufacturers' brochures. The history of penicillin allergy must be regarded seriously and such patients should not receive penicillin or its derivatives on an outpatient basis.

Tetanus

Tetanus is a disease characterized by severe tonic contractions of skeletal muscles and generalized convulsive seizures, caused by tetanus toxin produced by *Clostridium tetani*, a gram positive, spore-forming anaerobic bacillus. Spasm of the muscles of mastication produces trismus (inability to open the mouth), which gives the disease its common name of "lockjaw." Tetanus occurs as a complication of traumatic injury or in septic deliveries, as either puerperal tetanus or tetanus of newborn infants (tetanus neonatorum). Tetanus organisms and spores are commonly present in feces. Barnyard accidents, fecal contamination and animal bites have a relatively high risk of tetanus.

As a complication of injury, tetanus has a mortality rate of approximately 20 per cent,[19] and immediate hospitalization is required in all patients suspected of having tetanus. The disease is not contagious, since symptoms are caused by the toxin rather than the bacillus *C. tetani*. The toxin is distributed by the blood stream to the nervous system, where it has a high degree of affinity, especially for motor nerves.

The incidence of tetanus has been greatly reduced by widespread active immunization with DPT vaccine in childhood, and tetanus toxoid immunizations given to adults. Tetanus may result from trivial injury or may even occur in the absence of any known injury in patients who have not been immunized with tetanus toxoid. Tetanus can also occur as the result of massive contamination and inadequate débridement in patients who have previously been immunized. Persistence of low grade immunity may be present for as long as 21 years after previous tetanus toxoid immunization, but a level of immunity adequate to cope with overwhelming infection requires additional protection. However, the routine use of tetanus boosters after every trivial injury is not recommended because of the occasional occurrence of allergic reactions, which are usually manifested by fever and malaise. The exact interval at which booster doses of tetanus toxoid should be given is debated and recommendations are changed frequently following conferences and reports by authorities. At the present time booster doses are recommended every six years by the armed forces and every ten years by the Public Health Service.[5] Additional booster doses are usually given for minor wounds at intervals of 6 to 12 months, as recommended by the American College of Surgeons,[9]* although the PHS Advisory Committee[5] (1971) stated that it is unnecessary to use booster doses more often than every five years.

Tetanus antitoxin is used to produce immediate serum antibody protection in patients with a high risk of tetanus who have no history of tetanus immunization, or who have not received tetanus toxoid within the past 6 to 10 years. Human immune serum (Hyper-tet) is highly preferable to the older forms of antiserum, which were prepared in domestic animals. Equine tetanus antitoxin should be administered only in remote areas where human tetanus immune globulin is totally unavailable. In the rare event in which equine globulin must be used, careful skin and conjunctival testing should be performed as described in the manufacturers' brochures.

An outline of recommended tetanus prophylaxis is shown below:

1. Previously immunized individuals.

---

*Posters and reprints of the guide to tetanus prophylaxis of the American College of Surgeons may be obtained from: Committee on Trauma, 55 East Erie St., Chicago, Illinois 60611.

a. For patients with wounds in which a relatively *low likelihood* of tetanus is present and who have previously received a complete series of tetanus toxoid or DPT inoculations, give: tetanus toxoid 0.5 cc, IM, unless the patient has received a booster within the previous 12 months.

2. For individuals with no previous tetanus immunizations.

   a. Prior to injury:

      (1) Children: DPT (diphtheria, pertussis, tetanus) toxoid 0.5 ml IM given monthly for three months, followed one year later by a booster dose and another dose at school entry.

      (2) Adults: DT or tetanus toxoid alone, given in doses and intervals similar to those described in *2a(1)*.

   b. For patients with wounds in which a *low likelihood* of tetanus is present, give meticulous débridement, start the series of active tetanus immunizations described above *(2a)* and consider the use of penicillin or tetracycline for seven to ten days.

   c. For patients with wounds having a relatively *high likelihood* of tetanus, use meticulous débridement and give:

      (1) tetanus toxoid 0.5 ml, IM, and

      (2) human tetanus immune globulin, 400 units, IM, and

      (3) penicillin or tetracycline for seven to ten days followed by completion of toxoid immunization course as described in *2a*.

Rabies

Rabies is an acute disease of the nervous system caused by a specific virus of the large class of miscellaneous neurotropic viruses. It is virtually 100 per cent fatal in man, though chronic infections occur in bats, skunks and other animals. All warm-blooded animals are susceptible to the disease. Rabies in man is usually the result of the bite of an infected dog, skunk or bat. The biting animal should be confined as soon as possible after the bite and observed for signs of rabies.

After an incubation period of 10 to 90 days or more an infection becomes manifested by local pain, headache, apprehension, excessive salivation, sore throat, difficulty in swallowing (which causes "hydrophobia") and fever. Muscular spasm and seizures occur subsequently. Patients with rabies or suspected rabies must be hospitalized and treated with great care. Secondary infection of attending personnel should be avoided.

Because of the long incubation period, treatment of rabies is unique in that active immunization can successfully be performed in most cases *after* the patient has been infected. Rabies prophylaxis should usually be undertaken when a person has been bitten by a wild animal, or by a domestic animal under unexpected circumstances, especially when the animal cannot be retained for observation. About 20 per cent of untreated humans bitten by rabid animals will develop rabies. The danger of rabies is increased when the bite is large or on the face, and treatment should be started prior to knowledge of the results of laboratory tests in such patients. Rabies is extremely uncommon in dogs and cats in cities within the United States, probably as the result of extensive rabies vaccination programs for pets. It is generally unnecessary and even unwise to embark on a rabies prophylaxis program for patients bitten by these domestic animals within city limits, unless the animal was unusually aggressive or otherwise abnormal.

The World Health Organization recommends that rabies prophylaxis with duck embryo vaccine (DEV) be given to patients who were exposed to rabies. The recommendations are shown in

Chapter 26 and are summarized as follows:

1. For mild exposure, such as a lick on mucosa or abraded skin and for a single bite on the trunk or leg, start treatment immediately if the animal is known to have rabies, or if it becomes ill during a ten day period of observation. DEV alone may be used, except in bites of wild animals, in which case rabies antiserum should be added.

2. For severe exposure, such as bites of the head, neck and arm or multiple bites elsewhere, the treatment with DEV is the same as for mild exposure, and rabies antiserum is also added.

When rabies prophylaxis is given as recommended by the World Health Organization,[24] it is extremely rare for the disease to develop.

Bites of animals suspected of being rabid should be washed vigorously with 20 per cent soap or a quaternary ammonium disinfectant, and should not be sutured unless absolutely necessary.

DEV treatment is usually given in a series of 14 daily subcutaneous doses of 1.0 ml each in different sites, usually on the abdomen and back.

The following modifications of the rabies treatment program are recommended in special circumstances: only five doses are usually given if the biting animal appears healthy after the fifth day, and treatment is subsequently continued only if the animal is later proved to be rabid. However, after the bite of a wild animal, *two* daily doses should be given for the first seven days, and one daily dose thereafter for the next seven days. In cases in which rabies antiserum is indicated, antiserum is given both locally and at sites distant from the bite, as indicated in the brochure which accompanies the serum. Up to one-half of the antiserum should be used to infiltrate the wound.

DEV has been associated with a very low risk of anaphylaxis, encephalitis and myelitis. On the other hand, rabies antiserum has caused both local allergic reactions and serum sickness. Neither agent is free of risk, and, unfortunately, rabies can develop in spite of intensive use of prophylaxis. The use of antiserum probably interferes with antibody formation in response to vaccine. Therefore, if antiserum is administered, booster doses of DEV are recommended 10 to 20 days after the initial series is completed.

Individuals such as veterinarians, who are likely to be exposed to rabies, should be protected by a series of three or four prophylactic injections during a period of six months, followed by booster doses every one to two years. The serum antibody titer of vaccinated individuals can be tested on specimens sent to the Center for Disease Control in Atlanta, Georgia.

The use of rabies prophylactic treatment must be individualized for each patient, since anxiety, pain and risk are factors which plague the patient and his community. But it is generally wisest to *overtreat* rather than *undertreat* if there is a question of rabies, since the risk of permanent complications or death from DEV and antiserum are relatively low.

Human Bites and Animal Bites

Human and cat bites are notoriously liable to be infected, and ordinarily they should not be closed by suture. The occurrence of any 3–5 mm transverse laceration at the metacarpal phalangeal joint should be suspected of being a human bite regardless of the history obtained. Careful irrigation, débridement, and dressing are indicated, but the wound should not be sutured when it is first inspected. Cat bites are more commonly puncture wounds than lacerations, and rarely require closure. The mixed infections which result from bites of cats or humans are usually composed of anaerobes, aerobes and spirochetes. Systemic antibiotic prophylaxis is indicated with penicillin or tetracycline in these bites. Local antibiotic treatment is relatively ineffective, and is not employed in this type of injury in our clinic. Dog bites

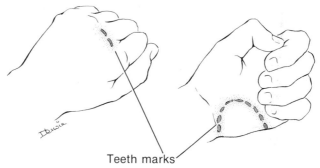

Ibicia

Teeth marks

Figure 4–3 Human bites. A particularly dangerous wound, because of the high incidence of sepsis. Should be irrigated, debrided and treated with systemic antibiotics. Do not close with sutures.

are relatively less likely to become infected, although prophylactic systemic antibiotics are indicated if the bites are extensive. In general, dog bites can be cleaned, irrigated, debrided and sutured, and they have a relatively low incidence of infection. In most towns and cities, dog bites must be reported to the police, and the possibility of rabies prophylaxis must also be considered.

RECOGNITION OF INFECTION

Infection in surgical patients may be located at the primary wound or at a metastatic location, or it may be disseminated. Infection may be present in the classic form of *calor, rubor, tumor,* and *dolor.* However, when sepsis is located in deep tissues in a distant site, symptoms may be puzzling and bizarre. Infection in surgical patients may be a complication of clean surgery or it may represent persistent infection in a contaminated wound. Infection in surgical patients may also be unrelated to the operation, as in nosocomial or hospital-acquired infections. In any case, when the patient is under the care of a surgeon, it is his responsibility to suspect, identify and initiate proper therapy for the infection, and to obtain consultation and referral if necessary.

Most infections incurred in the outpatient clinic can be detected if the wound is inspected on the first or second

day following closure. Ideally, the patient should return to the clinic for observation of the incision by a physician. But if this is impossible, another reliable observer must be entrusted with the responsibility. It should be emphasized, however, that a brief inspection by a physician is worth much more than a report by an untrained layman. Early return visits occasionally present a problem, unless the clinic staff is entirely familiar with the routine. Occasionally personnel have unwittingly removed sutures on the second day or scrubbed the sutured wound with soap and water. It is unfortunate if hospital routine requires a full charge to be made for a simple inspection of the wound, but this may be necessary in order to obtain adequate postoperative observation. A brief record should be made at the time the wound is inspected. If the wounding agent was blunt and considerable force was used, inflammation and pain may be present around the incision. Only a trained physician can distinguish these signs from early infection. And even the wisest physician will occasionally require additional follow-up visits in order to be certain that the wound is healing well.

A more difficult problem is presented by patients who are seen in the clinic following discharge from major surgery in the hospital. The diagnosis of abdominal abscess—pelvic, subhepatic, subphrenic, and so on—may be difficult if the surgeon attending the patient in the clinic is a different person from the attending surgeon in the hospital. If the patient does not continue to improve following discharge from the hospital, the possibility of infection should be raised. Diagnostic x-rays may be helpful, including plain films and laminograms, and air fluid levels should be looked for. Barium studies may reveal shifts of the intestinal tract around intra-abdominal abscesses. The presence of fever, night sweats, failure to gain weight, or weight loss are possible signs of infection. The patient with suspicious signs should be asked to record his temperature four times per day and bring the record back for inspection at each clinic visit. Infections may involve areas distant from the operative field, and may be as bizarre as meningitis or reactivated tuberculosis. The most important consideration in diagnosing a postoperative infection is to consider the *possibility* that infection is present.

Wound abscess following major surgery is ordinarily relatively easy to recognize. It is therefore uncommon for the patient to appear in clinic with a previously undiagnosed wound infection. However, in obese patients or in patients with organisms of low pathogenicity, wound infections may become apparent at periods of 4 weeks to 13 years or more following surgery.

Patients with chronic draining infections should be considered as possibly having one or more of the following classic causes: unrecognized cancer, osteomyelitis, fistula proximal to a point of obstruction, retained foreign body (e.g., sponge), tuberculosis, fungus, or epithelial-lined sinus tract. Recognition of infection inevitably requires specific smears and cultures for micro-organisms. The foul odor of anaerobic infections with clostridium species can easily be recognized by a surgeon who has had a previous experience with these organisms. In every case, however, confirmation by bacterial smear and culture is important for scientific and legal reasons. The culture should be retained long enough to determine if the antibiotic selected was therapeutically effective. It is unnecessary to test bacterial sensitivity to antibiotics in each case, but the culture should not be discarded until the clinical result is known. In unusual, delayed, or recurrent infections the acid-fast stain and culture for TB is particularly important. Cultures for fungi should also be taken when an unusual infection is encountered.

Diabetes is occasionally discovered at the time of an infection. At least one urine specimen should be tested for glucose in patients who develop a wound infection, and a postprandial blood glucose should, ideally, be performed in these patients. Other predisposing causes of infection are hypertension, old age, obesity, malignancy, peripheral ischemia and diseases with inherent immuno-suppression such as leukemia, lymphoma, Hodgkin's disease, lupus erythematosus, and immunoglobulin deficiencies.[16] If the patient presents any clinical indications of multisystemic disease, further investigation is warranted.

Infections with β-hemolytic streptococcus frequently produce a diffuse red color in the skin near the wound, called "surgical scarlatina." Some strains of β-strep do not produce an erythrogenic toxin, and some patients have previously developed antibody to the toxin, so the characteristic erythema is not present in all patients. An abscess containing creamy yellow, relatively odorless pus is usually found to be due to *Staphylococcus aureus*.

TREATMENT OF INFECTION

Treatment should take into consideration the cause of the infection, the organism involved, the general health of the patient, the location and extent of the infection and the social environment of the patient.

Infections treated in the Outpatient Department should be restricted to those which do not present a serious risk of fatality or long-term morbidity. In borderline situations it is always wiser to hospitalize a patient for the first few days of treatment than to risk incurring progression of infection in the event that outpatient treatment is inadequate.

The most important immediate decisions which must be answered are: (1) is the infection fluctuant—and therefore suitable for drainage? (2) if drainage is needed, can it be performed in the Outpatient Department, or is hospitalization required? and (3) should antibiotics be given?

Incision and Drainage of Abscess ("I and D")

Experience is the best guide to the presence of fluctuance and the indication for drainage. Compression of a suspected abscess with two fingers will sometimes reveal fluctuance—a clue to the presence of infection. Aspiration of the suspected abscess with a needle will often provide a guide to the depth of the abscess as well as to the proof of its existence.

A relatively superficial abscess on the trunk or extremities can usually be drained with local anesthesia by an in-

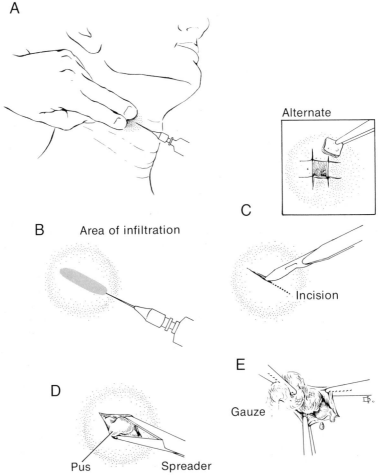

A

B Area of infiltration

Alternate

C

Incision

D

Pus Spreader

E

Gauze

Figure 4–4 Incision and drainage of abscess: A. Fluctuance detected by palpation and localized by aspiration. B. Intradermal anesthesia. C. Drainage by incision in skin lines or with cruciate incision. (A gridiron incision used to unroof carbuncle is shown in inset as an alternate incision.) D. Wound edges are spread and clamp inserted to break up loculations of pus. E. A gauze wick is inserted, packed tightly enough to control bleeding from the depths of the abscess. It should be removed on the following day and reinserted loosely, to promote drainage. A small rubber drain may also be inserted, but will usually have to be sutured in place.

cision in the direction of the natural skin lines. A cruciate incision is often necessary to obtain adequate drainage for deep abscesses and for those which are recurrent. Cruciate or gridiron incisions are usually mandatory for carbuncles, which present with multiple points of purulence, draining a mass of abscesses separated by fibrous septae.

Anesthesia

For a single incision or small cruciate incision, local anesthesia is easily given in the dermis with a 25 gauge needle. If the abscess is nearly ready to rupture, ethyl chloride spray is usually adequate. For drainage of carbuncles, a field block is usually best. General anesthesia is best for incision and drainage on the face and neck,[3] especially in children. Special techniques for infections of hand and feet are described in Chapters 13 and 22.

Packing and Irrigation

The wound should be loosely filled with $1/8''$–$1''$ wide cotton wick, which is removed gradually at 24–48 hour intervals. It should be "packed" tightly only to control bleeding. A "packed" abscess should have all wick removed in 24–48 hours, and a loose wick should then be inserted. Plain cotton or iodoform are probably equally beneficial clinically, but iodoform is generally preferred except in patients with iodine sensitivity. Irrigation of wounds with saline, 2 per cent hydrogen peroxide or hypochlorite solutions helps to break up residual abscesses and stimulates formation of granulation tissue. Irrigation is facilitated if a small rubber tube or drain has been inserted for dependent "through-and-through" drainage. Irrigation of most wounds can begin 24–48 hours after I and D. If a wick is present in the wound, irrigation is relatively ineffective. The visiting nurse, clinic nurse or doctor should first remove the wick, irrigate the wound and then re-insert a new wick, slightly looser than the previous one.

Nonsurgical Treatment

Infections frequently begin in small, superficial sites—a furuncle ("pimple") of the face, or a small paronychia on the finger, or minor folliculitis in nasal, axillary or other body hair. Topical antibacterial treatment with "Camphophenique" is often effective in arresting these small infections before they become serious. Topical antibiotic ointments containing bacitracin, polymyxin B or neomycin are somewhat more hazardous, because of the risk of drug sensitivity, but they are effective and are generally quite safe.

Incision and drainage may be deferred to an optimum time or avoided completely in some instances. Poorly localized major infections, suppurative thrombophlebitis, and phlegmon of the extremities should be treated initially by rest, heat, moisture, and elevation. Antibiotics may be added if the infection is serious, or the patient is in poor general health. The patient and the afflicted part are put at rest, with activities limited to a minimum. Thus mechanical disruption of tissue planes is avoided and micro-organisms remain localized instead of disseminated. Moist heat appears to promote localization of infection and certainly makes the patient more comfortable. An effective, safe way to obtain moist heat for an infected area on an extremity is by wrapping the area in a wet towel and inserting the wrapped, moist extremity into a plastic bag. Body heat raises the temperature within the bag to 37°+ and maintains this temperature safely. A variety of clean plastic bags are now available in grocery and drug stores. The bag should be closed with Scotch tape or adhesive tape, not a rubber band.

The infected extremity should be elevated 6 to 12 inches on soft pillows, thus promoting egress of lymph. The patient should be watched closely for lymphangitis, which is recognized as a red

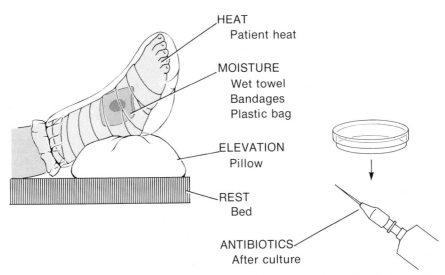

Figure 4–5 Nonsurgical treatment for infections which are not suitable for drainage. Rest, heat, moisture, elevation, and antibiotics if infection is serious. Watch for lymphangitis, which should be treated with antibiotics.

streak 3–5 mm in width along the extremity, usually overlying the major veins. Lymphangitis indicates the possible presence of β-hemolytic streptococcus and is an indication for use of systemic antibiotics.

Infection in a Sutured Laceration or Biopsy Incision

Wound infections usually require the removal of sutures and cultures, and the insertion of a loose wick or drain. If the sutures are promptly removed, these infections will produce a slightly wider scar than is obtained by primary closure. However, if effective treatment is delayed by a timorous doctor or a careless patient, serious infections may develop.

Sebaceous Cysts and Epidermal Inclusion Cysts

These may be removed intact or may be treated as an abscess. Ideally, sebaceous cysts should be removed electively in a manner similar to biopsy of a small skin tumor. However, the cysts frequently become infected or rupture; clean, complete removal then becomes impossible. If such a cyst is opened deliberately or inadvertently, the epithelial lining should be removed by curettage. The growth of granulation tissue which follows will lead to healing with only a small residual scar in most cases. Recurrence is relatively uncommon if the cavity is carefully irrigated and curetted and if healing is allowed to occur gradually by secondary intention.

Late Infection Following Major Surgery

Abdominal surgery may be followed by development of abscess in the subhepatic or subphrenic spaces, in the wound, pelvis, lesser sac, mesentery, retroperitoneal gutters, and in solid viscera such as liver and kidneys. Each type of major surgery has late septic complications, such as an infected subdural space, empyema, endocarditis and osteomyelitis. The alert surgeon will watch for unexpected tenderness, erythema, fever, pain, and leukocytosis.

He will perform appropriate studies and—most important—consider re-hospitalization and consultation. Each such infection must also be reported to the hospital's Infection Committee. A search should be made for the source by a review of the operative note, examination of reports of cultures taken in the OR, and discussion with all members of the operative team.

Specific Organisms

Staphylococcus, β-hemolytic streptococcus and *E. coli* appear to be the most common organisms recovered from infections in outpatients, in contrast to the relative predominance of Enterobacter, Klebsiella, Pseudomonas and Candida in inpatients. If systemic antibiotics are indicated, the selection of a drug should be based on antibiotic sensitivities and by current statistical studies in the clinic. Guidelines currently used for initial selection of antibiotics for outpatients are shown in Table 4–1.

A smear and culture of all infections should be carried out, since bizarre infections may occur in outpatients. The diagnosis may be missed completely unless the organism is seen on smear and proper cultures are set up. For example, black pustules may be seen in anthrax but also occur from *Aspergillus niger*. *Erysipelothrix* is an unusual infection which occurs in butchers and fish handlers. Cultures required for gonococcus must be low in oxygen and high in CO_2. Anaerobic *tissue* specimens are usually needed to detect bacteroides and clostridium species.

A brief list of infections which should be suspected under specific circumstances is shown below:

Bright red, poorly localized infection with little or no pus: Streptococcal *erysipelas* (β-streptococcus).

Abscess with creamy yellow, odorless pus: *Staphylococcus aureus*.

Immunosuppressed patients: Bacteroides (suspect if foul odor).

Tissue crepitation: *Clostridium welchi* or *septicum* (gas gangrene, foul odor) or gas-producing *E. coli.*

Periorbital suppuration in diabetic patient: Mucormycosis.

Chronic skin infections with considerable induration and inflammation but little pus: Blastomycosis (especially of scrotum); histoplasmosis, actinomycosis.

Relatively painless infections of fingers and toes: secondary pyogenic sepsis in patients with neuropathy due to diabetes or leprosy.

Chronic suppuration with little or no erythema, fever and tenderness in submaxillary or supraclavicular areas: Tuberculosis.

Chronic parotid abscess: Actinomycosis.

Painless ulceration of lips, external genitalia or perianal area: Syphilis (chancre).

Chronic paronychia: Atypical mycobacterium (tropical fish fancier), or fungus.

Reddish-purple subacute infection *Erysipelothrix rhusiopathiae.* Especially common on hands of humans who work with fish, swine and cattle. Microaerophilic gram positive rod.

Recurrent boils: Penicillinase-producing *Staphylococcus aureus*; if alpha-strep, consider SBE; also consider self-induced infections, especially in hospital personnel.

Purulent discharge or abscess in any site in a sexual deviate: Gonococcus.

Axillary or groin abscess: Cat-scratch fever, bubonic plague, lymphoma.

Chronic fever and weight loss associated with formation of small abscesses: Tularemia, brucellosis.

Drug addicts with severe fever and local abscesses at injection sites: Malaria, tetanus and staphylococcal endocarditis.

Each community and state has specific requirements for reporting infections, but in general a call to the county health department is wise regarding any bizarre infection.

TABLE 4–1   SUGGESTED THERAPY OF MICRO-ORGANISMS ENCOUNTERED
IN OUTPATIENT DEPARTMENTS

GRAM POSITIVE COCCI
  Staphylococci
    Penicillin-sensitive   Penicillin; erythromycin
    Penicillin-resistant   Cloxacillin, dicloxacillin or oxacillin; cephalothin;
                                                   erythromycin

  Streptococci
    Pyogenes-Group A (β-hemolytic)   Penicillin; erythromycin; sulfa
    Enterococci (α-hemolytic)   Penicillin + streptomycin; ampicillin; erythromycin
    Anaerobic and microaerophilic   Penicillin; Chloramphenicol; bacitracin; zinc
                                                   peroxide (Meleney)
  Pneumococci   Penicillin; erythromycin

GRAM NEGATIVE COCCI
  Neisseria
    Meningitides (aerobe)   Actual infection treated in hospital (penicillin
                                                   20×10^6 units per day $\times$ 7 days)*
    Gonorrhea (intracellular; fastidious need for Penicillin; tetracycline
    low oxygen, 2–10% CO_2, temp. 30–38.5° C)

GRAM NEGATIVE RODS**
  Hemophilus
    Influenzae   Ampicillin; chloramphenicol
    Ducreyi (chancroid)   Sulfa; streptomycin

  Corynebacterium
    Diphtheriae   Prevention is done in OPD with DPT series.
                                                   Infection is treated in hospital with antitoxin and
                                                   penicillin.
    "Diphtheroids"   Usually saphrophytes—no antibiotic treatment
                                                   needed unless septicemia develops

  Enterobacteriaceae (aerobic)
    E. coli   Ampicillin, sulfa or tetracycline; kanamycin
    Klebsiella   Kanamycin; gentamicin
    Aerobacter   Kanamycin; gentamicin
    Salmonella   Ampicillin; chloramphenicol
    Shigella   Ampicillin; chloramphenicol
    Serratia   Kanamycin; gentamicin
    Proteus   Kanamycin; gentamicin
    Alkaligenes   Test for sensitivity
    Herella   Kanamycin

  Pseudomonas (aerobic)   Gentamicin; colistin (For topical use: Polymyxin
                                                     B or Furacin)

  Brucella   Hospitalize for streptomycin and tetracycline

  Pasteurella
    Pestis—plague (aerobe, but also a facultative Hospitalize for chloramphenicol, tetracycline or
      anaerobe)   streptomycin
    Tularensis (aerobe)   Hospitalize for tetracycline or streptomycin

  Bacteroides (anaerobe or microaerophilic)   Tetracycline for moderate infections;
                                                     chloramphenicol or clindamycin (Cleocin) for
                                                     severe infections (Pearson)

  Streptobacillus moniliformis (facultative anaerobe)   Hospitalize and treat with penicillin

GRAM POSITIVE RODS
  Bacillus anthrax (aerobe; spores)   Hospitalize for penicillin or chloramphenicol

  Clostridium (anaerobic; spores)
    Tetanus   Prevent with tetanus toxoid or antiserum,
                                                   débridement and penicillin; treat infection in
                                                   hospital

TABLE 4–1 *Continued.* SUGGESTED THERAPY OF MICRO-ORGANISMS ENCOUNTERED IN OUTPATIENT DEPARTMENTS

Gas gangrene (perfringens, welchii, and so on)	Prevent with débridement. Treat infection in hospital with débridement and penicillin.
Botulism	Prevent with proper food preparation. Treat in hospital with tracheostomy, antitoxin and respiratory support.
Mycobacterium	
Tuberculosis (obligate aerobes, no spores)	Prevent with BCG, INH. Treat infection initially in hospital with INH, streptomycin and Ethambutol
Leprae (no synthetic medium for cultivation)	Treat with sulfones, PAS or Geigy B663 (Hill)
Actinomycetales	
Actinomycosis (anaerobe)	Penicillin G or V
Nocardosis (aerobe)	Sulfa
Listeria monocytogenes (aerobe but also a facultative anaerobe)	Penicillin; tetracycline
Erysipelothrix insidiosa (microaerophilic)	Penicillin; sulfa; chloramphenicol
SPIROCHETES	
T. pallidum (syphilis)	Penicillin; tetracycline
Yaws, bejel and pinta	Penicillin
Borrelia (relapsing fever)	Penicillin; tetracycline
Fusospirochetal disease (Vincent's angina- mixed oral infections with spirochetes and gram negative rods)	Penicillin

*Most strains are now sulfa-resistant, so families and personnel should receive high-dose, inpatient penicillin if significantly exposed, and no treatment if exposure is minimal.

**Treatment should be based on antibiotic sensitivities *in vitro.* Drugs listed are those which commonly are used or recommended at the University of Colorado Medical Center.

CHEMOTHERAPY

Antibiotics and Other Antibacterial Agents

Antibiotics are indicated for prophylaxis in cases with heavy potential contamination, or in which infection would be devastating to a repair.[7] In general, antibacterial chemotherapy should be reserved for treatment of specific, established infections, rather than in prophylaxis of infection. The use of antibiotics should be taken advisedly, considering the possibility of drug reaction. The patient and his family should be told the nature of possible drug reactions, so that therapy may be changed immediately if a reaction is noted. The antibiotics most widely used in prophylaxis of wound infections are the penicillins and tetracycline.

Penicillin

The natural and semisynthetic penicillins are bacteriostatic and bactericidal for multiplying bacteria at low concentrations. The penicillins act by inhibition of cell wall synthesis in bacteria. Relatively high concentrations of penicillin are well tolerated in most individuals. The major problems observed are the emergence of drug-resistant strains of bacteria—especially penicillinase-producing staphylococci—and drug sensitivity. A prior history of allergy to penicillin is, in general, a contraindication to the use of any of the penicillins in outpatient therapy.

1. *Penicillin G.* Useful against a wide variety of gram positive organisms, Neisseria and spirochetes. Many streptococci and staphylococci and all pneumococci, actinomyces, clostridia, and treponema are sensitive to penicillin. Resistance has appeared in staphylo-

cocci, many strains of which produce penicillinase, and in increasing numbers of gonococci. Emergence of resistance to penicillin G has not yet become a serious problem with other previously sensitive organisms. Because it is poorly absorbed by mouth, penicillin G is usually administered intramuscularly as procaine penicillin G in a dose of 1,200,000 units daily to outpatients, or as Benzathine penicillin G 1,200,000 units once a week. Adequate blood levels are difficult to maintain on an outpatient basis except for organisms highly susceptible to penicillin. A syndrome similar to serum sickness is a rare but serious side effect of penicillin therapy.

2. *Penicillin V.* Has a spectrum of activity and resistance similar to that of penicillin G. It is well absorbed by mouth and causes little gastrointestinal toxicity. For outpatient therapy of sensitive organisms, one week of therapy is generally advisable with 250–500 mg p.o. four times daily. It should be given on an empty stomach since food interferes with its absorption. Increasing numbers of relapses of gonorrhea following a course of penicillin have been observed during the past few years. Diligent follow-up information is therefore required to demonstrate cure in these patients. Long-term therapy is needed for actinomycosis, but outpatient therapy of this condition can be effective as long as the necessary surgical therapy has also been performed.

3. *Ampicillin (Penbritin, Polycillin).* A broad-spectrum penicillin with activity against gram positive cocci, and also against gram negative bacteria such as salmonella, shigella, *E. coli*, proteus, *H. influenzae* and *N. gonorrheae*. It is useful in the treatment of infections of the urinary tract, ear, nose, throat and lower respiratory tract, for typhoid carriers and other gastrointestinal infections. It should not be used in outpatient therapy of patients with a prior history of allergy to penicillin. It is not resistant to penicillinase and should not be used for staphylococci resistant to penicillin

G. Although ampicillin may be started empirically, a culture and sensitivity is indicated to guide further therapy. Ampicillin is available in oral and parenteral forms. The usual outpatient adult dose is 250–500 mg p.o. four times daily for one to two weeks. Superinfections with pseudomonas, Enterobacter or fungi may emerge during ampicillin treatment.

4. *Cloxacillin (Tegopen).* This, along with dicloxacillin (Dynapen) and oxacillin (Prostaphlin), is an oral semi-synthetic penicillin which is especially useful in the outpatient treatment of penicillinase-producing staphylococci. Methicillin and nafcillin are related drugs which must be given parenterally to achieve satisfactory blood levels, and they are therefore rarely used in outpatient therapy. Cloxacillin is well absorbed and well tolerated by mouth. It has a good spectrum of activity against pneumococci and streptococci. It is not the best drug for these organisms — penicillin G or V would be preferable. Cloxacillin is indicated as the initial drug in staphylococcal infections, especially if the infection was acquired in the hospital. Fortunately, most strains of staphylococci in the U. S. are still sensitive to Cloxacillin and the other semi-synthetic, penicillinase-resistant penicillins. The usual treatment is 250–500 mg four times daily for seven to ten days.

5. *Carbenicillin (Geopen).* A benzyl penicillin derivative which has recently been released for use. It is particularly useful in treatment of gram negative bacilli, especially pseudomonas, proteus and some of the rare organisms such as Herella and Serratia. Pseudomonas frequently develops resistance rapidly, and Klebsiella is usually resistant. Like the other penicillins, it is relatively free of renal toxicity, though blood levels increase rapidly in the presence of poor renal function. It must be administered parenterally, a feature which limits its use in outpatients. Carbenicillin is also effective against gram positive cocci, but it is not resistant to penicillinase. Paren-

teral outpatient therapy utilizes 1–2 gm IM every six hours. It is mainly used for urinary tract infections in this dose.

Cephalothin

Cephalothin (Keflin, Keflex) and cephaloridine (Loridine) are broad spectrum antibiotics structurally related to penicillin, derived from cephalosporin C. These antibiotics are produced by the fungus *Cephalosporium*. Although these agents are powerful bacteriostatic and bacteriocidal drugs, they are rarely used in outpatient therapy. The multiple daily doses of the parenteral forms required are usually not practical for outpatients. The oral form (Keflex) has recently become available, and—when used in large doses—it has reportedly been useful in treatment of respiratory and urinary tract infections. Patients with penicillin allergies should receive these drugs with caution, because of crossover allergy due to a structural similarity to penicillin. Nevertheless, a history of penicillin allergy is currently a major indication for the use of cephalosporin derivatives in inpatients at the UCMC. Pseudomonas is notably resistant to cephalosporin derivatives and super-infection with pseudomonas is common in patients treated with cephalosporins. Troublesome proteus or *E. coli* urinary tract infections may be treated with the cephalosporins in cooperative out-patients if sensitivity studies indicate that the organisms are sensitive.

Tetracycline, Chloramphenicol and Erythromycin

These are potent antibacterial agents which act by inhibition of protein synthesis.

1. Tetracycline. Tetracycline (Achromycin, Sumycin) and the tetracycline derivatives are bacteriostatic antibiotics which are mainly useful in treatment of gram negative infections. Minor infections with gram positive cocci may also occasionally respond to these antibiotics. Tetracycline is relatively less dangerous for short-term outpatient therapy than other broad spectrum antibiotics. It is particularly useful for treatment of bacterial infections of the biliary, respiratory or urinary tracts. It is also used in treatment of syphilis in patients who are allergic to penicillin. Chronic or intensive therapy has been associated with many problems, including staphylococcal enterocolitis, hepatic failure, deposition of tetracycline in bones and teeth, and abnormalities of skin, kidneys and blood. The most common problem is, however, nausea or diarrhea from mild gastrointestinal toxicity, which subsides when therapy is discontinued. The usual treatment is 250–500 mg four times daily for seven to ten days. It should be emphasized that tetracycline resistance is common in staphylococci and emerges rapidly during treatment.

2. Chloramphenicol (Chloromycetin). This drug is highly effective in the treatment of a broad spectrum of gram negative infections, but hematologic toxicity generally precludes its use in outpatient surgical infections. Hematologic toxicity may occur as an idiosyncratic fatal aplasia, but fortunately this is rare. It is more common to see a dose-related and time-related leukopenia occur gradually, subsiding when treatment is stopped. If chloramphenicol is believed to be indicated because of *in vitro* and *in vivo* studies, the manufacturer's brochure should be studied carefully and blood counts monitored frequently during therapy.

3. Erythromycin (Erythrocin, Ilotycin). This is a broad spectrum macrolide-type of antibiotic which is active against multiplying bacteria. Macrolides are complex chemicals containing a lactone ring, a deoxyamino sugar with a dimethyl amino group, and an unsaturated α, β ketone. These antibiotics are utilized in the form of esters. Erythromycin is bacteriostatic at low concentrations and bactericidal at high concentrations. It is relatively ineffective against gram negative infections, except *C. diphtheriae*, but is a very useful alternative to penicillin in many infections with gram positive cocci. It is well absorbed and well tolerated by mouth. Troublesome side reactions are very rare and ordinarily all side effects disappear when therapy is discontinued. Erythromycin is particularly useful in treatment of β-streptococcal infections, and for other penicillin-sensitive bacteria in patients who are allergic to penicillin. It is used in doses of 250–500 mg p.o. four times per day.

Streptomycin

Streptomycin is an antibiotic produced by *Streptomyces griseus*. It is useful against a broad spectrum of organisms not affected by penicillin. It is bactericidal by its effects on the cell wall, on nucleic acid formation and on protein synthesis. It is effective against salmonella, Klebsiella and many other gram negative organisms, but resistance may appear within 24 hours. The rapid emergence of resistant populations and toxicity for the eighth cranial (auditory) nerve have been major problems limiting the usefulness of streptomycin. The discovery of other broad spectrum antibiotics has essentially reduced the use of streptomycin to short courses in combination with penicillin G in mixed infections caused by unknown organisms, and in tuberculosis. It is given in doses of 0.5–1.0 mg IM daily with careful sequential studies of auditory and vestibular nerve function. The usual course for nontubercular infections is five days.

Kanamycin

Kanamycin (Kantrex) is a streptomyces-derived antibiotic with activity against a very broad spectrum of bacteria, including gram positive and gram negative cocci, and many gram negative rods. Most strains of enterobacter and *E. coli* and most strains of proteus are sensitive to kanamycin. It is also effective against salmonella, shigella and *E. histolytica*. Systemic therapy requires parenteral administration, and it is therefore difficult to use kanamycin in outpatients. It also produces renal and

eighth nerve toxicity, so careful monitoring is required. Oral therapy is used for preoperative sterilization of the bowel and treatment of sensitive gastrointestinal infections, since kanamycin is not absorbed from the GI tract. Clostridium, bacteroides and yeast overgrowth may occur and should be watched for in patients receiving kanamycin by mouth. Parenteral therapy may be given with doses of 0.5 gm IM each 12 hours and should be limited to five days. Oral therapy for preoperative bowel preparation is given with 1.0 gm per hour for four hours, followed by 1.0 gm every six hours for 36–72 hours. This method of outpatient bowel preparation has become the method most frequently used at the author's hospital.

Neomycin

Neomycin is an aminoglycoside antibiotic obtained from *Streptomyces fradiae*. It is bactericidal against a wide variety of gram positive and gram negative bacteria, including Proteus. It is useful as an oral, nonabsorbable antibiotic for preoperative preparation of the colon, and for other conditions requiring suppression of intestinal bacteria. It is also used in topical ointments and solutions for treatment of localized, accessible infections. Side effects occurring after oral administration include mild diarrhea, yeast or staphylococcal overgrowth, and renal toxicity if ulcerative lesions permitting absorption into the blood stream are present. It is a potent intestinal antiseptic, and should not be used for more than 36 hours. If symptoms suggesting enterocolitis appear, the patient should be hospitalized promptly. If staphylococcal enterocolitis is demonstrated, treatment may require methicillin and restoration of normal flora with oral lactobacillus (Lactinex) or fecal enemas. Neomycin is used by mouth in doses of 1.0 gm per hour for four hours, then 1.0 gm every four hours for 24–36 hours. Topical neomycin is available in ointments, alone and in combination with polymyxin B and bacitracin (Neosporin).

Colistin

Colistin (Coly-mycin) is a polypeptide antibiotic which is bactericidal by absorption into specific receptor sites in gram negative organisms. It also prevents chromosomal recombination. Since its mechanism of action is different from other antibiotics, its spectrum of action is also different. It is uniquely effective against *Pseudomonas aeruginosa*, and is also effective against a wide variety of other gram negative bacilli. Unfortunately, it is not absorbed from the GI tract, and requires parenteral therapy (2.5 mg per kg per day in two to four divided doses, deep IM). Neurotoxicity should be watched for, but outpatient therapy is possible. The patient should receive one dose daily in the clinic and his subsequent doses can be given at home from a trained member of his family or from a visiting nurse.

Polymyxin B

Polymyxin B (Aerosporin) is a bactericidal antibiotic derived from *B. polymyxa*. It is effective against most of the troublesome gram negative bacilli, except Proteus. It can be used effectively against Pseudomonas, Klebsiella, Aerobacter and *E. coli*, but systemic use or absorption may produce significant renal toxicity. It must be given parenterally in systemic therapy, and frequent checks of renal function are required during therapy. Polymyxin B is a useful and relatively safe topical antibiotic used in treatment of accessible localized infections. It is available in combination with bacitracin (Polysporin) and bacitracin and neomycin (Neosporin).

Gentamicin

Gentamicin (Garamycin) is an amino glycoside antibiotic with a broad spectrum of activity against gram negative and gram positive organisms. Cross-resistance is rare. It has drawbacks similar to the other parenteral antibiotics, and is used infrequently in outpatient therapy.[13]

Bacitracin

Bacitracin is a bactericidal polypeptide antibiotic derived from *B. subtilis*. It is highly effective against gram positive organisms, but because of renal toxicity its use is restricted to topical chemotherapy, usually in ointments, in combination with polymyxin B (Polysporin) and polymyxin B and neomycin (Neosporin).

Amphotericin B

Amphotericin B (Fungizone) is a potent polyene antifungal antibiotic derived from a streptomyces species. It is supplied as a solubilized desoxycholate salt, and may be applied topically, administered by mouth, or—for systemic administration—given parenterally. It has significant renal toxicity[2,12] and is usually administered intravenously only to inpatients. However, long-term therapy may be performed intermittently in the Outpatient Clinic for diseases such as meningitis or draining abscesses due to coccidioidomycosis, blastomycosis, cryptococcosis and other systemic fungi. Amphotericin B can also be instilled into spinal fluid or bladder for localized fungal infections.

Mycostatin

Mycostatin (Nystatin) is a nonabsorbable antifungal agent used predominantly in treatment of oral and intestinal candidiasis.

Sulfa Drugs

Sulfisoxazole (Gantrisin) is one of several derivatives of sulfanilamide which are useful in systemic antibacterial therapy. The "sulfa" compounds act by competitive inhibition with the essential metabolite p-amino benzoic acid, which is necessary for synthesis of folic (pteroyl glutamic) acid. Folic acid is a co-enzyme required in synthesis of many nucleic and amino acids. Sulfisoxazole is useful in outpatient treatment of Group A β-hemolytic streptococcus, *E. coli*, Nocardia and lymphogranuloma venereum infections. It is rarely used in acute streptococcal infections because penicillin is more potent, but it is useful in chronic suppression of recurrent streptococcal infections. It is also useful in suppression of chronic urinary tract infections. The effectiveness of sulfisoxazole may be more apparent clinically than *in vitro*. It is well tolerated, inexpensive and relatively potent in acute urinary tract infections such as cystitis[8] and prostatitis. In these cases, symptomatic relief can be accelerated with phenazopyridine (Pyridium), a topical mucosal analgesic excreted through the urinary tract. Phenazopyridine is given by mouth in tablets of 200 mg three times daily. Sulfisoxazole is effective in long-term therapy with 500 mg four times daily, although acute infections should be treated with twice this dose for the first few days.

Sulfathalidine and *Sulfasuxidine* are nonabsorbable sulfadiazine derivatives used for intestinal antisepsis, especially in preparation for surgery of the colon. They appear to be less effective but are also less dangerous than kanamycin and neomycin. *Azulfidine* is a well-tolerated nonabsorbable sulfa derivative which is commonly used in chronic therapy of ulcerative colitis.

Nitrofurans

Nitrofurans are synthetic antimicrobial compounds which interfere with anaerobic and aerobic carbohydrate metabolism in bacterial cells. A broad spectrum of activity is seen, and resistance rarely appears. Topical nitrofurazone (Furacin) is a highly effective antibacterial agent, useful in secondarily infected excoriations and burns. Most patients tolerate it well, though approximately 1 per cent develop atopic allergic reactions. Nitrofurantoin (Macrodantin, Furadantin) is excreted rapidly in the urine and is a highly effective antibacterial agent for many gram negative bacillary infections. Its use is limited partially by nausea, and it is also considerably more expensive than sulfisoxazole. The adult dose is 50–100 mg four times daily. The drug is satisfactorily absorbed and better tolerated when given with milk. Furazolidone (Furoxone) is used in treatment of a variety of gastrointestinal infections, including giardiasis. The nitrofurans may cause anemia in patients with glucose 6-phosphate dehydrogenase deficiency, so Negros and patients of Eastern Mediterranean ancestry should be observed closely for hemolytic reactions. Mono-amine oxidase inhibition has also been reported in association with furazolidone, so sympathomimetic amines and tyramine-containing foods should not be given in conjunction with this drug. Chronic pulmonary fibrosis has been demonstrated in some patients treated with nitrofurantoin.

Metronidazole

Metronidazole (Flagyl) is a potent systemic trichomonacide, effective against these organisms in the vagina, in extravaginal sites and in the genitourinary tract. It is given by mouth in doses of 250 mg two to three times daily. Metronidazole has also recently been described as an effective agent in amebic abscesses due to *E. histolytica*. The manufacturer does not support this use of the drug at present, but reports from the field indicate that it is safer and more effective than emetine. It is currently being used in doses of 1–2 gm per day for seven to ten days as an amebicide.

Combinations

Combinations of antibiotics, or antibiotics and antibacterial agents may occasionally be selected injudiciously, producing antagonism instead of additive or synergistic benefits. In general, if infections appear to be resistant to therapy with single agents, consultation with a specialist in infectious diseases is recommended before beginning therapy with combinations.

Summary

Smear and culture of a purulent discharge or body fluid may provide the first clue to diagnosis, giving a rational basis for therapy. Follow-up should be diligent until convalescence is progressing smoothly, and the culture report confirms the initial impression. All patients placed on antibiotics must be seen regularly during the course of their therapy, since serious drug reactions may develop and relapses may occur when antibiotics are discontinued prematurely.

In general, the surgeon must be particularly diligent when any form of treatment of an abscess other than I and D is used. If the organism is unusual or the infection is not well localized, careful thought is needed to avoid overlooking a disease which requires more attention than can be given in a surgical outpatient clinic.

References

1. Brachman, P. D. (ed.): *Isolation Techniques for Use in Hospitals*. U.S. Public Health Service Publication No. 2054. Washington, D.C.: U.S. Government Printing Office, 1970.
2. Butler, W. T., Bennett, J. E., Alling, D. W., Wertlake, P. T., Utz, J. P., and Hill, G. J., II: Nephrotoxicity of amphotericin B. Early and late effects in 81 patients. *Ann Intern Med, 61*:175–187, 1964.
3. Crystal, D. K., Day, S. W., Wagner, C. L., and Kranz, J. M.: Emergency treatment in Ludwig's angina. *Surg Gynecol Obstet, 129*:755–757, 1969.
4. Dineen, P.: The exchange of skin bacteria between patients and hospital personnel. *Surg Gynecol Obstet, 125*:979–982, 1967.
5. Diphtheria and tetanus toxoids and pertussis vaccine. *Morb Mortal Wkly Rep.* 396–397, October, 1971.
6. Dobson, T., and Shulls, W. A.: A study of various surgical scrubs by glove counts. *Surg Gynecol Obstet, 124*:57–60, 1967.
7. Eaton, R. G., and Butsch, D. P.: Antibiotic guidelines for hand infection. *Surg Gynecol Obstet, 130*:119–122, 1970.
8. Gillespie, W. A., Lee, P. A., Linton, K. B., and Rowland, A. J.: Antibiotic resistance of coliform bacilli in urinary infection acquired by women outside hospital: A 12-year survey. *Lancet, 2*:675–677, September, 1971.
9. A guide to prophylaxis against tetanus in wound management. *Bull Am Coll Surg, 56*:22–23, June, 1971.
10. Hard, D., Postlethwait, R. W., Brown, I. W. Jr., Smith, W. W., and Johnson, P. A.: Postoperative wound infections: A further report on ultraviolet irradiation with comments on the recent (1964) National Research Council Cooperative Study Report. *Ann Surg, 167*:728–743, 1968.
11. Hill, G. J., II.: *Leprosy in Five Young Men*. Boulder: Colorado Associated University Press, 1970.
12. Hill, G. J., II, Butler, W. J., Wertlake, P. T., and Utz, J. P.: The renal histopathology in amphotericin B toxicity in man and the dog: A study of biopsy and postmortem specimens. *Clin Res, 10*:249, 1962.
13. Kessner, D. M., and Lepper, M. H.: Epidemiologic studies of gram-negative bacilli in the hospital and community. *Am J Epidemiol, 85*:45–60, 1967.
14. Kippax, P. W., and Thomas, E. T.: Surgical wound sepsis in a general hospital. *Lancet, 2*:1297–1300, 10 December, 1966.
15. Louria, D. B., Pool, J. L., Blevins, A., and Armstrong, D.: The treatment of infections in patients with neoplasia undergoing surgery. *Med Clin North Am, 50*(3):791–802, 1966.
16. May, J., Chalmers, J. P., Loewenthal, J., and Rountree, P. M.: Factors in the patient contributing to surgical sepsis. *Surg Gynecol Obstet, 122*:28–32, 1966.
17. Meleney, F. L.: Shambaugh, P., and Millen, R. S.: Systemic bacitracin in the treatment of progressive bacterial synergistic gangrene. *Ann Surg, 131*:129–144, 1950.
18. Pearson, H. E., and Harvey, J. P.: Bacteroides infections in orthopedic conditions. *Surg Gynecol Obstet, 132*:876–880, 1971.
19. Robles, N. L., Walske, B. R., and Tella, A. R.: Tetanus prophylaxis and therapy. *Surg Clin North Am, 48*:799–806, 1968.
20. Postoperative wound infections: The influence of ultraviolet irradiation of the operating room and of various other factors. *Ann Surg, 160*: Suppl. 1:1–192, August, 1964.
21. Thoburn, R., Fekety, F. R. Jr., Cluff, L. E., and Melvin, V. B.: Infections acquired by hospitalized patients. *Arch Intern Med, 121*:1–10, 1968.
22. Todd, J. C.: Wound infection: Etiology, prevention, and management, including selection of antibiotics. *Surg Clin North Am, 48*(4):787–798, 1968.
23. Walter, C. W.: *The Aseptic Treatment of Wounds*. New York: Macmillan, 1948.
24. *World Health Organization. Technical Report Series, 321.* Expert Committee on Rabies, 5th Report, 1966.

5

Tumors

By ERICK R. RATZER, M.D.

INTRODUCTION

The initial management of patients with tumors will be covered in this chapter, as well as several areas of special concern. This chapter will specifically deal with tumors of the skin, oral cavity, and soft somatic tissues, plus the work-up of a patient presenting with a neck mass, and the indications and technique of cervical esophagostomy. Various aspects of outpatient tumor surgery will also be presented in other chapters.

The characteristics of a good history, physical examination and proper interpretation of laboratory studies will be described, all of which provide strong clues regarding the diagnosis. The most important single step in outpatient tumor surgery is biopsy, and this chapter will discuss the steps which lead to this maneuver. Once the definitive histologic diagnosis is made, it is possible for the responsible practitioner to make recommendations for further treatment.

The subject of cancer is discussed in more detail in the valuable texts prepared by Ackerman, Dargeon, Martin, Moore, Nealon and Pack (see chapter references).

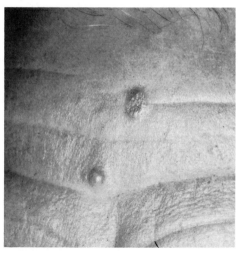

Figure 5-1 Example of lesion suitable for excisional biopsy in the Outpatient Department: basal cell carcinoma of forehead.

BIOPSY

Indications

Definitive Treatment

There are clinical situations when a histological diagnosis is not mandatory in order to proceed with definitive therapy. An example is a lesion of the skin of the cheek which can be excised and closed primarily without leaving a significant cosmetic defect (Fig. 5-1). Occasionally, histological examination may dictate further treatment, as — for example — when the lesion is a melanoma. But if the lesion is benign or an adequately excised cancer, no further treatment is necessary.

Diagnosis

A lesion large enough to require cosmetic reconstruction after excision presents another problem (Fig. 5-2). In

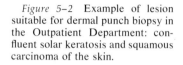

Figure 5-2 Example of lesion suitable for dermal punch biopsy in the Outpatient Department: confluent solar keratosis and squamous carcinoma of the skin.

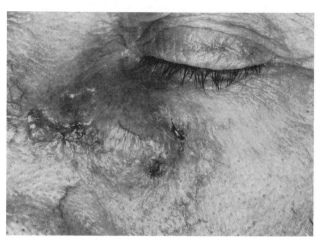

order to properly advise the patient, a histologic diagnosis obtained with a small dermal punch is frequently helpful. While there is a theoretical objection to spreading cancer with an incisional biopsy, this threat has probably been exaggerated in regard to patients with curable tumors.

Pre-Biopsy Record of Information

It is impossible to illustrate biopsy techniques in a manner that will apply to every clinical condition. However, guidelines applicable in most situations are suggested here and modifications can be made as needed.

Medical record keeping seems to be an enigma to most physicians and as a result, much of it is done poorly. Accurate information is often important in making management decisions on patients, and better records may make these decisions easier.

The first step in a biopsy is the accurate recording of a description of the lesion in the chart. The exact size, consistency, color, mobility and sensitivity are described. In some tumors, the auscultatory findings may also be important. The use of drawings or anatomical stamps with the lesion diagrammed is enthusiastically endorsed (Fig. 5–3 *A* and *B*).

Types of Biopsy

There are several types of biopsies; the particular clinical setting usually determines the selected type:

1. Incisional
2. Excisional
3. Punch (incisional or excisional)
4. Needle (tissue or aspiration)
5. Curettage
6. Scraping of surface lesion⎤for
7. Fluid aspiration ⎦cytology

Incisional Biopsy. An incisional biopsy (Fig. 5–4) is the removal of part of a lesion for histologic examination, leaving the remainder to be controlled by definitive therapy. Whenever possi-

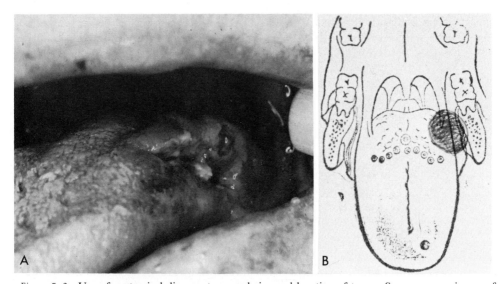

Figure 5–3 Use of anatomical diagram to record size and location of tumor. Squamous carcinoma of the tongue (*A*), Stage T_1; N_0; M_0 (*B*). Biopsy performed in OPD. Patient refused definitive surgery; he received Co^{60} therapy, but induration persisted, and neck node developed. He underwent resection ("Commando") and is now free of tumor five years later.

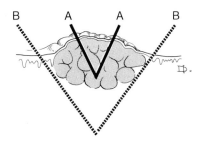

Figure 5-4 Incisional (*A*) and excisional (*B*) biopsy.

ble, a section of normal tissue adjacent to the tumor should be included in the specimen. A cup biopsy forceps can also be used for incisional biopsy (Fig. 5–5).

There is a possible objection to incisional biopsy in a potentially curable tumor because of the theoretical chance of spreading tumor by the biopsy. Although this objection may be valid, the value of an exact diagnosis when planning definitive treatment is a significant benefit which outweighs the danger of spreading tumor cells. If danger of spreading the cancer exists at all, the degree to which it is present probably parallels the ability of the cells to spread in the absence of external trauma. This

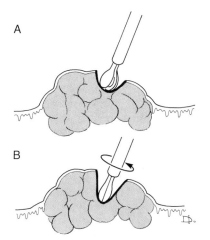

Figure 5-5 Cup biopsy forceps used for incisional biopsy.

danger is minimal if definitive care is carried out within a week or two of the biopsy.

Excisional Biopsy. An excisional biopsy (Fig. 5–4) is the complete removal of the lesion for a histologic diagnosis. This type of biopsy provides the advantage of definitive one-stage treatment in many instances while the diagnosis is being made. Complete excision of benign tumors or, in many cases, complete excision of malignant tumors is all that is necessary. Except for removal of sutures, one procedure does the job.

Punch Biopsy. This has advantages for both the patient and the physician. It is a simple technique to master and requires minimal anesthesia, equipment, and post-biopsy care. However, it does require a pathologist who has enough experience and is willing to make a diagnosis from a small segment of tissue.

Needle Biopsy. There are two types of needle biopsy: with the Vim Silverman technique a core of tissue is actually removed (Fig. 5–6), and the other technique is an aspiration biopsy, in which cells are sucked into the syringe. When a core of tissue is obtained it is submitted for fixation and staining as are other excisional biopsies. Aspiration specimens are stained and examined for cytology in a manner similar to the cervical "pap smear."

Curettage Biopsies. These are infrequently used in the general surgery outpatient area, but are applicable more often in gynecologic and orthopedic procedures.

Scrapings. Scrapings from surface lesions can be used to make a diagnosis, but the cooperation of the pathologist is very important when this method is utilized, since the diagnosis is usually based on cytology.

Fluid. The needle aspiration of fluid for cytologic examination is used most frequently in patients with ascites and effusions in the pleural and pericardial spaces. The use of aspiration in the proper clinical situations can make the diagnosis of metastatic cancer easier, perhaps saving the patient from a major

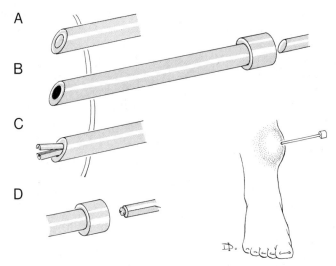

Figure 5–6   Vim Silverman needle biopsy technique. *A*. Skin is punctured with a No. 11 blade and needle is inserted with obturator in place. *B*. Obturator is removed. *C*. Biopsy forceps introduced through the hollow needle. *D*. Needle advanced to tip of forceps, shearing off the entrapped tissue. Forceps, containing a core of tissue, are then removed.

surgical procedure to diagnose an incurable malignancy.

Anesthesia

Prior to inducing anesthesia, the area designated for biopsy and its immediate surroundings are washed thoroughly for two to three minutes with soap and warm water. After drying, the area is washed again with G.S.I. solution.

Most biopsies can be performed under local anesthesia. Topical sprays can occasionally be used, but the best anesthesia is achieved with local injection; (my preference is 1 per cent lidocaine without epinephrine). Between 5 and 10 ml will be sufficient for most procedures. A 25 gauge needle is used to raise a skin wheal next to the biopsy site, followed by infiltration of the entire area using a 20 or 22 gauge needle.

Draping should expose the site to be operated upon, but should cover the surrounding area. The most versatile drape for local excisions is a sterile circumcision sheet.

Preservation of the Specimen

Once the specimen has been obtained, it must be properly preserved in order to present it to the pathologist in optimum condition. Solid segments of tissue should be placed in 10 per cent formalin for fixation. No specimen should be allowed to dry out, nor should it be crushed. Specimens for cytologic examination are air-dried and then immediately placed in 95 per cent alcohol.

The importance of proper labeling of all specimens must be stressed. This responsibility belongs to the surgeon and no one else. The transportation to the pathologist of the properly labeled specimen in the correct solution is usually done by the outpatient administrative staff. However, a wise surgeon may wish to carry the specimen to the pathologist personally.

As a general rule, frozen section diagnosis of outpatient biopsies is not performed. However, a frozen section insures that a diagnosis will be made on the tissue submitted, allowing further biopsies to be performed, if necessary, without requiring a second anesthesia. Quick knowledge of the diagnosis also expedites treatment decisions.

After completing the procedure and sending the properly labeled specimen to the Pathology Department one more record-keeping task remains to complete the job: the operative note. Some institutions require these to be dictated, but most hospitals specify that the surgeon enter it directly on the chart. This information is very important and should be accurate and complete. When several physicians rotate through Tumor Clinics, accurate records assume even greater importance. A complete operative note should contain:

Date and time of operation
Preoperative diagnosis
Postoperative diagnosis
Operation, including gross estimate
   of margin
Surgeon's name
Anesthesia used
Estimated blood loss
Drains
Postoperative condition

It is also a good idea to indicate the follow-up plans for the patient.

SKIN

Both benign and malignant lesions of the skin and its appendages have common clinical presentations and are approached similarly. These lesions include tumors of hair follicles, sweat glands, and apocrine glands. Therefore, although many histologic types of skin tumors are encountered in a variety of anatomic settings, guidelines can be set down to cover almost all of the problems which are presented to the outpatient surgeon.

The most common areas of the skin that require biopsy examination are on the head, neck and hands. The upper extremities, the trunk and the lower extremities are operated upon less frequently.

The epidermis, dermis (including its nerves, arteries, veins), hair follicles, apocrine glands, and sweat glands give rise to all the benign and malignant tumors encountered in the skin, except for metastatic deposits, which will be dealt with separately (see Chapter 25). None of the benign tumors and almost none of the malignant tumors require more than adequate local excision for treatment. The exceptions to this general rule are malignant melanomas and the rare malignant tumors associated with palpable regional lymph nodes.

Squamous cell carcinomas are more apt to metastasize to regional lymph nodes than basal cell carcinomas, but this is relatively rare, except in the case of carcinoma of the lip. It may not be proper to include lip lesions with other skin lesions, since their behavior is often different.

Presenting Complaints

The two most common presenting complaints of skin lesions are "a growth," or a "sore" (ulceration). Warts, nevi, keratoses, squamous cell carcinomas, basal cell carcinomas, hemangiomas, fibromas and so forth usually present as "abnormal growths." Carcinomas and keratoses are more apt to be ulcerated.

Pain and interference with normal function are infrequent complaints.

Physical Findings and Differential Diagnosis

The physical findings will obviously vary with the lesion. Certain lesions have classic appearances, while others which look alike can be differentiated under the microscope. Verruca vulgaris is an example of the former, while senile keratosis and basal cell carcinomas are examples of the latter.

In many cases it is impossible to determine benignity or malignancy of a particular lesion from physical appearance alone. For this reason, biopsy must usually be performed to establish a definitive diagnosis.

Ulceration, induration, diffuse local spread of a pigmented nevus, and enlarged regional nodes are all signs which suggest malignancy, but infection can also produce these findings.

Anesthesia

Many good local anesthetics, all equally satisfactory, are available today. My preference is for 1 per cent lidocaine without epinephrine.

In achieving anesthesia for skin and subcutaneous tissue operations, 2 per cent lidocaine is not required. Use of a more concentrated solution actually limits the amount of anesthesia which can be used. Longer-lasting anesthesia is obtained from stronger solutions, but long-acting anesthesia is not necessary for most outpatient operations. Epinephrine constricts cutaneous blood vessels, decreasing bleeding from the wound and prolonging anesthetic action by decreasing the rate of absorption of the anesthetic agent. However, bleeding should be controlled at the time of surgery, thus avoiding the risk of delayed bleeding when the effect of epinephrine is dissipated.

In most cases, after the operation site has been prepared and draped, a 25 gauge needle on a 5 cc syringe is used to raise a dermal wheal with the local anesthesia. The small needle is replaced with a 22 or 20 gauge needle and the entire operative field injected just beneath the skin. A wheal involving the injected skin should be apparent. If the solution is injected too deeply into the subcutaneous tissue the wheal will not be visible, nor will anesthesia necessarily occur.

Prior to administering any local anesthetic a history for possible allergic reaction must be obtained. Also, gentle aspiration should be performed prior to any injection, to guard against intravascular injection.

Techniques of Excision

It is not possible to outline in detail every conceivable operation on the skin and subcutaneous tissues. The four most common local excisions are:
1. Nevus
2. Ulcerated lesion (cancer, keratosis)
3. Inclusion cyst
4. Lipoma

Nevus

These pigmented lesions are found most commonly on the face and neck, although some patients have them everywhere. The important points in excision are: (1) 2–3 mm margin, (2) line of excision parallel to lines of tension (Langer's lines), and (3) closure that will obliterate all dead space.

Ulcerated Lesion

The same principles apply here as for the removal of a nevus.

Inclusion Cyst

Excision of these tumors in the subcutaneous tissues is simple if certain principles are followed:
1. Almost all of these tumors communicate with the skin through a duct. In fact, plugging the duct is usually the first step in the formation of the lesion. The initial skin incision should be placed to avoid the skin opening, or the tumor may be accidentally entered. An ellipse of skin taken over the center of the tumor will avoid this.
2. Sharp dissection is carefully performed around the tumor to avoid cutting the capsule.
3. All of the capsule must be removed to avoid recurrence.
4. A drain may be needed if obliteration of all the dead space is not possible. If the tissues cannot be brought together without tension, the skin may be closed over a drain and a pressure dressing applied.

Lipoma

An incision parallel to Langer's lines should be used for excision of lipomas. If the color of the lipoma and the surrounding normal subcutaneous tissue are the same, as they often are, the texture of the tumor will have to be used to determine where to cut. The tumor has a firm, indurated consistency compared to normal fat.

Follow-up Procedures

All patients who undergo local excisions of tumors should be instructed on after-care of their wounds. Incisions should be kept clean and dry until the sutures are removed.

Provisions for postoperative discomfort must be made. The patient should always have the name and telephone number of the surgeon in case he develops unexpected problems.

Limitations in activity, if any, should be explained. Most incisions around the face and neck do not limit activities as do those crossing a joint or located on the sole of the foot.

The time to remove skin sutures depends on the location of the wound and the type of closure. Wounds with a good blood supply heal faster than those with a reduced supply, but whether the decision to remove the sutures should be based on this fact is debatable.

Sutures can be removed from the face and neck in five days, from the scalp and trunk in seven days, and from the extremities in ten days. If subcutaneous sutures are used the skin sutures can come out two days earlier than if they are not used. The early removal of sutures is important in decreasing visible scar formation on the skin. One additional postoperative visit after the sutures are removed is all that is usually required in benign conditions, and this can be scheduled three weeks after the sutures are removed.

Malignant conditions may require arrangements for further therapy. For instance, patients with melanomas should be admitted for further work-up and possibly more surgery. Periodic follow-ups of skin cancers should be arranged — preferably every three months for an indefinite period.

ORAL CAVITY

The mouth can be involved in a large number of benign and malignant growths. Almost all these growths are easily treated if diagnosed when small. The mouth is readily available for examination but it is commonly overlooked as a routine part of the physical. However, the mouth is endowed with a sensitive tactile system, and small irregularities are noticed early by the alert patient.

Technique of Routine Examination

A complete examination of the mouth requires a tongue blade, a finger cot and a light. The finger cot is not essential but it is certainly more esthetic. A systematic approach is desirable to avoid omissions.

With the mouth open wide and the tongue in its normal anatomical position the lips are examined, followed by inspection of the buccal mucosa bilaterally, the upper and lower gingiva, the soft and hard palates, the tonsillar fossa and the oropharyngeal wall posteriorly. The tongue blade is then used to hold the edge of the tongue aside, exploring the floor of the mouth and the inner aspect of the gingiva on each side. The junction of the posterior aspect of the middle third of the tongue with the anterior tonsillar pillar should always be checked as this is the most common site of cancer of the tongue (Fig. 5–3 *A*).

The lips, floor of the mouth, and tongue, in addition to any suspicious areas in other sites, should routinely be palpated. Mirrors are needed to examine the nasopharynx and larynx.

Types of Lesions

Tumors occurring in the mouth arise from the mucosal lining, the submucosa and minor salivary glands located in the submucosa. The overwhelming preponderance of malignant oral lesions arise from the mucosa and are epidermoid carcinomas. Adenocarcinomas of the minor salivary glands occur but are uncommon, accounting for 1 to 2 per cent of the malignancies. Sarcomas from the submucosa of the tongue and soft palate are extremely rare.

Inflammatory ulcerations are the most frequently encountered benign oral conditions. Inclusion cysts and fibromas occur not infrequently.

The most common site of oral cancer is the lower lip, followed by the tongue, floor of the mouth, tonsillar fossa or lateral pharyngeal wall. Often large tumors involve contiguous structures and it is impossible to determine the exact site of origin.

Presenting Complaints

Mouth lesions are usually noticed first by the patient because of one of three common symptoms: (1) a lump or tumor, (2) pain, or (3) bleeding, in that order of frequency.

Lump or Tumor

Since the oral cavity is generously endowed with sensory nerves in addition to the tongue, which can roam almost everywhere anterior to the facial arch, early recognition of even a small tumor or mucosal irregularity by the patient is insured.

Pain

Pain associated with a mouth lesion almost always indicates a secondary infection. This in turn implies a larger lesion that has outgrown its blood supply, followed by development of necrosis and infection. Small, painful ulcerated lesions are often viral in origin (herpetic ulcers). Foreign body inclusions with secondary infection and induration can be confused with tumors.

Bleeding

Bleeding is rarely the initial or solitary symptom of an oral lesion. When cancer is present, for example, bleeding is almost always associated with an ulcerated, painful tumor.

Occasionally benign vascular tumors such as hemangiomas will present with blood-tinged sputum.

Physical Findings

The physical findings of oral tumors are: (1) tumor, lump or irregular patch, and (2) ulcer.

Some clinicians classify mucosal patches into white patches and red patches, the former usually benign and the latter occasionally malignant. Leukoplakia, a white patch, is a premalignant lesion; however, the exact natural history of leukoplakia is not clearly understood. The harmless type of leukoplakia cannot be distinguished clinically from the premalignant form.

Differential Diagnosis

The more common benign and malignant oral conditions are listed below:

Benign	Malignant
1. inflammatory ulceration	1. squamous cell carcinoma
2. epulis	2. adenocarcinoma
3. hemangioma	3. sarcoma
4. granuloma	4. lymphoma
5. cheilosis	
6. leukoplakia	
7. mucocele	
8. verruca	
9. papilloma	

These lesions may or may not have characteristic gross appearances which will give the examiner clues as to the true diagnosis. However, since the patient pays a terrible price if a malignancy is missed, great care should be exercised in making recommendations without a tissue diagnosis. Many apparently innocuous lesions are found to be cancers.

Since it is not necessary to perform a biopsy on every lesion which develops in the mouth, a three week period of observation and conservative management seems safe for those lesions which appear benign. If there is no improvement after that period of delay, immediate biopsy is recommended.

Techniques of Biopsies

Either incisional or excisional biopsies are acceptable for diagnosis of most oral lesions. The clinical setting will determine which type to use.

Incisional Biopsy

The definitive treatment of oral cancer and a great many benign oral conditions requires anesthesia and major surgery. Therefore, the use of incisional biopsy to establish histologic diagnosis seems justified and expedient.

One per cent lidocaine without epinephrine is satisfactory for local anesthesia. A 2 cc syringe and a 25 gauge needle are used and the anesthesia is infiltrated submucosally.

If a small cup forceps is used (Fig. 5–5), the pain of the needle and the pain of a small nip are comparable. Therefore it may be permissible to eliminate the former.

No special preparation of the biopsy site with antiseptic is necessary — the mouth is a garden of bacteria and impossible to sterilize. It is not necessary to give antibiotics to the patient after the biopsy.

The following instruments should be available for use:

1. Knife
2. Scissors
3. Toothed forceps — "pickups"
4. Several types of forceps for biopsy, e.g., cup jaw, alligator jaw

In addition, absorbable suture should be available to control the bleeding which occasionally occurs. This is exceedingly rare, however, as oral rinsing with cold water for a few minutes almost always controls the ooze. It is also rare to expose bone with incisional biopsy, but if this occurs the bone must be covered with soft tissue to prevent osteomyelitis. This will require approximation with sutures.

Excisional Biopsy

A few oral lesions can be removed locally as excisional biopsies, and if this is possible it should be done (Fig. 5–7 *A* and *B*). The major requirement is that enough normal tissue be present around the lesion to permit approximation by sutures without tension (Fig. 5–8).

The Lip Shave (Fig. 5–9 *A, B,* and *C*)

Solar keratosis and *in situ* carcinomas of the lower lip are found with some frequency in men who spend a great deal of time out-of-doors. Patients with invasive epidermoid carcinoma of the lower lip also frequently have adjacent areas of keratosis or *in situ* carcinoma. In these patients, removal of the involved tissue can be achieved with a lip shave, achieving an excellent cosmetic result.

The procedure can be done under local or general anesthesia.

One per cent lidocaine without epinephrine is used to anesthetize the submental nerves bilaterally as they emerge from the submental foramen. Supplemental injections of 2 to 3 cc at the lateral commissures insure complete anesthesia for the entire lower lip.

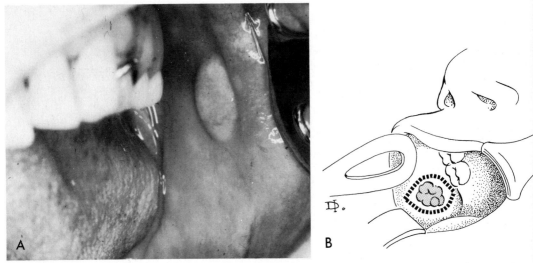

Figure 5–7 Intraoral lesion suitable for excisional biopsy in Outpatient Department. *A*. Small tumor of buccal mucosa, found to be a benign fibroma after excision. *B*. Technique of exposure and elliptical lines of excision.

The entire lower half of the face and upper neck are washed for three minutes with soap; this is followed by the application of an antiseptic solution. However, since the oral cavity is entered during the procedure it is impossible to maintain a sterile field.

The drapes should isolate the lower lip and leave the nose uncovered to allow easier breathing. The eyes should be covered and every maneuver explained to the patient before it is done. One or two gauze 4″ by 4″ sponges are placed in the mouth to prevent blood from trickling into the pharynx during the operation.

A total lip shave will be described, but it is emphasized that less than the total

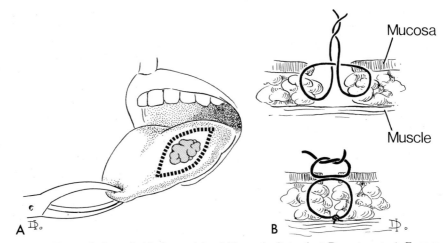

Figure 5–8 Tongue lesion suitable for excisional biopsy in Outpatient Department. *A*. Exposure and elliptical lines of excision. *B*. Two-layer closure of tongue with buried 3–0 chromic in muscle and 3–0 chromic catgut in mucosa.

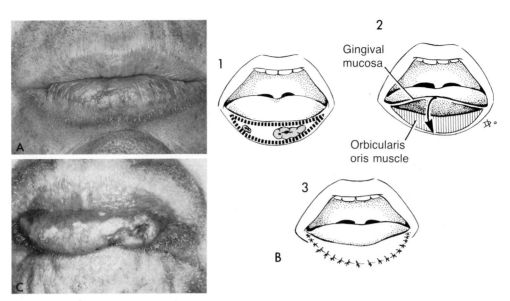

Figure 5–9 Lip carcinomas treated in Outpatient Department under local anesthesia. *A. In situ* carcinoma with adjacent leukoplakia, treated with lip shave. *B.* Lip shave technique. Submental nerves are blocked bilaterally with 2 to 3 cc of 1 per cent plain lidocaine. Similar injections are given at commissures of the mouth. (1) Lines of excision. (2) Buccal mucosa is undermined to prepare a flap for advancement. (3) Closure of defect with 5–0 nylon sutures. *C.* Invasive carcinoma and adjacent leukoplakia, treated with V-excision and lip shave.

can be done if only a part of the vermillion border is involved by a lesion suitable for removal in this way. It is not recommended that the normal vermillion portion be removed.

The initial incision is along the entire border of the vermillion portion and the skin of the lower lip from commissure to commissure. The incision is carried down to the orbicularis oris muscle.

Small dissecting scissors are then used to undermine the mucosa in the plane above the orbicularis oris muscle posteriorly toward the sulcus between the anterior gingiva and the anterior buccal mucosa. The extent of the undermining depends on the posterior extent of the lesion because the normal mucosa must be freed to the same width as the lesion to allow advancement. The lesion should not be resected until all the undermining has been accomplished. Once this is done, the involved lip mucosa is resected.

Bleeding may or may not be a problem, depending on whether or not the labial artery or vein is entered during the undermining maneuver. A large amount of hemorrhaging must be controlled by clamp and ligation, but small oozing is best ignored as it will stop when the mucosa is advanced and sutured.

Four–0 or 5–0 nonabsorbable simple sutures are used to approximate the mucosa to the skin of the lower lip. There will be some inversion of the lip, but this is minimal after complete healing. No drains are needed. An antibacterial ointment is applied to the wound, and the tube is sent home with the patient to be applied three times a day.

The patient is instructed to eat whatever he wishes, but initially jello, soups and other soft foods are preferred. Percodan is given every four hours for pain. A cold wet washcloth can be applied for 15 minutes every two hours to reduce swelling and give comfort. The sutures are removed in ten days.

When the patient returns for his follow-up visit, the pathology report must be available and should be explained to the patient. Further plans can then be made for definitive treatment, follow-up, or discharge from care, depending on the report.

TUMOR MASS IN THE NECK

Introduction

The correct evaluation of a patient who presents himself with a mass in the lateral neck is not difficult if certain points are kept in mind and proper diagnostic maneuvers are performed. Lateral neck masses are those beneath or lateral to the sternocleidomastoid muscles plus those at the angle of the mandible. Masses in the midline of the neck are usually related in some way to the thyroid gland, i.e., adenoma of the thyroid or thyroglossal duct cyst.

History

The length of time the mass has been present is helpful in the differential diagnosis. If it has been present several months or even years and has remained the same size, it is very apt to be a benign process. An enlarging mass of recent origin is strongly suspicious of cancer. Associated complaints referable to the head and neck area are important, especially hoarseness, sore throat, dysphagia, or painful sore in the mouth. However, often the mass itself is the only complaint.

Social history should be investigated. The patient should be asked if he has a history of heavy smoking or heavy drinking. The former habit allegedly predisposes to lung cancer, which can present as cervical lymph node enlargement. Smoking also is commonly associated with cancer of the upper alimentary and respiratory passages. The exact role alcohol plays in causing these cancers is not clear, but almost all epidermoid cancers of the upper respiratory and alimentary passages are associated with excess use of alcohol.

Physical Findings

The location of the mass is an important clue to its etiology as well as to the location of the primary tumor in the case of a metastatic lymph node. The consistency of the tumor may also be helpful in the diagnosis. A rock-hard mass is very likely to be cancer, especially if it is fixed to the adjacent tissue, whereas a soft mass may be a cyst or a lipoma.

Oral, pharyngeal, and hypopharyngeal cancers metastasize to cervical lymph nodes as a natural course of the disease. The sites of metastasis can frequently guide the examiner to the primary site.

Submental area
  lip
  anterior floor of the mouth
Submaxillary gland area (level I)
  floor of the mouth
  tongue—anterior two-thirds
Carotid bulb area (level II)
  soft palate
  tonsil and pharyngeal wall
  nasopharynx
  parotid gland
  scalp
  base of tongue
  pyriform sinus
  larynx
Midjugular (level III)
  pyriform sinus
  larynx
  thyroid
Lower jugular (level IV)
  larynx
  pyriform sinus
  thyroid
  lung
  cervical esophagus
Posterior cervical triangle (level V)
  thyroid
  scalp

The head and neck should be examined very carefully before removing any mass in the neck. If the mass is metastatic from primary cancer of the head and neck, open biopsy may compromise the possibility of cure from subsequent

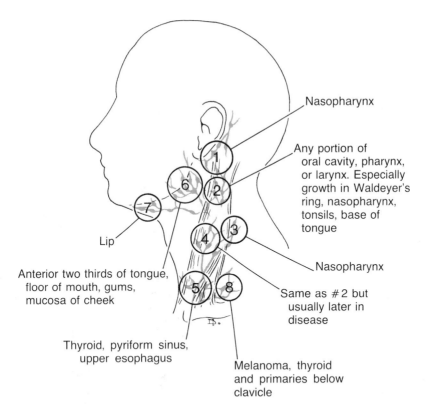

Nasopharynx

Any portion of
oral cavity, pharynx,
or larynx. Especially
growth in Waldeyer's
ring, nasopharynx,
tonsils, base of
tongue

Nasopharynx

Same as # 2 but
usually later in
disease

Lip

Anterior two thirds of tongue,
floor of mouth, gums,
mucosa of cheek

Thyroid, pyriform sinus,
upper esophagus

Melanoma, thyroid
and primaries below
clavicle

Figure 5–10 Lymph nodes of the neck and most likely sites of primary tumor. (1) Nasopharynx. (2) Oral cavity, Waldeyer's ring (nasopharynx, tonsil, base of tongue), pharynx, larynx. (3) Nasopharynx. (4) Same as (2), but usually later in disease. (5) Thyroid, pyriform sinus, upper esophagus. (6) Tongue (anterior two-thirds), floor of mouth, gums, buccal mucosa. (7) Lip. (8) Melanoma, thyroid and primaries below clavicle.

therapy, especially if a radical neck dissection is needed.

The scalp, skin of the head and neck, the mouth, nasopharynx, pharynx and hypopharynx must be examined closely.

All patients should have a chest film as part of the work-up. Contrast studies of the upper alimentary and respiratory passages can be useful, but they yield little as a screening procedure. Laryngogram, pharyngogram, cervical esophagogram and sinus films give little information in the asymptomatic patient which cannot be obtained more easily by a good examination. Silent cancers in the paranasal sinuses almost never present as a cervical mass.

Technique of Biopsy

Needle Biopsy. Whenever possible, if the cervical mass is suspicious for

cancer, the diagnosis should be sought using a needle biopsy (Fig. 5–6). The subsequent operative field is not violated and if the primary site is still obscure, further diagnostic studies can be performed—i.e., direct laryngoscopy, biopsy of nasopharynx, biopsy of the base of the tongue, and perhaps even a tonsillectomy.

1. The skin overlying the mass is prepared with soap and water for 2 inches, and this is followed by application of antiseptic solution.
2. One per cent lidocaine without epinephrine is used with a 25 gauge needle to raise a skin wheal.
3. The skin is punctured with a No. 11 knife blade. This prevents the needle from carrying any skin into the mass which could be interpreted as epidermoid cancer.

4. The Vim-Silverman needle is inserted and the biopsy taken. (A hollow No. 15 needle can be used and the mass aspirated.)

5. The Vim-Silverman needle specimen is placed in formalin. An aspirated specimen is squirted onto a slide, and then placed in ether-alcohol preparation (Pap fixative solution).

If a neck mass appears to be metastatic cancer, and a primary site is not readily apparent, a biopsy should be performed on the base of the tongue, along with a direct laryngoscopy and a biopsy of the nasopharynx. If these are negative, open biopsy of the neck mass is then in order.

Open Biopsy

1. The operative site is prepared in the same manner as for needle biopsy.
2. The site is draped to outline the sterile field.
3. One per cent lidocaine without epinephrine is used for anesthesia.
4. The incision should be placed parallel to Langer's lines and whenever possible in a position where it can be excised along with the specimen if a radical neck dissection is done subsequently.
5. Once the platysma is incised, the mass usually comes into view.
6. Sharp dissection is used to remove the mass in toto without cutting into it or rupturing it.
7. A ½ inch Penrose drain is placed after hemostasis is achieved.
8. The platysma and skin are closed with 4–0 nonabsorbable sutures.
9. A pressure dressing is applied. No antibiotics are used.

Follow-up. The pathological diagnosis will determine if further therapy is needed. The sutures can be removed in five days.

CERVICAL ESOPHAGOSTOMY

Cervical esophagostomy[8] is an operation associated with minimal risks that can be useful for many patients who require prolonged tube feedings. This operation can be substituted for gastrostomy or jejunostomy in patients who are candidates for these procedures unless there is total obstruction in the lower cervical esophagus, thoracic esophagus, proximal stomach or duodenum.

Indications

This procedure can be used for tube feedings except when there is obstruction of the alimentary tract *below* the cervical esophagus. The predominant use has been in treatment of head and neck cancers, when prolonged tube feedings may be required. It is impossible in some patients to pass a tube beyond an obstruction in the upper airway or cervical esophagus. In others, the prolonged use of a feeding tube reduces irritation and marked discomfort of the upper alimentary and respiratory passages.

Crusting of mucus on a nasal tube can cause painful irritation of the nasal mucosa, and mouth breathing secondary to obstruction of the nose can dry out the mucous membranes of the oral and upper air passages. In some patients an indwelling catheter near or on an oral or oropharyngeal suture line may interfere with healing, especially if extensive radiation therapy has been used previously.

Two other types of patients may benefit from this procedure. Occasionally, patients receiving radiation therapy to the pharynx or larynx develop severe irritation of these passages and are unable to swallow satisfactorily. A cervical esophagostomy allows feedings without having the catheter running directly through the irritated area. The second group includes patients unable to swallow because of extensive and unresectable oropharyngeal cancer. Very often these unfortunate persons survive for weeks with their tumor confined to the primary site or the neck, the disease remaining localized above the clavicles to the end. A cervical feeding tube enables them to maintain hydration and caloric intake until hemorrhage, sepsis, or some other event terminates the problem.

Finally, there is a sizable group of patients who have no obstruction in their digestive tracts and in whom gastrostomy has in the past been the preferred method of maintaining hydration and nutrition. These patients lack the normal means of moving food from their mouths to their stomachs. Almost exclusively they suffer from neurological disorders of various etiologies. This group of patients has the highest complication rate with gastrostomy, perhaps because they invariably need them permanently and have them in place for longer periods of time. Cervical esophagostomy can accomplish the same objective without significant morbidity.

Anesthesia

This operation can be done safely and satisfactorily under local anesthesia. However, local anesthesia deep in the neck is not always easy to achieve. If it is used, great care and gentleness is required for the dissection, pausing whenever necessary to supplement the anesthesia.

Position of the Patient

The position is important. We prefer to have the head turned away from the operative side and the neck slightly extended. The extension can be achieved by placing a small sandbag beneath the shoulders.

Technique

Regardless of which side of the neck is chosen as the site of the operation, the surgical procedure is essentially the same. The anatomy is almost identical except that the thoracic duct is more constant and larger on the left than its counterpart on the right. Injury to the major lymph vessels, hemorrhage and

recurrent nerve damage are the major complications. They can be avoided by obtaining good exposure and by taking reasonable care. We prefer an incision located one and a half to two finger breadths above and parallel to the clavicle (Fig. 5-11 *A*). We begin the incision 0.5 cm medial to the anterior border of the sternocleidomastoid muscle and carry it laterally 5 to 6 cm. Usually this places the most lateral point over the junction of the sternal and clavicular heads of the sternocleidomastoid muscle. The skin and platysma are divided, and hemostasis is then obtained.

The actual placement of the skin incision may vary according to individual preference, but it should allow easy access to the cervical esophagus below the inferior thyroid vessels. The area above these vessels presents a more difficult dissection and there is a greater risk of complications.

Once hemostasis has been obtained, we divide the sternal head of the sternocleidomastoid muscle (Fig. 5-11 *B*) to expose the carotid sheath and its contents—the internal jugular vein, the carotid artery and the vagus nerve (Fig. 5-11 *C*). The strap muscles—sternohyoid and sternothyroid—are medial to the plane of future dissection and can be retracted without difficulty if necessary. Occasionally their lateral edges must be cut to increase exposure.

Blunt dissection is next carried out between the carotid sheath and the trachea to expose the prevertebral fascia. This dissection is done using a hemostat or the finger tip (Fig. 5-11 *D*). The thyroid is often superior to this plane of dissection, but not infrequently the lower pole must be retracted superiorly and medially for exposure. Once the prevertebral fascia is identified, the space is enlarged superiorly and inferiorly to allow insertion of deeper retractors. It is at this point in the procedure that injury to the thoracic duct can occur. This is not common and will cause no problem if it is recognized and the duct securely ligated with nonabsorbable suture. If a lymph leak develops post-

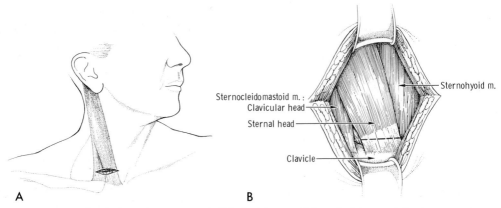

Figure 5–11   Cervical esophagostomy. *A*. Skin incision parallel to clavicle, overlying lower portion of sternocleidomastoid muscle. *B*. Line of division of clavicular head of sternocleidomastoid muscle.

Illustration continued on opposite page.

operatively, conservative management usually fails, and prompt return to the operating room for identification and ligation of the damaged lymph vessel is recommended.

Damage to the inferior thyroid vessels can also occur here, but again this should be infrequent, especially if blunt dissection is used. The recurrent laryngeal nerve should be specifically identified and protected whenever hemorrhage in this area requires control.

Once the prevertebral fascia is reached it is possible to feel the trachea anteriorly and medially (Fig. 5–11 *E*). The esophagus is right behind it, between the trachea and the vertebral bodies. In this position the esophagus is flattened from anterior to posterior and it may be difficult to recognize. However, a little traction medially on the trachea allows exposure of the longitudinal muscular wall of the esophagus and thus permits the placement of traction sutures into esophageal musculature. Tension on the traction sutures permits a scissors or a knife to be used to divide the various muscle layers down to the mucosa. Once the mucosa has been identified and opened, a nasogastric tube is threaded down into the stomach and secured in place by one or more pursestring sutures placed in the esophageal wall (Fig. 5–11 *F*). The

traction sutures may be used to reinforce the pursestring by tying them to each other, one set of ends above the tube and the other below. When passing the tube, some resistance may be felt at the esophagogastric junction, but this can be overcome with gentle pressure and twisting of the tube. We use a bulb type syringe and try to aspirate gastric contents.

It is conceivable that the recurrent laryngeal nerve can be damaged at this point in the operation, but if blunt dissection is used this should not occur. We estimate that the nerve is seen about one-third of the time, and in those instances it is very easy to protect. None of our patients has had the recurrent nerve damaged as a result of this operation.

Once the esophageal pursestring sutures are secured, the tube is immediately sutured securely to the skin of the neck to prevent accidental dislodgement.

The tube can be brought out through the lateral aspect of the incision or through a separate stab wound. We usually omit specific drainage, as the tube itself is a good wick. Occasionally, when the feeding tube lies on or very close to the carotid artery, this vessel is protected by a one-half inch gauze pack left in place for two or three days. The end of the pack is brought out through the

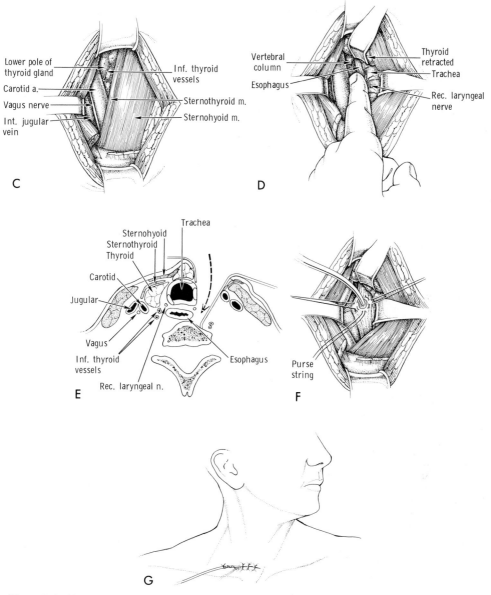

Lower pole of
thyroid gland

Carotid a.

Vagus nerve

Int. jugular
vein

Inf. thyroid
vessels

Sternothyroid m.

Sternohyoid m.

C

Vertebral
column

Esophagus

Thyroid
retracted

Trachea

Rec. laryngeal
nerve

D

Trachea

Sternohyoid
Sternothyroid
Thyroid

Carotid

Jugular

Vagus

Inf. thyroid
vessels

Rec. laryngeal n.

Esophagus

E

Purse
string

F

G

Figure 5–11 (Continued) *C.* Deep neck structures exposed by division of sternocleidomastoid muscle.
D. Exposure of prevertebral fascia. *E.* Sagittal section of neck at level of sixth cervical vertebra. *F.* Nasogastric tube in place in cervical esophagostomy. *G.* Fixation of tube by braided suture.

lateral corner of the incision. There is
no available tissue to obliterate the
"dead space" in this wound, so all that
we do is close the platysma and skin.

Antibiotics are recommended in the
postoperative period for five to seven
days.

Dependable fixation of the tube to
the skin is extremely important and cannot be stressed enough. It is discouraging, to say the least, to have the tube
accidentally pulled out on the first day
or two after surgery. We frequently
secure the tube in a manner similar to

that of a tracheostomy tube. Heavy suture (00) placed through the skin and braided around the tube also is effective (Fig. 5–11 *G*), but suture will cut through the skin over a period of time.

A sinus tract is well formed after two weeks, and the tube can then be removed and replaced without problem or risk to the patient. When the tube is no longer needed, it is removed and the fistula closes within 48 hours.

Complications

Potential complications include hemorrhage, lymph leak, damage to the recurrent laryngeal nerve, infection, and permanent fistula formation. However, we have had no serious intraoperative or postoperative complications which can be attributed to the cervical esophagostomy.

SOFT TISSUE MASSES

There are few problems in clinical medicine which cause as much confusion as the management of a patient presenting with a large soft tissue mass. Small soft tissue tumors rarely cause diagnostic problems as they are readily accessible to local excisional biopsy and histologic diagnosis. Lipomas, fibromas, hemangiomas, and so on, are representative of this group.

The problems arise when a patient presents with a large mass, often very firm, that cannot be resected without general anesthetic and major surgery. Even local excision for a benign tumor is a major undertaking in these large growths, not to mention the radical excision necessary if the tumor is malignant. Most of the tumors under discussion have arisen from the mesodermal elements, but they may include bone or cartilage.

Anatomical Sites

These soft tissue tumors can present wherever mesodermal elements are present, but the more common sites are:

1. Lower extremities
2. Trunk
3. Retroperitoneal area

Presenting Complaints

Painless swelling is the most common complaint. The fact that pain is absent lulls many patients into a false sense of security and they ignore the mass until it becomes very large.

Pain can be a complaint, but not often. It is likely to occur in retroperitoneal tumors which can achieve large size without detection because of their inaccessible location.

Occasionally a soft tissue mass can achieve a size large enough to interfere with function. Motion of the knee can be compromised by a popliteal mass, for example, or a retroperitoneal tumor can produce obstruction of the inferior vena cava.

Physical Examination

It is rarely possible to make a definitive diagnosis from physical examination since the consistency, mobility, and size of the tumor are not reliable tests of benignity or malignancy.

The exact anatomical location should be diagrammed and the dimensions recorded: this is important when evaluating the patient for major ablative surgery. The proximity of important structures often determines the extent of these procedures.

If the tumor is within a muscle, the exact muscle involved should be determined, as well as adjacent ones that may be involved.

Laboratory Studies

It is not practical to order an extensive work-up for metastatic disease before the histology of the tumor is known. However, all patients with large soft tissue tumors should have:

1. Roentgenogram of the tumor

2. Chest film

If the tumor turns out to be malignant, liver function tests should be added before any major ablative procedure is done. A liver scan should be ordered only if liver function tests are abnormal. A laparotomy should be done before hemipelvectomy for anaplastic sarcoma, but not for low grade sarcoma.

Biopsy

Planning for definitive treatment requires a tissue diagnosis. Whenever possible, this is accomplished by needle biopsy under local anesthesia (Fig. 5–12 *A-E*). The technique is the same as for needle biopsy of a neck mass.

Case Report. L. W. is a 61 year old female who was initially admitted to Colorado General Hospital for the treatment of biliary cirrhosis secondary to bile duct stricture. On her admission it was noted that she had a tumor of 28 to 30 cm diameter in the region of her right buttock. The tumor was firm and slightly movable. Interrogation at that time revealed that this tumor mass had been present for at least 36 months, but the significance of it had been overshadowed by the patient's liver problem. Plain roentgenological views of the mass indicated calcification was present.

Because of the definite possibility of a malignancy it was decided to try to obtain a

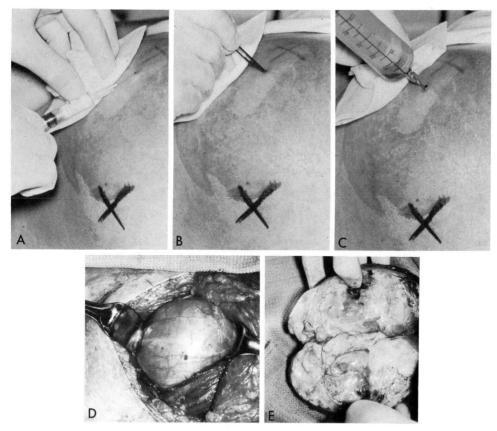

Figure 5–12 Management of a large soft tissue tumor; 60 year old woman with a large mass in the right buttock that was present for several years, growing slowly. *A.* Infiltration with local anesthesia. *B.* Skin incised with a No. 11 scalpel. *C.* After aspiration biopsy was performed, the pathologic condition reported was liposarcoma. Patient was then admitted to hospital for definitive surgery following preoperative radiation therapy. *D.* Liposarcoma exposed under general anesthesia. *E.* Cross-section of resected tumor.

tissue diagnosis with a needle biopsy. Between 25 and 30 cc of liquified fatty material were obtained on aspiration, and histologic examination revealed that the tumor was a liposarcoma.

The patient therefore received preoperative radiation therapy, and six weeks after the completion of treatment had a resection of her liposarcoma.

Open Biopsy. When the tumor is small enough for an excisional biopsy, this is the procedure of choice. However, in large tumors, excisional biopsies are formidable procedures and are really not indicated when amputation would be necessary if the tumor were malignant. Therefore, incisional biopsy must be done. Whenever possible, frozen section should be obtained prior to closure of the wound to determine if a diagnosis has been established. The exact histologic type is not as important as the fact of its benignity or malignancy. This saves the surgeon the dilemma of later receiving a diagnosis of "fibrous tissue compatible with capsule."

A generous wedge of tumor and complete hemostasis should be obtained. The wound should be closed without dead space and without drainage. Nonabsorbable sutures are recommended.

Follow-up

The tissue diagnosis on the permanent sections is usually available in 24 hours and plans for further treatment can be formulated then, if necessary.

The sutures are removed from extremity wounds in ten days, and from trunk wounds in seven days. The delay of 24–48 hours does not alter the end results of therapy for cancer. If the biopsy shows that the lesion is benign, the patient is spared the pain and expense of an elaborate and unnecessary work-up.

TUMOR CLINIC

Long-term follow-up of all patients is mandatory following surgery for cancer.

A registry of all tumor patients should be established in each hospital. Stable funding, secretarial assistance and staff coverage for these clinics is essential for successful recall of patients and intelligent, sequential recording of information. The general surgical Tumor Clinic in most hospitals will follow patients with cancers of the head and neck, breast, thyroid, lung, gastrointestinal tract and soft tissue sarcomas, including melanomas. Most specialty clinics follow the patients with cancer who were operated upon by their inpatient services.

The interval for follow-up will vary depending on the prognosis at surgery and the length of time since operation. For most cancers, monthly follow-up is indicated for three months, followed by visits at three month intervals for the remainder of the first postoperative year. The visits may be at six month intervals for the next four years, and then at yearly intervals. Patients should be strongly advised to return sooner if any of the typical warning signs[2] of cancer appear, such as:

1. Unusual bleeding or discharge
2. A lump or thickening in the breast or elsewhere
3. A sore that does not heal
4. Change in bowel or bladder habits
5. Hoarseness or cough
6. Indigestion or difficulty in swallowing
7. Change in size or color of a wart or mole

The nature of the follow-up examination will vary with the type of tumor which the patient had. In all cases, the operative incision and regional lymph nodes must be examined. The breasts, other node-bearing areas, neck and abdomen should also be examined. A pelvic and rectal examination is recommended at six month intervals, along with a Pap smear in women over age 30 and a proctoscopy in men and women over age 35. A chest x-ray is usually indicated at six month intervals for patients who have been operated upon for cancer, except cancers which recur locally almost exclusively, such as cervix and skin. Melanomas and sarcomas frequently reappear as silent pulmonary metastases.

The first indication of recurrent or metastatic cancer should be an indication for prompt, thorough evaluation of the patient for possible reoperation, or intensive radiation therapy, since if cure is still to be achieved, no time can be wasted. The chemotherapist (Chapter 25) should also be consulted at this point, so that if chemotherapy or hormones are indicated, this form of treatment may be started before the patient is terminal.

An interdisciplinary tumor conference is an effective means for stimulating interest in patients with tumors, and provides a useful opportunity to obtain consultation for patients with unusual problems.[9]

References

1. Ackerman, Lauren V., and del Regato, Juan A.: Cancer; Diagnosis, Treatment, Prognosis. St. Louis, C. V. Mosby, Co., 1962.
2. American Cancer Society, "Cancer Facts for Women," New York, 1964.
3. Dargeon, Harold W.: Tumors of Childhood, A Clinical Treatise. New York, Paul B. Hoeber, 1960.
4. Martin, Hayes: Surgery of Head and Neck Tumors. New York, Paul B. Hoeber, 1957.
5. Moore, Condict: Synopsis of Clinical Cancer. St. Louis, C. V. Mosby Co., 1962.
6. Nealon, Thomas F., Jr. (ed.): Management of the Patient with Cancer. Philadelphia: W. B. Saunders Co., 1965.
7. Pack, George T., and Ariel, Irving M. (eds.): Treatment of Cancer and Allied Diseases. Volumes I–VI, VIII, and IX. New York, Paul B. Hoeber, 1958–1964.
8. Ratzer, Erick R., and Morfit, H. Mason: Cervical Esophagostomy. Surg. Clin. N. Amer., *49*:1413–1420, 1969.
9. Ratzer, Erick R. (ed.): Recurrent malignant melanoma. Tumor Conference from the University of Colorado Medical Center. Rocky Mountain Med. J., *67*:42–46, April, 1970.

6

Metabolism and Endocrinology

By GEORGE J. HILL, II, M.D.

BIOCHEMISTRY AND PHYSIOLOGY FOR THE OUTPATIENT SURGEON

Body composition, metabolism and physiology are important aspects in the preoperative evaluation of patients. The surgeon should recognize deficiencies which can be corrected, for many patients can be prepared for surgery more economically as outpatients than as inpatients. Chronic vitamin deficiencies, anemia, and obesity are examples of metabolic lesions which can frequently be improved prior to hospitalization for elective surgery. Awareness of patients' biochemical and endocrine status will also expedite their hospital course and lead to a more successful result from surgery.[16]

This chapter reviews the characteristics of body composition which may be assessed in ambulatory patients. Metabolic defects commonly seen in out-patients will be discussed. The surgical aspects of the endocrine organs will be reviewed, with emphasis on the features which are pertinent in outpatients.

BODY COMPOSITION AND METABOLISM

Normal Values (Table 6–1)

The mass of the different components of the body has been determined by a variety of indirect means. A considerable amount is now known about the composition of "typical" men, women and children in a variety of clinical situations. It is therefore important to be aware of reports which are available in this field by authorities such as Moore (1959)[14] and Shires (1971).[18]

The red cell mass and blood volume can be measured with considerable accuracy in outpatients using isotope dilution analysis of Cr^{51}-labeled red blood cells. Most major hospitals offer this service in the hematology, diagnostic radiology or pathology departments. Dilution analysis of Evans blue dye is a cumbersome but accurate nonisotopic method for measuring plasma volume (and when hematocrit is known, calculation of total blood volume is then a simple arithmetical manipulation). A commercial device (Volemetron) that performs the same measurement rapidly is available, using I^{131}–labeling of plasma proteins.

Abnormalities in physiology and metabolism are frequently detected by chemical analysis of serum, body fluids, blood cells, and cells of specific organs and tissues (Table 6–1). The acid-base balance of the individual is a reflection of overall metabolic compensation in health and disease. The most convenient tests of acid-base balance are the arterial blood gas studies and pulmonary function tests shown in Table 6–2. Body surface area may be estimated from the values listed in Table 6–3.

Abnormal Body Composition

Weight

The patient should always be weighed as the first step in an elective routine physical examination and in subsequent interval follow-up examinations. Obesity is common in the United States, so a loss in weight may be missed if weight is recorded only after weight loss has commenced. Unexplained weight loss of significant degree is frequently due to cancer, but a vast number of other diseases also cause loss in weight. Psychological factors may cause severe weight loss, even though the patients may not be aware of a decrease in appetite. The presence of a psychosis is usually recognized without undue difficulty by the physician or members of the patients' family. However, neuroses and external psychic stresses may require considerable probing to uncover. It is obviously important to be aware of these factors rather than to plunge directly into an expensive and possibly fruitless work-up for the cause of weight loss. Chronic infection, metabolic diseases, arteriosclerosis, peptic ulcer and endocrinopathies are other common causes of weight loss which are seen in surgical clinics. Ideal weights for men and women of various ages are shown in Table 6–4.

Water

Retention or loss of body fluids should be detected and treated appropriately prior to elective surgery. Net retention of water is usually the result of cardiac, renal or hepatic decompensation, but may also result from the physical effects of blockage in lymphatic or venous drainage. Water intoxication can be self-induced, accidental or iatrogenic (through excessive intravenous fluid administration). Less common are endocrine disorders such as Cushing's syndrome, exogenous steroid hormone administration, and inappropriate ADH secretion in oat cell cancer of the lung. Peripheral edema may occur in chronic

(Text continued on page 134)

TABLE 6-1 Body Composition — Normal Values (Adult)

Body water 47–80% of body weight (approximately 50% in healthy young people)
  Intracellular 30–40% of body weight
  Extracellular 20% (5% plasma volume; interstitial fluid 15%) of body weight
Serum osmolarity (the sum of anionic, cationic and nonionic molecules present) approximately 300 mOsmoles (285–310)/liter
Blood volume 6.0–9.0% of body weight

Serum and Plasma Values

Ammonia nitrogen (P)		56–122 mcg/100 ml
Amylase (S)		80–160 Somogyi units
Bicarbonate (P)		22–26 mE/L
Bilirubin (S)	Direct	0.1–0.4 mg/100 ml
	Indirect	0.2–0.7 mg/100 ml
	Total	0.3–1.1 mg/100 ml
Calcium (S)		8.8–11.0 mg/100 ml
		4.5–5.5 mEq/L
		(Approx. 50% is ionized)
CO$_2$ capacity (S)		55–75 vol %
		20–33 mE/L
CO$_2$ content (S)		24–30 mE/L (20–27 in Denver)
Chloride (S)		96–106 mEq/L
Cholesterol	Esters	68–76% of total
	Total	150–250 mg/100 ml
Cortisone (P)		6–16 mcg/100 ml
Creatinine (S)		0.7–1.5 mg/100 ml
Fatty acids (S)		190–420 mg/100 ml
Fibrinogen (P)		160–420 mg/100 ml
Glucose (blood)		58–100 mg/100 ml
Immunoglobulins (S)	IgG	800–1500 mg/100 ml
	IgA	50–200 mg/100 ml
	IgM	40–120 mg/100 ml
Iodine, protein-bound (S)		3.5–8.0 mcg/100 ml
Iron (S)		75–175 mcg/100 ml
Lactic acid (blood)		6–16 mcg/100 ml
Lactic dehydrogenase (S)		0–320 m I.U./ml
Magnesium (S)		1.5–2.5 mEq/L (1.8–3.8 mg/100 ml)
Phosphatase (S)	acid	1.0–5.0 King Armstrong Units
	alkaline	30–85 King Armstrong Units
Phosphate, inorganic (S)		2.2–4.5 mg/100 ml (0.6–1.1 mEq/L)
Potassium		4.1–5.6 mEq/L
Protein, total (S)		6.0–8.2 gm/100 ml
albumin		3.5–5.5
globulin		2.5–3.7
α1 globulin	1.0–0.4	
α2 globulin	0.3–0.9	
β globulin	0.5–1.2	
γ globulin	0.7–1.7	
Prothrombin time (blood)		50–100%
Sodium (S)		136–145 mE/L
Transaminase		
SGOT		0–19 m I.U./ml
SGPT		0–17 m I.U./ml
Urea nitrogen (blood)		7–24 mg/100 ml
Uric acid (S)		1.5–8.0 mg/100 ml

TABLE 6–1 *Continued* BODY COMPOSITION — NORMAL VALUES (ADULT)

Vitamin B$_{12}$	200–800 picograms/ml
Vitamin C	0.4–1.5 mg/100 ml

BLOOD CELLS AND HEMATOLOGY

RBC males	4.6–6.2 million/cu mm
females	4.2–5.4 million/cu mm
WBC	5,000–10,000/cu mm
Reticulocytes	0.5–1.5%
Platelets	150,000–450,000/cu mm
PMNs	54–62%
Band forms	3–5%
lymphocytes	25–33%
monocytes	3–7%
eosinophiles	1–3%
basophiles	0.1%
Hematocrit	
males	40–54%
females	37–47%
Hemoglobin	
males	14.5–18.1 gm/100 ml
females	12.3–16.7 gm/100 ml

URINE

Ammonia	11–115 mEq/24 hrs
Calcium	100–300 mgm/24 hrs
Catecholamines	0–0.08 mgm/gm creatinine
Creatinine	0.4–2.6 gm/24 hrs
	(15–25 mg/kg/24 hrs)
Creatine	0–200 mg/24 hrs
male	(5.1–8.8% of creatinine)
nonpregnant female	(4.8–18% of creatinine)
5-hydroxy indoleacetic acid	
(5 HIAA)	less than 16 mgm/24 hrs
17-hydroxycorticoids	
male	5–15 mg/24 hrs
female	4–10 mg/24 hrs
17-ketosteroids	
male	10–20 mg/24 hrs
female	5–15 mg/24 hrs
Pituitary gonadotrophins	
male	6.5–13 mouse units
female	6.5–53 mouse units
postmenopausal	>104 mouse units
Porphyrin, uro	0–60 mcg/24 hr.
copro	100–300 mcg/24 hr (male)
copro	75–275 mcg/24 hr (female)
Potassium	30–150 mEq/24 hrs
	(66–90% of dietary intake)
Protein	0
PSP	
20 min	greater than 30% excretion
60 min	greater than 60% excretion
Sodium	40–350 mEq/24 hrs
	(88–100% of dietary intake)
Titratable acidity	18–64 mEq/24 hrs
Urobilinogen	0.1–1.5 Ehrlich units/2 hrs
Vanilmandelic acid (VMA)	11–25 mg/gm creatinine
Urea nitrogen	2.7–18.7 gm/24 hrs

TABLE 6–2　Respiratory Function and Blood Gas Values (Adults)

Arterial Blood Gas
- pH　　　7.35–7.45
- pCO_2　34–45 mmHg
- pO_2　　75–100 mmHg
- Oxygen content　　15–23 vol. %
- Oxygen capacity　　16–24 vol. %
- Oxygen saturation　94–100 %
- CO_2 content　　　45–55 vol. %

Pulmonary Function (from Comroe)

Vital capacity
Male	[27.63–(0.122 × age in years)] × height in cm
Female	[21.78–(0.101 × age in years)] × height in cm

Respiratory rate　　11–14/min

Tidal volume　　　450–600 ml

Minute volume
Males	3.1–3.9 × body surface area
Females	3.2–3.4 × body surface area

Basal oxygen consumption　135–145 ml/min/sq meter of body surface

Maximum breathing capacity
Males	[86.5–(0.522 × age in years)] × surface area in sq meters
Females	[71.3–(0.474 × age in years)] × surface area in sq meters

Forced expiratory volume
1 sec	75–83% of total vital capacity
3 sec	97% of total vital capacity

TABLE 6–3　Body Surface Area (M^2) as a Function of Height and Weight*

Height (inches)	Weight (pounds) 90	100	110	120	130	140	150
48	1.21	1.27	1.34	1.40	1.46	1.51	1.57
50	1.23	1.30	1.36	1.42	1.48	1.54	1.60
52	1.25	1.32	1.38	1.45	1.51	1.57	1.62
54	1.27	1.34	1.41	1.47	1.53	1.59	1.65
56	1.29	1.36	1.43	1.49	1.55	1.62	1.67
58	1.31	1.38	1.45	1.51	1.58	1.64	1.69
60	1.32	1.40	1.47	1.54	1.60	1.66	1.72
62	1.34	1.42	1.49	1.56	1.62	1.69	1.75
64	1.36	1.44	1.51	1.58	1.65	1.71	1.77
66	1.38	1.46	1.53	1.60	1.67	1.73	1.79
68	1.40	1.47	1.55	1.62	1.69	1.75	1.82
70	1.41	1.49	1.57	1.64	1.71	1.78	1.84
72	1.43	1.51	1.59	1.66	1.73	1.80	1.86
74	1.45	1.53	1.61	1.68	1.75	1.82	1.88
76	1.46	1.55	1.62	1.70	1.77	1.84	1.90
78	1.48	1.56	1.64	1.72	1.79	1.86	1.93

TABLE 6–3 *Continued* BODY SURFACE AREA (M²) AS A FUNCTION OF HEIGHT AND WEIGHT*

	160	170	180	190	200	210	220
60	1.78	1.84	1.89	1.95	2.00	2.05	2.10
62	1.81	1.86	1.92	1.97	2.03	2.08	2.13
64	1.83	1.89	1.94	2.00	2.05	2.11	2.16
66	1.85	1.91	1.97	2.03	2.08	2.13	2.18
68	1.88	1.94	2.00	2.05	2.11	2.16	2.21
70	1.90	1.96	2.02	2.08	2.13	2.19	2.24
72	1.92	1.98	2.04	2.10	2.16	2.21	2.27
74	1.95	2.01	2.07	2.13	2.18	2.24	2.29
76	1.97	2.03	2.09	2.15	2.21	2.26	2.32
78	1.99	2.05	2.11	2.17	2.23	2.29	2.34

*Values for intermediate heights and weights may be obtained by interpolation. (e.g., 125 lbs., 56″ = 1.52 M²).

TABLE 6–4 IDEAL WEIGHTS (POUNDS)

MEN

Height Feet	Inches	25–29	30–34	35–39	Age 40–44	45–49	50–54	55 up
5	4	134	137	140	142	144	145	146
	5	138	141	144	146	148	149	150
	6	142	145	148	150	152	153	154
	7	146	149	152	154	156	157	158
	8	150	154	157	159	161	162	163
	9	154	158	162	164	166	167	168
	10	158	163	167	169	171	172	173
	11	163	168	172	175	177	178	179
6	0	169	174	178	181	183	184	185
	1	175	180	184	187	190	191	192
	2	181	186	191	194	197	198	199

WOMEN

Height Feet	Inches	25–29	30–34	35–39	Age 40–44	45–49	50–54	55 up
5	0	118	121	124	128	131	133	134
	1	120	123	126	130	133	135	137
	2	122	125	129	133	136	138	140
	3	125	128	132	136	139	141	143
	4	129	132	136	139	142	144	146
	5	132	136	140	143	146	148	150
	6	136	140	144	147	151	152	153
	7	140	144	148	151	155	157	158
	8	144	148	152	155	159	162	163
	9	148	152	156	159	163	166	167
	10	152	155	159	162	166	170	173
	11	155	158	162	166	170	174	177

anemia, such as that due to carcinoma of the cecum. Edema may also occur in patients with protein loss from polypoid lesions of stomach or colon. Excessive net water retention is usually manifested by Hct↓, [Na]↓, [Cl]↓ in venous blood.

Water loss (dehydration) may occur from the gastrointestinal, genitourinary or respiratory tracts, or through the skin. GI losses in surgical patients are exemplified by chronic diarrhea resulting from a partially obstructed intestine, from vomiting due to gastric outlet obstruction, from GI tract fistulas, and from villous adenomas or hypertrophic gastritis. Loss of water from other causes is rarely seen in surgical outpatients, though patients with chronic high output renal failure, fever or permanent tracheostomies should be watched closely for signs of dehydration. Insensible loss of water through the skin is a serious problem in patients with burns and in unacclimatized persons in hot environments. Water loss is manifested by Hct↑, [Na]↑, and [Cl]↑ in venous blood.

Acid-base Balance and Changes in Serum Electrolytes

Most alterations in acid-base balance in outpatients are compensated. They will not usually be detected unless the surgeon is alert to the possibilities and does the proper tests to detect the biochemical lesions.

1. Respiratory Acidosis. Chronic obstructive respiratory disease or acute airway obstructions produce hypoxia, hypercarbia and acidosis (arterial pO_2↓, pCO_2↑ and pH↓; urinary pH usually acid). Treatment for severely decompensated patients includes placement of an endotracheal tube by the oral or nasal route, followed by creation of a tracheostomy with placement of a cuffed tracheostomy tube. Oxygen should be given only after the airway is controlled, since administration of oxygen may remove the only remaining respiratory drive. When the airway is controlled, a ventilating bag or respirator can be used to remove CO_2 by hyperventilation, and to administer an increased concentration of oxygen in inspired air. If the patient had shown bradycardia and obtundation prior to establishment of the airway, administration of $NaHCO_3$ intravenously (44–88 mEq) is advisable to correct the metabolic acidosis present due to hypoxemia. Arterial blood gases should be drawn before and after intubation and use of the respirator or ventilating bag. Patients with chronic respiratory acidosis frequently compensate successfully with metabolic alkalosis (through renal excretion of acid), and have a normal blood pH, in spite of the high pCO_2.

2. Respiratory Alkalosis. Severely injured casualties frequently exhibit mild respiratory alkalosis on arrival in the Emergency Room.[1] Several causes are apparent: anxiety, chest wall injury and pulmonary contusion stimulate a high rate of breathing, and automatic respiratory compensation also occurs for the metabolic acidosis which results from tissue injury and poor perfusion. Arterial blood shows pH↑, and pCO_2↓. pO_2 may be ↓ or normal. It is important to remember that the alkalosis of traumatized patients should not be treated with metabolic acids. Instead, the causes must be determined and treated specifically. Increasing the concentration of inspired oxygen and judicious use of narcotics to alleviate pain will usually lead to a more appropriate rate and depth of respiration.

3. Metabolic Acidosis. Acute metabolic acidosis will occur from tissue injury and poor perfusion. This condition is seen in traumatized patients, patients with ischemic necrosis of limbs or intestines, after irregular rewarming following frostbite, and in a variety of other situations with low blood flow. Tissue injury causes a measurable increase in circulating levels of lactic acid, as the result of a shift from aerobic to anaerobic glycolysis in skeletal muscle. When recovery is delayed, aerobic conversion of lactate to pyruvate by the Krebs cycle does not occur at a normal rate, and an increase is seen in the ratio of lactate to pyruvate. A high or increasing lactate-pyruvate ratio in the blood is a poor prognostic sign in patients with acute metabolic acidosis.

Chronic metabolic acidosis may occur as the result of retention or addition of metabolic acid, or by loss of base. Renal retention of acid occurs in patients treated with carbonic anhydrase inhibitors such as topical sulfamylon, and in patients with chronic renal failure. "Subtraction" acidosis is seen in patients with chronic diarrhea or fistulas distal to the stomach (pancreatic, biliary or small bowel). Chronic metabolic acidosis is associated with hyperchloremia and a decreased blood bicarbonate level, but blood pH is usually normal because of compensation by respiratory excretion of CO_2, and by renal excretion of acid, predominantly in NH_4^+ ions. Thus, venous blood shows $[Cl]\uparrow$, $[HCO_3]\downarrow$; arterial pH is normal; urine pH is acid. If an acidotic patient has a paradoxically alkaline urine, a renal acidifying defect should be suspected.

4. Metabolic Alkalosis. The problem of acute post-traumatic metabolic alkalosis begins when the injured patient is first seen in the Emergency Room. Metabolic alkalosis does not become apparent until one to three days after severe injury, when the patients are under treatment on the inpatient wards. However, a major factor in the cause of post-traumatic alkalosis begins during the initial resuscitation, when large amounts of lactated saline solutions and citrated blood are administrated. Lactate and citrate are metabolized during the next few days, and provide a significant burden of base for the normal respiratory and renal excretory systems to handle. Alkalosis in these traumatized patients is detrimental because oxyhemoglobin dissociation is less effective, and cerebral perfusion is diminished in the presence of an elevated blood pH.

Peptic ulcer is the usual cause of chronic metabolic alkalosis in surgical patients. Chronic use of antacids produces "addition" alkalosis, which may cause the formation of renal calculi and secondary hyperparathyroidism—the "milk-alkali" syndrome. "Subtraction" alkalosis becomes a serious problem in patients with vomiting from chronic gastric outlet obstruction. Loss of gastric acid in these patients produces hypochloremic, hypokalemic alkalosis, measured by $[Cl^-]\downarrow$, $[K^+]\downarrow$, and $[HCO_3^-]\uparrow$ in venous blood. Acid-base balance is maintained by conservation of H^+ by renal excretion of K^+ as the predominant cation. If vomiting occurs over a long period of time, failure of the renal compensating mechanism eventually occurs, followed by a rapid increase in metabolic alkalosis. This dangerous situation can be detected because the urine becomes acid at this time, as the result of severe depletion of potassium, so that K^+ can no longer be excreted instead of H^+. A patient with long-standing gastric outlet obstruction who has a paradoxically acid urine is in precarious condition. Prompt therapy with intravenous saline and stronger acids (NH_4Cl, glutamic acid or arginine HCl) is usually required in such patients (see later, *Mixed Acid-base Imbalance.*)

5. Mixed Acid-base Imbalance. An isolated defect such as respiratory acidosis or metabolic alkalosis is actually seen on only rare occasions in clinical medicine. As indicated above, compensatory mechanisms immediately begin to regulate each lesion in acid-base balance. Metabolic acidosis usually leads to increased respiratory rate (respiratory alkalosis); on the other hand, a lesion producing respiratory alkalosis is compensated for by retention of metabolic acids, and so forth.

In addition, it is common to encounter mixed acid-base imbalance clinically because patients frequently have lesions which tend to produce more than one type of acid-base disturbance. For example, a patient may present with severe chronic obstructive pulmonary disease (respiratory acidosis) and pyloric obstruction from peptic ulcer (metabolic alkalosis). Or a child may be seen on a hot summer's day with severe dehydration from fever and lack of water intake (metabolic acidosis), complicated by severe diarrhea (subtraction-type of metabolic alkalosis).

Obviously, a careful history, examination and use of good judgement regarding the etiology of the illness is of great importance in such patients. A simplistic view of treatment based on laboratory results alone would be devastating. Also, since errors occasionally occur in even the best laboratories, each piece of data should be examined in the total context of the patient and all other available information regarding his illness.

Electrolytes

1. Sodium. Net retention and net loss of sodium ions both tend to produce a reduction in serum sodium concentration. *Loss* of sodium as a cause for hyponatremia is so rare in surgical patients that it should be documented before treatment is given with NaCl. In most cases hyponatremia is due to *retention* of both sodium and water. Occasionally, chronic GI loss or sodium-loss nephropathy will produce a deficit in sodium. Rarely, a severe dietary restriction of sodium, combined with chronic loss in perspiration, GI tract or urine will produce a sodium deficit. Diuretics will also cause loss of sodium ion, and the patient with puzzling hyponatremia should be queried carefully regarding his use of medications. The question of sodium-loss nephropathy may easily be studied in outpatients by collection of serial 24-hour urine samples for sodium. After several days with a normal diet, the patient is placed on a diet severely restricted in NaCl. Normally, urine Na will immediately drop to 2–3 mEq per 24 hours. A salt-losing nephropathy will block this conservation in Na, and urinary Na excretion will continue unchanged.

Sodium retention is induced by adrenal cortical hormones, especially aldo-sterone. Sodium retention usually occurs from cardiac, hepatic or renal failure. It is usually treated with diuretics, expecially furosamide (Lasix), Aldactone or hydrochlorthiazide (Hydro-diuril). Intractable sodium retention may also be treated successfully in some instances by diuresis induced with rapid infusion of 100–300 ml of 3 or 5 per cent NaCl. The patient should be placed in the observation unit overnight for this treatment.

2. Potassium. Relatively wide variations occur in serum levels of potassium, which is the predominant intracellular cation. Accuracy of measurement is impaired by hemolysis of red cells, and the technique of analysis also has a relatively high absolute error. Potassium is an important ion in membrane function, especially in acid-base transfers in the kidney. The $K^+ : Ca^{++}$ ratio is of great importance in myocardial function, especially in the presence of digitalis. Loss of K^+ subjects the heart to the danger of cardiac irritability and digitalis toxicity. Hyperkalemia [$K^+ \uparrow$], on the other hand, diminishes the strength of cardiac contraction, which can lead to asystole, followed by anoxic-induced ventricular fibrillation. The cardiac effects of potassium are essentially opposite to those of calcium.

Potassium loss is a serious problem in chronic diarrhea or GI fistulas. Hypokalemia is frequently produced by excessive use of diuretics, though this loss can be controlled by administration of liquid potassium salts (KCl elixir; K-Triplex) if the physician remembers to give the correct instructions to his patient. In patients who take diuretic tablets infrequently, potassium supplementation with a glass of orange juice is usually satisfactory. Urinary potassium loss also occurs from endogenous or exogenous adrenal cortical hormones, especially aldosterone. Hypokalemia [$K^+ \downarrow$] of unknown origin should therefore raise the question of an adrenal cortical tumor, whereas hyperkalemia [$K^+ \uparrow$] is seen in adrenal insufficiency. The body's stores of potassium can be estimated in outpatients by potassium determination on a solution of hemolyzed red cells in distilled water. If the volume of red blood cells and distilled water was accurately measured, the intracellular RBC potassium concentration can be calculated with ease by a simple algebraic relationship.

3. Bicarbonate. The bicarbonate-carbonic acid system is the major buffering apparatus of the body. Venous blood bicarbonate is determined by a variety of methods, which have a wide range of normal values. The test is relatively inaccurate, depending on the laboratory and the method used. Since the purpose of measurement of HCO_3^- in patients is to assess the acid-base balance, we prefer to measure arterial pH, pCO_2 content directly and simultaneously with a polarographic gas electrode. The CO_2 content, HCO_3^- and pH are directly related to each other through the Henderson-Hasselbalch equation, as described in standard textbooks of biochemistry and outlined in Shires (1971). Regulation of bicarbonate was discussed in the previous section, *Acid-Base Balance.*

4. Calcium. The concentration of serum calcium is predominantly under the control of the parathyroid glands, the effect of parathyroid hormone being to increase serum calcium concentration, which thereby increases urinary excretion of calcium. Serum phosphate concentration is decreased by parathyroid hormone, which impairs renal tubular reabsorption of phosphate. Calcium is also regulated by thyrocalcitonin (also known as calcitonin), a hormone manufactured by the "C" cells of the thyroid gland, which lowers serum calcium. Thyrocalcitonin is ordinarily a major control mechanism for calcium only in patients with medullary carcinoma of the thyroid, a tumor derived from the "C" cells. Recent evidence suggests that thyrocalcitonin may also be the cause of hypocalcemia in acute pancreatitis, since thyrocalcitonin is released from the thyroid gland by stimulation by glucagon, which can escape from the acutely inflamed pancreas.[17] Hypercalcemia also occurs in some patients with hyperthroidism.

Hypercalcemia occurs in a variety of diseases in addition to hyperparathyroidism; sarcoidosis and metastatic cancers are the other major causes of hypercalcemia observed by surgeons. Of metastatic cancers, the most frequent cause of hypercalcemia is carcinoma of the breast with bony metastases. However, hypercalcemia can also occur in patients who have no demonstrable bony metastases, and in other cancers such as adenocarcinoma of the colon and lung. A parathyroidlike hormone secreted by the tumor has been implicated in some of these patients.

Hyperparathyroidism is caused by parathyroid adenoma, parathyroid hyperplasia and carcinoma of the parathyroid gland. Hypercalcemia produced by hyperparathyroidism may cause chronic illness or an acute crisis which warrants emergency parathyroidectomy. The chronic disease is associated with nonspecific and occasionally bizarre symptoms, including nausea, diarrhea, constipation and mental disturbances. Chronic hyperparathyroidism also causes bony resorption (osteitis cystica) recognizable as cystic lesions of the bone, fractures and resorption of lamina dura, and renal calculi. The acute crisis is manifested by profound lethargy, coma, cardiac irritability, and can be fatal.[23] Although the symptoms of hyperparathyroidism are nonspecific and may be inconstant, a consistent finding of *hypercalemia* should be considered due to hyperparathyroidism unless another cause for the abnormality can be found.

Hypocalcemia is frequently a difficult, long-term complication of radical surgery for carcinoma of the thyroid, and of jejunoileostomy performed for control of obesity. Mild hypocalcemia for one to six months is a frequent problem after other forms of thyroid surgery, especially when performed for hyperthyroidism. It can usually be controlled with oral tablets of calcium lactate or liquid calcium chloride, but may require the addition of vitamin D. Mental sluggishness, premature senility and constipation may occur in chronic hypoparathyroidism, even though serum calcium does not fall low enough to produce periorbital tingling, numbness in the fingers, muscle cramps or tetany. Subclinical hypocalcemia may be detected by the Chvostek or Trousseau sign, or by rapid onset of paresthesias during voluntary hyperventilation. Approximately 50 per cent of the calcium in serum is bound to albumin, and it is the unbound (ionized) fraction which is responsible for most of the effects of calcium which are described in this portion of the text. In patients with significant degrees of hypoalbuminemia, the ionized calcium level obviously takes on greater significance; this determination formerly was usually made indirectly by the nomogram provided in standard textbooks of biochemistry, but increasing numbers of hospitals now provide the determination of ionized calcium as a routine laboratory procedure.

5. *Magnesium.* The control mechanisms for magnesium in the body are poorly understood, but the level of this ion in the blood apparently follows that of calcium to a great extent. Magnesium is predominantly an intracellular cation, serum concentrations being only 1.5–2.5 mEq/L. Magnesium is of major importance in the long-term supplementation of patients with extensive small bowel resection, and jejunoileostomies for obesity. Hypomagnesemia produces muscular cramps, delirium, seizures and other mental changes. Magnesium sulfate or magnesium chloride is an effective emergency parenteral treatment for seizures due to eclampsia of pregnancy, and oral magnesium salts are given to supplement the diet of patients with chronic magnesium deficiency.

6. *Trace Elements.* Other cations are of relatively less significance in surgical outpatients. The role of zinc in wound healing is still under investigation and is hotly debated. It may have some role in local application for leg ulcers due to venous stasis, but these lesions have been treated with almost every poultice known to man and are still an unsolved problem. Iron is necessary for hemoglobin formation and should be given to surgical outpatients when deficiency exists. Anemia from chronic blood loss may not be correctible until the causal lesion is resected. However, if iron deficiency anemia is the result of menstrual bleeding in a woman, or lack of iron in the diet of a nursing infant, oral treatment with ferrous salts (gluconate or sulfate) should be administered for 30–45 days prior to admission for elective surgery. Iron must be given on an empty stomach, since it is not absorbed well in the presence of food or an alkaline pH.

7. *Proteins.* Serum proteins, which are predominantly anions, account for approximately 16 milliosmols (5 per cent) of the total ionic strength of plasma. Removal of fibrinogen as fibrin lowers the oncotic pressure in serum slightly, compared with plasma. Albumin, fibrinogen and the immunoglobulins make up approximately 75 per cent of the circulating plasma proteins. Conjugated globulins such as glycoproteins, lipoproteins, mucoproteins and metal-binding proteins constitute most of the final 25 per cent of the plasma proteins.

Albumin is synthesized only in the liver, at a rate of approximately 25–50 gm per day. The globulins are also all formed in the liver, except for gamma globulin which is formed by lymphocytes and plasma cells. Serum protein synthesis is impaired by a variety of diseases, including cirrhosis and cancer, and by antimetabolites. Serum protein can be lost from the GI tract by failure of digestion (loss of gastric or pancreatic enzymes) and by loss from diarrhea, from Menetrier's disease, or villous adenoma of the colon. Massive losses of serum proteins (predominantly albumin, because of its relatively small size) may occur in the nephrotic syndrome, and moderate losses of gamma globulin may occur in multiple myeloma. Both of the latter diseases have surgical complications, so the surgeon may be forced to contend with serious hypoproteinemia in the postoperative period.

One of the most remarkable achievements of the past decade in surgical metabolism has been the use of intravenous administration of protein hydrolysate, glucose, vitamins, minerals and small amounts of plasma which permit dogs and humans to synthesize proteins, fat and skeleton. Dudrick (1968)[4] achieved positive nitrogen balance, weight gain, and normal growth and development on a well-balanced intravenous "diet" administered through a central venous catheter. Dudrick's technique has been used widely and the results confirmed in many other laboratories and clinics. This alternative or supplement to oral feeding, termed "hyperalimentation," can be used for outpatients. The protein hydrolysate and hypertonic glucose solutions are commercially available, e.g., Aminosol and 50 per cent glucose ampoules. The surgeon who desires to use this technique must be experienced in the placement and maintenance of central venous cathethers (see Chapter 3). He should also be familiar with the methods and hazards of hyperalimentation and give pertinent instructions to his patients and the professional staff.

Protein solutions of various types are available for intravenous therapy. All are expensive, and if not sterilized, they carry the risk of viral (serum) hepatitis. "Plasmanate" (5.0 gm protein per 100 ml in hypotonic saline) or concentrated serum albumin are the best proteins for intravenous administration to outpatients. Single units of type specific, frozen or fresh plasma may be used for specific indications on the recommendation of a hematologist.

8. *Other Anions.* Phosphates, sulfates and organic acids are present in a total of approximately 8 mEq/L in plasma. The concentration of these anions increases in a variety of metabolic diseases, especially renal failure. Since many are di- or tri-valent, they contribute significantly to the buffering power of the blood. Blood levels of these ions, are, however, of relatively little significance in the surgical outpatient clinic.

Nonionic Substances in Blood

1. *Glucose.* Both hyperglycemia and hypoglycemia provide a multitide of problems for the surgeon. In most cases, the diagnosis is known, and the patient has an internist who will advise and assist in the regulation of glucose metabolism during the pre- and postoperative period. It should be remembered that far more deaths occur in surgical patients from *hypo*glycemia due to overzealous use of insulin than result from *hyper*glycemia.

Hyperglycemia. It is of great importance for the surgeon to remember that occasionally patients appear in the surgical clinic because of complication of hitherto undiagnosed diabetes mellitus. Infection or diabetic foot ulcer with neuropathy are the most common problems of this type. A relatively painless but badly infected foot is a typical diabetic lesion. Any patient with an infection should, therefore, have his urine sugar checked, and all known diabetics must be watched closely for ketoacidosis when they develop infections. Let us emphasize that a *positive* urine sugar in an outpatient should be considered as an indication that the patient has diabetes mellitus unless some other cause can be found; there are very few false positives (e.g., IVP dye). Diabetics should in general receive more careful attention to cultures, antibiotics, and follow-up than nondiabetics in all outpatient procedures. The diabetes mellitus which follows pancreaticoduodenectomy usually is relatively simple to manage, with 20–40 units of NPH insulin daily.

Hypoglycemia. Reactive hypoglycemia is a common, nonpathologic accompaniment of the irregular and irrational dietary habits of many people. Nevertheless, the surgeon will be alert to the possibilities of beta cell (insulin-secreting) adenomas in all patients with symptoms of hypoglycemia. It is remarkable that many patients with these tumors are diagnosed only after a long history of psychiatric evaluations and fainting spells, even when hypoglycemia was suspected or known to exist. Liver glycogen stores become depleted in many chronic diseases. The outpatient surgeon should therefore be prepared to reduce insulin or oral hypoglycemic drug doses in diabetics who become emaciated because of cancer, or complications of other diseases.

2. *Urea and Creatinine.* Ordinarily urea is measured only in transit from the liver, where it is produced in protein catabolism, to the kidneys, where it is excreted. Urea is usually measured as blood urea nitrogen (BUN), although serum urea nitrogen (SUN) or total protein nitrogen (NPN) provide essentially the same information; all measure the degree of azotemia present. Urea accounts for most of the nitrogen excreted daily. The amount excreted fluctuates greatly with the nitrogen balance achieved by protein anabolism and catabolism. Approximately 30 grams of urea are excreted daily by normal adult humans. Urea accounts for approximately 90 per cent of the 24 gm of nitrogen excreted on a normal or high protein diet. The additional, relatively constant 3 gm of urinary nitrogen is accounted for by ammonia, uric acid, creatine and creatinine plus small amounts of amino acids, hippuric acid and indican. After injury or during starvation, protein catabolism releases nitrogen in the form of amino acids, which are utilized in energy consumption through gluconeogenesis. The outpouring of nitrogen, predominantly as urea, in the absence of protein intake is referred to as negative nitrogen balance. Positive nitrogen balance is an accompaniment of the convalescence from injury or operation, so patients who return to the surgical clinic for postoperative follow-up may have a relatively low urinary nitrogen output. Urinary nitrogen excretion may be as low as 3 gm per day for as long as one to two months in convalesence from major trauma, depending on the length of the period of protein anabolism. Nitrogen excretion gradually rises as the patient regains his normal muscle

mass and is normal in the final phase of convalescence, when adipose tissue is synthesized.

When urea is administered intravenously it acts as an osmotic diuretic and formerly was used extensively for this reason to reduce brain edema.

High levels of BUN may occur from pre-renal lesions — most commonly dehydration, from intrinsic renal disease or from postrenal urinary tract obstruction. Azotemia is also a hallmark of decreased renal excretion of metabolic acids and of potassium, which causes lethal cardiac arrythmia when present in high concentrations. As an indicator of renal function, BUN is not as specific as creatinine. However, BUN is quicker and easier to measure, and the determination of BUN is less subject to intrinsic error than creatinine. BUN is filtered through the glomerulus and is passively reabsorbed in the renal tubules, whereas creatinine — in man — is excreted almost solely by glomerular filtration.

Glomerular filtration rate (GFR) in man is approximately equal to the rate of creatinine clearance. GFR is therefore estimated by calculation of creatinine clearance (Ccr), using the equation:

$$C = \frac{U \cdot V}{P}$$

C = Clearance (ml/min)
U = Urinary creatinine excretion (mg/100 ml)
V = Volume of urine (ml/min)
P = Plasma creatinine concentration (mg/100 ml)

The test is simple to perform in outpatients, requiring only a 24-hour urine collection and one (or preferably two) serum (plasma) creatinine determinations. The main problem is to perform the calculation properly! The normal rate of creatinine clearance in an adult man is approximately 100–150 ml/min. Creatinine excretion is relatively constant in a given individual, so a 24-hour output of creatinine should be used to assess the accuracy of 24-hour urine collections for other purposes, such as excretion of protein and hormone metabolites.

3. *NH₃*. Ammonia is produced in the gut by protein-splitting bacteria, in the liver (in the process of deamination of amino acids), and in the kidney, where it is used as a vehicle of H^+ excretion as NH_4^+. Excretion of NH_4^+ conserves other cations, such as Na^+, K^+ and Ca^{++}. The hepatic production of NH_3 normally is followed promptly by conversion to urea, which is then excreted by the kidney. Ammonia produced by bacteria in the GI tract is also metabolized in the liver. This important function of the liver does not occur properly if the portal circulation is diverted from the liver or if hepatic failure is present. Portal-systemic shunts and cirrhosis are therefore common causes of increased blood levels of NH_3. These patients frequently exhibit asterixis, confusion and coma. It is believed that NH_3 is not the sole cause of hepatic coma, but a high or increasing blood ammonia level is usually a sign of impending coma. The coma-producing effects of a high protein diet in these patients can be improved or controlled by reduction of dietary protein to 70 gm or less, and by elimination of protein-splitting bacteria with nonabsorbable sulfa drugs or neomycin.

4. *Lipides*. Blood lipides are particularly important in two types of surgical diseases: (1) the atherosclerotic-hypertensive diseases of aging, and (2) the familial hypercholesterolemias. The measurement and control of serum cholesterol in patients over age 50 is of relatively little surgical importance. The effects of dietary cholesterol are relatively irreversible by late middle age, except by massive alteration in diet. The surgical problems related to atherosclerosis in middle aged and older patients are the technical repair or removal of diseased vessels and organs, including placques in coronary arteries, aorta, peripheral arteries of the trunk, limbs, kidneys and brain, and atherosclerotic aneurysms of great and small vessels. Patients with familial hypercholesterolemias frequently appear to be benefitted by reduction in serum cholesterol by dietary means, by cholestyramine resin, or by ileal bypass.[2] When serum cholesterol is lowered significantly in these patients, placques sometimes resorb from soft tissues, and coronary artery disease appears to be improved or stabilized.

Cholesterol is excreted by the liver as one of the components of bile. It is formed by decomposition of RBCs, and it is also synthesized in the liver as a precursor of bile salts. Bile salts are the salts of glycocholic and taurocholic acids; they are of enormous importance in digestion: emulsifying fats, stimulating pancreatic enzymes and intestinal motility, and aiding the absorption of fat-soluble vitamins, such as vitamin K. And the bile salts are responsible for solubilizing and transporting cholesterol. Bile is concentrated in the gallbladder, and it is here that cholesterol usually tends to precipitate and form stones. Gallstones are composed of precipitated cholesterol, pigment and calcium carbonate in various concentrations, but cholesterol accounts for more than 90 per cent of the weight of most human gallstones. Cholesterol and the bile salts are responsible for most of the color in feces, so acholic (white) stools are the classic sign of obstruction of the biliary tree. Cholesterol is normally reabsorbed in the distal ileum, along with vitamin B_{12}, and this vitamin must therefore be administered parenterally to patients who have undergone the ileal bypass operation for hypercholesterolemia.

Other blood lipides of surgical importance are the triglycerides, free fatty acids and alcohols. The triglycerides, known as neutral fats, are esters of glycerol with fatty acids. Fats and fatty acids are insoluble in water, transported in blood in chylomicrons as β-lipoprotein, and bound to albumin. The albumin-bound lipides are the non-esterified fatty acids (NEFA's), also known as free fatty acids (FFA's). NEFA's are a rapidly-transported form of energy, which have a half-life in plasma of only two or three minutes. Their level fluctuates greatly with various states of stress and disease. Epinephrine, norepinephrine, growth hormone and ACTH cause NEFA levels to rise, whereas glucose and insulin reduce blood NEFA levels. Natural fats are complex mixtures of triglycerides, which are in dynamic equilibrium in living tissues. Fats occur in a spectrum from oils and soft fats to hard fats and waxes. Softness is imparted by short length and desaturation in fatty acids. Oleic and linoleic acids are examples of relatively short, unsaturated fatty acids which contain 17 carbon atoms. It is still uncertain which of the fatty acids are essential for humans, but linoleic acid apparently cannot be synthesized by man, so small quantities of it should be provided for optimum maintenance on a totally artificial diet. Hydrolysis of fats to glycerol and fatty acids may occur by enzymatic degradation, or by saponification, as occurs when calcium soaps are precipitated in the peritoneal cavity in patients with acute pancreatitis.

Ethanol is an alcohol which is of considerable interest and importance in surgery. Like glycerol, it is classified as a lipide, but it is metabolized as a carbohydrate. Ethanol is the antecedent cause of many surgical lesions, including traumatic injuries, cirrhosis of the liver and its complications, pancreatitis and acute hemorrhagic gastritis. Chronic addiction to alcohol interferes with proper preoperative preparation and postoperative convalescence—problems range from failure to return for scheduled appointments to acute delirium tremens. Acute intoxication with ethyl alcohol is a significant cause of automobile accidents, the leading single cause of traumatic deaths in this country. The "social" drinker may easily achieve a blood level of 0.1 per cent (100 mg/100 ml) of ethanol, which is the legal definition of intoxication for drivers in many states. Ethanol interferes with glucose tolerance, and conversely glucose ingestion apparently lowers the blood level of ethanol. Although the "happy" state of inebriation is generally recognizable by physicians, the precise concentration of alcohol in the blood can only be determined by a laboratory test. Since the test is simple, inexpensive and accurate, we encourage more frequent use of blood alcohol determinations in evaluation of acutely ill patients, especially when the question of head injury, ketoacidosis or intoxication by other drugs has been raised. Alcohol must not be used for skin preparation when drawing a specimen for blood alcohol determination. It has been frequently pointed out that ethanol is a high energy-yielding substance, producing 7 cal. per gram when fully oxidized. Nevertheless, the side effects of alcohol are so undesirable that virtually the only therapeutic use of ethanol in surgical patients is to prevent the development of delirium tremens in patients with chronic alcoholism who require emergency operations.

Metabolism of fats consists of the utilization of glycerol and the fatty acids in the Krebs (tricarboxylic acid) cycle to form CO_2 and H_2O. Glycerol is handled directly as a carbohydrate. The fatty acids, on the other hand, are broken into 2-carbon units, bound to coenzyme A, and then metabolized in the Krebs cycle. When fatty acids are presented to the liver at an excessively high rate or in the presence of a diminished rate of glucose metabolism, the acetyl-co-A fragments accumulate and condense in pairs as acetoacetic acid. This is the first step in ketogenesis, which produces ketoacidosis in diabetics and starved patients who metabolize fat in the absence of glucose. It is of interest that although glucose is metabolized to form fats and proteins, and proteins can be utilized as a new source of glucose, the formation of fatty acids from glucose is a one-way street—for all practical purposes, fatty acids cannot be converted back to carbohydrates.

Blood Cells

1. Red Blood Cells (RBC's). Red cells are responsible for 98 per cent of oxygen transport, and hemoglobin in the red cells is the most important buffer in the blood. Red cells contain large amounts of carbonic anhydrase, the enzyme which catalyzes the reversible reaction between CO_2 and H_2O to form carbonic acid, thus permitting easy transport of CO_2 in the blood. Synthesized in the bone marrow, RBC's normally lose their nuclei when released into peripheral blood. There they have a half-life of 28 days in normal individuals, and less than that in patients with a variety of diseases, including infection, trauma on defective heart valves, and hemolytic diseases. Approximately 60 per cent of the red cell is water, and most of the rest (35 per cent) of its substance is hemoglobin. Red cells are usually exceedingly uniform in appearance and are approximately 6μ in greatest diameter.

Hemoglobin is an iron-containing protein composed of four heme molecules joined to a specific globulin, globin. Each heme molecule consists of four substituted pyrrole rings bound to iron, which is in the ferrous (Fe^{++}) state. Pyrrole rings are five-membered rings, containing four carbons and one nitrogen atom; in hemoglobin the rings are substituted with methyl, vinyl and propionic acid groups. Hemoglobin is a medium-sized globulin, with a molecular weight of 66,700. It is approximately the same size as prothrombin and only half as large as most gamma globulins. Each globin molecule consists of two polypeptide subunits, the α-chain and the β-chain, which are important in the cause of sickle cell anemia (see below). Hemoglobin binds oxygen loosely, combining with oxygen in passage through the lungs. Part of the oxygen is released in transit through the tissues, where oxyhemoglobin dissociation is favored by the higher CO_2 pressure, lower pH and warmer temperature.

Red cell formation is controlled by erythropoietin, a hormone which is released by the kidneys. Hypoxia is the main stimulus to production of erythropoietin and thereby to formation of RBC's.

Any excessive level of RBC's in the peripheral blood is referred to as polycythemia and is commonly seen in chronic obstructive airway disease and other diseases in which chronic hypoxemia occurs, such as tetralogy of Fallot. Polycythemia vera is a condition of unknown etiology in which excessive red cell formation occurs. Patients with this condition also have a high blood platelet count, sometimes in excess of 1,000,000 per cm. The platelets are defective and may allow troublesome bleeding to occur in surgery. Preoperative preparation of patients with all types of polycythemia should include normalization of the hematocrit with venesection and replacement by saline or plasma (by plasmapheresis or Plasmanate). Patients with polycythemia should be bled regularly to keep the hematocrit at 55 per cent or less to prevent spontaneous thrombosis, pulmonary hemorrhage and hemochromatosis. P^{32} is also used to poison medullary hematopoiesis in patients with polycythemia vera.

Autotransfusion is the ideal form of blood transfusion in elective surgical operations. For this reason, preoperative removal and storage of one to four pints of blood is recommended prior to major elective surgery. This blood can be withdrawn in the outpatient clinic or blood bank. The volume of each pint of blood removed should be replaced simultaneously with 500 ml of saline or lactated Ringer's solution. The patients will reconstitute their shed RBC's rapidly if iron stores are maintained with 5 ml of Imferon given IM at the time of each venesection. Removal of one to two pints per week will not deplete the red cell mass excessively in most patients. However, each patient should have a hematocrit performed on the day on which venesection is planned.

Congenital diseases of the red cells have important implications for surgery. Spherocytosis is a familial disease in which the normal biconcave shape of the red cells is absent, apparently as a result of a deficiency in enolase, the enzyme which converts 2-phosphoglycerate to phosphoenol pyruvate. This deficiency diminishes the energy production available in the red cell by anaerobic glycolysis. The spherocytic red cells are trapped and destroyed at an increased rate in the spleen. Anemia is observed in the patients, and they may also develop heme-pigment gallstones and jaundice. Splenectomy should be done when the diagnosis is made, and cholecystectomy, too, if stones are present.

Sickle cell anemia is one of many diseases due to abnormal hemoglobins. Sickle cell anemia is a congenital disease caused by the presence of hemoglobin S instead of normal hemoglobin (hemoglobin A). It is an autosomal (i.e., not sex-linked) genetic disease which occurs almost exclusively in Negroes. Hemoglobin S, like other abnormal hemoglobins, is the result of amino acid substitution in one of the polypeptide chains of globin. In the case of hemoglobin S, valine is substituted for glutamic acid in the β-chain. Hemoglobin-S chains polymerize at low pO_2. The RBC's thereupon become sickle-shaped and move sluggishly in small vessels. Infarction may occur in viscera such as spleen, kidneys, bowel, brain and bone. Severe abdominal pain occurs in sickle "crisis" and may require laparotomy to rule out infarction. A careful family history should be taken prior to any elective surgery in blacks, searching for familial occurrence of sickle cell disease. Sickle cell disease (homozygous) or trait (heterozygous) can be diagnosed easily by hemoglobin electrophoresis. Patients with hemoglobin S should be advised to live at altitudes under 8000 feet, not to fly in unpressurized planes, and they should be kept particularly well-oxygenated during surgery. Although sickle cell crisis is more common and more severe in homozygous individuals, it has been reported in heterozygotes as well.

Acute intermittent porphyria is an hereditary disease in which severe crises of abdominal pain occur, related to a congenital defect in heme production. Patients with this disease have an excessive production of δ-amino levulinic acid (DAL) and porphobilinogen, probably because of excessive amounts of DAL synthetase and dehydrase in the liver. The patients excrete urine containing increased amounts of porphobilinogen and its precursor, δ-amino levulinic acid. The urine of these patients may turn red spontaneously or on exposure to light. Since the abdominal pain in porphyria usually is not caused by a lesion which can be remedied by surgery, and since porphyria is exacerbated by anesthetics such as the barbiturates, careful observation rather than immediate surgery is indicated in patients with acute porphyria who develop abdominal pain.

Hematin is the oxidized form of heme. It is relatively insoluble in acid, and precipitates in the renal tubules of patients who have free circulating hemoglobin due to hemolysis of a mismatched transfusion. The tubular necrosis which follows transfusion reaction may be alleviated in part by liberal administration of $NaHCO_3$ to alkalinize the urine and diminish the precipitation of acid hematin.

2. White Blood Cells (WBC's). Several types of circulating leukocytes exist, each with somewhat different functions, and all of which have implications for surgeons. The most numerous, *polymorphonuclear leukocytes* (PMN), are phagocytes which engulf and (usually) destroy bacteria and other small foreign bodies. Attracted by serum opsonins, they begin to arrive at the site of injury within minutes, and later are joined by mononuclear cells. PMN's have a short half-life, probably less than 24 hours, and become increasingly segmented as they age. Their numbers can be increased rapidly; when released in large numbers from bone marrow they appear as "band forms" which lack the usual segmentation of mature PMN's. The presence of "band forms" is frequently a good indication of the presence of infection in the body. This change in segmentation of PMN's is referred to as a "shift to the left" in the differential leukocyte count, because traditionally the PMN's and band forms are listed at the left side of the table of WBC percentages. The control of leukocyte maturation and release is under intense investigation at the present time, and present evidence suggests that a hormone (leukopoietin) may be important in this regard. Pyogenic bacteria are usually destroyed by PMN's. However, large numbers of intact intracellular gonococci are present in gonorrhea. This suggests that multiplication rather than destruction may be taking place. Intracellular multiplication also may occur in tuberculosis and leprosy.

Eosinophiles are PMN's containing eosinophilic granules. These cells increase greatly in allergic diseases — up to 40 to 50 per cent of peripheral leukocytes are eosinophiles in some cases. A high percentage of eosinophiles often points to a diagnosis of an allergenic disease, such as an infestation by amoebae or parasites. In patients with eosinophilia and abdominal pain who have a history of residence in areas where parasitic diseases are common, a cautious trial of drug treatment based on appropriate laboratory tests may be indicated instead of immediate exploratory surgery. It should be remembered that parasitic diseases are common in the tropics, and in many other areas where sanitation is inadequate. Poor hygiene is a problem in economically deprived subtropical and temperate communities and in the arctic, where permafrost prevents filtration and dispersal of waste. Echinococcal disease and trichinosis are widespread problems in dogs and other carnivores in the arctic and these diseases are easily transmitted to unwary humans.

Basophiles are PMN's containing black-staining granules, which are believed to be circulating mast cells, associated with heparin formation. Other than this, our knowledge of their exact function in health and disease is incomplete.

Mononuclear cells include lymphocytes and monocytes. *Lymphocytes* are small mononuclear cells with relatively little cytoplasm, which have a polyfunctional role in immunology. The circulating lymphocyte is one of a variety of lymphocytes which are histologically similar; others are present in spleen, marrow, thymus and lymph nodes. The age, life expectancy and exact function of the lymphocytes in each area are not known with certainty. It does, however, appear that some small lymphocytes are long-lived, multiplying cells. They play an important role in antibody synthesis, in transfer of antigenic information, and in the inflammation which occurs in chronic immunity. The lymphocyte appears to be the effector of rejection of homografts and of control of chronic infections such as tuberculosis. When properly stimulated by antigen, the small lymphocyte enlarges and acquires eosinophilic (pyroninophilic) staining material; it then synthesizes new DNA and may either divide or become multinucleated. *Monocytes* are large mononuclear cells with round or kidney-bean-shaped nuclei. They appear to act as transferrers of antigenic information, and are increased in numbers in patients with chronic infections.

Plasma cells are rarely observed in peripheral blood of normal individuals. The plasma cells have a distinctive nuclear conformation, segmented like the spokes on a wheel. Their function apparently is the synthesis of gamma globulin, and they are usually seen only in tissue sections.

3. *Platelets.* Megakaryocytes in bone marrow give rise to these tiny (2–3 microns), angular cytoplasmic fragments which are of vital importance in coagulation. Thromboplastin is released from platelets in the first stage of clotting. Platelets accumulate quickly at the site of any bleeding, and are present in tumor metastases. Deprivation of platelets may occur as the result of excessive loss in external or internal bleeding, or in bacteremia, parasitemia[8] and other types of consumption coagulopathy. A large number of serious acute illnesses have now been associated with disseminated intravascular coagulation (DIC). DIC is rarely encountered in outpatients, but may be seen in septicemia, massive trauma (especially with fat embolism) and metastatic cancer. When platelets are incorporated into

microthrombi, the platelet count falls[7] and fibrin split products appear in the peripheral blood. Evaluation of a patient for possible presence of DIC should include platelet count, prothrombin time, clotting time, clot retraction, clot lysis at 37°C, fibrinogen and fibrin split products. If bleeding is due to DIC, heparinization may be required to control the consumption of platelets and fibrin. Hospitalization is required to initiate this treatment. On the other hand, if prothrombin deficiency is observed, outpatient treatment may be sufficient, using vitamin K and correction of the underlying cause for decreased prothrombin time. Platelets contain serotonin (5-hydroxy tryptamine), a potent vasoactive substance which is also secreted by carcinoid tumors.

Blood clotting is of obvious importance to the patient with a surgical lesion, such as an injury or a disease for which surgery will be needed. Briefly, normal clotting is a dynamic process in which clot formation and clot lysis occur constantly. The equilibrium normally leads to clot formation in the presence of tissue injury and bleeding, in a sequence which is outlined in Figure 6–1. The most common conditions leading to increased bleeding in surgical outpatients are thrombocytopenia, prothrombin deficiency, capillary fragility, exogenous heparin administration, and hemophilia (an hereditary deficiency in antihemophiliac globulin). Surgery should not be undertaken electively in any of these patients in the Outpatient Department. If emergency surgery in a "bleeder" is required, consultation with experienced hematologists should be obtained immediately. Heparin is a mucoitin sulfuronic acid which is a powerful thrombin antagonist. It is ineffective by the oral route, and is given subcutaneously, IM, or IV. The usual daily dose is variable, depending on the effect desired and the patient's tolerance. Doses range from 200–600 mg (2000–6000 international units) per day. Depo-heparin is the most commonly used heparin preparation in our Outpatient Clinic.

Diet and Nutrition

Although every physician quickly develops his own notions about the optimum diet and the value of specific foods, a review of some pertinent data may be of help to doctors in counseling their patients. A "balanced" diet will be discussed and illustrated. The suggested requirements for water, calories, carbohydrates, fats, proteins, mineral and vitamins will be outlined briefly. The composition of foods is presented in detail in Watt and Merrill.[22]

A Balanced Diet

An adequate diet should include foods in four main categories in addition to condiments, oils, sugars and other types of foods which are less essential. The essential aspects of the diet are:

a. Milk and dairy products. Two cups

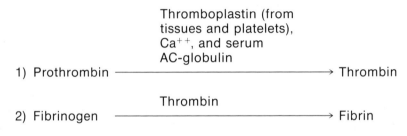

Figure 6–1   Coagulation diagram.

daily for adults; 3 to 4 cups for children, teenagers and pregnant women; 6 cups for nursing mothers.

b. Meats and eggs. At least 2 servings daily; soybeans and nuts can substitute if taken in large amounts.

c. Vegetables and fruits. At least 4 servings daily, including: yellow or green leafy vegetables for vitamin A; citrus fruit for vitamin C.

d. Cereals and bread (whole grain). At least 4 servings daily.

Water

The homeostatic economy of the body requires water for internal movement of substances by diffusion and circulation. Water is a necessary vehicle for transportation of food and for excretion of waste products by the gastrointestinal and urinary systems. Water must also be available for evaporation in regulation of body temperature. Conservation of water is assisted by the integument, by reabsorption in the air passages, and by concentration in kidneys and gastrointestinal tract. Water conservation is highly developed in some species, such as the camel—which can obtain water by oxidation of its fatty "hump"—and by the mouse, which can live almost indefinitely in closed burrows by obtaining water from seeds, and by its intense conservation in respiratory, renal and gastrointestinal systems. Adaptation also occurs in man, as seen in decreased water excretion in perspiration during adaptation to a hot environment.

The daily requirements for water are extremely variable, depending on age, general health, body surface area, and environmental conditions. Approximately 2000 ml is sufficient for normal adults in temperate climate zones. Increased respiratory rate, fever, or diminished reabsorptive mechanisms will increase the need for water. Water requirement may be calculated precisely by metabolic balance, utilizing factors such as daily weight, serum osmolarity, urine specific gravity, deuterium-labeled water and hematocrit. However, clinical signs of increasing or decreasing body water are also important. These signs include turgor of skin and soft tissues, moisture of the mucous membranes, and frequency of urination. In outpatients, clinical judgment regarding the patient's water balance must be skillfully rendered, since the laboratory tests are usually not requested or interpreted correctly until the physician suspects an abnormality on clinical grounds.

Water is available in the form of liquids, such as drinking water, other dietary fluids, and intravenous fluids; in solid foods, and as water of oxidation released by combustion of foods or body tissues. A 3000 cal. diet contains approximately 450 ml of water in solid food and releases approximately 400 ml more during combustion. Combustion releases approximately 0.3 ml per gram of protein, 0.5 ml per gram of carbohydrate, and 1.0 ml per gram of fat.

Water content of solid food can generally be estimated from the relative moisture and texture of the food. Exact values are given in Watt and Merrill.[22] Values range from more than 90 per cent in many fresh and canned fruits and vegetables to values of 5 to 10 per cent in dried foods. Desiccated and powdered foods generally consist of less than 5 per cent water. Meats are approximately 50 per cent water; bread is about 30 per cent water; and fat is about 10 per cent water.

Calories

The usual caloric intake for a 70 kgm male with moderate exercise should be approximately 3000 cal. per day. For heavy exercise, up to 6000 cal. may be required. A balanced diet providing 2000 cal. will be satisfactory for sedentary conditions, but if less is provided than is required, negative nitrogen balance will occur due to catabolism of muscle protein for energy. Oxidation provides 4 cal./Gm of carbohydrates, 4 cal./Gm of protein and 9 cal./Gm of fat. Anaerobic glycolysis releases only 21 per cent of the energy of glucose, since it is less efficient than aerobic metabolism for energy production.

Caloric contents of 100 gram and 1 pound edible portions of foodstuffs are given in Watt and Merrill and summarized in Table 6–5. Energy available ranges from 783 cal. in salt pork to 1 cal. in black coffee. Foods with a high fat content provide the most energy, e.g., mayonnaise, bacon, butter and heavily sweetened dessert pastries. The energy available in nuts, seeds and soybean flour is remarkably high (421–598 cal./100 gm). Medium calorie

TABLE 6–5 CALORIC CONTENT OF SOME COMMON FOODS*
(cal. per 100 grams edible portions)

High Calorie (>400 cal/100 gm)		Medium Calorie (100–400 cal/100 gm)		Low Calorie (<100 cal/100 gm)	
DAIRY PRODUCTS					
Butter	716	*Cheese* Swiss	370	*Milk* whole, cow	65
Chocolate sweet	528	*Cheese*		skimmed, cow	36
Salad dressing		Cottage, creamed	106	*Yoghurt* from whole milk	62
Roquefort	504	*Cream* (half & half,			
Mayonnaise	718	milk & cream)	134		
		Ice Cream rich	222		
MEATS, EGGS AND NUTS					
Almonds	598	*Beef*, choice grade, trimmed	301	*Beef & vegetable stew,* canned	79
Bacon, cooked	611	*Bluefish*, fried	205	*Chow mein*, canned	38
Fat, cooked	729	*Chicken pot pie*	235	*Lobster*, cooked	95
Peanuts	564	*Chicken*, cooked		*Oyster stew*, commercial,	
Pork		light meat	166	with milk	84
total edible	553	*Eggs*, hard boiled	163	*Soup*, chicken,	
salt	783	*Haddock*, fried	165	consomme, canned	9
Pumpkin seeds	553	*Ham*, cooked	289	prepared with milk	73
Suet, beef kidney,		*Liver*, beef, cooked	229	with rice, prepared	
fat, raw	854			from dehydrated mix	20
VEGETABLES AND FRUITS					
Potato chips	568	*Cherries*, with extra heavy syrup	112	*Apples*, raw	58
Popcorn, without oil and salt	456	*Jelly*	273	*Asparagus*, cooked	20
Soybean flour		*Olives*		*Celery*, raw	17
full fat	421	ripe	129	*Cherries*, raw	58
		ripe, Greek style	338	*Corn*, kernels, cooked on cob	91
		Potatoes, fried	268		
		Prunes, raw, soft	255	*Fruit cocktail,* canned, with light	
		Soybeans, cooked	130	syrup	59

TABLE 6–5   CALORIC CONTENT OF SOME COMMON FOODS* *(Continued)*
(cal. per 100 grams edible portions)

High Calorie (>400 cal/100 gm)		Medium Calorie (100–400 cal/100 gm)		Low Calorie (<100 cal/100 gm)	
VEGETABLES AND FRUITS					
				Onions, boiled	29
				Oranges, raw	49
				Peas, cooked	71
				Potatoes, boiled in skin	76
				Soybean "milk"	33
				Tomatoes, raw	26
CEREALS AND BREADS					
Cookies, chocolate chip	516	*Baby food barley cereal*	348	*Farina*, cooked	42
Crackers, saltine	433	*Biscuits*	369	*Oat cereal*, cooked	62
Pie, pecan	418	*Bread*, whole wheat	243	*Wheat cereal*, cooked	45
Rolls, Danish	433	*Cake*, chocolate with icing	369		
		Crackers, graham	384		
		Macaroni, cooked, tender	111		
		Pancakes, made with egg and milk	225		
		Pie, apple	256		
		Pie, strawberry	198		
		Pudding, vanilla	111		
		Rice, white cooked	109		
		Rolls, whole wheat	257		
		Sugar, granulated	385		
BEVERAGES					
		Spirits, (gin, whisky, etc.) 80 proof	231	*Beer* (alcohol 4.5% by volume	42
				Coffee	1
				Cola	39
				Wine, (table; alcohol 12% by volume)	85

*Adapted from Watt and Merrill.

yields are obtained from foods with high carbohydrate or protein content, such as beef, cheese, fish, sweetened fruits, and breads. Low calorie yield is seen in raw or cooked, unsweetened fruits and vegetables, and cooked cereals. For balanced diets with low calories, variety and sufficient protein can be obtained from such foods as milk, yoghurt, lobster, commercial stews and soybean "milk." Significant differences in calorie yield due to methods of preparation are illustrated by the various types of olives, cherries, potatoes and corn shown in Table 6–5. There appears to be little practical difference between the caloric content of various spirits, wines and beers, since the caloric content of 8 oz of beer is approximately the same as that of 4 oz of table wine and 1 oz of 80 proof whisky.

Carbohydrates

Simple sugars of six carbon atoms, (e.g., glucose, fructose and galactose), disaccharides (e.g., maltose, lactose and sucrose), or polysaccharides (e.g., starch) are subjected to oxidative phosphorylation in the Krebs cycle, or are metabolized to lactic acid by anaerobic glycolysis. Pentoses such as ribose can be utilized, but produce relatively little energy. In oxidative energy production, CO_2 and H_2O are produced. The anaerobic pathways lead to production of CO_2 and lactate. Lactate is ordinarily metabolized further when the temporary period of hypoxia is past and sufficient oxygen is again available. Carbohydrates are predominantly stored in the form of glucose, present in all of the body tissues, and in glycogen, which occurs mainly in liver and skeletal muscle but is also present in many other tissues.

Foods also include other carbohydrates such as D-xylose and cellulose, which cannot be assimilated by humans. D-xylose is therefore used as a tracer substance for GI tract function; it is absorbed but excreted through the kidneys without metabolic degradation. Cellulose is neither degraded nor absorbed and therefore serves as an important source of bulk in the diet, a factor which is necessary for normal function of the colon. Disaccharides must be hydrolyzed before they can be utilized, and intestinal lactase deficiency is considered to be a cause of milk intolerance in the postgastrectomy "dumping" syndrome.

Several other types of abnormal carbohydrate metabolism are important in surgery. These include: lactate accumulation in metabolic acidosis; glycogen storage disease with splenomegaly and hypersplenism; diabetes mellitus (with renal, vascular and ocular complications); and excessive production of insulin and glucagon in islet cell tumors of the pancreas.

Carbohydrate content of common foods ranges from 0 per cent in meat, fish and chicken to 99.5 per cent in granulated sugar. Low carbohydrate content is seen in eggs (1 per cent), cheese (2 to 3 per cent), and most cooked vegetables, which have less than 10 per cent, usually less than 5 per cent. Cow's milk is also low in carbohydrate (5 per cent), although of course condensed sweetened milk has a high carbohydrate content (54 per cent). Beer and wine are surprisingly low (4 per cent), compared with fresh fruits (10 to 15 per cent) and nuts (20 per cent). Custard is a low carbohydrate dessert (11 per cent), compared with cookies (60 to 80 per cent) and candy (up to 95 per cent in butterscotch). Nougat and caramel have the lowest carbohydrate content of the common candies (39 per cent). Prepared breads and cereals have a wide range of carbohydrate content (generally 50 to 80 per cent), with a maximum in corn flakes (91 per cent). The fibre content of our foods is remarkably low, being far less than 1 per cent in the common starchy foods, and only 1.6 to 2.6 per cent in such foods as soybeans, peanuts and almonds.

Proteins

Amino acids are joined together within the ribosomes to form polypeptides, which—when an arbitrary molecular weight of 5000 has been reached—are called proteins. The two major types of proteins synthesized in the body are enzymes and structural proteins. Protein anabolism is directed by a complex series of events stimulated by androgens and growth hormone, and catabolism occurs continuously. Catabolism releases amino acids for reuse, as well as for energy production in cases where fats and glycogen cannot be used at an adequate rate. Far more reserve energy is present in fat than in glycogen, since only 1600 cal. can be liberated by the glycogen in an adult human liver. On the other hand, each kilogram of muscle can yield 1000 cal. through gluconeogenesis from its content of protein. Of the approximately 22 naturally occurring amino acids, eight* are required in human diets and six others are "semidispensable."** The other amino acids are either nonessential in humans or can be synthesized in sufficient amounts from the essential amino acids if adequate protein intake is provided. Casein, the protein of milk and cheese, is an excellent source of all of the essential amino acids and is a well-balanced source of 18 others, lacking only hydroxyproline. A mixture of animal and vegetable proteins is generally preferable to a restricted diet, however.

The most convenient dietary sources of proteins are, of course, meats, poultry and fish. Cooked meats, including beef, bacon, chicken and cod, usually contain 30 to 35 per cent protein by weight. Raw whole eggs are 13 per cent protein, which is moderately higher than enriched breads (8–10 per cent). Baby food cereals are generally deficient in protein (6 per cent with rice cereal), although high-protein baby food cereal is available, containing 35 per cent protein. Cooked beans (8 per cent), soybeans (10 per cent), almonds (19 per cent) and peanuts (26 per cent) are all considerably higher than milk, cream and yogurt, each of which contains only 3.5 per cent protein. Saltine crackers (9 per cent) are surprisingly high in protein, compared to spaghetti (3 per cent). Medium raw pork is only 10 per cent protein, but is 52 per cent fat. Candy contains 2 per cent protein or less. Most fresh fruits and vegetables contain less than 1 per cent protein, although raisins are 2.5 per cent protein and the edible portion of breadfruit is 5.9 per cent protein.

A convenient source of amino acids for intravenous use in outpatients is 5 per cent dextrose in Aminosol. Dietary protein supplements are available commercially as Sustekal, Vivonex-100† and Instant Breakfast.

Protein formation is essential in sur-

---

*Isoleucine, leucine, lysine, methionine, phenylalanine, threonine, tryptophan and valine. However, recent evidence suggests that valine and phenylalanine may be synthesized in man from their ketoacids.

**Arginine, cystine, glycine, histidine, serine and tyrosine.

†Vivonex-100 is an elemental, bulk-free diet which is stated by the manufacturer to contain *(in six 80 gm packets, which should be diluted to 1800 ml)*:

		Caloric contribution
Available nitrogen, as purified amino acids	5.88 gm	8.5%
Fat (safflower oil—linoleic acid)	1.33 gm	0.7%
Carbohydrate (glucose and glucose oligosaccharides)	406.8 gm	90.8%
Calories	1800	

Vitamins—measured amounts of 16 vitamins, including A, B_{12} and C

Minerals—measured amounts of 8 cations and 6 anions, including sodium (2385 mg), potassium (2105 mg), calcium (798 mg) and magnesium (156 mg). 1800 ml supplies 133 mEq of sodium and 54 mEq of potassium

"Six packets supply 1800 Kilocalories and the known daily nutritional requirements. . . . The above vitamins and minerals have been included in amounts which follow the general guidelines for adults and young adults as set forth in the National Research Council Recommended Daily Allowances." (Eaton Laboratories Division, Norwich Pharmacal Company, Norwich, N.Y. 13815)

Vivonex-100 HN has recently been released for use. It is stated to contain 3.4 times the nitrogen in the recommended daily intake of Vivonex-100 Standard Diet.

gical patients, with polymerization and cross-linking of collagen occurring to give strength to the healing wound. Specific deficiencies occur in diseases such as lathyrism and vitamin C deficiency. On the other hand, excessive formation of collagen causes a multitude of complications, including failure of tendon repairs, common duct strictures, and recurrent bowel obstructions due to adhesions. High doses of corticosteroids have occasionally been reported to interfere with excessive formation of collagen, and for this reason dexamethasone has been used to prevent recurrent adhesions and fallopian tubal fibrosis.

Fats

The class of biochemical compounds which will dissolve in organic solvents is complex. It includes: the triglycerides and their constituents (the fatty acids and glycerol); sterols, such as cholesterol and the steroid hormones; alcohols; and the lipides of the nervous system, such as sphingomyelin. The surgeon is particularly concerned with the most common of the fats, the triglycerides, for these are the main constituents of adipose tissue. Adipose tissue is poorly vascularized and is easily subject to infection, yet it is, per gram, the most important source of energy in the body. The free fatty acids are energy sources which are rapidly mobilized in response to stress, through hormonal systems utilizing insulin and epinephrine. Surgical diseases and operations specifically involving the fatty tissues include cosmetic removal of subcutaneous fat in excessively obese patients, jejunoileostomy for control of obesity, lipomas, liposarcomas and lipidystrophy of the mesentery. Fat interferes locally with wound healing, although the fatty tissues of the body are essential reserves in convalesence from severe injury.

Fat is usually thought of as the dietary derivation of certain meats such as pork and bacon, which are approximately 50 per cent fat. However, a similar proportion of fat is obtained from peanuts (48 per cent), almonds (54 per cent) and many other nuts. The largest proportion of fat in any common food is raw beef kidney fat (suet) which is 94 per cent fat. Cooked lean beef, on the other hand, contains only 7 per cent fat, which is considerably less than cake (9 to 20 per cent) and candy (10 to 40 per cent), or even cream (12 per cent in "half and half"). Whole milk contains 3.5–4.0 per cent fat, which is about the same as cooked chicken light meat (3 per cent), soybeans (5 per cent) or codfish (5 per cent). Saltine crackers are remarkably high in fat (12 per cent), which is the same as whole eggs. Most raw fruits and vegetables contain less than 1 per cent fat, but some cereals are considerably higher; bread contains up to 4 per cent fat, and baby food oatmeal contains 5.5 per cent fat.

Considerable concern has recently been expressed regarding the potential danger of a high fat intake in the diet of normal adults, and the special danger of high fat intake in patients with hyperlipoproteinemia.

It is likely that little can be done to produce massive reversal in body fat distribution in most outpatients who are seen in surgical clinics with problems of obesity, atherosclerosis or xanthomas. Nevertheless, it is entirely reasonable to make dietary suggestions which may prevent *progression* of disease, and which may reduce the likelihood of similar disease developing in younger members of the household who share the diet. If the patient has accepted dietary instructions with interest and follows the recommendations carefully, it is likely that he would profit by dietary counseling from a dietitian or an internist specializing in this field. On the other hand, if the patient shows little inclination to study his own problem objectively and to participate in the planning of his diet, it is unlikely that he will be able to exert sufficient self-discipline to alter his fat metabolism significantly.

It is generally believed that a high fat intake should be avoided, and that the caloric contribution of fats in the diet should be no greater than 35 per cent. Dietary fats should be relatively high in unsaturated fatty acids, and cholesterol intake should be reduced as much as possible. It has recently been reported that multiple xanthomas were completely eliminated by eight years of careful dieting by a patient with type-2-hyperlipoproteinemia.[15] In this case, the unsaturated/saturated fatty acid ratio in the diet was approximately 1.5/1.0, and the total caloric intake was maintained at 2500 cal. per day.

Table 6–6 shows the total fat, fatty acid and cholesterol content in several common foods. It is apparent from cursory examination of this table that many surprises are in store for those who begin to evaluate the fat content of their diet. A serious student of this problem should utilize a more complete reference such as Watt and Merrill.[22]

As would be expected, most fresh fruits and vegetables are extremely low in total fat, saturated fatty acids and cholesterol. Canned beans, for example, contain only 3 per cent fat. A higher fat content is available in some vegetables, such as avocados and soybeans, which still preserve a relatively high unsaturated/saturated (U/S) fatty acid ratio. On the other hand, coconut meat has a *high* saturated fatty acid content (30 per cent). Meats range from a high of 85 per cent fat with salt pork and 52 per cent with whole pork or bacon to a low of 4 per cent with venison. Beef and lamb have 21–25 per cent fat and a U/S ratio of approximately 1.0. Chicken (12 per cent), veal (12 per cent) and fish are lower in fat content. But fish have considerable variation in fat content, as illustrated by the 4 per cent fat in humpback salmon and 16 per cent fat in Chinook salmon.

All "shortening" is high in fat, but considerable variation is possible in the U/S ratio by careful selection, as shown in Table 6–5. Vegetable oils have a high unsaturated fatty acid content, safflower oil being 11.0/1.0, and also providing the highest amount of the essential fatty acid, linoleic acid. On the other hand, butter, which is 81 per cent fat,

has a U/S ratio of only 0.62. The use of fats and oils in cooking clearly converts cooked breads and vegetables to a higher fat content, as illustrated by bread vs. biscuits (3 per cent vs. 17 per cent fat) and mashed vs. French fried potatoes (4 per cent vs. 14 per cent). Salad eaters can clearly see the difference in fat content of the ingredients, by noting that cottage cheese is 4 per cent fat, whereas most salad dressings are 50 per cent fat. However, dietary salad dressings provide significantly lower fat content (6 per cent).

Of all commonly eaten foods, the cholesterol content of egg yolks is highest—1.5 per cent by weight. Only beef brains, with more than 2.0 per cent cholesterol, are higher than egg yolks. It is usually forgotten that egg *whites* have virtually *no* fat, however. Other foods with significantly high cholesterol are shellfish (0.2 per cent), liver (0.3 per cent) and butter (0.25 per cent). Margarine is much lower in cholesterol than butter, with no cholesterol in vegetable margarine, and only 0.065 per cent cholesterol in margarine which is two-thirds animal in orgin. The common meat, fish and fowl are all approximately the same in cholesterol content, with 0.060 to 0.070 gm cholesterol per 100 gm of edible food.

Minerals

The importance of sodium, potassium, calcium, magnesium and iron was stressed above. Copper and cobalt are required in enzymes which facilitate oxidative phosphorylation. On the other hand, lead and mercury are poisons which cause symptoms mimicking the acute surgical abdomen and brain tumors.

Few natural foods are truly high in content of sodium and potassium. Man has a profound craving for salt, however, and prepared foods are frequently salted to an astonishing degree. The concentration of sodium, potassium, phosphorus, iron and magnesium in common foods can be found in Watt and Merrill.[22] The summary presented in this text

TABLE 6–6 Fat Content of Some Common Foods
Total Fat; Saturated and Unsaturated Fatty Acids; Cholesterol

Food	Amount In 100 Gm of Edible Portion			
		Fatty Acids		
	Total fat (gm)	Saturated (gm)	Unsaturated (gm)	Cholesterol (gm)
Almonds, roasted	57	5	51	.070
Avocados	17	3	10	
Bacon, cooked	52	17	30	
Beans, canned	3	1	1	
Beef, choice, trimmed	25	12	12	
Biscuits				
made with lard	17	6	10	
made with vegetable shortening	17	4	12	
Bread, white	3	1	2	
Butter	81	46	29	.250
Chocolate candy	35	20	14	
Cheese				
Swiss style	28	15	10	
American style	32	18	12	.100
Cottage, creamed	4	2	1	.015
Chicken, cooked with vegetable shortening	12	3	8	.060
Coconut meat, fresh	35	30	2	
Crackers, saltine	12	3	8	
Eggs, chicken, raw				
whole	12	4	6	.550
whites	trace			0
yolks	31	10	15	1.5
Fat, cooking				
vegetable	100	23	72	
animal & vegetable	100	43	52	
Ice cream	13	7	4	
Lamb	21	12	9	.070
Lard	100	38	56	.095
Margarine	81	18	60	0–65
Oils				
corn	100	10	81	
cottonseed	100	25	71	
safflower	100	8	87	
Milk				
whole	4	2	1	0.011
skimmed	2	1	1	
Pancakes made with egg and milk	7	3	5	
Peanuts	48	10	34	
Pork	52	19	27	
Potatoes				
mashed, with milk and butter	4	2	1	
french fried	14	3	10	

TABLE 6–6   Fat Content of Some Common Foods (*Continued*)
(Total Fat; Saturated and Unsaturated Fatty Acids; Cholesterol)

Food	Amount In 100 Gm of Edible Portion			
		Fatty Acids		
	Total fat (gm)	Saturated (gm)	Unsaturated (gm)	Cholesterol (gm)
Salad dressing				
Roquefort, regular	52	11	39	
special dietary	6	3	2	
Salmon				
King (Chinook)	16	5	5	.070
humpback (pink)	4	1	1	
Salt pork	85	32	44	
Soup, creamed chicken, prepared with milk	4	1	2	
Soybean "milk"	20	6	5	
Veal	12	6	5	0.090
Vension	4	3	1	
Yoghurt, made with whole milk	3	2	1	
Zweibach	9	2	6	
Foods With High Cholesterol Content				
Brains				>2.000
Egg yolk				1.500
Liver				.300
Caviar				>.300
Lobster				.200
Oysters				>.200

refers to concentration of these ions in mgm per 100 gm of edible food.

It is generally recognized, of course, that sodium content is high in bacon, corned beef and saltine crackers. These foods have sodium contents of slightly more than 1000 mg/100 gm of food. It is, however, rarely remembered that many other common foods also have high sodium concentrations, although they do not taste particularly salty. Examples are cheddar cheeses (1136 mg), Italian-style salad dressing (2092 mg) and puffed oats dry cereal (1267 mg). Baby foods generally have high sodium concentration, and may reach 300–450 mg/100 gm in cereals and meats. Truly salty foods, of course, have expectedly high sodium concentration, with smoked herring (6231 mg), lightly salted dry cod (8100) and soy sauce (7325) leading the list. (For comparison, table salt contains 37,758 mg per 100 gm).

Salt is usually added in preparation of most canned vegetables, raising the concentration from 1 mg or so to 200–300 mg/100 gm. Special diet-pack canned foods are available, with sodium concentrations of 3 mg or less per 100 gm. Most fresh fruits and nuts are also low in sodium, as illustrated by bananas (1 mg) and dried almonds (3 mg). Preparation of food in the home usually involves addition of either sugar or salt. For example, white bread contains 507 mg sodium per 100 gm, whereas chocolate cake contains only 294 mg. And whole milk contains 50 mg sodium whereas cottage cheese contains 229. Lightly cooked meat, fish and fowl contain only 24–70 mg sodium per 100 gm, until it is "salted to taste." A moder- ately restricted sodium diet (2.0 gm; 87 mEq) is shown in Table 6–7. More stringent diets (500 or 1000 mg) are available in manuals published by the

TABLE 6–7   87 mEq Sodium Diet (2000 mg)
University of Colorado Medical Center
Dietary Department

SALT SHOULD NOT BE USED ON ANY FOODS OR IN THE PREPARATION OF FOODS EXCEPT AS ALLOWED. ALL SALT SUBSTITUTES FOR PATIENTS MUST BE APPROVED BY THE PHYSICIAN.

	ALLOWED	AVOID
BEVERAGES:	Coffee, coffee substitutes, tea; 3 cups daily of whole or skim milk (if more milk is desired use low sodium milk), cocoa made from cocoa powder and milk allowance; fruit juices, lemonade, Kool-Aid, carbonated beverages in moderation	Cultured buttermilk, malted milk; low calorie carbonated beverages which use sodium base sweeteners; instant cocoa mixes
BREAD:	4 slices daily of salted yeast bread or rolls (if more bread is desired use low sodium bread); quick breads made with sodium-free baking powder or potassium bicarbonate and without salt, or made from low sodium dietetic mix; barley, cornmeal, cornstarch, flour; melba toast, graham crackers, low sodium crackers	Waffles, pancakes or quick breads made with baking powder, baking soda, or salt; commercial mixes; self-rising cornmeal or flour; any crackers except those allowed
CEREAL:	Unsalted cooked cereals; puffed rice, puffed wheat, shredded wheat; and any other low sodium dry cereal; cornmeal, barley	Dry cereals except those allowed
CHEESE:	Unsalted cottage cheese, unsalted American cheese	All other cheese
DESSERT:	Tapioca; unflavored gelatin (use fruit and fruit juices with gelatin), commercial low sodium gelatin, low sodium rennet dessert powder or tablets; unsalted fruit pies; desserts using milk allowance and other allowed food items	Commercial sweetened gelatins containing sodium; pudding mixes; other commercial desserts or dessert mixes
EGGS:	1 per day if desired, prepared any way without salt	No more than 1 per day
FATS:	4 teaspoons per day of salted butter or margarine (if more is desired use unsalted butter or margarine); $1/2$ cup cream; unsalted fat or oil for cooking; unsalted salad dressing and unsalted mayonnaise; unsalted nuts	Bacon and bacon fat, salt pork; commercial salted salad dressings, salted nuts
FRUITS:	Fresh, canned, dried, or frozen fruits, fruit juices, unsalted tomato juice; apples, melons and berries may be used if they do not cause distress	Regular canned tomato juice; crystallized or glazed fruit, and those containing salt or sodium compounds
MEAT, FISH AND POULTRY:	5 ounces daily (2 servings) of fresh beef, chicken, duck, lamb, pork, quail, rabbit, fresh tongue, turkey, veal; beef or calf liver allowed not more than once in two weeks; fresh	Brains or kidneys; canned, salted or smoked meat such as bacon, bologna, chipped or corned beef, frankfurters, ham, kosher meats, luncheon meats, salt pork, sausage, smoked

TABLE 6–7 87 mEq Sodium Diet (2000 mg) *(Continued)*

	ALLOWED	AVOID
	fish such as bass, bluefish, catfish, cod, eels, flounder, haddock, halibut, rockfish, salmon, sole, trout, tuna, whitefish; unsalted canned tuna or salmon	tongue; packaged frozen fish; canned, salted or smoked fish such as anchovies, caviar, salted or fried cod, herring, canned salmon or tuna (except low sodium dietetic), sardines; shellfish such as clams, crabs, lobsters, oysters, scallops, shrimp
POTATO AND SUBSTITUTE:	White or sweet potato, macaroni, noodles, spaghetti and rice	Instant mashed potato, commercial potato products, potato chips
SEASONINGS:	Most spices and herbs may be used including garlic powder, onion powder, and pepper	Regular salt at the table or in cooking (except as allowed); celery salt, garlic salt; onion salt; monosodium glutamate, meat tenderizers, Accent; dried parsley flakes, celery seeds
SOUPS:	Unsalted broth, unsalted cream soups made with milk allowance and allowed foods; low sodium canned soup	Bouillon cubes, salted commercial soups
SWEETS:	White sugar; home-made candy without salt, or special low sodium candy; jam, jelly or marmalade, honey; hard candy without salt or sodium compounds	Commercial candies made with salt or sodium compounds and milk or eggs; large amounts of brown sugar, molasses, syrups
VEGETABLES:	2 to 3 servings daily of any fresh, frozen, or canned vegetables	Sauerkraut and those which cause distress
MISCELLANEOUS:	Cream of tartar, sodium-free baking powder, potassium bicarbonate, yeast; cocoa, unsweetened baking chocolate; unsalted nuts, *salted* peanut butter, unsalted popcorn; unsalted catsup; lemon juice; extracts of almond, lemon, peppermint, and vanilla; vinegar	Regular baking powder, baking soda (soda bicarbonate); salted gravy or white sauce; Worcestershire sauce, Kitchen Bouquet, soy sauce, prepared mustard or horseradish, chili sauce, pickles, olives; Dutch processed chocolate; pretzels and snack foods; any foods prepared in a salt brine

General Rules:

1. *Read labels carefully* and avoid products containing salt, sodium, and NaCl unless allowed on your diet.
2. If snacks are desired between meals, use foods allowed on the diet not exceeding the amount permitted per day.
3. *Do not use* unprescribed medicines such as alkalizers, antibiotics, cough medicines, laxatives, pain relievers, and sedatives containing sodium.
4. *Do not use* water which has been treated in water-softening equipment with sodium compounds.

SUGGESTED MEAL PLAN

Breakfast	*Lunch*	*Supper*
Orange juice	Salt free chicken noodle	Salt free roast beef
Salt free Cream of Wheat	soup with salt free	Baked potato with 1 tsp.
with ½ cup cream	crackers	salted butter
Soft cooked egg	Salt free baked fish	Regular carrots
1 slice salted toast	Salt free potatoes	Lettuce and tomato salad
1 tsp. salted butter	Frozen peas	with salt free dressing
1 cup milk	1 slice salted bread	1 slice salted bread
Sugar–jelly	2 tsp. salted butter	1 tsp. salted butter
Coffee or tea	Canned peaches	Salt free vanilla pudding
	1 cup milk	(using ½ cup milk
	Sugar	allowance)
	Coffee or tea	2 squares graham crackers
		½ cup milk
		Sugar
		Coffee or tea

American Heart Association, 44 East 23 Street, New York City, New York 10010.

Potassium content of most foods is changed relatively little in the course of preparation. The naturally occurring potassium concentration, is, however, quite variable. For example, meats have potassium concentrations of 200–400 mg/100 gm. On the other hand, potassium concentration of eggs (129) and milk (144) is considerably less than that of meat. And almonds (773) are unexpectedly high. Most vegetables and fruits have potassium concentrations between 100 and 200 mg/100 ml, although some are higher—bananas contain 370 mg/100 gm, which is higher than cooked bacon! Some of the high sodium foods are comparatively low in potassium, as illustrated by Italian dressing (15) and smoked herring (157). Alcoholic beverages are generally low in both sodium and potassium, although table wine has 92 mg potassium per 100 gm.

Calcium is generally a well-tolerated and useful addition to diets, especially in children and lactating or pregnant women. Unfortunately, many of the foods with high calcium content also have high concentrations of substances which are generally not as valuable or well-tolerated—particularly sodium, saturated fats or cholesterol. However, for those who are in specific need of calcium, for bone formation or for treatment of hypoparathyroidism, it is important for the surgeon to know which foods provide significant amounts of calcium. In general, calcium content is good in dairy products, sea foods, and foods prepared from these raw materials. Calcium concentration of milk is 118 mg/100 gm; biscuits contain 209 mg, white bread 98 mg, and caramel 148 mg/100 gm. Although most fruits and many vegetables are low in calcium (0.3–10 mg/100 gm), beans contain 50 mg/100 gm and collards 188 mg. Egg yolks are a good source of calcium (141 mg), although whole eggs are considerably less (54), since egg white contains only 9 mg/100 gm. Almonds are surprisingly rich in calcium (234 mg/100 gm). Seafood is especially rich in calcium, with sardines containing 437 mg/100 gm, and kelp 1093 mg. Fish flour contains the astonishing quantity of 4610 mg/100 gm. For those rare patients who must receive calcium deficient diets, the most useful foods will be fresh fruits, vegetables such as potatoes (9 mg/100 gm), starches such as spaghetti (8) and most terrestrial meats and fowl (11 mg/100 gm).

Magnesium is abundant in many nuts (225–270 mg/100 gm), chocolate (292 mg) and soybeans (265). Moderate amounts are found in many other vegetables. Magnesium is relatively low in milk (13), meats (12–15) and fish (25–30).

Iron is generally found in sufficient quantities in meats (3–4 mg/100 gm) and seafood. Iron concentration is particularly high in braised kidneys (15 mg/100 gm) and egg yolk (5.5). As with many other substances needed in the human diet, almonds are rich in iron (4.7 mg/100 gm). On the other hand, milk contains only a trace of iron, and children who are fed predominantly on milk will develop a profound iron-deficiency anemia.

Vitamins

Although vitamins are obviously of general importance to surgical patients, three are of particular interest: vitamins C, B_{12} and K.

Vitamin C (ascorbic acid) is a powerful reducing agent. It is essential for wound healing, and must be supplemented vigorously in chronically neglected, debilitated patients or those who are undergoing a prolonged series of operations while receiving little dietary intake. Treatment may consist of 500–1000 mg per day. Scurvy is the classic disease produced by deficiency of this water soluble vitamin. Wound healing can be impaired by ascorbic acid deficiency in the absence of the classic signs of pyorrhea and cutaneous sores. Blood levels of ascorbic acid can be easily and accurately determined in any chemistry laboratory.

Citrus fruits are the most notable source of ascorbic acid, but many other fruits, berries and vegetables such as cabbage or kohlrabi are equally high in ascorbic acid content. Liver, onions and okra also provide substantial amounts of ascorbic acid. The ascorbic acid content of most foods is shown in Watt and Merrill.[22]

Vitamin B_{12} (cyanocobolamin) is a necessary coenzyme for synthesis of many amino acids. Vitamin B_{12} is widely distributed in meats and fish, especially in liver. It is not commonly found in fresh vegetables. Natural sources are documented in detail in a U. S. Government document on the subject (Home Economics Research Report[12]). It is believed that much of the Vitamin B_{12} utilized in human beings is synthesized by intestinal bacteria and absorbed in the terminal ileum.

In the absence of a specific glycoprotein ("intrinsic factor") secreted by the parietal cells of the stomach, B_{12} is not absorbed, and pernicious anemia develops. Pernicious anemia is a disease characterized by severe megaloblastic anemia and peripheral neuropathy. Patients with pernicious anemia have achlorhydria and a high incidence of carcinoma of the stomach. Unfortunately, they frequently have been given folic acid in the form of a multivitamin preparation. Folic acid will control the anemia, but it does not prevent development of neuropathy. It also masks the presence of pernicious anemia, so that the potential danger of gastric carcinoma is not recognized. It is important for surgeons to be aware of the dangers of B_{12} deficiency, and of the need for correction of this deficiency with B_{12} rather than with folic acid.

B_{12} must be given to patients who have had a total or nearly total gastrectomy, and to patients with ileal bypass (since B_{12} is absorbed in the terminal ileum). B_{12} deficiency develops slowly, occasionally becoming apparent only after many months or years. The patient may by then have moved to the care of another doctor. B_{12} is administered in injections of 100 mcg intramuscularly every month. Since only 1 mcg per day is required to maintain adequate levels of the vitamin, it has been said that vitamin B_{12} is the most potent therapeutic agent known to man.

Vitamin K is synthesized by intestinal bacteria and obtained in the diet from green leafy vegetables. It is a fat-soluble vitamin which is absorbed from the GI tract and used as a coenzyme in hepatic production of prothrombin. Surgeons may unintentionally interfere with vitamin K formation by alteration of intestinal bacterial flora with nonabsorbable antibiotics. The coumarin drugs, warfarin (Coumadin) and Dicumarol, block hepatic synthesis of prothrombin. The action of these drugs is potentiated by phenylbutazone (Butazolidine), which is frequently used in treatment of superficial phlebitis, bursitis or muscular pain. Many other drugs increase or decrease the action of the coumarin drugs, so patients receiving these drugs should be cautioned to consult their physician before accepting any other medication. Prothrombin formation is also impaired in patients with a variety of biliary and hepatic diseases, including cirrhosis and common duct obstruction. Vitamin K may be replaced by oral (Synkayvite) or parenteral (Synkayvite, Aqua Mephyton, Konakion) therapy. In general, Aqua Mephyton (vitamin K_1 oxide) is preferred, because jaundice has been observed in infants treated with synthetic vitamin K (Synkayvite), and the possibility of nonicteric liver damage is considered a potential danger of Synkayvite.

Intravenous Therapy

A wide variety of replacement and supplemental solutions are commercially available and can be used in the Outpatient Clinic. Many institutions have recently noticed increasing numbers of cases of septicemia associated with the use of intravenous therapy. The solutions used should therefore be examined carefully to be certain that no sediment or particles are present, and questionable solutions should be cultured but not administered to patients. Meticulous aseptic technique should be used for venipunctures; plastic catheters should be used as a route for infusion only when necessary; and catheters and needles should be removed from the veins as soon as possible.

The components of intravenous solutions commonly used are outlined in Table 6–8. Additional information regarding intravenous fluids and blood substitutes can be obtained in the monographs by Shoemaker and Walker (1970)[19] and Gruber (1969).[6]

The selection of a site for intravenous infusion is dictated by the type of therapy to be used, by the urgency of the situation, and by the patient's anatomy. In general, I prefer to use peripheral veins of the upper extremity for slow, elective infusions. The vein can thereby be watched closely for evidence of extravasation, phlebitis or infection, and the patient can assist with these observations.

A series of so-called "scalp vein" needles will take care of most of the needs for intravenous infusions in surgical outpatients. Phlebitis and infection do not appear to be as common or rapid in onset when needles are used as when plastic intravenous catheters are employed. A 19 gauge scalp vein needle in a hand or forearm vein is an excellent route for blood, plasma or isotonic glucose and electrolyte solutions. The internal bore of this needle is as large as a standard 18 gauge needle. The short length of a scalp vein needle actually allows flow to occur more rapidly than occurs through standard $1\frac{1}{2}$ inch long needles, and much more rapidly than with plastic catheters, which are usually 3 to 36 inches long! The differential rate of flow is most apparent when viscous solutions such as packed red cells are being infused. When solutions run slowly because of spasm of peripheral veins, intravenous injection of 0.5–1.0 ml of procaine or lidocaine through the tubing will often speed things up nicely, and simultaneously relieve the patient's discomfort.

Intravenous catheters must occasionally be used, because a secure route is necessary if percutaneous venipuncture attempts have failed. When venous cannulation of this type is necessary, I prefer to use as short a catheter as possible, thereby avoiding unnecessary trauma to the vein, and reducing the impediment to flow which is caused by long tubing. A medium (16) or large (14) gauge catheter is usually used, preferably of the needle-through-catheter type (Rochester, Buffalo, Angiocath, E–Z Cath, among others) instead of a catheter-through-needle (e.g., Intracath), to avoid the risk of shearing off the catheter with the needle. A silastic catheter is theoretically preferred, but it is difficult to advance this type of catheter very far in most peripheral veins, and silastic catheters have a tendency to kink or be cut easily. A polyethylene catheter is therefore usually best for most patients.

If a cut-down is needed on a elective basis, I usually use the basilic vein at the antecubital fossa, as shown in Hill (1969).[10] For administration of hypertonic solutions, or in emergency placement of intravenous catheters, superior vena cava cannulation by the subclavian approach is usually more appropriate (see technique in Chapter 3).

ENDOCRINOLOGY

Endocrinology is the science of hormones—chemicals which are produced in the body, circulate through the blood stream, and produce effects elsewhere in target organs. Hormones are produced in specific endocrine glands, in other organs and tissues, and in some tumors. The surgeon is particularly interested in tumors of the endocrine glands, for these are frequently benign and are curable when operated upon early enough. The surgeon must be aware of the nature of hormones normally produced through-

TABLE 6–8 COMPOSITION OF INTRAVENOUS SOLUTIONS*

INTRAVENOUS SOLUTION	Glucose Gm/100 ml	COMPOSITION mEq/L					pH	Comment
		Na	K	Cl	Ca	Lactate		
5% Dextrose injection, U.S.P.	5.0	0	0	0	0	0	4.0	isotonic
10% Dextrose injection, U.S.P.	10.0	0	0	0	0	0	4.0	hypertonic
20% Dextrose injection, U.S.P.	20.0	0	0	0	0	0	4.0	hypertonic
50% Dextrose injection, U.S.P.	50.0	0	0	0	0	0	4.0	hypertonic
5% Dextrose and 0.2% NaCl injection, U.S.P.	5.0	34	0	34	0	0	4.0	hypertonic
5% Dextrose and 0.45% NaCl injection, U.S.P.	5.0	77	0	77	0	0	4.0	hypertonic
5% Dextrose and 0.9% NaCl injection, U.S.P.	5.0	154	0	154	0	0	4.0	hypertonic
Lactated Ringer's (Hartmann's solution) with 5% dextrose	5.0	130	4	109	3	28	5.0	hypertonic
Lactated Ringer's injection, U.S.P.	0	130	4	109	3	28	6.5	slightly hypotonic
Ringer's injection, U.S.P.	0	147.5	4	156	4.5	0	5.5	isotonic
Sodium chloride injection, U.S.P.	0	154	0	154	0	0	5.5	isotonic
0.45% Sodium chloride in water (1/2 normal saline)	0	77	0	77	0	0	5.5	hypotonic
Sodium lactate injection, U.S.P. (M/6 sodium lactate)	0	167	0	0	0	167	6.0	slightly hypertonic
5% alcohol, 5% dextrose in water	5.0	0	0	0	0	0	4.5	5.0 ml absolute ethyl alcohol per 100 ml

TABLE 6–8   Composition of Intravenous Solutions* (Continued)

Intravenous Solution	Glucose Gm/100 ml	Composition mEq/L Na	K	Cl	Ca	Lactate	pH	Comment
6% Gentran 75 (Dextran 75) in 0.9% sodium chloride solution	0	154	0	154	0	0	5.0	hypertonic Dextran mol. wt. 75,000, similar to colloid effect of albumin
10% Gentran 40 (Dextran 40) in 0.9% sodium chloride	0	154	0	154	0	0	5.0	hypertonic. Dextran mol. wt. 40,000
5% sodium bicarbonate in water	0	595	0	0	0	0	7.5	HCO_3^- 595 mEq/L
5% Travamin (protein hydrolysate injection, U.S.P.-Casein), 5% dextrose	5.0	35	19	20	5	0	5.0	also Mg 2 mE/L PO_4^{3-} 30 mE/L and amino acids

approximate amounts (mg/100 ml)

leucine (410)	isoleucine	260	methionine	130
valine (310)	phenylalanine	200	histidine	130
lysine (310)	threonine	190	tryptophane	35

*Adapted from August 1971 Brochure of Travenol Laboratories, Morton Grove, Ill. 60053

out the body, and of the deficiency states which exist in the absence of these hormones. The hormones produced by malignant tumors of endocrine and nonendocrine tissues frequently present serious problems, since the patients may be in more distress from the effects of the hormones than from the tumors themselves.

It is not easy to recognize excess hormone production in its early stages. Many wise physicians have missed the early stages of conditions such as thyrotoxicosis, Cushing's syndrome, insulin-secreting adenomas of the pancreas, and hyperparathyroidism—all of which are obvious to medical students when in florid state. Yet each of these diseases and many others can be cured by surgery. It is therefore important to consider endocrine disorders in the differential diagnosis of a variety of seemingly routine complaints. Examples include changes in complexion, fatigue, headache, dizziness, weight gain, weight loss, and so on. Since most of these complaints are screened initially by internists, surgeons are frequently spared the embarrassment of having erred in the initial assessment. But surgeons may be the first to have the opportunity to make the diagnosis of an endocrine disorder. Examples of several endocrine lesions in which the primary presentation has been a surgical problem are shown in Table 6–9.

It is wise to obtain prompt consultation with a competent internist or endocrinologist for each patient in whom an endocrine disorder is strongly suspected, whether it is excessive or insufficient hormone production. The studies listed below represent a summary of current methods used in screening for endocrine diseases. The tests and diseases are further amplified elsewhere in relation to the specific organs involved.

Pituitary

Chromophobe adenomas are the most frequent pituitary tumors, representing two-thirds of the neoplasms of that gland. They usually do not cause excessive secretion of pituitary hormones. Enlargement of the sella turcica produces compression of the optic chiasm, bitemporal hemianopsia and headaches. Compression of the posterior pituitary lobe causes reduction in secretion of ADH and diabetes insipidus, which is manifested by increased urinary frequency and thirst. *Eosinophile adenomas* represent about one-third of anterior pituitary tumors. They secrete growth hormone, causing gigantism if they arise in childhood, and acromegaly if they arise in adults. Enlargement of the sella occurs, though not as disproportionate to the size of the skull as is seen in chromophobe adenomas. *Basophile adenomas* represent only 1 to 2 per cent of pituitary tumors. They secrete ACTH and cause Cushing's syndrome. Most patients with Cushing's syndrome can be successfully treated with adrenalectomy, but up to one-fifth of these patients will later require pituitary irradiation or hypophysectomy.[5] Basophile adenoma should be particularly suspected in adrenalectomized patients who develop hyperpigmentation of the skin in spite of adequate steroid replacement therapy. Since these adenomas are slow-growing and do not cause enlargement of the sella, they are difficult to detect except at surgery or at autopsy.

Tests of pituitary function which may be performed with accuracy in outpatients include:

1. Urinary volume, concentrating power and 24-hour excretion of 17 ketosteroids and 17 hydroxycortico steroids. All specimens should be checked for accuracy of collection by performance of creatinine excretion, which remains relatively constant. Concentrating power is assessed by measuring specific gravity on the first voided specimens in the morning, following deprivation of water overnight.

2. ACTH and growth hormone bioassay—not routinely available in most

TABLE 6–9   SURGICAL PRESENTATIONS OF ENDOCRINOPATHIES

INITIAL PRESENTATIONS	ENDOCRINE LESIONS
Peptic ulcer Renal calculi Pancreatitis Kidney transplant recipient	Hyperparathyroidism
Mass in neck Excessive weight loss	Hyperthyroidism
Mass in neck	Calcitonin-secreting thyroid cancer
Orthopedic problems related to excessive bone growth	Pituitary eosinophilic adenoma
Urinary frequency from dysfunction of posterior pituitary and decreased release of ADH	Pituitary chromophobe adenoma
Compression fracture of spine Peptic ulcer Atrophy of skeletal muscle	Cushing's syndrome (adrenal hyperfunction or pituitary basophile adenoma)
Peptic ulcer, virulent (gastrin-secreting adenoma—the Zollinger-Ellison syndrome) Seizures (from hypoglycemia in insulin-secreting adenoma) Coma (insulin- or glucagon-secreting adenoma)	Pancreatic islet cell adenoma
Intestinal obstruction Gastrointestinal bleeding Abdominal mass, with or without abdominal pain	Carcinoid
Amenorrhea Sterility in females Clitoral hypertrophy	Androgen hypersecretion (adrenal or ovarian tumors; adrenal-genital syndrome; Stein-Leventhal ovaries)
Abdominal mass (males or females) Gynecomastia and nipple discharge (males or females) Question of pregnancy (females) Testicular mass (males)	Female gonadotrophin hypersecretion (choriocarcinoma of trophoblast or testis)
Cough, palpable lymph nodes, chest pain or abnormal chest x-ray	Antidiuretic hormone hypersecretion (oat cell carcinoma of lung)
Hypertension or fever in patients with neuro-fibromatosis or medullary carcinoma of thyroid	Pheochromocytoma

hospitals but will become more easily available during the next few years.

3. ACTH test. Four, 6 or 8-hour infusion of 25–40 units of ACTH intravenously, with 24-hour collection for steroids the day before, during and after the day of ACTH infusion. Plasma cortisols can be obtained before and at the end of infusion and on the following day.

4. Metopirone (metyrapone) test. This drug blocks 11-beta hydroxylation of corticosteroids in the adrenal gland, and thereby leads to increased secretion of ACTH by normal individuals. The response in a patient with normal pituitary and adrenal glands is an increase in production of urinary metabolites measured as 17-ketosteroids and 17-hydroxycortico steroids.

5. Lateral skull x-ray with measurement of size of sella turcica.

Thyroid

Hyperthyroidism does not commonly produce symptoms which bring the patient initially to a surgeon. If a surgeon suspects hyperthyroidism in a patient whom he is evaluating for some other reason, he should arrange for a full evaluation by an endocrinologist.

Thyrotoxicosis usually is the result of diffuse thyroid hyperplasia. Thyrotoxicosis from an adenoma is extremely unusual, though "hot" nodules are occasionally seen on scan.

The usual initial therapy for most patients with hyperthyroidism is medical—destruction of the gland with I^{131} or I^{125}, or reduction in circulating thyroxine levels with propylthiouracil. Surgery is usually reserved for those who do not accept propylthiouracil well (because of failure to take the drug or untoward side effects from the therapy), and in those who should not receive a therapeutic dose of radioactive iodine (such as prepubertal children and women in the child-bearing age group). Occasionally, patients are referred for surgery who cannot be controlled with medical therapy. These patients represent the group at highest risk from surgery. In general, however, most patients with thyrotoxicosis can be rendered euthyroid prior to surgery.

Final preparation for thyroid surgery is best performed by seven to ten days in the hospital, where the patient can be kept quiet, with sequential observations of pulse, weight, temperature and caloric intake. If necessary, outpatient preparation can be performed, however. The patient should receive his usual doses of propylthiouracil (approximately 50–100 mg/day), plus Lugol's solution, 30 drops per day in divided doses. The iodine and iodide in Lugol's solution reduces vascularity of the hyperactive gland. Exophthalmos is rarely benefited by thyroidectomy, and usually becomes worse postoperatively. Every effort should therefore be made to treat exophthalmic goiter medically, including possible use of immunosuppressive agents to reduce secretion of the gamma globulin (long-acting thyroid stimulating hormone — LATS) recently incriminated in hyperthyroidism.

Colloid goiter in euthyroid patients is usually operated upon for cosmetic reasons or to rule out the presence of cancer. This disease is more common in geographical regions in which the diet is deficient in iodine. Since a goiter may extend posterior to the sternum, a chest x-ray must be obtained preoperatively.

The best management of a thyroid nodule is still debated between internists and surgeons. It has been reported that well-differentiated papillary or follicular carcinoma can be suppressed with high doses (180 mg or more) of thyroid hormone per day. Nevertheless, we believe that surgical treatment is preferable. A percutaneous Vim-Silverman needle biopsy can be performed in the Outpatient Clinic, with convalesence overnight in the observation ward. If the nodule is superficial and easily biopsied, report of an adenoma probably justifies medical therapy. But if carcinoma is found, surgery is indicated. Our hospital has received two patients in the past four years who had massive, slowly growing local recurrences of papillary carcinoma of the thyroid which were eventually fatal. The type of operation performed will vary with the gross and microscopic findings at exploration. For biopsy-proven follicular or papillary carcinoma, total lobectomy of the involved lobe and subtotal lobectomy of the contralateral lobe appear to be indicated. A careful neck exploration should be performed for metastases, and a modified neck dissection should be done if tumor is found in the nodes. In less well-differentiated tumors, a larger margin of surgical excision is necessary for success, although in undifferentiated cancer of the thyroid the results of excision are no better than are achieved by tracheostomy and radiation therapy. Medullary carcinoma, a functioning tumor of the thyroid "C" cells, may occur by itself or in a familial disease associated with pheochromocytoma (Sipple's syndrome).

Patients may develop postoperative hypoparathyroidism of a significant degree, but it may be missed if it develops slowly. Chronic, severe, hypoparathyroidism has been reported in a large percentage of patients following thyroidectomy for a variety of reasons. In such patients, mental sluggishness, constipation or premature aging should be signs which warrant obtaining serum calcium and urinary calcium determination.

Hypothyroidism should be recognized and treated prior to performance of elective surgery for other diseases. Since the signs may be subtle, it should be remembered that hypothyroidism is a common late complication of I^{131} treatment for thyrotoxicosis, or of hypophysectomy—if the patient does not take thyroid hormone. Thickened tongue, mental sluggishness, viscid peripheral edema and heart disease should alert the surgeon to study his patient and to arrange for proper therapy to be given.

Tests of thyroid function in outpatients include:

1. Basal metabolism. Used with decreasing frequency in recent years because of the relative ease and greater accuracy of other tests.

2. Plasma bound iodine (PBI). This test is invalid in patients who have received iodine in any form in recent weeks, including I^{131}, iodine surgical skin prep, or iodine-containing radiopaque dyes, as in IVP or gallbladder x-rays.

3. I^{131} uptake in neck. The normal value is 30 per cent in 24 hours. Abnormal values range from greater than 40 per cent in hyperthyroidism to less than 10 per cent in hypothyroidism.

4. I^{131} scan (searching for differentiation between "hot" and "cold" areas in the gland and outside the gland—in which case metastatic cancer of the thyroid is suspected).

5. Red cell T^3 uptake.

6. Chest x-ray: looking for metastases, substernal thyroid, or evidence of heart disease secondary to hyper- or hypothyroidism.

7. Lateral x-ray of trachea.

8. Barium swallow with view of larynx and trachea.

Parathyroid

Diagnosis of hyperparathyroidism has been made earlier in the course of the disease in recent years. It is now rare for patients to present with hypercalcemic crisis or endstage multisystem disease resulting from long-standing hyperparathyroidism. Consistent elevation of serum calcium is a sufficient indication for parathyroid exploration if other causes have been ruled out. Other causes include sarcoidosis, metastatic cancer, chronic renal disease, vitamin D intoxication, multiple myeloma, hyperthyroidism, and milk-alkali syndrome. Obviously, a thorough general medical and endocrinological work-up should be done before parathyroid exploration is carried out. The surgeon should review the information and ask for confirmatory tests in questionable cases, and for tests which will help localize the lesions if they are available. The most common of these additional tests are barium swallow (looking for impingement by a posteriorly situated adenoma), radioactive selenium scan (now considered relatively ineffective), and selective percutaneous thyrocervical arteriography (probably the best technique now available for localization of an adenoma).

Tests which may be used in outpatients are:

1. Serum calcium, repeated until at least three elevated values are obtained.
2. Serum phosphorus (should be low; if both Ca and P are elevated, hyperparathyroidism due to adenoma is less likely than if P is subnormal).
3. Urinary calcium (24-hour excretion, while on 200 mg calcium diet). Excretion of more than 200 mg per day indicates an increased rate of turnover of calcium and is consistent with hyperparathyroidism. Excretion of more than 200 mg per day also will occur in other types of hypercalcemia, such as metastatic cancer and multiple myeloma.
4. Barium swallow (look for indentation by adenoma).
5. Chest x-ray (to rule out sarcoidosis and metastatic carcinoma).
6. BUN and creatinine. If these values are elevated, consider the possibility of parathyroid hyperplasia due to chronic renal disease, rather than adenoma. But renal failure can also develop in longstanding hyperparathyroidism, owing to recurrent formation of calculi.
7. Selective thyrocervical arteriography.
8. X-rays of bones: long bones, hands and teeth. Look for cysts, fractures, reabsorption ("motheaten" bones), or absent lamina dura.

Hyperparathyroidism may be due to any of several pathologic conditions. Parathyroid adenomas were formerly found as the cause in up to 80 per cent of patients, with hyperplasia occurring in most of the remainder. Parathyroid carcinoma ranges from 1 to 4 per cent in various hospitals. Hyperplasia is now found increasingly in hospitals which manage chronic renal failure and have a large number of renal transplant recipients. Of adenomas, three-fourths are tumors of chief cells (eosinophilic), and approximately half of the rest are water-clear cells. Adenomas may be multiple or recurrent, and patients must be followed permanently following para-

thyroidectomy for signs or symptoms of either recurrent hyperparathyroidism or other endocrine adenomas.

Pancreas

Abnormalities in carbohydrate metabolism may be dramatic in patients with hormone-secreting tumors of the pancreas. Most of these patients are seen initially by internists, psychiatrists or endocrinologists, and are referred to surgeons only after a long work-up has been performed. Since hyperactivity of normal islets may be difficult to distinguish from adenoma, patients are often remarkably late in undergoing laparotomy. It should be remembered that patients with β-cell (insulin-secreting) adenomas do not necessarily exhibit Whipple's triad. In Tompkins' series of ten insulin-secreting adenomas, three did not have the classic pattern of blood sugar less than 50 mg/100 ml with symptoms, and symptoms which were relieved by administration of glucose. The accuracy and safety of selective celiac arteriography has increased remarkably in past years, and patients with a question of adenoma should undergo this study. Alpha cell glucagon-secreting adenomas are very rare, but can also be localized by arteriography. Patients with the Zollinger-Ellison syndrome (δ-cell adenoma) are usually seen early by surgeons because of the severity of their ulcer diathesis. If possible, patients suspected of this diagnosis should also undergo arteriography, although occasionally the complication of gastrointestinal perforation or hemorrhage requires emergency surgery. Most of the procedures for study of small, functioning pancreatic tumors require inpatient care. However, arteriography can easily and safely be performed in outpatients if a period of close observation follows the procedure.

The tests which can be performed on outpatients include:

1. Fasting blood sugar.
2. Glucose tolerance test, with careful observation for reactive hypoglycemia.

If symptoms of hypoglycemia develop, a blood sugar should be drawn immediately for documentation.

3. Serum insulin (immunoreactive insulin, or—less satisfactory—insulin-like activity).

4. GI series, with small bowel follow through, looking for indentation into barium column, widened C-loop of duodenum, peptic ulcer, or anterior displacement of duodenum.

5. Selective celiac arteriography, with venous phase also studied for "tumor blush" in pancreas or liver, or displacement of arteries around a tumor nodule.

6. Serum gastrin immunoassay (not yet routinely available in most hospitals).

Adrenal

Functioning adrenal cortical tumors may produce Cushing's syndrome (glucocorticoids) or Conn's syndrome (aldosterone). Adrenal medullary tumors – pheochromocytomas – secrete epinephrine and other catecholamines, causing episodic hypertension and fever. Pheochromocytomas can also occur in other areas of the body, especially in the retroperitoneum at the bifurcation of the aorta—the organ of Zuckerkandl. Arteriography is therefore an important part of their work-up. Patients with adrenal tumors are almost invariably referred to surgeons after a prolonged medical work-up, which usually involves a period of hospitalization for study.[13] If the possibility of one of these lesions arises in a surgical outpatient, a simple series of tests may be utilized for screening purposes. Most patients admitted for surgery will already have undergone these tests:

1. Fasting blood sugar (elevated by epinephrine and corticosteroids).

2. Urinary excretion of ketosteroids and ketogenic steroids (24-hour collections, with volume and creatinine recorded).

3. Plasma cortisol.

4. ACTH test (see Pituitary gland).

5. Decadron suppression; effect of 4–12 mg per day of decadron on steroid excretion. If ACTH-induced hyperplasia is present, steroid output will decrease to normal during decadron administration. If adenoma is present, output will usually decrease somewhat. Functioning adrenal cortical carcinoma usually does not alter output when decadron is given.

6. Metapirone test to determine the effectiveness of adrenal-pituitary homeostatic balance. (See Pituitary gland.)

7. Glucose tolerance test.

8. Serum Na and K. Sodium is variable and potassium is low in Cushing's syndrome; potassium is especially low in Conn's syndrome. The effect of adrenal steroids can also be seen in urine: sodium is retained and potassium is excreted in higher than normal amounts.

9. Blood pressure (elevated in Cushing's syndrome and pheochromocytoma).

10. Urinary catecholamine and VMA excretion for suspected adrenal medullary tumor. False positive is seen when bananas are present in diet.

11. Selective distal aortography and adrenal arteriography and venography.

The outpatient surgeon must be alert to the possibility of a crisis of insufficient adrenal hormone production associated with any surgical procedure in patients who have received therapy with cortisone or its derivatives, in patients with tuberculosis or metastatic cancer,[9] and in patients treated with Rauwolfia derivatives, which deplete nerve ending granules of catecholamines.

Carcinoid

Patients with the carcinoid syndrome exhibit, to a varying degree, one or more of the following signs and symptoms: (1) cutaneous flushing—constant or intermittent, (2) diarrhea, (3) dyspnea, with or without asthma, (4) palpitations and cardiac arrythmias, (5) neurosis or psychosis, (6) fluid retention, (7) abdominal mass and (8) abdominal pain. Functioning carcinoid tumors occur mainly in the midgut (ileum, appendix and cecum). They usually secrete serotonin, and occasionally other hormones such as bradykinin, ACTH and insulin. The diagnosis of a functioning carcinoid tumor is confirmed by an elevated level of urinary 5-hydroxy indole acetic acid (5 HIAA). The normal excretion of 5 HIAA is ≤ 16 mg per day. Most patients with functioning carcinoids will excrete amounts larger than this—up to 1000 mg or more per day in some cases. Occasionally 5 HIAA excretion is only slightly increased, 5 hydroxy tryptophane being the metabolite excreted by the tumor. Not all patients with carcinoid tumors develop the carcinoid syndrome, since some carcinoids do not produce hormones. Serotonin is detoxified in the liver, so hepatic or pulmonary metastases are usually present in patients who have the syndrome. A rare exception to this rule exists with primary or metastatic carcinoids of the ovary, which can produce the syndrome because venous drainage of the ovary bypasses the liver. Carcinoids are slow-growing tumors and usually metastasize late in the natural history of the disease. Most patients are cured by resection of the primary tumor. The most common site is the appendix; bronchial adenomas of the carcinoid type are usually cured by lobectomy or a sleeve resection of the bronchus. Palliative resection of tumor metastases has been performed in some patients with carcinoid syndrome, and cardiac surgery has also been performed in cases where the myxofibrous reaction produced pulmonic stenosis. Usually the treatment is pharmacological, using serotonin antagonists, cytotoxic agents or palliative drugs.[11] Hepatic artery infusion with 5-fluorouracil should be considered in patients who do not respond to systemic therapy.

Ovary and Placenta

The outpatient evaluation and treatment of lesions of the female organs is discussed in detail in Chapter 20. The endocrinological problems considered are predominantly related to sterility, amenorrhea and neoplasms. The studies which can conveniently and accurately be performed in outpatients to assess function in the pituitary-ovary-placenta relationships are:
1. Pregnancy tests—qualitative.
   a. A-Z test.
   b. Gravidex test.
2. Chorionic gonadotrophin (24-hour urine)—quantitative. If positive postpartum, choriocarcinoma must be ruled out.
3. Vaginal cytology for percent cornification. Squamous cells denote estrogen effect. A routine pap smear is performed, and the differential count is made on this specimen: cornified cells, precornified cells and basal cells.
4. Daily temperature record for estimation of date of ovulation.
5. Vaginal mucous test for estimation of date of ovulation.
6. Urinary ketosteroids and ketogenic steroids, to rule out adrenal tumor in patients with presumed polycystic (Stein-Leventhal) ovaries.

Testis

Tumors and questions of fertility are the major endocrinologic aspects evaluated regarding the testicles in outpatients. The diseases and studies are also discussed in Chapter 19. In summary, the studies appropriate in outpatients are:
1. Semen analysis (for volume of semen, sperm count—done in a hemocytometer—and sperm morphology on a stained, dry specimen).
2. Chorionic gonadotrophin—urinary. Should be performed in all males with gynecomastia. Unless an obvious, treatable cause is found for gynecomastia, a nonpalpable choriocarcinoma of the testis must be ruled out. Choriocarcinoma of testis may cause unilateral or bilateral gynecomastia. Other neoplasms, such as seminomas, teratomas and embryonal cancers of the testis may also secrete hormone and give positive CGT tests.
3. Urinary ketosteroids and ketogenic

steroids. Normal male production of ketosteroids is 10–20 mg per day.

4. Buccal smear. Testicular atrophy is one sign of Kleinfelter's syndrome, which is due to the XXY chromosome abnormality. These patients have a buccal smear which shows Barr bodies (female chromatin pattern).

5. Testicular biopsy. This test can be performed under local anesthesia with proper sedation, in the operating room associated with the Emergency Room, or in the main operating room. The patient can be released from the hospital later in the day.

Summary

Although definitive proof of an endocrinopathy usually requires hospitalization for completion of studies, endocrine diseases must first be suspected in ambulatory patients. The proper screening tests must be obtained to determine if further studies are warranted. An alert surgeon is sure to have his curiosity rewarded by the occasional discovery of patients with thyrotoxicosis, hyperparathyroidism, Cushing's syndrome, the Stein-Leventhal syndrome, or other endocrine diseases. If the disease is discovered while it is still localized and curable, this diligence should permit restoration of the patient to a normal life.

References

1. Berman, I. R., Moseley, R. V., Doty, D. B., and Gutierrez, V. S.: Post-traumatic alkalosis in young men with combat injuries. Surg. Gynecol. Obstet., *133*:11–15, 1971.
2. Buchwald, H., Frantz, I. D., Jr., and Gebhard, R. L.: Effect of ileal bypass versus ileal excision on cholesterol synthesis and whole blood cholesterol concentration in the rabbit. Surgery, *64*:126–133, 1968.
3. Comroe, J. H., et al.: The Lung: Clinical Physiology and Pulmonary Function Tests. Chicago, Year Book Medical Publishers, Inc., 1962.
4. Dudrick, S. J., Wilmore, D. W., Vars, H. M., and Rhoads, J. E.: Long-term total parenteral nutrition with growth, development and positive nitrogen balance. Surgery, *64*:134–141, 1968.
5. Glenn, F., and Mannix, H., Jr.: Diagnosis and prognosis of Cushing's syndrome. Surg. Gynecol. Obstet., *126*:765–776, 1968.
6. Gruber, U. F.: Blood Replacement [Translated by L. Oxtoby and R. F. Armstrong]. New York, Springer, 1969.
7. Hill, G. J., II, and Longino, L. A.: Giant hemangioma with thrombocytopenia. Surg. Gynecol. Obstet., *114*:304–312, 1962.
8. Hill, G. J., II, Knight, V., and Jeffery, G. M.: Thrombocytopenia in vivax malaria. Lancet, *1*:240–241, 1964.
9. Hill, G. J., II, and Wheeler, H. B.: Adrenal insufficiency due to metastatic carcinoma of the lung: Case report and review of Addison's disease caused by adrenal metastases. Cancer, *18*:1467–1473, 1965.
10. Hill, G. J., II: Central venous pressure technique. Surg. Clin. N. Amer., *49*:1351–1359, 1969.
11. Hill, G. J., II: Carcinoid tumors: Pharmacological therapy. Oncology, *25*:329–343, 1971.
12. Home Economics Research Report No. 13, "Vitamin B-12".
13. Melby, J. C.: Assessment of adrenocortical function. N. Eng. J. Med., *285*:735–739, 1971.
14. Moore, F. D.: The Metabolic Care of the Surgical Patient. Philadelphia, W. B. Saunders Co., 1959.
15. Palmer, A. J., and Blacket, R.: Regression of xanthomata of the eyelids with modified fat diet. Lancet, *1*:66–68, 1972.
16. Schumer, W.: Metabolic considerations in the preoperative evaluation of the surgical patient. Surg. Gynecol. Obstet., *121*:611–620, 1965.
17. Shieber, W., Kingsbury, R., and Baue, A. E.: The role of the thyroid gland in the hypocalcemia of acute pancreatitis. Surg. Forum, *22*:333–334, 1971.
18. Shires, G. T.: Fluid and electrolyte therapy. In Kinney, J. M., Egdahl, R. H., and Zuidema, G. D. (eds.): Manual of Preoperative and Postoperative Care. Philadelphia, W. B. Saunders Co., 1971.
19. Shoemaker, W. C., and Walker, W. F.: Fluid-Electrolyte Therapy in Acute Illness. Chicago, Year Book Medical Publishers, Inc., 1970.
20. Skillman, J. J., Awwad, H. K., and Moore, F. D.: Plasma protein kinetics of early transcapillary refill after hemorrhage in man. Surg. Gynecol. Obstet., *125*:983–996, 1967.
21. Tompkins, R. K., Hardacre, J. M., Tzagournis, M., and Greider, M.: Definitive diagnosis of insulin-secreting tumors of the pancreas. Surg. Gynecol. Obstet., *125*:1069–1074, 1967.
22. Watt, B. K., and Merrill, A.: Composition of foods; raw, processed, prepared. Washington: U. S. Dept. of Agriculture, 1963. (U. S. Dept. of Agriculture. Agriculture Handbook no. 8).
23. Wilson, R. E., Bernhard, W. F., Polet, H., and Moore, F. D.: Hyperparathyroidism: The problem of acute parathyroid intoxication. Ann. Surg., *159*:79–93, 1964.

7

The Nervous System — Neurosurgery

By THOMAS K. CRAIGMILE, M.D.

NECESSARY FACILITIES AND EQUIPMENT

Although fewer and less specialized instruments are usually employed in the surgical treatment of trauma and other acute neurological lesions than in the more intricate and difficult cases, certain ones are essential. Every experienced surgeon has his favorite instruments, but the neurosurgical house officer and the general surgeon who must deal only occasionally with an acute disorder of the nervous system

171

require only certain basic instruments to perform creditably. These include:

1. Basic neurosurgical instruments and supplies (Fig. 7–1)
2. Craniotomy instruments
3. Laminectomy instruments
4. Equipment for angiography (Fig. 7–2)

The electrosurgical unit, suction, tantalum or silver hemostatic clips with the appropriate appliers, bone wax, Gelfoam, and cottonoid sponges are indispensable for the proper conduct of cranial and spinal operations. The operating table must be fully adjustable and the use of a three point headholder often facilitates the establishment and main-

tenance of proper position in cranial cases. The use of the surgical microscope is occasionally helpful. Serial film changing devices are necessary for adequate angiography, and a pressure injector must often be used when transfemoral or transbrachial techniques are employed.

The neurosurgical operating room should be large, uncluttered, and windowless. The use of an adjacent anesthesia room avoids unnecessary sources of contamination and confusion. When the operating room lighting is adequate, headlights, lighted retractors, and other supplemental sources of illumination are rarely necessary. If

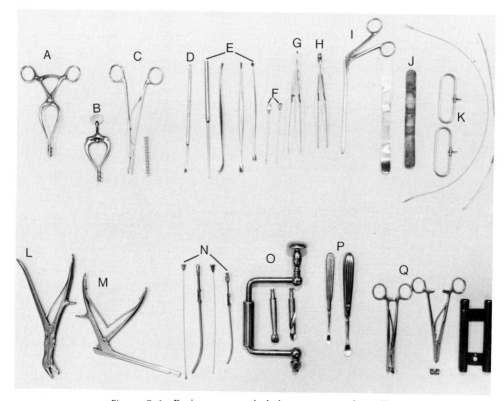

Figure 7–1 Basic neurosurgical instruments and supplies.

A Weitlander self-retaining retractor
B Jansen mastoid retractor
C Weck clip applicator and clips
D Dura separator
E Penfield dissectors
F Ventricular needle and stylet
G Bayonet forcep
H Bipolar bayonet forcep
I Pituitary rongeur

J Ribbon retractors
K Gigli saw, guide wire and handles
L Duckbill rongeur
M Schlesinger rongeur
N Neurosurgical suction tips and stylets
O Hudson drill with Cushing burr and perforator
P Osteotomes
Q Raney clip appliers and clips

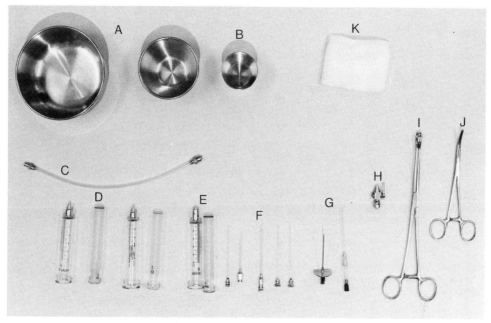

Figure 7–2 Equipment for angiography.

A Solution bowls
B Medicine cup
C Adapter tubing
D Syringes, 10 ml, plain tip
E Syringe, 10 ml, Luer lock

F Spinal needles with obturators
G Cournand needle
H Stopcock, Luer lock
I Sponge forcep
J Kelly clamp

the theater does not contain wall-mounted radiographic tubes, portable x-ray equipment should be available.

ANCILLARY DIAGNOSTIC STUDIES

Skull Films

Routine radiographic studies of the skull are usually made after the preliminary clinical evaluation of the patient with an acute craniocerebral injury or with acutely increased intracranial pressure due to a suspected space-occupying lesion (Fig. 7–3). The most helpful film projections are the anterior-posterior, Towne, lateral stereoscopic and base views. Other special views and tomographic studies are occa-

sionally needed to provide detail not visualized in routine examinations. Except in those extraordinary circumstances when the patient cannot be moved from his bed because of attached orthopedic traction appliances, the films should be made in the radiology department. Portable skull films are almost invariably of poor technical quality, and disclose only the most glaring abnormalities.

In the patient who has sustained a cranial injury, one may observe several changes which influence management. These include a simple fracture overlying or interrupting the course of an arterial or venous channel, a depressed fracture, displacement of a calcified pineal or, rarely, calcified choroid plexuses, pneumocephalus, or the presence of an unsuspected intracranial foreign body. Pathological intracranial calcification, displacement of normally

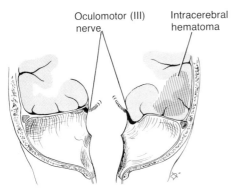

Oculomotor (III) nerve   Intracerebral hematoma

Figure 7–3 Compression of oculomotor nerve in uncal herniation. Pupillary inequality in acute craniocerebral injury is commonly caused by temporal lobe hematoma, causing compression and traction on the oculomotor (III cranial) nerve. Pupillary inequality is usually a late sign of trauma to the brain, and its development is often preceded by bradycardia and depression in consciousness. Coma usually follows, accompanied by cessation in all extraocular motor function. Isolated extraocular muscle palsy is rarely seen in trauma, except in orbital or periorbital injuries.

calcified structures, proliferative or lytic cranial lesions, or inflammatory changes in the paranasal sinuses or mastoid air cells may be seen in patients with neoplasms or abscesses. General and local radiographic changes associated with increased intracranial pressure vary according to age. They include separation of cranial sutures, increased convolutional markings, diffuse or focal changes of the sella, destruction of the clinoid processes, and areas of thinning of the cranial vault or sphenoid wing.

Spine Films

Since unnecessary transport of a patient who has had a recent spinal injury is to be avoided, preliminary portable anterior-posterior and lateral x-rays should be made on the Emergency Room table or the ambulance litter. Subsequent films to assess the effectiveness of measures to reduce a fracture-dislocation may be made without moving the patient from his Foster frame or circular bed. All other spinal studies, including those in persons suspected of having acute intraspinal tumors, abscesses, or hematomas or acute herniations of the intervertebral discs, should be conducted in the radiology department. Anterior-posterior, lateral, and oblique views are taken routinely. They may be supplemented by views made in flexion or extension or by tomograms in special instances. Visualization of the relationship of the sixth cervical vertebra to the seventh is a commonly encountered problem in a heavy person with a compact neck in whom there may be considerable paraspinal muscle spasm. This difficulty may often be overcome by careful traction upon the upper extremities, the direction of pull being 45° anterior to the longitudinal axis of the body.

In the patient who has suffered acute trauma, particular attention must be directed to alterations in the relationship between vertebral bodies, pedicles, and articular facets and to the configuration of fractures—including spicules which may encroach upon the spinal canal and its contents. When an intraspinal mass lesion is considered, destructive lesions may be observed in the vertebral bodies or pedicles. Similar changes may involve the laminae and spinous processes but are less readily evident. Hemangiomas and osteitis deformans produce typical structural changes. Focal widening of the canal usually accompanies only the more slowly growing neoplasms. Often no abnormality can be seen in spinal roentgenograms in the presence of an acute intervertebral disc herniation. Occasionally there will be a reduction in the intervertebral space (which is not invariably at the level of nerve root compression), and osteophytes which contribute to the neural compromise may occur in the cervical region. Subluxation secondary to spondylitis may be a factor in cervical nerve root and cord compression, while spondylolisthesis and spondylolysis are often present in those with lumbar disc syndromes.

Echoencephalography

Echoencephalography is a useful screening diagnostic aid in the presence of those supratentorial lesions causing lateral distortion of the septum pellucidum and third ventricle. It can be carried out with little hazard except in those cases in which clinical deterioration is occurring so rapidly that even the slightest delay in surgical decompression may be critical.

Brain Scanning and Electroencephalography

The need to establish quickly the exact nature of the lesion in the injured patient or in the person with rapidly increasing intracranial pressure secondary to a tumor or abscess usually precludes the use of radioisotope scanning or electroencephalography as diagnostic aids. When the patient's condition is stable or the progression of neurological change is slow, both tests may be informative. A peripherally disposed arc of increased uptake overlying one or both cerebral hemispheres on the scan may be seen in the presence of a subdural hematoma. Intracerebral areas of heightened activity ordinarily suggest that the lesion is a rather vascular neoplasm, although such abnormalities may be due to infarcts, abscesses, intracerebral hematomas, arteriovenous malformations or giant aneurysms. A slow wave electroencephalographic focus may be due to any one of several common destructive processes involving the cerebral hemispheres. Of the extracerebral lesions, hematomas infrequently produce localized dysrhythmias. More frequent causes are peripherally situated tumors, subdural empyema and cortical vein thrombosis.

Cerebral Angiography

Cerebral angiography is the radiographic study which provides the most specific diagnostic information with the least immediate or potential hazard, in a wide aggregation of both supra- and infratentorial lesions which demand prompt attention. Included are the cases of suspected epidural, subdural and intracerebral hematoma, tumor, abscess, aneurysms and other vascular malformations, and instances of intracranial or extracranial vascular occlusion. In many cases the pathological nature of the disorder can be established along with its anatomic site. Changes in vascular configuration suggest or confirm herniation through the tentorial incisure or foramen magnum, or beneath the falx, while an accurate measurement of ventricular size may be made from both arterial and venous studies. Angiography ordinarily produces little or no alteration in intracranial hydrodynamics and pressure relationships — a notable safety feature compared with pneumography.

The suspected presence of an acute intracranial hematoma or, rarely, a swiftly enlarging abscess is the only reason for performing angiography in an institution which does not have a well-equipped and adequately staffed neurosurgical unit. When the circumstances are less urgent, the patient with an intracranial lesion should be transferred to a hospital with proper neurosurgical facilities. Angiography should not be performed under suboptimal conditions for patients who are not critically ill, since the result is usually a substandard examination which must be repeated later under more suitable conditions.

Cerebral angiography should ordinarily be performed as one of the final steps in the orderly investigation of a neurological disorder when the earlier clinical and laboratory examinations indicate that it will establish or, occasionally, exclude a diagnosis more effectively and safely than any other method. In no event should it be carried out as a routine diagnostic screening maneuver. The study should be performed only upon the order of one well qualified in neurological diagnosis and under his direction so that essential views may be made and unnecessary ones avoided.

Not infrequently, in the individual with an acutely expanding intracranial process, decline in neurological function is so rapid that routine systematic investigation must be abandoned and only the most specifically informative evaluations made. In such instances, rapidly repeated clinical examinations will indicate the necessity for haste, and routine skull films can be taken and angiography performed while the operating room is being prepared for the anticipated operation. A decision to proceed with extraordinary haste is a difficult one for the inexperienced surgeon, but may be lifesaving.

Principal contraindications to angiography are: (1) an extremely rapid clinical deterioration of the patient with a suspected acute hematoma, (2) severe arterial hypertension, and (3) a demonstrated sensitivity to the contrast medium.

In the patient with quickly advancing signs of an acute expanding process, there is simply not sufficient time to permit angiography, although the examination would supply information helpful in planning the operation. This situation presents the only absolute contraindication.

When angiography is deemed essential to establish a diagnosis in the patient with extraordinarily elevated blood pressure, antihypertensive drugs should be administered. A previous allergic reaction to an orally or intravenously administered iodine compound does not always portend intolerance to an iodine-containing contrast medium. Advanced age alone is not a contraindication, nor is a previous complication of angiography not attributed to hypersensitivity to the contrast material.

The techniques and typical findings in arteriography are illustrated in Figures 7–4, 7–5 and 7–6.

CRANIOCEREBRAL INJURIES

Acute epidural hematoma is illustrated in the arteriogram in Figure 7–7. Emergency evacuation may be performed by twist drill aspiration (Fig. 7–8), but if time permits, a limited craniectomy

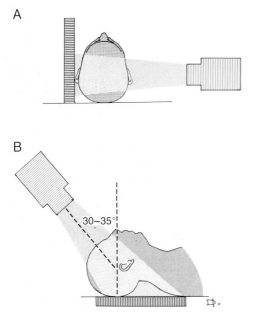

A

B

Figure 7–4 X-ray tube placement in biplane carotid angiography. The patient is supine, with the nose pointed directly anterior. Films are taken simultaneously in lateral and anterior-posterior projections. *A.* Lateral projection. The tube is centered immediately superior to the ear. *B.* AP projection (modified Towne position). The tube is 30–35° off the vertical, and is centered on a point immediately superior to a line which passes through both ears.

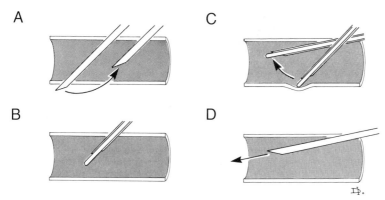

Figure 7–5 Needle placement in carotid angiography. An 18 gauge spinal needle is used for carotid arteriography, modified by removal of the distal 5 mm of the needle tip.

A. Needle is inserted into arterial lumen. If it is initially passed through the artery, it is withdrawn slightly until good arterial pulse of blood indicates that it is within the lumen.

B. Obturator is then introduced in the needle.

C. Hub of needle is then depressed, so that needle is directed superiorly. If needle is close to back wall of artery, obturator protects intima from injury, as shown.

D. Contrast material is injected after obturator is withdrawn.

Conray (meglumine iothalamate) 60 per cent is currently used for arteriography in our Clinic. X-rays are taken during the definitive injection five minutes after a test dose of 1 cc. For arteriogram, a 7 cc dose is injected rapidly from a 10 ml syringe. Simultaneous lateral and AP x-rays are taken, beginning midway in the injection. The first six x-rays are taken at 30 second intervals, and the next five at 1 second intervals. Needle is left in place until technical adequacy of the x-rays has been determined. Firm compression over a gauze sponge is used after the needle is withdrawn, until all bleeding ceases.

should be performed (Fig. 7–9). The differences between acute and chronic subdural hematomas are shown diagrammatically in Figure 7–10. The method of evacuation of chronic subdural hematoma is shown in Figure 7–11. Patients with acute spinal cord injuries should receive immediate stabilization with

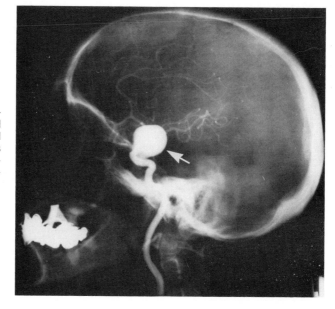

Figure 7–6 Large internal carotid aneurysm. Patient had visual field defect and impaired visual acuity. Giant aneurysms such as this (arrow) rarely bleed. They commonly cause compression of adjacent neural structures.

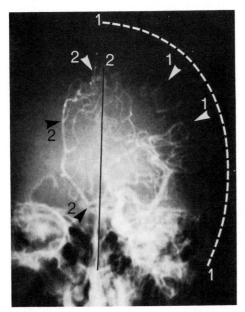

Figure 7–7 Acute epidural hematoma. Carotid arteriogram in a 68 year old man with an acute epidural hematoma. There is marked displacement (arrow 1) of the middle cerebral arterial group from the inner table of the skull (dotted line), with an extreme transfalx herniation of the brain, as demonstrated by a 3.0 cm shift of the anterior cerebral artery (arrow 2). Craniotomy was immediately performed, but was unsuccessful.

Crutchfield tongs (Fig. 7–12). Compound depressed skull fracture requires prompt decompression (Fig. 7–13).

ACUTELY INCREASED INTRACRANIAL PRESSURE DUE TO TUMORS AND OTHER SPACE-OCCUPYING LESIONS

Diagnosis

Frequently patients with rapidly growing cerebral tumors or other lesions producing obstruction to the normal circulation of cerebrospinal fluid within the ventricular system will be seen because of clinical findings of acutely in-

creased intracranial pressure. The illness may seemingly be of exceedingly brief duration but the history may reveal a significantly longer period of prodromal headache, loss of visual acuity, diplopia, impaired intellectual function, dysphasia, varying motor and sensory abnormalities or seizures. Careful inquiry should be made concerning recent paranasal sinus, or mastoid, pulmonary or systemic infections which could be a primary locus responsible for abscess formation.

A sudden increase in the intensity of symptoms produced by a supratentorial tumor — in addition to simply rapid growth of the neoplasm — may be due to reactive swelling of the adjacent brain with accompanying necrosis, formation of a neoplastic cyst, and bleeding from an abnormally fragile vessel supplying the tumor. When the mass compromises the ventricular circulation, precipitous

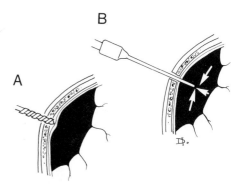

Figure 7–8 Twist drill aspiration of acute hematoma. Emergency aspiration of acute epidural or subdural hematoma may be performed in the emergency room or at the bedside if necessary. Skin is prepared in the midpoint of the cranium, immediately superior to temporalis muscle, placing the drill hole superior to the major trunk of the middle meningeal artery. *A.* A small incision is made, and the drill is inserted through the skull and dura. *B.* After drill tip has entered hematoma, it is removed and a 15 gauge brain cannula is passed in to evacuate the hematoma.

The most reliable lateralizing signs in coma due to acute epidural hematoma are: 1. Hematoma is on the same side as the dilated pupil, if there is pupillary inequality, or 2. Hematoma is on the side of obvious external trauma to the head.

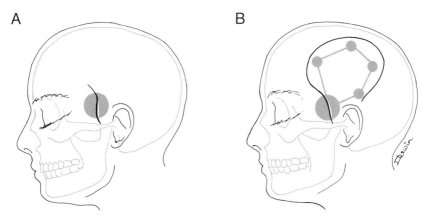

Figure 7–9 Incision and possible extension for craniectomy. *A*. Scalp incision and extent of bone removed in subtemporal craniectomy. *B*. Method of combining subtemporal craniectomy and osteoplastic craniectomy for the evacuation of acute epidural or subdural hematomas.

deterioration results from obstruction within the third or fourth ventricle, at the level of aqueduct of Sylvius, or at the foramina of Magendie or Luschka. Such obstruction may follow either direct tumor occlusion, compression or herniation at the tentorium or foramen magnum. In the presence of an abscess, sudden decline may be due to rapid enlargement of the primary lesion, edema of adjacent cerebral tissue, or cerebral or cerebellar herniation.

Some degree of impairment of the sensorium is often apparent, and the patient may be profoundly obtunded. Nuchal rigidity may be present, due to cerebellar herniation. Bradycardia, arterial hypertension and depressed respiratory activity are common, and one may observe anisocoria secondary to oculomotor compression by a herniating uncus (Fig. 7–3). Generally, increased intracranial pressure may be manifested by papilledema and unilateral or bilateral abducens palsies. There may be varying abnormalities of motor func-

Figure 7–10 Configuration of brain in acute and chronic subdural hematoma. In the acute lesion (left), the cerebral convexity is maintained. After about three weeks, the hematoma assumes a lentiform configuration (right), and the cerebral deformity is concave.

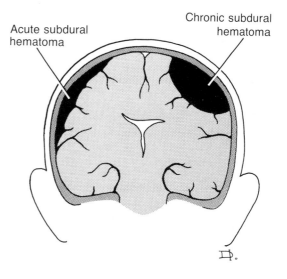

Acute subdural hematoma

Chronic subdural hematoma

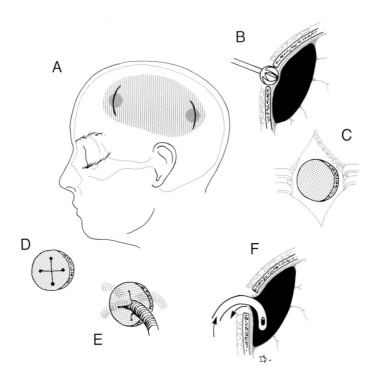

Figure 7–11 Evacuation of chronic subdural hematoma. Chronic hematoma should be evacuated on the day that it is diagnosed, since deterioration may occur rapidly at any time.

A. Shaded area shows the extent of hematoma in this patient, and location of burr holes. Hematoma was localized by preoperative angiography.

B. Burr hole is made through the skull, but not through dura. Cushing burr and Hudson brace are the preferred instruments.

C. Dura is exposed at bottom of burr hole. Bone fragments are removed by irrigation before proceeding. Hematoma is usually recognized at this point by bluish discoloration deep to dura.

D. Cruciate incision made in dura with a 15 Bard-Parker blade, following electrocoagulation of the line of the incision. Ends of incision are additionally coagulated to shrink the dura and increase exposure.

E. A 12 French soft rubber catheter is inserted.

F. Subdural space is evacuated by irrigation with normal saline. Wound is closed in layers.

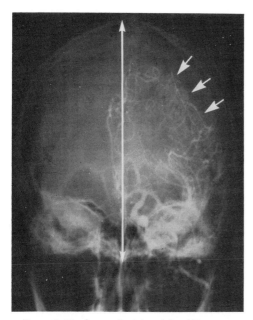

Figure 7-12 Large chronic subdural hematoma. Depression of the middle cerebral arterial branches, and lateral displacement of anterior cerebral artery to the opposite side (arrows). Configuration of the vessels indicates that this hematoma is more than three weeks old. (Brain is concave and hematoma is lenticular.)

zation usually demands the use of angiography or ventriculography, and often both studies are necessary (Figs. 7-14 and 7-15). Emergency decompression of the ventricular system in the casualty ward or at the bedside can be done simply through a twist drill opening and may be lifesaving. Occasionally a mass of reduced vascularity, as seen on the angiogram, indicates the presence

A

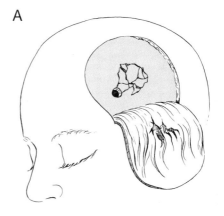

B

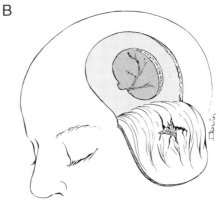

tion in the extremities and the plantar response may be one of extension on one side or both.

The general physical examination should be thorough in an effort to recognize evidence of focal or systemic infection or of metabolic disorder. Laboratory evaluation should include a complete biochemical survey and studies to detect specific toxic substances if a history of exposure is elicited.

Radiographs of the skull may disclose displacement of a calcified pineal gland, an abnormal intracranial calcification, a cranial destructive lesion or evidence of inflammation within the paranasal sinuses or mastoids. Radiographic evidence of generally increased intracranial pressure may be present. If the patient's condition permits and the test can be made without undue delay, radioisotope scanning may disclose an area of abnormal uptake. Precise locali-

Figure 7-13 Treatment of compound (open) depressed skull fracture. *A.* The burr hole is placed immediately adjacent to the fracture. *B.* Bone fragments are carefully removed. The cranial defect is debrided and the edges smoothed with a rongeur. Dural defects should be repaired with graft of temporal fascia or pericranium. Scalp margins should be debrided to remove contused or grossly contaminated areas.

Open fractures should also be treated with antibiotics and tetanus prophylaxis. Closed depressed fracture may be treated by elevating or repositioning the bone fragments.

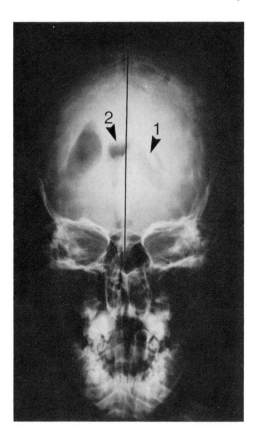

Figure 7–14   Brain abscess. Marked lateral and downward displacement of right lateral ventricle (arrow 1), and shift of third ventricle to patient's left (arrow 2), in a 10 year old boy with large parietal lobe abscess.

Figure 7–15   Left parietal glioma. Left carotid angiogram in a 15 year old girl who had developed headache and hemiparesis one week after a fall from a bicycle. Brain scan was strongly positive. Angiogram demonstrates a large anterior parietal stain (arrow 1). There is typical pathological vessel formation and marked downward displacement with stretching of the posterior temporal artery (arrow 2). With operation and external radiation therapy, the girl demonstrated temporary improvement.

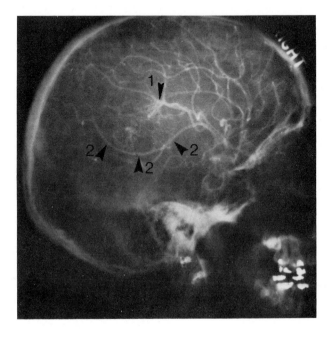

of a neoplastic cyst or an abscess which may, in urgent circumstances, be decompressed by a brain cannula inserted through a twist drill hole in an emergency or treatment room while the operating suite is being readied for a definitive surgical procedure. During ventriculography, the ventricular cannula will occasionally enter a tumor cyst or abscess, thereby fortuitously locating the lesion and effecting its decompression.

Treatment

The preferred treatment of most intracranial tumors, and certainly those producing life-threatening increases in intracranial pressure, is surgical excision. Often the involvement of vital neural or vascular structures by a tumor prohibits its complete excision and, in such cases, partial excision of the neoplasm combined with removal of the bone flap to effect decompression may be the only feasible choice. If a tumor obstructing the circulation of cerebrospinal fluid cannot be completely removed with reasonable safety, one of several shunting procedures may be carried out to decompress the ventricular system. Postoperative radiotherapy is a valuable adjunct in the management of several malignant and a few benign intracranial tumors. The employment of chemotherapeutic agents has thus far met with little practical success, but will surely play a more valuable role in the future.

Although there is some disagreement in the matter, the safest primary definitive surgical treatment of a brain abscess is usually simple tapping of the cavity, careful aspiration of its contents, and gentle irrigation with an antibiotic preparation. It is important to remember that many abscesses are multilocular and more than one insertion of the exploring cannula may be necessary to completely evacuate the contents of the various compartments. The abscess capsule is usually impermeable to systemically administered antibiotics, but antibiotics are important to prevent dissemination of infection secondary to operative contamination of the subarachnoid or subdural space. Repeated tapping of the abscess is usually required, and the progress of the treatment can be radiographically monitored by injecting a radiopaque substance (Thorotrast or Barosperse) into the lesion at the completion of the initial aspiration. In some cases, excision of the abscess capsule and its contents may be necessary if clinical or radiographic evidence of a significant mass lesion persists after a series of aspirations has been made. This can often be accomplished with little or no increase in the residual neurologic deficit and frequently results in significant return of function.

Convulsive seizures frequently accompany supratentorial neoplastic or inflammatory processes. Anticonvulsant medication should therefore be prescribed and continued once the diagnosis is established.

ACUTE SUBARACHNOID HEMORRHAGE

Diagnosis

Acute subarachnoid hemorrhage is usually due to rupture of an intracranial aneurysm, a cerebral vascular malformation, hypertension, or a defect in a sclerotic vessel. Less common sources of bleeding are intracranial and intraspinal tumors, intraspinal vascular lesions, and inadequately controlled anticoagulation therapy. Both intracranial and spinal trauma may, of course, be accompanied by varying degrees of subarachnoid hemorrhage, but bleeding into the thecal space in these instances is ordinarily insignificant in the overall evaluation and treatment of the primary injury.

Spontaneous hemorrhage is commonly followed shortly by severe, throbbing, generalized or fronto-occipital headache. Nausea and vomiting are usual symptoms, and photophobia is common. Thoracic or lumbar back pain or lower extremity radicular pain may be initial symptoms when the source of bleeding is intraspinal, but rarely when the lesion lies within the cranium. The state of consciousness may be altered from minimal drowsiness to deep coma. The lucid patient may be aware of some stiffness of the neck which usually appears some hours after the first manifestations of the hemorrhage. Focal cerebral symptoms may include motor or sensory abnormalities, difficulty in verbal expression or visual defects. Seizures may accompany cortical or intracerebral lesions, but are uncommon when the bleeding is confined to the subarachnoid space. Vascular abnormalities of the spinal cord may produce variable motor or sensory dysfunctions along with sphincter disturbances.

History. A careful history taken at the time of the first evident bleeding episode may disclose premonitory symptoms which were not recognized or were ignored. These include headache, often migrainous in nature, focal or general-ized seizures, and variable or transitory motor, sensory and speech disorders.

Intracranial aneurysms which are frequently encountered arise from the anterior communicating (Fig. 7–16 *A*), internal carotid, posterior communicating, middle cerebral, and basilar arteries. Less commonly involved are the arteries supplying structures within the posterior fossa. Sites of origin are usually bifurcations of major vessels. Giant aneurysms may bleed, but more frequently they disclose their presence by compromising adjacent neural structures and producing appropriate localizing manifestations. Arterial and arteriovenous malformations (Fig. 7–16 *B*) may occur in any portion of the cerebral or spinal circulation. Vascular malformations in the areas of distribution of the internal carotid arteries are the most common. Aneurysms of the venous sinuses are rare, predominately involving the vein of Galen. They may produce obstruction of cerebrospinal fluid pathways more often than other sites.

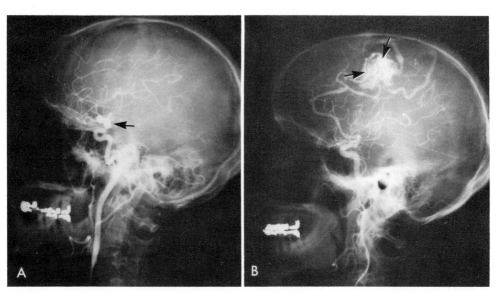

Figure 7–16 Arteriography in acute subarachnoid hemorrhage. *A.* Right carotid angiogram demonstrates large anterior communicating aneurysm (arrow), which was the site of hemorrhage. *B.* Left carotid angiogram demonstrates asymptomatic central arteriovenous malformation (arrows).

The anterior communicating aneurysm was suspected as the cause of bleeding, because a malformation such as that in *B* would cause localizing signs and arteriogram would show intracerebral hematoma. At operation, the aneurysm *(A)* was found to be the source of hemorrhage.

Most aneurysms appear at the site of congenital deficiency in the media of an artery. Incidental autopsy discovery or rupture of aneurysms is rare in children but occurs rather uniformly in the various age groups after the age of 20. Other etiological factors are trauma, infected emboli, arteriosclerosis and syphilis.

Examination of the patient with subarachnoid hemorrhage will disclose a sensorium which may vary from normal to profound coma. Blood pressure, pulse and respiratory rates are often not in an abnormal range but may be greatly altered when the degree of bleeding has been great and the intracranial pressure proportionately raised. Such changes are ominous prognostic signs. Middle cerebral and — less frequently — anterior cerebral aneurysms may bleed into the cerebral parenchyma as well as the subarachnoid space with resultant focal motor, dysphasic, sensory and visual deficits. Intrapontine hemorrhage from a basilar aneurysm may produce a variety of localizing neurologic changes, while signs of an intramedullary or a cord-compressing lesion may be in evidence when the abnormality has an intraspinal location. Nuchal rigidity, along with other manifestations of meningeal irritation, may be present at the onset but is often delayed. When hemorrhage has been severe, papilledema may appear early. Aneurysms may be classified on the basis of the patient's age, stage of consciousness and integrity of neurological function. This classification is a useful guide in the selection of patients for surgery.

Lumbar Puncture. In the acute phase, lumbar puncture will almost always confirm the diagnosis of subarachnoid bleeding. Cerebrospinal fluid is usually grossly hemorrhagic, with fluid ranging from a pink discoloration to what occasionally appears to be almost undiluted blood. Alterations in the appearance of the CSF due to injury of a vessel at the time of puncture ordinarily disappear promptly with the escape of a small quantity of fluid, while discoloration secondary to spontaneous hemorrhage persists. Should there be any uncertainty concerning the source of the bloody discoloration, the fluid must be centrifuged and the supernatant layer examined for xanthochromia. Such a color change, due to the presence of hemoglobin from lysed cells or bilirubin, is an indication that the hemorrhagic changes in the fluid existed prior to the puncture. Manometric pressure usually ranges from a small elevation to one of 300 to 400 millimeters of water. In extreme instances, however, the pressure rise may be to 600 millimeters or even greater. The hazards of lumbar puncture when the bleeding is contained within the subarachnoid space are ordinarily not great, but when there is clinical evidence of associated intracerebral hemorrhage a small bore needle should be employed and only a small amount of fluid removed. Removal of excessive quantities of CSF in the presence of an intracerebral mass could result in catastrophic incisural or foraminal herniation. Obviously, the Queckenstedt's test should never be performed when the CSF is bloody. In the period immediately following the hemorrhage, the cerebrospinal fluid may contain several hundred to as many as three million red blood cells per cmn with the leukocyte and protein content increased in proportion to the severity of the bleeding. The glucose content may be normal but is often reduced. When examination of the CSF is made some days after bleeding has occurred, the fluid is usually xanthochromic. The red blood cells are crenated and much reduced in number. The protein remains elevated while the glucose level returns to normal. Leukocytosis persists for some time. Depending upon the severity of the original hemorrhage and the absence of recurrent bleeding, gross xanthochromia disappears within a period of several days to three or four weeks.

Treatment

Primary care of the patient who has sustained a subarachnoid hemorrhage is directed toward prevention of further bleeding, which may be fatal or may increase the extent of neurologic deficit. A program of absolute bed rest must be employed, with avoidance of any exertion. If the state of consciousness permits, the head of the bed should be elevated. When the patient is unconscious, pulmonary complications can best be prevented by maintaining the bed on a level plane and frequently changing the patient's position. He should not be permitted to lie supine for more than short periods. Secretions should be gently and promptly removed from the respiratory tract. When parenteral fluid administration is required, fluid intake and electrolyte content should be physiologic. Blood pressure, if elevated above normal values, should be reduced with antihypertensive agents to minimize the possibility of additional bleeding. Repeated lumbar puncture may reduce the intensity of headache, but this technique is of little value in effectively removing erythrocytes from the cerebrospinal fluid. Narcotics and sedatives should be avoided. Anticonvulsant agents are not routinely used prior to surgery but should be employed if seizures occur.

Once the diagnosis of spontaneous subarachnoid hemorrhage has been made, specific diagnostic studies should be made to establish the nature and location of the lesion if the patient's condition permits. Occasionally roentgenograms of the skull will disclose displacement of a calcified pineal or calcification within an aneurysm, but usually plain x-rays are of little value. Similarly, brain scans, electroencephalograms and echoencephalograms rarely give helpful specific diagnostic information. Their routine use is not warranted. Curious aberrations in the electrocardiogram may follow subarachnoid hemorrhage and other intracranial disturbances, but surgical treatment is ordinarily not altered by these EKG changes.

If it appears that the patient will survive the initial bleeding episode, and if a severe neurological defect is not present which precludes surgery, angiography should be carried out promptly. Since aneurysms and other blood vessel malformations are frequently multiple, or may be fed by more than one arterial source, the carotid and vertebral circulation should be visualized bilaterally. Episodes of recurrent bleeding are common within one to two weeks of the original hemorrhage. Therefore, when a surgically correctible defect is found, and the general neurological status is acceptably intact, a definitive operation should be made without undue delay. A major contraindication to early surgery is the angiographic finding of significant spasm in the vessels from which the aneurysm arises. Appearance of such arterial constriction is an unfavorable prognostic sign and surgery should ordinarily be deferred until repeated angiography indicates that spasm has disappeared or materially lessened. Although early definitive surgical intervention is usually not advisable when there is appreciable impairment of consciousness or profound dysphasia or hemiparesis, an exception occurs when angiography discloses an intracerebral hematoma which accounts for the clinical deficit. In this instance, the clot should be evacuated as quickly and simply as possible. If the aneurysm can be readily identified, it should be dealt with at the time. Otherwise, definitive treatment should be postponed until swelling and hemorrhage recede and the neurological state improves.

The surgical treatment of intracranial aneurysms and other malformations is beyond the scope of this treatise, but certain principles may be pointed out. The ideal form of therapy of an accessible aneurysm is its exclusion from the parent vessel by the application of a metal clip or ligature to the aneurysm neck. When the size, location, or configuration of the lesion makes such treatment undesirable, other means may be utilized. These include reinforcement of the aneurysm wall with an adhesive plastic, fine-mesh gauze, or muscle, and induction of thrombosis within the aneurysm by electrical or magnetic force, by injection of animal bristles, or by reduction of blood flow through the lesion by extracranial carotid artery ligation. The use of hyperventilation and hypotensive anesthesia, osmotic agents to reduce brain volume, and the removal of cerebrospinal fluid during surgery has made the surgical approach to intracranial vascular abnormalities less formidable and reduced the morbidity and mortality accompanying operation. Hypothermia, once popular as a surgical adjunct, now enjoys less favor. Of cardinal importance in evaluating the patient with an arteriovenous malformation is the decision regarding the possibility of operation without creating an unacceptable neurological defect. Simple surgical occlusion of feeding vessels produces only temporary reduction in the size of the malformations. Complete excision of all the involved vessels is necessary for a cure. The employment of biplane, stereoscopic angiography is an invaluable aid in the intelligent planning of operations for arteriovenous malformations. Both myelography and spinal cord angiography may be necessary to accurately assess the configuration of intraspinal angioma. In the past, surgical treatment of these malformations consisted mainly of decompressive laminectomy, radiotherapy and ligation of readily accessible supplying arteries. All of these methods were rather uniformly ineffectual. Now the use of improved microsurgical techniques and bipolar coagulation for hemostasis permits complete excision of some angiomas with little or no increase in cord dysfunction. Percutaneous artificial embolization may be helpful in eradicating other less accessible lesions, but long-range observation of such cases has shown some favorable results to be temporary.

Vascular abnormalities of the nervous system are among the most formidable and treacherous confronting the surgeon. Surgery in such cases should be performed only in properly equipped hospitals providing capable assistants and expert anesthesiologists.

ACUTE OCCLUSIVE AND HEMORRHAGIC VASCULAR DISORDERS

Diagnosis of intracranial occlusive disease is usually first suspected by a history of stroke, with or without eventual recovery. The diagnosis should be confirmed by arteriography (Fig. 7–17). Treatment may include vasodilators or vascular surgery, including thrombectomy or embolectomy. In general, surgery is recommended only for patients with stable neurological status, although early operation is recommended in some centers if it can be started within the first 30 minutes after the stroke. Intracerebral occlusion of the thalamic artery may cause severe pain, a situation which is fortunately uncommon, since treatment is generally ineffective.

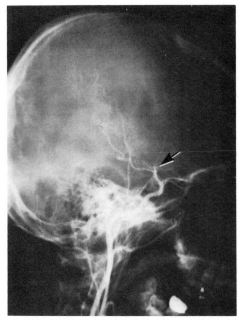

Figure 7–17 Acute thrombosis of internal carotid artery in a child. Thrombosis occurred at point marked by arrow. Almost all acute spontaneous occlusive carotid lesions in children occur intracranially, in contrast to the extracranial thrombosis which is common in adults. This child had a previous contralateral spontaneous internal carotid thrombosis from which she had recovered. She presented with hemiparesis at the time of this x-ray and again recovered spontaneously.

Occlusive extracranial disease presents a similar history, with the additional feature of intermittent small strokes which are now believed to be due to small emboli released from ulcerated placques in the carotid vessels. Other common syndromes are intermittent vertigo associated with basilar artery occlusion, and amaurosis fugax (temporary blindness) which can be caused by micro emboli of the arterial supply of the optic nerve and retina. Direction of blood flow is important in patients with arteriosclerosis obliterans, for cerebral vascular insufficiency may occur due to a "steal" of blood from the carotid to the subclavian artery, with retrograde flow down the affected carotid. Treatment is planned after carotid and vertebral arteriography is performed: this form of surgery inevitably requires careful neurological consultation, for the hazard of hemiplegia is significant following arteriography and surgery.

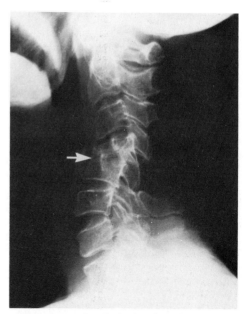

Figure 7–18 Cervical spine distortion from arthritis and failure of attempted fusion. Distortion of cervical spine, due to extensive osteoarthritis. Previous laminectomy elsewhere led to instability. An anterior interbody fusion at C_{4-5} (arrow) did not prevent continued deformity, and paraparesis developed. Extensive injury to cord occurred and no benefit could be achieved from reoperation.

ACUTE SPINAL CORD INJURIES

Spinal cord injuries may occur from direct or indirect trauma, or, rarely, from acute worsening of chronic bony degeneration (Fig. 7–18). The outcome is dependent upon the severity of trauma, since complete recovery may occur if only contusion has occurred, or in the presence of compression which can be relieved. On the other hand, paraplegia will be permanent if the cord has been severed (Fig. 7–19). Early operation may be hazardous if the spine is not displaced and function begins to return within a few hours after injury. On the other hand, surgery may be necessary to establish the diagnosis of a completely severed cord, thus allowing realistic plans for long-term care to be made. If there is a question of a bony spicule or other foreign body impinging on the cord, operation is obviously indicated.

Spinal fusion may be helpful in rehabilitation, even if the cord is found to be completely severed.

The patient with a suspected spinal cord injury should be stabilized by a firm board and transported with the head held firmly between the hands of an assistant who is not simultaneously engaged in lifting the patient's body. The head should be supported by sandbags to prevent rotation, flexion or extension until a surgical facility is reached. The diagnosis should be suspected by a history of injury to the head, neck or back in which pain, tenderness, dysesthesia, paresis, anesthesia or plegia are present. A comatose patient with a head injury should also be suspected of a cervical spine injury. An incidence of as high as 50 per cent cervical spine or cord injuries has been reported in such patients.

Properly supported patients may re-

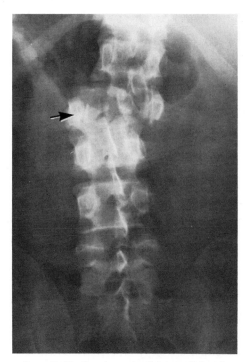

Figure 7–19 Lumbar spine fracture-dislocation. Extreme fracture dislocation of L_{1-2} (arrow) due to fall from scaffolding. Also, multiple fractures of lumbar spine transverse processes, with avulsion of left L_3 transverse process. At operation, complete transection of conus medullaris was found.

cover completely (Fig. 7–20) following stabilization with Crutchfield tongs, using the technique shown in Figure 7–21. The tongs should be applied in the Emergency Room but the weight should be removed when the patient is transported, to avoid excessive traction being applied inadvertently in case the litter is jostled accidentally.

ACUTE SPINAL CORD COMPRESSION DUE TO INTRASPINAL MASS LESIONS

Etiology

The rapid onset of symptoms and signs of spinal cord compression is usually

due to an intraspinal metastatic tumor and the involvement is almost invariably confined to the epidural space. On the other hand, intradural neoplasms are ordinarily primary and progress much more slowly. Common primary sites of metastatic tumors which spread to the spine are the prostate, breast, thyroid, lung, kidney and lymphatic tissue. Rarely will a malignant bone or other connective tissue neoplasm encroach primarily upon the spinal canal. Meningiomas, neurofibromas and other benign tumors are uncommon in an epidural location and usually result in gradually increasing symptoms. Infrequent causes of spontaneous acute cord compression are epidural abscess and hematoma, tuberculous spondylitis, and engorged, often partially thrombosed, vascular malformations of the spine and spinal cord (Fig. 7–22). Benign tumors of

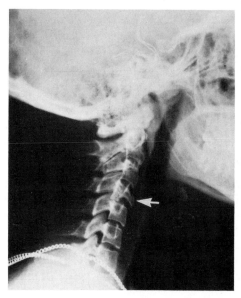

Figure 7–20 Cervical spine fracture. Twenty year old woman injured in auto accident. There is marked compression and comminution of the fourth cervical vertebral body (arrow), and loss of normal cervical lordosis due to cervical paraspinal muscle spasm. No neurological injury was sustained. With careful initial management, skeletal tong traction, and, later, a cervical brace, complete recovery occurred.

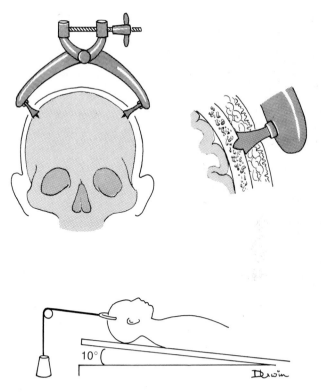

Figure 7–21 Use of Crutchfield tongs for cervical spine injury. *A*. Proper positioning of Crutchfield tongs. The skin is prepared and incised with a scalpel superior to each ear. The special Crutchfield drill (not shown) is used to prepare conical defects in the outer table of the skull, half way through the diploë. The points of the tongs are then inserted into the defects. The tongs are secured by force applied with a wing nut. When firmly in place, proper position is maintained with a lock nut. Tension on the tongs should be checked daily, because of a tendency to loosen.

B. Traction is applied in the long axis of the body, with bed elevated 10°. Ten to 30 pounds of traction (depending on the size of the patient) are applied for reduction. Alignment can ordinarily be maintained with 7–15 pounds. For the first few days, a circular bed such as a Foster or Stryker frame should be used. Patient should not be transported in this type of traction, because force of traction may vary accidentally.

nerve roots (Fig. 7–23) and cauda equina (Fig. 7–24) are less common than malignant tumors (Fig. 7–25). Physical compression of the cord by the mass lesion is ordinarily not the only factor responsible for its dysfunction. Both reduced arterial flow and, particularly, impaired venous drainage contribute significantly. Thoracic and lumbar areas are involved more frequently than cervical.

Diagnosis

Pain is often the first symptom. It may be confined to the involved area of the spine, but radiation into the areas of distribution of irritated nerve roots is common. Discomfort is often worse at night and is usually aggravated by motion of the spine, coughing and sneezing, straining or exertion. The patient soon becomes aware of diminishing motor function below the level of involvement and a sensory defect of corresponding extent. Urinary retention and constipation often appear early.

Sensory and motor changes below the level of compression may be symmetrical or irregular, depending upon location of the mass within the spinal canal and the

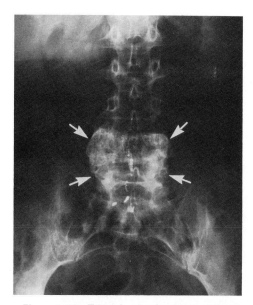

Figure 7-22 Extensive hemangioma of fourth lumbar vertebra. Compression by hemangioma (arrows) caused acute paraparesis. Hemorrhage had not occurred. Treatment by surgery and external irradiation led to nearly complete recovery.

the mass but about its relationship to the meninges as well (Figs. 7-24, 7-25). In the presence of a complete subarachnoid space block the conventional myelogram will delineate only the caudad extent of the compression, and subarachnoid instillation of Pantopaque by cisternal puncture may be helpful when the upper limits of the mass cannot be ascertained clinically or from the plain radiographic studies. Removal of cerebrospinal fluid may rapidly accentuate the degree of cord compression, and the surgeon should ordinarily proceed with decompressive laminectomy immediately upon completion of the diagnostic study.

Recovery of spinal cord function following removal of a benign lesion which has produced gradual compression may be virtually complete even if compression has been severe. On the other hand, the cord withstands sudden

nature of circulatory compromise. In cases of acute compression, muscle tone is usually diminished and deep reflexes are diminished or absent in contrast to those cases in which the compression is a gradual one. When the onset is rapid, segmental motor neuron changes are seen less frequently. The cephalad extent of the lesion is usually one to three segments above the level of the sensory deficit. Disseminated sensory deficits are less common in acute compressions. Focal spinous process tenderness may be of some value in establishing the site of involvement.

A destructive process of the vertebral bodies or pedicles may be seen in the roentgenograms (Figs. 7-22, 7-23). Lesions of the laminae and spinous processes are ordinarily less evident. Lumbar puncture, with analysis of the cerebrospinal fluid and performance of the Queckenstedt test, should not be made as an independent procedure but only as a prelude to myelography, since the latter study provides more precise information not only as to the level of

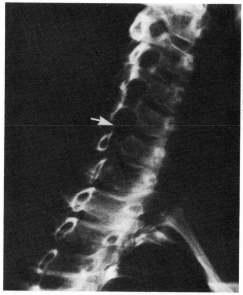

Figure 7-23 Cervical nerve root and cord compression from neurilemoma. Cervical spine radiograph of a 36 year old woman presenting with symptoms of C_6 nerve root compression. There is marked erosion of the C_{5-6} intervertebral foramen (arrow). This lesion later produced cervical cord compression as well. This benign tumor was operable, with sacrifice of the nerve root involved.

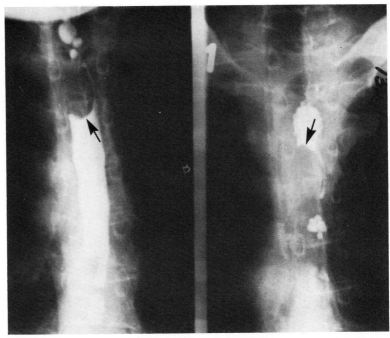

Figure 7–24 Paraparesis from intraspinal neurilemoma. Myelogram which demonstrates a large intraspinal neurilemoma producing severe paraparesis in a 60 year old woman. The superior and inferior margins of the tumor are indicated by arrows. Recovery of neurological function was complete following resection of the tumor.

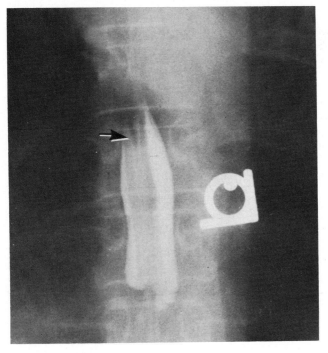

Figure 7–25 Paraplegia due to Hodgkin's disease. Complete myelographic subarachnoid space block in a 45 year old man who became acutely paraplegic from Hodgkin's sarcoma invading the spinal canal at midthoracic level. The irregular configuration (arrow) of the Pantopaque column is typical of that seen in epidural tumors. He was operated upon within one day after onset of symptoms, and had a complete temporary recovery following surgery and external irradiation. Symptoms, including paraplegia, later recurred and reoperation was without benefit.

compromise poorly. Little recovery can be anticipated in the patient with an acute neoplastic or other compressive lesion if dysfunction is allowed to progress to complete loss of motor and sensory modalities. Therefore, the need for speed in carrying out the essential diagnostic studies cannot be emphasized too strongly. Surgical decompression must be prompt when undue delay would permit irreversible functional changes to occur.

Treatment

Complete and lasting restoration of function often follows prompt and thorough evacuation of the epidural hematoma or abscess. Surgical treatment in the latter case must be augmented by local and systemic administration of the appropriate antibiotics. Surgical excision of the arteriovenous malformation, when performed by one skilled in the treatment of such problems, may not only alleviate the immediate compression but will often prevent subsequent insult to the cord from bleeding or thrombosis. Excision of metastatic neoplasms is usually incomplete but should be as extensive as possible to afford the most enduring palliation. Radiation therapy combined with cytotoxic agents may prolong the beneficial effects of surgical decompression.

ACUTE HERNIATION OF THE INTERVERTEBRAL DISCS

Acute herniation of an intervertebral disc is a specific type of spinal cord compression which is considered in Chapter 12. The principles of diagnosis and treatment are similar to the aspects of cord compression mentioned in the preceding section. It should be remembered that although lumbar and cervical herniations are most common, thoracic disc herniation may also occur. Most patients with herniated discs can be treated conservatively with bed rest, unless bladder, bowel or peripheral neuropathy occur, or if pain is recurrent or intractable.

INJURIES OF THE PERIPHERAL NERVES

Etiology

Peripheral nerve trauma, extremely common on the battlefield, occurs much less frequently during peacetime. Mechanisms of injury include laceration with anatomic interruption of the nerve trunk, contusion in either closed or compound injury, compression, stretching, avulsion and injection.

Lacerations are usually inflicted by knives or other sharp objects, by firearm missiles and by falls through windows. Contusions may be caused by a variety of injuries, particularly those occurring on the highway and from high velocity missiles. Patients under anesthesia are especially prone to incur compression nerve injury from improper positioning. Alcoholics frequently sustain compression neuropathy, particularly involving the radial and common peroneal trunks, because of the prolonged assumption of an abnormal posture while intoxicated. In these patients, the neurotoxic effects of alcohol are a contributing element. Most often the radial nerve becomes impinged between fragments of a long bone fracture, with resulting compression. Stretching and avulsion injuries often accompany auto and motorcycle accidents and falls from considerable heights (Fig. 7–26). An antibiotic is usually the offending agent in injection injuries, and the sciatic nerve is the one most frequently involved. The most common peripheral nerve lesions, except during wartime, are those of the median nerve due to entrapment beneath the transverse carpal ligament and the late ulnar palsy which usually results from chronic injury due to adhesion formation about the nerve at the elbow.

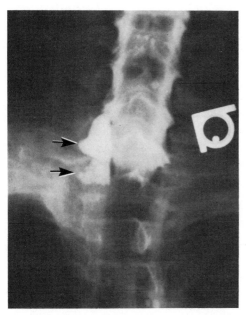

Figure 7-26 Cervical nerve root avulsion. Myelogram demonstrates avlusion of C_8 and T_1 roots. Contrast medium extends into dural pouches (arrows) at the level of avulsions. Injury was sustained in an 85 foot fall from an oil well derrick. Severe motor defect in right extremity, and extremely severe, chronic burning pain in arm and forearm were present.

Symptoms and Findings

The diagnosis of peripheral nerve injury, except when the state of consciousness is impaired, may often be made from the patient's description of a loss of sensation and inability to perform certain movements and can be confirmed by the appropriate motor, sensory, and reflex examination. Evaluation is more arduous when a major plexus or more than one peripheral nerve is involved and when there has been extensive associated injury to tendons, muscles and long bones. Electromyographic and conduction velocity studies are of little diagnostic and no prognostic value immediately following injury.

Treatment

Although associated muscle and tendon injuries should be surgically cor-

rected at the time of the injury, suture of nerve lacerations should ordinarily be delayed and not performed as an emergency procedure. There is some disagreement as to the optimum time of repair of a lacerated peripheral nerve, but most authorities favor an interval of three to four weeks following the injury. At this time there is heightened metabolic activity of the neuron and maximum regenerative capacity of the axon. Thickening of the epineurium and perineurium have occurred, thereby facilitating placement and retention of sutures. Swelling and inflammation of surrounding injured tissue have receded and the longitudinal extent of nerve injury can be better evaluated at this time.

Adherence to certain technical principles will facilitate peripheral nerve repair. The involved extremity should be prepared and draped in such a way that extensive dissection proximal and distal to the injury is possible. This is particularly important when the nerve must be freed from surrounding tissues to permit closure of a gap caused by significant loss of nerve tissue through contusion or neuroma formation. The use of the operating microscope or other magnification is useful in both dissection and repair. Débridement of the sectioned nerve ends is best done with a razor blade while the nerve is supported on a firm plastic cutting board. All scarred, contused or lacerated tissue should be excised by serial section until a well-defined fascicular pattern is visualized. Nerve ends should be apposed with the least possible tension using fine vascular silk suture through the perineurium only, and hemostasis should be immaculate. Injection of normal saline into the nerve on each side of the suture line may be helpful in aligning fascicles. Application of a silastic cuff about the site of anastomosis is believed to prevent distortion of axonal patterns and invasion of extraneural connective tissue at the suture line. The degree of range of motion permissible in adjacent joints without producing disruption of the anastomosis should be determined before the wound is closed. When the nerve is apposed under tension, the extremity should be immobilized in a plaster splint for about four weeks. Particular care should be exercised to avoid pressure upon an anesthetic area from a poorly fitting cast.

Closed peripheral nerve injuries rarely require surgical treatment. Therapy is directed toward prevention of contractures, maintenance of range of motion, avoidance of injury to anesthetic areas and, when necessary in cases in which spontaneous recovery does not occur, a variety of orthopedic proced-ures for the transfer of tendons and stabilization of joints.

In addition to the selection of an optimum time for neurorrhaphy and performance of a technically satisfactory surgical procedure, several other factors influence the prognosis in peripheral nerve trauma. Recovery is generally much better in children than in adults. The outcome is usually better in the distal injuries than in those situated closer to the spinal cord. Prognosis is poorer when the injured nerve contains both motor and sensory elements. Other factors which adversely affect recovery are the co-existence of diabetes, alcoholism or impaired nutrition.

8

The Integument—
Plastic and Reconstructive Surgery

By R. C. A. WEATHERLEY-WHITE, M.D.

THE REPAIR OF INJURIES

Principles of Wound Healing

The fundamental aim of the surgeon faced with a disruption of the integument is to ensure that the wound heals as rapidly as possible and with the minimum of complications. This axiom, seemingly self-evident, is valid for the optimum care of all injuries whether they are simple incised lacerations or major wounds involving loss of tissue, crush or burns. Too often, however, in the emergency situation, principles of tissue management are neglected, with the predictable consequences of decreased tensile strength and unsightly hypertrophic scarring.

The process of wound healing is complicated, and a detailed description would be out of place in this context. For a review of the intricate responses of the body to injury, Schilling's monograph is complete and up to date.[16] However, a brief summary is pertinent to a discussion of the factors known to inhibit wound healing.

Immediately following injury and sur-

196

gical repair, a nonspecific inflammatory response takes place, the object of which is to enhance the circulation to the wound. Phagocytes remove clot, necrotic tissue and bacterial inhabitants of the injured skin, and undifferentiated cells from the circulation migrate into the injury to undergo metamorphosis into fibroblasts. Endothelial budding takes place in the capillaries adjacent to the injury, and these anastomose across the interface of the wound to produce microvascular continuity. At this stage (one to three days following injury) the only tensile strength to the repair resides in the sutures holding the wound edges together, with some weak assistance from fibrin and mucopolysaccharide ground substance deposited at the interface.

The main constituent giving strength to the healed wound is collagen, produced by the proliferating fibroblasts in three to ten days following injury. Although collagen production is at a maximum at the end of this period, there is still relatively little strength to the wound. It is the co-valent cross-linking of single strands of tropocollagen into the triple helices of mature collagen and the orientation of these molecules which provide the ultimate tensile strength to the healed wound. This alignment process takes several weeks and is dependent largely upon tension. Finally, the scar tissue produced by this sequence of events softens and matures over a number of months until there is little histologic evidence of previous injury.

In our present state of knowledge, it can be stated that there is an optimum rate of wound healing. Apart from some controversial studies involving the deposition of powdered cartilage in the wound,[15] there is no evidence that the surgeon's dream—the acceleration of wound healing—can be accomplished. All we can do is avoid known inhibitory factors.

These inhibitory factors may be conveniently subdivided into systemic and local influences. There will be little time in the acute care of the injured patient to diagnose, let alone restore to normal, systemic deficiencies known to affect adversely the normal progress of wound healing. In elective outpatient procedures, however, these deficiencies should be investigated and treated as carefully as they are before major operations, for they will have an equivalent adverse effect.

The two main systemic factors involved in the inhibition of wound healing are anemia and protein deficiency. It is known that skin grafts rarely "take" when the hematocrit is less than 35 per cent; this specific clinical situation serves well as an experimental model for wound healing in general. Dunphy[5] has pointed out that the principal cause of delayed wound healing is a decreased oxygen tension at the site of the wound; certainly correction of a pre-existing anemia is necessary to avoid this situation. Hypoproteinemia will result in a decreased number of proliferating fibroblasts, with a consequent shortage of collagen, the single most important constituent of the healed wound. Other systemic factors known to be implicated in healing include the deficiency of vitamin C and the trace element zinc, and recently Peacock has given us insight into the biomechanics of collagen cross-linking through his experimental use of beta-amino-proprionitrile, the active agent in lathyrism, a connective tissue disease.[14]

It is, however, the local factors which are most directly under the control of the operating surgeon and are, unfortunately, the most abused. Of these, infection is the prime offender. In the presence of infection, not only will cellular proliferation of all types cease, but tissue already laid down will necrotize. The recurrence rate of repaired inguinal hernias is over 50 per cent when there has been an operative infection; many times the surgeon involved in the care of burns has seen apparently well-taken skin grafts "melt" when adjacent granulating tissue becomes grossly infected.

Hematoma in the wound not only will

provide the substrate for bacterial growth, but will in itself, by virtue of its space-occupying nature, produce tension on the wound edges and attenuate the capillary blood supply to the interface, thus causing a decreased tissue pO_2 at the critical location. Hematoma must be recognized immediately, drained, irrigated, and if possible any active bleeding identified and terminated.

Undue tension on the wound per se will unquestionably harm the quality of healing. Its short-term effect is the jeopardy of blood supply; it has long-term effects on the cross-linking and alignment of mature collagen fibers. Not only will the wound brought together under tension and held in place only by means of tight constricting sutures heal with an unsightly spread scar (an important factor on the face), but the tensile strength in the wound will be measurably decreased.

Arterial insufficiency and venous stasis (both resulting in decreased tissue pO_2) are most commonly seen by the plastic surgeon engaged in the preparation of a skin flap for transfer. Frequently, injured patients will manifest a "flap" partially separated from its source of blood supply; in this case, an individual surgical judgment will have to be made as to the viability of the tissue.

Control of local factors known to inhibit wound healing involve the Halstedian principles of surgical technique first introduced to the medical student in the "dog lab" and reinforced, hopefully, throughout surgical residence. These include rigid asepsis, immaculate hemostasis and gentle handling of tissue.

There is no excuse for slipping a pair of gloves over unwashed hands and, with face unadorned by a mask, suturing a laceration whose edges have been perfunctorily dabbed with antiseptic solution. These techniques would not be tolerated in the operating room, and outpatient care should be no less immaculate.

A thorough (five minute) wash of the adjacent skin with pHisoHex or any of the surgical soap solutions can be regarded as an adequate skin preparation. Copious irrigation of the wound itself with sterile saline solution will serve to flush out debris carried into the wound at the time of injury. Following injection of a local anesthetic, the wound should be inspected carefully and any foreign material not removed by irrigation picked out. Retained foreign bodies (glass fragments, shreds of clothing, road dirt, and so on) will either cause immediate infection or, if walled off by a fibrous capsule, may necessitate secondary removal.

Ragged wound edges are best trimmed to straight lines to effect a neat linear scar, and any devitalized or grossly contaminated tissue must be débrided to prevent infection (Fig. 8–1). These measures may result in a modest tissue deficit, the suturing of which would be

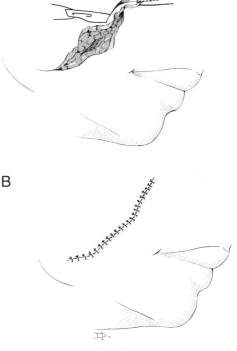

A

B

Figure 8–1 Trimming the ragged or devitalized skin edge to produce a clean linear closure.

possible only under some tension. This undesirable situation may be averted by the judicious undermining of adjacent skin for a centimeter or so at a level between the underside of the dermis and the subjacent fat, separating the fibrous septa which are holding the wound edges apart. The laceration may then be closed in layers (to minimize dead space) and the skin sutured with fine silk or nylon under little or no tension. When a major loss of tissue has occurred, the surgeon will have to decide whether wide undermining will allow the wound to be closed directly, or whether a skin graft will be needed to resurface the defect. In general, if the skin sutures are seen to blanch the skin when it is brought together, closure is under *too great tension*, and alternative methods must be sought.

Hemostasis must be absolute, and particular care must be paid to potentially serious bleeders when epinephrine has been used in the local anesthetic injected. Severed vessels which are constricted under the influence of the agent so as not to show obvious bleeding at the time of repair, may well "cut loose" several hours after the patient has been discharged from the Emergency Room. Immobilization and a firm pressure dressing will help prevent hematoma formation. All sutured lacerations should be inspected the following day to detect hematoma or infection so that appropriate measures may be taken to forestall their known inhibitory effect on healing.

Handling of tissue should be gentle and superimpose no additional necrosis to that of the injury itself. The use of skin hooks rather than forceps on skin edges is recommended, and after a little practice this useful instrument can be handled with a surprising dexterity. Placement of hemostats on bleeders should be accurate and precise, and as little tissue taken with the open vessel as possible. Fine catgut ligature is preferred to use of the cautery. Skin suture should be of as fine a material as will

hold the apposition securely, and should be placed close to the wound edge. Many fine sutures are preferable to a few gross "bites."

When these simple measures, which occupy little additional time and effort, are taken the optimum rate of wound healing will be attained and both surgeon and patient rewarded by the development of an unobtrusive and firmly healed scar. When neglected, such a favorable result will be fortuitous, and more commonly the end-point will be either an infected wound or at the very least an unsightly hypertrophic scar with little tensile strength.

Common Emergency Room Situations

The first responsibility of the surgeon called to examine an injured patient in the Emergency Room is *not* to treat the region apparently injured, but to ensure that there are no associated injuries which threaten the well-being of the patient or even pose a hazard to life. The history of the means by which injury occurred, if available, is of paramount importance. Facial abrasions sustained when thrown 50 feet by a speeding car carry more obvious implications of associated injury than do the same abrasions incurred in a fist fight.

Measurement of vital signs should be a routine procedure on admission to the Emergency Room, and it should be noted that soft tissue injuries to the head and face rarely, if ever, cause circulatory collapse, even when bleeding is profuse. If shock is apparent, a diligent search for causative factors such as pelvic fractures, blunt abdominal trauma causing lacerations to liver or spleen, or pneumothorax, should be undertaken before proceeding with repair of facial lacerations. Physical examination should be complete, and in cases of injury to the face and scalp should include a neurological evaluation.

Facial Lacerations

It is perhaps in dealing with facial lacerations that the technical skills and patience of the reparative surgeon are most obviously rewarded, for deforming scars which might be acceptable in other locations are always "on display" for the constant inspection of the patient and his associates. Such scars may be a source of psychological disturbance to the patient and they are frequently avoidable by attention to details of wound healing as outlined in the foregoing section.

The adequacy of blood supply to the face is an advantage from two standpoints, both related to wound healing. The incidence of infection is lessened to the point of being a rarity unless there have been gross errors of technique, and the entire healing process takes place in a shorter time space than in areas where the blood supply is less abundant.

The so-called "golden period" (within which lacerations can be safely sutured) of three to four hours following injury is at least doubled, allowing time for evaluation of more serious associated injuries. There is no reason, however, why facial lacerations should not be repaired meticulously under local anesthesia while the patient is being observed for signs of intraperitoneal bleeding; or a combined surgical approach can be taken to multiple injuries so that the plastic surgeon deals with the face while another team is operating on a different area. Where circumstances absolutely preclude the early repair of facial lacerations, these may be dressed with frequently changed moist compresses until surgery is accomplished, preferably within 48 hours. In such cases, broadspectrum antibiotic coverage is used and a rather more extensive débridement of the wound edges employed.

Fine suture (5-0, 6-0, or 7-0 silk or nylon) is for the repair of the skin, and owing to the rapid healing response, it may be removed earlier than is customary to prevent "stitch marks." One acceptable approach is to remove alternate sutures three days following repair, the remainder 48 hours later; a bolder method is to remove all of the sutures at three days, and to support wound edges with steri-strips or muslin soaked in collodion.

When a facial injury is necessarily closed under some tension, because of tissue loss, the most advantageous method of repair is the intradermal subcuticular "pull-out" suture (Fig. 8–2). Either nylon or fine monofilament wire may be used and the free ends taped to the skin rather than employing lead shot or heavy knots. This suture may be left for two or three weeks to hold the edges together until the reparative processes, delayed by tension, take over; yet it will not cause the ugly scarring that would inevitably accompany conventional skin sutures if left in place for that length of time.

Automobile Accidents

Some of the most technically awkward lacerations to the face come about as the result of automobile and motorcycle accidents. The force of injury may well cause fractures of the facial skeleton which are obscured by the rapid onset of edema; stereoscopic x-ray in the

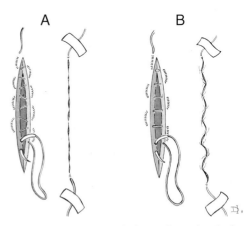

Figure 8–2 The technique of a subcuticular pull-out closure, using wire or nylon. To obtain a straight scar it is necessary to go back slightly with each suture.

Waters position (a 30° occipitomental view) will best show such fractures. Management of these fractures requires a general anesthetic and operating room care, in which case the soft tissue injuries can be repaired simultaneously. Many injuries involving soft tissue alone are so extensive that admission of the patient to the hospital is appropriate; a good rule of thumb is that if the repair will take two hours or more, or if skin grafting for tissue loss is required, then the situation is best handled on an inpatient basis.

Even those limited injuries suitable for outpatient repair may well pose a reconstructive challenge. Lacerations will frequently be of a "bursting" nature, in which soft tissue has been rapidly compressed over a bony prominence. Such lacerations will be jagged, irregular, and accompanied by massive contusion of adjacent tissue, not seen in incised injuries. Contamination of the wound with foreign material is common, and road dirt may be "ground in" to such an extent that irrigation alone will not remove it. Such potential contaminants must be removed by firm scrubbing with a brush, or even by cutting away the involved tissue.

It is readily apparent that injuries of this nature require more extensive débridement than usual to accomplish primary healing without infection; loss of tissue will consequently be greater. It may be possible by undermining and mobilization of adjacent tissue to restore continuity without undue tension; if not, a skin graft will be necessary.

The temptation to achieve primary reconstruction with the use of an ingeniously planned flap must be resisted. When a wound is contused and contaminated, the most meticulous surgical reparative technique may result in the development of an unsightly hypertrophic scar. If the use of the knife has been limited to the injured area, such disfigurement is amenable to a secondary revision several months later. If the wound has been extended by "relaxing incisions," or the creation of a flap, these incisions may also undergo hypertrophy, making a subsequent revision infinitely harder.

In general, surgical débridement and repair of complex injuries to the soft tissue of the face should be adequate and simple, aimed at achieving healing as quickly as possible. Elaborate reconstructions have no place in the primary treatment of such injuries, for these procedures are best electively performed in the well-healed wound, where there is no accompanying tissue destruction.

Bites

The ordinary dog bite is an extremely common injury, and it is estimated that approximately one-half million persons are treated yearly in Emergency Rooms throughout the U.S.A. for this problem. Such injuries are seen most frequently on the hands or face and commonly occur in children, who are more prone to pet or tease unfamiliar dogs than are adults. In fact, a completely unprovoked attack by a dog is a rarity, and should arouse grave suspicions of rabies infection in the animal.

Dog bites may range in severity from small punctures to major avulsions of tissue requiring general anesthesia and operating room care; however, the majority are quite suitable for treatment in the Emergency Room. Many have advocated leaving these wounds open to heal by granulation, but it is this author's firmly held opinion that a dog bite is relatively clean, and if strict attention is paid to the principles of wound débridement and copious irrigation, they may all be closed primarily. Following a thorough skin prep as described, the wound is sutured loosely, dressed with moist compresses which can be changed at home, and the patient given tetanus toxoid and antibiotic coverage. It must be acknowledged that even with meticulous care about 10 to 15 per cent of dog bites become infected, with the consequent necessity of opening the repair to relieve purulent collection; however, to condemn 85 to 90 per cent of these people to slow granulation and a mandatory scar revision would seem an unnecessarily conservative approach. Awkward bites on the face in small children have customarily been handled on an inpatient basis with a general anesthetic used to secure an immobile operating field; however, the recent advent and use of ketamine anesthesia has extended the scope of outpatient repair.

The most serious complication of a dog bite is of course rabies, a reportable disease which kills 10 to 25 individuals in this country yearly. Every physician involved in Emergency Room care should understand the indications for initiating prophylactic treatment against this disease. Recently the World Health Organization has published guidelines to assist in making this decision. (See also Chapter 4, and Chapter 28, Table 28-2.) These guidelines may be abstracted as follows:

1. When the attacking dog is shown by postmortem examination to have the disease.
2. When a clinical diagnosis of rabies is made by a veterinarian.
3. When an unprovoked attack is made, and the dog escapes or is killed without postmortem.

Treatment consists of *not* suturing the wound, but injecting hyperimmune rabies serum in the adjacent tissue, while commencing a 14 to 21 day course of rabies vaccine. It must be remembered that wild animals such as bats, skunks, foxes and squirrels may also carry rabies.

Human bites generally occur in the heat of passion, either amorous or belligerent, and should include, by definition, knuckles skinned on the teeth of an adversary. The principal complication of such bites is massive secondary infection due to the large quantities of pathogenic bacteriae—streptococcus, staphylococcus and spirochetes—which are normal inhabitants of the human, as opposed to the canine mouth. Such injuries should never be sutured primarily, but admitted to the hospital where intensive local and systemic treatment aimed at eradicating infection may be instituted.

The recent growth of camping and related outdoor activities has led to an increased incidence of snake bite. Several thousand people a year are bitten by poisonous snakes, and whereas the actual mortality is low (10 to 20 per year) the local complications, such as tissue necrosis, are severe. The vast majority of poisonous snakes belong to the croatalidae family, which includes the rattlesnake, the cottonmouth moccasin and the copperhead. Such snakes are residents of almost every state, but have not to date been found in Alaska, Hawaii, or Maine or at altitudes above 7,000 feet.[13]

The principal problem is to decide whether the patient has been bitten by a poisonous or an innocuous snake. Ideally the snake should be killed and brought in for identification using the charts available in most Emergency Rooms. Poisonous snakes have fangs, and a double puncture rather than the marks of serrated teeth is pathognomonic of the bite of a croatalida. Local reaction—pain and swelling—is severe and instantaneous, and systemic symptoms such as nausea, vomiting, chills, fever, dizziness and tachycardia develop rapidly.

Treatment consists of the application of a loose tourniquet to impede lymphatic flow, cruciate incisions through the bite with suction, and the local and systemic injection of polyvalent antivenin. Packing the injured extremity in ice has received unfortunate publicity and is to be condemned as an extremely hazardous and ineffective procedure. The systemic absorption of venom is delayed rather than prevented, and several serious injuries (including the complete loss of an arm below the elbow) have been reported as a direct result of injudicious hypothermia.

The coral snake, found in the Gulf states, Arizona and New Mexico, is the most deadly of all snakes found in the

U.S.A. This snake produces a lethal neurotoxin, and although an antivenin is manufactured in Brazil, it is not generally available in this country. Consequently its bite is invariably fatal.

The most common biting spider is the black widow, found principally in outhouses, garages and basements. Only the female is dangerous, and she may be recognized by her globular jet-black body and the characteristic red or yellow "hour-glass" mark on the belly. There is usually some local discomfort at the time of the bite; this is rapidly followed by generalized muscle spasms. These patients may present in the Emergency Room with belly pain and spasm, and the differential diagnosis of an acute abdominal crisis such as a perforated duodenal ulcer may be hard to rule out. Treatment consists of relief of pain, injection of antivenin and the use of intravenous calcium gluconate and other muscle relaxants.

Specific Problem Situations

There are certain regions of the face which, due to their unique anatomic or functional characteristics, require special consideration when injured.

1. Eyebrows and Eyelids. Facial lacerations, particularly those resulting from automobile accidents in which the unbelted rider may be ejected through a shattered windshield, will frequently involve the adnexal structures of the eye. The globe itself, due to the protective "blink reflex," is less commonly injured; however, in any through-and-through laceration of the eyelid the globe should be examined by an ophthalmologic surgeon. The sequelae of unrecognized and untreated injuries to the globe are disastrous, and if only for medico-legal reasons consultation should always be obtained in these situations.

Lacerations through the eyebrows are repaired in the customary manner appropriate for facial lacerations. The brow itself should not be shaved, less from the standpoint of hair not growing back (a rarity) than from the fact that correct alignment of the laceration will be easier with the hairs in place to serve as a guide. However, when hair adjacent to a laceration is deliberately left in situ, not only must the area be prepped with additional thoroughness to prevent infection, but care must be taken not to invert hair-bearing skin into the repair.

Lacerations of the lids themselves may be superficial or through-and-through, involving skin, orbicularis muscle, tarsal plate and conjunctiva. When these lacerations do not involve any absolute loss of tissue they are simply repaired in layers, care being taken to re-approximate each anatomic structure separately and in correct position. The "key" suture is in the gray line immediately behind the lashes; correct positioning of this stitch will align the other structures. The conjunctiva is repaired next using fine (6-0) catgut with the knots away from the globe; the other structures are sutured in sequence from inside out with the skin repair last.

Two adnexal structures deserve special mention. A deep horizontal laceration of the upper lid may divide the levator palpebrae muscle or its tendinous attachment to the tarsal plate. This filmy muscle may be hard to identify in the bloody mess of an acute injury, yet a diligent search must be made, for if left unrepaired, ptosis of the upper lid, requiring an elaborate secondary procedure for its correction, may develop. Lacerations through the medial portions of the lid margins may divide the canalicular system providing drainage of tears. An injury to the upper canaliculus may be fairly safely ignored, as it contributes only 10 per cent of the drainage of lacrimal secretions. If, however, a laceration through the margin of the lower lid is seen to be medial to the punctum, a search must be made for the cut ends of the divided inferior canaliculus. A fine polyethylene or silastic catheter is threaded through the punctum, across the divided canaliculus, and into the lacrimal sac just below the attachment of the medial canthal ligament to the periosteum of the nasal bones. If this precaution is ignored, and soft tissue repaired without regard to the canaliculus, scarring of this structure will prevent proper internal drainage of tears with consequent epiphora.

Tissue losses of up to one-quarter of the lid margin may be repaired directly without distortion of the palpebral fissure.[12] Both skin and conjunctiva must be undermined laterally in order to move the residual tissue in a medial direction; too much pull on the canalicular system is undesirable. Losses of up to one-third of the margin of either upper or lower lid may be similarly repaired with the added maneuver of dividing the appropriate branch of the lateral canthal ligament. A small horizontal incision is made just lateral to the eye and the Y-shaped ligament exposed. Division of the upper bifurcation for tissue losses of the upper lid, and the lower branch for losses of the lower lid, will permit additional mobilization of the entire lid for tension-free closure. The main attachment of the ligament to the lateral orbital rim should not be incised before it divides into upper and lower portions, for a major deformity of the palpebral fissure will result. Losses of greater than one-third of either lid will require a more elaborate reconstruction than should be performed in the Emergency Room. Major losses of skin alone will require either a graft or a local flap for their resurfacing; such reconstructions are described in a subsequent section of this chapter.

2. The Ears. The pinna of the ear is a subtle structure characterized by three-dimensional curves. Reconstruction is hard and frequently disappointing because of the inability to restore surgically the original delicacy of contour. Lacerations of the ear will commonly be jagged and irregular, and avulsing injuries may cause exposure of the cartilage owing to loss of surface skin.

Simple lacerations are repaired in layers with fine chromic catgut for the cartilage, using the folds of the ear as landmarks to achieve anatomic alignment. The ear is dressed with moderate pressure, using moist cotton or gauze fluffs packed both in front of and behind the ear itself to reduce the possibility of hematoma formation. Hematoma is a common sequel of ear injuries whether or not the skin has been lacerated, and should be aspirated promptly and the ear redressed with a pressure dressing as described. If hematoma recurs following aspiration, a formal incision and drainage using a short length of rubber band for the drain will be needed. Recognition of the problem is essential, for undrained hematoma of the pinna will result in destruction of cartilage and a "cauliflower ear," a deforming and preventable condition.

When more serious injuries necessitate débridement of devitalized skin, cartilage will be exposed. There is little laxity to the skin of the ear; consequently a decision will have to be made whether to excise the exposed cartilage to achieve tension-free closure or to employ alternative means of achieving coverage. Cartilage denuded of its nutrient skin should never be left exposed, for the inevitable consequence will be progressive chondritis resulting in a major destruction of the architecture of the ear. Depending on the location of the exposed cartilage and the deformity which would result from its excision, as much as half a centimeter may be removed. Otherwise a primary skin graft will be needed for coverage.

Major losses of a portion of the pinna may be dealt with in the following manner (Fig. 8–3 *A, B, C*). The ear is debrided to viable and uncontaminated tissue and "laid back" against the adjacent postauricular scalp. An incision is made in this area directly under the cut margin of the ear, spread slightly, and the skin of the ear sutured in two layers to the postauricular scalp. This may be elevated in a later stage and a skin graft placed behind the pinna to replace lost tissue. If the loss has been relatively small, the scar tissue may be enough to provide adequate "stiffness" to the ear.

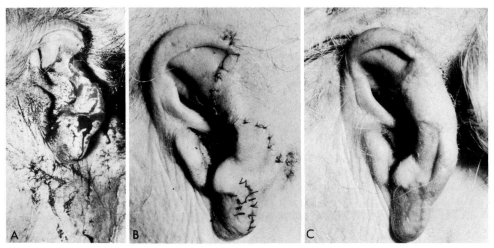

Figure 8–3 *A.* Raccoon bite of the ear with multiple lacerations and loss of a major portion of the pinna. *B.* Debrided and with a postaural skin flap sutured to defect. *C.* Flap divided and ear elevated from scalp with split-thickness skin graft.

If the loss has been greater, added structural support in the form of carved costal cartilage or a silastic prosthesis may have to be implanted before raising the ear. Such a reconstructive procedure will require a general anesthetic and inpatient care, but the preparatory maneuvers can be carried out in the Emergency Room.

3. *The Lips.* Lacerations of both upper and lower lip are common and frequently involve loss of tissue. Small lacerations of the inner aspect of the lips do not require suturing, but with a clear liquid diet and frequent peroxide mouthwashes they will heal spontaneously and rapidly. Through-and-through injuries must be repaired in layers; if the laceration crosses the skin-vermilion border,

correct anatomic alignment of this feature is highly important. The vermilion margin is marked with a dye (methylene blue, brilliant green or India ink) *prior* to injection of the local anesthetic, for this will blanch and distort both skin and mucosa and make recognition of the border difficult. The initial suture is placed at the pre-marked border (Fig. 8–4); alignment of other structures, mucosa, muscle and skin, follows in sequence. Failure to observe this precaution will frequently result in a "step deformity" which will need a later revision.

When tissue is missing because of the injury, losses of up to one-quarter of the lip may be sutured primarily without significant deformity; greater degrees

Figure 8–4 When the lip is lacerated through and through, the key stitch aligns the skin vermilion border correctly.

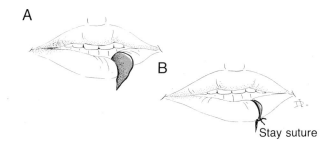

of loss will require a reconstructive procedure too elaborate for the Emergency Room.

4. Injuries to the Facial Nerve and Parotid Duct. Deep lacerations of the cheek will frequently involve two important structures, the facial nerve and the parotid duct.

A careful preoperative examination of muscular activity of the face will reveal any injury to the branches of the facial nerve. If the laceration is anterior to a line dropped from the lateral canthus of the eye, then only fine peripheral branches are involved. These need not be repaired, as their function will almost always regenerate. When major branches of the facial nerve appear to be interrupted on the basis of the neurological examination, only operative exploration will identify a loss of continuity. It is the author's conviction that repair of these structures should be carried out primarily—however, a procedure of this type requires lighting, equipment and teamwork best supplied by the Operating Room.

Failure to identify and repair a divided parotid duct will result in persistent leakage of saliva through the skin repair. The duct runs in a straight line between the tragus of the ear and the commissure of the lips; a deep laceration of the cheek across this line should raise the suspicion of an injury to this structure. Intraoral probing of Stensen's duct will determine whether there has been an interruption of continuity; if so it should be repaired with fine catgut over a polyethylene catheter extending into the oral cavity and fixed to the buccal mucosa. This may be withdrawn after a week.

Lacerations of the parotid gland itself (located between the lobule of the ear and the angle of the mandible) may cause a temporary fistulous leak; these, however, usually subside spontaneously, although a collection of salivary fluid will occasionally require aspiration. Radiation therapy has been recommended to suppress parotid activity if the accumulation is persistent.

Thermal Injuries

Burns have been classified traditionally according to the depth of injury into first degree, second degree and third degree; a more descriptive term for the latter two categories would be "partial-thickness" and "full-thickness" burns. In partial-thickness burns, only the more superficial layers of the dermis are destroyed, and if kept free from infection will heal spontaneously with skin of good quality. Full-thickness burns have by definition lost the entire depth of the dermis including the stratum germinativum, and if ungrafted, will heal only by scarring and contracture. Thus an early recognition of the depth of the burn should be attempted, for on this factor will depend not only the prognosis but also the eventual management of the burn.

If the skin is charred or dead white, with thrombosed capillaries evident on the de-epithelialized surface, then the burn is almost certainly full-thickness in depth. If intracutaneous blebs are present, implying that the dermal circulation is intact, then the burn is probably only of partial thickness. Not all burns are so clear-cut, however, and in addition there may be a mosaic pattern of areas of mixed partial- and full-thickness burns present. Although supra-vital dyes and thermography have been used experimentally to determine the depth of a burn, the single most useful clinical test remains the retention of sensation to pinprick in a burn of partial thickness.

In addition to recognition of the depth of the burn, assessment of the surface area involved is crucial, for on this will depend, among other things, the program of fluid replacement therapy. The "rule of nines" is a reasonably accurate guide for the relative areas of different parts of the body; the head being 9 per cent, each surface of the trunk 18 per cent, each arm 9 per cent and each leg 18 per cent. The proportions in the infant or small child are different in that the head is relatively larger and the legs smaller.

An important decision facing the

examining physician in the Emergency Room is, "Can the burn be treated on an outpatient basis or is it serious enough to warrant admission to the hospital?" In general, our criteria for admission are as follows:

1. Any burn of greater extent than 10 per cent, or 5 per cent in a small child or old person (burns are tolerated poorly on the extreme ends of the age spectrum) represents a threat to life on the basis of fluid loss and should be admitted.

2. Any full-thickness burn will require grafting and should be admitted, although with limited areas of loss, admission need not be effected until the dead eschar is separated and the burn ready for surgical coverage.

3. Burns of the hands, face or perineal region are hard to care for at home and should all be admitted to the hospital.

Standards for admission will be more liberal in the case of children, and if there is the suspicion that the parents are not equipped to deliver conscientious and effective care at home, the child should always be taken into the hospital.

Minor burns not meeting the above criteria may be treated on an outpatient basis. First-degree burns manifesting erythema only may be quite painful and can be treated with an analgesic ointment and discharged. Partial-thickness burns of limited extent should be washed gently but thoroughly with pHisoHex, all contaminants removed from the surface, blisters aspirated and cultured and the areas dressed with a fairly bulky dressing. Furacin mesh-gauze is a very suitable material to place next to the wound itself. It must be remembered that the arbitrary classifications of burns are *not* static, and that if a partial-thickness burn becomes infected, it may well be converted into a full-thickness loss which will require a skin graft for coverage. Consequently the burn should be inspected and re-dressed daily until there is evidence of healthy re-epithelialization. Sterile technique should always be used for the dressing changes, and prophylactic penicillin employed systemically for the same reason, that of prevention of infection.

The remainder of this section will deal with the important sequence of measures to be taken when an acute major burn is first brought into the Emergency Room. Burn centers will have their own Standard Operating Procedures for the receiving area; in the Emergency Rooms of the average general hospital the admission of a major burn is an event associated with some degree of urgency and excitement, consequently a "check list" is vital to ensure that therapeutic and diagnostic measures follow a logical sequence without forgetting any important aspects of management.

These measures are listed as follows:

1. Airway. The integrity of the airway is of prime importance in any acute injury and burns are no exception. Flashburns to the face, neck or upper chest should always suggest the possibility of an intraoral burn which may involve the glottis and vocal cords. Stridor, retraction and a rising respiratory rate will confirm these suspicions, and if there is upper airway obstruction due to the burn, then a tracheostomy or nasotracheal intubation should be performed. It must also be remembered that small children have not only a narrower trachea but also a more reactive laryngeal mucosa than the adult; consequently the sequence of events leading to total obstruction occurs in an accelerated manner requiring greater alertness on the part of the responsible physician.

2. Fluids. Any burn of greater than 10 per cent of the body surface is potentially hazardous on the basis of fluid loss and hypovolemic shock. Consequently the early administration of fluid replacement is mandatory. Insertion of a polyethylene catheter into the subclavian vein not only will allow a convenient route for rapid fluid administration but will also allow constant monitoring of the central venous pressure. Either normal saline or lactated Ringer's solution in dextrose may be used for initial treatment until the exact fluid requirements are derived. All administered fluids should be by the intravenous route at this early stage, for oral fluids may merely dilate the stomach to be vomited later.

3. *Urine Output.* Hourly measurement of the urine output and specific gravity is the most useful way to assess the effectiveness of fluid replacement, as well as to detect at the earliest possible moment impending renal failure. If the urine output begins to dwindle, and the specific gravity to rise, then the patient is being underhydrated and will need an increased rate of fluid administration. Changes in the urine will provide proof of impending hypovolemic shock well before any change in the pulse or blood pressure. Consequently insertion of a Foley catheter to allow easy measurement of these indices is one of the important early measures to take in the acute management of the severely burned patient.

4. *Charting.* Having assured the patency of the airway, established an intravenous line and urinary drainage, a more leisurely assessment of the burn itself can be made. A detailed description should be charted of both depth and extent in the permanent record using the criteria outlined previously. On the basis of the severity of the burn a fluid plan should be evolved, recognizing that this will always need modification according to the individual's unique response to the burn as measured by urinary output, specific gravity, hematocrit and central venous pressure. However, the Brooke Army Formula:

0.5 cc plasma × body weight in Kg × % of the burn (up to 50%)

+

1.5 cc electrolyte (saline or Ringer's) × weight × % burn

+

Daily maintenance fluids

for the first 24 hours' needs has proved successful in preventing gross mis-management of fluid therapy and serves as a useful preliminary plan.[1]

5. *Other Measures.* Before transferral from the Emergency Room to the burn or intensive care unit, the patient should be sedated, the burned areas cleansed, and whichever form of topical antibacterial therapy is in vogue commenced. Currently in our unit we are using dressings soaked in 0.5 per cent silver nitrate as described by Moyer,[10] but sulfamylon, gentamicin and silver sulfadiazine all have their devotees. A discussion of the relative merits of these agents is out of place in this context, except to say that none of them will substitute for devoted and laborious wound care. Prophylactic penicillin is added to the intravenous fluids until cultures of specific organisms dictate a change of antibiotic.

If these measures are taken promptly and in sequence, culpable disasters due to errors of omission can be avoided, and the patient admitted to the hospital in optimal condition for appropriate inpatient care.

Injury by cold represents the opposite end of the thermal spectrum, and frostbite in civilian practice is not as common, nor are the sequelae as devastating, as a burn injury.

Our experience at the University of Colorado Medical Center is based on the review of 113 patients admitted over the past ten years,[8] and implies that the physical appearance of the acutely injured part bears no correlation whatsoever with the extent of tissue ultimately lost. Thus no "first, second or third degree" system can be evolved on the basis of physical examination; of greater value as a prognostic indicator is a detailed knowledge of the duration of exposure, the ambient temperature and wind speed during exposure, (Table 8-1) and the type of protective clothing worn. The injury is a product of the tissue temperature reached and the time period that the tissue remains frozen. The rate of heat loss will determine the ability of the body to "self-warm" a cooled part with increased blood flow;

TABLE 8–1   CHILL FACTOR CHART

WIND SPEED (MILES/HOUR)	THERMOMETER READING (°F)									
	40	30	20	10	0	−10	−20	−30	−40	−50
	EQUIVALENT TEMPERATURE (°F) — THE CHILL FACTOR									
calm	40	30	20	10	0	−10	−20	−30	−40	−50
5	37	27	16	6	−5	−15	−26	−36	−47	−57
10	28	16	4	−9	−21	−33	−46	−58	−70	−83
15	22	9	−5	−18	−36	−45	−58	−72	−85	−99
20	18	4	−10	−25	−39	−53	−67	−82	−96	−110
25	16	0	−15	−29	−44	−59	−74	−88	−104	−118
30	13	−2	−18	−33	−48	−63	−79	−94	−109	−125
35	11	−4	−20	−35	−49	−67	−82	−98	−113	−129
40	10	−6	−21	−37	−53	−69	−85	−100	−116	−132
		Least Danger			*Greater Danger*			*Great Danger*		

hence an individual protected by insulated clothing will sustain a lesser injury than the same individual whose socks and feet are soaked by tramping through the snow in indoor shoes, or who has removed his gloves in an effort to start his car stalled on an isolated mountain pass.

When patients present in the Emergency Room with an acutely frozen extremity, the part is usually white, hard and lacking in sensation. If enough time has passed for the part to be partially thawed out, there may be edema, cyanosis, blisters and a varying degree of return of sensation.

Emergency Room treatment consists of immediate rewarming of the part in a water bath whose temperature is precisely 40° C. A cooler bath will not be as effective, a hotter one will increase the metabolic demand on the tissue and cause additional necrosis. Narcotics may be necessary during this often painful procedure which should be prolonged until return of blood flow to the part is seen. Rapid rewarming reduces the duration of time during which the tissue is at subviable temperatures, and is the *only* therapeutic maneuver which has to date been shown clinically effective in reducing or preventing the gangrene of frostbite. It should be accomplished in the Emergency Room.

All patients in whom tissue damage is suspected should be admitted to the hospital, where the subsequent treatment will depend on whether one believes the necrosis of cold injury a direct result of thermal cellular assault, immediate and irreversible, or a slow process due primarily to intravascular aggregation and infarction. Our own laboratory studies imply that frostbite injury is potentially reversible if the microcirculation is kept patent. We are currently using intravenous infusion of Pluronic F-68 (a co-polymer of polyoxyethylene and polyoxypropylene glycol), which is a nontoxic surface-active agent known to stabilize both the endothelial lining and the red cell membrane as an adjuvant to rapid rewarming. Use of this agent is still in the experimental stage.

Whether or not drugs are used in an

attempt to augment the capillary circulation, the treatment for frostbite consists of supportive measures designed to prevent infection. The extremities are elevated, the patient kept on bed rest, and sterile dressings changed daily. *No* attempt at surgical débridement should be made, for preferably the nonviable tissue should separate spontaneously.

ELECTIVE RECONSTRUCTIVE PROCEDURES

The ascending spiral of hospital costs in recent years has forced conscientious physicians to consider a wider use of the Outpatient Department rather than inpatient operating room care for certain elective surgical procedures. "Unnecessary" hospitalizations should be avoided as long as this can be done without jeopardizing the optimal care of the patient. Many reconstructive procedures of limited extent are performed under local anesthesia and thus lend themselves ideally to outpatient care; in some institutions brief procedures under a general anesthetic are performed and the patients discharged after a period of observation in the recovery room.

What are some of the types of procedures most suited to surgery on an outpatient basis? They include excision of skin lesions, both benign and malignant.

Skin Lesions

Basal Cell Carcinoma

Basal cell carcinoma is the commonest skin malignancy, and arises in the connective tissue beneath the dermis. Its etiology is related to solar radiation and consequently is found most frequently on the exposed portions of the body—face and the dorsum of the

hands—of fair-skinned persons of middle age who spend a great deal of time out-of-doors. It is rarely, if ever, found in Negroes and in general, the darker the complexion the less prone the individual is to basal cell carcinoma (presumably a protective genetic adaptation). It is more common in males than in females and very rare in adolescents, the youngest case in the author's experience being 15 years of age.

Basal cell carcinomas are divided both clinically and histologically into several types but all have in common masses of deeply staining basophilic round cells with palisading of their nuclei at the periphery. The most common form is the papular basal cell carcinoma which may present as a nodule or a small ulcer with a rolled pearly edge (Fig. 8–5). It is slow-growing, circumscribed and may be ignored for several years by the patient since it is painless. Other types of basal cell carcinoma include the cystic lesion, and the sclerosing and morpheic types which manifest an ill-defined indurated surface and marked subdermal extension. The rare pigmented basal cell carcinoma is important in that it is

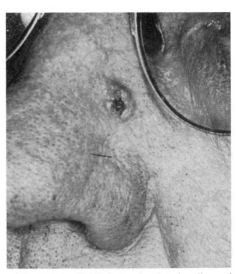

Figure 8–5 Typical papular basal cell carcinoma, with pearly rolled edges. (From the collection of S. E. Blandford, Jr., M.D.)

hard to differentiate clinically from a malignant melanoma.

Basal cell carcinoma is a local lesion and extends only by direct invasion, never by metastasis via the blood-stream or lymphatics. Consequently the treating physician is required only to ensure adequate local removal. Treatment modalities have included surgical excision, radiation therapy, electro-dessication and topical chemotherapy. The recurrence rate following adequate treatment from any of these means is low (2 to 5 per cent); however, it is strongly recommended that surgical excision be employed for the following reasons:

1. A surgical specimen will be obtained from which may be defined not only histologic confirmation of the diagnosis but, most important, the adequacy of surgical resection. Some of these tumors are multifocal, and some manifest subdermal extension not apparent to clinical examination. When the pathologic specimen reveals tumor extending to the margin of resection, a re-excision must be performed with complete clearance from the pathologists of a margin adequately free of tumor.
2. When recurrence of basal cell carcinoma is noted following surgical resection, the re-excision may be limited to the area of recurrence; when recurrence occurs following radiation, the entire radiated area must be re-excised. This will often involve removal of a great deal of tissue with the consequent necessity of performing an elaborate reconstruction to prevent a major deformity.
3. Surgery is preferred to radiotherapy when adjacent structures may be damaged by radionecrosis. These regions include the lids and canthal regions, the nose, the external ear, the lips and the hands.

An adequate surgical excision usually entails a 5 mm margin around the clinically evident lesion; *all* specimens should be submitted for histologic examination and a re-excision performed if sectioning shows evidence of inadequate resection. All patients in whom basal cell carcinomas have been removed should be examined at six-month intervals for the rest of their lives—to recognize recurrence and to diagnose the appearance of new lesions. The patient with one basal cell carcinoma is constitutionally and environmentally liable to develop others. For the same reason such patients should be advised to avoid deliberate sun-bathing, and to protect the exposed parts with clothing or an ultraviolet screening lotion when solar exposure is inevitable.

Most basal cell carcinomas are small, and excision and direct closure can be accomplished without deformity by placing the long axis of the elliptical incision in the natural tension lines of the face when this is the region involved (Fig. 8–6). However, when the lesion is larger owing to patient neglect, the resection may entail sacrifice of so much skin that simple closure under tension would result in a major disfigurement.

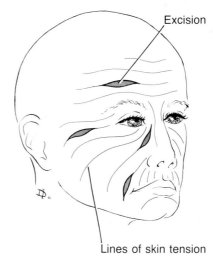

Figure 8–6 Elliptical excisions of facial lesions are made with their long axes in the direction of wrinkles in the aged or lines of tension in the younger patient.

In these cases, there is controversy over whether to merely resurface the area with a skin graft, or to employ a local flap for immediate reconstruction of the deformity. The proponents of grafting hold that, whereas the cosmetic appearance is less satisfactory, recurrence is easier to detect than when tissue adjacent to the tumor is "buried" under a flap. Those, including the author, who prefer direct reconstruction of the deformity, feel that with a histologically adequate margin of resection, the recurrence rate of basal cell carcinoma is so low that the best possible means of achieving a normal appearance should be employed. Specific examples of local flaps will be described in a later part of this section.

Squamous Cell Carcinoma

Squamous cell carcinoma, also occurring commonly on the face and hands, is hard to differentiate clinically in its initial stages from basal cell carcinoma (Fig. 8–7). It is, however, rapidly growing, highly invasive, liable to metastasize through lymphatic channels, and therefore requires a more aggressive surgical approach. Prone to occur in radiated tissue, it is a frequent and tragic aftermath of injudicious radiotherapy for benign lesions such as acne and hemangioma. The tumor is usually less well defined than a basal cell carcinoma, and local induration is marked. Growth is rapid and may be characterized by ulceration and bleeding or by the development of an irregular cauliflower-like excrescence.

The majority of squamous cell carcinomas can, if diagnosed early, be excised locally with primary closure. Because of the higher degree of invasiveness noted in these tumors, the margin of excision should be wider than for basal cell carcinoma, and should include at least 1 cm of histologically clear tissue. For the same reason, the extent of the resection is best judged by frozen section.

Lymph node dissection, which is outside the scope of outpatient surgery,

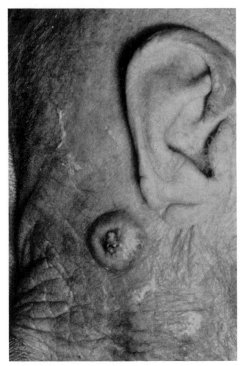

Figure 8–7 A squamous cell carcinoma, rapidly growing and with marked adjacent induration. (From the collection of S. E. Blandford, Jr., M.D.)

should be carried out in continuity when nodes are clinically involved. Serious consideration should be given to a delayed prophylactic node dissection when the lesion is recurrent or has an anaplastic histologic appearance, or when the patient is under 45 years of age.

When the extent of resection makes primary closure a deforming procedure, the same controversy exists as to whether to perform a primary reconstruction or to resurface the defect with a skin graft. Each case must be judged entirely on its own merits; the early and well-circumscribed lesion can be safely reconstructed when frozen section gives evidence of adequate resection. In long-standing lesions with diffuse indurated edges it would seem more prudent to accept the temporary deformity of a skin graft; if there is no evidence of recurrence within a year the grafted area can be excised and a delayed reconstruction performed if frozen section demonstrates no further tumor cells in the specimen removed. Lifetime follow-up of each patient is of course mandatory.

Keratoacanthoma is a rapidly growing benign lesion which greatly resembles squamous cell carcinoma in its physical appearance; however, its rapid growth is followed by equally rapid resolution. The experienced clinician may be able to make the differential diagnosis and await disappearance of the tumor with equanimity; others less confident of their acumen (including the author) prefer the security engendered by excisional biopsy and histologic section (Fig. 8–8 *A* and *B*).

Nevus and Malignant Melanoma

Nevi, or moles, are pigmented skin lesions which may be flat or elevated, hairless or hair-bearing. Although the exact etiology of these lesions is controversial, the most generally accepted theory is that they arise from neural elements within the dermis. They are extremely common, it being estimated that each individual bears an average of 15 nevi on his or her body.

Nevi are classified histologically into intradermal, junctional and compound nevi.[3] The intradermal nevus is the common mole of adulthood and characteristically is brown or black, with a raised surface which frequently bears hairs (Fig. 8–9). The clinical importance of this physical description is that melanoma rarely if ever arises from an intradermal nevus.

The junctional nevus, common in childhood, is so named because the mass of melanotic cells comprising the lesion resides at the junction between the dermis and the epidermis. Most preadolescent junctional nevi mature at puberty into adult intradermal nevi; however, as malignant melanomata arise almost exclusively from junctional nevi, it is important to recognize their physical characteristics. Junctional nevi are flat or only slightly raised, may vary in color from light brown to black, are hairless and commonly have a less well-defined edge than the intradermal nevus, the margin "blending" into the adjacent skin.

Compound nevi are a histologic combination of the two with a darker raised central intradermal portion surrounded by a flat "areola," usually paler in color and representing the junctional part of the lesion.

The indications for removal of nevi are twofold, cosmetic and prophylactic. An obvious intradermal nevus of the face, dark, raised and hairy, represents a disfigurement which can well be improved by careful surgical excision. A small ellipse is planned aligning the long axis with the known tension lines (see Fig. 8–6) and, after undermining the incisional edges to relieve tension, is sutured with fine silk or nylon, the sutures being removed on the third or fourth postoperative day to prevent stitch marks. As the principle object of this procedure is cosmetic, care must be taken to ensure an inconspicuous scar less offensive than the original lesion. The specimen should, of course, be consigned to the pathology department for section and histologic confirmation of the benign nature of the lesion.

The junctional nevus, because of its malignant potential, should be watched carefully. In addition, it would seem proper to excise prophylactically junctional nevi in areas of chafing and potential irritation from belt, collar, or brassiere, for it has been shown that continued trauma may precipitate melanomatous change in the junctional or, rarely, the compound nevus. For the same reason, measures other than formal surgical excision should *never* be employed. Electrodesiccation or cryotherapy must not be performed. A high proportion of patients with malignant melanoma will present a history of previous improper treatment of this type, the trauma quite possibly precipitating the malignant change.

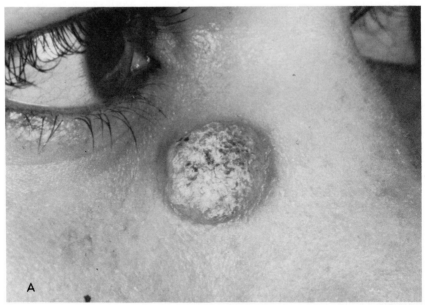

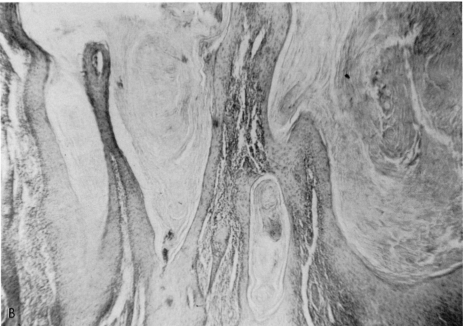

Figure 8–8 *A*. Keratoacanthoma clinically resembles squamous cell carcinoma. *B*. Microscopically it is easily distinguished by the lack of mitotic cells and the hyperkeratotic plugs. (From the collection of S. E. Blandford, Jr., M.D.)

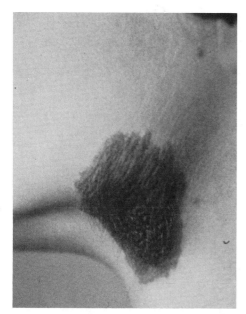

Figure 8-9   A typical intradermal nevus, raised, hairy and with a uniform color.

Malignant melanoma (Fig. 8-10 *A* and *B*) is a highly malignant lesion which frequently metastasizes early. Definitive treatment consists of wide and deep excision (a margin of 5-10 cm is acceptable) and en-bloc lymphatic dissection in continuity, if possible. This procedure cannot be done satisfactorily on an outpatient basis. The poor prognosis of the patient can, however, be improved by the early recognition of malignant changes in an established pigmented lesion. These signs include:

1. Enlargement of the lesion or satellite formation
2. A change in pigmentation—either lighter or darker
3. Crusting, ulceration or bleeding
4. Pain or itching, and local inflammation
5. Melanuria

Any new or established pigmented lesion which demonstrates one or more of these physical changes should undergo excisional biopsy with a margin of at least 1 cm and be submitted for frozen section, to determine if melanoma is present. Pigmented lesions of the soles of the feet, the palms and genitalia should be excised, for these lesions have

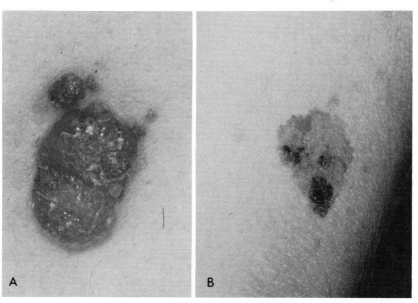

Figure 8-10   Malignant melanomas: *A*. showing satellite formation and adjacent inflammation, and *B*. showing typical irregularity of both edges and pigmentation. (From the collection of S. E. Blandford, Jr., M.D.)

a distinct predilection for junctional activity and melanoma formation.

Hemangiomas and Lymphangiomas

Hemangiomas are benign tumors of vascular origin, principally occurring in or just beneath the skin. They are common, with an overall incidence of 10 per cent, and the sex ratio shows a predisposition for females over males by 3:1.[7] As 50 per cent of these tumors occur in the head and neck region, mostly evident at or just after birth, they are highly visible and commonly a source of great anxiety to the parents. Consequently an understanding of their natural history is important for planning effective and logical treatment. Hemangiomas are divided both clinically and pathologically into two principal types— capillary hemangiomas and cavernous hemangiomas. Occasionally lesions show features of each type.

Capillary hemangiomas (port-wine stain, nevus flammeus, angioma simplex) are characterized histologically by masses of densely packed abnormal capillaries, usually lined with adult endothelial cells, located within or immediately below the dermis. Clinically they present as a smooth discoloration, ranging from deep pink to livid purple, with a sharp margin cleanly delineated from the adjacent normal skin. They occur principally on the face, located usually on only one side and following the distribution of one or more branches of the trigeminal nevus. The congenital nature of these lesions, together with an anatomic distribution limited to one of the fetal facial processes, suggests that it is a developmental rather than a neoplastic entity.

Although some faint capillary hemangiomas spontaneously resolve during the first few years of life, the majority remain unchanged, growing with the other facial structures and retaining their color. Malignant degeneration has never been reported and the problem is entirely cosmetic. However, the disfiguring nature of these lesions is such that merely ignoring capillary heman-

giomas as a harmless accident of birth is an inadequate approach.

Various methods of treatment have been employed. Radiation of any kind is to be condemned absolutely, for not only is it entirely ineffective against the mature endothelial cells, but the short-term hazards of alteration of growth of facial structures and the long-term sequelae of radiodermatitis and skin cancer are well known.

An opaque make-up may be used with great success in camouflaging the lesion where it is of similar texture to the adjacent skin. This is psychologically more suited to the female than the male patient, and has the disadvantage of requiring constant re-application, especially when the individual tends to sweat with activity.

Relatively small lesions may be excised and closed either directly, using the lines of skin tension, or with the aid of a local flap. The majority of these hemangiomas are, however, quite extensive, and the resurfacing involved might well lead to a greater disfigurement than the original lesion.

A rather unique and successful approach to the problem was evolved by Conway.[4] This consists of the tattooing of pigment into the superficial layers of the dermis to conceal the underlying angioma. Inorganic pigment is sterilized and carefully mixed to match the individual complexion of the patient. The principal pigment used is white (titanium oxide) and small amounts of red, yellow, brown and green are added judiciously by trial and error to achieve an exact color match. A surgical instrument—the Dermajector—has been modified from the crude equipment of the tattoo parlor, and this can be attached to the cord of a conventional Stryker motor. Following induction of local anesthesia, the pigment, mixed with sterile saline, is "painted" onto the skin surface and driven into the dermis by the repeated needle punctures of the Dermajector. The entire operation should, of course, be conducted as a sterile surgical procedure.

Frequently, two or three procedures,

several months apart, are necessary to achieve the desired degree of opacity for camouflage of the hemangioma. Never perfect, the results are usually satisfactory, particularly to the male who does not wish to be seen applying make-up in the men's room.

Rarely, a capillary hemangioma of the face is accompanied by hemangiomas of the cerebral cortex and retinal vascular lesions. This syndrome — Sturge-Weber's disease — should be thought of whenever a patient with a facial hemangioma demonstrates seizure activity.

Cavernous hemangiomas are the commonest benign tumors of childhood, and are histologically characterized by vascular channels of large size, lined with embryonal endothelium. They will present as raised, compressible lesions with a bluish or red discoloration, and may range in size from a small nodule to a gross lesion involving most of the face or an extremity. Also of embryonal rather than neoplastic origin, they may not become evident until the latent vascular "lakes" become continuous with the systemic circulation, usually by the end of the first month of life.

The surgical treatment of cavernous hemangioma is almost never an emergency and when possible a course of "watchful waiting" should be adopted by the surgeon and urged on the parents.

Statistically 80 per cent of cavernous hemangiomas will undergo spontaneous involution (even when growth of the lesion in the early months of life occurs at an alarming rate); 10 per cent will regress to the point where surgical resection is limited and relatively easy; and 10 per cent, usually fed by a major vessel, will require early operation. Involution usually occurs during the second or third year of life, is hastened by infection or the injection of sclerosing agents such as sodium morrhuate, hot water, or hypertonic saline solution, and is heralded by the appearance of gray atrophic patches in the epithelium overlying the hemangioma.

It is readily apparent that conservative treatment of these lesions is justified in the majority of cases. Radiation is again to be condemned in the young child, and the indications for surgery should be clearly understood. These include recurrent bleeding (an uncommon problem usually due to the child picking at the lesion), pain caused by a phlebolith, and persistent ulceration. If a bruit is heard within a rapidly growing lesion, it usually signifies the presence of an arteriovenous fistula of significant size. This will preclude spontaneous involution and is an indication for early surgery.

In general only the smallest hemangiomas, or those which have incompletely resolved, are amenable to outpatient care. In these cases, the principles of excision of skin lesions as previously described apply; most hemangiomas are so richly vascular that effective hemostasis is the pre-eminent surgical consideration; this is best obtained in the operating room.

Cavernous hemangiomas appearing after infancy should be resected, for not only are they unlikely to involute, but they are hard to distinguish from hemangiopericytoma, a malignant lesion which must be widely excised for control of local spread.

Lymphangioma is a true neoplasm of lymph vessels, and resembles hemangioma in that it is compressible and frequently exhibits a bluish discoloration of the overlying skin. It frequently involves the tongue and lips, causing macroglossia and macrocheilia respectively, and is common anywhere on the upper half of the body. It may be noticeable at birth or acquired in later life, and it will not involute. When noted, it should be excised in order to make a definitive diagnosis ruling out lymphangiosarcoma, from which it cannot be clinically distinguished.

Scars and Keloids

The ideal scar is an unobtrusive fine line, supple in texture, and producing no functional or esthetic deformity. When a surgical incision is properly planned with regard to lines of skin tension and executed with gentle handling of tissue, and the normal wound healing sequence proceeds without complication, the end result will usually be an acceptable scar. Injuries requiring suture may well, owing to circumstances such as tissue crushing or contamination, produce a scar which is thick, red and unsightly. When a scar has been infected, or allowed to granulate slowly, a hypertrophic scar will be the rule rather than the exception. Scars of this nature, particularly on the face where they are a source of embarrassment to the individual, will be referred for elective reconstruction frequently suitable for the Outpatient Department.

The natural tendency for a scar is to contract somewhat along its longitudinal axis. For this reason an incision should never be planned directly across a flexion crease, for it will usually form a "bridle" which either limits full extension or at the least gives rise to an objectionably noticeable scar. Areas where this precaution should be noted include the inguinal crease, the antecubital, volar wrist and popliteal regions, the axilla, the neck and the nasolabial folds. Injuries are not as discriminating as the wise surgeon, and lacerations in the "wrong direction" may cause scar contractures even when repaired perfectly.

Massive contractures such as commonly follow burns which have been allowed to granulate will frequently require release and a skin graft to resurface the resultant bare area. Contractures of a lesser degree will respond well to a Z-plasty, one of the basic techniques in the plastic surgeon's armamentarium.

The Z-plasty, whose origins are obscure,[9] consists essentially of the transposition of two triangular flaps (Fig. 8–11). The principal functional purpose of the Z-plasty is to increase the length of the skin in a desired direction at the expense of the width. The central portion of the Z is the contracture, which may be excised or incised depending on the characteristics of the tissue. Two side incisions of the same length as the central portion are made, generally at an angle of 60° to the axis of the scar,

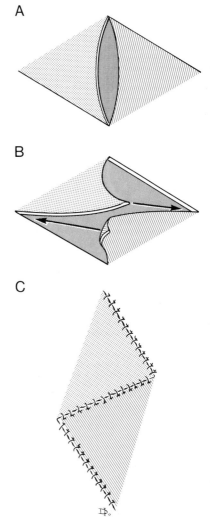

Figure 8–11 The Z-plasty, consisting of the transposition of two triangular flaps to lengthen the axis or change the direction of a contracted scar.

creating two triangular flaps which, after undermining, are transposed. It is the interposition of the width of these triangles which provides lengthening of the previous axis of the scar, and thus release of the contracture. The simple Z-plasty is suitable for the release of all contractures of modest dimensions, the greatest elongation possible being one-third of the original scar. When the bridle to be released is lengthy, requiring the transposition of large flaps, a series of Z-plasties along the length of the excised scar may be effectively employed with a less obtrusive result.

Another justifiable use for the Z-plasty is to change the direction of a scar. Lacerations of the face across the lines of tension may be thrown into prominence because their immobility in the presence of expressive muscular activity is noticeable. Examples are vertical scars of the forehead, scars across the nasolabial crease, and vertical scars between lower lip and chin. Their egregious characteristics may be reduced by a carefully planned Z-plasty, switching the main axis of the scar through 90° as shown in the illustration. The degree of cosmetic improvement resulting from this simple maneuver is often remarkable.

Linear scars of the face, even when well healed, are highly visible and in certain cultures carry unfortunate social connotations. The long scar of an innocently acquired "windshield laceration" may suggest the stigma of knife-fighting and prostitution in an adolescent Spanish-American girl. Breaking up this scar by means of multiple Z-plasties not only will reduce the visual impact of the scar, but will imply surgical intervention rather than that of the wielder of a switch-blade or razor.

An alternative method of breaking up the straight line of a long linear scar to render it less conspicuous is the "W-plasty."[2] If camouflage is required, rather than change of direction per se, then this is probably a better method than the multiple Z-plasty. W-plasty subjects the adjacent tissue to less pull than does multiple Z-plasty. Triangular sections, equilateral and with the sides 1 cm in length are taken along with the scar to be removed (Fig. 8–12). Sections larger than 1 cm will be too conspicuous, and smaller sections will be ineffective. This may be done by eye or by means of a pre-set pattern; if done by eye, the ends must be carefully plotted and the same number of triangles cut on each side. This procedure, first described by

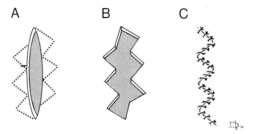

Figure 8–12   The W-plasty, an effective method of breaking up a prominent linear scar.

Borges, is a very valuable means of scar revision.

The degree of hypertrophy of a scar usually depends on the length of time taken for the wound to heal. Infected or granulating wounds, or incisions closed under extreme tension, will nearly always become thick, reddened and subject to breakdown and itching. Maturation of these scars into a flat, supple structure which is asymptomatic is always delayed and may never occur, in which case surgical revision will be necessary. However, the intense reaction of these scars may be suppressed and maturation hastened by the local use of steroids.

Steroid-impregnated adhesive tape (Cordran tape), when applied directly to the scar and left in place 24 hours a day, will often, over the course of months, achieve a fair degree of improvement. For the more troublesome scar, triamcinolone (Aristocort, 15 mgm per cc) may be injected directly into the scar tissue at monthly intervals until regression has taken place.[7] The same agent may be deposited into the superficial 5 mm of the scar without pain by the use of the French-designed Derma-jet, which works on an "air-rifle" principle and blasts a bolus of fluid into the skin by pressure alone. When 1.5 cc of triamcinolone is mixed with 0.5 cc of 1 per cent Xylocaine and 0.5 cc of Wydase, the administration is painless and effective. This is the method preferred by the author for the suppression of the moderately hypertrophic scar.

The most objectionable type of scar tissue formation is keloid. Commonest to Negroes and swarthy whites, but by no means limited to them, it is regarded by some as the ultimate degree of scar hypertrophy. As the true keloid will not respond to the limited measures described above for suppression of hypertrophic scar, a distinction would be practical. Keloid scar exists when:

1. The scar tissue extends beyond the confines of the original injury and invades the adjacent normal skin.
2. There has been no precipitating cause for scar hypertrophy such as infection or tension, or when the reaction is out of proportion to the stimulus.
3. A similar reaction has occurred before in the same individual—the "keloid former."
4. Histologic or tissue culture differentiation can be made.

Whereas a scar, hypertrophic from a known causative factor, can frequently be excised and closed meticulously to achieve a permanent "hair-line incision," the keloid treated in this manner will tend to recur. Treatment of keloids in the past has generally consisted of excision of the lesion, direct suture and immediate radiotherapy (2000 R in four daily divided doses) commencing the day of surgery. However, as this level of irradiation will produce dermal atrophy in the adjacent normal skin, the author prefers an intermediate and less hazardous step—that is, excision of the keloid and closure after deposition of triamcinolone into the edges of the wound. Treated in this manner, over 50 per cent of keloid scars are significantly improved; the remainder will need re-excision and the more powerfully suppressive effect of radiation as outlined.

Mowlem[11] has pointed out that retained foreign bodies often serve as a nucleus for keloid formation. For this reason, no buried suture material is used; the layers are closed with pull-out sutures of nylon or wire. Ideally neither ligatures nor the cautery should be used for hemostasis, cessation of flow being obtained by leaving clamps longer than usual on the cut ends of blood vessels and then "twisting" them, or by the use of compresses soaked in dilute (1:200,000) epinephrine solution.

Skin Grafting in the OPD

The taking of a skin graft is generally regarded as a fairly major procedure requiring a general anesthetic and admission to the hospital. Certainly the successful coverage of large areas of skin loss can best be attained by the close attention to the patient and his wound that this environment provides. However, within certain limitations, it is entirely possible to resurface smaller areas of loss with a skin graft taken under local anesthesia and followed on an ambulatory basis.

Certain areas of the body lend themselves better than others to this economical approach. Grafts on the trunk are hard to immobilize, owing to constant motion, and need to be observed closely; grafts on the lower extremities should *never* be treated in an ambulatory manner, for the poor venous return of the legs dictates that the grafts be immobilized with a pressure dressing and the legs elevated for at least ten days. Relatively limited areas of skin loss on the head, neck and upper extremities are ideally suited for coverage by skin grafting on an outpatient basis.

Skin grafts are classified anatomically according to the thickness of the graft. Split-thickness skin grafts consist of the epidermis and part of the dermis. As the deeper layers of the dermis are left behind, the donor site will heal spontaneously by epidermal regeneration. They may be cut either freehand (Fig. 8–13, *A* and *B*), using a skin grafting knife, or by a mechanical dermatome. The new Davol battery-powered dermatome is suitable for use in the Outpatient Department. The entire cutting head is

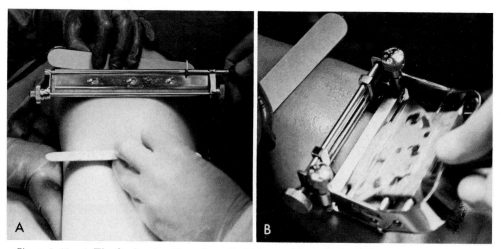

Figure 8–13 A. The freehand cutting of a split-thickness skin graft; immobilization of the donor part by an assistant is essential. *B.* Use of the Brown electric dermatome.

sterile and disposable, and the motor unit may be wrapped in a sterile polyethylene bag provided with each head piece. A suitable donor site for the split-thickness skin graft is the inner aspect of the upper arm, which is anesthetized by field block. The soft tissues of the arm are pressed taut against the humerus to present a flat surface to the blade, and the graft is taken. The donor site is dressed with scarlet-red gauze next to the raw surface, and covered with sponges and a Kling bandage.

The full-thickness skin graft consists of the epidermis and the entire thickness of the dermis. Cut by hand, it requires that the donor site be sutured closed, thus limiting the extent of the graft. Favorable locations for taking a full-thickness skin graft include the postauricular region, the upper eyelid in elderly people and the supraclavicular skin. The full-thickness skin graft will neither contract nor develop unsightly pigmentation; hence it is an ideal graft to resurface skin loss on the face. This is particularly so when the raw area involves the lower lid or the skin adjacent to the mouth. In these areas, minor degrees of contracture meet no resistance and thus cause significant distortion.

The survival and successful healing of skin grafts depend on the development of vascular communications between the graft and its recipient bed. The graft is initially sustained by diffusion alone. Capillary endothelial budding occurs at the interface to restore blood flow between recipient site and skin graft within 36 hours. Any factor which tends to disrupt these tenuous early vascular anastomoses will predispose to failure of the graft. The most important of these are "shearing," or sliding of the graft on its bed, hematoma formation which will elevate the graft, and infection.

Dressing techniques must therefore minimize these factors, providing both compression and immobilization to ensure rapid adherence of the graft. The "tie-over bolus dressing" (Fig. 8–14) has stood the test of time and is particularly suited for outpatient care as it will immobilize the graft while allowing movement in the grafted part.

The skin graft, taken as described, is laid in place on the recipient site and tacked at its four corners. Silk sutures are placed at one-inch intervals, the ends being left long enough to tie over the dressing. The graft is then trimmed so as to fit the defect exactly, and a fine running nylon suture is used to approxi-

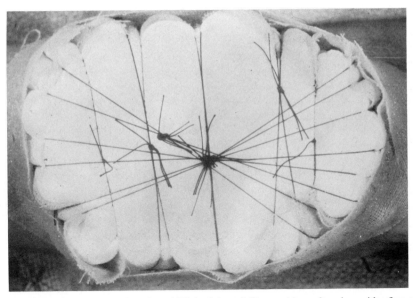

Figure 8–14   The tie-over bolus dressing which both immobilizes a skin graft and provides firm compression to minimize hematoma.

mate the edge of the graft to the borders of the defect, after irrigation under the graft. The dressing is then built up, using wet cotton, fluffs or sterile foam rubber (Reston, manufactured by the 3M Company, is a recent and very suitable material). The long ends of the sutures are then laid over the dressing to secure firm coaptation of the graft to its bed and yet allow motion in the grafted part without shearing. The whole area is wrapped in a bulky compression dressing. Pain, fever, purulent odors or bleeding imply the necessity of a dressing change, and may salvage a jeopardized graft.

The Reverdin or "pinch-graft" is popularly taught to surgical trainees as a simple method of obtaining skin under local anesthesia. However, the resultant scarring of both donor site and grafted area make it an unacceptable substitute for the methods described above.

The Use of Local Flaps

The other method of resurfacing a defect, alluded to many times in the preceding portion of this chapter, is by means of a flap. The flap, sometimes referred to as a "pedicle graft," is the earliest known reconstructive procedure, and originated with the Hindu tile cutters, who used forehead tissue to replace noses punitively amputated for adultery. The free graft (usually skin) is transplanted without blood supply and depends for its survival upon development of vascular anastomoses with the recipient site. The flap, in contrast, carries with it its own blood supply. The flap consists of skin, dermis and fat, and is always left attached (at least temporarily) with a vascular pedicle to maintain tissue respiration. The skillful design of a flap retains great fascination for the plastic surgeon, for when artistically executed the results are usually far superior to the more pedestrian and easily executed free skin graft. Sir Harold Gillies characterized this appeal when he titled one of the chapters in his outstanding text, "Flap Happy."[6]

Indications.   The use of a flap rather than a graft for resurfacing a defect is indicated in the following instances:

1. When a weight-bearing surface,

or an area constantly subjected to minor trauma, is involved.

2. When a further reconstructive procedure, for example, tendon transfer or bone graft, is contemplated at the site.

3. When major vessels, nerves, bone without periosteum or tendon denuded of paratenon are exposed.

4. Where a bulky defect would leave significant deformity if merely resurfaced with skin alone.

5. Where the recipient site is of poor vascularity—for example, in radiated tissue.

6. Flaps are in general preferred to grafts for resurfacing defects of the lower half of the face (i.e., below the level of the eyes) where a graft, subject to changes of pigmentation and texture, would tend to present a "patchy" appearance.

Classification. Flaps are usually classified under two principal headings: local flaps where the tissue to be transferred lies adjacent to the defect, and flaps from a distant source. Distant flaps—the cross-leg flap and those flaps transferred by means of an intermediary carrier such as the wrist—are operative procedures outside the scope of a discussion of outpatient surgery and properly belong in the operating room. Many local flaps are entirely suited to outpatient care, for immobilization and frequent inspection will not be as critical in determining the outcome.

Advancement Flap. The simplest flap is the advancement flap, where incisions in the axis of the desired tissue shift, undermining to provide mobility, and the natural elasticity of the skin will permit movement of tissue into an adjacent location (Fig. 8–15). Frequently "back-

A

B

Figure 8–15 The advancement flap.

C

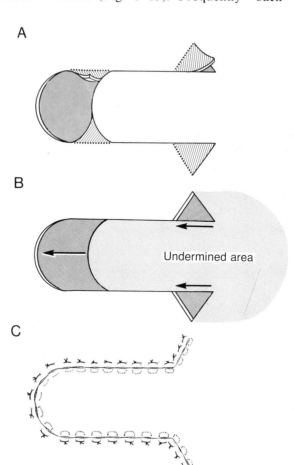

cuts" into the base of the pedicle will be required to allow the tissue to expand pantographically, or small triangles can be excised laterally to the flap to compensate for the disparity of length along the axis of closure. An example of the advancement flap is where the tissue of the cheek, incised and undermined generously, is advanced to resurface a defect at the side of the nose (Fig. 8–16 *A* and *B*).

Rotation Flap. The rotation flap utilizes a long, curving incision to allow the tissue to rotate about a pivot point (Fig. 8–17 *A, B, C*). Where the adjacent tissue is lax, as in the glabellar region between the eyebrows, the resultant defect may be closed primarily. Where easy closure of the defect is precluded by unyielding tissue, it is best resurfaced with a skin graft of appropriate size.

Interpolation Flap. The interpolation flap again is rotated about a pivot point, but it is taken from a suitable region near, but not immediately adjacent to, the defect (Fig. 8–18 *A, B, C*). The flap must therefore be "jumped" over intervening

tissue and should be planned so that the defect created by elevation and transfer of the flap can be closed directly. This requires a careful selection of donor sites in which the axis lies in a natural crease and the tissue is lax enough to permit nondistorting closure. Common sites for the interpolation flap include the use of lax upper lid skin to resurface defects of the lower lid as in the canthal flap (Fig. 8–19 *A, B, C*), and the nasolabial region to restore defects of the lower part of the nose (Fig. 8–20 *A, B, C*).

Technique. Most local flaps are applied directly with the raw surface of the flap laid on the defect. Where the base of the flap lies at some distance from the defect, part of the flap will serve as a bridge, which if unsurfaced, will provide a raw area liable to infection. A closed system can be provided either by grafting the underside of the flap or "tubing" the pedicle by sewing the edges of the flap together to provide a seam down the axis of the pedicle. Care must be taken not to do this under too great

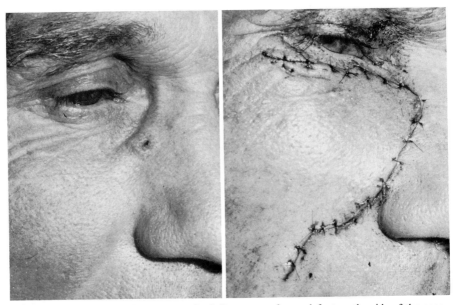

Figure 8–16   Use of an advancement cheek flap to resurface a defect on the side of the nose.

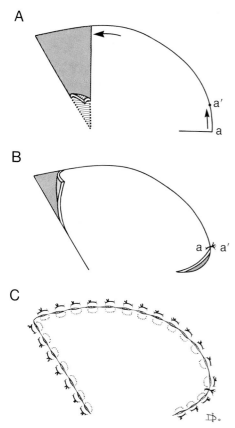

Figure 8–17 The rotation flap pivots tissue about a fixed point.

a defect of the medial canthus involving both upper and lower lids.

All flaps of whatever type have this in common: the secret of success lies in meticulous planning. Ideally a pattern of the defect is made and the operative steps planned in reverse until a template corresponding to the outline of the tissue to be transferred is traced on the skin of the donor site. Care must be taken to include the base of the pedicle in the pattern which must be cut a little longer and wider than the defect to allow for shrinkage of the transferred tissue.

"Delaying" a Flap. Much has been written about the supposed ideal dimensions of flaps in an attempt to introduce mathematical certainties into an imprecise field. The vagaries of individual circulatory patterns depend on the age of the individual and the location and direction of the flap. "Safe" length: width ratios are therefore almost meaningless. Rather than to incise the whole of a planned flap, and upon undermining find that the tip is avascular, it is better to incise and undermine only part of the flap and determine whether the circulation is sufficient to allow extension of the flap. If at any time during the preparation of the flap for transfer, dermal bleeding is dark and capillary filling slow, it is mandatory to return the flap to its original site in order for it to recover from circulatory assault. The oxygen debt in the tissue will enhance collateral circulation through the base of the pedicle—the principle of "delaying" a flap—which will permit the eventual transfer of a

tension, causing compression of the nutrient vessels, and the underside of the flap may be defatted to allow easy closure of the tube. An example of this technique is shown in Figure 8–21 (*A* to *E*), where a small tube pedicle from the forehead is used to reconstruct

Figure 8–18 The interpolation flap, which is jumped over intervening tissue.

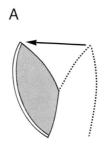
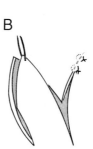
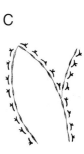

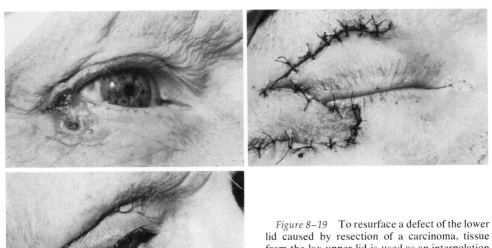

Figure 8-19 To resurface a defect of the lower lid caused by resection of a carcinoma, tissue from the lax upper lid is used as an interpolation flap.

pedicle too long and narrow to be formed in a single stage.

Enemies of flap survival other than incorrect planning include hematoma, which will "balloon" the flap and stretch the already marginal blood supply. For this reason, hemostasis must be pre-cise, and gentle pressure must be applied to the flap, although pressure must not be so great as to further embarrass the circu-lation. Various modalities have been used experimentally to enhance the circulation in a flap of dubious viability. These include hypothermia, hyperbaric

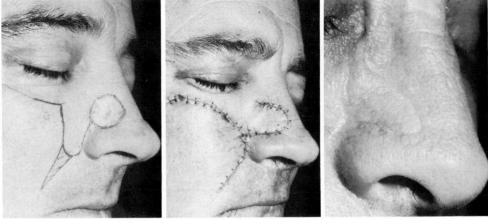

Figure 8-20 Defects of the lower nose may be replaced effectively by means of a nasolabial inter-polation flap.

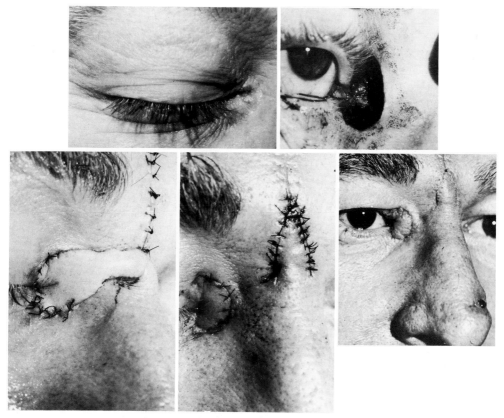

Figure 8–21 A small tube pedicle based on the glabella and taken from the central forehead is used to reconstruct a sizeable defect of the medial canthus caused by removal of a recurrent basal cell carcinoma.

O_2, and antisludging agents such as low molecular weight Dextran. None will substitute for correct planning.

Tissue handling must be gentle in the extreme, the tip of the flap being held with skin hooks or stay sutures through the dermis rather than crushing forceps. Suture technique of the flap to the recipient site is important and must cut off as little of the dermal circulation as possible. The "half-buried mattress suture," being parallel to the dermal plexus, is the least noxious in this regard (Fig. 8–22) and should be employed in preference to other sutures.

When these considerations are followed with care, the successful preparation and transfer of flaps become routine, and the dismaying sight of a partially necrotic flap, incapable of fulfilling the reconstructive role for which it was designed, may be avoided. Gillies defines plastic surgery as a "constant battle between beauty and blood supply," and nowhere is this more pertinent than in the design and execution of flaps.

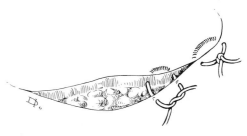

Figure 8–22 The half-buried mattress suture described by Halsted; this technique is most appropriate when blood supply to the skin edge is jeopardized.

References

1. Artz, C. P., and Reiss, E.: The Treatment of Burns. Philadelphia, W. B. Saunders Co., 1957.
2. Borges, A. F.: Improvement of anti-tension scar lines by the W-Plasty operation. Br. J. Plast. Surg., *12*:29–33, 1959.
3. Conway, H. C., Hugo, N. E., and Tulenko, J. F.: Surgery of Tumors of the Skin. Springfield, C. C Thomas, 1966.
4. Conway, H. C., and Montroy, R. E.: Permanent camouflage of capillary hemangiomas of face by intradermal injection of insoluble pigments (tattooing): indications for surgery, N. Y. State J. Med., *65*:876–885, 1965.
5. Dunphy, J. E.: On the nature and care of wounds. Ann. R. Coll. Surg. Engl., *26*:69–87, 1960.
6. Gillies, H. D., and Millard, D. R.: The Principles and Art of Plastic Surgery. Boston, Little, Brown and Co., 1957.
7. Griffith, B. H.: The treatment of keloids with triamcinolone acetonide. Plast. Reconstr. Surg., *38*:202–208, 1966.
8. Knize, D. M., Weatherley-White, R. C. A., Paton, B. C., and Owens, J. C.: Prognostic factors in the management of frostbite. J. Trauma, *9*:749–759, 1969.
9. McGregor, I. A.: Fundamental Techniques of Plastic Surgery. Baltimore, Williams and Wilkins Co., 1962.
10. Moyer, C. A., Brentano, L., Gravens, D. L., Margraf, H. W., and Monafo, W. W.: Treatment of large human burns with 0.5% silver nitrate solution. Arch. Surg., *90*:812–867, 1965.
11. Mowlem, R.: Hypertrophic scars. Br. J. Plast., Surg., *4*:113–120, 1951.
12. Mustardé, J. C.: Reconstruction of eyelids and eyebrows. In Grabb, W. C., and Smith, J. W.: Plastic Surgery. Boston, Little, Brown and Co., 1957.
13. Paton, B. C.: Bites—Human, dog, spider and snake. Surg. Clin. N. Amer., *43*(2):537–553, April, 1963.
14. Peacock, E. E., and Madden, J. W.: Some studies on the effects of B-aminopropionitrile in patients with injured flexor tendons. Surgery, *66*:215–222, 1969.
15. Prudden, J. F., Wolarsky, E. R., and Balassa, L.: The acceleration of healing. Surg. Gynecol. Obstet., *128*:1321–1326, 1969.
16. Schilling, J. A.: Wound healing. Physiol. Rev., *48*(2):374–423, 1968.
17. Stark, R. B.: Plastic Surgery. New York, Harper and Row, 1962.

9

The Eye — Ophthalmology

By JAMES R. CERASOLI, M.D.

INTRODUCTION

The ability of the physician to formulate a diagnosis and proceed with treatment is the basis for training in all fields of clinical medicine, but is especially difficult in ophthalmology because physicians tend to feel awkward when treating eye problems. As in other specialties, in ophthalmology a methodical approach is necessary in order to arrive at a proper diagnosis, and this will include a history, examination, and appropriate laboratory tests. This chapter will describe the evaluation and treatment of eye complaints in the Outpatient Clinic or office. For a more complete review of ophthalmology and methods of treatment utilized in hospitalized patients, a definitive text such as that of Newell (1965) should be consulted.

ANATOMY

Seven bones form the bony orbit (Fig. 9-1 A). The zygoma, maxilla and frontal bones form the orbital rim, which is the strongest part; the thin bones of the inner walls fracture easily, especially those in the floor and medial wall. The sphenoid bone contains the optic canal through which pass the ophthalmic artery and the optic nerve. Located temporally to this canal is the supra-orbital fissure through which pass into the orbit cranial nerves III and IV, and

229

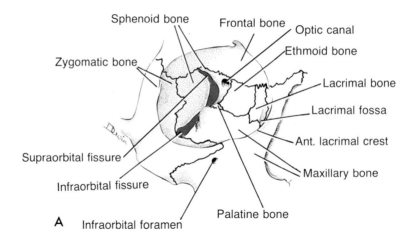

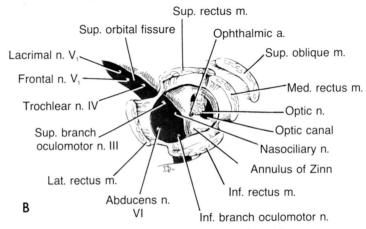

Figure 9–1   *A.* Bony orbit. *B.* Posterior orbit.

first division of V and VI. In the orbital apex syndrome, cranial nerve II and part or all of the cranial nerves passing through the superior orbital fissure may be affected (Fig. 9–1 *B*). In contrast to this syndrome, the superior orbital fissure syndrome does not involve cranial nerve II. If the second division of cranial nerve V is involved along with the other cranial nerves passing through this area, a localization in the cavernous sinus can be made.

Periosteum (periorbita) lines the orbit as a continuation of the dura mater.

Originating from the annulus of Zinn which encircles the optic canal and part of the superior orbital fissure are the four rectus muscles (medial and lateral, superior and inferior). Pain caused by movement of the eye in patients with optic neuritis may be explained by the proximity of the origin of these muscles to the optic canal. The rectus muscles insert in the globe anteriorly to the equator approximately 5.5 to 7 mm from the limbus. Above the annulus of Zinn originate the superior oblique and levator palpebrae muscles, while the inferior oblique muscle takes its origin from the inferior orbital rim near the anterior lacrimal crest. The two oblique muscles insert posteriorly to the equator on the temporal aspect of the globe. A cone-shaped compartment is formed by the recti muscle sheaths behind the globe where the injection of local anesthetic is placed for a local block of the orbit. Adipose tissue fills in the posterior orbit.

The eyeball measures approximately 24 mm in all diameters and has three layers composed of sclera, uvea and retina (Fig. 9–2). The outer scleral layer is a protective shell with a corneal window anteriorly. The middle vascular layer, or uvea, consists of choroid, ciliary body and iris, while the retina makes up the third inner layer. The lens lies behind the iris suspended by zonules. The ciliary body epithelium secretes aqueous humor into the posterior chamber and flows into the anterior chamber between the lens and iris through the pupil, exiting from the eye through the trabecular meshwork located in the angle of the anterior chamber and finally into Schlemm's canal.

A loose layer of connective tissue called Tenon's capsule encloses the eye from the limbus to the optic nerve. Conjunctiva lies external to Tenon's and reflects from the eyeball onto the lids in the upper and lower fornices. It contains mucous, sebaceous and accessory lacrimal glands which secrete the tear layers. Located upper temporally in the orbit near the rim, the lacrimal gland secretes tears reflexly which flow into the superior and inferior punctum at the inner canthus with each blink. Tears exit into the nose via the canaliculi, into the lacrimal sac and then into the lacrimal duct, and from there into the inferior meatal area in the nose (Fig. 9–3).

The orbit is separated into anterior

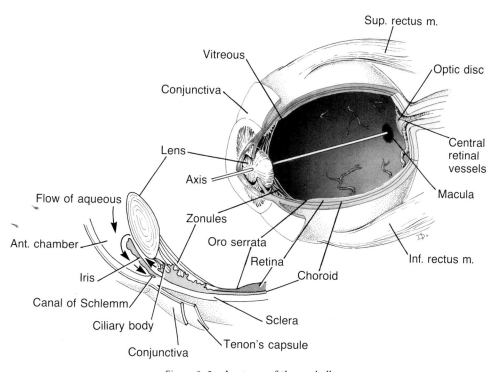

Figure 9–2 Anatomy of the eyeball.

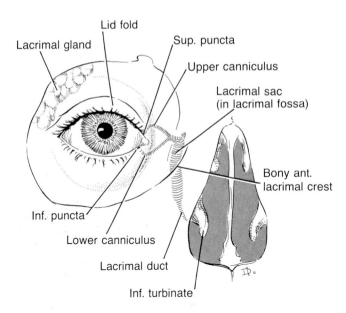

Figure 9–3   Lacrimal system.

and posterior compartments by the orbital septum, which extends as a connective tissue layer from the bony rim to the tarsus of the upper and lower lids. A defect in the orbital septum allows posterior orbital fat to prolapse into the anterior compartment. A fibrous tarsal plate provides stability to the lids when blinking (Fig. 9–4). The upper tarsal plate measures approximately 10–12 mm in width as opposed to 5–6 mm in the lower lid. The levator palpebrae muscle inserts largely into the upper

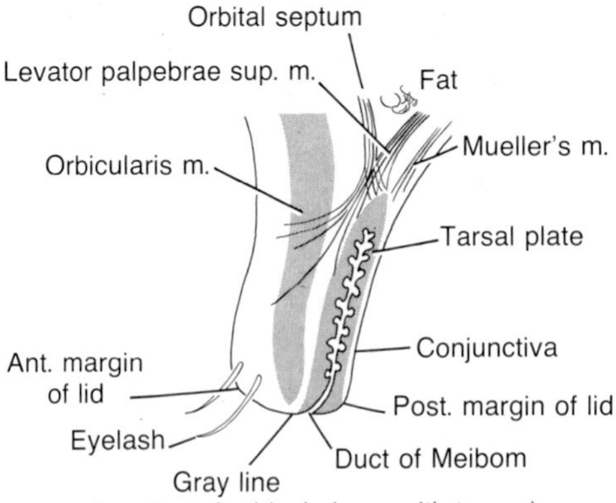

tarsus and the strands which extend into the skin form a lid fold in the upper lid. Mueller's muscle, a sympathetically innervated smooth muscle, lies between the palpebral conjunctiva and the levator palpebrae muscle.

PHARMACOLOGY

Some of the following medications should be readily available for diagnosis and treatment (Fig. 9–5):

1. Topical Anesthetic. Proparacaine (Ophthaine, Ophthetic) is a minimally irritating topical corneal anesthetic with a rapid onset of action (15 seconds) which lasts approximately 15 minutes. Pain, photophobia and blepharospasm from a superficial foreign body or corneal irritation are relieved with one topical application, allowing the physician to examine the eye comfortably. Side effects rarely occur with its use. It should be refrigerated when used infrequently.

2. Topical Antibiotics. A broad-spectrum preparation of neomycin, bacitracin and polymycin (Neo-polycin,

Figure 9–4   Anatomy of eyelid.

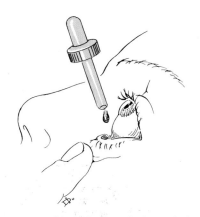

Figure 9–5 Method of introducing topical medications: (1) Have patient look up. (2) Slightly evert lower lid. (3) Place drop in lower cul-de-sac. (4) Do not touch eye or lashes with dropper.

Neosporin) is used prophylactically after the removal of foreign bodies and in the treatment of unknown conjunctival infections while awaiting a culture report. A local allergic reaction to neomycin may occur.

3. *Cycloplegics.* Homatropine (2 and 5 per cent) is a parasympatholytic drug which paralyzes the ciliary body and dilates the pupil. Its action relieves pain from ciliary body spasm such as that which occurs in traumatic iritis from an injury, or after removal of a corneal foreign body. Its duration of action (24 hours) does not inconvenience the patient as do the longer acting cycloplegics atropine and scopolamine. Uncommonly in older patients an attack of acute narrow angle glaucoma may be precipitated (see section on Glaucoma).

4. *Mydriatics.* Phenylephrine 10 per cent is a sympathomimetic drug which dilates the pupil and is useful for examining the fundus. Its effect begins in approximately 30 minutes and lasts approximately 3 hours. It also may precipitate an attack of narrow angle glaucoma (see section on Glaucoma).

5. *Glaucoma Treatment.* Ophthalmologists use parasympathomimetic drugs (pilocarpine and echothiophate iodide) which constrict the pupil, lower intraocular pressure and facilitate accommodation. Only echothiophate iodide (Phospholine Iodide) is used in the treatment of accommodative esotropia, but both medications are used for chronic glaucoma.

Glycerol, Diamox and mannitol lower the intraocular pressure by an osmotic action. One of these osmotic agents (preferably IV mannitol, 20 per cent, 1 gm/Kg) combined with the frequent topical use of pilocarpine 4 per cent usually breaks an attack of narrow angle glaucoma. The pupil becomes miotic and the intraocular pressure normal.

6. *Steroids.* The use of topical steroid preparations should be avoided because of the ocular side effects of glaucoma, cataracts and corneal ulcers. Patients tend to use these preparations unsupervised for the treatment of viral conjunctivitis and nonspecific corneal irritation because of the symptomatic relief provided.

LOCAL ANESTHESIA

The first division of the trigeminal nerve enters the orbit through the superior orbital fissure and provides the sensory innervation to the orbit and upper lid (Figs. 9–6 and 9–1 *B*). The supraorbital nerve is a branch of the ophthalmic division and exits through the supraorbital foramen in the superior rim. The infraorbital nerve, a branch of the maxillary division, exits through the infraorbital foramen in the lower rim. Xylocaine (1 or 2 per cent) with epinephrine infiltrated in either area gives excellent local anesthesia for the upper or lower lid. Sometimes the medial and lateral canthal areas of the upper and lower lids may require additional infiltration because of overlapped innervation from other branches of the ophthalmic and maxillary division of V. Xylocaine injected into the muscle cone gives akinesia and anesthesia for globe and orbital structures. This type of retrobulbar injection may be complicated by a hemorrhage and rarely by occlusion of the central retinal artery.

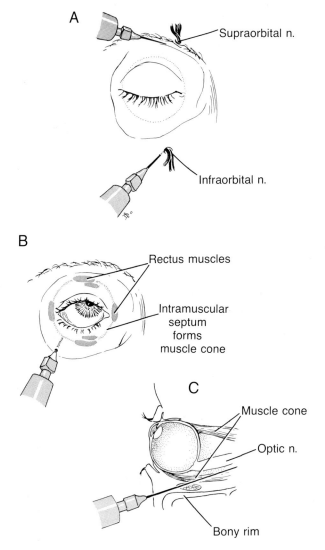

Supraorbital n.

Infraorbital n.

Rectus muscles

Intramuscular
septum
forms
muscle cone

Muscle cone

Optic n.

Bony rim

Figure 9–6 Methods of local anesthetic blocks. *A.* Technique for local anesthesia for upper and lower lids: (1) Use a 24 gauge needle to infiltrate 1–2 cc of 2 per cent xylocaine in the area of the supraorbital or infraorbital nerve near periosteum. (2) To block the VIIth nerve innervation of the orbicularis muscle, an additional injection must be given temporally by infiltrating an area from the brow to the zygomatic imminence.

B and *C.* Technique for retrobulbar block: (1) Palpate lower temporal orbital rim as patient looks up and nasal. (2) Insert 23 gauge needle of less than 2 inches length in the space between the eyeball and bony rim. (3) Once the eyeball is cleared by the needle tip, direct the needle toward the center of the annulus of Zinn, which is approximately the middle of the posterior orbit. This will place the needle in the muscle cone. (4) Never insert the needle a full 2 inches into the orbit because the anesthetic agent can be accidentally injected into the bony optic canal and compress the optic nerve. (5) Approximately 2 cc of 2 per cent xylocaine injected into this space will give excellent orbital anesthesia and akinesia.

EYE EXAMINATION

A physician can examine the eye adequately with a visual acuity chart, a bright hand light, an ophthalmoscope and a Schiøtz tonometer. This section will outline the steps in an eye examination.

1. Vision. The corrected visual acuity is the most important part of the eye examination. For acute eye problems, the examiner must rely on the patient's glass prescription as the best correction. A difference in acuity between the two eyes or poor vision in both eyes requires an explanation. Normal vision (20/20 in both eyes) indicates the central visual apparatus is intact which includes the cornea, lens, vitreous, macula and the visual pathway to the lateral geniculate nuclei. The peripheral vision is tested monocularly by a finger-counting confrontation technique as part of the vision exam. Each quadrant is examined as the patient fixes on the examiner's eye. The patient and the examiner should see the fingers in approximately the same peripheral position. A gross field defect should have quantitative perimetry and its etiology should be explained by the eye examination or a neurological examination.

2. *Pupils.* The afferent and efferent pathways of the light reflex which include the iris, visual apparatus and autonomic nervous system are intact if the pupils are equal in size and react briskly and equally to a light stimulus when tested both directly and consensually. Consider the pupils abnormal if they are unequal in size or if the light reaction is poor or absent. Their cause must be explained since the prognostic significance of these findings varies greatly. Some common causes of abnormal pupils are eye medications, third nerve paralysis, Horner's syndrome, Adie's tonic pupil, tertiary syphilis and trauma to the iris. A Horner's syndrome consists of ptosis, miosis and anhidrosis with apparent enophthalmos which results from a lesion in any one of the three neurons forming the sympathetic pathway from the hypothalamus to the eye. In Horner's syndrome, the pupil responds like a postganglionic, sympathetically denervated structure which is hypersensitive to weak dilutions of topical epinephrine (1 : 1000) and will dilate, whereas the normal pupil will not. Topical cocaine dilates the normal pupil by preventing the re-uptake of norepinephrine at the effector site. In Horner's syndrome, topical cocaine will not dilate the affected pupil since norepinephrine is not secreted in the denervated situation. Cocaine (4 per cent) compared to epinephrine (1 : 1000) gives more reliable results when testing for Horner's syndrome. The subject of the physiology of the eye is discussed in detail by Moses (1970).

In the tonic pupil or Adie's syndrome, parasympathetic denervation of the pupil occurs because of a lesion in ciliary ganglion. Clinically the abnormal pupil is larger than normal and the reaction to a light stimulus is poor or absent. Topical application of a weak cholinergic agent (methacoline 2.5 per cent) constricts the affected pupil but not the normal pupil. Recognition of this common syndrome is important because it is a benign condition and should be differentiated from a third nerve paralysis. In most cases the history and other neurologic findings help differentiate a third nerve paralysis from other causes of abnormal pupils. Pilocarpine (4 per cent) will constrict a pupil which is dilated because of third nerve paralysis. Many patients have unilateral or bilateral dilated, poorly reacting pupils caused by mydriatic medication placed in the eye that a patient usually fails to relate to the examiner. Pilocarpine (4 per cent) will not constrict these pupils.

The Argyll Robertson pupil seen in tertiary syphilis consists of an intact near-reaction while the light reaction is poor or absent. Both pupils are usually miotic and irregular in shape. They may dilate very poorly in response to any mydriatic. In paresis or in latent lues, the patient may have, instead of an Argyll Robertson pupil, a fixed dilated pupil.

Abnormal pupils secondary to trauma can usually be recognized. A small defect in the pupillary sphincter causes a partially dilated pupil with a very irregular margin. In some cases, a defect in the iris stroma (iridodialysis) may occur. The history, examination and use of appropriate topical medications help differentiate these different causes of abnormal pupils.

3. *Extraocular Muscles.* (Fig. 9–7.) The third, fourth, and sixth cranial nerves are evaluated when a patient follows a light into the eight fields of gaze. Old photographs and the history help distinguish an acute external ophthalmoplegia (extraocular muscle paresis) from a decompensated congenital muscle imbalance. The degree of diplopia increases in the field of action of the acutely paretic muscle. Mechanical limitation from an orbital floor fracture or mass may simulate a muscle paresis. A forced duction test consists of moving the eye in all positions of gaze

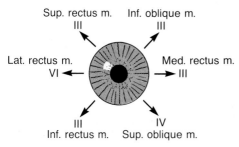

Sup. rectus m.   Inf. oblique m.
III   III

Lat. rectus m.   Med. rectus m.
VI   III

III   IV
Inf. rectus m.   Sup. oblique m.

Figure 9–7   Testing eye muscle movements.

with a tooth forceps to determine if mechanical limitation is present. This test is easily performed after several drops of topical anesthesia with ophthane or cocaine. The eye is grasped with a 0.5 mm toothed forceps near the limbus in front of the muscle tested. The test is positive (mechanical limitation is present) when the eye cannot be moved fully with the forceps.

4. *Anterior Segment of the Eye.* The lids, lacrimal apparatus, conjunctiva, cornea, anterior chamber, iris and lens may be grossly evaluated with a bright hand light. Fluorescein dye placed in the tears helps in locating small foreign bodies and corneal epithelial abrasions. The dye stains the disturbed corneal epithelium a bright green after the excess is blinked away with the tears.

Blood in the anterior chamber (hyphema) may settle inferiorly as a red clot or may, if extensive, obscure the iris detail. Usually inflammatory cells in the anterior chamber, like those in an iritis, cannot be seen with a hand light, but a flush of the perilimbal vessels is usually present. Tremulous movements of the iris (iridodonesis) occur when the lens partially dislocates (subluxation) or totally dislocates (luxation). Also, the depth of the anterior chamber appears deeper or irregular compared to its normal fellow eye.

5. *Posterior Segment of the Eye.* Ophthalmoscopic evaluation of the vitreous, disc, macula, retina and retinal vessels should be done through a dilated pupil. One drop of neosynephrine (10 per cent)

works well. A monocular visual loss or central scotoma may be explained by changes in any of the posterior structures. Scars, hemorrhages or tumors in the macular area can cause a marked visual loss. Abnormalities in the peripheral area such as hemorrhages, inflammation, scars, vascular abnormalities, tumors and retinal detachments are other common causes of monocular visual loss.

Early signs of papilledema are bilateral blurring of the disc margins, hyperemia of the disc and loss of venous pulsation. The presence of splinter hemorrhages and elevation of the disc margins establish the diagnosis. The vision remains normal but the blind spot enlarges on testing the central fields. In optic neuritis the disc may appear similar to that seen in papilledema, but it is usually unilateral and vision is decreased with the presence of a field defect.

6. *Glaucoma.* A screening measurement of the intraocular pressure with a Schiøtz tonometer for hypotony or glaucoma should be done on patients who have had trauma or possible acute angle closure glaucoma attack (see Fig. 9–8 and Table 9–1). An intraocular pressure of 10–22 mm of mercury that is bilaterally equal is normal. A low intraocular pressure may be the only clue to a posterior rupture of the globe. If the optic disc looks suspiciously cupped, the measurement should be repeated another day because one isolated measurement of the intraocular pressure will miss 50 per cent of patients with chronic open angle glaucoma.

A large irregular central cup should alert the examiner to possible chronic glaucoma (Fig. 9–9). A comparison of the diameter of the central cup to the diameter of the disc gives a cup/disc ratio (C/D). If the cup/disc ratio is 0.3 or greater, the intraocular pressure should be checked.

Acute or narrow angle glaucoma is differentiated from chronic or open angle glaucoma by gonioscopy. An ophthalmologist must make this evaluation

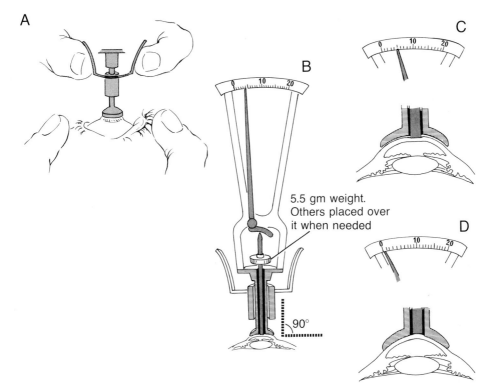

5.5 gm weight.
Others placed over
it when needed

90°

Figure 9–8 Use of Schiøtz tonometer. For conversion numbers see Table 9–1. (1) Patient recumbent. (2) Cornea anaesthetized. (3) Patient fixates with opposite eye. (4) Lids held open with no pressure on eyeball. (5) Tonometer reading is converted to mm of mercury by chart supplied with instrument (see Table 9–1). (7) Tonometer readings 0–2.5 with 5.5 gm or any weight are inaccurate and additional weights must be added until the tonometer reading is greater than 2.5.

by examining the appearance of the angle of the anterior chamber. In acute glaucoma there is a sudden rise in the intraocular pressure (usually greater than 50 mm of mercury) associated with sudden severe pain, loss of vision and an injected irritable eye with a dilated pupil. Usually a clinical diagnosis is easily made. Delay in treatment of the glaucoma may result in permanent loss of vision after several hours (see section on Pharmacology). In contrast, chronic glaucoma occurs bilaterally with an insidious loss of the peripheral fields over many years while good central acuity is maintained with few symptoms or none.

TRAUMA

For a definitive review of the problems of trauma to the eye and its supporting structures, the reader is referred to the standard text by Paton and Goldberg (1968).

1. Foreign Bodies. Foreign body complaints from flying metal fragments and blast injuries require orbital x-rays. To distinguish an intraocular from an orbital foreign body, a localization may be performed using a Sweet's radiological technique (Pendergrass), or a radiopaque contact lens may be placed on the cornea. Most inaccessible orbital foreign bodies need not be removed, but

TABLE 9–1   Schiøtz Conversion Table*

Schiøtz Reading	5.5 gms	7.5 gms	10 gms	15 gms
0.0	41.5 mm Hg	59.1 mm Hg	81.7 mm Hg	127.5 mm Hg
0.5	37.8	54.2	75.1	117.9
1.0	34.5	49.8	69.3	109.3
1.5	31.6	45.8	64.0	101.4
2.0	29.0	42.1	59.1	94.3
2.5	26.6	38.8	54.7	88.0
3.0	24.4	35.8	50.6	81.8
3.5	22.4	33.0	46.9	76.2
4.0	20.6	30.4	43.4	71.0
4.5	18.9	28.0	40.2	66.2
5.0	17.3	25.8	37.2	61.8
5.5	15.9	23.8	34.4	57.6
6.0	14.6	21.9	31.8	53.6
6.5	13.4	20.1	29.4	49.9
7.0	12.2	18.5	27.2	46.5
7.5	11.2	17.0	25.1	43.2
8.0	10.2	15.6	23.1	40.2
8.5	9.4	14.3	21.3	38.1
9.0	8.5	13.1	19.6	34.6
9.5	7.8	12.0	18.0	32.0
10.0	7.1	10.9	16.5	29.6

*To use the Table:
  1. Determine scale reading on Schiøtz tonometer.
  2. Find reading on Conversion Table under column titled Schiøtz Reading.
  3. Determine intraocular pressure in mm Hg by reading under column with appropriate wt. used.

an intraocular foreign body should be referred to an ophthalmologist for management. It is helpful for him to know the kind of metal composing the foreign body, since iron and copper are

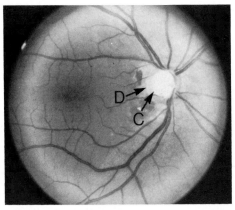

Figure 9–9 Glaucoma cupping of optic nerve. *C.* Optic cup. *D.* Optic disc.

extremely toxic to the eye while some inert materials are best left undisturbed. Magnetic foreign bodies are easier to remove with a magnet and therefore have a better prognosis than other types.

Superficial foreign bodies of the tarsal conjunctiva and cornea may be located by use of fluorescein staining, a bright light and magnification. After topical corneal anesthesia, the foreign body may be wiped away with a moist, sterile, cotton-tip applicator. This may be unsuccessful if the foreign body is deeply imbedded in the corneal stroma. In this case, it should be referred to an ophthalmologist who can remove it under high magnification with a sharp needle or spud.

Sand and dirt particles lodge in the tarsal conjunctiva of the upper lid and, to the patient, feel like corneal foreign bodies. They cause streaklike, diffuse staining of the cornea and can be removed by everting the upper lid and wiping away with a sterile, moist, cotton-tip applicator (see Fig. 9–10). A topical broad-spectrum antibiotic should be used prophylactically on the eye. Daily follow-up examinations are necessary until the corneal epithelium no longer stains with fluorescein because these abrasions frequently result in corneal ulcers which require emergency management. An untreated corneal ulcer may perforate the cornea with loss of the eye. These infections are difficult to treat because of corneal avascularity.

Large corneal abrasions, whether due to a foreign body or other trauma, require the same precautions as outlined above. Two oval eye pads taped firmly to splint the lid relieve symptoms and allow the corneal epithelium to regenerate more quickly. The epithelial defect usually regenerates in 24 to 48 hours.

2. Lacerations of the Lids. A lid laceration should alert the physician to possible intraocular damage. Multiple lid lacerations may appear as avulsed tissue. Usually little or no tissue loss occurs and the lid fits together like a jigsaw puzzle. The physician should copiously irrigate the debris from the laceration, but try not to débride tissue unless truly necrotic (the excellent blood supply to the lid usually prevents necrosis). Superficial lid lacerations which do not involve the lid margin or canalicular area are easily repaired with interrupted 6–0 silk sutures. A deep laceration involving the orbital septum can be recognized when orbital fat prolapses into the wound; the deep layers should be closed anatomically with 5–0 or 6–0 absorbable sutures. If skin avulsion does occur, the most satisfactory sites from which to take a skin graft are the opposite upper lid or the site behind the ear. Extensive loss of tissue requires a bridge flap from the uninvolved lid.[1]

Exposure and tearing problems may result from poorly repaired lid lacerations through the margin. Since the lower canaliculus drains the majority of tears into the nose, lacerations through this area require meticulous repair and are best referred to an ophthalmologist. Lacerations through the upper canaliculus and lid margins are repaired as diagrammed (Fig. 9–11). Lid notches may occur if these lacerations are not exactly approximated, and corneal irritation with pain and decreased vision may develop.

3. Laceration of the Eyeball. Pigmented uveal tissue found in a corneal or scleral laceration establishes this diagnosis. The laceration requires immediate repair by the ophthalmologist. Both eyes should be patched lightly without further manipulation and the patient instructed to remain quiet. Squeezing

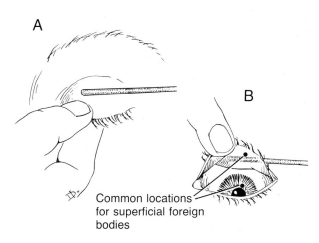

Figure 9–10 Technique of everting lid and removing foreign body. (1) Anesthetize cornea. (2) Patient looks down. (3) Lid everted as shown. (4) Foreign body located and removed.

Common locations for superficial foreign bodies

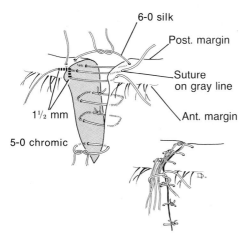

6-0 silk

Post. margin

Suture
on gray line

1½ mm

Ant. margin

5-0 chromic

Figure 9–11 Repair of laceration of lid. (1) Place the posterior lid margin suture first and leave its ends long for traction while placing the other sutures. (2) Repair the tarsal and orbicularis laceration with 5-0 chromic. (3) Complete the gray line and anterior margin suturing with long ends so that the knots can be pulled away from the cornea as illustrated.

of the lid, coughing and unnecessary movements will increase the intraocular pressure and cause further prolapse of the intraocular contents.

4. Contusion Injuries to the Eye. Blunt trauma about the eye causes serious intraocular injury in approximately 15 per cent of all cases. A methodical examination differentiates the routine black eye from one which has a serious intraocular injury. Rupture of the sclera, traumatic glaucoma, blood in the anterior chamber or vitreous, dislocation of the lens, traumatic cataracts, retinal detachment, retinal hemorrhage and injury to the optic nerve with permanent loss of vision can occur if not properly treated.

5. Orbital Fractures. Proper x-ray examination helps make the diagnosis when orbital fractures are suspected. A routine orbital series of x-rays should include an anterior-posterior view, a lateral view, a Waters' projection and a submental view. These views may be interpreted as normal even when there is clinical evidence of a fracture, in which case further study by tomography

should be done. A blow-out fracture incarcerates the inferior orbital contents into the floor defect, thus mechanically limiting elevation and depression of the eye and causing vertical diplopia. Injury to the infraorbital nerve in this area causes hypesthesia to the lower lid area. Optimally the fracture is repaired within one or two weeks after the injury when the swelling has subsided. If misdiagnosed, organization of the tissues in the fracture site occurs and makes repair difficult. A blow-out fracture is best repaired through an orbital approach with a silastic or methylmethacrylate implant inserted to cover the defect after the incarcerated tissue is retracted.

The trimalar fracture usually involves the zygomatic-maxillary suture, zygomatic-frontal suture, and arch of the zygoma. A nondisplaced trimalar fracture requires no further treatment; however, displacement causes flattening of the cheek bone and occasionally temporo-mandibular joint problems. Repair is accomplished by wiring two legs of the tripod at the zygomatic-frontal and zygomatic-maxillary sutures after open reduction of the displacement. Isolated fractures involving only the orbital rim do not require repair. Orbital emphysema may occur from a fracture in the ethmoid sinus or the orbital floor, and treatment requires time for the orbital air to slowly reabsorb, during which time the patient should be given a broad-spectrum antibiotic and instructed not to blow his nose for several weeks.

A fracture in the optic canal is difficult to diagnose using x-rays alone. Tomograms sometimes help. Edema of the intraosseous portion of the optic nerve occurs and may result in permanent visual loss if not decompressed early by a neurological approach. Surgical treatment of this edema should not be undertaken if vision is poor on the initial examination; this diagnosis should be considered and surgery contemplated only if the vision has been reported on an initial examination and later deteriorates.

6. Radiation. Ultraviolet light from

an arc welder's machine or prolonged exposure to the snow or sandy beaches causes corneal epithelial changes. Severe pain, photophobia, and blurred vision occur five to ten hours after the insult. Fluorescein stains the cornea in a stippled pattern. One application of a topical anesthetic gives instant relief; however, its chronic use can inhibit epithelial regeneration and can cause corneal scarring. A firm dressing on both eyes and mild sedation provide relief for the patient until the epithelium regenerates. Usually no residual corneal problems occur.

7. Chemical Burns. Any caustic material in the eye requires rapid and copious irrigation with any solution at hand. The patient may blink his eyes under water as an initial treatment at home or at work. Thereafter, the physician should use a topical anesthetic, irrigating the eye with 2 to 3 liters of normal saline or balanced Ringer's lactate using a bulb syringe or IV tubing. To remove particular matter in the cul-de-sacs of the upper and lower lids, a cotton-tip applicator may be used. The damage resulting to the eye from a chemical burn depends upon the type, concentration and duration of the chemical in the eye; lye burns heal poorly while acid burns cause relatively less damage.

Mace and tear gas corneal injuries are self-limiting and usually leave no residual corneal defects. The eye may be irrigated with 0.4 per cent sodium sulfite solution or normal saline after application of a topical anesthetic. The propellant used in mace may cause a contusion injury if ejected near the patient's eye.

INFLAMMATION OF THE EYE

In the differential diagnosis of a red eye, conjunctivitis, iritis, scleritis and acute glaucoma must be considered. Certain guidelines for these entities can be set (see Table 9–2), although their differentiation may puzzle the examiner if a methodical history and eye examination are not done. Acute glaucoma requires emergency treatment and a delay in diagnosis can result in permanent loss of vision. Corneal ulcers cause the patient to complain of pain and a foreign body sensation, and vision is usually decreased; on examination a corneal opacity is usually noted. A dendritic ulcer of herpes simplex may be seen only after staining the cornea with fluorescein. All corneal ulcers require scrapings for gram stains, culture and sensitivities to establish the diagnosis. Treatment with antibiotics is started according to the results of the bacteriology studies.

Orbital cellulitis usually is caused by a sinus infection or trauma, and the inflammation can quickly spread to the cavernous sinus because of the orbital venous drainage into this area. These patients should be hospitalized and treated with appropriate antibiotics after culture and sensitivity studies. In dacryocystitis inflammation occurs over the lacrimal sac, and with pressure over this area, pus can be expressed through the lower punctum. These infections tend to be chronic because of obstruction in the nasal lacrimal system. After antibiotic treatment, a dacryocysto-rhinostomy re-establishes a drainage system into the nose which cures the epiphora and prevents recurrent infections.

COMMON LID PROBLEMS IN THE OUTPATIENT CLINIC

Lagophthalmos or inability to close the lids usually results in corneal exposure and occurs after a seventh nerve paresis or proptosis of the globe. Short-term management with frequent topical methyl cellulose drops, ointment and patching at night works very well. If

TABLE 9-2 Differential Diagnosis of a Nontraumatic Inflamed Eye

	Conjunctivitis	Iritis	Scleritis	Acute Glaucoma
Vision	Normal	Normal or mild blur	Normal	Decreased
Discharge	Mucoid or pus	Tearing from photophobia	Tearing from photophobia	Tearing from photophobia
Congestion	Lids and superficial conjunctival vessels	Circumcorneal and conjunctival	Deep scleral vessels	All vessels
Pain	Foreign body sensation, sandy or mild	Moderate to severe	Severe	Severe
Cornea	Normal	Probably clear Keratic precipitate present*	Normal	Cloudy
Anterior Chamber	Normal	Probably clear Cells present*	Normal	Shallow
Pupil	Normal	Usually miotic	Normal	Dilated
Intraocular Tension	Normal	Usually decreased	Normal	Increased
Treatment	Culture and smear Appropriate topical antibiotics	Cycloplegia Topical steroids qHs Treat systemic disease	Cycloplegia Treat systemic disease Analgesia Topical steroids qHs	Osmotic agents 1) Intravenous: Diamox, mannitol, urea 2) Oral: glycerol, pilocarpine 4% topically Surgery

*Can be seen with biomicroscope.

A

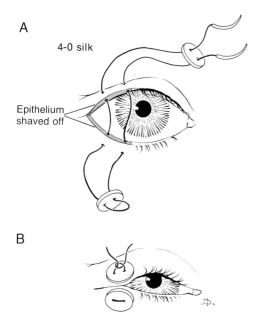

4-0 silk

Epithelium shaved off

B

Figure 9–12   Temporary tarsorraphy.

corneal exposure problems develop during long-term management, partial closure of the lids is necessary with a tarsorrhaphy. A temporary tarsorrhaphy is accomplished by excising a thin layer of both lid margins in the lateral canthus and placing a 4–0 silk mattress suture through the lid, as demonstrated in the diagram (Fig. 9–12).

Lid margin carcinomas require pathological diagnosis prior to surgical management. A basal cell carcinoma is removed en-bloc with frozen sections at the time of surgery to show clear margins. Small lesions which involve less than 30 per cent of the lid can usually be closed primarily (Fig. 9–11). A lateral cantholysis may be necessary to close larger lesions.[6] Very large defects must be closed with bridge flaps from the upper or lower lid (see Chapter 8). Squamous cell carcinoma of the lid is uncommon and requires extensive surgery with a node dissection.

Subconjunctival hemorrhages alarm the patient but usually cause no eye damage. They may indicate systemic problems such as hypertension or clotting deficiencies and should alert the physician.

Chalazions are chronic granulomatous inflammations of the meibomian gland whose etiology has not been established. Hordeolums are acute inflammations of glands of the lid margin. Both can be managed with frequent warm soaks and topical antibiotics. A hordeolum may be incised if pointing. If the chalazion does not regress with conservative management it may be curetted through an incision which overlies it. No sutures are necessary.

Conclusion

A methodical history, eye examination and appropriate laboratory tests are essential in evaluating any eye problem. Commonly overlooked in this procedure is the test for visual acuity, which undoubtedly is the most important part of the examination. It is difficult to advise the physician which eye problems to treat and which to refer to an ophthalmologist, since this depends on so many factors, but one of the most important of these is a correct diagnosis.

References

1. Hughes, W. L.: Reconstructive Surgery of the Eyelids. St. Louis, C. V. Mosby Co., 1954.
2. Moses, R. A.: Adler's Physiology of the Eye: Clinical Application. St. Louis, C. V. Mosby Co., 1970.
3. Newell, F. W.: Ophthalmology: Principles and Concepts. St. Louis, C. V. Mosby Co., 1965.
4. Paton, D., and Goldberg, M. F.: Injuries of the Eye, the Lids and the Orbit: Diagnosis and Management. Philadelphia, W. B. Saunders Co., 1968.
5. Pendergrass, E. P.: The Head and Neck in Roentgen Diagnosis. Springfield, Ill., C. C Thomas, 1956.
6. Smith, B., and Cherubini, T. (eds.): Ophthalmic Plastic Surgery. International Ophthalmology Clinics: *10*(1), Spring, 1970.

10

Ear, Nose, Throat and
Sinuses — Otorhinolaryngology

I. EAR
  A. Examination
    1. History
        a. Hearing loss
        b. Pain
        c. Vertigo
        d. Tinnitus
        e. Otorrhea
    2. Techniques of examination
    3. Hearing tests — Weber and Rinné
    4. Vestibular function
  B. Congenital lesions
    1. Preauricular cysts
    2. Accessory auricles
    3. Angioma
    4. Bat ears
  C. Traumatic conditions
    1. Hematoma
    2. Lacerations
    3. Frostbite
    4. Foreign bodies and cerumen
    5. Traumatic rupture of the tympanic membrane
  D. Tumors
    1. Sebaceous cysts
    2. Fibroma
    3. Cutaneous horn
    4. Senile keratoses
    5. Keratoacanthoma
    6. Papilloma
    7. Exostoses
    8. Adenoma
    9. Carcinoma
  E. Inflammatory conditions
    1. Perichondritis
    2. Chondrodermatitis nodular helicis chronicis
    3. External otitis
    4. Acute otitis media
        a. etiology
        b. myringotomy
        c. convalescence
    5. Serous otitis media
    6. Chronic otitis media
  F. Ear piercing for earrings

II. NOSE
  A. Examination

  B. Congenital lesions
    1. Dermoid cysts
    2. Inclusion cysts
    3. Nasoalveolar cysts
    4. Atresia
        a. Anterior choanal atresia
        b. Posterior choanal atresia
  C. Traumatic conditions
    1. Types of injuries
    2. Fractures
        a. Anesthesia
        b. Reduction of fracture
        c. Packs
        d. Postoperative care
  D. Epistaxis
    1. Etiology
    2. Treatment
        a. Packs
        b. Injection
        c. Ligation
  E. Nasal polyps
  F. Foreign bodies
  G. Nasal myiasis
  H. Nasal furunculosis
  I. Rhinoliths
  J. Epithelial papilloma
  K. Nasopharyngeal angiofibroma
  L. Nasal carcinoma

III. PARANASAL SINUSES
  A. Examination
  B. Nasoantral irrigation
  C. Oromaxillary fistula
  D. Nonsecreting cysts
  E. Carcinoma

IV. LIPS
  A. Congenital lesions
    1. Cleft lip
    2. Labial pits
    3. Hemangioma
  B. Traumatic lesions
    1. Abrasions
    2. Lacerations
  C. Tumors
    1. Lip ulcers and squamous carcinoma
    2. Mucocoele
    3. Verruca vulgaris

By GERALD M. ENGLISH, M.D.

INTRODUCTION

This chapter contains a description of those surgical procedures that can be performed on outpatients either in the Emergency Room or in the office. These surgical problems constitute a large percentage of those encountered in the daily practice of otolaryngology.

Diagnosis depends upon the ability to examine the head and neck carefully and accurately, and often the success or failure of therapy depends upon these clinical skills.

THE EAR

Examination

A good history is especially important in deciding what is relevant in the patient's account of his otologic problem. Hearing loss, tinnitus, vertigo, pain and drainage are the symptoms that lead patients to seek help. These symptoms may either distress the patient or he may ignore them, depending upon his age, intelligence, psychologic state, education and occupation.

Hearing loss may be sudden or slow in onset, unilateral or bilateral, and progressive or stable. Wax occluding the ear canal or pressing against the tympanic membrane produces a sudden deafness that leads the patient to seek help quickly. On the other hand, the slow, insidious, progressive hearing loss produced by otosclerosis may not stimulate the patient to consult a physician until deafness is well advanced. Questioning a close relative may help in establishing the time of onset and rate of progression of hearing loss when the patient is vague in his replies. The association of deafness with symptoms of pain, vertigo, tinnitus and otorrhea may be very helpful in making the proper diagnosis. Common causes of hearing loss such as noise, trauma and ototoxic drugs should be included in the history.

A fluctuating hearing loss with episodes of vertigo followed by symptom-free intervals is characteristic of Meniere's disease.

Pain may be due to diseases within the ear or it may be referred from other structures (Fig. 10–1). Most inflammatory disease affecting the external or middle ear will produce pain and often the most severe pain will be caused by inflammations of the external ear. Pain arising from otitis media is often severe and it usually subsides dramatically when there is a release of the inflammatory exudate from the middle ear space. Relief of pain is just as dramatic with a rupture of the tympanic membrane as with a myringotomy or spontaneous drainage through the Eustachian tube. Continuing pain, in spite of therapy, or recurring pain, after a symptom-

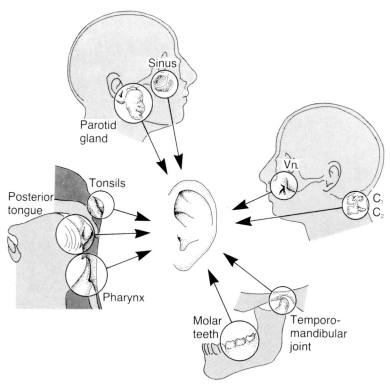

Figure 10–1 Referred otalgia. Referred otalgia is a common problem. Several diseases involving the maxillary sinus, parotid gland, pharyngeal tonsil, base of the tongue, hypopharynx, larynx, molar teeth, upper cervical nerves, and maxillary division of the trigeminal nerve are depicted. These areas must be carefully examined in any patient who complains of ear pain and has no apparent ear disease.

free interval, often indicates a more serious problem. Referred ear pain may arise from the molar teeth, the pharynx, the posterior tongue, the palatal tonsils, the paranasal sinuses, the parotid gland, the temporomandibular joint, and herpetic lesions of the fifth cranial nerve or upper cervical nerves.

The term vertigo should be reserved for the symptom of an hallucination of motion.[1] When the environment moves and the patient feels stationary, it is called "objective vertigo" and when the patient feels he is turning in a stationary environment, it is called "subjective vertigo." Symptoms of dizziness, light headedness, unsteadiness or fainting are usually associated with cardiovascular or psychoneurotic disorders and rarely arise from inner ear diseases. The relationship of the attack of vertigo to various activities may give some clue to its cause. Vestibular disease will often cause an attack when the patient is quiet or when the head is placed in certain positions. Sudden changes in posture may produce momentary attacks of unsteadiness or dysequilibrium in patients with cardiovascular insufficiency. The duration of the attack will often help determine its cause. Vertigo that lasts several minutes to hours and subsides to recur again after a symptom-free interval is characteristic of Meniere's disease. The prolonged attack that subsides after several days or weeks, followed by vertigo with certain head positions, often indicates irreversible vestibular damage. When both vestibular end organs are slowly damaged, as with streptomycin, the patient may have only a slight balance disturbance, but have great difficulty walking in the dark or on uneven surfaces. Nausea and vomiting often accompany an acute vestibular disturbance and these symptoms may direct the patient's or physician's attention away from the vestibular disorder.

The word tinnitus indicates a subjective symptom of ear or head noise, and these sounds are often characterized as whistling, blowing wind, bells, sea shell sounds and throbbing or pulsating noises.

Tinnitus may be associated with many ear disorders, and is often increased when the patient is tired, worried or under stress. It is usually more troublesome at night when the patient is trying to sleep. Objective or audible tinnitus may arise from tumors within the ear, vascular lesions, foreign bodies and temporomandibular joint disease.

Otorrhea may arise from many problems involving the ear. Any inflammatory condition in the ear canal or middle ear, whether acute or chronic, will cause a variable amount of ear drainage. The appearance, odor and amount should be noted. Watery or mucoid secretions are produced by chronic inflammations of the middle ear or inflammation of the ear canal. Purulent drainage is associated with acute inflammatory diseases and foul-smelling material may indicate suppuration of bone.

Careful examination of the entire ear will help avoid errors in diagnosis. The pinna must be gently palpated and inspected before inserting the speculum into the ear canal. Superficial lesions, small pits, areas of swelling and tenderness, excoriation of the epithelium, and scars should not be overlooked. By gently pulling the pinna upward and backward and stretching the tragus forward the external meatus and canal can be seen. In many children and in a few adults this simple maneuver will expose the meatus, external canal and tympanic membrane. Reflected light from the headmirror is a good source of illumination. In most patients an aural speculum large enough to avoid unnecessary pain and possible trauma to the ear is required for this part of the examination. The battery-powered otoscope or reflected light from the headmirror may be used for examining the ear. Cerumen or other debris must be carefully removed to allow complete inspection of the entire canal and tympanic membrane. A cerumen curette, a Day hook or a Baron suction are useful instruments for this purpose. Eustachian tube patency can be determined by altering air pressure in the ear canal with a pneumatic speculum or by having the patient perform a Valsalva maneuver to inflate the middle ear. Movement of the tympanic membrane with either technique indicates a patent Eustachian tube.

Hearing tests are essential for the proper evaluation of ear disorders. An audiometric examination performed in a sound room is ideal; however, this is not always possible. Tuning fork tests, such as the Weber and Rinné, are dependable when performed correctly; they are easy to perform and will help distinguish a conductive from a sensorineural hearing loss (Table 10–1). The 512, 1024, and 2048 cycle per second forks are the most practical for these tests, which should be performed near the patient's threshold of hearing.

Air conduction and bone conduction can be tested with a tuning fork. The test for air conduction measures the ability of the ear to transmit an airborne sound through the entire ear to the temporal lobe of the brain, and is performed by holding a vibrating tuning fork near the external auditory canal. The test for bone conduction measures the ability of the inner ear and hearing nerve to receive and utilize a sound stimulus without air conduction sound transmission; it does not depend upon the external auditory canal or the middle ear. The handle of the tuning fork is held directly on a portion of the skull and the vibrations reach the inner ear directly. The tuning fork can be placed on the mastoid bone, the forehead, the closed mandible or the upper teeth.

The Weber test is performed by holding the handle of the vibrating tuning fork against a midline point of the patient's forehead or the upper incisor teeth (Fig. 10–2). The patient is then asked where he thinks the sound is loudest. The patient with a conductive hearing loss will usually hear the louder sound in the ear with poorer hearing. Plugging the external auditory canal with a finger produces a conductive hearing loss and the tuning fork will be heard better in this ear. This technique may be used by the examiner to determine the reliability of this test. The Weber test will refer to the patient's better hearing ear when there is a nerve or perceptual deafness and when there is a significant difference between the nerve functions of the two ears.

The Rinné test is used to detect either a conductive or a perceptual hearing loss and is performed in the following manner. A vibrating tuning fork is held beside the ear and then placed behind the ear over the mastoid bone (Fig. 10–2). The patient is asked whether the sound is louder in front of the ear or behind it. When the fork is heard louder behind the ear, that is, on the mastoid bone, bone conduction is better than air conduction, and the patient has a conductive hearing loss. When the air conduction sound is heard louder than the bone conduction sound, the patient either has normal hearing or a nerve deafness.

Tests for vestibular function should also be performed. Spontaneous and positional nystagmus should not be overlooked. Frenzel glasses may help the examiner detect the nystagmus. The caloric test is a simple method of determining vestibular function, requiring little equipment, and allowing the physician to test the two ears separately.

TABLE 10–1   SUMMARY OF TUNING FORK TESTS

TEST	NORMAL HEARING	CONDUCTIVE HEARING LOSS	SENSORINEURAL HEARING LOSS
Weber	Equal	Loudest in poor ear	Loudest in better ear
Rinné	*AC better than BC**	BC better than AC	AC better than BC

*AC—Air conduction
**BC—Bone conduction

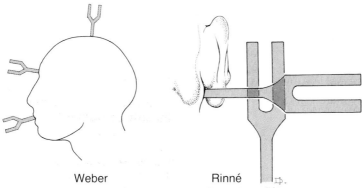

Weber   Rinné

Figure 10–2 Hearing tests: Weber and Rinné. Tuning fork tests, such as the Weber and Rinné, are useful in differentiating and detecting the various types of hearing loss.

Before these tests are performed, the ears should be examined for perforations of the tympanic membrane; if present, the ears must not be irrigated with water. Foreign bodies or cerumen plugs should be removed to insure proper stimulation of the labyrinth. It is preferable to start with a mild stimulus since this produces little subjective vertigo and no nausea and vomiting. Stronger stimulation may be required for the patient with a relatively insensitive labyrinth. The patient's head is tilted back (Fig. 10–3) at an angle of 60° and 0.2 cc of ice water (0° C) is placed in the external canal while the eyes are observed for nystagmus. The direction and duration of

nystagmus should be recorded, the direction being determined by the direction of the quick component, which is normally away from the stimulated ear. The duration should be one and a half to two minutes. After a five minute interval the opposite ear is stimulated and the response from this side recorded. The direction of nystagmus should be away from this ear and the duration of nystagmus comparable to the other side. When no response is detected, a larger volume of ice water (5 cc) is injected into the ear canal and the responses recorded. If there is still no response, 30 cc of ice water are injected into each ear canal over a 30 second period and if this

Figure 10–3 Caloric test. Vestibular function can be tested by placing a small quantity (0.2 cc) of cold or hot water near the tympanic membrane for 30 seconds. Horizontal nystagmus lasting for 60 seconds indicates a reacting vestibular system.

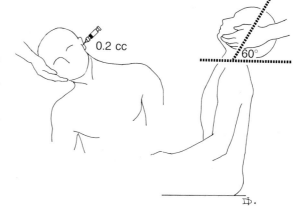

stimulus produces no nystagmus it may be concluded that the vestibular system is not functioning. Those patients with vestibular disorders will usually report that the vertigo produced by caloric testing is quite similar to their usual symptom of vertigo.

Congenital Lesions

Minor variations in the size and shape of the auricle are not uncommon. These are not anomalies, but simply variations from the normal and require no treatment. True malformations are often associated with other anomalies of the ear and face. These patients should have a complete and careful evaluation before any surgical therapy is undertaken.

Preauricular Cysts

The preauricular cyst or fistula (Fig. 10–4) is a congenital lesion arising from a defective union of the first and second branchial arches as they form the auricle. Usually, a small opening or cyst can be identified anterior to the helix or tragus. From this opening, a long branched tract extends under the skin. If the tract becomes obstructed or infected a cyst may develop. Many are asymptomatic and require no treatment; however, pain,

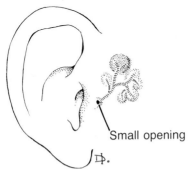

Small opening

Figure 10–4 Preauricular sinus or cyst. A small opening in the preauricular area may be an indication of an extensive preauricular sinus and cyst. Multiple branches are quite common and all of these must be excised if surgical treatment is to be successful.

drainage or an enlarging mass are indications for surgical excision. The operation can be performed with general or local anesthesia, and a small segment of skin surrounding the cyst opening should be included. Branching tracts make it difficult to define the complete extent of the fistula, and an injection of methylene blue into the fistula stains the tracts and makes it easier to excise them. One should remember that the methylene blue might not enter the smaller branches of the tract and these small unstained channels must also be removed. The dye may spread into surrounding normal tissue and this should be spared. The operation must be performed with care since the tract may extend deep into soft tissue and lie close to branches of the facial nerve. When the cyst is infected, antibiotics should be used before and after surgery.

Accessory Auricles

These small firm skin elevations often contain elastic cartilage (Fig. 10–5). They may be either single or multiple, and occur anterior to the tragus along the ascending crus of the helix or on the cheek along a line between the tragus to the angle of the mouth. Accessory auricles may be excised with local anesthesia, and the dissection should include the elastic cartilage that extends into the underlying soft tissues. Branches of the facial nerve may be closely related to these structures and these branches must not be injured or excised during surgery.

Angioma

These congenital tumors are rather common, often involving the auricle and other areas of the face and neck. Two types of angioma occur in the auricle. Capillary hemangiomas consist of capillary-sized vessels in the form of a "spider nevus" or flat mass with a "port wine stain" appearance. The "spider nevus" is usually not a problem and either no treatment at all or coagula-

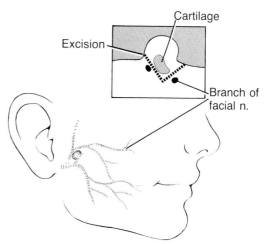

Figure 10–5 Accessory auricle. *A*, Accessory auricles usually contain a small piece of cartilage and may be close to the facial nerve. *B*, Excision must be performed carefully to avoid facial nerve injury.

tion of the central vessel is all that is necessary. Since large, flat "port wine stain" tumors may increase in size and become disfiguring, these patients require extensive treatment and should be sent to a specialist in plastic surgery (see Chapter 8).

Cavernous hemangiomas or "strawberry tumors" consist of raised masses of large blood-filled spaces. They enlarge rapidly during the first years of life and produce severe cosmetic deformities. These patients should be referred for treatment (Chapter 8).

Bat Ears

Protruding auricles are not uncommon. Minor degrees of protrusion require no treatment, but the markedly protruding auricle causes embarrassment and it should be corrected. The operation should not be performed on outpatients.

Traumatic Conditions

The auricle is frequently injured and this may result in hematomas, lacerations or tissue loss. These injuries must be treated promptly and adequately to reduce subsequent deformities.

Hematoma

Extravasation of blood between the perichondrium and cartilage will result in cartilage necrosis and severe deformities. Ischemic necrosis results from the interference with the blood supply to the cartilage from vessels within the perichondrium. "Cauliflower ear" is the deformity produced by this process. A large, bluish swelling involving the auricle is the characteristic appearance of this problem.

Treatment consists of evacuating the blood as soon as possible (Fig. 10–6). When a patient with a small hematoma is seen shortly after the injury, needle aspiration may be all that is necessary. Larger hematomas and those of longer duration will require an incision and evacuation of the hematoma. This procedure should be performed with careful aseptic surgical technique since any bacterial contamination may produce a severe perichondritis. Antibiotics are useful in preventing this complication. A tight pressure dressing is placed over the ear for 48 hours to prevent future accumulations of blood. Moistened cotton can be molded to the contours of the ear to insure adequate pressure. Drains in the incision must not be left more than 48 hours because of the risk of infection. Local or general

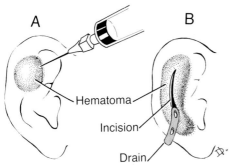

Figure 10–6 Treatment of hematoma of the auricle. Subperichondrial hematomas of the auricle can be *(A)* aspirated or *(B)* incised and drained. Aspiration may have to be repeated several times and should be used for small hematomas. The incision of a hematoma must be adequate in length and should be made through the perichondrium. Drainage can be obtained by placing a small rubber drain beneath the perichondrium. A pressure dressing should be placed on the ear for at least 72 hours.

anesthesia may be used depending upon the age of the patient and the extent of the injury.

Lacerations

These injuries may extend through the skin, the perichondrium and the cartilage, and occasionally the entire auricle is severed from the head. These injuries require meticulous surgical repair. Control of bleeding, cautious débridement of de-

vitalized tissue, and removal of all foreign materials is essential. Careful approximation of tissues with fine sutures is important and these sutures should not pass through the cartilage. Exposed cartilage must be covered and skin flaps from the postauricular area can be used for this purpose (Fig. 10–7). Antibiotics will help prevent infection and pressure dressings will help prevent accumulations of blood or serum. The auricle has been successfully resutured to the head in a number of patients with severe injuries. A partial success is well worth the time and the effort involved.

Frostbite

The unprotected position of the auricle and its lack of subcutaneous tissue predispose it to this injury. Severity of trauma is dependent on the duration and degree of exposure. At first the auricle has a white appearance and is cold to the touch. Later, a stage of hyperemia and edema follows. The ear becomes swollen with fluid-filled "blebs" forming beneath the skin. Treatment consists of allowing the ear to return to body temperature and analgesics for pain. Dressings and other manipulations of the auricle must be avoided since this may cause further injury. Should gangrene or aseptic necrosis develop, the patient should be hospitalized and referred to a specialist for treatment.

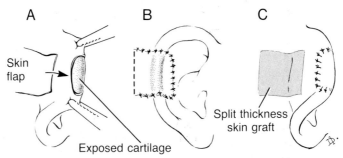

Figure 10–7 Protection of cartilage. Exposed cartilage must be covered to prevent perichondritis and loss of the cartilage. *A.* A full-thickness postauricular skin flap has been elevated. *B.* The skin flap is then sutured to the skin edges of the auricular defect. *C.* After adequate healing, the auricle is freed from the flap and any postauricular defect covered with a split-thickness skin graft.

Foreign Bodies

A wide variety of objects have been removed from the ear canal. Children are more apt to insert a foreign body than an adult. Small stones, beads, cotton balls, beans and erasers are the objects most frequently found in the ear. Insects fly or crawl into the ear canal and cause great discomfort while alive.

All foreign materials should be removed from the ear and the major difficulties of this procedure can be overcome by a few simple techniques. First, the patient must be comfortable since he must remain immobile. Injuries to the tympanic membrane or ossicular chain can occur if the patient moves. A local anesthetic injected around the external meatus will provide excellent anesthesia, although children who are very apprehensive may require a general anesthetic. Second, insects that are still alive must be killed before attempting to remove them. A small cotton tampon moistened with ether and placed in the ear canal for 5 to 10 minutes will stupify the insect, and sterile mineral oil instilled into the canal will kill it.

Either a small cerumen curette or a Day hook is a useful instrument for removing foreign bodies. A Baron finger control suction and Hartmann alligator forceps may also be used. Any manipulations in the external canal may elicit a cough reflex, making removal of the foreign body difficult. A local anesthetic will block this reflex in addition to relieving pain.

Removing foreign bodies by irrigation is risky. If there is a pre-existing perforation of the tympanic membrane, the irrigating solution may enter the middle ear and produce an acute inflammation. Occasionally the force of the irrigating solution will rupture a thin tympanic membrane to produce a conductive hearing loss and middle ear infection. Unless the tympanic membrane can be seen, it is best to remove foreign bodies without irrigation. The trauma of extracting a foreign body is preferable to the complications of irrigation.

Foreign bodies that are large or in contact with the tympanic membrane are more difficult to extract. Some foreign bodies are hygroscopic and swell to completely occlude the ear canal. Edema and inflammation of the external canal may make it nearly impossible to remove the foreign body, and occasionally these patients require a general anesthestic and an endaural incision before the foreign body can be removed.

Excessive cerumen is a problem for some patients. Soft moist cerumen can be removed with the curette without too much difficulty (Fig. 10–8). Cotton-tipped metal applicators can be used to cleanse the ear canal of debris. Hard impacted cerumen can be softened by using a few drops of mineral oil in the ear two or three times each day for a day or two before removing it. The hard wax plug can be removed with instruments, but occasionally a local anesthetic is necessary to insure the patient's cooperation and comfort. Irrigation should be used only in those patients with an intact

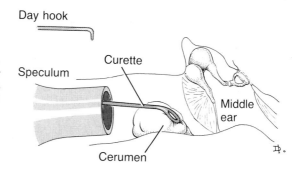

Day hook

Speculum   Curette

Middle ear

Cerumen

Figure 10–8 Cerumen removal from external auditory canal. Cerumen or other foreign bodies should be removed with a curette and direct vision. A Day hook may be used instead of the curette.

tympanic membrane. Water injected through a perforation into the middle ear may cause an acute otitis media, and vigorous irrigations can perforate an atrophic drum.

Traumatic Rupture of Tympanic Membrane

These injuries result from blows to the ear with a cupped hand, instrumentation of the ear, blast injuries, diving, water skiing, forceful inflation of the Eustachian tube when the membrane is thin, rapid descent in unpressurized aircraft and basal skull fractures. Welders develop a perforation from hot metal fragments flying into the ear canal. These perforations fail to heal due to cauterization of the edges of the perforation. The symptoms are pain, hearing loss, tinnitus and occasionally some bleeding from the ear.

Treatment is quite simple and consists of aspirating the blood and debris from the ear canal. This is necessary to determine if there are injuries to the tympanic membrane. The ear should not be irrigated or the clot in the middle ear disturbed. Ear drops have little value and may do some harm. Usually the perforation heals slowly over a period of weeks and the patient's hearing returns to normal. During this interval the patient should be advised to avoid getting water in the ear. Swimming should be discontinued and the external meatus filled with cotton. Vaseline should be smeared over the cotton and auricle before showering and shampooing the hair. This simple technique will prevent water from entering the middle ear and help to prevent acute otitis media, which will delay healing of the perforation and perhaps lead to more serious problems. If the perforation has not closed in 10 to 12 weeks, the patient should be sent to an otologist for evaluation and surgical repair of the tympanic membrane.

Tumors

Most ear tumors arise from the skin or its appendages; however, bone, cartilage or neural tissues may be involved. Early diagnosis is important to avoid extensive tissue loss, functional impairment and death. Both benign and malignant tumors occur in the ear, and the diagnosis will depend upon a histopathologic examination of a biopsy specimen.

Sebaceous Cysts

These cysts (Fig. 10–9) are common around the ear. They are usually located on the posterior surface of the lobule, the postauricular sulcus and the skin overlying the mastoid process. Soft and nontender, they are easy to diagnose, though they may become infected and then may be confused with a furuncle. Treatment consists of total excision of the cyst with its walls intact. This technique insures complete removal. A margin of skin about the external opening should be removed with the cyst. Local anesthesia is usually adequate for this surgical procedure.

Fibroma

Fibromas are firm, discrete tumors that are nontender. They grow slowly and

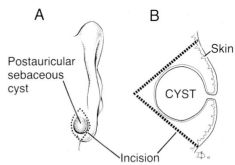

Figure 10–9 Sebaceous cyst of the ear. The postauricular sulcus and lobule (A) are the most common sites for sebaceous cysts near the ear. The incision should include a margin of normal tissue (B) and should be placed in the postauricular sulcus (A).

occasionally occlude the external meatus. Surgical excision is indicated when the mass occludes the canal or creates a cosmetic problem. Keloids result from trauma to the ear and are a form of fibroma. They occur most frequently in dark-skinned people, particularly Negroes, arising as pedunculated tumors on the lobule following ear piercing. Surgical excision followed by 500 R of irradiation to prevent recurrence is the most satisfactory treatment.

Cutaneous Horn

This rough, hard, brownish colored tumor occurs on the rim of the helix in older patients who have a long history of exposure to inclement weather. Surgical excision of this hornlike tumor will improve the patient's appearance.

Senile Keratoses

These flat, raised, yellowish-brown lesions appear on the auricle in elderly persons. They produce few if any symptoms and are treated much the same as anywhere else on the body, with topical lanolin cream or excision.

Keratoacanthoma

This rare lesion is potentially malignant. The tumor may grow rapidly at first and then slowly regress in size to leave a retracted scar. Excisional biopsy is necessary to be sure a carcinoma is not developing.

Papilloma

Papillomas occur on the auricle and in the external canal. The etiology may be viral or a response to chronic irritation of the skin. They may become malignant and should be excised completely. Obstruction of the external canal with a conductive hearing loss may result from these tumors.

Exostoses

These are common benign tumors of the external canal. They are usually symptomless unless they obstruct the external canal or interfere with wax and epithelial debris passing from the canal. Many patients with this tumor have a history of swimming in cold water.[2] This sessile tumor arises from the canal wall near the tympanic membrane, and there may be more than one tumor mass. When they interfere with hearing or are associated with repeated infections from retained debris, surgical excision is necessary and the patient must be referred to an otologist for treatment.

Osteomas are usually solitary and pedunculated. They may obstruct the canal or allow an accumulation of debris within the canal that leads to repeated infections. Surgical excision should be performed by an otologist.

Adenoma

These tumors arise from the cerumen glands of the canal skin. They have a marked tendency to recur and may become frankly malignant. Wide surgical excision is necessary to prevent recurrence and this should be done by a specialist in ear surgery.

Carcinoma

Squamous cell carcinoma, basal cell carcinoma and adenocarcinomas occur on the auricle. The squamous carcinomas are the most common and comprise about 75 per cent of malignant tumors of the auricle. Fifteen per cent are basal cell carcinomas and 10 per cent are adenocarcinomas. The clinical course of these tumors varies, but 20 per cent of patients with these tumors will have metastatic disease when they are first seen.[7] The diagnosis is not difficult to make if a biopsy is obtained.

The treatment of carcinoma of the auricle depends upon the location and size of the tumor. Very small lesions may be excised in the clinic; however, larger lesions should be treated by more radical surgery. This may entail excision of the underlying cartilage or amputation of the entire auricle. Obviously, these procedures are beyond the scope of this text.

Inflammatory Conditions

Perichondritis

Inflammation of the perichondrium (Fig. 10–10) may occur when the cartilage has been exposed or injured by trauma, surgery, frostbite, burns or infection introduced during aspiration or incision of a hematoma. Occasionally a superficial infection of the auricle or canal will spread to the perichondrium. Pus collecting between the perichondrium and the cartilage causes a necrosis of the cartilage resulting in a marked deformity of the ear. This infection should be treated promptly with a broad-spectrum antibiotic. Any purulent drainage should be sent to the laboratory for culture and sensitivity tests. When an abscess forms it should be incised and drained. The incision should be delayed until definite fluctuation is detected. Premature incisions will only spread the infection. In a few patients, the pain and swelling may continue despite these measures and more extensive surgical therapy will be required. This treatment should never be performed outside the hospital.

Chondrodermatitis Nodularis Helicis Chronicis

This small, painful, tender nodule arises from the upper margin of the auricle (Fig. 10–11). It is more common in men than women and is thought to arise from exposure to cold temperatures. Patients often have difficulty sleeping because of the pain when the ear comes in contact with a pillow. A local anesthetic is sufficient for the excision of this lesion with a small wedge of underlying cartilage, which usually results in a cure.

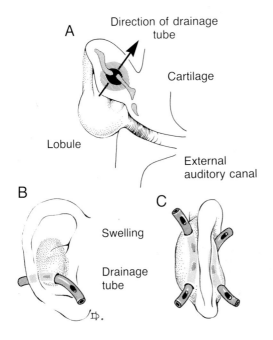

Figure 10–10 Perichondritis. Perichondritis should be treated by incision and drainage. *A.* When there has been destruction of the cartilage, the tube should be inserted through the auricle *(B).* Drainage tubes placed on both sides of the auricle beneath the perichondrium *(C)* can be used to evacuate an abscess.

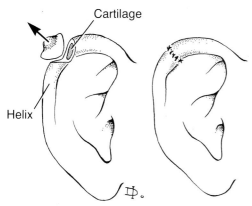

Figure 10–11 Chondrodermatitis nodularis helicis chronicis. Surgical excision of this painful helical nodule must include part of the underlying cartilage.

External Otitis

Furunculosis is a circumscribed external otitis that arises from a staphylococcal infection of a hair follicle. These infections may be multiple and may recur over long periods of time. The first symptoms are tenderness in the external meatus and pain that is increased with jaw movements. As the infection progresses, the pain becomes more severe and hearing loss results from edema occluding the external meatus. Examination reveals a red swollen area in the cartilaginous part of the ear canal. Manipulations of the auricle will cause a great deal of pain. Enlarged tender postauricular lymph nodes may simulate an acute mastoiditis. These nodes may displace the auricle forward and make it difficult to differentiate this condition from a mastoid infection. A mastoid x-ray will usually help clarify the problem. However, it is unusual for mastoiditis to cause pain and tenderness of the auricle unless there is an associated perichondritis. Lymphadenitis is unusual in acute mastoiditis and ordinarily the tenderness in mastoiditis is localized over the mastoid process. When the tympanic membrane can be seen, it will appear normal in furunculosis and it is abnormal in mastoiditis. Antibiotics should be used and the furuncle incised and drained when it localizes. A wick moistened with bacitracin ointment may be gently inserted into the external canal. This will allow drainage and prevent the accumulation of purulent debris in the canal.

Diffuse external otitis is quite common and may be associated with skin disorders such as eczema, neurodermatitis and seborrheic dermatitis. Hot, humid climates and bathing or swimming are often associated with this disorder. Trauma is an important factor and scratching the ears, unskilled irrigations of the canal, and vigorous drying with a soiled towel must be avoided. Occasionally, pus draining from a chronic otitis media will produce a diffuse inflammation of the canal, and this possibility can be excluded by a careful examination of the tympanic membrane. Meticulous cleaning of the canal is essential when treating this problem, and cotton-tipped metal applicators, suction, and small curettes are useful for this purpose. The patient must keep his ear dry during shampooing and showering by occluding the external canal with cotton and applying Vaseline over the meatus and auricle. Ear drops are of little value when debris in the canal will not allow the medication to reach the inflamed areas. Antibiotic ear drops may sensitize the canal and aggravate the problem. Topical steroids are of some value. Burrow's solution (1:17) or a saturated solution of boric acid in ethyl alcohol helps relieve the itching and pain. A cotton or ribbon gauze wick placed in the canal will facilitate drainage and allow the ear drops to reach inflamed areas.

Those patients who fail to respond to treatment should be referred to an otologist for treatment.

Acute Otitis Media

Acute otitis media is one of the commonest diseases in children. In general, this disease results from a bacterial infection of the middle ear (72.8 per cent).

The remainder (27.2 per cent) are thought to be viral in etiology. Hemenway and Smith (1970)[3] have reviewed the etiologic agents in acute otitis media, and their data are presented in Table 10–2.

The patient's age must be considered in the etiology of this disease. Children under the age of six often have *Hemophilus influenza* cultured from the ear; whereas, patients over age six rarely have this organism. Children under six should receive an antibiotic that will eradicate *D. pneumoniae, H. influenza,* and a group A β-hemolytic streptococcus. The antibiotics of choice in this situation are ampicillin, tetracycline, or erythromycin and sulfisoxazole. Those over six respond well to oral potassiumphenoxymethyl-penicillin or erythromycin. *Hemophilus influenza* is rarely involved in these patients.

When pus is present in the ear canal, this should be obtained for culture and sensitivity tests. A gram stain will help determine the best antibiotic for immediate use.

Myringotomy is indicated in those patients with severe pain, marked bulging of the tympanic membrane, severe toxemia, poor response to antibiotic therapy, a persistent conductive hearing loss and apparent or impending complications. This simple procedure involves little risk to the patient when performed skillfully. Adequate anesthesia is essential and sedation is frequently necessary in small children. Meperidine and pheno-

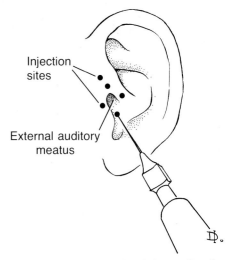

Figure 10–12 Anesthesia of the ear. Local anesthesia of the external auditory canal, tympanic membrane and middle ear can be obtained by injecting the external meatus and canal with a local anesthetic.

barbital 1 mgm each per pound of body weight is injected 30 minutes before the procedure is begun. A local anesthetic solution of 1 per cent lidocaine HCl, (Xylocaine) and epinephrine (1:100,000) is infiltrated around the external canal at 12, 3, 6 and 9 o'clock positions (Fig. 10–12). About 0.5 cc of the solution is slowly injected at each site. Blanching of the canal occurs with the injection due to the vasoconstrictive action of epinephrine. The myringotomy incision is made in the inferior portion of the drum (Fig. 10–13) whose anterior inferior

TABLE 10–2   Etiologic Agents in Acute Otitis Media
(1048 Specimens)

Organism	Positive Cultures	Per Cent*
Diplococcus pneumoniae	451	43.0
Hemophilus influenza	273	26.1
β-Hemolytic streptococcus	118	11.3
Staphylococcus aureus	24	2.3
Streptococcus viridans	12	1.1
Neisseria catarrhalis	7	0.7
Other	4	0.4
Negative for bacteria	285	27.2

*Infrequently more than one organism was cultured from the same specimen.

RIGHT EAR

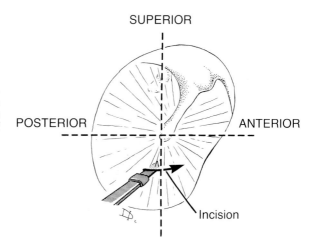

Figure 10–13 Myringotomy. Incision of the tympanic membrane (myringotomy) can be performed with local anesthesia. The incision should be made in the inferior-anterior portion of the drum head.

quadrant is farthest from the middle ear ossicles and the facial nerve, because injury of these structures can have serious consequences and must be avoided. A circular incision is better than a radical one since the latter may extend into the annulus of the tympanic membrane and cause troublesome bleeding. Magnification of the ear will help prevent accidents during the operation and a Zeiss operating microscope is quite useful for this purpose.

After myringotomy, the patient should be instructed to keep water out of the ear until the membrane has healed. Sterile cotton placed in the ear and changed frequently when soiled will prevent pus draining out of the ear onto the face and clothing.

Analgesics, bed rest, mild sedation and antipyretics will make the patient more comfortable during his convalescence. The patient should return in 72 hours. If symptoms persist, a change in antibiotic may be indicated on the basis of sensitivity tests. This patient should be examined again in three or four days. Fever after seven days of treatment is nearly always an indication for myringotomy. A middle ear fluid specimen should be cultured and sensitivity tests performed. If the patient is doing well after 72 hours, he can be examined in 10 or 12 days and then periodically until the drum appears normal and the hearing is normal. Any patient with signs or symptoms of continuing infection must be hospitalized and observed for the complications of otitis media.

Serous Otitis Media

This clinical condition is characterized by an accumulation of nonpurulent fluid in the middle ear. The only consistent symptom is a conductive hearing loss. The onset of hearing loss may be gradual or sudden, in one or both ears. Hearing may be better in the supine position than when the patient is erect.

Several etiologic factors have been implicated in this disease. Unresolved acute otitis media either from inadequate therapy or a failure to develop immunity is a common cause of middle ear fluid. Obstruction of the Eustachian tube from enlarged adenoids, infection, neoplasm, trauma or allergy may result in a middle ear effusion. Diseases of the palate including clefts, submucous clefts, paralysis or trauma are frequently complicated by serous otitis media.[4]

Examination reveals a dull, retracted tympanic membrane with a prominent malleus. An air-fluid meniscus or bubbles may be seen in the middle ear. Pneumatic otoscopy reveals a tympanic membrane that moves poorly or not at all. Audiometry and tuning fork tests will indicate a conductive hearing loss.

Treatment is directed at removing the fluid from the middle ear. Catheterization of the Eustachian tube may produce edema in the tube and cause more fluid accumulation. Auto inflation of the middle ear may be helpful and this should be repeated several times each day for several days. Myringotomy and insertion of a polyethylene tube (Fig. 10–14) through the tympanic membrane is an effective means of treatment. The anesthetic and technique are the same as described for acute otitis media. A small polyethylene tube inserted through the myringotomy after evacuation of the fluid allows ventilation of the middle ear. Local anesthesia is usually sufficient except for small children or uncooperative patients. The polyethylene tube can be removed after several weeks and during this time the patient must avoid any water in the ear. Oral decongestant therapy of pseudoephedrine HCl (Sudafed) is useful in many patients. Patients who do not respond to these techniques must be reexamined to be sure an unsuspected etiology has not

been overlooked. This is particularly true in the adult with serous otitis media. An unsuspected nasopharyngeal tumor may be responsible for the problem and a mistake in diagnosis will produce serious consequences. Occasionally, mastoidectomy will be indicated in some of those patients who do not respond to treatment.

Chronic Otitis Media

There are two distinct types of chronic otitis media.[5] Each has a somewhat different etiology, clinical course and potential for serious complications. The benign form is due to recurrent or continuing infection in the middle ear and is associated with a perforation of the pars tensa portion of the tympanic membrane. The dangerous variety is associated with cholesteatoma formation in the pars flaccida area of the tympanic membrane. The pars tensa may be normal in these patients and a small perforation or retraction pocket in the pars flaccida overlooked; since serious complications may develop from this condition, these patients should be referred to an otologist.

The middle ear mucosa can be inspected through the perforation. Its appearance changes during various stages of the disease—in acute infections, it will appear thickened and edematous, and during quiescent periods it will appear normal. These changes are important indicators for the various methods of treatment. Patients with mucosal changes and otorrhea suggesting an infection should be treated with antibiotics. Culture and sensitivity tests are important in this situation since the bacterial flora may vary with each infection. Resistant organisms may develop with prolonged use of antibiotics. Swimming must be avoided and care should be taken to avoid water entering the ear during bathing and hair washing. Occlusion of the external meatus with cotton followed by a liberal application of Vaseline will effectively prevent water

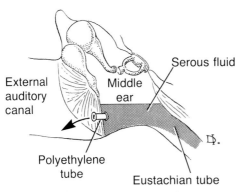

Figure 10–14 Insertion of polyethylene tube. A flanged tube is inserted through the tympanic membrane into the middle ear space. This tube drains the serous fluid from the middle ear and allows air to enter the middle ear.

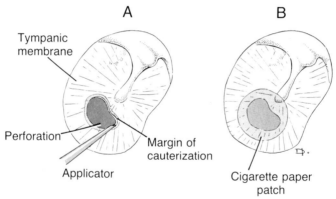

Figure 10–15 Patching the drum. A central perforation will often heal with cauterization of the edges of the perforation *(A)* and application of a paper patch *(B)*. A small amount of trichloracetic acid on a metal applicator is touched to the perforation margins *(A)*.

from entering the middle ear. Many perforations will close if recurrent infections can be prevented. Those perforations that do not heal may require tympanoplasty and reconstruction of the sound-conducting mechanism (Fig. 10–15).[6] Cholesteatomas are potentially dangerous and should be treated by an otologist. Failure to recognize this problem could result in irreversible deafness, facial nerve palsy, meningitis and intracranial abscesses.

Ear-piercing for Earrings

The popularity of pierced ears varies considerably, but many women ask their physicians to perform this minor procedure (Fig. 10–16). The operation should be inexpensive, simple, safe and effective. A 16 gauge needle with the hub removed is an ideal instrument for piercing the ear lobe. The needle and a plain gold "stud" are placed in ethyl alcohol for 15 minutes. The ear lobe is

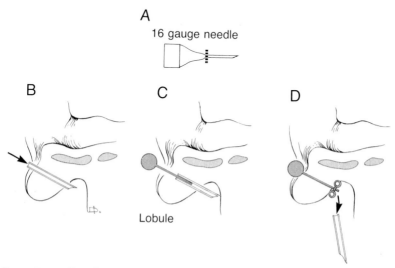

Figure 10–16 Ear-piercing. A simple method of ear-piercing with a 16 gauge needle.

washed thoroughly with germicidal soap and water. An antiseptic solution is then applied to the ear and the lobe anesthetized with lidocaine HCl and epinephrine (1:100,000) solution. After piercing sites are selected and the 16 gauge needle pushed through the ear lobe, the earring is then threaded into the barrel of the needle and pulled into proper position. The patient should be instructed to clean the ear lobes with ethyl alcohol swabs several times each day for several days. A topical antibiotic ointment will also help prevent infections. The earring should not be removed or changed for 7 to 10 days. At this time, a well-epithelialized tract should exist and the earrings can be removed or changed as desired. Should infection occur, the earring must be removed immediately and systemic antibiotics prescribed. Keloids may occur and require treatment, particularly in dark-skinned persons.

NOSE

Examination

Inspection and palpation of the nose during the nasal examination will yield a great deal of information that might be missed when trauma is involved. Palpation can reveal a fracture that might not

be detected with an x-ray examination. When a deformity is suspected, a previous photograph should be used for comparison.

Several basic instruments are necessary for examining the interior of the nose. Reflected light from a headmirror gives excellent illumination of the nasal cavity and allows the freedom of both hands for various manipulations. A nasal speculum inserted into the nares can be used to dilate the nares without discomfort for the patient. Tilting the patient's head from side to side and upward and downward will give a good view of the entire interior of the nose.

When mucosal edema or congestion hamper the examination, a decongestant should be used. A solution of cocaine hydrochloride (0.5 per cent) and ephedrine sulfate (1 per cent) sprayed into the nasal cavity or inserted on cotton pledgets shrinks the mucous membrane. A bayonet forceps is a good instrument for accurate placement of cotton pledgets (Fig. 10–17). The cotton pack should be left in place for four to five minutes and should not be uncomfortable for the patient. When the cotton is removed, the examiner will have good visualization of the nasal cavity in those patients with edema of the mucous membrane. The cocaine-hydrochloride solution will also anesthetize the nasal membrane and make subsequent intranasal manipulations less painful.

Secretions or blood may interfere with

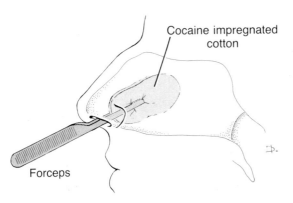

Cocaine impregnated cotton

Forceps

Figure 10–17   Nasal decongestion. Nasal decongestion can be obtained by inserting a cotton pledget saturated with an appropriate material, such as ephedrine 1 per cent or cocaine hydrochloride 0.5 per cent.

the examination and should be removed by a Fraser suction with a fingerhole control.

Congenital Lesions

Dermoid Cysts

These cysts often indicate their presence with a small moist sinus opening in the midline of the nose near its bone-cartilaginous junction. Caseous material may discharge from this opening from time to time. The cyst often extends into the nasal septum, and excision of the superficial portion will allow a recurrence of the cyst. Since an adequate excision often includes an exploration of the septum to insure complete removal of the cyst, the operation should not be performed in the office or Outpatient Department.

Obstructed sebaceous glands cause cysts and these may be excised using local (Xylocaine) anesthesia. A small ellipse of skin should be excised with the cyst.

Inclusion Cysts

These cysts occur along the lines of junction of segments of the face, at the sides of the nose and the philtrum of the upper lip. They can be excised with the use of local anesthesia. The incisions should be placed in natural skin lines to minimize unsightly scars.

Nasoalveolar Cysts

A smooth swelling in the floor of the nose is the usual presentation for these lesions. Unerupted incisor teeth may confuse the examiner, and an x-ray of this area will help to clarify the problem. These lesions should be removed in the operating room.

Atresia

This condition consists of a closure of one or both nasal openings. It may be partial or complete, congenital or ac-quired. Atresias may occur at either the anterior or posterior choanae.

Anterior Choanal Atresia

Congenital atresia of the anterior apertures of the nasal passage is a rare condition. This situation occurs when the medial and lateral nasal folds fail to absorb in the embryo. More frequently, anterior atresia is an acquired condition due to destruction of the normal cartilage and skin by injury or chronic inflammatory diseases such as lupus, syphilis or leprosy. Scar tissue contracts to decrease one or both nasal openings. Cosmetic deformities are often associated with the atresia, and these defects may be very disfiguring. Reconstructive procedures should not be performed until the underlying disease has been eradicated. A surgeon trained in rhinoplasty should be consulted for repair of these problems.

Posterior Choanal Atresia

Atresia of the posterior choanae (Fig. 10–18) is not very common and is usually congenital in origin, although it may not be recognized immediately after delivery. The infant may have serious respiratory difficulties when sucking at the breast or bottle, and he usually keeps the mouth open continually during sleep.

Congenital atresia may be unilateral or bilateral. When it is unilateral, the infant will have less difficulty during feeding. This problem can be corrected later in life; however, the patient with bilaterial atresia must be detected as soon as possible and treated immediately. Some method of providing an airway during feeding is essential since the child may suffocate if the problem is not detected. The diagnosis can be made by: (1) observing persistent nasal obstruction that does not improve with suctioning of secretions or decongestant drops; (2) passing a thin plastic catheter through the baby's nose into the pharynx; and (3) obtaining x-rays of the newborn in-

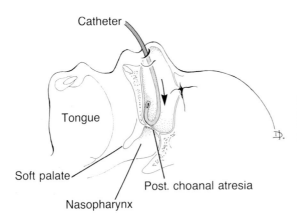

Catheter

Tongue

Soft palate

Nasopharynx

Post. choanal atresia

Figure 10–18   Posterior choanal atresia. Posterior choanal atresia can be detected by passing a small rubber catheter into the nose. The obstruction will be apparent when the catheter reaches the posterior choana.

fant's nose. A radiopaque liquid instilled into the nose can be seen on the x-ray against the occluding membrane.

In 90 per cent of cases, the atresia will consist of a bony occlusion.[7] This bony obstruction must be completely removed along with a portion of the posterior septum. This operation should not be performed by an inexperienced surgeon.

Traumatic Conditions

Injuries to the nose are very common, and usually result from blows or falls. Abrasions and contusions from subcutaneous hemorrhage may obscure an underlying injury and make the diagnosis difficult. External lacerations (Fig. 10–19) often extend through the bone and cartilage into the nasal cavity. Inspection and palpation are important diagnostic techniques when evaluating a patient with nasal trauma. Nasal deformity, subcutaneous emphysema or crepitus, and mobility of the nasal bones indicate a fracture. Examination of the nasal interior is often unsuccessful because edema or blood clots obscure it. The clots should be removed by suction and the edema reduced with a decongesting solution. Dislocations, fractures or subperichondral hematomas (Fig. 10–20) of the nasal septum may produce deformities that obstruct the airway or alter the appearance of the nasal

contour. These septal problems must not be overlooked.

Fractures of the nose may be either simple or compound with varying degrees of deformity. Often, the mucous membrane has been torn by depressed bone fragments penetrating the interior of the nose. There may be associated injuries to the orbit and its contents, the lacrimal apparatus, the ethmoid sinuses and brain, the maxillary sinus and the teeth. A roentgen examination will aid in the diagnosis and the choice of therapy. Complicated nasal fractures should always be treated by a surgeon who is familiar with these problems.

Anesthesia must be obtained before reducing the fracture. Cotton packs moistened with 4 per cent cocaine hydrochloride are inserted into the nose to anesthetize and shrink the mucous membrane. These packs should be placed along the course of the anterior nerves, over the sphenopalatine ganglion and along the floor of the nose. Infiltration anesthesia with 1 per cent Xylocaine containing epinephrine hydrochloride (1:100,000) is started by raising a wheal beside each ala (Fig. 10–21). A 2 inch 25 gauge needle is inserted through the wheal along the lateral wall of the nose to its root just medial to the inner canthus of the eye. The solution is deposited along this tract as the needle is withdrawn. This injection will anesthetize fibers of the infratrochlear, infraorbital and anterior alveolar nerves. The second

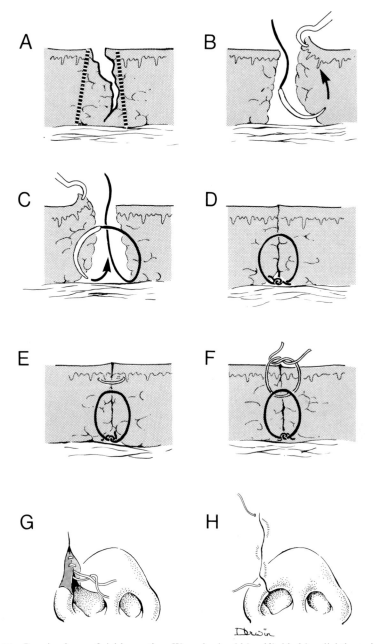

Figure 10–19 Repair of superficial laceration. Wounds should be débrided by slightly undercutting the skin edges *(A)*. This provides the optimal surface for suture repair. The wounds are undermined slightly and the deep layers approximated with fine nylon subcuticular sutures *(E)* or interrupted sutures *(F)*. The interrupted sutures should be removed in three days, but the subcuticular suture may be left in place much longer. A laceration of the nose is repaired using these techniques *(G* and *H)*.

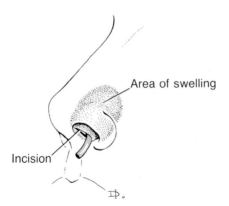

Figure 10–20 Septal abscess or hematoma. Septal abscess or hematoma should be incised and drained. After adequate anesthesia, a vertical incision is made into the area of swelling under direct vision. The incision is made through the mucosa and perichondrium and the blood or pus evacuated. A small rubber drain is inserted through the incision beneath the perichondrium and a pack inserted into the nose.

injection is made through the nostril by passing the needle through the intercartilaginous sulcus between the upper and lower lateral cartilages. The needle is passed upward over the lateral dorsal portion of the nasal bone to the root of the nose and the anesthetic solution is deposited in the subcutaneous tissue as the needle is withdrawn. This injection anesthetizes the external nasal nerve and the terminal branches of the nasociliary nerve. Similar injections are made on the opposite side. The membranous septum and nasal spine are injected on each side, and the previously inserted nasal packs are then removed. This technique, when performed properly, will give excellent anesthesia and allow the surgeon to manipulate the nose with little discomfort for the patient.

The Asch forceps is ideal for reducing

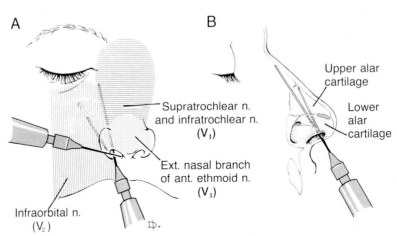

Figure 10–21 Anesthesia of the nose. The nose is anesthetized by injecting a local anesthetic solution as shown in this illustration. The infraorbital branch (1) of V_2 is injected by inserting the needle beneath the lower alar cartilage and passing it close to the infraorbital foramen. This foramen can be located by palpating the cheek. The supratrochlear and infratrochlear branches of V_1 can be anesthetized by inserting the needle along the base of the nasal pyramid up to the medial canthus of the eye (2). As the needle is withdrawn a small amount of anesthetic is deposited between the skin and periosteum of the nasal bones. The base of the columela can be anesthetized (3) by inserting the needle into the subcutaneous tissues about the anterior maxillary spine. This is particularly important for reducing fractures of the floor of the nose and anterior nasal spine. The external nasal branch of the anterior ethmoid nerve is blocked by inserting the needle through the groove between the upper and lower alar cartilages (4). Additional anesthesia of the supratrochlear and infratrochlear nerves is obtained by passing the needle over the dorsum of the nose between the skin and periosteum of the nose up to the root (glabella) of the nose, and anesthetic solution deposited in this area.

nasal fractures; however, a small hemostat or bayonet forceps can be used (Fig. 10–22). Fragments can be pushed into alignment with the intranasal lever action of the forceps while the other hand molds the bones into proper position. An upward anterior force applied to the undersurface of the nasal bones with the forceps with external manipulation produces the desired reduction of

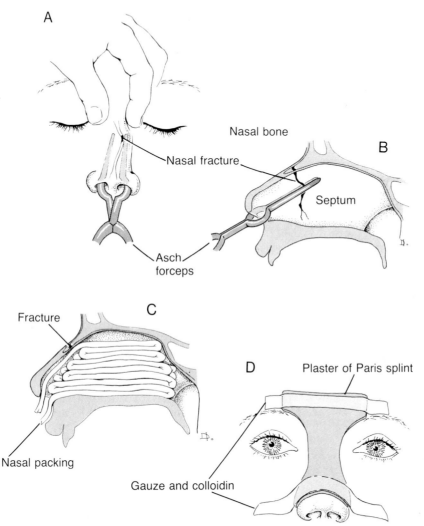

Figure 10–22 Nasal fracture reduction. *A.* The Asch forceps is inserted carefully into the nose on each side of the nasal septum. Using an upward and anterior force and palpation of the nose, the fractured segments can be guided into accurate realignment.

B. The nasal septum can also be straightened by applying pressure on both sides with the Asch forceps. When extreme comminution is not present, the bones and cartilages will remain reduced so that intranasal packs *(C)* and an external splint *(D)* can be applied for adequate support.

C. The nasal pack is placed gently and carefully into the nose from the nasal floor to its roof. Vaseline gauze ¹/₂″ impregnated with an antibiotic is used. Both ends of the pack are brought out through the anterior naris to avoid dislodgement of the end of the pack into the pharynx. Placement of the pack into the fracture line or beneath the nasal mucosa can be avoided by inserting it with direct visualization.

D. Plaster of Paris is trimmed and gently molded to the nasal pyramid. This lightweight splint is then held in position over the forehead and cheek with gauze strips and colloidin.

the fracture. Normally, it is necessary to insert the forceps into both nasal cavities, one blade on each side of the septum, to obtain a satisfactory reduction. When there is a unilateral displaced fracture, one blade of the forceps is inserted intranasally with the other blade on the external surface of the nose. External molding is required to obtain a good reduction.

Injuries of the nasal septum must not be overlooked. Alignment of fragments and drainage of hematomas will prevent serious deformities at a later date. A septum buckled out of position can be straightened with the Asch forceps by applying pressure against the two sides of the septum. A simple incision through the mucosa and perichondrium with evacuation of the blood and clots will prevent ischemic necrosis of the septal cartilage. These incisions should be left open to allow drainage—packing material should not be inserted in them.

After the fractures have been aligned, any external lacerations should be carefully inspected, irrigated with a sterile normal saline solution, and all foreign material removed. The wound edges should be carefully approximated with fine nonabsorbable sutures such as 5-0 monofilament nylon.

Intranasal packs of one-half inch petroleum (Vaseline) gauze impregnated with an antibiotic ointment are inserted after reduction of the fracture (Fig. 10–22 C). This pack should be removed in 48 to 72 hours. Plaster of Paris gauze is one of the best of several possible materials that can be used to make an external nasal splint (Fig. 10–22 D). It can be easily molded over the skin and provides support for the nasal bones while preventing hematoma and edema formation. A layer of coarse mesh gauze impregnated with nonflexible colloidin placed across the forehead and the cheeks holds the splint in place. A small piece of folded gauze is placed under the nares and held with adhesive tape to absorb blood or mucus draining from the nasal openings. This "snuffer" should be changed frequently.

While the nose is packed, antibiotics should be given to reduce infection. An orally administered decongestant and appropriate analgesics will add to the patient's comfort.

Splints should be removed in 5 to 10 days depending upon the degree of comminution and displacement of the fracture. Edema and eccymosis subside slowly and may require three or four weeks to completely disappear. The nasal skeleton is rather unstable and vulnerable to injury during the first eight or ten weeks after fracture and the patient should be advised to avoid any activities that could result in trauma to the nose.

Epistaxis

Nasal bleeding is always disturbing to the patient and may become serious when not treated promptly and adequately. Hemorrhage usually results from a rupture of the small vessels that lie within the mucous membrane of the nose. Epistaxis can be classified into four types: anterior, posterior, superior and generalized. Localizing the bleeding point helps to determine the bleeding vessel. The anterior ethmoid artery supplies the anterior and anterosuperior portion of the nose, whereas the remainder of the nose is supplied by the sphenopalatine and posterior ethmoid arteries (Fig. 10–23). Kiesselbach's plexus, located at Little's area in the anterior septum, is composed of vessels from both sources as well as labial branches from the upper lip.

Epistaxis has a varied etiology, a large number of local and systemic conditions contributing to the problem (Table 10–3). Trauma, infection, hypertension and other circulatory disorders, as well as neoplasms, coagulopathies and many miscellaneous conditions are some of the important causes.

Almost all epistaxis in children occurs in the anterior septum in Little's area, whereas about 50 per cent of adults bleed from the posterior nose. Posterior

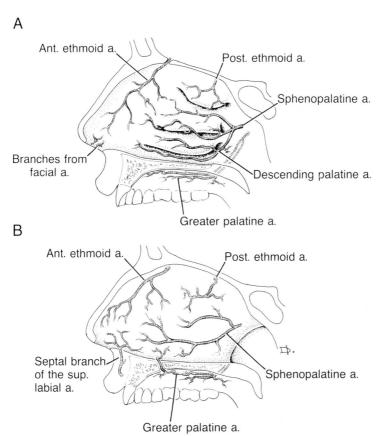

Figure 10–23 Blood supply of the nose. There is a rich blood supply to the interior of the nose, the vessels arising from several sources and entering the nose in various locations. The posterior portion of the lateral nasal wall is supplied by the sphenopalatine from the maxillary artery and the posterior ethmoid from the ophthalmic artery *(A)*. The anterior lateral nasal wall receives its blood from the anterior ethmoid which is also a branch of the ophthalmic artery. The vestibule is supplied by small branches from the facial artery and the nasal septum *(B)* is supplied by essentially the same vessels. The anterior septum also receives a branch from the superior labial artery. A very vascular area (Little's) on the anterior septum is supplied by all the vessels that supply the nose except the posterior ethmoid. This site is often injured and is a common site of bleeding.

bleeding is usually caused by a spontaneous rupture of a blood vessel and is not associated with trauma. Many of these patients have a systemic disease that contributes to the nasal bleeding.

A history of the duration and amount of blood loss is important when evaluating a patient with epistaxis. When there is a small blood loss it is usually easily controlled and little treatment will be required. However, most patients will have had epistaxis for some time and quite often they have been bleeding intermittently for several days before

they seek help. The patient is often frightened and an injection of morphine sulfate will help calm him. During this time, a history of illness, trauma, medications or bleeding disorders should be obtained. A good indication of the bleeding site can be obtained by asking whether the blood was first noticed coming from the anterior nose or posteriorly into the pharynx.

When both patient and doctor are gowned, the patient should sit up and lean slightly forward to prevent blood running down his throat and to make the

TABLE 10–3 Differential Diagnosis of Epistaxis

I. Trauma
   A. Blows to the nose with or without fractures
   B. Nose picking
   C. Surgical trauma
   D. Nasogastric tubes
   E. Foreign bodies
   F. Septal perforations

II. Inflammation
   A. Acute rhinitis and sinusitis
   B. Chronic or atrophic rhinitis
   C. Acute systemic infections
      1. Rheumatic fever
      2. Scarlet fever
      3. Measles
      4. Typhoid and paratyphoid fever
      5. Rickettsial diseases
      6. Pertussis
      7. Diphtheria
      8. Leprosy
      9. Malaria
   D. Granulomatous diseases
      1. Syphilis
      2. Rhinoscleroma
      3. Tuberculosis
      4. Lupus erythematosis
      5. Sarcoidosis
      6. Wegener's granulomatosis and lethal midline granuloma
   E. Allergic disorders
      1. Henoch-Schönlein's purpura
      2. Allergic polyps

III. Cardiovascular and Circulatory
   A. Hypertension
   B. Atherosclerosis
   C. Hereditary hemorrhagic telangiectasis
      (Rendu-Osler-Weber disease)
   D. Increased venous pressure
      1. Bronchitis, asthma or other chronic lung disease
      2. Cardiac failure
      3. Pulmonary or neck tumors

IV. Neoplasms
   A. Carcinoma of the nose, sinuses or nasopharynx
   B. Papilloma
   C. Angiofibroma

V. Coagulopathies
   A. Anticoagulant therapy
   B. Hemophilia
   C. Thrombocytopenia
   D. Prothrombin deficiency—alcoholic cirrhosis of the liver
   E. Leukemia
   F. Aplastic anemia
   G. Polycythemia

VI. Miscellaneous
   A. Rhinoliths
   B. Irradiation
   C. Parasites and myiasis
   D. Chemical and drug poisoning
      1. Salicylates
      2. Phosphorus
      3. Cyanide gas
   E. Caisson disease
   F. Violent exertion

examination easier. The clots can be removed from the nose with suction or by having the patient gently blow his nose. If the bleeding is profuse it may be necessary to insert a cotton pledget soaked with 4 per cent cocaine hydrochloride solution. Gentle pinching of the alae for 10 to 15 minutes will usually reduce the bleeding sufficiently to allow examination and the localization of its site of origin. Most often the blood will be coming from a small vessel on the anterior septum—Kiesselbach's plexus. Lidocaine hydrochloride 1 per cent (Xylocaine) with 1:100,000 epinephrine hydrochloride U.S.P. injected into the submucosa with a 25 gauge needle will provide the anesthesia and vasoconstriction that are necessary for further manipulations. Cotton moistened with 1:1000 epinephrine solution applied to this area will often stop the bleeding. This cotton pack should be left in place for at least five minutes and pressure on the ala will increase its effectiveness. Such techniques may have to be repeated one or more times before the bleeding is controlled. Usually the vessel involved will be standing out from the mucosa and the next step is to permanently thrombose this vessel. After anesthetizing the area with a topical application of cocaine hydrochloride solution or an injection of lidocaine hydrochloride (Xylocaine), electrocautery or chemical cautery with trichloracetic acid (10 per cent) can be used. Occasionally, the attempts to coagulate the vessel will start the nose bleeding again and the whole process will have to be repeated.

Epistaxis originating from the posterior part of the nose is more difficult to evaluate and treat. This variety of epistaxis is often caused by a systemic disease, and these patients should be admitted to the hospital for an investigation of these problems.

To determine the bleeding site, the mucous membranes must be shrunk with a cocaine-ephedrine or epinephrine solution and the interior of the nose carefully inspected. Decongestant solutions must

be used with care in patients with hypertension or other cardiovascular diseases. A suction tip inserted along the floor of the nose will help to locate the bleeding site. When the bleeding vessel is approached by the suction tip, blood will cease to flow into the nasal cavity. The most common bleeding site is located beneath the inferior turbinate on the lateral nasal wall. A small pledget of cotton saturated with a decongesting solution placed beneath the inferior turbinate at this site will often stop the bleeding.

Occasionally, this small pack will solve the problem; however, a larger pack is usually necessary. Several types of posterior nasal packs can be used (Fig. 10–24). Packs made of gauze or a vaginal tampon work quite well. The pack should be held securely in place by tying strings from the pack across the columella of the septum. Pressure necrosis of the columella can be prevented by using a small gauze pad beneath the knotted strings. A number 12 or 14 French Foley catheter with a 30 cc bag makes a good posterior nasal pack. After inserting the catheter through the naris until the tip has passed beyond the posterior naris into the nasopharynx, the bag is filled with 5–10 cc of water or air. The catheter is gently pulled forward until the inflated bag is lodged in the posterior choana. The catheter should be secured to the cheek with adhesive tape. Too much traction may pull the catheter from the nose and this trauma may increase the amount of bleeding.

Usually an anterior pack must be inserted when a posterior pack is used (Fig. 10–22 C). The most suitable material is one-half inch Vaseline gauze. An antibiotic ointment applied to the gauze, oral antibiotics, and an oral decongesting agent will reduce the odor, rhinorrhea and the danger of infection associated with these packs.

Nasal packs should be removed after 48 to 72 hours. This period should be adequate for the control of the bleeding and allow enough time to investigate the

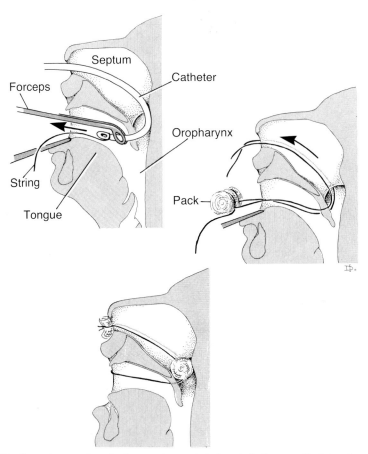

Figure 10-24 Posterior nasal pack. A posterior pack is inserted after anesthetizing the nose. A small rubber catheter (No. 10 French) is passed through the nose into the oropharynx where it is grasped and pulled through the mouth with a forceps *(A)*. A pack is fashioned from a roll of gauze with three 18 inch lengths of string tied about it. The pack is then tied to the catheter with one of the strings and the catheter and string pulled through the nasopharynx, nasal cavity and external naris. This procedure is repeated on the opposite side. With steady traction on the nasal strings and pressure from the index finger, the pack is directed into the nasopharynx *(B)*. The third string is left hanging from the mouth and taped to the cheek to allow easy removal of the pack *(C)*.

patient's illness. Hypertension or a coagulopathy must be treated before removing the packs.

Padrnos (1968)[8] advocates the use of a pterygomaxillary injection for the treatment of epistaxis (Fig. 10-25). This technique is quite useful in the patient with a posterior nose bleed and will reduce the necessity for packs. The greater palatine foramen is located medial and adjacent to the last molar tooth. A 25 or 27 gauge needle one and a half to two inches in length can be inserted through the foramen one-half to three-fourths of an inch into the pterygomaxillary canal. An injection 1 to 1.5 cc of 1 per cent lidocaine with 1:100,000 solution of epinephrine into the canal will compress the vessels and reduce the amount of circulating blood to the nose. Quite often this injection will control the bleeding and make packing unnecessary.

When these measures fail to control nasal bleeding, appropriate vessel ligation may be indicated. The anterior

Figure 10–25 Pterygopalatine injection. A pterygopalatine (pterygomaxillary) injection is a useful technique for controlling posterior epistaxis and obtaining anesthesia of the posterior nose, palate and parts of the nasopharynx. A shallow dimple is usually visible next to the third molar tooth. This serves as a convenient landmark for inserting a 25 gauge needle 2½ inches in length which can be inserted easily at an angle of 50°. The needle is passed into the pterygopalatine fossa about 1 inch, and 1–1.5 cc of anesthetic solution with 1:100,000 units of epinephrine is deposited before the needle is withdrawn. This solution will temporarily tamponade the descending palatine artery and frequently control a posterior epistaxis. If this injection fails to stop bleeding, it provides some anesthesia for the insertion of a posterior nasal pack.

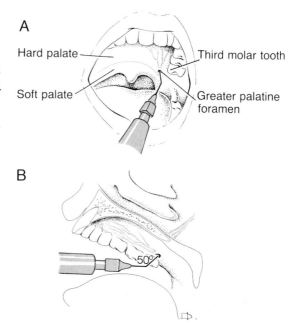

ethmoid, sphenopalatine and external carotid arteries may be ligated. Localizing the bleeding site is important when deciding which vessel should be ligated. Allen (1970)[9] has used a transmaxillary approach for ligating branches of the sphenopalatine artery. This operation has been successful in a large number of patients in whom nasal packs were ineffective. Those patients who need vessel ligation should be hospitalized and referred to an otolaryngologist for surgery.

Nasal Polyps

These non-neoplastic tumors are composed of edematous hypertrophied nasal mucosa that arises from a chronic inflammatory process. Often bilateral, these masses occur singly or in numbers and may be either pedunculated or sessile. A smooth, glistening, grapelike lesion that is grey-white in color is the typical appearance of the nasal polyp. They must be differentiated from a squamous carcinoma, papilloma, angiofibroma, hemangioma, glioma, meningioma or encephalocoeles.

Successful treatment must include therapy for the underlying allergic or infectious problems. Polyps can be removed with a snare and Green or Takahashi forceps (Fig. 10–26 *A*), but unless the above etiologic factors are controlled they will inevitably recur. Underlying chronic sinus infections may require hospitalization and surgical treatment.

Allergy treatment may require a thorough investigation of the patient's hypersensitivity status and referral of these patients to an allergist is usually necessary.

Unilateral polyps should always be approached with caution. These lesions have many of the characteristics of an allergic or inflammatory polyp but biopsy often reveals a more serious condition. Injudicious excision may lead to severe bleeding, CSF rhinorrhea or failure to diagnose a neoplasm. All tissue removed should be sent to a pathologist for histopathologic diagnosis.

Injections of polyps with a depository steroid preparation will control many of them for long periods of time. Depo-Medrol 0.5–1.0 cc injected directly into

A

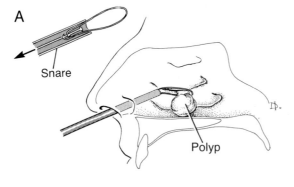

Snare

B

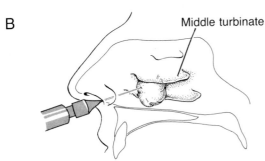

Polyp

Middle turbinate

Figure 10–26 Removal of nasal polyp. *A.* After anesthetizing the nose with tetracaine 2 per cent or cocaine 10 per cent, a nasal snare is slipped around the polyp and transected. The polyp is then removed with a forceps. Usually more polyps will be seen after the initial ones have been removed. These should be excised in a similar fashion. *B.* The nasal polyp is visualized and a 25 gauge needle inserted into the polyp. A small amount of steroid solution (Depo-Medrol) is injected into the polyp. Usually 0.25–0.5 cc is sufficient for this purpose.

the polyp (Fig. 10–26 *B*) frequently produces a marked reduction in size with subsequent improvement in the nasal airway. This procedure may have to be repeated at weekly intervals before a more or less permanent resolution of the polyp occurs. Topical anesthesia with a cocaine hydrochloride solution (4 per cent) is all that is necessary for this procedure and often the injection can be performed without anesthesia.

Antrochoanal Polyp

Antrochoanal polyps arise from abnormal mucosa within the maxillary sinus. The gradually enlarging polyp passes through the natural ostium of the sinus into the middle meatus of the nose. It extends backward into the posterior choana where it can be seen quite easily with a mirror. Occasionally, the polyp will become large and present below the soft palate. The polyp will have a smooth, translucent, slightly yellowish appear-

ance, and is associated with a radiopaque maxillary sinus from which it arises.

Once the diagnosis is made, the treatment consists of surgical excision of the maxillary sinus disease through a Caldwell-Luc incision, an operation which should not be performed in the Outpatient Department. Squamous carcinoma must be suspected until the entire specimen has been examined microscopically, since most carcinomas of the maxillary antrum are associated with squamous hyperplasia, and biopsy of the surface is frequently reported as benign.

Foreign Bodies

Many animate and inanimate foreign bodies, including anything small enough to enter the nose, have been found in the nose. Since most foreign bodies are placed in the nose by the patient, children are the most frequent offenders. Foreign bodies are usually easy to localize; however, x-rays may be of value in some instances. The exact location should be ascertained before any attempts are made to remove it. Usually the foreign body can be removed through the anterior naris without a general anesthetic, although in some cases this is inadvisable.

A forceps may be used to grasp an object with a rough surface. A curved probe may be adapted to remove smooth objects such as beads or marbles (Fig. 10–27) by passing the curved part of the probe behind the object and gently pulling it forward. When objects such as beans or peas have been in the nose long enough to swell and soften, a suction tip is a useful instrument to use for removing them. Enlarged objects may have to be fragmented before removal. The uncooperative patient may require a general anesthetic before the foreign body can be removed. There is always the danger that a foreign body can be dislodged from the nose and aspirated. A cuffed endotracheal tube or a finger in the nasopharynx will help prevent such a disaster. Quite often, small children will insert several objects into the nose and multiple foreign bodies should always be suspected.

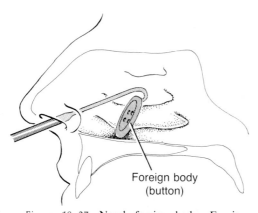

Figure 10–27 Nasal foreign body. Foreign bodies are frequently inserted into the nose. Such objects should be removed with care under direct vision or they can be dislodged into the nasopharynx, larynx, trachea or bronchi. A small hook is a useful instrument for removing some objects, but a suction or a forceps may also be used. Topical anesthesia can be obtained with either a cocaine or tetracaine solution.

Nasal Myiasis

Nasal myiasis occurs when the common blow fly (screw worm) or the green bottle fly deposits its eggs in the nasal cavity. Such flies inhabit warm dry climates at low altitudes, with the screw worm fly *(Cochliomyia americana)* predominanting in North America. The eggs hatch within 24 hours after being deposited in the nose. Mucous membranes may be destroyed, exposing bone and cartilage. Usually this condition is associated with local nasal disease or systemic diseases (diabetes mellitus) in patients living in unsantiary conditions. The symptoms are those of an acute rhinitis or sinusitis and include rhinorrhea with an offensive odor, pain or headache. Rhinorrhea may be quite profuse, unilateral with a bloody mucopurulent appearance. The worms cling tenaciously to the tissues of the nose, but must be removed. Any associated pyogenic infection should be treated with antibiotics.

Nasal Furunculosis

These superficial abscesses may occur in any part of the nose, but the most common site is the nasal vestibule. *Staphylococcus aureus* is the most common infecting organism. Bacteria may enter through minor injuries to the tissues produced by picking the nose or plucking the hairs from the vestibule of the nose. Diabetes mellitus may be associated with recurrent furunculosis.

Furuncles in the nasal vestibule, nasal apex or upper lip are potentially dangerous since the infection may spread into the cavernous sinus through veins that drain directly into the sinus from these areas. This serious complication will be evident by the conjunctival chemosis, edema of the lids, proptosis, limitation of extraocular movement, papilledema and decreased visual acuity.

Most abscesses around the nose will respond to systemic antibiotic therapy.

Cultures from the area will reveal the infecting organism and sensitivity studies will indicate the antibiotic best suited for the infection. Oxacillin or methicillin are the antibiotics of choice for a *Staphyloccus aureus* infection. Heat and topical bacitracin-neomycin ointment will relieve much of the discomfort. The abscess should not be squeezed or manipulated since these maneuvers may enhance the possibility of intracranial spread of infection. When the abscess becomes localized with an obvious fluctuant "head," it should be incised (Fig. 10–28) carefully and gently to avoid a cavernous sinus extension of the infection.

Rhinoliths

This term is applied to foreign bodies that have remained in the nose for some time and have become coated with calcium and magnesium salts. The nucleus may consist of bacteria, blood, pus, inspissated mucus or a small undetected foreign body. A mass with a rough exterior and a brown color is characteristic of these foreign bodies. They are often unilateral and vary considerably in size. The consistency may be either soft, crumbly, hard or brittle. A unilateral fetid nasal discharge and airway obstruction are the usual symptoms. The treatment is removal with topical, local or general anesthesia.

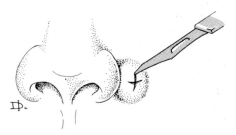

Figure 10–28 Incision of facial abscess. An area of cellulitis or an abscess of the face should be drained through a cruciate incision. Manipulation of these infections may allow pus to enter the cavernous sinus and produce thrombosis of this structure.

Epithelial Papilloma

Papillomas of the nose may be single or multiple. They are pink in color, firm, pliable and tend to bleed when manipulated. The septum and inferior turbinate are the commonest sites of origin and the diagnosis may be missed if the specimen is not submitted for histopathologic examination.

A pedunculated mass of papilloma can be removed with a snare. Multiple papillomas require wide surgical excision and any recurrences should have complete excision followed by radiation therapy. Malignant degeneration is common.

Nasopharyngeal Angiofibroma

Angiofibromas arise in the posterior nose and nasopharynx of the pre-adolescent male.[10] They are firm, bluish red tumors that produce symptoms of nasal obstruction, rhinorrhea and epistaxis. These benign tumors may become very large and extend into adjacent areas such as the maxillary sinus, pterygomaxillary fossa, infratemporal fossa, sphenoid sinus, orbit and middle cranial fossa. Patients with large tumors may complain of failing vision, exophthalmos, proptosis, swelling of the cheek and nasal deformity. A biopsy of the tumor may produce disastrous consequences in the patient from massive bleeding. A patient with this tumor should be admitted to the hospital for diagnosis and treatment.

Nasal Carcinoma

Squamous cell carcinoma is the most common malignant neoplasm of the nose and paranasal sinuses and is difficult to treat. Unilateral nasal obstruction and a sensation of pressure and rhinorrhea may be the only symptoms. The discharge can be serous, serosanguinous or purulent. Pain, when present, is apt to be worse at night or when the patient is lying down.

Careful examination of the nose will often reveal a tumor and biopsy with histopathologic examination of the specimen will assure the diagnosis. Such a carcinoma requires carefully planned surgical and irradiation therapy.

Esthesioneuroblastoma is an unusual tumor arising from the olfactory epithelium high in the nasal cavity. Common symptoms are one-sided nasal obstruction with associated rhinorrhea and epistaxis. A history of repeated polypectomy is quite common. Usually there is a rapid recurrence of the "polyp" and if this tissue has not been examined by a pathologist, the diagnosis will be missed.

Small tumors may be difficult to see. They are usually located on the septum or the superior turbinate. The tumor may spread by infiltration or metastasis. Large lesions often extend into the ethmoid and frontal sinuses, the orbit and the face through the nasal bones. Exophthalmos, increased lacrimation, headache, and masses about the nose occur when the tumor extends in these areas. Treatment consists of irradiation and surgery.

Several other malignant tumors may arise in the nose. Lymphoma, adenoid cystic carcinoma, malignant melanoma, chondrosarcoma, liposarcoma, and fibrosarcoma have all been detected in the nose. Biopsy is essential to make the diagnosis and even the innocent "polyp" should be submitted for histopathologic examination. Many patients have not received prompt treatment for a serious disease because tissues removed from the nose were discarded, a practice to be avoided.

PARANASAL SINUSES

These spaces consist of the maxillary, ethmoidal, frontal and sphenoidal air cavities on each side. The specific functions of the sinuses are unknown. They often harbor diseases that are overlooked.

Examination

Direct inspection of the sinuses is not ordinarily possible and some indirect method of examination is required when a disease is suspected.

The signs and symptoms of sinus disease are often subtle and easily missed. Disease may be restricted to a single sinus or it may be present in several on either one or both sides.

Pain is usually located over the affected sinus and is often increased with coughing, sneezing, bending over or walking. It may be referred to other areas and often decreases with rest in bed. Maxillary sinus pain is characteristically localized over the cheek and occasionally radiates along the upper alveolus, teeth or gums near the affected sinus. It may also be referred to the supraorbital nerve and mistakenly interpreted as arising from the frontal sinus. Occasionally the pain will be referred to the ear, and this pain is usually located in front of the ear with a normal tympanic membrane. Ethmoidal pain is located over the bridge of the nose and inner canthus of the eye, and may be associated with a feeling of tenderness of the globe that is aggravated by moving the eye. This pain is often referred to a small area on the parietal eminence of the skull. Sphenoid disease usually produces an occipital or vertex headache; there may be pain behind the eye but the globe itself is not tender. Sometimes this pain is referred to the mastoid process. Frontal pain is localized to the forehead and is usually associated with a generalized headache. This pain often starts an hour or two after rising in the morning and decreases later in the afternoon. So-called "sinus headaches" are usually not associated with sinus disease. Patients with this symptom should be investigated for other diseases.

Other symptoms of sinus disease include malaise, anorexia, mental dullness, forgetfulness and a slight elevation of temperature. In acute inflammations, rhinorrhea consisting of mucoid or mucopurulent material is seen. These patients usually have airway obstruction. Chronic inflammations produce few nasal symptoms. The sense of smell is usually lost and vocal resonance may be altered. Epistaxis is mild and may occur repeatedly; especially when the maxillary sinus is involved. An unpleasant-tasting postnasal drip may be noticed by the patient when the inflammation becomes less acute.

Flushing and swelling of the cheek, eyelids and forehead is sometimes seen in maxillary, ethmoid and frontal sinus infections. Swelling of the eyelids is more often associated with ethmoiditis in children. Tenderness in these areas is usually associated with a closed infection or abscess formation. Supraorbital nerve tenderness is often associated with maxillary sinus infections, whereas gentle tapping over the frontal sinus or pressure on its floor just above the inner canthus causes exquisite pain when the frontal sinus is involved.

Examination of the nose often reveals a generalized redness and swelling of the mucous membrane. Shrinking this congested membrane with a topical decongestant will make it much easier to see the signs of sinusitis. A localized area of swelling and redness with pus coming from the drainage area of the sinus usually means disease in that sinus. Chronic sinusitis may be accompanied by a hypertrophic or atrophic rhinitis.

Nasopharyngeal examination with a small mirror or nasopharyngoscope will often reveal a pool of pus on the upper surface of the palate or pus trickling over the posterior end of the inferior turbinate. Pus coming from the region of the sphenoid ostium or sphenoethmoid recess indicates an infection in these sinuses.

Swelling of the lateral pharyngeal lymphoid tissue or pus coming down the lateral pharyngeal gutter indicates a sinus infection on that side. These findings may also be detected in patients who have a carcinoma of the paranasal sinuses with a superimposed infection.

Transillumination of the sinuses as a method of examination has been recommended for many years, but in my experience has not been very reliable. Standard x-ray views are more valuable, but must be taken with proper positioning of the head. All radiopaque articles must be removed, including dentures, hairpins, wigs or "pony tails" of hair. A textbook of radiology or otolaryngology should be consulted for the proper radiographic techniques. Air fluid levels, opacification, mucosal thickening and bone destruction may be seen on the x-ray and these findings, when correlated with the patient's symptoms and signs, are of great value in making a diagnosis.

Nasoantral Irrigation

This simple procedure (Fig. 10–29) is useful for treating maxillary sinusitis and for obtaining purulent secretions from the sinus for culture and sensitivity tests. The preferred route is through the thin bone separating the maxillary sinus and nasal cavity in the inferior meatus. This area is anesthetized by packing the meatus with cotton soaked in 4 per cent cocaine hydrochloride solution. A small amount of lidocaine hydrochloride with 1:100,000 solution of epinephrine hydrochloride can be injected into the nasal vestibule near the pyriform crest and the anterior end of the inferior turbinate. This injection will provide good anesthesia and decrease the amount of bleeding when the sinus is punctured. A 2½ inch disposable 18 gauge spinal needle can be used for this procedure. This needle is placed beneath the inferior turbinate approximately 1.0 centimeter behind its anterior tip. Steady pressure on the needle will force it through the antronasal wall into the sinus. The needle should be directed slightly upward, but it should not be inserted with such force that it traverses the sinus and enters the orbit or the lateral sinus wall. A 50 cc glass syringe is then attached to the needle with a rubber tube and adapter. It is essential to aspirate before irrigating the sinus. Either pus or air will indicate proper placement

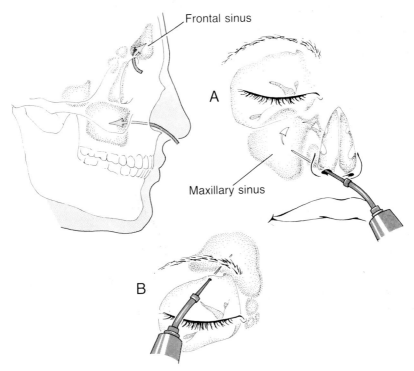

Figure 10-29 Sinus trephination. *A.* Irrigation of the maxillary sinus is a technique that can be performed with local anesthesia. The interior of the nose is packed with cotton saturated with cocaine hydrochloride solution (4 per cent). A small amount (0.5–1.0 cc) of local anesthetic (Xylocaine) with 1:100,000 of epinephrine is then injected into the floor of the nasal vestibule and anterior end of the inferior turbinate. Within a few minutes the inferior meatus of the nose will be anesthetized and a 2 inch 16 gauge disposable needle can be pushed through the inferior nasoantral wall into the maxillary sinus. The needle must be carefully controlled to avoid its misplacement into the orbit or lateral wall of the antrum. A syringe is then attached to the needle and the sinus aspirated. Air or pus entering the syringe usually indicates entry into the sinus. Warmed sterile saline is injected in the sinus. Excessive pressure may cause severe pain or may fracture the roof of the sinus into the orbit. Air should not be injected into the sinus, since it may cause an air embolus. *B.* Trephination of the frontal sinus can be performed with local anesthetic. Xylocaine with epinephrine is injected along the medial floor of the frontal sinus. The sinus floor is usually quite thin and easily punctured. A small incision is made through the skin, subcutaneous tissue, muscle and periosteum. A trocar or a 16 gauge needle is then forced through the bone into the frontal sinus. When the bone is too thick, a small drill may be used to enter the sinus. Aspiration with a syringe will usually reveal purulent material when the sinus is infected. A small polyethylene tube is then inserted through the wound into the sinus to allow drainage of secretions.

of the needle. When air or pus cannot be aspirated, it means the needle tip is either not in the sinus or it is filled with solid material such as polypoid mucosa or neoplasm. Warmed sterile, normal saline solution is then injected into the sinus and collected in a basin as it flows from the nose. Excessive syringe pressure must be avoided when irrigating the sinus, and it is important to avoid injecting air into the sinus since this can

cause an air embolism. Secretions from the sinus should be cultured. The irrigations may have to be repeated every two or three days before the infection is controlled, and subsequent irrigations should yield less purulent material.

In patients with chronic sinusitis, a fine polyethylene tube can be placed in the sinus through the lavage needle and left in place for two to three days. It can be attached to the cheek with ad-

hesive tape and an appropriate antibiotic injected into the sinus three or four
times a day. These locally applied antibiotics may help eradicate an infection
that otherwise might not improve with
the usual medical treatment. Systemic
antibiotics, decongestants, heat, humidification of the air, bed rest and analgesics
are all helpful. I usually treat the acute
sinusitis patient with systemic antibiotics for 24 hours before attempting
an antral irrigation; this reduces the
risks of the irrigation spreading the infection.

Uncomplicated acute frontal sinusitis
should be treated medically for 24 to 48
hours before any surgical intervention
is considered. When the infection is
not controlled by medical therapy or
there are signs and symptoms of complications, it may be necessary to drain the
sinus surgically (Fig. 10–29 C). Drainage
can be accomplished through an external incision ¼ of an inch below and
parallel to the medial end of the eyebrow.
This incision should be made straight
through to the bone. The superficial
tissues are retracted away and a small
hole is made with a drill or trocar. This
opening into the sinus should be large
enough to accommodate a small polyethylene tube. A suture placed through
the skin and around the tube will hold it
securely in position. Pus from the sinus
should be submitted to the laboratory
for culture and sensitivity tests. Gentle
irrigation of the sinus with warmed
sterile normal saline will help relieve the
patient's symptoms. The irrigating solution should drain through the nasofrontal duct if mucosal edema or inspis-
sation secretions do not obstruct it. The
operation should take only a few minutes
and can be performed with either local
or general anesthesia.

Before antibiotics were available,
numerous complications developed from
even minor operations on the frontal
sinus, so it is important that frontal
sinus trephination not be performed
without concomitant antibiotic therapy.
Frontal sinus infections usually respond
rapidly to this treatment and the drain-

age tube can be removed after four or
five days. Patency of the nasofrontal
duct can be determined by injecting a
small quantity of colored fluid into the
sinus and observing whether or not
this fluid passes through the duct into
the nose.

Oromaxillary Fistula

Several of the upper molars are in
intimate contact with the floor of the
maxillary sinus. Large sinus cavities
are separated from the apices of these
teeth by a thin plate of bone, and in some
instances the root of the tooth may extend into the sinus. Extraction of these
teeth may produce an oromaxillary
fistula (Fig. 10–30).

Blood in the nasal cavity and air
escaping from the tooth socket are the
initial symptoms of an oromaxillary
fistula. Oral liquids may escape from the
nose. Sinus infection will become apparent in a few days and this problem
produces pain and tenderness over the
sinus and a profuse, foul-smelling rhinorrhea. Pus draining from the extraction
site and a foul taste are characteristic
of this problem.

Many fistulae will heal rapidly with
conservative therapy, especially when
they are detected early. Culture and sensitivity tests of secretions will help determine the choice of antibiotics. Systemic and local antibiotic therapy with
nasal decongestants for a two week
period will often allow the fistula to
close.

Several surgical procedures have been
devised for the treatment of large or
persistent fistulae. A buccal or palatal
mucosal flap combined with resection
of part of the alveolus may be required
to close a fistula. These operations
should not be performed on outpatients.

Nonsecreting Cyst

The floor of the maxillary sinus is the
most common site for these cysts,

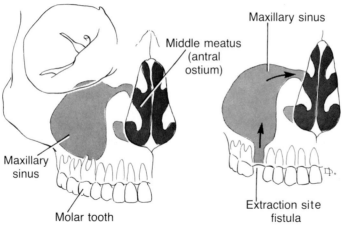

Figure 10–30 Oroantral fistula. The roots of molar teeth may project into the maxillary sinus *(A)*. Extraction of such a tooth may result in an oroantral (oromaxillary) fistula with food particles and other foreign material entering the sinus. An infection usually develops, causing profuse rhinorrhea.

which are smooth and round and contain a small amount of clear yellow fluid. These cysts are usually asymptomatic and have little significance. Surgical treatment is usually not indicated unless another problem becomes apparent.[11]

Carcinoma

Squamous cell carcinoma is the most common malignant neoplasm of the paranasal sinuses. This tumor accounts for almost 60 per cent of these problems.[7] Adenocarcinomas, cylindromas, various sarcomas, lymphomas, intracranial tumors (meningiomas) and the occasional metastatic tumors account for the remainder. Carcinomas of the paranasal sinuses do not produce consistent clinical manifestations, and quite often the diagnosis is not made until the disease is in an advanced stage. These patients are often treated for an inflammatory disease that does not respond to medical therapy. A high index of suspicion that an underlying malignant process may be involved will help to avoid this delay in diagnosis. A biopsy is necessary to make a diagnosis, and it should be performed as early as possible. The management of these tumors is beyond the scope of

this text, since the patients cannot be treated in the Outpatient Department. They must be admitted to the hospital and treated by a physician familiar with these problems.

LIPS

Congenital Lesions

Cleft Lip. Cleft lip is the most common congenital defect in this area. These abnormalities are frequently associated with an alveolar cleft or cleft palate. The surgical treatment of these defects is beyond the scope of this book and such problems should be referred to a specialist for treatment.

Labial Pits. These small slits usually occur in the lower lip and are thought to arise from improper development of the mucocutaneous junction of the lip. They produce a partial double lip and can be treated by local excision and advancement of labial mucosa. Careful approximation of the tissues with fine sutures to reduce scar formation is important.

Hemangioma. These tumors may produce gross deformities and require intensive therapy. Only the smaller lesions should be treated by local excision in the office, clinic or outpatient department.

Traumatic Lesions

Injuries of the face are quite common and the lips may be involved separately or in conjunction with other areas. Tissues in these areas usually heal rapidly and are relatively resistant to infection due to a rich blood supply. Careful repair reduces scar formation and cosmetic deformities.

Abrasions. These injuries usually require a minimum of treatment. All foreign material must be removed and simple cleansing with soap and water will often suffice. When foreign particles of dirt, stones or other debris are imbedded in the tissues, they must be removed mechanically. A fine forceps or number 11 Bard-Parker knife blade may be used to remove implanted foreign material. Antibiotics are usually not necessary, but tetanus toxoid should be administered.

Lacerations. Puncture wounds of the lips made by teeth are common. Two important considerations should be kept in mind:—first, thorough cleansing of the wound to avoid infection, and second, careful approximation of tissues to prevent excessive scar tissue. These wounds usually bleed freely and hemostasis may require ligation of larger vessels. Lacerations through the entire thickness of the lip must be repaired by approximating each layer carefully. Mucosa, muscle, subcutaneous tissue and skin should be approximated in layers and irregular edges carefully removed before the repair is started. The vermillion border and mucocutaneous border should be aligned as accurately as possible. Failure to accomplish this will result in an obvious cosmetic defect. Avulsion injuries may require flaps or grafts for closure of the defect and these injuries should be treated in the operating room by an experienced surgeon.

Tumors. Small ulcers are quite common on the lower lip, particularly in individuals who are exposed to intensive sunlight. Since it is virtually impossible to differentiate a benign or malignant lesion from the clinical appearance alone, a biopsy of the lesion is often necessary to make a diagnosis. A small lesion, under 1 cm in diameter, can be excised with a margin of normal tissue, whereas in larger lesions biopsies should be performed in several areas with a small cup forceps. Malignant lesions (squamous carcinoma) can be treated with surgery or irradiation, and benign lesions should be treated with a bland ointment and avoidance of local trauma.

Mucocele. Mucous retention cysts present as small, circumscribed, elevated translucent lesions of the mucosa. They may rupture, drain a small amount of thick mucoid material, collapse and then slowly reform. They develop from an obstruction or injury of the duct of a small accessory salivary gland with a subsequent accumulation of saliva within the tissues. Local anesthesia and surgical excision usually result in a cure.

Verruca Vulgaris. These soft, sessile, papillary lesions are usually only a few millimeters in size. Local excision results in a cure, but spontaneous regression may occur. A virus infection is thought to be the cause of this lesion.[12]

Papilloma. A papilloma is a benign epithelial neoplasm that can occur anywhere in the oral cavity. When it develops on exposed surfaces it is rough and scaly, whereas if it develops within the oral cavity it is soft and pliable. Papillomas do not undergo malignant transformation and rarely recur when adequately excised.

Fibroma. These are elevated pedunculated or sessile lesions that occur as a response to local trauma. They vary in size from a few millimeters to a few centimeters. Lip biting is a common cause of this lesion, and local excision is the preferred treatment; however, when contributing factors are not removed the tumor often recurs.[12]

Inflammatory Conditions

Furuncles. Furuncles about the lips and face are usually due to staphylococcal infections and differ little from furuncles elsewhere on the body. Facial movements and an almost uncontrolled tendency to squeeze these lesions often result in a spread of infection with a larger area of cellulitis. The "dangerous zone" of the face consists of the upper lip and nose and infections from this area may spread into the cavernous sinus, resulting in thrombosis. This serious problem must be constantly borne in mind when treating infections arising in this area.

Carbuncles. A large area of swelling from cellulitis with pus draining from many small openings is characteristic of this problem. The lips are frequently involved. After culture and sensitivity studies, antibiotics should be administered in large doses. Heat, rest, intravenous fluids and analgesics will give the patient relief from his symptoms.

Cellulitis. Streptococci or other pathogens may enter the skin through a small wound to produce the redness, swelling and tenderness that are characteristic of cellulitis. An underlying sinus or dental disease should be suspected when these findings are located in an appropriate area. Treatment consists of bed rest, hot moist compresses and antibiotics. Penicillin is the most effective antibiotic for this infection and it should be used routinely unless the patient is allergic to it.

Erysipelas. The lips and face are common sites for erysipelas. Streptococci enter through small openings in the skin to produce a rather characteristic lesion. Often, the nose is the primary site of infection, with the lesion gradually extending onto the cheek, lips and forehead. The lesion may have a "butterfly" configuration with elevated red edges. Older people are most frequently affected during the spring and fall months of the year. This infection responds very rapidly to penicillin therapy and most of the patients can remain ambulatory.

FACE

The common congenital lesions, tumors and infections of the face in general are similar to the problems described for the lips.

Injuries

Lacerations. (Figure 10–31). These wounds bleed freely and heal rapidly because of the rich blood supply to the face. Infections will not be a problem if the wound is carefully cleaned and debrided before repair. Several structures may be involved in facial lacerations that require consideration. The seventh cranial nerve may be transected, the parotid duct severed, the paranasal sinuses entered, the medial canthal ligament detached and the lacrimal apparatus injured with a facial laceration. Failure to recognize such coexistent injuries can lead to serious complications. These problems require immediate attention and should not be handled in the Outpatient Department by an inexperienced surgeon.

Uncomplicated lacerations can be treated with local anesthesia. Meticulous cleansing and débridement of the wound should be performed before repairing

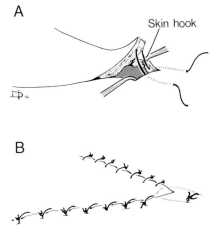

Figure 10–31 Corner suture. Gilles' corner suture for facial laceration.

the laceration. A nonabsorbable suture such as 5–0 monofilament nylon or silk should be used on the skin. A few vertical mattress sutures will help prevent inversion of the wound edges. The deeper layers of the wound should be carefully approximated with fine catgut sutures. Small rubber drains or a piece of sterilized rubber band inserted into the wound will prevent fluid accumulations and subsequent infection; a light pressure dressing left undisturbed for three or four days is usually sufficient. Pain and swelling usually indicate an infection and the dressing should be removed and inspected. Antibiotics, hot compresses and improved drainage of the wound will usually control any infection and allow healing.

Burns. Thermal, electrical and chemical agents cause burns of the face. These are handled in the same way as burns involving other areas of the body. See Chapter 8.

Fractures of the Maxilla and Zygoma (Figure 10–32). Fractures of the maxilla and zygoma are caused by blows to the cheek from a fall, a fist, or a hard object. Moderately severe blows may produce a separation of the zygomaticofrontal suture. Severe blows can produce a fracture of the zygoma, maxilla and orbit.[13]

Pain, swelling, anesthesia of the distribution of the infraorbital nerve (lower lid, lateral nose and upper lip), diplopia and pain on opening the mouth are the usual symptoms of these fractures. Comparison of both sides of the face will reveal flattening of the involved cheek, displacement of the lateral palpebral ligament, retraction of the lower lid, ecchymosis of the cheek, lids, conjunctiva and sclera, and decreased mobility of the globe. Bimanual palpation will reveal depressions and irregularities that are not present on the opposite side of the face.

The Waters' view is the most useful x-ray for evaluating fractures of the zygomaticomaxillary complex. The stereoscopic method is of value. This view shows the outlines and contours of

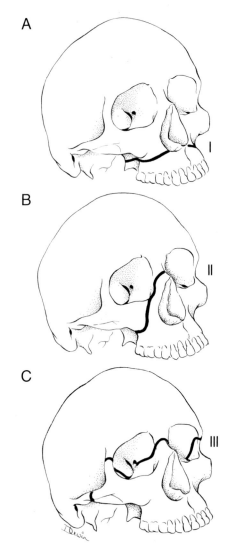

Figure 10–32 LeFort classification of midface fractures. LeFort classification of fractures of the maxilla. LeFort I (transverse or Guérin fracture). LeFort II (pyramidal fracture). LeFort III (craniofacial disjunction.)

the zygomaticomaxillary complex with a minimal superimposition of other structures. A submento-vertex view will demonstrate the zygomatic arches quite well. Planograms may be required to demonstrate irregularities of the orbital floor. Irregularities of the infraorbital margin and lateral wall of the maxilla, separation of the zygomaticofrontal

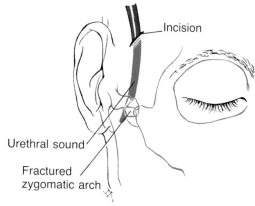

Figure 10-33 Reduction of fractured zygomatic arch. An incision is made through the skin, subcutaneous tissue and temporalis fascia. A small urethral sound is passed through this incision beneath the fracture and the fragments manipulated into position with the other hand.

suture, and clouding of the maxillary sinus are present in almost all these fractures.[14]

Zygomatic arch fractures can usually be reduced with the Gilles' operation (Fig 10-33). After shaving the hair from the temporal area a small (2 cm) vertical incision is made behind the hair line. The incision is carried through the subcutaneous tissue and the temporal fascia overlying the temporalis muscles. A heavy elevator is inserted between the temporalis fascia and the muscle in the temporal fossa medial to the zygomatic arch. Using a lever force with a roll of bandages placed on the skull above the incision as the fulcrum, the arch can be guided into position. The opposite hand should be used to palpate the arch through the skin and assist in the reduction. Gentle pressure on the arch will demonstrate its stability after reduction. The wound is then closed in layers. The patient and his attendants should be instructed to avoid any pressure on the side of the fracture. If there are no complications, the patient can be discharged from the hospital in two or three days; however, even minimal trauma or pressure may dislocate the fracture. Pain and a recurrence of trismus usually mean the fracture has been dislocated.

Fractures of the Mandible. Fractures of the mandible make up about two-thirds of all facial fractures. Dingman and Natvig (1964)[13] have classified mandible fractures according to location (Fig. 10-34). Most of these result from automobile accidents, fights or sports trauma. The common symptoms of fractures of the mandible are pain on motion of the jaw; tenderness over the fracture site; inability to open the mouth; swelling and facial asymmetry; discoloration of adjacent tissues; deformity of the mandible; abnormal mobility of the jaw; grating, cracking, and grinding sounds as the jaw is moved; drooling of saliva from the mouth; and offensive breath.

When one or more of the characteristic findings are evident, a tentative diagnosis of mandibular fracture should be made. Malocclusion is a reliable sign in patients with teeth. This may be more apparent with marked dislocation of the fracture and less evident with minimal dislocations. Binaural manipulation of

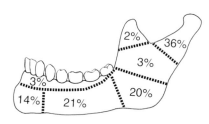

Figure 10-34 Fractures of the mandible. Frequency of fractures in various parts of the mandible. Midline fractures occur in less than 1 per cent of these injuries. (Adapted from Dingman, R. O., and Natvig, P., Surgery of Facial Fractures, Philadelphia, W. B. Saunders Co., 1964).

the mandible will usually produce movement and pain at the fracture site. Crepitus is not a very reliable sign for the diagnosis of a fracture. However, abnormal mobility of the mandible with deviation to one side when opening the mouth is a reliable indication of a fracture. Difficulties with eating and speech and swelling at the fracture site are quite common, but they do not necessarily indicate the presence of a fracture.

X-rays should be obtained in all patients with suspected fractures of the mandible. Fractures of the body and angle are usually detected on standard films, but the condylar processes are quite difficult to see and special stereoscopic views or tomograms may be necessary to delineate fractures of these processes. Dental x-rays and occlusal films sometimes help locate fractures of the symphysis, alveolus or the teeth. Postreduction x-rays are necessary to determine the effectiveness of reduction.

Fractures of the mandible are not emergencies, but the patient should have reduction and immobilization as early as his general condition permits. If treatment is delayed too long (seven to ten days) healing processes may make reduction more difficult.

Fractures of the mandible are often associated with intraoral lacerations. The oral cavity should be suctioned free of blood clots and secretions and then carefully inspected for foreign bodies such as teeth, fragments of bone and other debris. Aspiration of foreign bodies or gastric secretions may produce serious complications. Tracheostomy may be necessary to insure an adequate airway and it should be performed immediately whenever it is indicated. Nearly all patients with a mandible fracture will require hospitalization and surgical reduction of the fracture. A Barton bandage (Fig. 10–35) can be applied to hold the mandible in position until the patient can be moved to a hospital or until his general condition permits reduction.

Multiple Facial Fractures. Multiple facial injuries are usually quite obvious.

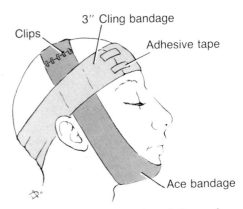

Figure 10–35 Barton bandage. A Barton dressing is an effective means of immobilizing a fractured mandible.

The clinical findings are those associated with the various facial bones involved in the fracture. Severe edema, periorbital ecchymosis, malocclusion, lacerations of the skin and oral mucosa, partial or complete airway obstruction and mobility of the fragments on palpation may be present, depending upon the severity of the fracture. Clear fluid coming from the nostrils or wounds should always be suspected as spinal fluid. Pulsation of the fluid, an increased flow with the head in a dependent position, or compression of both jugular veins will help identify a cerebral spinal fluid leak. A simple chemical test for sugar will help confirm the diagnosis of this problem.

Radiographic examinations will help to determine the severity and location of these fractures. Patients with these fractures must be admitted to the hospital for treatment. The treatment of facial fractures may be safely delayed for several days; however, treatment should not be postponed once the patient's condition stabilizes.

Injuries to Teeth. Dental injuries may occur independently or coexist with fractures of the mandible. The exposed anterior teeth are most often injured but injuries are not limited to these teeth. Several types of injury may occur with a simple chip fracture of a tooth, a crown broken off at the gum line, or avulsion of

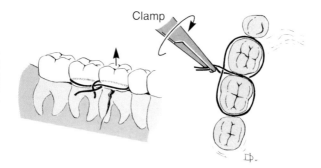

Figure 10–36 Dental wiring. Stainless steel 20–30 gauge wire is passed around two teeth and the ends twisted together. This is an excellent method for holding one or two teeth in alignment.

one or more teeth. Fragments of teeth that will serve no useful purpose in stabilizing a fracture can be removed either at the time of reduction or after the fracture has healed. Teeth that are tender to palpation or loosened may heal spontaneously without subsequent necrosis. They should be retained, although very loose teeth or those attached to a small segment of alveolar bone will require support by ligating them to adjacent teeth or by using arch bars (Fig. 10–36). Reimplantation of evulsed teeth is occasionally successful, but usually is not advisable in patients with fractures.

Dislocation of the Mandible

Dislocation of the mandible, particularly the first occurrence, may be very distressing to the patient. It usually results from yawning, although recurrent dislocations may occur during the act of eating, speaking or laughing. These spontaneous dislocations may be unilateral or bilateral with the mandible protruded in an anterior open bite position. Physical violence or trauma usually produces medial or lateral dislocation and is nearly always associated with fractures or severe temporomandibular joint injuries. Chronic dislocation results in deformity and malfunction of the mandible. These problems can be avoided by prompt diagnosis and treatment. X-ray examination of the temporomandibular joint and condyles before and after reduction will reduce the risk of missing an associated fracture.

Moderate sedation to relieve apprehension and relax the musculature will help the operator manipulate the dislocated mandible into its proper position (Fig. 10–37 *A*). With the patient in a sitting position and the head supported, the operator faces the patient and places the thumbs inside the mouth on the occlusal surfaces of the teeth or the alveolar ridges if the patient is edentulous. Pressing downward on the posterior area, elevating the anterior area and pushing the mandible backward allows the condyle to slip over the articular eminence into its normal position. This usually gives the patient immediate relief of symptoms. When there is severe muscle spasm or the patient is unable to cooperate, a general anesthetic and muscle-relaxing drug will be required.

Johnson[15] in 1958 described another method of reducing acute dislocations of the temporomandibular joint (Fig. 10–37 *B*). This method consists of preparing the preauricular area of the face with an antiseptic solution on either side. This is to be used as the site for injection and even though the dislocation is bilateral, only one side requires injection. A depression over the glenoid fossa is readily apparent because the heads of the condyles are locked anterior to the articular eminences. About 2.0 cc of lidocaine hydrochloride solution is drawn into a syringe with a 25 gauge needle, which is then inserted into the subcutaneous tissue over the glenoid fossa depression. This anesthetic solu-

A

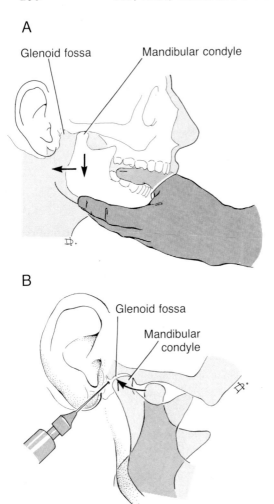

Glenoid fossa   Mandibular condyle

B

Glenoid fossa

Mandibular
condyle

Figure 10–37 Reduction of dislocated mandible. *A.* Reducing a dislocated mandible can be accomplished by inserting the thumbs over the last molar teeth and exerting a downward force. When the condyle is below the anterior tubercle, a slight posterior force will complete the reduction.

B. Johnson's technique for reducing a dislocation of the condyle is a simple and often effective method of treatment. A small 25 gauge needle is inserted through the skin and subcutaneous tissue in the shallow depression created by the anteriorly displaced condylar head. Xylocaine is injected into this site (1.5–2.0 cc) and the needle withdrawn. Within a few minutes the dislocated mandible will return to its normal position.

tion is injected slowly as the needle is directed inward and slightly anterior toward the head of the condyle. When the head of the condyloid process is contacted, the needle is slightly withdrawn and the remaining solution injected into the tissues surrounding the glenoid fossa. Johnson[15] reported that the dislocations were reduced spontaneously without manipulation in about one minute. I have used this technique in many patients and found it satisfactory. Occasionally, I have injected both sides and found that spontaneous reduction occurred in some patients in whom a single injection had failed. After

an acute dislocation, patients may be unable to occlude the posterior teeth for several days. The patient should avoid overextending the joint for several months because repeated injury of the joint may cause permanent damage and produce a recurring or chronic dislocation.

MOUTH

Congenital Lesions

Fordyce Spots. These small yellowish white granules may occur in clusters or plaquelike areas. The buccal mucosa along the occlusal planes, the lips and the retromolar areas are the most common sites. Almost 80 per cent of the population have these harmless developmental lesions, consisting of submucosal sebaceous glands which increase in size with age, but should not be excised.

"Tongue Tie." Although this condition is known to exist, it is quite rare and almost never interferes with speech. The lingual frenulum appears short or taut and restricts movement of the tongue upward to the lower alveolar ridge. Surgical correction of a shortened frenulum can be accomplished in a number of ways. A child who is uncooperative or frightened may require a general anesthetic, but most children can be operated upon with a local anesthetic and physical restraints. A small wedge excision of the frenulum (Fig. 10–38) will increase the mobility of the tongue in these children. Hemostasis may require ligation of vessels. An absorbable suture material is preferred because it loosens and falls free in a few days. The child's articulation problems usually continue after frenulectomy unless his tongue and speech habits are retrained.

Glossoptosis. Pierre-Robin syndrome consists of micrognathia, glossoptosis and cleft palate. Micrognathia and glossoptosis are responsible for episodic respiratory obstruction in some newborn infants, involving cyanosis and stridor during feeding or when the infant is supine. The airway can usually be improved by placing the infant in the prone position. Glossoptosis interferes with deglutition, and aspiration during feeding is common. These infants fail to thrive and have repeated respiratory infections. As the infant becomes weaker from feeding problems, the respiratory obstruction becomes more severe and may result in death unless treatment is instituted early.

The most satisfactory method of treatment utilizes feeding by gavage or gastrostomy and fixing the tongue in an anterior position until the mandible develops sufficiently. A temporary glossopexy is the most effective method of relieving the airway obstruction and improving oral feeding. The micrognathic mandible usually catches up with the other facial structures by the end of the first year of life and spontaneous improvement results.

The Duhamel[16] operation has been a most satisfactory method of treatment (Fig. 10–39). It is a simple procedure that can be done at the bedside and gives immediate results.

A 2–0 silk suture is passed through each side of the posterior tongue and threaded through a small caliber silicon tube resting across the base of the tongue. This tube prevents the suture from pulling through the tongue. Each end of the suture is brought out along the floor of the mouth beside the tongue and passed through the anterior mandible with a cutting needle. The ends of the suture are tied snugly across the front of the mandible, holding the tongue in the desired position, and they may be left in place for several weeks.

Cysts. Many cysts occur in the oral

Figure 10–38 "Tongue tie." This procedure should be performed only on those patients who cannot protrude the tongue beyond the incisor teeth. The operation will not benefit patients with paresis or paralysis of the tongue. Local anesthesia is usually sufficient. Sutures are placed above and below the anticipated incision without obstructing the submaxillary duct orifices and the frenum is incised.

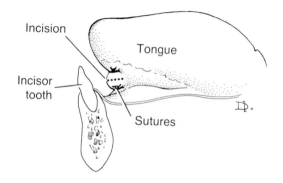

A   B

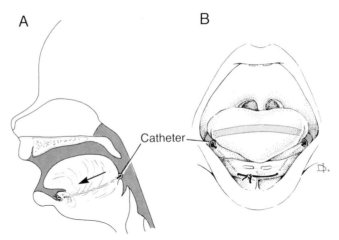

Catheter

Figure 10–39   Glossopexy. The glossoptosis associated with micrognathism (Pierre Robin syndrome) may cause severe respiratory distress. A simple and effective method of supporting the tongue in an anterior position is illustrated. A small rubber or polyethylene tube is threaded over a large (No. 1 or 2) nonabsorbable suture. This tube should be placed at the base of the tongue, and each end of the suture passed through the floor of the mouth under the mandible and tied securely. The position of the tongue can be altered by the amount of tension on the sutures.

cavity, mandible or maxilla, and some of these arise in the area of fusion of the facial processes. The median palatal, median alveolar, globulomaxillary and nasoalveolar cysts are examples of such developmental cysts. The nasopalatine cyst arises from remnants of the naso-palatine duct. Follicular cysts arise from the enamel organ or tooth follicle, and epithelial rests adjacent to a tooth may produce a radicular or residual cyst. Because these cysts involve the maxilla and mandible most of them should be treated in a hospital by a surgeon trained in the management of these problems.

Salivary Glands

Ranula (Figure 10–40).   These cysts develop in the sublingual salivary gland from an obstruction of the ducts of this gland. They are usually located on one side of the frenum of the tongue and may become quite large. Aspiration or incision and drainage will give temporary relief, but recurrences are common. Total excision through a neck incision may be necessary for recurrent cysts.
Salivary Calculi.   Calculi can form

in all the salivary glands or ducts. The submaxillary gland and its ducts are the most common sites with 80 to 85 per cent of stones occurring in these areas. The remaining 15 to 20 per cent occur in the parotid and sublingual glands or ducts.

The cause of these calculi is unknown, but they probably develop around a small

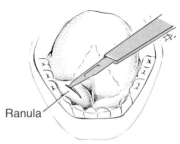

Ranula

Figure 10–40   Incision of ranula. Ranulas are cystic structures located in the floor of the mouth on each side of the tongue. After incising the cyst and evacuating the seromucus contents, part of the dome should be removed and the cyst mar-supialized. A shallow gutter beside the tongue may persist after treatment.

nidus of bacteria or other foreign material. Composed mostly of calcium carbonate and phosphate, they can be either single or multiple.

They will cause symptoms when they become large enough to block the duct or induce stasis of secretions with a subsequent infection of the gland. The involved gland becomes swollen and tender, the mouth becomes drier than usual, especially after eating. Pressure on the swollen gland may force saliva or pus around the stone through the duct opening into the mouth. Frequently, the calculus can be felt during palpation of the involved duct. A lacrimal probe inserted into the duct will often help localize the exact position of the calculus by the rough grating sensation that will be apparent when the probe comes into contact with the calculus. Care must be taken not to force the calculus further back into the duct or gland with the probe. Since about 20 per cent of calculi are radiolucent and are not visible on x-rays, a sialogram should be obtained in these patients.

Occasionally, a calculus will pass from the duct spontaneously. Dilating the orifice of the duct with a lacrimal probe and gently dislodging the calculus may allow the stone to pass into the mouth.

When the stone does not pass spontaneously or cannot be removed with dilatation and a probe, surgical extirpation is necessary (Fig. 10–41). Local anesthesia is usually sufficient for this procedure. The calculus must be fixed by grasping either it or the duct distal to the stone with a forceps. A suture around the duct will prevent the stone from passing further back into inaccessible areas of the duct or the gland. An incision made along the duct in its long axis and dissected downward allows exposure of the calculus and its extraction. Pressure on the gland often makes this procedure easier by bringing the stone into a more accessible position. Multiple stones are common in the submaxillary duct and should not be overlooked. The sublingual artery, lingual nerve, lingual vein and hypoglossal nerve are in close proximity to the submaxillary duct and must be avoided during surgery. The stones that lie near the hilum of the submaxillary parotid gland require an external incision, dissection and removal. Recurrent stones, dilatation of the duct system, calculi within the gland or chronic inflammation of the gland are the indications for gland excision. These procedures should not be performed on outpatients.

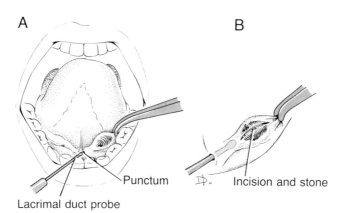

A

B

Punctum

Incision and stone

Lacrimal duct probe

Figure 10–41   Submaxillary duct stone. Submaxillary duct stones can be removed with local anesthesia. The duct is occluded with a clamp or forceps *(A)* and a lacrimal duct probe inserted through the punctum into the duct. The stone is located and a small linear incision is made directly over the stone *(B)*. One or more stones can be removed in this manner.

Salivary Gland Tumors. The parotid gland is the salivary gland most frequently involved by both benign and malignant tumors. The submaxillary gland and sublingual gland are less often affected, but tumors in these glands are more likely to be malignant than those that occur in the parotid gland.

Mixed tumor and papillary cystadenoma lymphomatosum (Warthin's tumor) are the two most common benign tumors of the salivary glands. Mucoepidermoid carcinomas, squamous cell carcinomas, adenocarcinomas and malignant melanomas are the usual malignant tumors of these glands.

These neoplasms are also occasionally found in the minor salivary glands located in the mucosa of the pharynx, palate and larynx.

A biopsy is necessary for diagnosis; however, sialography is an important technique that will often determine the exact location of the tumor, and it should be performed before a biopsy is made. Very often the biopsy will entail an extensive operative procedure and these operations should not be performed on outpatients.

Traumatic Lesions

Hematoma. Submucosal collections of blood are quite common. Clotting disorders are occasionally associated with hematoma formation. However, trauma is a more common etiology. Unless the hematoma interferes with respiration or swallowing it should be left alone. Respiratory distress may necessitate a tracheostomy.

Lacerations. Small lacerations usually require no surgical treatment. More extensive injuries should be carefully debrided of devitalized tissue, irrigated with sterile saline and repaired with fine sutures. Palatal, lingual and tonsilar lacerations are common in children who fall with a toy or "stick" in the mouth. Copious bleeding is common. These children are usually frightened and a general anesthetic may be needed to repair the laceration. Careful approxima-

tion of the tissues will help prevent scar formation and loss of function.

Bleeding from around a tooth usually stops spontaneously. A loose tooth should not be disturbed, but partially extracted or fractured teeth should be removed, particularly when there is any danger that they may be aspirated by the patient. Lacerations of alveolar mucosa should be repaired with fine sutures.

Oral hygiene is important after any injury to the mouth. Hydrogen peroxide $1\frac{1}{2}$ per cent or buffered sodium peroxyborate monohydrate (Amosan) solutions should be used within the oral cavity every two hours. Normal saline and a pleasant tasting mouthwash (Cēpacol) will make the patient more comfortable.

Burns. Mucosal injuries may result from thermal, chemical or electrical agents. Chemical agents such as lye, ammonia, Clorox, Lysol, potassium permanganate and iodine solutions may be accidentally ingested or used in a suicide attempt. Children under age 5 make up 60 per cent of these patients and 80 per cent are under age 15.[17] The extent and degree of injury are important and may not be apparent when the patient is first examined. Oral burns without an esophageal injury occur in 25 per cent of these injuries and esophageal burns without an oral injury occur in 75 per cent of patients. The level of injury must be determined accurately. Esophagoscopy should be performed, although the scope should not be inserted beyond the area of the first burn.

All these patients must be admitted to the hospital. They require intravenous fluid therapy and should receive nothing by mouth until the extent and the degree of injury have been determined. A nasogastric tube or beaded string should be carefully inserted into the stomach. Induced vomiting may produce aspiration pneumonia, particularly in the comatose or obtunded patient. Neutralizing substances such as dilute acetic acid, aqueous sodium bicarbonate (2 per cent), or milk may be of value, but must be administered within three hours of ingestion to be effective. Shock is not uncommon and must be corrected with IV fluid therapy. Antibiotics and steroids help to reduce stricture formation.[18] Esophageal dilation may be required, but should never be performed by someone who is not completely familiar with the technique and its hazards.

Foreign Bodies. Accidental ingestion or inhalation is the most common cause of a foreign body in the food and air passages, although occasionally a disturbed person may attempt suicide by this means. Some foreign materials may be imbedded as a result of trauma and all patients with injuries of the oral cavity should be examined carefully to be certain that a foreign body is not overlooked. Usually a foreign body lodged in the gastrointestinal tract is not an emergency, whereas a laryngeal, tracheal or bronchial foreign body may cause severe respiratory distress. These latter patients may require tracheostomy or bronchoscopy for relief of this problem; however, ill-advised attempts to remove a foreign body may cause more trouble than the foreign body itself.

Small sharp foreign bodies usually lodge in the tonsil or lateral pharyngeal wall. These are usually obvious and can be removed with a forceps or clamp under direct vision. A topical anesthetic spray such as lidocaine hydrochloride 4 per cent will relieve some of the discomfort, reduce the gag reflex, and make extraction easier. Larger articles may become lodged in the valleculae, lingual tonsils or pyriform recesses. The ones that can be seen without special instruments should be removed.

Foods may contain bones or other objects. Adults who chew poorly, swallow hastily, and have poor dentition may accidentally ingest such objects. This may cause acute distress that simulates an acute coronary occlusion. Children may swallow an object that is carried in the mouth and this may go unnoticed for some time. Vegetable objects such as nuts and seeds are the most common objects aspirated in children.

Foreign bodies that enter the esophagus, larynx or tracheobronchial tree should be removed carefully and as promptly as possible. These procedures usually require hospitalization and endoscopic treatment.

Benign Tumors

Many benign and malignant tumors occur in the oral cavity, pharynx, esophagus, larynx or tracheobronchial tree. Biopsy and histopathologic diagnosis are essential before starting any form of therapy. Small lesions should be excised with a margin of normal tissue and biopsy in several areas should be performed on the larger ones (see Chapter 5). Some of the tumors not discussed in that chapter are presented here. Carcinoma of the mouth is discussed in Chapter 5.

Epulis. These growths are usually associated with ill-fitting dentures, extraction wounds or small extruding sequestra of bone. They are soft, red, painful masses of granulation tissue that bleed easily when manipulated. A surface ulcer is quite common, but usually the surface is covered with stratified squamous epithelium. Excision or curettage is necessary for the larger tumors, but the origin of the problem should be treated directly by correcting the denture, removing a sequestrum of bone or closing the mucosa over an extraction site to prevent recurrence of the lesion.

Giant Cell Reparative Granuloma. These tumors occur most frequently on the gingiva or soft tissue of an edentulous ridge. The mandible is more often involved than the maxilla, and most of the patients are over age 20. Males are affected slightly more often than females and a history of trauma such as tooth extraction is quite common. Pedunculated or broad-based, these tumors have a smooth surface and are bluish red in color. They are sometimes lobulated and bleed quite easily when manipulated. X-rays are usually negative, but occasionally the underlying bone may be radiolucent. Local excision with a small margin of normal tissue will prevent recurrence of the tumor.

Pyogenic Granuloma. These tumors occur in both sexes and in nearly all age groups. The gingiva is the most common location, but the lips, tongue, oral mucosa and nasal mucosa may be involved. They may be pedunculated or broad-based and an ulceration of the smooth surface is common. The tumor bleeds easily when manipulated. Treatment of this benign tumor consists of surgical excision. Excision should include a small margin of healthy tissue.

Granuloma Gravidarum. Gingivitis of pregnancy is a common condition and a small number of these patients develop this tumor on the gingival surface. These tumors are histologically identical with the pyogenic granuloma. They appear during the first trimester of pregnancy and often spontaneously regress after delivery. Recurrence at the same site during subsequent pregnancies is not uncommon. Those tumors that do not regress should be excised after delivery. Excision may be necessary during pregnancy when the tumor becomes large or when bleeding is a problem.

Irritation Fibroma. This is probably the most common tumor of the oral cavity and is identical to the fibroma involving the lip.[12] Characteristically, it is an elevated, pedunculated or sessile lesion paler than the surrounding tissue and varying in size from a few millimeters to a few centimeters. These tumors are often associated with local trauma or irritation. Treatment consists of excision and eradication of the source of irritation.

Hemangiomas. Capillary and cavernous hemangiomas may be seen at any age in either sex. Most of them arise from congenital malformations that become apparent at a later age. They may be elevated or submerged, circumscribed or diffuse, and red or bluish in color. Characterized by a smooth surface and variations in size, they are normally soft and compressible and may blanch with pressure. The tongue and cheek are the most common sites, but hemangiomas may occur anywhere in the oral cavity. Although large tumors may interfere with speech and mastication, and minimal trauma may cause considerable bleeding, they grow very slowly or not at all, and rarely become malignant.

Fibrosis and spontaneous regression may occur with internal bleeding or thrombosis of vessels. Superficial lesions should be removed surgically; cryosurgery has been found useful for larger or deeply seated tumors.

The juvenile hemangioma occurs in children shortly after birth up to about three years of age. The lip, oral cavity, parotid and submaxillary glands are the most frequent sites of involvement, usually presenting a clinical picture of a firm, slowly growing mass with a normal mucosal surface. Surgical excision is the treatment of choice, but spontaneous regression may occur and a period of observation is indicated before attempting any treatment. Small superficial lesions may be excised in the clinic or Outpatient Department, but if they are larger the patients should be hospitalized and surgery performed in the operating room by an experienced surgeon.

Lymphangiomas. The oral cavity and tongue are common sites for these tumors. Superficial tumors present as a cluster of colorless, soft masses on the mucosa. Deeper tumors cause a diffuse enlargement and, when the tongue is involved, there may be a loss of surface structures such as the papillae. These tumors rarely undergo malignant degeneration. Since they do not respond to radiation, surgical excision is the treatment of choice.

Neurofibroma and Schwannoma (Neurilemoma). These two tumors are distinct entities, but because of their many similarities they will be considered together. The tongue, lips, palate and cheek are the usual sites for these tumors. Small, sessile, smooth surfaced tumors or circumscribed nodules that grow slowly and produce few if any symptoms are the usual presentation of these tumors. Local excision is the preferred treatment.

Granular Cell Myoblastoma. This benign soft tissue tumor may occur anywhere on the skin or mucous membranes or in the gastrointestinal tract. In the oral cavity, one of the more common sites of origin, the dorsal and lateral surfaces of the tongue are the usual locations for this tumor. A small, slightly elevated, smooth-surfaced growth under the mucous membrane is characteristic of this lesion. Surgical excision of the lesion produces a cure.

Plasmacytoma. This extramedullary plasma cell tumor occurs most frequently in males, the usual sites of occurrence being the nasal cavity, nasopharynx, tonsil, pharynx tongue, paranasal sinuses and larynx. There is no distinctive clinical feature for this tumor; it may be characterized by a diffuse or pedunculated swelling. Bone involvement (multiple myeloma) may not develop until years after the soft tissue tumor has been discovered, but this problem is so frequent that a bone survey should be made when a soft tissue tumor has been diagnosed. Local recurrence without development of multiple myeloma is not uncommon.

Surgical excision or electrocoagulation are usually adequate to eradicate the local lesions.

Leiomyoma. This rare tumor composed of smooth muscle cells can occur in the oral cavity. It is usually small and grows very slowly. Excision results in a cure in most patients.

Benign Mixed Tumors. These tumors arise from accessory salivary glands or mucous glands in the oral cavity, palate, pharynx, nose or nasopharynx.[19] Males are more often affected than females and these tumors are most common between the fourth and sixth decades of life. About half remain localized and grow quite slowly; the others may grow rapidly and require a major surgical resection. Small tumors can be locally excised, but these patients must be followed carefully for a long period of time because the tumor often exhibits a greater malignant potential than when it occurs in a major salivary gland.

Inflammatory Conditions

Oral infections are very common and most of them can be treated medically. Only those infections that require surgical therapy are included in this section.

Periapical Abscess. These abscesses develop suddenly and are associated with swelling, pain, redness of the overlying mucosa or skin, elevation of the tooth, sensitivity of the tooth on percussion, and occasionally an elevated temperature. The tooth may appear normal or it may have a deep carious lesion. Duration and location of the abscess will determine where the abscess "points." When it points within the mouth, it may appear on either the buccal or lingual surfaces.

X-rays may reveal either no abnormalities or a radiolucent area about one or more teeth.

Treatment consists of surgical drainage and antibiotics. Extraction of the tooth or surgical incision will allow drainage of the pus and relief of pain. When the tooth has not been removed, dental consultation should be requested for further treatment.

Ludwig's Angina. Cellulitis of the floor of the mouth and neck due to an infection with a hemolytic streptococcus is a serious complication of acute pharyngitis or inflammation of the mouth. The patient is usually in great distress. Movements of the tongue cause severe pain and the patient often deprives himself of food and fluids. Speaking and breathing may become almost impossible. Salivation is increased and the inability to swallow causes saliva to run freely from the mouth. The most striking clinical feature is a hard brawny swelling between the chin and the neck. Bimanual palpation reveals that this swelling occupies the floor of the mouth and sublingual spaces. Fluctuation is rarely noted because the pus is located deep from the surface.

Intravenous antibiotics are indicated

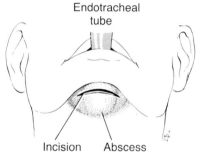

Figure 10–42 Ludwig's angina. A submental abscess should be incised, the pus evacuated and a drain inserted. The incision is made beneath the mandible and a small hemostat inserted into the abscess cavity and opened gently.

during the acute stage. When the condition does not respond to this treatment, incision and drainage must be considered. General anesthesia and oraltracheal intubation are necessary (Fig. 10–42). A midline submental incision or sublingual oral incision will usually expose the abscess which should be opened widely with a blunt instrument. Rubber drains should be inserted and left in place until drainage ceases, the swelling has subsided, and there is no danger of respiratory obstruction. Fever and toxemia usually subside after draining the abscess and the patient recovers quite rapidly. Cultures of the abscess will assist in the selection of appropriate antibiotics. Intravenous fluids should be continued until the patient can take adequate oral feedings, and antibiotics should be administered until the drains have been removed and the signs of inflammation have subsided. A total of ten days of antibiotic therapy is usually sufficient.

OROPHARYNX AND NASOPHARYNX

Most of the diseases occurring in this region can be diagnosed with simple techniques and inexpensive equipment.

With a little practice and experience, a clinician can become quite adept at these procedures. A thorough systematic approach will help the examiner avoid costly mistakes. In general, it is best to begin with the lips and proceed backward, including the buccol-oral mucosal surfaces, teeth, tongue, floor of the mouth, tonsils, palate and pharynx. The nasopharynx, hypopharynx and larynx must also be included. Materials necessary for the examination are a headmirror, tongue blades, and several handmirrors for the nasopharynx and larynx.

Good light is essential for examining these areas and the best light source is a headmirror. First, place the mirror with its opening over the left eye and focus the beam of light on the patient's forehead. Movements of the mirror direct the light to the desired location and both hands remain free for manipulation. Inspect the lips, then have the patient open his mouth and examine all buccal and oral surfaces. Either a metal or disposable wooden tongue blade can be used for this purpose. I have found the large number 9 laryngeal mirror an effective "retractor" for exposing areas of the oral cavity that are ordinarily difficult to see. Do not forget to inspect the openings of the salivary ducts. Have the patient extend his tongue and carefully examine all of its surfaces as well as the gum margins and teeth. If active dental disease is suspected, a sharp tap on the questioned teeth will usually indicate which are involved. Movements of the palate should be symmetrical and an active gag reflex should occur when the base of the tongue, soft palate and pharynx are stimulated. Much of the pharynx can be seen by gently pulling the patient's tongue forward with a gauze pad. Instructing the patient to "relax" his tongue helps with this part of the examination. The nasopharynx, hypopharynx and larynx are examined after the inspection of the oropharynx. Mirrors of the proper size are required to reflect light into these areas.

Nasopharyngeal Examination

An indirect mirror technique is used for this examination (Fig. 10–43). A headmirror and lamp serve as the light sources. Gentleness and patient cooperation are essential for success.

A small mirror introduced through the mouth behind the palate gives a good view of the nasopharynx and posterior choanae of the nasal cavity. A tongue blade is introduced into the mouth and the tongue gently pushed downward. A warmed mirror is then slipped along the tongue blade behind the uvula and palate. Light can be reflected from the headmirror onto the nasopharynx. Rotation of the mirror by moving the handle along its long axis gives a panoramic view of the nasopharynx.

When the palate interferes with examination, small catheters should be inserted through the nose into the pharynx, grasped, and pulled forward to retract the palate. This allows better visualization of the nasopharynx with the mirror.

An electrically lighted nasopharyngoscope can be used when the other techniques fail; however, it should be used by a specialist who is familiar with the instrument.

Peritonsillar Abscess

Quinsy or peritonsillar abscess (Fig. 10–44) usually arises during the third or fourth day after the onset of an acute follicular tonsillitis; occasionally there is no antecedent tonsillar infection. Most of the patients are adults; however, peritonsillar abscesses are more common in children than is generally recognized.

When there is a preceding acute tonsillitis, the patient reports that all his

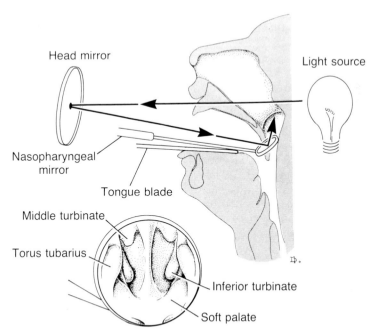

Figure 10–43 Nasopharyngeal examination. Nasopharyngeal examination is performed by inserting a warmed No. 1, 2 or 3 mirror into the oropharynx. With the tongue depressed, the mirror is inserted along the depressor behind the uvula and the nasopharynx inspected. The nasopharyngeal vault, the adenoid mass, the posterior ends of the middle and inferior turbinates and the Eustachian tube orifices can be seen.

A

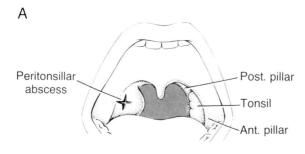

Peritonsillar abscess

Post. pillar

Tonsil

Ant. pillar

Figure 10–44   Peritonsillar abscess. The incision is made near the anterior pillar through the area of greatest fluctuance. Local anesthesia is usually quite adequate for this operation.

B

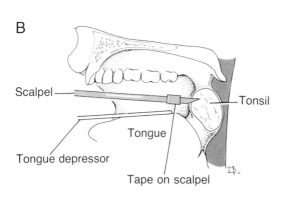

Scalpel

Tonsil

Tongue

Tongue depressor

Tape on scalpel

former symptoms are intensified. The pain becomes almost unbearable and radiates to the ear. Malaise, fever, dysphagia, indistinct speech, trismus, drooling of saliva and a foul breath are common symptoms. Examination reveals the whole chain of cervical lymph nodes to be enlarged and tender on the involved side. The soft palate and uvula are often edematous and deviated to the opposite side. The affected tonsil may appear to be displaced backward and inward with an exudate or large necrotic ulcer on its surface. The surrounding mucosa is usually red and markedly thickened with edema. Fluctuation or softening can sometimes be detected with a probe or tongue blade. A yellow spot on the anterior pillar may indicate that the abscess is ready to rupture, but more often the abscess is too deep and its capsule too thick for this sign to be evident.

When the abscess has not ruptured spontaneously, it should be incised and drained. Antibiotics should be used, but they do not take the place of surgical

therapy. If these patients are hospitalized and treated with intravenous fluids and antibiotics, most of them will be ready for discharge 24 to 48 hours after surgical treatment.

Good illumination is absolutely essential. The patient should be placed in an upright position with the head supported. General anesthesia may be quite hazardous because of the risk of aspirating pus into the trachea and should be used with care; a surface anesthetic of cocaine hydrochloride solution or 2 per cent lidocaine hydrochloride is often sufficient. An incision should be made at the center of the most edematous portion of the anterior pillar after depressing the tongue as much as possible; a small clamp with sharp points is then thrust one-half to three-quarters of an inch into the chosen site. The blades of the clamp are opened widely to allow the pus to escape. A knife may be used for this procedure, but the blade should be covered with adhesive tape except for the terminal one-half inch. A gush of pus from the abscess indicates success.

However, the first attempt occasionally fails when the incision enters the tonsil rather than the abscess and another incision in a more lateral position is indicated. There is a dramatic relief of pain within a few hours after a successful incision.

Recurrent peritonsillar abscesses are common and in general it is advisable to perform a tonsillectomy four to six weeks after the infection has subsided.

Tonsillectomy for peritonsillar abscess has been advocated by some authors.[20] However, this procedure should probably be reserved for those patients with an impending pharyngomaxillary infection.

Retropharyngeal Abscess

Most of these infections (Fig. 10–45) occur during the first year of life. Infected adenoids or a nasopharyngitis are the usual sources of infection. Hemolytic and nonhemolytic streptococci or a *Staphylococcus aureus* are often responsible for these abscesses.

A history of a preceding upper respiratory infection in a child who refuses to take food, holds the neck stiffly and has a moderate elevation of temperature should alert the physician to the possibility of a retropharyngeal abscess. Slight swelling of the posterior pharyngeal wall a little to one side of the midline may be the only indication of this condition. As the abscess increases in size, the breathing becomes noisy, the cry muffled and a croupy cough develops. A lateral x-ray of the neck will help in making the diagnosis, since widening of the retropharyngeal space is usually apparent. Palpation of the posterior pharyngeal wall may reveal fluctuation.

After applying restraints, the child's head should be lowered and a mouth gag inserted. A vertical incision is made over the point of maximum swelling. The procedure can be made much easier by the use of good illumination, suction and assistants who help hold the child. A sharply pointed clamp should be inserted into the abscess and opened. The opening must be made large enough to allow drainage and prevent a reaccumulation of pus. Good suction will prevent aspiration of the pus. Surgical treatment should be supplemented with antibiotic therapy. The patient usually recovers quite rapidly after treatment; however, severe dyspnea may ensue and tracheostomy may become essential.

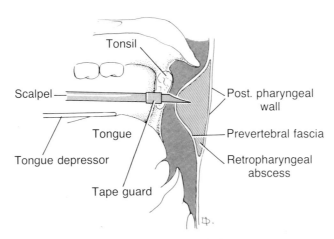

Figure 10–45 Retropharyngeal abscess. Retropharyngeal abscess may cause severe respiratory distress. A scalpel with a "tape guard" is used to incise the abscess. The guard prevents laceration of the prevertebral wall, and the incision is made vertically in the midline. If pus does not escape from the wound a small pointed hemostat is inserted into the wound and the tissues spread apart.

Carcinoma

Malignant neoplasms should always be suspected whenever a mass or ulcerated lesion is detected in the pharynx or nasopharynx. A biopsy will usually assist in making the diagnosis; however, those tumors that arise in the nasopharynx are difficult to see and are often missed. These patients often have impaired hearing from obstruction of the Eustachian tube and a secretory otitis media. They may also have pain over the distribution of the second division of the fifth cranial nerve and asymmetry of the palate.

Irradiation and surgery are usually required for these tumors and these procedures are beyond the scope of this text.

LARYNX

Indirect Laryngoscopy

A laryngeal mirror and headmirror are used for this examination (Fig. 10–46). The most common light source is a standard lamp placed at the patient's left side. The examiner and patient sit facing each other, the patient sitting all the way back in his chair with his head

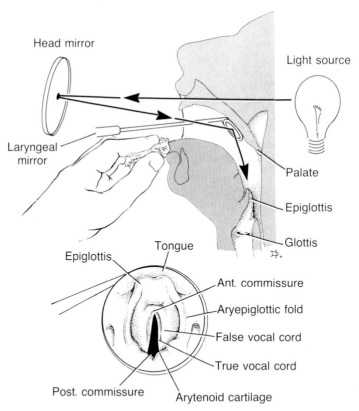

Figure 10–46 Indirect laryngoscopy. Indirect laryngoscopy can be mastered with the proper equipment, a little patience and practice. The patient's back should be straight, the body bent slightly forward at the waist. The mouth is opened wide and the tongue pulled forward with the fingers. A warmed mirror is then inserted into the oropharynx and directed downward. The base of the tongue, epiglottis, oropharynx, hypopharynx and larynx should be visualized. If the entire larynx is not seen the examination is not complete. This is particularly true of the anterior commissure, and a direct examination may be indicated.

and shoulders forward and his back straight. The patient should point his chin up, open his mouth and protrude his tongue. Either the examiner or patient should grasp the tongue with a piece of gauze and pull it out as far as possible without causing pain. Gentleness, patience and reassurance will make the examination much easier for both the examiner and the patient. A laryngeal mirror of the proper size warmed so that it will not fog from the patient's breath is passed into the pharynx without touching the tongue. If gagging occurs the mirror should be withdrawn and the pharynx sprayed with a topical anesthetic such as Cetacaine. After the back of the mirror has been placed against the uvula and palate, it should be tilted slightly forward and the uvula and soft palate pushed backward. These maneuvers will allow visualization of the base of the tongue, the valleculae, the epiglottis and the larynx. Movements of the mirror will give a good view of all parts of the larynx. Ask the patient to say "Eee" and this should bring the cords into apposition in the midline. All parts of the larynx must be visualized or the examination is not complete. Also, remember that the structures seen on the mirror are reversed in position.

Direct Laryngoscopy

Direct laryngoscopy (Fig. 10–47) is indicated in the following cases: in young children, and adults in whom the indirect examination is unsuccessful; for biopsy of lesions; for removal of foreign bodies; and for insertion of an oral endotracheal tube. Either general, local or topical anesthesia can be used. Preoperative sedation should be given one hour before the procedure is carried out. A combination of a barbiturate (Nembutal), narcotic (morphine sulfate), and tranquilizer (Vistaril) will give good

Figure 10–47 Direct laryngoscopy. Topical anesthesia or a superior laryngeal nerveblock is usually adequate for this procedure. The laryngoscope is inserted on one side of the mouth and directed to the base of the tongue. The tongue is retracted upward without exerting any pressure on the incisor teeth. The base of the tongue and epiglottis should be carefully inspected before inserting the laryngoscope into the larynx. The laryngoscope is then brought gently onto the midline of the tongue and the tip of the epiglottis. The posterior commissure, arytenoids, aryepiglottic folds, pyriform sinuses and hypopharynx are visualized. With extension of the head, the tip of the laryngoscope is advanced toward the base of the epiglottis. When the epiglottis is elevated, the entire glottis will be seen. A methodical, unhurried and relaxed approach to this procedure will make it much more comfortable for the patient and more rewarding for the examiner.

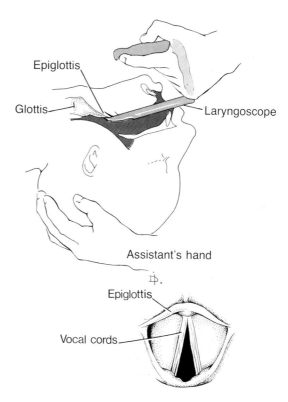

Epiglottis

Glottis

Laryngoscope

Assistant's hand

Epiglottis

Vocal cords

relaxation and sedation. Intravenous Innovar drip has been used successfully, but should never be used by an inexperienced physician. The examination should be conducted in a quiet darkened room. Relaxation and cooperation of the patient is very important and a calm, reassurring, unhurried and gentle approach by the examiner will facilitate the procedure.

The patient is placed on the operating table in the supine position with the head and shoulders extending beyond the end of the table. An assistant sits on the right side of the patient, his right arm placed underneath the patient's neck with the right hand on the left side of the patient's face and his left hand placed on the occiput and vertex of the patient's head. This technique stabilizes the patient's head and allows controlled movement of the head into the various positions necessary for the examination. By extending the head, the mouth, pharynx, larynx and trachea are brought into a straight line that facilitiates insertion of the laryngoscope. Either a battery-powered or fiberoptic light source can be used and the light should be checked before inserting the laryngoscope. Insert the laryngoscope under direct vision over the dorsum of the tongue, placing a finger between the barrel of the laryngoscope and the patient's teeth to avoid an injury to the teeth or lips. The tip of the laryngoscope should be placed beneath the edge of the epiglottis and the entire scope lifted forward. Do not tilt the laryngoscope on the teeth. Advance the scope forward beneath the epiglottis until the larynx is in view. If the larynx is not completely anesthetized it will be in spasm (10 per cent cocaine introduced through the scope as a spray or on a swab will reduce the spasm). After carefully inspecting all parts of the larynx, slowly withdraw the scope under direct vision. A biopsy should be performed on any suspicious lesions. Failure to visualize all areas of the larynx, hypopharynx or base of the tongue can lead to serious mistakes in diagnosis.

Larynx Fractures

The most common cause of a laryngeal fracture is blunt trauma to the neck from automobile accidents. Quite often, multiple injuries result from such accidents and the laryngeal injury may be overlooked. The patient who has an airway problem may undergo a tracheostomy with no further thought given to the possibility of a laryngeal injury until decannulation is attempted. By this time, it may be too late for a definitive repair and the patient will have to accept either poor laryngeal function or further corrective surgery. A laryngeal injury should be suspected in any patient who needs a tracheostomy or has a history of neck trauma.

The symptoms most often produced by a laryngeal injury are increasing airway obstruction with dyspnea and stridor, dysphonia or aphonia, cough, hemoptysis or hematemesis, neck pain, and dysphagia or odynophagia. The clinical signs of an injury involving the upper airway are deformities of the neck, including swelling, subcutaneous emphysema, laryngeal tenderness, and crepitus of the thyroid cartilage and cricoid cartilage or hyoid bone. X-rays of the neck and chest must be obtained to detect laryngeal fractures, tracheal injuries or a pneumothorax.

A diagnosis of fractured larynx should be made as early as possible. Indirect and direct laryngoscopy should be performed on any patient in whom laryngeal injury is suspected. An endotracheal tube must be inserted with great care because it may be misplaced through a fracture site into the neck and completely obstruct the airway. A careful tracheostomy placed below the second tracheal ring is a much better way to insure a competent airway. If a cricothyrotomy has been done, it should be replaced with a tracheostomy as soon as the patient's condition permits. Laryngeal fractures should be reduced and immobilized as soon as the patient's condition has stabilized. Chronic stenosis can be avoided if reduction and fixation are carried out within seven to ten days. These procedures should not be performed on outpatients by surgeons unfamiliar with the principles and techniques of laryngeal surgery.

Tracheostomy

Obstruction of the airway is one of the most common medical emergencies. Any available physician should be able to act quickly and expertly to prevent a death or the complications that may occur. Bronchoscopy, oral-tracheal intubation, laryngotomy and tracheostomy are the four techniques that can be used to establish an airway and the indications for each technique depend upon the circumstances in which the emergency is encountered.

Bronchoscopy and oral-tracheal intubation require special skills and equipment but either technique will alleviate the immediate problem and allow the physician to perform a tracheostomy under more favorable circumstances The techniques for these two procedures are presented in Chapters 15 and 26. When these methods are not possible a tracheostomy or laryngotomy may be required as the initial method of therapy and a knowledge of these surgical techniques is essential.

Although most of the diseases causing airway obstruction are reversible with appropriate therapy, the airway must be established first, and the physician's attention should not deviate from the primary goal of a patent airway without which life will not be sustained. Several broad categories of diseases causing upper airway obstruction are presented in Table 10–4. Since the glottic aperture of the larynx is the narrowest part of the upper airway, many diseases in this area cause some degree of respiratory distress.

The diagnosis of airway obstruction is usually apparent. Inspiratory dyspnea and stridor result from air passing through the narrowed airway. Retractions of the suprasternal notch, epigastrium, supraclavicular areas and intercostal spaces arise from the increased effort needed to pull air through the restricted airway. Such retractions serve as cardinal signs of airway obstruction, and are not usually associated with cardiac or pulmonary diseases. Hoarseness or a "croupy" cough may be present. The respiratory and cardiac rates will be increased, and restlessness, apprehension and uncooperative behavior are common. Cyanosis occurs rather late and unless the airway is improved unconsciousness and respiratory-cardiac failure will develop, possibly indicating a terminal situation.

Laryngotomy. Superior tracheostomy or coniotomy (Fig. 10–48) is a very useful technique for severe obstruction of the airway. Hemenway (1961)[21] has enumerated the advantages of this technique. No special training or equipment is required and the procedure can be performed almost anywhere. An adequate airway can be established in a few seconds with this innocuous procedure at any time the patient's condition indicates an obstruction.

Surgical Technique. When the patient's condition is deteriorating rapidly, no anesthesia, skin preparation or draping is necessary. Otherwise a small amount of local anesthesia (lidocaine HCl) can be injected, the skin cleansed with alcohol and a few drapes applied around the neck. The face should not be covered because the surgeon must constantly observe it for signs of deterioration during the operation. After the space between the cricoid and thyroid cartilages is identified, the neck is extended, but not until the surgeon is ready to make his incision, because extension of the neck may cut off the only remaining available airway. A vertical skin incision is made over the cricothyroid membrane if time permits and a knife is available, but this incision is not always necessary. Any sharp object (knife, nail file, screw driver or piece of glass) is forcefully inserted between the thyroid and cricoid cartilages into the larynx. The instrument is then turned

TABLE 10–4   Differential Diagnosis of Airway Obstruction

I. Congenital Anomalies
   A. Glossoptosis — Pierre Robin syndrome
   B. Laryngotracheomalacia
   C. Laryngocele
   D. Laryngoesophageal clefts

II. Inflammations
   A. Laryngotracheobronchitis
   B. Epiglottitis
   C. Parapharyngeal abscesses
   D. Angioneurotic edema

III. Trauma
   A. Fractures
      1. Facial
      2. Laryngeal
      3. Cervical
      4. Chest
   B. Hematoma
      1. Oral
      2. Pharyngeal
      3. Laryngeal
      4. Cervical
   C. Burns
      1. Ingestion of caustics
      2. Inhalation of fumes, chemicals, smoke, steam.
   D. Postoperative
      1. Endoscopic injury
      2. Intubation injury
      3. Abdominal surgery
   E. Postirradiation
      1. Perichondritis
   F. Nasogastric intubation
   G. Foreign bodies

IV. Neoplasms
   A. Oral
   B. Pharyngeal
   C. Laryngeal
   D. Thyroid
   E. Cervical

V. Neurologic
   A. Cerebrovascular accidents
   B. CNS depressants
      1. Barbituates
   C. Skull trauma
      1. Hematoma
      2. Fractures
   D. Arnold-Chiari malformation
   E. Myasthenia gravis
   F. Eclampsia
   G. Cervical cord tumors and injuries

VI. Miscellaneous
   A. Laryngospasm
   B. Cricoarytenoid arthritis

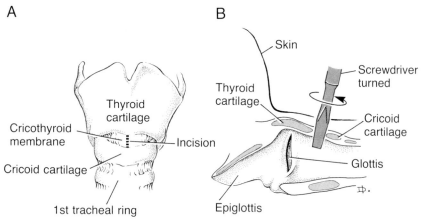

A

B

Skin

Screwdriver
turned

Thyroid
cartilage

Thyroid
cartilage

Cricothyroid
membrane

Cricoid
cartilage

Incision

Glottis

Cricoid cartilage

1st tracheal ring

Epiglottis

Figure 10–48 Coniotomy. Coniotomy or cricothyroidotomy is used to establish an airway quickly when a tracheostomy is not possible. The cricothyroid membrane is located by palpating the thyroid and cricoid cartilages. A sharp object is then guided between these two structures to perforate the membrane into the upper trachea. This simple procedure will provide an adequate airway until tracheostomy can be performed.

90 degrees to hold the incision open. This hole is well below the vocal cords and is usually below most obstructive lesions. The instruments may be left in place or replaced with a rigid tube if one is available. A permanent airway, usually by tracheostomy, should be established as soon as possible, but can be deferred until the proper facilities are available. Some bleeding will be encountered but this is usually not excessive and will not endanger the patient's life. Injuries to the cricoid cartilage and subsequent laryngeal stenosis have been overemphasized. Hemenway (1961)[21] emphasizes that large cricoid lacerations heal well with antibiotic treatment.

Tracheostomy is the procedure of choice when time and adequate facilities are available. Success depends upon a reasonable degree of surgical skill, a knowledge of neck anatomy, adequate surgical instruments, competent assistants, and good light and suction. Whenever possible the procedure should be performed in the operating room. Insertion of an oral-tracheal tube or bronchoscope will usually alleviate the airway obstruction and create more favorable conditions for the operation. Quite often, it is necessary to perform a tracheostomy on the ward or in the Emergency Room and under these circumstances the surgeon should be very careful that the necessary equipment and assistants are available to prevent a serious complication or disaster.

Tracheostomy: Surgical Technique (Figure 10–49). Oxygen should be administered if available and sedatives or premedications should *not* be given to the patient. A few words of explanation and reassurance will often relieve the patient's apprehension and increase his cooperation during the operation. Even small children become more cooperative since they realize all too well how desperately ill they are.

The skin of the neck is then painted with a suitable antiseptic and the area draped with sterile towels. The face must be left uncovered so that the patient's condition can be constantly observed throughout the procedure. If a respiratory crisis develops before the tracheostomy is completed, a laryngotomy should be performed immediately and the tracheostomy completed when the patient's condition improves.

General anesthesia should not be administered unless an endotracheal tube or bronchoscope is in place. Local anesthesia is adequate when injected

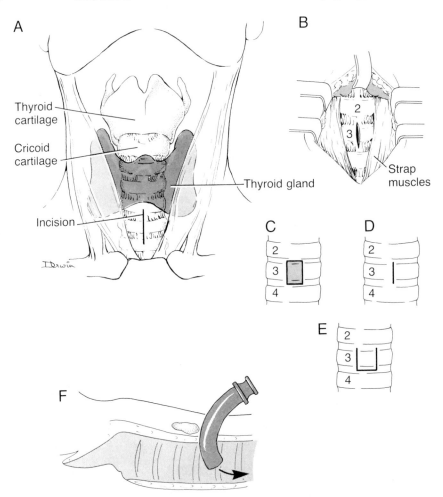

Figure 10–49 Tracheostomy. A vertical incision is made in the midline between the sternomastoid muscles *(A)*. The "strap" muscles are separated and the thyroid gland elevated and retracted superiorly *(B)*. The tracheal rings must be identified and an incision is made through the third tracheal ring. Several different tracheal incisions can be made *(C, D,* and *E)*, and a tracheostomy tube inserted *(F)*.

subcutaneously between the suprasternal notch and the lower border of the thyroid cartilage. Anesthesia is not necessary in patients with advanced stages of asphyxia.

Both the transverse and vertical midline incisions have been used in the past. The transverse incision has been recommended as the better tracheostomy incision for cosmetic reasons. However, when tracheostomy is an emergency procedure and is being done under less than ideal circumstances, the vertical midline incision is best. There will be

less bleeding from this incision, and coughing and swallowing will produce less shearing force on the tube with resulting extubation. If desired, a vertical scar can be revised later with a Z-plasty. The vertical midline incision should extend from the inferior border of the cricoid cartilage to just above the suprasternal notch. All dissection must be kept strictly in the midline. The skin edges should be retracted and the incision deepened until the isthmus of the thyroid gland is exposed. Sometimes the isthmus may be retracted upward or downward by cutting the fibrous connective tissue between the gland and the trachea—Cooper's ligament. When the isthmus cannot be retracted sufficiently, it must be cut between clamps and each side of the incised gland must then be ligated with a silk suture. These techniques result in good exposure of the trachea. *Lateral dissection must be avoided.* Tracheal rings are easily identified by palpation; however, in infants and small children the trachea is small, soft and difficult to recognize. In this case, the soft tissues are dissected from the upper tracheal rings.

A tracheal hook is helpful at this stage of the operation. This instrument should be used to stabilize the trachea and pull it more superficially for better exposure. An incision into the trachea is then made with a No. 11 Bard-Parker blade at least one tracheal ring below the cricoid cartilage and above the fifth tracheal ring. Large 1–0 or 1 silk sutures can be placed on each side of the tracheal cartilage selected for incision. These sutures make good tracheal retractors during incision and insertion of the tube. They should be left in place and taped to the chest for the first 72 hours after surgery or until a tract between the trachea and skin has developed. If the tube should be coughed out or accidentally misplaced, these sutures can be used to pull the trachea up into the wound and guide the tube back into the trachea. The patient usually coughs when the trachea is incised and the surgeon must not allow the knife blade to penetrate the posterior tracheal wall and enter the esophagus. A cruciate incision may be made or a small piece of tracheal cartilage removed to facilitate insertion of the tracheostomy tube. A Trousseau dilator or hemostat may be used to hold the incision open while the tube is inserted. A tracheostomy tube of appropriate size should be selected and carefully checked for any defects before it is inserted. The tube must be held securely in place with a finger until a tape is well–tied about the neck. This will prevent the patient from coughing the tube out of the trachea.

Hemostasis can be obtained during the procedure if time permits; however, bleeding vessels can be clamped and tied after the tube is in place. When there are more pressing circumstances many of the preceding steps may be omitted if absolutely necessary, but serious complications are more common when the operation is done too quickly.

The wound should never be sutured tightly about the tracheostomy tube, since a tight closure will predispose the patient to subcutaneous emphysema. Two or three 4–0 silk sutures can be used to approximate the lateral portion of the skin edges. However, one-half or two-thirds of the wound should be left open. A four-by-four gauze pad dressing should be placed beneath the flanges of the tube over the wound.

The postoperative management of a patient with a tracheostomy is very important. Careful, continuous observation is mandatory and special nurses may be necessary. Antibiotics should be given since an open wound often becomes infected and the operation may have been performed without absolutely sterile techniques. The tube should be checked repeatedly to be certain that it remains in the trachea. An extra tube of the same size should be taped to the patient's bed as an available replacement for a dislodged or obstructed tube. If it cannot be reinserted immediately another tracheostomy set should be obtained, the wound opened quickly and the tube reinserted. The outer tube should not be changed for three to five days. During this time granulation tissue will form about the tube, creating a fistula that makes reintroduction of a tube relatively easy. The inner cannula should be removed and cleaned as often as necessary.

Frequent suctioning is very important to keep the tube and tracheobronchial tree free of secretions. Secretions may accumulate that obstruct the airway or dry out to form crusts. This problem may cause or aggravate existing pulmonary difficulties. A sterile suction catheter of suitable size with a finger control should be inserted into the lower trachea. This usually stimulates coughing and as the catheter is withdrawn the finger control is occluded. This technique will effectively remove secretions and cause a minimal amount of distress for the patient.

Humidification of the patient's room will help keep tracheal secretions thin and reduce crusting. Oxygen may be needed if the patient's pulmonary function is impaired.

A simple explanation of the procedure and a little reassurance will help reduce many of the patient's anxieties. The patient should be told that he can talk by occluding the tube with a finger and that help is available when needed.

There are several special problems associated with airway obstruction in infants and children. Congenital anomalies, certain inflammatory conditions and foreign bodies are common in these patients. Holinger and Johnson (1950)[22] have discussed the significance of the small glottic aperture in infants. They emphasize that 1.0 mm of mucosal swelling can reduce the infant's glottic airway by 65 per cent! Perhaps the best way to handle an airway problem in an infant or small child is to insert a bronchoscope into the trachea. This relieves the immediate problem and allows a tracheostomy to be performed in a more routine manner. Also, some infants are too weak to withstand tracheostomy as a primary operation and these patients should have their anoxia corrected before any operative procedure is attempted. The rigid bronchoscope makes the trachea much easier to identify and reduces some of the risks of surgery. Postoperative care must be carried out more carefully than with adults because tubes are often dislodged and the child is helpless when such difficulties occur. In addition, the small lumen of the tracheostomy tube is easily occluded with crusts and secretions.

Complications. Tracheostomy is not an innocuous operation.[23,24] Many complications have been reported and these are generally classified as occurring during the procedure, during the postoperative period or later during convalescence. The patient may suddenly deteriorate before the airway is established. This situation must be recognized and an immediate laryngotomy performed. Many of these patients can be revived and the tracheostomy completed after resuscitation. Severe bleeding may occur from engorged neck veins, the thyroid isthmus, an anomalous vessel (thyroid ima) or a high innominate vein. Careful dissection in the midline will help the surgeon avoid the carotid sheath and vessels. Laceration of an innominate vein can lead to death from an air embolus. Improper positioning of the tube outside the trachea will increase the patient's respiratory distress. An incision into the posterior wall of the trachea and esophagus can lead to mediastinitis and a tracheoesophageal fistula. Sudden cardiac arrest or respiratory failure must be treated with immediate resuscitation measures. A rapid reduction of blood carbon dioxide levels may produce apnea. This problem can be reversed by artificial respiration until the carbon dioxide and oxygen levels are adjusted. Pneumothorax is not uncommon, especially in children, and results from cutting the dome of the pleura or from interstitial emphysema. Infections of the wound, neck and mediastinum will usually respond to appropriate antibiotic therapy and good postoperative care. Expulsion of the tube from coughing or improper handling should be promptly recognized and managed. Pulmonary atelectasis can be prevented by frequent suctioning, and crusting of blood or mucus reduced by adequate humidification, hydration of the patient and cleansing of the inner tube.

Tumors

Papillomas, chondromas, myomas, myxomas, chemodectomas, neurofibromas and angiomas are the usual benign neoplasms that occur in the larynx.

These tumors usually produce hoarseness if they occur on the vocal cords; however, the patient may remain asymptomatic until the tumor becomes large enough to cause dyspnea or swallowing difficulties. The diagnosis can often be made by an indirect mirror examination of the larynx. The tissue type of the tumor can be determined only by a biopsy that is obtained during a direct examination of the larynx. These patients should be treated by a laryngologist.

Most malignant neoplasms of the larynx are squamous cell carcinoma. These tumors are highly curable when detected early and treated aggressively. Hoarseness, airway obstruction, sore throat, difficulties with swallowing or referred otalgia are usually symptoms produced by these tumors. The diagnosis can usually be made by mirror examination of the larynx plus direct examination and biopsy. Treatment varies from irradiation therapy to surgical excision of the tumor or a combination of these two methods of treatment. There is a wide variety of surgical procedures that are used for these tumors, and in many instances a conservative operation can be used that preserves the functions of the larynx. These operations should be performed only by a surgeon familiar with the techniques and problems these procedures entail.

Esophagoscopy

The patient who is to have esophagoscopy should have an empty stomach. Preoperative sedation should be given at least one hour before esophagoscopy. For the average adult, a narcotic (morphine sulfate 10 mg), atropine (0.4 mg) and a barbiturate (Nembutal 100 mg) are satisfactory. General or topical anesthesia can be used. Cocaine hydrochloride (10 per cent solution) or tetracaine (2 per cent solution of Pentocaine) should be administered 5 to 10 minutes before inserting the esophagoscope. The patient's position is the same as that described for laryngoscopy.

The assistant should elevate and extend the head at the beginning of the procedure. The scope should be held with the right hand. The upper lip is retracted with the third and fourth fingers of the left hand while the tube is stabilized with the thumb and index fingers of the same hand. The scope is passed over the tongue into the oropharynx under direct vision. The tip is pushed along the right pharyngeal wall behind the right arytenoid cartilage into the right pyriform sinus. At the bottom of the pyriform sinus the instrument comes to a full stop. This is the cricopharyngeus muscle that usually remains closed and opens only with swallowing. By raising the tip of the scope anteriorly with the left thumb and pointing it at the suprasternal notch, a small lumen will appear. If the patient is asked to swallow, sometimes a small opening may be revealed through which the scope can be inserted. The danger of perforation is greater at this point than anywhere else and great care must be exercised to avoid this complication. A small flexible lumen (Fig. 10–50) finder gently passed through the esophagoscope will often elicit a swallow reflex and descend into the esophagus. This instrument also serves as a valuable guide for inserting the esophagoscope. Once the lumen appears the scope can be easily inserted into the upper esophagus. Patient cooperation and relaxation are extremely important and will make the procedure much easier and less dangerous. After the scope reaches the upper esophagus the patient's head is lowered so that the lumen is in view and does not disappear. The scope is passed into the thoracic esophagus and the head is moved slightly to the right. The scope is aimed at the patient's left anterior iliac spine as the surgeon looks for the hiatal opening. A small slit in an oblique line between 4 and 10 o'clock or a small rosette indicates the opening. The lumen finder may be used to identify the esophageal hiatus and a moderate amount of pressure with the tube mouth will allow passage of the scope into the stomach. A change in the color of the mucosa, a

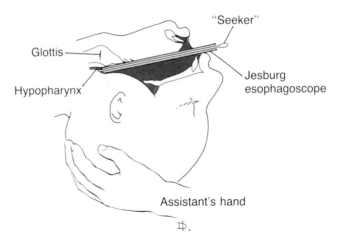

Figure 10–50 Esophagoscopy. Esophagoscopy is performed with the patient in the supine position, using either local or general anesthesia. The technique is relatively simple, but should be learned by performance under the guidance of an experienced surgeon.

gush of gastric fluid and the appearance of gastric rugae will be apparent when the scope enters the stomach. As the scope is withdrawn the esophagus should be carefully inspected and a biopsy should be done on any suspicious lesions.

No oral feedings should be allowed for at least four hours after the procedure, and the patient must be examined for neck tenderness and subcutaneous emphysema. The immediate onset of pain that radiates into the upper mediastinum or back often indicates a perforation. A white blood count will reveal a marked leukocytosis before fever develops. Perforations of the esophagus are serious and should never be overlooked, for immediate hospitalization is required for definitive care.

References

1. Hemenway, W. G., and Black, F. O.: Some thoughts on peripheral vestibular disorder. Ann. Otol. Rhinol. Laryngol., 76:509–518, 1967.
2. Fowler, E. P., Jr., and Osmun, P. M.: New bone growth due to cold water in the ears. Arch. Otolaryngol., 36:455–466, 1942.
3. Hemenway, W. G., and Smith, R. O.: Treating acute otitis media. Postgrad. Med., 47:110–115, 1970.
4. Armstrong, B. W.: Chronic secretory otitis media: Diagnosis and treatment. South. Med. J., 50:540–545, 1957.
5. Shambaugh, G. E.: Surgery of the Ear. Philadelphia, W. B. Saunders Co., 1967.
6. English, G. M., Hildyard, V. H., Hemenway, W. G., and Davidson, S.: Autograft and homograft incus transpositions in chronic otitis media. Laryngoscope, 81:1434–1447, 1971.
7. Ballenger, J. J.: Diseases of the Nose, Throat and Ear. Philadelphia, Lea and Febiger, 1969.
8. Padrnos, R. E.: A method for control of posterior nasal hemorrhage. Arch. Otolaryngol., 87:181–187, 1968.
9. Allen, G. W.: Ligation of the internal maxillary artery for epistaxis. Laryngoscope, 80: 915–923, 1970.
10. English, G. M., Hemenway, W. G., and Cundy, R. E.: Surgical treatment of invasive angiofibroma. Arch. Otolaryngol., 96:312–318, 1972.
11. Hemenway, W. G., and Lindsay, J. R.: Malignancies of the paranasal sinuses. Arch. Otolaryngol., 70:61–64, 1959.
12. Bhaskar, S. N.: Synopsis of Oral Pathology. St. Louis, C. V. Mosby Co., 1965.
13. Dingman, R. O., and Natvig, P.: Surgery of Facial Fractures. Philadelphia, W. B. Saunders Co., 1964.
14. English, G. M., Cundy, R. E., and Hemenway, W. G.: Orbital fractures. Laryngoscope (in press, 1972).
15. Johnson, W. B.: New method for reduction of acute dislocation of the temporomandibu-

lar articulations. J. Oral Surg., *16*:501–504, 1958.

16. Oeconomopoulos, C. T.: The value of glossopexy in the Pierre-Robin Syndrome. N. Eng. J. Med., *262*:1267–1268, 1960.

17. Daly, J. F., and Cardona, J. C.: Acute corrosive esophagitis. Arch. Otolaryngol., *74*:629–634, 1961.

18. Johnson, E.: A study of corrosive esophagitis. Laryngoscope, *73*:1651–1696, 1963.

19. Stuteville, O. H., and Corley, R. D.: Surgical management of tumors of intraoral minor salivary glands: Report of eighty cases. Cancer, *20*:1578–1586, 1967.

20. Grahne, B.: Abscess tonsillectomy: Seven hundred twenty-five cases. Arch. Otolaryngol., *68*:332–336, 1958.

21. Hemenway, W. G.: The management of severe obstruction of the upper air passages. Surg. Clin. N. Amer., *41*(1):201–212, February, 1961.

22. Holinger, P. H., and Johnston, K. C.: Factors responsible for laryngeal obstruction in infants. J.A.M.A., *143*:1229–1232, 1950.

23. Beatrous, W. P.: Tracheostomy (tracheotomy). Its expanded indications and its present status. Based on an analysis of 1,000 consecutive operations and a review of the recent literature. Laryngoscope, *78*:3–55, 1968.

24. Head, J. M.: Tracheostomy in the management of respiratory problems. N. Eng. J. Med., *264*:587–591, 1961.

11

Musculoskeletal System: Fractures and Dislocations

By LELAND G. HAWKINS, M.D.

INTRODUCTION

This chapter is primarily concerned with fractures and dislocations which are treated on an outpatient basis. It is based on the author's experience as chief of the fracture service at Denver General Hospital.

Our service is responsible for the primary emergency care of approximately 7000 patients a year with significant injuries to the locomotor system. In 1970, 2000 of these patients presented with fractures or dislocations. Five hundred and fifty were admitted to the hospital and 1350 were treated entirely on an outpatient basis. The patients were divided ethnically as follows: Anglo-Saxon 46 per cent, Hispano-American 30 per cent, and Negro 17 per cent. The distribution of injuries and the relative numbers admitted are shown on Tables 11–1 and 11–2.

The primary physician must treat all tissues of the extremities, including the skin, tendons, ligaments, muscles, joints, nerves, veins, and arteries. To isolate the management of the bone injury would be a disservice to the patient, because the end result depends upon restoration of function of each of the tissues in the extremity.

The primary physician evaluates each patient in the Emergency Room. For patients with musculoskeletal injuries, a consultation form is completed in duplicate—one record is for the chart and the other is for the physician's office file. The form is brief, but emphasis is placed on evaluation of all tissues (Table 11–3). Ideally, the extremity physician should be trained to handle each tissue included on the encounter form.

Today, in our training centers, care too often remains segmented. In the future, all tissues of the locomotor system in the traumatized patient should be managed by one physician who has a solid background in the basic sciences.

TABLE 11–1 DISTRIBUTION AND
MANAGEMENT OF FRACTURES*
DENVER GENERAL HOSPITAL
FRACTURE SERVICE
DEC. 1, 1969 TO DEC. 1, 1970

UPPER EXTREMITY	Closed	Open	Admission
Clavicle and scapula	115	2	19
Shoulder	90	0	11
Humerus	64	3	12
Elbow	50	4	8
Forearm	260	1	41
Wrist	51	0	10
Hand	322	17	26
Total	952	27	127

LOWER EXTREMITY	Closed	Open	Admission
Pelvis	57	2	40
Hip	104	1	96
Femur	66	2	60
Knee	95	7	35
Tibia and fibula	144	9	59
Ankle	190	4	37
Foot	157	3	5
Total	813	28	332

*Open fractures associated with gunshot wounds are not included.

This chapter is designed to be a practical reference for physicians treating patients with injured extremities who may not otherwise be fully acquainted with these types of injuries nor their management. The initial pages emphasize the soft tissue injuries which frequently accompany fractures and dislocations. Commonly missed fractures and dislocations are then discussed. Instructions for the application of several types of plaster dressings are included. The drawings will permit prompt access to the information. Although outpatient management is frequently not as convenient as inpatient treatment and shortages of operating room time and bed space may often be encountered, it is nevertheless possible to maintain a high level of medical care, and it may greatly expedite patient care.

SKIN

The condition of the skin overlying a fracture or dislocation may dictate a course of management which will appear to be at variance with standard orthopedic practice. The primary physician must recognize the common associated skin injuries accompanying fractures and dislocations and appreciate, from the outset, how they may alter fracture management. All patients with skin injuries should receive tetanus protection (Table 11–4). Most wounds can be handled in the Outpatient Department except those which require formal débridement in the operating room or which overlie a fracture requiring hospital management.

TABLE 11–2 DISLOCATIONS
DENVER GENERAL HOSPITAL
FRACTURE SERVICE
DEC. 1, 1969 TO DEC. 1, 1970

UPPER EXTREMITY		Number
Sternoclavicular Acromioclavicular	}	20
Shoulder		59
Elbow		40
Wrist		6
Hand		20
	Total	145

LOWER EXTREMITY		Number
Hip		6
Knee		8
Ankle		17
Foot		5
	Total	36

TABLE 11–3

PRIORITY	Age	Ht.	Wt.	T	BP	P	Accident Date		Type	
I							Time		Place	
II										
III										

History, Exam, Present Problem   Confidential or additional information on back.

──────────────── DIAGNOSIS/PROBLEM ────────────────

FRACTURE Location	1.		☐ Simple	☐ Comminuted
	2.		☐ Open	☐ Closed
	3.		☐ Stable	☐ Unstable
Type of Reduction				Degrees Angulated
Type of Retention				Percent Displaced
Type of Anesthesia				
Skin				
Nerve				
Artery				
Joint				
Ligament				
Tendon				

ADDITIONAL PROCEDURES   ── LAB & X-RAY ORDERS ──

☐ Crutches ☐ Sling ☐ Cast Instruction Sheet

─ DRUG ORDERS ─ ── STRENGTH ── ── SIG. ── ── QUAN. ──

REFER/ DESTINATION	EST. LENGTH OF DISABILITY
RETURN VISIT DYS. MOS. Clinic	
WKS. PRN	

Signature	No.		
Current Address	Phone	Date	Facility Cl./Serv.
Medicaid/Insurance Ident.		Name	
Medicare	Rate		Sex
	Stat.	Site	Outc.	D.H.H. No.	Birthdate

☐ Comp. ☐ Liab. ☐ BC ☐ BS ☐ CI

DEPARTMENT OF HEALTH AND HOSPITALS
ORTHOPEDIC HEALTH CARE VISIT FORM

Responsible Party

CHART COPY   Appt. Time   D.H.H. No.   Clerk and Time
Med. Rec. 115 (Rev. 3/71) DHH

TABLE 11–4   TETANUS PROTECTION

PREVIOUS IMMUNIZATION	NO IMMUNIZATION
Tetanus toxoid	Hypertet
0.5 cc IM	250–500 units IM
Booster needed every ten years	

TABLE 11–5   BETADINE SOLUTION

Betadine solution is the most effective topical germicide for use in treating open fractures. It kills bacteria (including antibiotic-resistant organisms), fungi, viruses, protozoa and yeasts. It is bactericidal, not merely bacteriostatic, and maintains germicidal activity in the presence of blood, pus, serum and necrotic tissue. It has a more prolonged germicidal action than ordinary iodine solutions, and forms a golden-brown film when topically applied that delineates treated areas. It can easily be washed off skin and natural fabrics. (Editor's note: The superiority of Betadine brand iodophor over other topical organic iodine preparations has not been conclusively demonstrated.)

Abrasions

Abrasions (Fig. 11–1) overlying mid-shaft fractures of both bones of the forearm in an adult illustrate the way skin damage may alter management of the fracture. This bone injury usually requires open reduction and internal fixation but the multiple tears in the epidermis make a perfect medium for superficial infection. It is too risky to proceed with any type of surgery through this potentially contaminated area. Infection may follow the open reduction. Therefore, initially I take great care in obtaining a satisfactory reduction and maintaining the reduction with length and alignment because I may never be able to fix the fracture internally. Wound care requires repeated dressing changes to prevent further skin necrosis and allow early skin healing. Anesthesia may be required to avoid pain during the removal of the plaster and rescrubbing of the wound with iodophor sponges (Table 11–5). Repeated careful re-

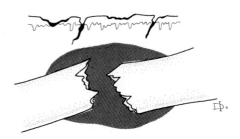

Figure 11–1   Abrasions overlying fractures.

reduction and application of plaster is usually necessary. Before the plaster is applied, the abrasion is scrubbed vigorously and covered with a sterile fine mesh gauze, followed by a layer of gauze sponges. Finally, a circular dressing of Webrile, Kling or Kerlex bias-cut stockinette or sheet wadding is lightly applied (Fig. 11–2). In one week these dressings are removed, using anesthesia if necessary. Drainage or superficial

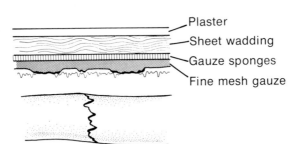

Plaster
Sheet wadding
Gauze sponges
Fine mesh gauze

Figure 11–2   Circular dressings for abrasions.

infection alters the above routine. More frequent dressing changes may be necessary until the wound is clean, with continuous Bunnell's soaks that are changed every eight hours (Table 11–6). Once the skin is entirely healed the surgeon can consider open reduction and internal fixation of the fracture.

TABLE 11–6 BUNNELL'S SOLUTION (MODIFIED FOR USE AT DENVER GENERAL HOSPITAL)	
Benzalkonium chloride 10%	200 cc
Glacial acetic acid	212 cc
Glycerin	8000 cc
Water, distilled qs ad	10 gal
D & C Red #39	1.0 gm

Tension on Overlying Skin

The fracture or dislocation which has placed *tension on overlying skin* (Fig. 11–3) should be reduced promptly to prevent necrosis. The lateral displacement and external rotation of the foot associated with a trimalleolar fracture often stretches the skin over the irregular fracture surface of the distal tibia. Simple linear traction and internal rotation of the foot relieve this tension. Another example is the tension on skin over the dislocated body of the talus after a fracture dislocation of the talus. Simple fingertip pressure moves the talar body into a position which reduces the skin tension.

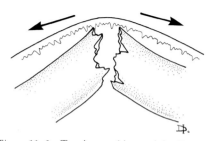

Figure 11–3 Tension on skin overlying fracture.

Blisters

Fracture *blisters* (Fig. 11–4) are usually avoided by covering the extremity promptly with a well-molded firm circumferential dressing. Blisters should be covered by a sterile dressing and well-molded plaster. The presence of blisters indicates poor venous outflow and edema due to widespread underlying subcutaneous hemorrhage. They are not a contraindication to surgery unless they rupture and become secondarily infected.

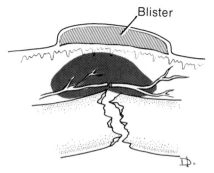

Figure 11–4 Fracture blisters.

Contusions

Complete necrosis of skin and adjacent subcutaneous tissue occasionally develops after a *severe contusion* (Fig. 11–5). The precarious circulation at the periphery of the contusion may be compromised if precautions are not taken to prevent pressure and swelling. These developments may cause or increase the area of necrosis by further compromising the circulation. Elevation, soft dressings, and a water mattress or floatation bed are necessary in these circumstances.

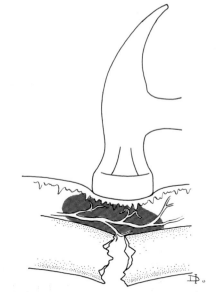

Figure 11–5   Contusion with skin necrosis associated with fracture.

Missile Wounds

A low-velocity *missile wound* with associated fracture such as that inflicted by a .22, .38 or .45 caliber missile (Fig. 11–6) needs simple skin débridement, soft dressings and antibiotics. By following this routine one rarely encounters a deep infection. The tract need not be debrided nor the missile removed initially. When the fracture is comminuted, plaster dressings and nonoperative methods of treatment are frequently satisfactory.

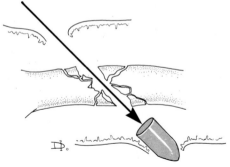

Figure 11–6   Missile wound with associated fracture.

Lacerations and Puncture Wounds

All *lacerations* or *puncture wounds* (Fig. 11–7) in the area of a fracture which result in communication between the skin surface and fracture hematoma are considered open fractures. The most frequent open fracture is the open distal fingertip injury, and open fracture of the tibial shaft is next in frequency. Intravenous antibiotics (Table 11–7) must immediately be started in the

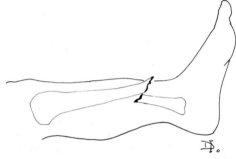

Figure 11–7   Laceration overlying fracture.

TABLE 11–7 RECOMMENDED ANTIBIOTIC COVERAGE FOR OPEN FRACTURES

ORGANISM	ROUTE	PATIENT DRUG SENSITIVITY	DRUGS	RECOMMENDED DOSE FOR 70 kgm PATIENT
Gram +	Intra-venous	Sensitive to penicillin	cephalothin (Keflin)	1–2 gm IV piggy-back q 4 hrs
		None	nafcillin (Unipen)	1–2 gm IV piggy-back q 4 hrs
	Oral	Sensitive to penicillin	cephalexin (Keflex); or	250–500 mg tabs q 6 hrs
			erythromycin (Erythrocin, Ilotycin)	250–500 mg tabs q 6 hrs
		None	dicloxacillin (Dynapen)	250–500 mg tabs q 6 hrs
Gram −	Intra-muscular	None	kanamycin (Kantrex)	15 mg/Kg/day divided q 12 hr doses
			gentamicin (Garamycin)	2.5–4.5 mg/Kg/day divided q 8 hr doses
	Oral	Sensitive to penicillin	cephalothin (Keflex)	250–500 mg tabs q 6 hrs
		None	ampicillin (Omnipen, Penibritin, Polycillin, etc.)	250–500 mg tabs q 6 hrs

Emergency Room, and continued intra-operatively and postoperatively. Beta-dine-soaked sterile dressings are applied to the open fracture prior to the patient's arrival in the operating room. The incidence of infection is low if the wound débridement is carried out in the operating room within two to three hours after the injury. Antibiotics are administered for ten days and primary wound closure is accomplished when possible. A laceration or puncture wound in continuity with a fracture which is debrided in the Emergency Room should not be closed with sutures.

VASCULAR INJURY

Vascular injury (Fig. 11–8) is the single most important aspect of trauma to the extremities, and it demands immediate recognition by the primary physician. An extremity can be deprived of arterial blood supply for only five hours. Irreversible changes then occur in the muscles, nerves, arteries and skin.

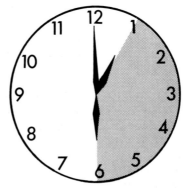

Figure 11–8 Vascular injury associated with fracture must be treated within five hours.

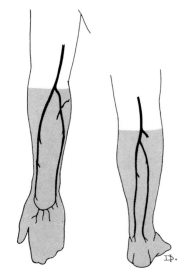

A vascular surgeon should be called before arteriograms are obtained, so that precious time is not lost. We do not usually attempt to repair arteries distal to the bifurcation of the brachial artery nor distal to the trifurcation of the popliteal artery (Fig. 11–9).

Figure 11–9 Injuries distal to bifurcation of brachial and trifurcation of popliteal arteries are not usually repaired.

Vascular Insufficiency

Vascular insufficiency is recognized by the following aspects of the physical examination:

First, the peripheral pulses of one extremity are quickly compared to the pulses of the opposite extremity.

Second and more important, the promptness of capillary refill after pressure on the nail beds is assessed (Fig. 11–10).

Third, early ischemia to muscles causes severe pain when the muscle belly is stretched, while early nerve ischemia causes progressive distal sensory loss and paralysis in the extremity. An artery which is under tension, as in a fracture dislocation of the ankle, may leave the foot cold and pulseless until the dislocation is reduced (Fig. 11–11). A rapidly expanding hematoma suggests partial laceration of an artery (Fig. 11–12). The completely transected artery will clamp down, preventing continued blood loss. Undermined skin flaps demarcate slowly over several days, with necrosis resulting from venous stasis.

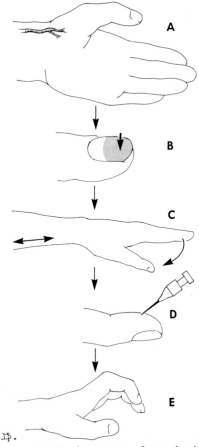

Figure 11–10 Assessment of vascular injury. *A.* Pulse. *B.* Capillary refill. *C.* Passive stretch. *D.* Sensory loss. *E.* Motor loss.

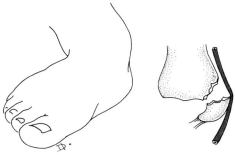

Figure 11–11   Arterial compression from fracture dislocation causes temporary ischemia.

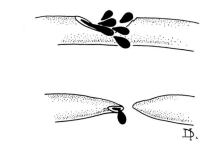

Figure 11–12   Rapidly expanding hematoma suggests partial laceration of artery.

Tight primary skin closure will increase the risk of necrosis in these situations. Arteriovenous fistula (Fig. 11–13) is rare; it is most frequently associated with stab wounds and low velocity gunshot wounds. A stethoscope may detect a bruit in these cases.

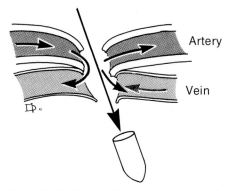

Figure 11–13   Traumatic arteriovenous fistula.

Aseptic Necrosis

In most cases, loss of arterial blood supply to bone cannot be recognized at the time of the fracture. *Aseptic necrosis* can be seen later by careful scrutiny of the x-ray. The three common fractures associated with a significant incidence of aseptic necrosis are the intra-articular fractures of the neck of the femur, the waist of the carpal navicular, and the neck of the talus (Fig. 11–14). In each case the proximal fragment partially or completely loses its blood supply at the time of injury. The long-range prognosis is guarded as related to the union of the fracture, the degree of pain and the loss of function of the involved joint.

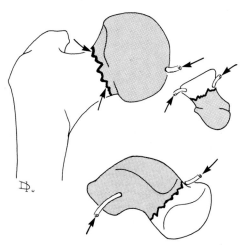

Figure 11–14   Common fractures associated with aseptic necrosis: femur, carpal navicular, and talus.

Fractures and Dislocations Commonly Associated With Vascular Injury

1. *A patient with a crush injury of the proximal tibia or knee*, with or without a significant tibial fracture, must not be treated as an outpatient because in 6 to 24 hours local hemorrhage and swelling may (Fig. 11–15) necessitate fasciotomy and arterial exploration.

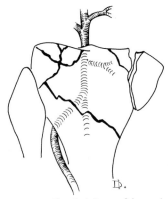

Figure 11–15 Crush injury of knee (proximal tibia), which frequently requires fasciotomy and arterial exploration.

2. *Dislocation of the knee* is a rare but significant injury, since it is associated with a tear or contusion of the popliteal artery in 50 per cent of cases. Ligamentous damage is of secondary importance to the arterial injury. Unnecessary delay in reduction and recognition of popliteal artery damage will result in amputation (Fig. 11–16). Restoration of blood supply must be prompt and effective.

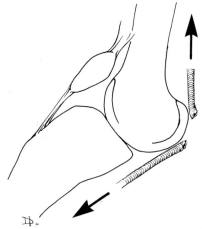

Figure 11–16 Dislocated knee is associated with popliteal artery injury in 50 per cent of cases.

3. The superficial femoral artery may be partially or completely lacerated at the time of *fracture of the mid or distal shaft of the femur.* Major arterial and venous injuries also accompany fractures of the pelvis. These injuries necessitate prompt surgical repair. Upper extremity fractures and dislocations are occasionally associated with arterial injuries (Fig. 11–17).

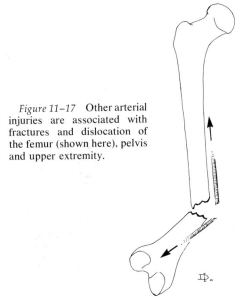

Figure 11–17 Other arterial injuries are associated with fractures and dislocation of the femur (shown here), pelvis and upper extremity.

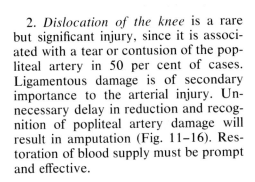

4. A child who has fallen on an outstretched arm and presents with marked deformity about the elbow is also likely to have an arterial injury. The deformity may be due to *dislocation of the elbow or supracondylar fracture* of the humerus (Fig. 11–18). The latter has a high incidence of vascular damage and associated hemorrhage which will usually not become significant during the emergency transport and splinting phase if the physician will keep the elbow extended and the forearm aligned and elevated. Signs of ischemia frequently develop after closed reduction. Venous drainage and arterial blood flow are then blocked by swelling and the flexed position of the elbow. The radial pulse is obliterated (Fig. 11–19). When reduction and a good radial pulse cannot be maintained with the elbow in more than 90 degrees of flexion, the brachial artery may be torn, divided, or in spasm. In this situation, skeletal overhead olecranon traction is immediately initiated. If capillary filling is good, and if straightening the thumb, index, and long finger does not cause pain in the forearm, the child can be observed closely, and exploration will not usually be needed. The pulse will return in a few days or weeks. The fracture can safely be reduced and retained during this period by overhead traction on a skeletal pin placed through the olecranon.

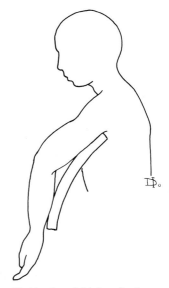

Figure 11–18 Arterial injury is also associated with dislocation of the elbow (shown here) or supracondylar fracture of the humerus.

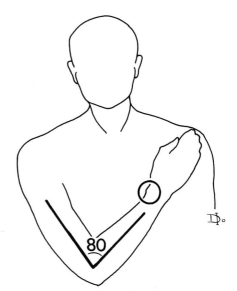

Figure 11–19 Postreduction immobilization of supracondylar fracture.

NERVE INJURY

The peripheral nerves are occasionally injured at the time of fractures and dislocations of the extremities. The primary physician needs to do little more than take all possible tension or angular forces off the nerves by reducing the fracture or dislocation. The nerve which is under tension or is ischemic benefits immediately by reduction and function returns within minutes, hours or days. A nerve contused by a direct blow or stretching (Fig. 11–20) has disrupted axons and requires weeks or months before peripheral function returns. The prognosis for a contused nerve with only motor or sensory function involvement is more optimistic. Late appearance of motor or sensory loss does not indicate a laceration unless the loss appears after closed reduction. In this situation, the nerve should immediately be visualized and released from the bone

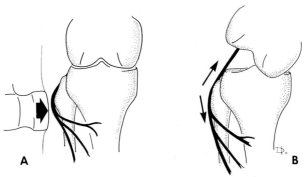

Figure 11–20 Peroneal nerve injury by external trauma *(A)* and during lateral collateral ligament injury *(B)*.

fragments. After contusion or laceration of a nerve, the use of plaster dressings, passive motion, elevation and splints will maintain the extremity free of contractures (Fig. 11–21). Occasionally a peripheral nerve is completely lacerated at the time of the fracture dislocation. If there is no return of function after a reasonable time has elapsed to allow for nerve regeneration, surgical exploration and neurorrhaphy may be necessary. If no function or only partial function returns after neurorrhaphy, tendon transfers may be used to eliminate the need for braces. Function can be greatly improved in this way for patients with injury to the radial nerve, the peroneal nerve, the median nerve and the ulnar nerve.

Dermatomes and Peripheral Nerve Distribution

A review of the peripheral sensory and motor losses associated with the nerves which are commonly damaged at the time of fractures and dislocations seems appropriate. Occasionally the peripheral losses do not coincide with the patterns of distribution shown for the separate peripheral nerves. Consideration must then be given to more central injuries. The peripheral distribution of the dermatomes is shown in Figure 11–22. A brachial plexus injury

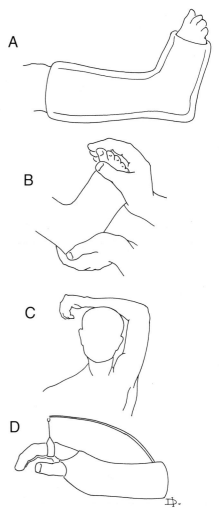

Figure 11–21 Prevention and treatment of peripheral nerve injuries associated with fractures by *(A)* plaster dressings, *(B)* passive motion, *(C)* elevation and *(D)* splints.

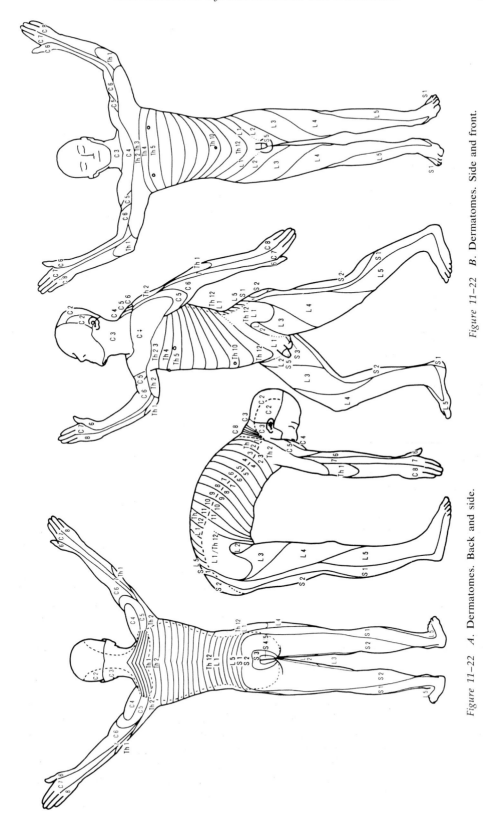

Figure 11–22 B. Dermatomes. Side and front.

Figure 11–22 A. Dermatomes. Back and side.

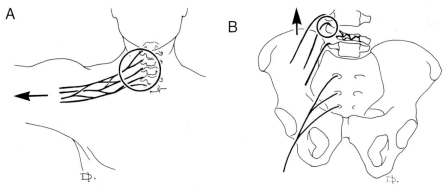

Figure 11–23   Brachial plexus and sciatic nerve injury.

(Fig. 11–23 *A, B*) can result from a severe stretch of the nerve roots as they exit from the neural canal. A single nerve root may be damaged in lumbar and sacral fractures. Knowledge of dermatome sensory distribution may therefore be useful in diagnosis.

Radial Nerve

The most frequent nerve injury in our service is *radial sensory and motor palsy* associated with closed fractures of the shaft of the humerus. The nerve rests on the posterior surface of the humerus, winding around distally to pass anterior to the elbow. It is directly contused at the time of the fracture (Fig. 11–24), but it is unusual for this nerve to be lacerated. Therefore, sensory and motor function can be expected to return within three to four months. The *radial nerve* is also susceptible to contusion in children with supracondylar fractures of the humerus. Observation for several weeks to three months is usually all that is necessary, since peripheral function will return in that time. The deep radial nerve passing through the supinator muscle is occasionally contused in fractures of the proximal radius. It also can be stretched when the radial head is dislocated at the time of a Monteggia fracture of the ulnar shaft. Out-

rigger wrist and finger extensor splints are needed in adult patients to keep the hand free from edema and contracture while nerve regeneration occurs.

Ulnar Nerve

The ulnar nerve courses deep in the muscles of the arm and forearm, and is exposed to trauma primarily at the shoulder, elbow and wrist (Fig. 11–25). A patient with an anterior dislocation of the shoulder will occasionally complain of paresthesias in the ulnar distribution. Normal motor and sensory functions usually return promptly after reduction of the dislocation. The nerve is more frequently traumatized by external forces at the elbow where it rests subcutaneously in the ulnar groove on the distal humerus. At the wrist, a volar dislocation of the distal ulna associated with a distal radial shaft fracture (the Galleazzi's fracture) may stretch or contuse the ulnar nerve.

Frequently ulnar motor function is lost in the hand after a patient with a Colles' fracture is placed in excessive flexion. The problem can be avoided by promptly releasing all dressings. Obviously, patients should always be checked to determine if ulnar motor or sensory loss has occurred after reduction of a Colles' fracture.

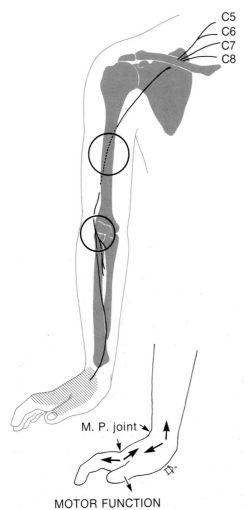

MOTOR FUNCTION
(EXTENSION WRIST AND THUMB)

Figure 11–24 Radial nerve injury in fracture of the humerus.

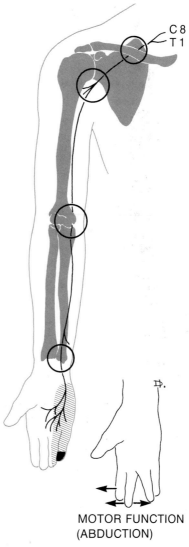

MOTOR FUNCTION
(ABDUCTION)

Figure 11–25 Ulnar nerve injury.

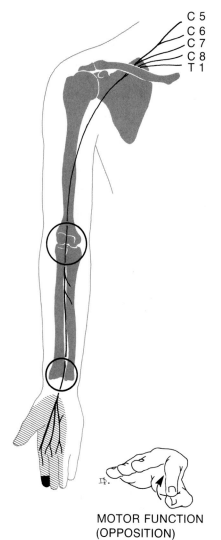

C 5
C 6
C 7
C 8
T 1

MOTOR FUNCTION
(OPPOSITION)

Figure 11–26   Median nerve injury.

Median Nerve

The flexor muscle group in the arm and forearm usually affords good protection to the median nerve from injury by bone fragments at the time of fracture and dislocation (Fig. 11–26). The proximal humeral fragment of a supracondylar fracture may tear through the intervening brachialis muscle and contuse the median nerve. Most flexor muscles in the distal forearm are represented by their respective tendons which may be stretched or contused by a fracture of the radius at this level. A more common median nerve injury occurs from hemorrhage, swelling and extreme flexion of the wrist in a reduced Colles' fracture. Prompt recognition and release of dressings may prevent an avoidable ischemic and neuropathic contracture of the hand. After leaving the forearm the nerve enters the limited space of the carpal canal. Volar displacement of the lunate into the carpal canal at the time of dislocation routinely creates pressure and ischemia in the median nerve. Prompt reduction will usually eliminate permanent nerve deficit.

Sciatic Nerve

The sciatic nerve rests on the acetabulum posterior to the hip joint (Fig. 11–27). In a posterior dislocation of the hip the femoral head breaks through the joint capsule and frequently stretches or contuses the adjacent nerve. The nerve may be lacerated if a posterior acetabular lip fracture fragment accompanies the dislocation. When recognized, prompt reduction of the dislocation is mandatory. Frequently the peroneal portion of the sciatic nerve is contused, while the adjacent posterior tibial portion is spared. If function does not return immediately after reduction, a prolonged period of disability is anticipated. This may necessitate a double upright brace with ankle spring assists, or a tendon transfer at a later date.

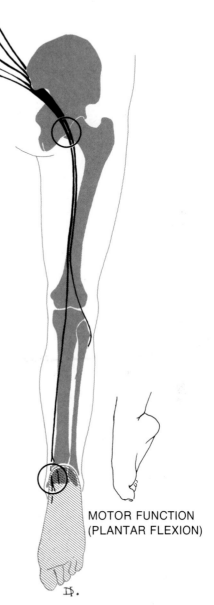

MOTOR FUNCTION
(PLANTAR FLEXION)

Figure 11–27 Sciatic nerve injury.

Posterior Tibial Nerve

The sciatic nerve divides at the junction of the middle and distal third of the femur into the posterior tibial and peroneal nerves (Fig. 11–27). Signs and symptoms of injury to this nerve frequently occur with subtalar dislocations and fracture dislocations of the ankle. Prompt reduction of these injuries usually results in early return of function.

Peroneal Nerve

This nerve passes lateral to the knee joint in contact with the biceps tendon which inserts into the proximal fibula. It winds around the subcutaneous surface of the fibula until it reaches the anterior compartment. The peroneal nerve is particularly vulnerable to trauma (Fig. 11–28) in its subcutaneous position adjacent to the head of the fibula. The nerve is stretched when the knee joint opens into a varus position, tearing the lateral collateral ligament, the biceps tendon, and the fascia lata from their insertion into the tibia. In its subcutaneous position the nerve is also exposed to direct external trauma, such as pressure from a mattress, an elastic bandage securing traction on the skin or a poorly padded plaster dressing. A direct blow causing a proximal fracture of the fibula may also damage the peroneal nerve.

LIGAMENTS AND CAPSULES

Certain ligamentous and capsular tears are frequently overlooked when there has been an associated fracture and dislocation. Once a spontaneous or manual reduction has been accomplished, the soft tissue damage is too often forgotten or not recognized. The local joint is painful and swollen with blood, and careful examination is difficult because of the patient's discomfort. In this situation,

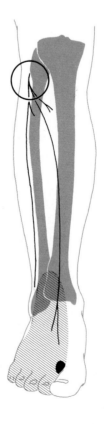

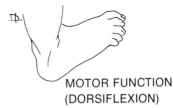

MOTOR FUNCTION
(DORSIFLEXION)

Figure 11–28   Peroneal nerve injury.

intra-articular injection of lidocaine may be used to produce satisfactory analgesia for examination. Thorough aspiration of the joint must be performed before lidocaine is injected. Uptake by the synovial membrane is prompt, and the total dose injected intrasynovially must be below toxic levels (1 mg per pound). A stress x-ray view provides verification and a permanent record of associated ligamentous damage or instability.

Common Injuries Associated with Fractures and Dislocations

A *tibial plateau fracture* (Fig. 11–29) can be associated with a torn collateral ligament on the opposite side of the knee from the fracture site. *Fracture of the lateral malleolus or distal fibula* (Fig. 11–30) may be associated with a torn medial collateral ligament of the ankle. Loss of stability may occur from avulsion of ligaments at their bony attachments. This is frequently seen when the anterior cruciate ligament avulses the *anterior tibial spine* (Fig. 11–31). The posterior cruciate ligament avulses bone from the posterior tibial surface. The medial and lateral ankle ligaments avulse bone from the *tips of the malleolus.* The collateral knee ligaments avulse bone from the *femur,* and *tibia* and *fibula.*

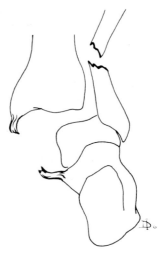

Figure 11–30   Lateral malleolus or distal fibula fracture associated with medial collateral ligament injury at the ankle.

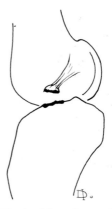

Figure 11–31   Avulsion of posterior tibial surface by posterior cruciate ligament.

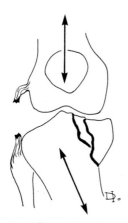

Figure 11–29   Stress x-ray for verification of instability and ligamentous injury associated with injury to a joint: tibial plateau fracture and associated collateral ligament injury.

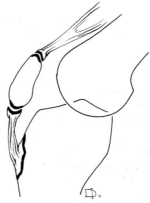

Figure 11–32   Patellar ligament avulses bone from patella and tibia.

The patellar ligament avulses bone from the *upper* and *lower pole of the patella* and the *tibial tubercle* (Fig 11–32). Radial deviation of the wrist avulses the *ulnar* styloid (Fig. 11–33). A fracture of the *shaft of the radius* may be associated with damage to the distal radial ulnar and ulnar carpal joints. A fracture of the *shaft of the ulna* may be associated with damage to the more proximal radial ulnar and radial humerus joints.

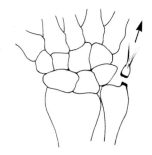

Figure 11–33   Ulnar styloid avulsion.

Treatment

The cartilaginous surfaces of the joints and intact soft parts usually lend enough stability to allow longitudinal capsular tears to heal with immobilization alone. The torn ligament or capsule may return to an anatomic position after reduction. Three weeks of immobilization is usually adequate for these injuries.

When transverse ligament and capsular tears heal there may be an increase in their length. This lengthening may be observed in the cruciate and medial collateral ligaments of the knee, the capsule of the elbow, thumb MP joint capsule and lateral ankle ligaments. All of these injuries may therefore be followed by recurrent dislocation or instability if the torn edges of the ligaments are not approximated surgically. Experimental ligament and capsule tears heal without laxity when their edges are anatomically repaired and adequately immobilized. Clinically, experience has demonstrated that treatment with adequate prolonged immobilization generally gives satisfactory results. Since a merely "satisfactory" result is not acceptable in young or athletic individuals, in these patients open surgical repairs of torn ligaments are routinely performed to assure that the ligament ends are approximated before immobilization is instituted.

MUSCLE TENDON UNIT INJURY AND ASSOCIATED FRACTURES

An interesting group of injuries occurs from violent muscle contraction or stress transmitted through the musculotendinous unit. The muscle tendon unit can rupture in various locations under such stresses. It is usually taught that the weakest point in this unit is the musculotendinous junction, as seen with ruptures of the Achilles tendon. Injuries classified as muscle strains occur when muscle fibers tear during violent muscle contraction. The pulled hamstring is a good example. However, avulsion fractures do occur at the origin or insertion of muscles. In the years prior to epiphyseal closure, avulsion fractures occur at the weak junction between an apophysis and adjacent metaphysis. An apophysis is a traction epiphysis not containing an articulating surface and it appears as a secondary ossification center on the roentgenogram. The force of muscular contraction is transmitted across the muscle origin or insertion to the adjacent epiphyseal plate. The epiphyseal plate contains a band of growing cartilage which then separates, allowing the apophysis to displace with the shortened muscle.

Medial Epicondyle of the Humerus

The *medial epicondyle of the humerus* (Fig. 11–34) is a small apophysis or secondary ossification center at the elbow. The medial epicondyle prior to epiphyseal plate closure may be displaced distally by the forearm flexor muscle mass which originates from it. Nonunion without impairment of function is the expected result when treated in plaster.

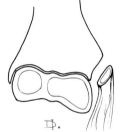

Figure 11–34 Avulsion of the medial epicondyle of the humerus by forearm flexors.

Anterior Inferior and Superior Iliac Spine

One of the four muscles in the quadriceps mechanism is the rectus femoris muscle, which takes origin from the *anterior inferior iliac spine* and inserts into the superior pole of the patella. A violent contraction of the quadriceps may avulse the anterior inferior spine and drag it into position anterior to the hip joint (Fig. 11–35). This may later lead to ossification anterior to the capsule of the hip, producing limitation of flexion of the hip. The sartorius or tensor fascia lata may avulse the *anterior superior iliac spine* or the leading edge of the anterior portion of the iliac crest. Both of these injuries are seen in young persons.

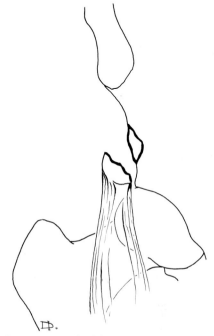

Figure 11–35 Avulsion of rectus femoris muscle origin from the anterior inferior iliac spine.

Ischial Tuberosity

The origin of the hamstrings is from the apophysis or secondary ossification center of the *ischial tuberosity*. This may be avulsed (Fig. 11–36). Nonunion can result from inadequate immobilization.

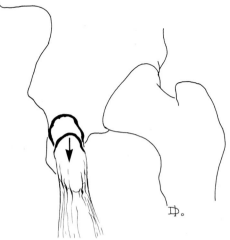

Figure 11–36 Avulsion of the apophysis of the ischial tuberosity by hamstrings.

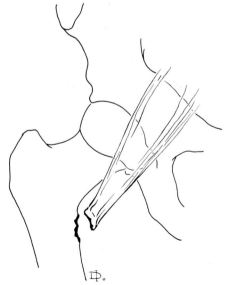

Lesser Trochanter

An avulsion may occur at the insertion of the iliopsoas tendon into the *lesser trochanter* of the femur (Fig. 11–37), and is called an apophysis. The lesser trochanter is displaced proximally, anterior to the head and neck of the femur.

Figure 11–37   Avulsion of the lesser trochanter by iliopsoas tendon.

Other Avulsion Fractures

In the adult large fragments of bone may be avulsed by violent muscle contraction; examples are seen in (Fig. 11–38) the transverse fracture of the patella, (Fig. 11–39) the upward displacement of the region about the insertion of the tendon Achilles on the *os calcis*, and (Fig. 11–40) the transverse fracture of the proximal and middle *olecranon*. These fractures frequently enter a joint and internal fixation of the displaced fragments may be necessary. However, minimally displaced avulsion fractures are best treated by immobilization and rest.

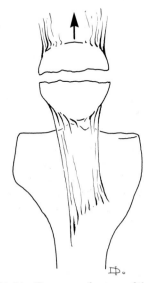

Figure 11–38   Transverse fracture of the patella.

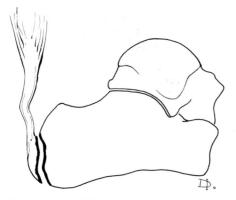

Figure 11–39   Displacement of the insertion of the Achilles tendon from os calcis.

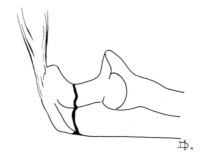

Figure 11–40   Transverse fracture of the proximal and middle olecranon.

Muscle Strain and Rupture

Muscle strains are intramuscular fiber tears associated with overlying fascial tears. They are simply treated by rest for two weeks, followed by progressive return to normal activity. The origin of muscle fibers from the periosteum of long bones is occasionally torn from the bone. This condition may be followed by the development of myositis ossificans, a condition which is poorly understood. The most common serious disease of the muscle-tendon unit in the older adult is rupture of the musculotendinous junction. This occurs at the junction of the Achilles tendon and the gastrosoleus muscle fibers (Fig. 11–41). Rupture also occurs in the quadriceps group just above the patella, and in the long head of the biceps distal to its exit from the bicipital groove of the humerus (Fig. 11–42). Surgical intervention is usually indicated in these cases.

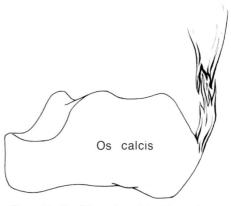

Os calcis

Figure 11–41   Disruption of Achilles tendon.

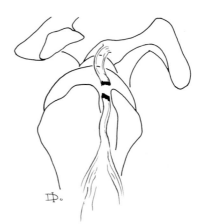

Figure 11–42   Disruption of tendon of long head of biceps.

SOFT TISSUE INJURIES ACCOMPANYING PELVIC FRACTURES

The patient with a fracture of the pelvis has usually sustained major blunt trauma which requires confinement in the hospital for an extended period of time. Prompt blood replacement is essential. The primary physician must be alert to the types of soft tissue damage which occur in these patients, requiring immediate recognition and surgical care. In 35 patients with pelvic fractures who required laparotomy (Table 11–8), the average blood replacement required was 4000 ml. Thirty of these patients had major injuries of intra-abdominal organs.[3] The only patient with a pelvic fracture who can safely rest at home is a patient who has had relatively minor trauma. Examples include a minimally displaced fracture of the ischial or pubic ramus with a normal hematocrit, a urine free of red blood cells, and stable vital signs. In these cases as the pain decreases activity is increased. Nonunion is distinctly unusual (Fig. 11–43).

DISLOCATIONS

Dislocations of the joints in the extremities are usually easily recognized. Most of these injuries can be reduced by closed methods. Exceptions exist when it is necessary to remove soft parts or remove fracture fragments interposed between joint surfaces prior to the reestablishment of the normal articular surfaces. This situation is commonly encountered after a metacarpal phalangeal dislocation of the little finger or index finger, in which the proximal phalanx is dorsally dislocated (Fig. 11–44). A successful closed reduction is prevented in these patients by volar plate interposition, and open reduction is therefore required.

Prompt reduction is recommended for all dislocations. The patient's severe pain

TABLE 11–8　ABDOMINAL INJURIES ASSOCIATED WITH PELVIC FRACTURES IN 35 PATIENTS WHO UNDERWENT LAPAROTOMY

Urinary tract		19
Ruptured bladder	13	
Ruptured urethra	6	
Gastrointestinal tract		13
Ruptured spleen	4	
Liver laceration	4	
Bowel laceration	3	
Ruptured gallbladder	1	
Pancreatic laceration	1	
Vascular injury		5
No major associated injury		5

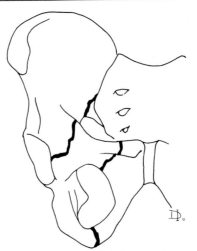

Figure 11–43　Pelvic fracture lines.

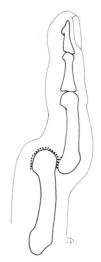

Figure 11–44　The irreducible metacarpal phalangeal dislocation.

is thus alleviated, and pressure and tension on the adjacent neurovascular bundle is relieved, preventing permanent distal vascular and neurologic loss. A long delay makes reduction more difficult because of local tissue edema and fibrosis, further hemorrhage, muscle spasm and contracture. Bone necrosis may occur if there is delay in reduction.

The primary physician can reduce most dislocated joints by placing manual traction on the extremity distal to the dislocation. Muscle spasm and local pain must be adequately controlled by sufficient analgesia. Relaxation then allows muscle and tissue stretching after traction is applied. After reduction, stability is obtained by the articular surfaces and soft parts. Surgical intervention may be required if the joint is unstable after reduction. Methods used include wire fixation across the joint, skeletal traction, ligament repair and plaster dressings.

Commonly Missed Dislocations

Every primary physician should be aware of the *commonly missed* dislocations. These include: posterior dislocation of the shoulder, volar dislocation of the carpal lunate, dislocation of the radial head associated with an ulnar shaft fracture and posterior dislocation of the hip associated with a femoral shaft fracture.

Posterior Shoulder Dislocation (Fig. 11–45). This condition should be suspected in a patient who presents with limited motion, crepitation and pain about the shoulder, who has a history of a recent seizure or a fall on the shoulder. The examination may be equivocal because of swelling and hemorrhage, and because the glenoid may be caught by the infracture which is present on the anterior aspect of the humeral head. The standard anterior-posterior and lateral shoulder x-rays may be reported as normal. The diagnosis is made by an axillary x-ray view of the shoulder, in which the posterior dislocation and the extent of the associated anterior infracture of the humeral head are recognized. Closed reduction and immobilization for three weeks is satisfactory for most patients if the diagnosis and reduction are accomplished promptly.

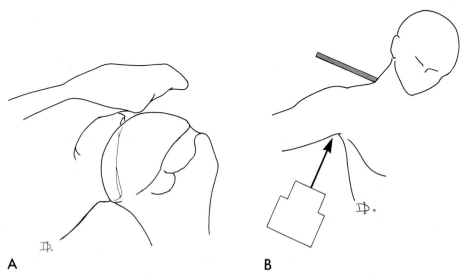

A   **B**

Figure 11–45   Posterior shoulder dislocation. *A.* Anatomy. *B.* Axillary x-ray technique.

Volar Dislocation of the Lunate. Primary physicians examining x-rays of the wrist need a review of the normal relationships of the carpal bones to avoid missing volar dislocation of the lunate. The diagrams demonstrate the normal position and the dislocated position of the lunate as seen on the lateral roentgenogram (Fig. 11–46). This bone can be reduced by placing traction on the hand with the wrist dorsiflexed. Pressure is then applied over the volar surface of the displaced lunate. The wrist is flexed while traction continues. The relationship between the lunate and the navicular may be disrupted and separated after reduction. Median nerve symptoms may be present, but they usually disappear after a prompt reduction. Another easily missed injury of the wrist is the transnavicular perilunar dislocation (Fig. 11–47). The capitate and distal pole of the navicular are dorsally displaced, leaving the lunate and proximal pole of navicular articulating with the distal radius. After reduction by straight traction the proximal and distal fragments of the navicular may be unstable and in unsatisfactory alignment. In this case open reduction and internal fixation is indicated to align and maintain the fragments. Malalignment of the carpal navicular fragment regularly results in nonunion.

Dislocation of the Radial Head. Dislocation of the radial head is often associated with a fracture of the ulnar shaft

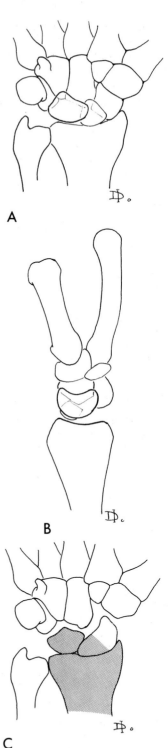

A

B

C

Figure 11–47 Transnavicular perilunar dislocation. *A.* AP view before reduction. *B.* Lateral prereduction view. *C.* Postreduction.

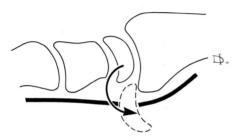

Figure 11–46 Dislocation of the lunate.

(Fig. 11–48). The primary physician will not miss this diagnosis if he obtains an x-ray of the joints proximal and distal to the fracture. X-ray of the elbow demonstrates volar or dorsal displacement of the radial head. Reduction is usually obtained easily and is begun by applying longitudinal traction to the extended elbow. Direct force is then placed over the radial head. Reduction is completed and maintained by flexing the elbow and keeping it flexed. The associated ulnar shaft fracture requires internal fixation. An isolated subluxation of the radial head ("nursemaid's elbow") cannot be recognized by x-ray. The patient presents with a history of having recently been lifted up in the air by the hand. The child keeps the hand in pronation and complains of pain in the extremity. He refuses to move the elbow. Treatment is simple. The physician grasps the child's hand and gently supinates the child's forearm. Immediate relief is obtained when reduction is completed and no further treatment is indicated.

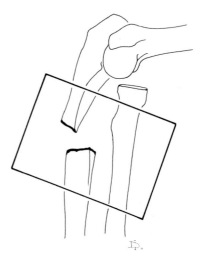

Figure 11–48 Dislocation of the radial head associated with fracture of ulna.

The isolated displaced angulated fractured radius in an adult is accompanied by varying degrees of disruption of the distal radial ulnar joint (Fig. 11–49). X-rays of the joints below the fracture are needed to recognize the distal injury. Internal fixation of the radius may aid in reduction of the distal radial ulnar joint, but does not protect against late development of painful degenerative arthritis.

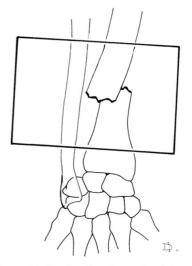

Figure 11–49 Displaced angulated fractured radius associated with disruption of distal radial ulnar joint.

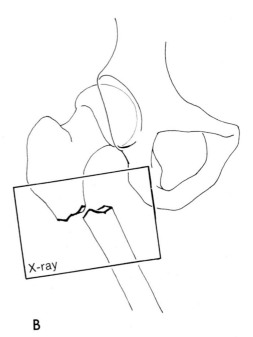

Posterior Dislocation of the Hip (Fig. 11–50). This is frequently associated with a femoral shaft fracture. The proximal femoral shaft fragment will be adducted in these cases. An x-ray of the joint above the fracture confirms the dislocation. Open reduction of the hip is performed because traction applied to the distal femoral fragment and leg may not be sufficient to obtain a reduction.

Common, Easily Recognized Dislocations

The common, easily recognized dislocations of the elbow, shoulder, hip, knee, subtalar and metatarsal tarsal joints will be considered next.

Figure 11–50 Posterior dislocation of the hip associated with femoral shaft fracture. *A*. Lateral view. *B*. AP view.

Posterior Lateral Dislocation of the Elbow (Fig. 11–51). This is a rather alarming deformity when seen initially. It may occur in all age groups following forced hyperextension of the elbow. There may also be an associated fracture of the radial head or coronoid process, and in the younger age groups, an avulsion fracture of the medial epicondyle. If the median nerve is stretched while the elbow is dislocated paresthesias occur which resolve with reduction. Intravenous lidocaine is excellent analgesia to aid the reduction. Traction is first applied on the forearm, with counter traction on the arm. The elbow is brought into extension and out of varus or valgus alignment to a neutral position. The reduction is accomplished by pressure applied over the olecranon while traction is maintained and flexion of the elbow is carried out. Further flexion to 90 degrees maintains the reduction. A posterior splint with cuff and collar is applied for three weeks. This allows capsular healing and prevents a lesser force from redislocating the joint. Return of normal motion may be slow, and residual loss of extension of the elbow may occur owing to capsular scarring. Recurrent dislocation is unusual.

Anterior Dislocation of the Shoulder. The most common dislocation seen on our service is anterior dislocation of the shoulder (Fig. 11–52). The patient comes to the Emergency Room holding the involved arm with his opposite hand, with the dislocated shoulder in a few degrees of internal rotation. Pain and muscle spasm are present. The glenoid is palpated through the deltoid muscle and the humeral head is palpated anterior and inferior to its usual position. The ulnar nerve and axillary nerve are commonly stretched in the axilla. The patient is placed supine on a cart (Fig. 11–53). Traction and counter traction are applied by securing the patient to the cart with a sheet wrapped around the axilla. Traction is gradually applied to the arm and maintained with the shoulder in about 30 degrees of abduction. If prolonged traction is required, it is helpful to wrap a sheet around the waist

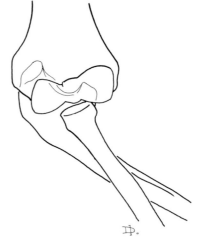

Figure 11–51 Posterior lateral dislocation of the elbow.

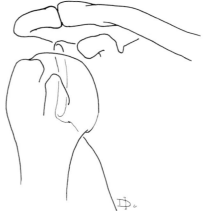

Figure 11–52 Anterior dislocation of the shoulder.

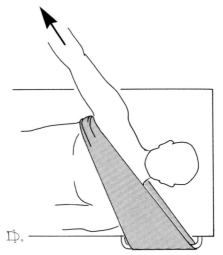

Figure 11–53 Reduction of anterior dislocation of shoulder.

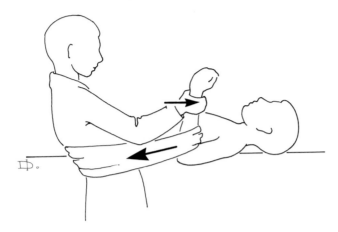

Figure 11–54 Alternate technique for reduction of anterior shoulder dislocation.

of the surgeon and the forearm of the patient (Fig. 11–54). Sufficient analgesia to relieve muscle spasm is accomplished with IV Valium and Demerol. Occasionally the glenoid rim will become an obstruction to reduction in a strong, muscular patient or in a patient with a large impacted fracture or infracture of the posterior aspect of the humeral head. In these cases, an interscalene block or general anesthesia is required. A sling and swathe or stockinette to prevent external rotation is advised for three weeks after the first dislocation. Any sensory and motor loss, if present, usually subsides after prompt reduction.

Posterior Dislocation of the Hip. A person sitting in a car which is involved in an accident frequently strikes his knee on the dashboard and dislocates his hip posteriorly (Fig 11–55). The force of the impact is transmitted along the shaft of the femur to the posterior aspect of the hip joint. The posterior capsule tears or the posterior acetabular lip fractures and the femoral head exits from the joint. As this happens an unknown amount of the articular cartilage of the femoral head is damaged (Fig. 11–56). When the patient is seen in the Emergency Room he is usually lying supine on a cart. He refuses to extend the involved hip, which is held in flexion, adduction and internal rotation. Sciatic nerve symptoms and signs may be present, and frequently do not resolve after reduction. Prompt reduction is indicated. Intravenous Valium and Demerol may

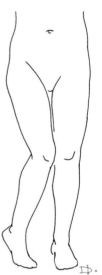

Figure 11–55 Posterior dislocation of the hip — position of the patient.

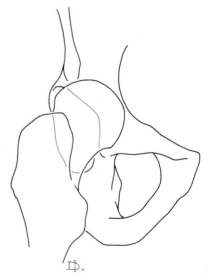

Figure 11–56 Posterior dislocation of the hip — anatomy (AP view).

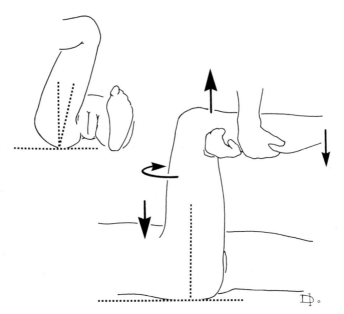

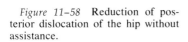

Figure 11–57 Reduction of posterior dislocation of the hip with assistance.

be sufficient for analgesia and relaxation. Reduction is accomplished simply if the primary physician can enlist the help of other personnel (Fig. 11–57). The pelvis is held on a stretcher while traction is applied to the femur with the hip flexed 90 degrees, adducted 10 to 20 degrees, and internally rotated 5 to 10 degrees. The knee is flexed to allow for a better hold on the leg when traction is applied. If no strong assistants are available, turn the patient prone, allowing the hips to flex over the side of the cart (Fig. 11–58). The knee is flexed

and pressure applied to the posterior calf. This produces traction along the shaft of the femur. A reduction can then be obtained by rotating the femur slightly. Occasionally these methods fail, and a muscle relaxant and general anesthesia are required. After reduction, active exercises are initiated, avoiding extremes of flexion. While resting, the patient maintains the hip in extension until the capsule is healed. Aseptic necrosis of the femoral head may follow this injury, so the patient should be followed closely for at least three years.

Figure 11–58 Reduction of posterior dislocation of the hip without assistance.

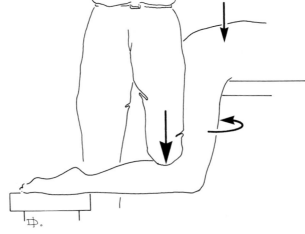

Knee Dislocation. The problem of knee dislocation is discussed in some detail so that the primary physician will not miss the associated vascular injury. *Anterior dislocation* (Fig. 11–59) follows hyperextension of the knee. First, the posterior capsule tears, followed by a tear of the posterior cruciate ligament. The tibia then slides forward on the femur and comes to rest anterior to the distal femur. A *posterior dislocation of the knee* (Fig. 11–60) occurs when force displaces the proximal tibia posterior to the femoral condyles. Complete dislocations may occur in both medial and lateral positions. The cruciate ligaments are torn in all of these injuries, although one collateral ligament may remain intact owing to rotation. Closed reduction of these dislocations is usually possible except in a posterior lateral dislocation when the femoral condyle buttonholes through the retinaculum and extensor mechanism. Open reduction is then required. The primary physician applies longitudinal traction which results in reduction, and then immediately concerns himself with the associated vascular injury. Immediate exploration of the popliteal space is recommended to verify and repair arterial damage if there is any question of the blood supply distal to the recently dislocated knee. In these cases the collateral ligaments are usually torn from their femoral insertion. Closed treatment of the collateral ligaments is adequate if the surgical repair is delayed. However, residual instability in the anterior posterior plane will leave the patient with an unstable knee.

Dislocation of the Talocalcaneal or Subtalar joint (Fig. 11–61). Usually medial in position, this dislocation produces marked deformity of the foot. Traction applied to the heel and forefoot in alignment with the tibial shaft brings about the reduction. If the reduction is stable a weight-bearing short leg plaster dressing should be worn for four weeks.

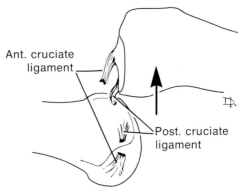

Ant. cruciate ligament

Post. cruciate ligament

Figure 11–59 Anterior dislocation of the knee.

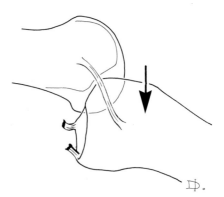

Figure 11–60 Posterior dislocation of the knee.

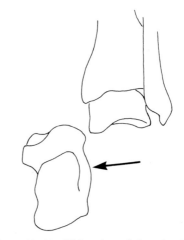

Figure 11–61 Dislocation of the talocalcaneal or subtalar joint.

Talonavicular Dislocation. The talo-navicular dislocation is unstable after reduction (Fig. 11–62). A K-wire across the joint is usually required to maintain the reduction. The navicular is frequently fractured. A short, non-weight-bearing plaster dressing is recommended for six weeks prior to removal of the K-wire. The early presence of residual pain directs the physician to recommend fusion of the joint.

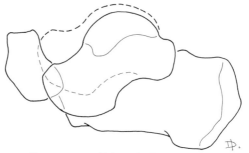

Figure 11–62   Talonavicular dislocation.

Tarsal-metatarsal Dislocations (Fig. 11–63). Dislocation between the base of the metatarsals and the tarsal bones is occasionally accompanied by a fracture at the base of one of the metatarsals. The associated tearing of the dorsalis pedis artery and gross swelling may obscure the deformity. Adequate roentgenograms are essential to establish the diagnosis. A closed reduction is obtained by traction and inversion force on the forefoot and local pressure over the base of the metatarsal. Steinmann pin fixation may be necessary to hold the reduction. Painful degenerative arthritis may follow this injury.

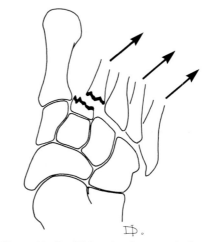

Figure 11–63   Dislocation between the base of metatarsals and tarsal bones.

FRACTURES

The physician treating a patient with a fracture should follow a logical course of thinking. We utilize an approach which we refer to as the *"four R's" of fracture therapy:*[5]

1. Recognition
2. Reduction
3. Retention
4. Restoration of Function

Different problems occur during each step in the patient's management. Additional information regarding the management of fractures may be obtained in the texts prepared by Blount (1955)[1] and Charnley (1967).[2]

Recognition of the fracture includes a description of the anatomic site, not merely the name of the bone. The fracture geography is outlined from roentgenograms. Is the fracture transverse, oblique, spiral, or comminuted (Fig. 11–64)? Is there a butterfly fragment?

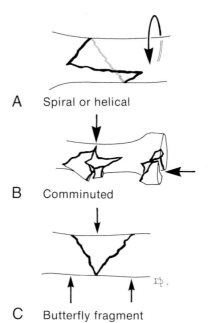

A   Spiral or helical

B   Comminuted

C   Butterfly fragment

Figure 11–64   Recognition of the fracture geography—types of fractures. *A.* Spiral. *B.* Comminuted. *C.* Oblique.

The fracture deformity is illustrated by the roentgenogram. Is there angulation, overriding, displacement, distraction, impaction, or rotation (Fig. 11–65)? *Reduction* or the removal of fracture deformity is planned in relation to the physician's plan for *retention* or maintenance of reduction. The final phase of fracture management is *restoration* of function, which is also the responsibility of the primary physician who treats a patient with a fracture. Fracture management is not complete when fracture union has occurred, but should continue until maximal rehabilitation of function is achieved.

Recognition

If the patient has multiple injuries, is unconsicous, has a language barrier, or is influenced by drugs or extreme pain, the doctor depends on a good physical and roentgenographic examination. Appropriate splinting is necessary before x-rays are taken, to prevent excessive pain and further damage to soft tissue. The splint must be applied in such a way that adequate x-rays can be obtained with the splint in place, and the splinting material must be easily penetrated by x-rays so that a fracture line will not be obscured. Well-padded balsa held to the extremity by a soft circular dressing is adequate for most fractures. A telescoping aluminum Thomas splint with Velcro straps and a windlass for traction is used for a fracture of the femur. This becomes extremely useful when a patient must be moved several times before arriving in his own bed.

The proper x-rays must be ordered to allow the radiologist and the primary physician to maintain a good diagnostic average. Anterior-posterior, lateral and oblique views of bones and joints are routinely obtained. I have also found that additional views often reveal a fracture or dislocation not seen on the routine roentgenogram.

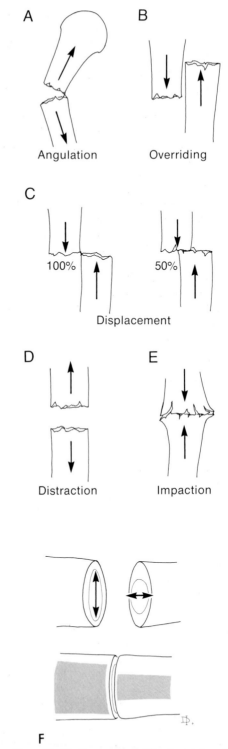

Figure 11–65 Recognition of fracture deformity *A.* Angulation. *B.* Overriding. *C.* Displacement. *D.* Distraction. *E.* Impaction. *F.* Rotation.

Special x-rays to detect fractures include:

1. *Axillary View of the Shoulder* (Fig. 11–66). Abduction of the shoulder in the supine or sitting position may be painful for the patient after injury to the shoulder, but the physician usually can gain adequate abduction for this film. It allows visualization and localization of fractures of the humeral head as well as clearly demonstrating the presence or absence of a dislocation.

2. *Multiple Views of the Radial Head* (Fig. 11–67 *A* and *B*). If routine films are normal in a patient with localized pain over the radial head, multiple views from full pronation to full supination may be helpful in identifying an undisplaced fracture.

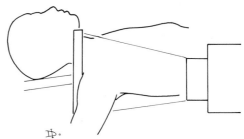

Figure 11–66   Axillary view of the shoulder.

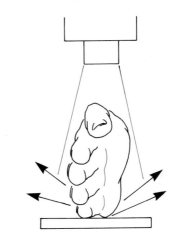

Figure 11–67   Multiple views of the radial head. *A*. Partial pronation. *B*. Full pronation.

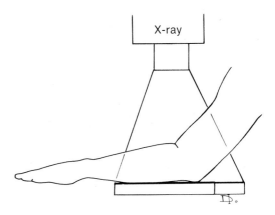

3. Navicular View of the Wrist (Fig. 11–68). Fracture of the navicular is regularly overlooked on standard AP, lateral and oblique views of the wrist. Localized tenderness over the navicular should alert the primary physician to avoid the casual diagnosis of sprained wrist. The long axis of the navicular is brought into view in the special x-ray technique shown here. When a diagnosis of fracture of the carpal navicular is suspected, the patient should be treated in plaster for two to four weeks. A repeat navicular view is then obtained. If a fracture is present, resorption of the fracture site will have begun and recognition is no longer a problem.

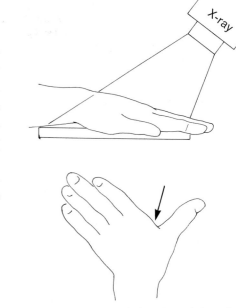

Figure 11–68   Navicular view of the wrist.

4. Carpal Tunnel View of the Wrist (Fig. 11–69). The bony margins of the carpal canal can be clearly visualized on a roentgenogram by requesting a carpal tunnel view. Fractures of the hook of the hamate and the distal pole of the navicular come into view with this technique. The carpal tunnel view should be obtained in patients with pain localized in this area.

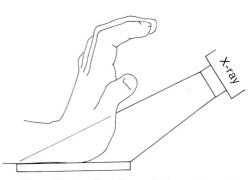

Figure 11–69   Carpal tunnel view of the wrist.

5. Posterior Oblique View of the Acetabulum (Fig. 11–70). This view aids in visualization of the posterior rim of the acetabulum, when tomograms are not available to visualize a fracture dislocation of the hip.

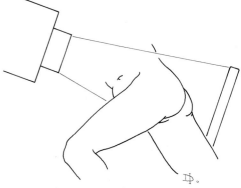

Figure 11–70   Posterior oblique view of the acetabulum.

6. Patellar or Sunrise View of the Knee
(Fig. 11–71).   A critical problem, after
an acute dislocation of the patella,
is the recognition of an osteochondral
fracture of the medial facet of the patella.
The relationship of the patella to the
femoral condyle may also be useful in
establishing the etiology of recurrent
subluxation of the patella.

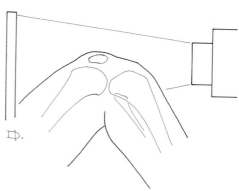

Figure 11–71   Patellar or sunrise view of the
knee.

7. Notch View of the Knee (Fig. 11–72).
The femoral condyles extend below
and posterior to the intercondylar notch.
Therefore, a loose body lodged in this
area may block the motion of the knee
but may not be seen clearly until the
notch view is obtained.

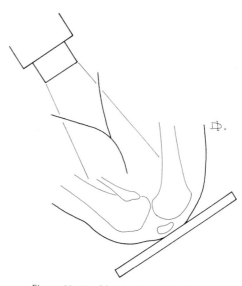

Figure 11–72   Notch view of the knee.

8. Ankle Mortise View (Fig. 11–73).
This may be a routine view of the ankle
in some hospitals. It demonstrates the
relationship of the medial malleolus
with the comma-shaped medial articular
surface of the talus, and the relationship of the distal tibial–fibular joint. An
oblique view of the ankle nicely demonstrates the inferior sag of the anterior
portion of a medial malleolus fracture.

9. X-ray of the Uninjured Extremity.
In children one must not forget that an
x-ray of the uninjured extremity will
show the normal relationship of the
epiphysis, secondary ossification centers,
apophysis and patterns of the epiphyseal
plates, if there is any doubt about the
normal anatomy.

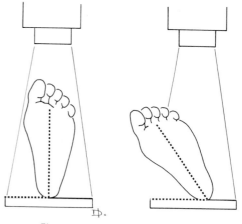

Figure 11–73   Ankle mortise view.

10. *"Fat Pad Sign" of Fractured Elbow.*
A lateral x-ray of the elbow which
demonstrates a positive "fat pad sign"
(radiolucency posterior to the olecranon
fossa) (Fig. 11–74) indicates a bloody
synovial effusion and raises the physician's index of suspicion regarding
fracture. If no fracture is seen, repeat
films two to three weeks later may reveal
the previously undetected fracture line.

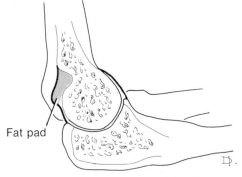

Fat pad

Figure 11–74　Lateral x-ray of the elbow.

Reduction

The second *"R"* of fracture therapy
refers to reduction of the fracture. The
primary physician must decide if reduction is necessary or possible. Obviously, the undisplaced fracture needs
no reduction, only protection from loss
of reduction.

Fractures Not Requiring Reduction.
The following fractures rarely need a
formal reduction. The first is a *comminuted fracture of the calcaneus* which
can rarely be reduced satisfactorily.
Immediate weight-bearing is begun in a
short leg walking plaster, and triple
arthrodesis is performed later if symptoms are prolonged and severe. The
metatarsal shaft fracture rarely requires reduction, because the soft tissues of the foot maintain a satisfactory
alignment and rotation. The *clavicle
fracture* maintains an intact sleeve of
periosteum and though widely displaced,
union is expected to occur. The most
common fracture of the forearm of children, a *torus fracture,* or outward buckling of the cortex, does not require reduction. This is also true of many *avulsion fractures* not involving the adjacent
joint function. Nondisplaced *stress
fractures* do not require reduction.

Indications for Open Reduction. At
the other end of the spectrum, generally
speaking, fractures which enter a joint
cartilage surface or cross a growing
epiphyseal plate require not only reduction but open reduction. Open reduction and internal fixation are required

in many cases to obtain and maintain
an anatomic position.

Methods. Traction in line with the
longitudinal axis of the long bone is the
most common method of reduction used
in overcoming fracture deformity. This
may cause the fracture to lose its intrinsic stability, and retention of this
position becomes difficult.

Analgesia is usually important in the
manipulations required to remove fracture deformity. In many cases intravenous meperidine (Demerol) will give
satisfactory analgesia. Intravenous diazepam (Valium) depresses a patient
to the point where some muscle relaxation is obtained. Valium also produces
temporary amnesia. This method is helpful in fractured tibia and ankle fractures
in the adult.

Fractures in the hand and foot are
managed by digital block or injection of
lidocaine directly into the fracture site.

I would like to suggest strongly that
IV block is a prompt, safe method of
anesthesia in the management of almost
all closed upper extremity fractures in
children and many adults.[4] It is very
satisfactory for outpatient use (see p.
351).

When a primary physician has adequate analgesia and a reduction is to be
performed he must understand and be
able to overcome fracture deformities
which are not relieved with simple traction. I have found that, in a young child,

INTRAVENOUS BLOCK TECHNIQUE

A blood pressure cuff is secured to the arm. A small scalp vein needle with attached five cubic centimeter saline syringe is inserted into the most distal vein that can be found and taped into place, usually on the dorsum of the hand. The arm is elevated for two minutes, the tourniquet elevated to 200 millimeters of mercury. Lidocaine one-third per cent is then injected in a dose of 0.25 cc per pound of body weight (Fig. 11–75). The needle is removed. After five minutes anesthesia is complete. The fracture or dislocation is reduced, and the plaster applied. The tourniquet is released. Normal sensation and motor function return within five minutes.

the periosteum is torn at the apex of the fracture deformity and may remain intact on the concave surface (Fig. 11–76). In a completely overriding, displaced *forearm fracture* this intact periosteum prevents a reduction when longitudinal traction is used alone. It is essential to exaggerate the deformity, push the distal fragment until the intact periosteum is tight, and bring the distal fragment into alignment with the proximal fragment. The fracture then hinges about the intact periosteum.

Metaphyseal fractures in the distal forearm or distal tibia in children commonly have rotational components. These require a specific rotational stress to bring about an anatomic reduction.

Intact collateral ligaments may stabilize a fracture fragment close to a joint. In the case of a transverse fracture of a proximal phalanx, the collateral ligaments of the metacarpal phalangeal joint of the index, long, ring or little finger allow no rotation or further flexion of the proximal fragments when held in 90 degrees of flexion. The distal fragments can now be brought into alignment with it. The dressing can be applied and immobilization maintained in this position until the fracture is stable.

The use of *Chinese finger traps* on the thumb and index finger or great toe can be useful when no assistance is available to hold an arm or leg while a carefully molded plaster is applied.

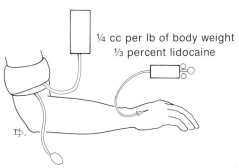

¼ cc per lb of body weight
⅓ percent lidocaine

Figure 11–75 IV block (intravenous lidocaine with arterial tourniquet).

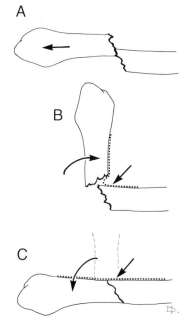

A

B

C

Figure 11–76 Forearm fracture with intact periosteum interfering with reduction.

Retention

The third *"R"* of fracture therapy includes the various methods of stabilizing the reduced fracture while healing takes place. Any immobilized part atrophies and new plaster dressings are indicated when looseness is apparent. The following types of retention are applied in the Emergency Room and are utilized until the fracture is stable enough to allow active exercises.

  1. *Hanging Arm Plaster. Materials:*
    1. Two rolls of 4″ plaster of Paris
    2. Webril or sheet wadding
    3. Stockinette for cuff and collar
    4. Four safety pins

Application (Fig. 11–77). The upper limit of the plaster does not have to reach the axilla or even extend above the fracture site but must immobilize the elbow at 90 degrees of flexion. The plaster extends distally across the wrist and palm but allows full metacarpal phalangeal motion. By shortening or lengthening the collar the angulation of the fracture is corrected in one plane. In the other plane angulation is corrected by moving the ring towards the palm or dorsal surface of the plaster. If more than two rolls of plaster are applied the weight may be excessive. This may serve to distract the fracture and is an undesirable feature of this technique. The patient must sleep sitting up in a chair the first few nights. Circumduction exercises are allowed early as pain subsides. When associated radial nerve palsies are present, active assist splints are applied to the plaster, helping to maintain contracture-free metacarpal phalangeal joints.

  2. *Plaster Leg Cylinder. Materials:*
    1. Benzoin or Ace adherent spray to secure tape to skin
    2. 3″ white tape rolls
    3. Stockinette to fit closely over the leg from groin to ankle
    4. Webril or sheet wadding to pad and protect the leg
    5. Three rolls of 6″ or 8″ plaster dressing

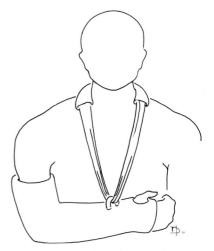

Figure 11–77   Hanging arm plaster.

· *Application* (Fig. 11–78). The stockinette is applied from the groin to the ankle. The lower half is turned and pulled above the knee, exposing the skin for application of the medial and lateral tapes. The tape, cut long enough to be turned back into the plaster when it is applied, prevents pistoning of the cylinder, a key feature in the successful use of this dressing.

3. *Short Leg Walking Plaster Dressing.*
Materials:
1. Stockinette
2. Sheet wadding or Webril to protect bony prominences
3. Three rolls of 4″ plaster and two rolls of 6″ plaster
4. Walking rubber heel

Application (Fig. 11–79). Stockinette is first applied from the knee to the toes. This is covered by additional sheet wadding or Webril to protect the malleolus, the heel and the peroneal nerve as it crosses superficial to the head of the fibula. This is uniformly covered with the rolls of plaster dressing from the tibial tubercle to the metatarsal phalangeal joint of the foot. A support under the forefoot during the application of the plaster helps maintain the ankle in neutral position and allows additional molding while the plaster is setting. The stockinette is folded back over the upper and lower margins of the plaster and these margins are buried in plaster. The walking heel is applied to the plaster in a line extending from the anterior surface of the tibia distally. Twenty-four hours later the plaster is dry and weight-bearing can be allowed. This utility dressing is safe in wet climates if a plastic bag is put over the entire cast and secured just below the knee.

4. *Long Leg Walking Plaster Dressing.*
Materials:
1. Stockinette
2. Sheet wadding or Webril to protect bony prominences
3. Three rolls of 4″ plaster, two rolls of 6″ plaster and two rolls of 8″ plaster
4. Walking rubber heel

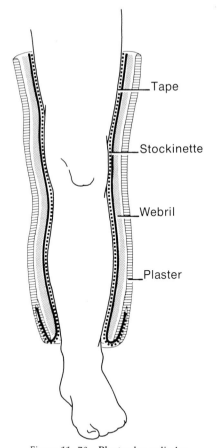

Figure 11–78　Plaster leg cylinder.

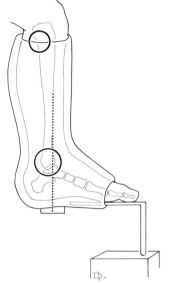

Figure 11–79　Short leg walking plaster dressing.

Application (Fig. 11–80). While the plaster is being applied for an acute tibial shaft fracture, reduction and retention of the fracture can be obtained if the knee is flexed 90 degrees and the leg hangs over the end of the table with gravity assisting in aligning the fragments. While the plaster hardens, the upper limits of this portion of the plaster can be narrowed and compressed in the AP direction. The knee is then extended to neutral and the thigh portion added with a smooth junction between upper and lower segments. Anterior-posterior molding at the knee while the upper portion hardens assures good contact and the immobilization which is needed for comfortable early weight-bearing. A heel and sole lift on the opposite shoe adds to a more balanced gait. When the leg is to be protected from weight-bearing a bent knee plaster is recommended. This type of dressing makes crutch walking and sitting more comfortable. The emphasis, in either case, must be to extend the stockinette, padding and plaster high on the thigh to assure adequate immobilization of the knee.

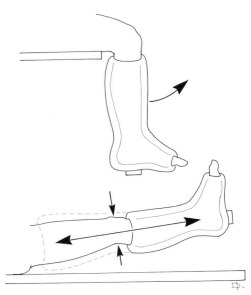

Figure 11–80 Long leg walking plaster dressing.

　　5. *Overhead Olecranon Skeletal Traction. Materials:*
　　1. Sterile Steinmann pin set, gloves and towel
　　2. Sling
　　3. Traction bow
　　4. Ropes, pulley, weights
　　5. Syringes and needles for lidocaine injection

Application (Fig. 11–81). The primary physician frequently must initiate skeletal traction in the Emergency Room, particularly in the widely displaced humeral fracture and the supracondylar fracture of the humerus in children. This technique will both reduce and retain the fracture. The insertion of wires for skeletal traction is carried out under sterile conditions. The skin is prepped with iodophor and draped with four towels, and the skin, muscles and periosteum are infiltrated with lidocaine. The Steinmann pin is inserted from the ulnar side to avoid damaging the ulnar

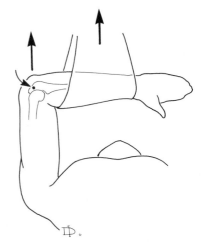

Figure 11–81 Overhead olecranon skeletal traction.

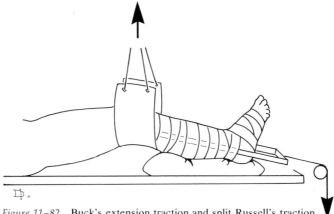

Figure 11–82   Buck's extension traction and split Russell's traction.

nerve, drilling the wire across two cortexes and the medullary canal and placing it close to the long axis of the humerus to avoid extending the elbow when traction is applied. A soft sling balances the forearm and supports the wrist. The elevation obviously aids in reducing swelling.

6. Buck's Extension Traction and Split Russell's Traction for Children. Material:
1. Ace wrap
2. Moleskin and ventform traction tape
3. Ropes, pulleys, weights, slings

Application (Fig. 11–82). Skin traction is applied in the Emergency Room prior to admitting the patient to the ward. In an adult with an intertrochanteric fracture or femoral neck fracture, Buck's extension traction will help reduce pain and muscle spasm when the leg is secured by the traction. The traction should not exceed five or six pounds because the skin will blister or the traction become loosened from the leg and slide down around the ankle.

The knee sling is added for children with femoral shaft fractures, lifting the thigh from the bed. This allows a vector force to come directly in line with the femur. Reduction of the fracture will then gradually occur.

The application of skin traction is successful if moleskin or a ventilated, spongy, hard-backed tape is available.

This material is secured to the skin by an elastic wrap applied carefully, protecting the skin from blistering over the malleolus and the heel. The elastic bandage is wrapped gently over the proximal fibula to avoid a peroneal palsy.

Restoration of Function

Restoration of function begins immediately after retention is applied. Edema and excessive swelling can be averted by elevating the extremity, decreasing risk of ischemia in the muscles of the hands and feet. Constant, prolonged elevation of the injured extremity is most important. Adequate elevation at night is assured with a simple sling applied on the upper extremity (Fig. 11–83). For elevation during the day the ambulatory patient is instructed to carry his hand on top of his head (Fig. 11–84). This is done for approximately one week. It frequently averts the need for bivalving the plaster. In the lower extremity a sling is suspended from the overhead bed frame (Fig. 11–85) which supports the plaster dressing. This supports the leg and foot at least two feet above the level of the chest.

Active motion of the muscles in an injured extremity should begin as soon as possible. When possible, circumduction or pendulum exercises should be

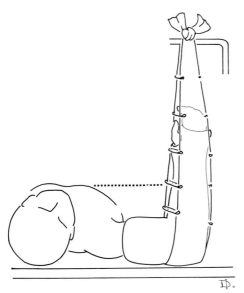

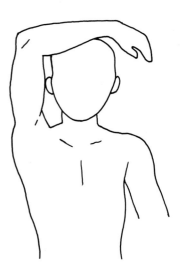

Figure 11–83   Elevation at night with a simple sling.

Figure 11–84   Elevation during the day with hand on head.

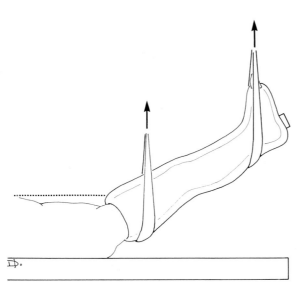

Figure 11–85   Elevation of the lower extremity from the bed frame.

used in all upper extremity fractures to obviate shoulder stiffness by preventing adhesions in the subdeltoid bursa (Fig. 11–86). In the lower extremity a walking plaster allows continued and constant motion of muscles and joints. This has been dramatically useful in the closed walking management of fractured tibia, as described in the tibial fracture section.

In the extremity with nerve deficit, full passive motion of joints is useful to prevent edema and contractures. Joint immobility is maintained and paralyzed muscles are not excessively stressed.

The duration of immobilization of a fracture is not decided on the first day. Changes in the plaster are necessary as swelling or atrophy progesss. I use direct palpation of the fracture site for assistance in the decision as to when to discard the plaster. Local motion, pain or edema indicates replacement of the plaster. The roentgenogram cannot be relied upon completely because frequently only minimal callus can be seen when the fracture is stable enough to begin adjacent joint motion. Fractures of the clavicle, olecranon, carpal navicular and phalanges are typical examples of fractures in which clinical judgment dictates the length of immobilization in plaster.

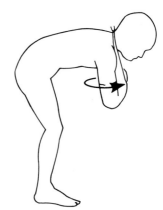

Figure 11–86   Circumduction or pendulum exercises for upper extremity fractures.

SPECIFIC FRACTURES

Scapula (Fig. 11–87)

A severe, direct blow to the shoulder region is required to fracture the scapula. This bone is mobile and well protected by the 17 muscles which originate or insert here. Underlying rib fractures must not be overlooked. Few fractures of the scapula require more than sling immobilization and early active exercises for the shoulder girdle. The return of function is usually quicker than expected. On the other hand, a downward displaced fracture of the acromial process may impede function of the rotator

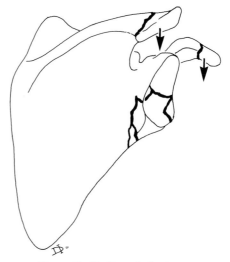

Figure 11–87   Scapula fractures.

cuff. This will require elevation and internal fixation. The widely displaced intra-articular (glenoid) fracture is a rare injury, occurring mainly in young patients, and may necessitate reduction.

Clavicle (Fig. 11–88 A)

The fractured clavicle in children may be severely displaced but will usually retain a sleeve of periosteum between the proximal and distal fragment. Union proceeds without incident along this periosteal sleeve if the patient is treated symptomatically with a figure-of-eight dressing (Fig. 11–88 B) until the fracture is stable by clinical examination. The roentgenographic evidence of solid union requires a prolonged period of time.

In the adult the displaced fracture of the clavicle has classically been managed by a figure-of-eight dressing. Open reduction has been followed by a high rate of nonunion. Damage to the closely approximated neurovascular bundle is rare but the possibility is greater when the first and second ribs are also fractured. A fracture extending obliquely through the distal third of the clavicle requires open reduction. The distal clavicular fragment is held securely in the acromioclavicular joint by the coracoclavicular ligaments. The proximal fragment swings into severe elevation through the trapezius and lies beneath the skin, simulating an acromioclavicular separation. In children the distal clavicle may break out of its periosteal sleeve and rest beneath the skin. Closure of this periosteum about the displaced clavicle is sufficient treatment for this condition.

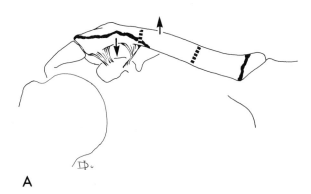

A

Figure 11–88 Clavicle fracture. *A.* Fracture lines. *B.* Figure-of-eight dressing.

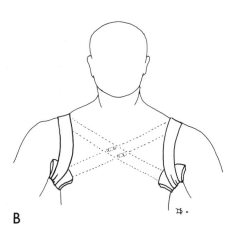

B

Humerus (Fig. 11–89)

The *greater tuberosity* may be displaced by the glenoid rim at the time of an anterior dislocation or subluxation of the shoulder. The attached portion of the rotator cuff containing teres minor, infraspinatus and supraspinatus will also be displaced. After reduction of the shoulder, a return of the tuberosity to its normal position should be demonstrated on two x-ray views. This proves that the cuff is not significantly torn. The injury is managed with a stockinette sling for four to six weeks, allowing bone and soft tissue healing to take place. On the other hand, the rotator cuff may be torn significantly in the direction of its fibers, beginning at the bicipital groove and extending toward the muscle fibers of the supraspinatus. In this case, the displaced greater tuberosity fracture does not return to an anatomic position, but remains posterior to the humerus. This requires open reduction and suturing of the rotator cuff.

The *lesser tuberosity fracture* of the humerus with its attached portion of the rotator cuff containing the subscapularis is occasionally displaced with posterior dislocation of the shoulder. If the displaced fragment is satisfactorily reduced a stockinette sling is the recommended treatment.

The *humeral head* is subject to anterior and posterior infractures, in conjunction with anterior and posterior dislocations of the shoulder. The glenoid rim, after producing this infracture, may become locked in the defect and make reduction of the shoulder more difficult. The axillary x-ray view is helpful in recognizing this injury. Operative treatment is not suggested for these defects unless the patient develops recurrent dislocations of the shoulder. The rare isolated *anatomic neck fracture* which leaves the head free of its attachments may require reduction if displacement is significant.

Surgical Neck of Humerus. A stable fracture without displacement is frequently seen in the osteoporotic patient.

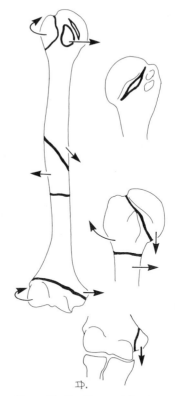

Figure 11–89 Humeral fractures.

A simple sling and early circumduction exercises are encouraged in these patients. If there is angulation and only 50 per cent displacement I place the patient in a light, hanging arm plaster. This is done because attempts at closed reduction often fail or create an unstable situation. Complete range of motion is not expected after union of the fracture, but pain is minimized by active early circumduction and external rotation exercises. Angular deformities frequently recur after closed reduction. If there is complete displacement the pectoralis major muscle is the deforming force and cannot often be dealt with except by olecranon skeletal overhead traction or open reduction.

A shoulder spica may be adequate when applied by those experienced in plaster work but this method is not recommended for routine outpatient use.

The correct alignment of a metaphyseal slip cannot be determined by x-ray in children younger than about four years of age, before the proximal secondary ossification centers of the humerus appear. In these patients the physician must depend upon the rotator cuff locking the epiphysis in an elevated position. The shoulder is swung into the pivotal position by lifting the humerus 180 degrees to a point where the arm is touching the ear and the forearm is resting on top of the head. Traction is applied. Reduction is obtained and the previously placed olecranon skeletal traction wire maintains the arm and shoulder slightly above the salute position. The child is kept in a supine position for two weeks.

The teenager with a mildly proximal angulated metaphyseal slip can be treated comfortably with a hanging arm plaster. Complete reduction is not expected. The double shadow of the epiphyseal plate in a young child may be mistaken for a fracture.

Humerus Shaft Fractures. Fractures in the proximal, middle and distal thirds of the humerus need not be classified as to their complexity. Gentle traction will reduce the angulation and a light, hanging arm plaster will maintain a satisfactory reduction if applied and managed correctly. (See section on hanging arm plaster technique.) Soft tissue interposition may prevent reduction of displacement. Inferior subluxation of the head of the humerus is commonly recognized during treatment but resolves itself when immobilization is discontinued. Mild angular deformities can be accepted. Two to three months may be required for adequate callus to mature and stabilize the fracture before immobilization is discontinued.

Supracondylar Fracture. The minimally displaced or angulated supracondylar fracture is frequently accompanied by an inordinate amount of swelling. Outpatient care is indicated only when an adequately applied posterior splint with a tight collar and cuff can be used. The displaced fracture is dramatic because of the deformity and hemorrhage which follow the injury. The radial and median nerves are frequently contused and the radial pulse may be absent. An axillary block or general anesthesia is utilized when swelling is not excessive. Reduction is accomplished by holding the patient's hand as if to shake it and then extending the elbow and applying longitudinal traction to dislodge the proximal humeral fragment from the brachialis muscle. The physician's fingertips are placed on the distal humeral fragment. Traction is maintained, the elbow is flexed and the distal fragment is pushed forward. The elbow is held in at least 110 degrees of flexion to stabilize the fracture and an x-ray is obtained. Rotation allows unacceptable varus and valgus angulation at the fracture site. If manual reduction is not anatomic or if swelling is excessive, overhead olecranon pin traction is applied to accomplish reduction and maintain a satisfactory alignment. Many of these fractures can be reduced and maintained using a posterior splint with short collar and cuff. At least 24 hours of observation in the hospital will usually permit an early detection of vascular insufficiency to the forearm. Prompt extension of the elbow and consideration of vascular exploration follows. Similar guidelines are appropriate in the adult patient with a displaced fracture.

The *medial epicondyle* is a traction apophysis which serves not only as the origin of the superficial forearm flexor muscle group but also as the proximal attachment of the medial collateral ligament of the elbow. Simple distal displacement of the fragment should be treated by immobilization. It will heal with a fibrous union which is free of epiphyseal plate disturbance and ulnar nerve symptoms. If the medial aspect of the joint is opened, as in a dislocation or extreme valgus deformity of the elbow, the fragment may come to rest in the joint. Removal is then required.

The adjacent trochlea with its irregular ossification center can be mistaken for a fracture. The opposite elbow should be x-rayed for comparison.

The lateral condylar fracture extends

into the articular surface of the capitellum or as far medially as the trochlea. It requires an anatomic reduction to prevent permanent deformity of the elbow. Closed reductions usually fail and are not recommended.

Forearm (Fig. 11–90)

The outpatient care of radial or ulnar shaft fractures in adults is recommended only for stable undisplaced fractures. A long arm plaster is applied to prevent pronation and supination of the forearm which may lead to loss of reduction.

A displaced, unstable fracture of both bones of the forearm in an adult cannot be managed on an outpatient basis because reduction cannot be maintained in plaster. Open reduction and internal fixation with compression plates is recommended.

The rule about obtaining roentgenograms of the joint above and below the fracture applies also in the forearm. Dislocation of the radial head with an ulnar shaft fracture and dislocation of the distal ulna with an isolated fracture of the radius must not be overlooked. These associated dislocations necessitate internal fixation of single bone fractures in the forearm.

The isolated significantly displaced fracture of either the radial shaft or ulnar shaft is best treated by plate fixation, as union of the ulna may be delayed and nonunion of the radius leaves the forearm with significant loss of function.

The *Colles' fracture* (Fig. 11–91) with its associated ulnar styloid avulsion presents a challenge in the last "*R*" of fracture therapy, restoration of function. In the elderly, osteoporotic patient the reduction is gained under IV lidocaine block, by traction and volar displacement of the comminuted distal radial fragment. Then, with the elbow flexed to 90 degrees, a ten-layer splint, previously measured, cut and moistened, is placed inside a stockinette. The splint extends to the metacarpal phalangeal joint on

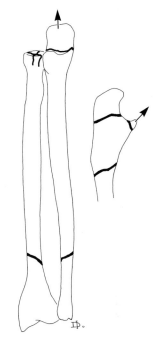

Figure 11–90 Forearm fractures.

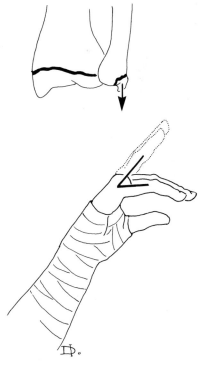

Figure 11–91 Colles' fracture.

the dorsum of the hand. It is brought around the elbow and then up along the volar surface of the forearm to reach the midpalmar area. The thumb and metacarpal phalangeal joints have complete freedom for active and passive motion. The wrist is in twenty degrees of flexion and ten degrees of ulnar deviation; too much flexion precipitates a median nerve compression. A mildly tight elastic wrap secures the splints to the arm and hand, which must be immediately and continuously elevated. The patient is given a night splint to maintain hand elevation during the sleeping hours. The Ace wrap is adjusted to secure uniform pressure as the hand and forearm swell or edema subsides. Immediate active finger and shoulder motion is started.

Perfect initial reduction may be lost in the elderly patient owing to the comminuted metaphyseal fragments. As swelling decreases better immobilization is obtained by a short arm circular plaster which is removed after five or six weeks. Restoration of function is stressed to the patient at all times. The young patient who has this fracture extending into the wrist joint needs a careful anatomic reduction maintained by skeletal wires in the second and third metacarpal and proximal ulna or radius. Open reduction may be indicated.

Forearm Fractures in Children. The undisplaced fracture without angulation becomes a simple matter of applying a short arm, well-molded plaster dressing and waiting for sufficient mature callus formation before removal of the plaster. A torus fracture or outward buckling of the cortex falls into the above category. It is the most frequent forearm fracture in children.

Children with angulated and displaced forearm fractures are managed as outpatients. Satisfactory reductions are obtained if analgesia is complete. This has been accomplished in our Emergency Room by the use of IV lidocaine block in closed fractures and dislocations of the forearm.

The *distal radial epiphyseal slip* in a child's forearm is a fracture along the zone of provisional calcification, frequently with a small metaphyseal fragment remaining attached to the dorsal surface of the epiphysis. The physician must use some care to avoid further damage to the epiphyseal plate. After satisfactory dense anesthesia, traction is applied in the direction of the distal fragment to loosen the two fragments. Increasing the deformity may be necessary. Then with direct pressure over the distal radial epiphysis (Fig. 11–92) and traction on the hand, the wrist is brought into extreme flexion. Usually the epiphysis then slides back toward its nor-

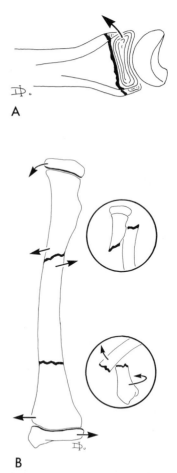

Figure 11–92 Radial fractures. *A.* Distal radial epiphyseal fracture in children. *B.* Other fractures of the radius.

mal position. Mild angular deformity and displacement is acceptable and is often advisable, since repeated manipulation may injure the epiphyseal plate. A well-molded short arm plaster will maintain this stable reduction. Immobilization for four to six weeks allows stable healing.

Fracture of Both Bones of the Forearm. Marked deformity is observed in angulated and completely displaced fractures at the middle and distal thirds of the forearm. After dense analgesia by IV lidocaine, a series of three maneuvers is performed. First, the fracture deformity is increased to 90 degrees of angulation. Second, mild traction is applied and the physician's thumb is placed at the apex or concavity of the deformity. The distal fragment is then moved distally to correct displacement and obtain adequate length. Third, the distal fragment is brought into alignment with the proximal fragment, the intact portion of the periosteum being used here as a hinge. After reduction it lends some stability to the fracture. The postreduction roentgenogram allows comparison of the thickness of the cortex proximal and distal to the fracture site, a discrepancy indicating rotational deformity which is unacceptable. Then the patient is placed in a long arm plaster with the forearm in a neutral position regarding pronation and supination. Eight to twelve weeks is usually an adequate period of immobilization. Weekly roentgenograms are obtained to check for recurrence of angular deformity.

Fractures of both bones in the proximal one-third of the forearm in children tend to angulate and open reduction may be required.

The volarly angulated undisplaced *fracture of the junction of the middle and distal one-third of the radius* in a child can present a problem in retention. Reduction is easily performed with IV block analgesia but often the fracture will tend to reangulate when the reducing force is removed. By overcorrecting the deformity the physician can snap the intact periosteum, or he

may place the forearm in full pronation and apply a well-molded long arm plaster. Both may aid in preventing recurrence of deformity. Weekly check films alert the physician to recurrence of deformity.

A radial neck fracture in a child with an angular deformity of less than twenty degrees is usually acceptable. Reduction is accomplished by direct pressure on the head of the radius associated with pronation and supination of the forearm. When the angular deformity is more than 50 degrees open reduction is necessary. Do not remove the radial head in children.

Wrist (Fig. 11–93)

Navicular. A young adult who has fallen on his outstretched hand will frequently present with pain in the wrist. A normal x-ray may lead to the erroneous diagnosis of a "sprained wrist." This patient should be placed in a short arm plaster for two to three weeks and the x-ray repeated out of plaster. Navicular views should be obtained. If a fracture is present, bone resorption will have occurred and the fracture will be visible for the first time. After the fracture has been recognized and the absence of displacement has been verified, a short arm plaster should be applied with thumb, index, and long finger immobilized. This will give adequate stability for healing. Prolonged plaster immobilization may be required to establish union. Aseptic necrosis of the proximal fragment usually leads to limited

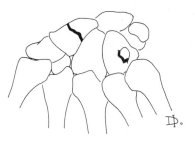

Figure 11–93 Carpal fractures.

wrist motion with pain at extremes if it is not promptly replaced by living bone. Wrist fusion may follow if symptoms are severe. Navicular fracture, when associated with a perilunar dislocation, may require internal fixation to stabilize the fracture during healing.

Hamate. The hook of the hamate can be fractured at its base. The carpal tunnel view will demonstrate the fracture. Simple recognition and immobilization are all that is usually required.

Triquetrum. A fracture of this bone results from a direct blow or in association with a transnavicular perilunar dislocation. Simple plaster immobilization is suggested.

Femur (Fig. 11–94)

Fractures of the femur in children and adults are not routinely handled on an outpatient basis. These fractures have a large associated blood loss and considerable pain with motion. It is almost mandatory to handle them in a hospital, where portable x-rays are easily obtained, and prolonged traction and bed care are available.

Small chip or avulsion fractures are the only femoral fractures which can be treated in the outpatient department.

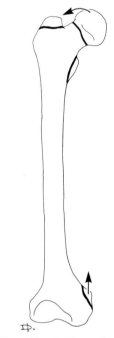

Figure 11–94   Femur fractures.

Patella (Fig. 11–95)

Most *patella fractures* result from a direct blow to the anterior aspect of the knee. If the articular surface is undisplaced and the adjacent extensor retinaculum is intact we place these patients in plaster cylinders and start early weight-bearing. After four to five weeks the fracture is united and quadriceps exercises are begun. The bipartate patella may be mistaken for a fresh fracture when there is a fibrous union in the upper outer quadrant between the patella and smaller secondary ossification center.

Widely displaced or highly comminuted fractures are treated by patellectomy, plaster and early weight-bearing.

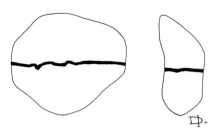

Figure 11–95   Patella fracture.

Tibia (Fig. 11–96)

Tibial Plateau. Anterior tibial spine fractures result from avulsion of bone by the anterior cruciate ligament. If extension of the knee brings the fragment back to its normal position a plaster cylinder is adequate treatment. Open reduction may be advisable if displacement is not reduced. The posterior cruciate ligament occasionally avulses a piece of bone from the posterior aspect of the tibial plateau, but more often the ligament is torn at its tibial attachment.

A fracture downward from the tibial articular surface into the *tibial plateau* without significant displacement is protected by a plaster cylinder dressing until soft tissues heal. Progressive active motion is then initiated. Protection from weight-bearing is necessary for six weeks in an unstable fracture. Since minimally displaced, simple fractures can be associated with extreme swelling and hemorrhage, careful observation is most important.

Associated collateral ligament injuries of the knee are common with tibial plateau fractures. A small avulsion chip fragment along the lateral tibial plateau and on the proximal fibula suggests a disruption of the lateral collateral ligament and iliotibial band. The younger patient with spreading of the plateaus or downward displacement of one plateau is treated by open reduction, followed by a cast brace to allow early motion and weight-bearing.

Tibial Shaft. Closed fracture of the shaft of the tibia is reduced in the Emergency Room and the patient is hospitalized to assure that elevation is maintained and swelling is not excessive, and to allow early weight-bearing under the direction of a physical therapist.

To obtain the reduction the supine patient is moved toward the end of the cart far enough to allow ninety degrees of knee flexion. The knee is allowed to flex over the end of the cart with the foot hanging free. The patient is given IV Valium and Demerol. After the fracture is reduced by traction on the foot, gravity

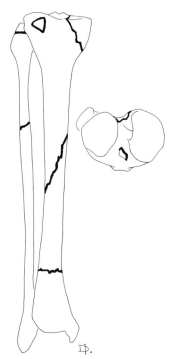

Figure 11–96   Tibial fractures.

maintains the reduction while the operator wraps the plaster dressing over two layers of sheet wadding. The ankle is maintained in a neutral position for most fractures. An equinus position of the foot helps prevent posterior angulation in the skier's boottop fracture. While the plaster sets, anterior and posterior pressure is applied to the plaster just below the knee, molding and narrowing it around the proximal portion of the tibia. This accomplished, the knee is extended to a straight position, avoiding hyperextension. The thigh and knee portions of the long leg plaster are then applied, molding carefully in the anterior posterior direction just below the patella. A walking heel is applied. There may be up to three-fourths of an inch of shortening, which is acceptable. However, angulation must be corrected by wedging the plaster. During the first few days the patient experiences intermittent dependent pain as he begins partial weight-bearing with crutches which are usually discarded during the third week. This long leg walking plaster is usually replaced in about two months by a short leg walking plaster. Most adults are removed from plaster after approximately three months.

Ankle

Lateral Malleolus (Fig. 11–97). Our most common lower extremity fracture is an isolated oblique distal fibula fracture. The fracture line is below the ankle anteriorly, then proceeds obliquely proximally and posteriorly. Lateral x-rays demonstrate the degree of displacement. There may be an associated medial ankle ligament injury. Reduction is accomplished with the patient sitting or lying on the edge of the cart. The involved leg hangs free in front of the operator with the knee flexed to 90 degrees. Reduction is accomplished by inverting the foot to tighten the lateral ligament and displace the distal fibular fragment distally. The operator's fingertips are then placed behind the distal fibula fragment and it is pulled forward and internally rotated to its former position. The forefoot is rested upon a support to prevent inversion and equinus when plaster is applied. The operator then has two free hands with which to apply the plaster and maintain the fibular reduction. A short leg plaster dressing is applied with a walking heel. A postreduction film is obtained and walking is encouraged as early as possible. The plaster is left on for six weeks. Nonunion is rare.

Posterior Malleolus. Vertical fracture of the posterior lip of the tibia is seen alone or in combination with other ankle fractures. The articular cartilage does not reach the posterior edge of the tibia and therefore, a large fragment must be present before the fracture line extends into the ankle mortise. Displacement can frequently be improved by local pressure or carrying the great toe into extreme dorsiflexion. When

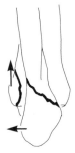

Figure 11–97   Ankle fractures. Lateral malleolus fracture.

there is upward displacement of the fragment which includes more than one-third of the articular surface, open reduction is recommended.

Medial Malleolus (Fig 11–98). Medial malleolus fractures which enter the ankle joint at the shoulder of the mortise remove the medial stability of the joint and create an irregular cartilage surface if they are not anatomically reduced. The infolded periosteum prevents an anatomic closed reduction. The anterior opening of the fracture line can often be improved by holding the foot in dorsiflexion before plaster application and therefore open reduction and internal fixation are given favorable consideration in all displaced medial malleolus fractures which cannot be reduced anatomically.

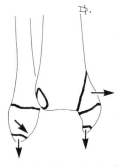

Figure 11–98   Medial malleolus fracture.

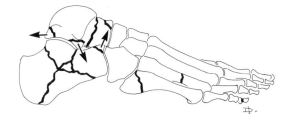

Figure 11–99   Fractures of the foot.

Foot

Calcaneal Fractures (Fig. 11–99). A calcaneal fracture most often follows a fall from a height. The bone has a thin cortex not suitable for internal fixation. I routinely apply a short leg walking plaster and begin weight-bearing as soon as tolerated. Weight-bearing will allow the remainder of the tissues in the leg and foot to maintain function and reduce atrophy while the fracture heals. The involvement of the subtalar joint often precipitates degenerative arthritis and fusion may be required. Also, following these fractures the normal lever arm of the tendo Achillis is altered and the patient has a persistent limp.

These patients must also be checked for an associated compression fracture of the spine.

Talus. Most fractures of the talus follow dorsiflexion or plantar flexion injuries. After traumatic plantar flexion of the ankle, the posterior tubercle of the talus is fractured from the body. Simple walking plaster is applied and no reduction is necessary. The neck of the talus is frequently fractured in dorsiflexion injuries. The subtalar joint is disrupted with displacement of the neck. A closed reduction may bring about the necessary anatomic reduction, by bringing the foot into extreme equinus. After a dorsiflexion injury the lateral process may be fractured. Other small chip fractures are frequently seen. A short leg, nonweight-bearing plaster

is used in these cases until fracture union occurs. Occasionally, open reduction and internal fixation may be indicated to maintain an anatomic reduction. If the neck fracture is displaced and associated with dislocation of the body of the talus from the ankle joint, attempts at closed reduction are unsuccessful. Aseptic necrosis complicates the management of displaced fractures of the neck of the talus.

Metatarsal. Transverse fracture of the base of the fifth metatarsal is the most common fracture of the metatarsals. It follows an inversion injury and avulsion of the tip of the metatarsal by the peroneus brevis tendon. Adequate, comfortable treatment is achieved with a short leg walking plaster for four weeks. Painless nonunion frequently follows treatment.

References

1. Blount, W. P.: Fractures in Children. Baltimore, Williams and Wilkins Co., 1955.
2. Charnley, J.: Closed Treatment of Common Fractures. Baltimore, Williams and Wilkins Co., 1967.
3. Hawkins, L. G., Pomerantz, M., and Eiseman, B.: Laparotomy at time of pelvic fracture. J. Trauma, *10*:619–623, 1970.
4. Hawkins, L. G., Storey, S. D., and Wells, G. G.: Intravenous lidocaine anesthesia for upper extremity fractures and dislocations. J. Bone Joint Surg., *52A*:1647–1650, 1970.
5. Miles, J. S.: Basic principles of fracture therapy. Surg. Clin. N. Amer., *41*:1453–1462, 1961.

12

Orthopedics

By SHELDON ROGER, M.D.

INTRODUCTION

This chapter deals with the common conditions of bones, joints and skeletal muscles which are seen in outpatient clinics, except fractures and dislocations and diseases of the hand, which are covered in Chapters 11 and 13 respectively.

Congenital and acquired diseases of children are discussed and described. The acquired diseases and injuries of adults are considered on a regional basis. Medications, manipulations and operations which are appropriate for the Outpatient Clinic are outlined.

CONGENITAL CONDITIONS

These conditions are commonly seen in outpatient clinics and in private practitioners' offices. Nonsurgical treatment is most commonly used.

Foot Deformities

Congenital Clubfoot

This condition presents with four deformities: plantar flexion of the ankle, inversion of the foot, adduction of the forefoot and internal rotation of the tibia.[1] The cause is thought to be a genetic defect. Differentiation from neuropathic causes and muscular diseases such as arthrogryposis should be made. In these instances, the deformity is usually bilateral.

The infant is often seen in the nursery. If there is no other contraindication, treatment should be initiated. Many infants will hold the affected foot in attitudes suggesting a clubfoot. Differentiation can usually be made by examination when it is noted that in the true clubfoot the deformity cannot be corrected passively.

Treatment. Forcible methods of manipulation have been abandoned in favor of gradual correction supplemented by plaster immobilization.[2] A method of gradual correction employing plaster is given here (Fig. 12–1). The leg, foot and ankle are sprayed with a spray type of Ace adherent. The assistant holds the extremity by the great toe. Two inch sheet wadding is employed and care is taken to make the cotton padding one layer thick. Excess padding will cause the cast to slip and will obscure landmarks. Plaster is applied and

A

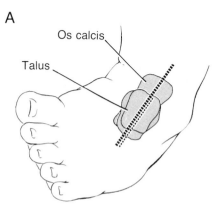

Uncorrected clubfoot deformity

B

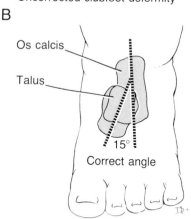

Corrected clubfoot deformity

Figure 12–1 Correction for clubfoot deformity. *A.* Uncorrected clubfoot deformity. The axis of the talus and axis of os calcis are superimposed, as seen on x-ray. *B.* Corrected clubfoot deformity. The axis of talus and os calcis has been unwound to the normal angle of 15–20°. Difficulty in correction should be assessed by radiograph. Ordinarily the varus deformity is corrected first, followed by correction of equinus.

the extremity grasped. In the first stages the adduction of the forefoot is corrected and the foot everted, maintaining the ankle in the equinus position. After the adduction and inversion deformities are corrected, the foot and ankle can be dorsiflexed. Initial casts are usually applied at weekly or biweekly intervals. When the foot is brought into dorsiflexion, pressure must not be applied only to the forefoot, as a "rocker bottom" foot may result with the hindfoot remaining in an equinus position and the forefoot in dorsiflexion.

The majority of clubfeet can be handled by gradual manipulation therapy as outlined. In some instances the equinus deformity of the heel persists in spite of the attempt at stretching. This may be due in many instances to medial insertion of the tendo Achillis heel cord. Lengthening or transplantation of the heel cord insertion may become necessary. Surgical treatment is not usually undertaken in the first six months of life.

After successful plaster correction reverse last shoes are prescribed, attached to a Denis-Brown night splint. Also, the mother is instructed in stretching exercises to be performed at diaper changes.

The status of the extremity is evaluated at follow-up visits during the first few years of life. Any indication of recurrence of the deformity is treated by resumption of plaster correction. In some instances additional surgical treatment is recommended for evidence of persistent muscle imbalance in the foot and ankle.

Metatarsus Varus

The diagnosis of this condition is made by examining the infant foot from a plantar view. The forefoot is seen to deviate medially from the hindfoot. In contrast to the clubfoot, the foot and ankle can easily be dorsiflexed. The heel is either in valgus or neutral, never in varus. There is often an accompanying internal torsion of the tibia.[3]

In very mild instances, stretching of the forefoot into a valgus (abducted) position by the mother at each diaper change will suffice. More often it is necessary to correct the deformity by application of several casts at biweekly intervals, molding the forefoot into an abducted position. A Denis-Brown night splint attached to reverse last shoes should be used after the plaster treatment to maintain the correction.

Treatment begun after the first six months of life often leads to a protracted course with poor and uncertain correction of the deformity. Unresponsive cases in the older child may require surgery.

Tibial Torsion

Most children who are brought into clinics because of toeing-in have this condition. Other common causes are metatarsus varus and pronated feet. The fetal position causes a torsion of the tibia which is apparent in most newborns. Rapid growth of the lower extremities usually "unwinds" the tibia into a normal appearing limb. In many of the infants in which the condition persists, sleeping in the prone position with the lower extremities internally rotated is often a factor in persistence of the deformity.

The condition can be diagnosed by placing the knee in a position with the patella pointing directly forward. It is then noted that the lateral malleolus is in an anterior position in relation to the medial malleolus. The normal position of the lateral malleolus is 15° to 20° posterior to the medial malleolus.

In the first two years of life, the use of a Denis-Brown night splint which holds both lower extremities in an externally rotated position is recommended. The appliance should be used during the sleeping hours, and it should be explained to the parents that the splint rotates the extremity at the hip joint. It does aid the natural growth processes, however, and will eventually achieve correction by "unwinding" the tibia.

In older children the use of an outer sole wedge will help keep the extremity in an externally rotated position during waking hours and thus not inhibit the natural growth tendencies. For the exceptional patient in whom the deformity persists, surgical treatment may be necessary, but this is not usually tried until all other measures have been exhausted or the child has reached the age of eleven or twelve years.

Calcaneovalgus Foot

In this deformity, which is recognized as the opposite of clubfoot, the ankle is quite mobile and the dorsum of the foot sometimes lies against the anterior aspect of the tibia. This condition is usually caused by intrauterine position, and almost always corrects itself spontaneously, unless associated with other neurologic problems (e.g., myelomeningocele).

Stretching exercises are shown to the mother, and the infant's foot and ankle are manipulated into the equinus and inverted positions at each diaper change.

Plaster treatment is indicated only for those feet in which the dorsal structures are tight, preventing manipulation of the ankle into the equinus position.

When weight-bearing is begun it is often necessary to employ shoes with medial heel wedges and medial Thomas heels, to prevent pronation of the hindfoot.

Flat Feet

One of the most common foot disorders of childhood is flat feet. It is recognized when the child is standing erect by an abnormality in alignment of the Achilles tendon, with a valgus attitude of the heel. Most youngsters normally appear to be flatfooted until one to two years of age, because of excess fat in the sole of the foot. If an older child has the deformity shown in Figure 12–2, it may be due to flattening of either the longitudinal (vertical) arch or the

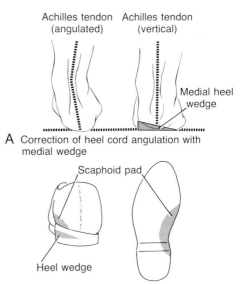

A Correction of heel cord angulation with medial wedge

B Scaphoid foot pad: position and shape

Figure 12–2 Medial heel wedge and scaphoid foot pad for flatfoot deformity. *A.* Correction of heel cord angulation with medial wedge. *B.* Scaphoid foot pad: position and shape.

transverse arch. The major deformity is usually flattening of the longitudinal arch. The aim in treatment is to prevent persistence of the valgus deformity, which leads to a flattened longitudinal arch. This can usually be achieved by application of a medial heel wedge and an interscaphoid pad. An attempt is thus made to make the youngster walk on the outer border of the foot and prevent the angulation of the Achilles tendon. Surgical treatment is rarely indicated, even for severe cases of flatfoot, because few of these patients are symptomatic.

Congenital Vertical Talus

In this condition, the infant is born with a deformity characterized by a rigid foot with equinovalgus hindfoot and a calcaneovalgus forefoot, with dislocation at the talonavicular joint.[4] This is differentiated from the other types of flat feet which usually become apparent when weight bearing is begun. The deformity is characterized by a convexity of the sole associated with tightness of the heel cord and prominence of the posterior portion of the os calcis.

Radiographs show a characteristic vertical position of the talus and a very *horizontal position of the os calcis.*

Treatment should be instituted early in infancy and usually requires operative measures.

Congenital Hip Dysplasia, Subluxation and Dislocation

The entities of hip dysplasia and subluxation will be discussed with the problem of congenital dislocation of the hip (Fig. 12–3). The latter problem usually requires inpatient treatment, while the other two problems are commonly handled in the clinic.

Congenital Hip Dysplasia

The child with the dysplastic hip is usually referred by the pediatrician. Limited abduction of the affected hip has been noted. With the thighs flexed ninety degrees, the affected extremity cannot be abducted. Occasionally the mother

has noted difficulty in abducting the thighs while diapering the infant.

Occasionally the affected extremity will remain in a higher position than the opposite member due to tightness of the adductor muscles and a pelvic tilt.

The condition is important in relation to differentiation from a true dislocation of the hip. On radiographs the acetabulum is underdeveloped and the acetabular index has an angle greater than 30–40°.[5] There does not appear to be lateral displacement of the femur. Delay in development of the ossification centers of the femoral head may be noted in comparison with the opposite hip.

Treatment consists of gradual correction of the adducted femur by the mother. In severe cases a Frijka pillow is employed for a period of several months. In those instances when a shallow acetabulum is seen on a radiograph without physical findings, no treatment is necessary, as this finding is probably a normal variant.

Subluxation of the Hip

Subluxation of the hip is probably a stage in the development of a true dislocation of the hip. Clinical and radio-

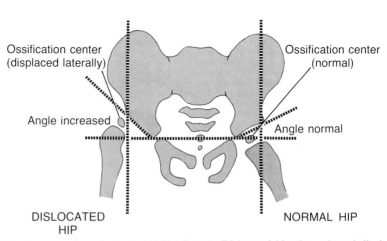

Figure 12–3 X-ray features of congenital hip disease. Dislocated hip shows lateral displacement of ossification center of femoral head and increased acetabular index angle. In dysplasia, the angle is increased, but the femur is not displaced laterally. In subluxation, the femur is malaligned with the acetabulum.

graphic signs are similar to those seen in hip dysplasia, with some exceptions. The adducted position of the femur in relation to the pelvis is almost always present. Asymmetrical thigh folds are usually seen. The trochanter on the affected side may appear more prominent.

On x-ray films there is usually widening of the cartilage space of the hip joint. With abduction of the hip there appears to be malalignment of the femur with the acetabulum.

Initial treatment is directed at passive stretching of the tight adductor muscles. Frijka pillow immobilization of the hips is used. Observation of the hip is indicated during the first year of life to assure proper retention of the acetabular-femoral head relationship.

Congenital Dislocation of the Hip

Main attention will be directed toward recognition of the condition, as almost all types of treatment include traction supplemented by manipulation or operative procedures.

The hip dislocation is not always present at birth but may develop in the first months of infancy or even later. Early recognition of the condition with prompt treatment is an important factor in avoiding treatment failures.

In the preceding discussion, clinical features were presented which aid the practitioner in making the diagnosis of hip dysplasia and subluxation. Most of these clinical findings are present in the frank dislocation, i.e., limited abduction at the hip joint, asymmetrical thigh folds and apparent tilting of the pelvis. In addition, the normal fullness to palpation of the femoral head distal to the inguinal ligament is absent. If the dislocation is bilateral the perineum will appear widened. A "clicking" sign may be felt when the thigh, which is held in the flexed position, is abducted. The sign has been described by Sharrard as a "visible or palpable movement, often erroneously described as a click." The femoral head sliding over the acetabular rim causes this sign.

In children who are walking, a gluteal limp is often present and is occasionally the presenting complaint.

Radiographic findings include those features noted in dysplasia and subluxation except that the femoral head is laterally displaced. The acetabular index is greater than 30–40°.

Treatment. Treatment measures include reduction of the femoral head into the acetabulum in an atraumatic fashion. The reduction, either by manipulative or operative means, is often preceded by a period of traction. Correction of the anteverted position of the femoral head is frequently necessary. In older children or in failures of other types of treatment, operative measures aimed at increasing the size, shape and direction of the acetabulum are often included.

Arthrogryposis

In this congenital condition the infant presents with contractures of major joints of the extremities. Abnormalities in the skeletal muscles have been described and are probably secondary to central nervous system changes. Bilateral dislocations of the hip are often seen along with ulnar club hands and club feet.[5]

Treatment of the lower extremities is aimed at correcting the contractures to the greatest possible extent without compromising the circulation. The clubbed deformities of the foot and ankle can be helped by patient and prolonged plaster applications, but recurrence is frequent. Bilateral hip dislocations are quite refractory to treatment and perhaps should be left *in situ*, resulting in the formation of false acetabuli. Bracing of the lower extremities will often give stability, enabling the patient to be self-ambulatory. In the upper extremities continuing attempts to maintain the wrist and thumb in functional positions should be employed. Plaster splints and braces are employed. The muscles of the shoulder girdle are usually quite weak.

Congenital Scoliosis

The most common cause of this condition is hemivertebra formation. Many of the congenital scolioses are stable and require no treatment other than observation. With the development of a severe curvature, correction and fusion may become indicated. Resection of the hemivertebra has been advocated by some.

Moe and Winter (1968)[6] advocate early fusion of two or three vertebrae when definite evidence of progression is apparent. As little as 5 degrees per year has been shown to be significant, since deterioration occurs rapidly in these children during the adolescent growth spurt.

CHILDHOOD ORTHOPEDIC DISEASES

Coxa Plana (Legg-Calvé-Perthes' Disease)

This disease of uncertain etiology affects children between the ages of five and fifteen. It is characterized by changes in the femoral head very suggestive of an avascular necrosis and subsequent replacement.

There is a heavy male predilection (4:1, male to female). The disease is usually unilateral.

Characteristically the onset is noted with the appearance of a limp not related to previous trauma. Pain is often present in the inner aspect of the thigh and knee. Occasionally a youngster will present with a clinical picture suggesting an inflammatory condition within the hip joint associated with low grade fever, acute pain in the thigh and painful limitation of motion.

Usual findings on examination include a hip flexion contracture and limitation of internal rotation of the hip joint. A pelvic tilt associated with thigh atrophy is frequently seen.

X-ray films will usually show widening of the cartilage space and thickening of the capsular shadows. These findings, even though present after the initial symptoms have subsided, should suggest the diagnosis and are signals for institution of treatment.

Later x-ray films will show increased density of the femoral head. Rarefaction and sclerosis adjacent to the capitol femoral epiphysis are frequently seen, accompanied by widening of the femoral neck.

Replacement of the femoral head is seen subsequently; lucent areas intermingled with radiodense segments are present. The outline of the femoral head may become enlarged and flattened, implying irreversible changes in the femoral head.

Treatment. In the early cases, when pain and spasm predominate, treatment by bed rest supplemented by mild traction may be indicated. Later in the course of the disease pain is not a dominant feature. The avoidance of weight bearing is important in order to protect the femoral head during the replacement process; many methods have been used, but immobilization is difficult because the patients are in the active age group. The isolation of the child by such treatment measures as bed rest and spica immobilization seems unwarranted.

Use of a suspension sling and crutches is a popular method to prevent weight bearing on the affected extremity and obviates the necessity of removing the youngster from social contacts. A Patten bottom, nonweight-bearing splint supplemented by a shoe lift on the opposite side will transfer much of the stress of weight bearing to the ischium.

Protection from weight-bearing stresses should be continued until there is adequate replacement of the femoral head.

The best functional and radiographic results are obtained in those children who exhibit an early age of onset. There also seems to be a favorable correlation with promptness in instituting treatment.

Synovitis of the Hip

The clinical picture in this condition is one of acute onset, usually without antecedent trauma, in which the child complains of groin, thigh or knee pain. Typical findings are limited hip motion, especially internal rotation. As in coxa plana the age group affected is between five and ten years. A temperature elevation is often present and the illness may follow an upper respiratory infection.

The intensity of the symptoms may cause concern about the possibility of a septic process. The absence of a peripheral leukocyte reaction and a minimal rise in the sedimentation rate will rule out the presence of this condition.

Treatment. Bed rest and traction will yield excellent pain relief. The restoration of free hip motion usually follows. Failure to regain full hip motion or recurrence of symptoms suggests that the youngster is suffering from the early stages of coxa plana.

Idiopathic Scoliosis

Idiopathic scoliosis is the most common type of scoliosis, amounting to approximately 80 per cent of scolioses seen in general practice. These curves commonly begin during the late juvenile period but are usually not discovered until adolescence. Typically the curve is a right thoracic or thoracolumbar curve measuring greater than 30° when first discovered. The female to male ratio is 9:1. Curves left untreated often progress rapidly during the adolescent growth spurt, bringing about severe cosmetic deformity and cardiopulmonary restrictive disease.

Early discovery is facilitated by bending the adolescent child at the waist and observing any rib hump, which develops secondary to rotational changes. Children examined in this way will show obvious deformity even when their curve is as small as 15°.

Curves under 40° can usually be treated successfully with a Milwaukee brace and an exercise program. Those between 40° and 60° may be helped by bracing, but if greater than 60°—in a skeletally immature child—they most commonly require posterior spinal fusion to obtain optimum results.

Cerebral Palsy

Cerebral palsy includes nonprogressive lesions of the central nervous system that interfere with the control of one or more limbs by paresis, incoordination or involuntary movement.[5] Causes are numerous but the majority of cases today are the result of intrauterine or birth trauma, the incidence being one to two per thousand. Clinically, five types exist: spastic, athetoid, rigid, ataxic and mixed, of which the spastic type accounts for about 60 per cent.

Prognosis and rehabilitation potential are extremely variable, depending on degree of both motor and intellectual involvement. Outpatient care must be directed at improving function and preventing deformity and complications such as scoliosis, contracture formation and hip dislocation.

Routine examination must be done to check range of motion, especially of hips, knees, ankles and hands. Hip abduction of less than 30° in extension is a sign of impending dislocation. Progressive or persistent equinus sets the stage for permanent bony deformity.

Guided therapy programs can help the child immensely. Surgery such as adductor tenotomy and Achilles tendon lengthening can supplement therapy. The key to care is prevention of problems, not restoration of complications.

DISEASES AND INJURIES CLASSIFIED BY REGION

Shoulder

Supraspinatus Syndrome (Fig. 12–4)

Included in this category are several conditions. The symptoms arise from attritional change in the rotator cuff. Degenerative changes occur from fric-

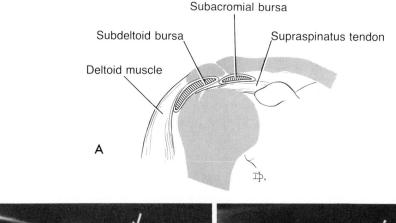

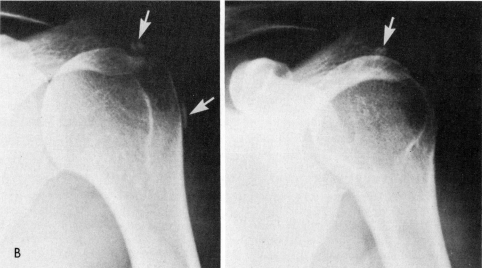

Figure 12–4 A. Diagrammatic representation of the relationship of shoulder bursae to the acromion and rotator cuff.

Figure 12–4 B. X-rays of calcified tendinitis of the shoulder. Calcification in the subdeltoid bursa and supraspinatus tendon, as shown. The lesions are most apparent in the externally rotated view (*left*), and may be almost impossible to detect when the shoulder is internally rotated (*right*).

tion of the rotator cuff and subdeltoid bursa against the acromion process. Fibrillation and fraying of the tendon fibers are seen initially, and calcaneous deposits in the bursa and tendon may form subsequently. Small rents or large tears may later occur in the area of degeneration. Subdeltoid bursitis, subacromial bursitis and tendinitis of the rotator cuff are impossible to differentiate clinically ·and arise following the initial degeneration of tendinous fibers in the rotator cuff. In calcaneous tendinitis calcific deposits may be seen in the region of the supraspinatus tendon adjacent to the greater tuberosity.

X-ray. Radiographs may show irregularity and sclerosis of the greater tuberosity of the humerus. More often, no abnormalities are seen on x-ray films. The presence of calcific deposits in the rotator cuff has been mentioned.

Clinical Picture. The patient is usually in the age group of thirty-five to fifty-five. Pain in the region of the shoulder with radiation into the lateral aspect of the arm is the presenting symptom. The patient has often noted discomfort in donning shirts or blouses; reaching for objects above his head has initiated pain. The discomfort is often minimal during the waking hours but may be quite intense at night. Acute calcific tendinitis may occur in adults of all age groups. The onset is often acute with severe pain. It is thought that deposits in the tendinous structures are not bothersome; however, when the adjacent bursal walls are involved and inflammation reaches tissues richly supplied with vessels and nerves, the condition becomes acute.

Examination of those patients who exhibit no limitation of passive motion will usually reveal a painful range of abduction between 80° and 120°, presumably caused by impingement of the inflamed area against the acromion. External and internal rotation of the shoulder in the abducted position will initiate a painful response.

Many patients will exhibit a painful limitation of motion, especially abduction and external rotation in the abducted position.

Treatment. If symptoms are mild and not accompanied by severe restriction of motion, the use of phenylbutazone (Butazolidine) may result in subsidence of symptoms in a three to five day period. Active abduction and rotational motions are encouraged to prevent ankylosis of the joint.

Failure of the anti-inflammatory agents or the presence of more severe symptoms should be treated by the use of intra-articular injections. Eight to ten cc of 1 per cent Xylocaine is used as a diluent, to which is added one-half cc of Hydeltra TBA (10 mgm/cc). After preparing the shoulder, the joint is entered through an anterior approach. During the injection the shoulder is maintained in the adducted position with neutral rotation. By "stepping off" the head of the humerus with the needle, entrance into the joint can be felt and the solution injected. If the joint has been entered, immediate improvement in discomfort will be noted, and the physician is also sure that the steroid will come in contact with the diseased area. If limitation of motion was present prior to the injection it should be improved considerably. The failure to regain almost full range of active motion suggests the presence of fibrous ankylosis of the joint. In some instances of subdeltoid bursitis, there may not be connection of the bursa with the shoulder joint. An additional injection is then made through a lateral approach, slightly below and anterior to the tip of the acromion.

Pain medications are prescribed, as occasionally severe pain is noted several hours after the injection. By limiting the amount of steroid injected it is felt that painful postinjection reaction can be reduced without limiting the efficiency of the treatment. The injection may be repeated at 10 to 14 day intervals.

Acute calcific tendinitis may require more frequent injections.

Bicipital Tendinitis

The patient with this condition usually presents with pain over the anterior of the shoulder joint. Because of the relationship of the bicipital tendon to the anterior capsule of the shoulder joint, the tendon is often involved with other inflammatory conditions of the shoulder. In addition, irritative symptoms may arise from inflammation of peritendinous structures in the region of the bicipital groove.

The shoulder pain accompanying this condition can sometimes be localized by stressing the forearm into supination with the elbow flexed. Injection of steroid into the anterior portion of the joint will usually relieve the condition due to the intra-articular location of the tendon. When symptoms can be accurately localized to the region of the bicipital groove, direct infiltration of the Xylocaine-steroid solution into the area will be successful.

Fibrous Ankylosis of the Shoulder

The origins of this condition are varied but most commonly ankylosis arises from immobilization of the shoulder in the adducted position or from painful conditions within the joint.

Even without direct injuries to the shoulder joint, injuries of the forearm and hand may cause painful limitation of shoulder motion unless the patient is instructed in active shoulder motion to prevent prolonged adduction of the shoulder joint.

Painful inflammatory conditions within the shoulder such as bursitis, supraspinatus syndrome and bicipital tendinitis may result in ankylosis of the joint if active exercise is not stressed. Fractures of the neck of the humerus may also lead to this unhappy finding, unless early active motion is instituted. Referred pain from cervical arthritis and cardiac disease may also lead to ankylosis of the shoulder.

The employment of gentle passive and active exercise by a skilled therapist will often suffice in the early stages of this disease. The importance of home self-administered treatment must be stressed to the patient. On some occasions, the use of ice packs prior to passive motion administered by the therapist will be more helpful than heat.

Failure to show progress often requires manipulative treatment done under general anesthesia. During the procedure, the joint is manipulated into a full range of motion. The maintenance of the range of motion regained depends on passive and active exercise carried out following the manipulative treatment.

Rupture of the Rotator Cuff

Rupture of the rotator cuff occurs through areas of degeneration of the supraspinatus tendon, and almost never occurs before the age of thirty-five. A fall or stress applied to the extremity in lifting or pushing an object is commonly the inciting cause. Partial ruptures of the rotator cuff occur frequently and are often undiagnosed. The pain associated with the injury usually subsides over a five to six week period. If ade-

quate deltoid function is maintained, little if any disability persists.

Evaluation of the acute injury usually reveals a range of abduction between 90° and 120° in which motion is quite painful. Motion may be associated with a clicking sensation.

Rest of the extremity in a sling for a seven to ten day period is indicated because functional impairment is minimal in the presence of adequate deltoid function. Abduction exercises are gradually instituted. Painful inflammatory change within the joint may necessitate injection into the joint to facilitate restoration of motion and diminution of pain.

Complete tears of the rotator cuff are associated with loss of abduction of the shoulder joint. Often the patient cannot initiate abduction, but if the first 20° of abduction are initiated passively he may be able to complete and maintain abduction by deltoid activity.

Differentiation from an incomplete rupture may sometimes be made by injecting Xylocaine into the shoulder joint. If the patient can then initiate abduction of the shoulder, the presence of an incomplete lesion is indicated.

The presence of a complete rupture in a patient in the younger age group usually requires surgical treatment. In older patients and in those in whom surgical treatment cannot be performed, amazingly good results can be obtained by splinting the extremity. The shoulder is immobilized for ten days, and this is followed by vigorous therapy, stressing deltoid strengthening.

Rupture of the Long Head of the Biceps

The rupture may be spontaneous or may follow a lifting episode. The patient presents with pain in the upper arm. "Bunching" of the muscle belly of the biceps into the distal portion of the arm is seen. Ecchymosis and swelling are seen in the anterior and medial aspect of the arm.

Because of amazingly little diminution of strength and no impairment of function in older individuals and those with sedentary activities, surgical treatment is not indicated. Supportive measures supplemented by the use of a sling are employed.

Elbow

Olecranon Bursitis

This condition is recognized by a saccular swelling over the posterior portion of the elbow. In the common irritative type of lesion the bursa is relatively nontender. Erythema and swelling in the region of the bursa and surrounding tissues may indicate the presence of gouty or septic inflammation.

When bloody or clear synovial fluid is aspirated from the bursa, 1 cc of Xylocaine and 1/2 cc Hydeltra TBA 10 mgm/cc should be instilled. A padded compression bandage is then applied.

If the aspirate is cloudy, a rheumatoid, gouty or septic involvement of the bursa may be present. Cultures and smears of the aspirate should be done to determine the presence and identification of the offending organism, after which the appropriate antibiotics may be employed. Rheumatoid or gouty involvement of the bursa can be successfully treated by instillation of steroids.

"Tennis Elbow"

The patient with this condition presents with pain over the lateral aspect of the elbow. The discomfort is accentuated whenever the wrist is actively dorsiflexed or stabilized by the extensor musculature. There is much doubt concerning the pathological lesion responsible for the syndrome; in addition to tennis players, the condition is frequently seen in golfers and bowlers. Tenderness is present over the lateral epicondyle of the humerus and extensor tendon immediately distally. Flexion force applied to the dorsiflexed wrist will cause pain in the region of the lateral epicondyle.

In mild cases the use of one of the anti-inflammatory drugs will yield relief. Injection of a solution of Xylocaine

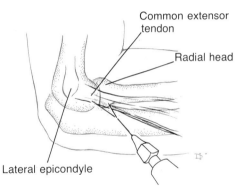

Figure 12–5 Injection for "tennis elbow." The area of maximum tenderness is palpated and injected. This is usually immediately adjacent to the origin of the common extensors from the lateral epicondyle of the humerus. The needle is carefully redirected into several points along the common extensors.

and steroid is the treatment of choice (Fig. 12–5). Four to five cc of 1 per cent Xylocaine with 1/2 cc Hydeltra TBA is injected into the extensor tendon at its site of origin from the lateral epicondyle. The joint is splinted for several days, after which active motion is encouraged. Several injections are given over a six week period if the symptoms persist; if they recur following injection treatment, surgical treatment is indicated.

Medial Epicondylitis ("Golfer's Elbow")

As with tennis elbow, the patient presents with pain, but in this instance, the pain occurs over the region of the medial epicondyle of the humerus.

Tenderness is present in the area of pain and usually extends somewhat distally.

Injection of the area as outlined earlier is employed (Fig. 12–6) and usually results in prompt subsidence of symptoms.

Rupture of Distal Biceps Tendon

This condition is much less common than rupture of the long head of the biceps. The presenting symptom is sudden onset of pain in the anterior elbow region during an episode of lifting. Swelling occurs in the antecubital fossa.

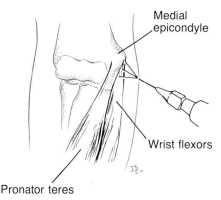

Medial
epicondyle

Wrist flexors

Pronator teres

Figure 12–6 Injection for medial epicondylitis ("golfer's elbow"). The injection is performed at several points around the area of maximum tenderness. This is usually immediately distal to the medial epicondyle of the humerus, within the origins of the wrist flexors and the pronator teres muscle.

Painful limitation of full flexion and extension is seen. The normal prominence of the biceps tendon in the antecubital space is absent. The muscle mass of the biceps is seen in a more proximal location in the arm.

Surgical treatment of the condition is indicated.

Wrist

Stenosing Tenosynovitis (De Quervain's)

The adductor pollicis longus and extensor pollicis brevis tendons traverse a synovial-lined sheath which is attached to the region of the styloid process of the radius. Inflammation of the synovial tissues results in the clinical condition described by De Quervain.

Excessive use of the wrist and thumb is the common causative condition. Pain over the radial aspect of the wrist is aggravated by grasping objects or clenching the fist. A cylindrical swelling is present over the radial aspect of the wrist. Pain can usually be elicited in the region of the swelling by forced ulnar deviation of the wrist with the thumb adducted and flexed into the palm.

Splinting of the forearm with the wrist in extension and the thumb in opposition is helpful in the acute phase of the condition. When symptoms are long standing, injection of a mixture of Xylocaine and Hydeltra into the distal end of the sheath will often cause diminution of symptoms (Fig. 12–7). If no lasting improvement is noted after several injections, surgical treatment is recommended.

Rupture of Extensor Pollicis Longus

Spontaneous rupture of the extensor pollicis longus tendon may occur where the tendon passes through a synovial sheath and over the distal end of the radius. The lesion is often seen following a fracture of the distal radius and occurs as a result of irregularity of the radius in the region of the fracture.

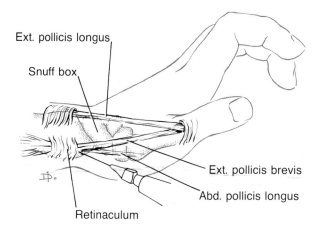

Ext. pollicis longus

Snuff box

Ext. pollicis brevis

Abd. pollicis longus

Retinaculum

Figure 12–7 Injection for stenosing tenosynovitis (de Quervain's). Injection is performed at the site of maximum swelling and tenderness, which is usually the retinaculum of the extensor pollicis brevis and abductor pollicis longus. The needle is inserted tangentially along these two tendons, entering the retinaculum as shown.

Surgical repair of the tendon is indicated.

Ganglions

These lesions are seen in many areas of the extremities but most frequently occur as a mass on the dorsum of the wrist (Fig. 12–8). Occasionally a ganglion will be noted arising from the volar aspect of the wrist adjacent to the radial artery. The origin is usually traumatic and follows an acute flexion or extension injury of the wrist. In the region of the wrist the lesion almost always arises from the capsule of the joint. Since dissection down to the capsule is necessary, surgery is the treatment of choice; it should be carried out in an adequate operating room employing either general or regional anesthesia.

Dissection is performed in the operating room under IV lidocaine anesthesia (Bier block), administered by an anesthesiologist. A bloodless field is achieved with a tourniquet, and the patient's condition is monitored carefully throughout the procedure.

No major structures other than the extensor tendons are observed in the dissection of a dorsal wrist ganglion. Volar ganglions should be carefully dissected away from the radial artery, and the median nerve should be identified and protected. Every effort is made to remove the ganglion intact, although we do not attempt to repair the rent left in the capsular origin of the ganglion.

Operating is done on an inpatient basis. The patient is allowed to leave the hospital after recovering from anesthesia, either on the same day or on the following morning.

Carpal Tunnel Syndrome

This syndrome results from compression of the median nerve in the carpal tunnel.[7] This channel is created by the transverse carpal ligament volarly and the carpus dorsally. The ligament arises proximally from the pisiform and prominence of the navicular and extends distally to the hamate and ridge of the greater multangular. Through the tunnel pass the median nerve and the flexor tendons of the fingers with their synovial sheaths. Since the walls of the tunnel are nonexpandable, any lesion within the channel may cause compression of the median nerve.

The most common pathologic finding is nonspecific inflammation and swelling of the synovial tissues. The syndrome occurs commonly in rheumatoid arthritis, owing to inflammation of the synovial tissues; encroachment by tissues involved in the healing process following a Colles' fracture has also been responsible. The syndrome occurs most commonly in postmenopausal women.

The symptoms are pain, numbness

A   View of volar ganglion

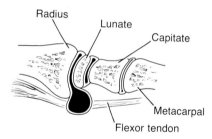

B   View of dorsal ganglion

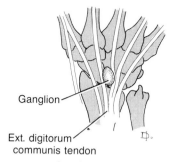

Figure 12–8 Ganglion. *A.* View of dorsal ganglion. The ganglion is shown in the most common location of ganglia of the wrist, presenting between the slips of the extensor digitorum communis, overlying the wrist joint. *B.* View of the volar ganglion. The most common location is on the radial aspect of the wrist, with the ganglion presenting just medial to the radial artery.

and tingling in the distribution of the median nerve. Frequently they will be most bothersome at night and typically will awaken the patient from sleep. The usual methods employed by the patient to alleviate the symptoms are shaking the hand and running warm water over the fingers.

On examination there may be visible swelling over the volar aspect of the wrist. The symptoms can usually be elicited by holding the wrist in acute flexion or extension for a one minute period. If hypesthesia is present in the distribution of the median nerve, the diagnosis can be confirmed and thereby differentiated from abnormalities in the cervical spine.

Tangential x-rays may show a bony abnormality within the tunnel. Usually the x-ray will be normal, however.

Splinting of the wrist and forearm with a volar appliance will often relieve the symptoms. If there is no medical contraindication, an oral steroid or phenylbutazone (Butazolidine) may be employed for three or four days.

When the syndrome follows a Colles' fracture, the treatment indicated above is usually all that is indicated. Under these circumstances, the condition is self-limiting and will often subside spontaneously after a five to six month period.

Injection of steroid into the tunnel will often cause alleviation of symptoms, but surgical division of the transverse carpal ligament is usually indicated.

Surgical treatment requires that the patient be admitted to the hospital and the operation be performed in the main operating room. Regional anesthesia (Bier block) is used, with a bloodless field achieved by using a tourniquet. Anesthesia is administered by an anesthesiologist, who monitors the patient's condition throughout the procedure. The patient is allowed to leave the hospital following recovery from anesthesia later in the afternoon or on the following morning.

The surgical technique employed is a longitudinal incision in the volar aspect of the distal forearm, slightly to the radial aspect of the midline. The incision is extended and angled medially in the transverse crease at the wrist and then extended longitudinally onto the palm, curving along the thenar eminence. The key to the dissection is identification of the median nerve, which is immediately radial and slightly deep to the palmaris longus tendon, covered by a thin fascia. The flexor carpi radialis tendon is immediately lateral (radial) to the median nerve, and is an important reference point in patients who have a congenital absence of the palmaris longus. The carpal tunnel, approximately 1½ cm long, must be divided completely. The proximal portion of the radial aspect of its origin is the easily palpable ridge on the navicular; its distal portion is the ridge on the greater multangular, which is easily palpable within the thenar eminence. The median nerve is carefully observed while the transverse carpal ligament is divided with fine dissecting scissors. The motor branch of the median nerve is protected by dissecting along the ulnar side of the median nerve. The entire dissection should be carried out from proximal to distal.

Hip

Trochanteric Bursitis

This condition is characterized by acute discomfort over the region of the greater trochanter arising from an inflammatory condition within the bursa (Fig. 12–9). Weight bearing on the affected extremity increases the pain, and the patient usually presents with a painful gait.

The bursa may be a focus of tuberculous infection. In this condition destructive changes are normally seen within the femur.

In the usual nonspecific inflammatory involvement of the bursa, symptoms can be alleviated with the use of anti-inflammatory agents or injection of steroids into the area.

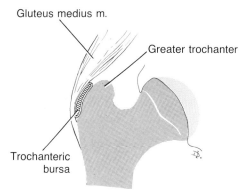

Figure 12–9 Anatomy of trochanteric bursa.

Iliopectineal Bursitis

This bursa overlies the iliopectineal eminence and lies posterior to the psoas muscle (Fig. 12–10). It lies somewhat superior to the capsule of the hip joint with which it sometimes communicates. Inflammation or swelling within the bursa may compress the femoral nerve and cause pain referred into the thigh.

In the acute picture, the joint is held in the flexed position with painful extension from this position.

The presence of sepsis within the bursa needs to be differentiated from a psoas abscess and intra-articular hip disease.

Ischial Bursitis ("Weaver's Bottom")

Ischial bursitis is a common painful condition due to inflammation in the ischial bursa. The condition may be relieved by injection of anti-inflammatory agents into the tender area overlying the ischial tuberosity. The relationship of the sciatic nerve is shown on the diagram (Fig. 12–11).

Knee

General Discussion

The knee joint, unlike the hip and ankle, depends upon integrity of the adjacent muscular tissues and ligamentous structures for stability and mobility. Because of its vulnerability, it is frequently the site of acute traumatic afflictions. A thorough history is of utmost importance in evaluating knee problems. The diagnosis can often be made on the basis of determining the direction of stress applied during the injury.

Inspection of the joint usually suggests the presence of an effusion, which is most prominent in the suprapatellar pouch. Atrophy of the thigh musculature suggests the presence of long-standing difficulty in the extremity. The range of motion within the joint is easily noted.

Evaluation of the integrity of the ligamentous structures is often difficult in the presence of an acutely painful knee but must be accomplished in order to determine the extent of the injury. Delay in making the diagnosis of a complete ligament rupture will often prevent successful surgical treatment.

Less urgency is necessary in making the diagnosis of a cartilage injury as delay in operative treatment will not affect the success of the end results.

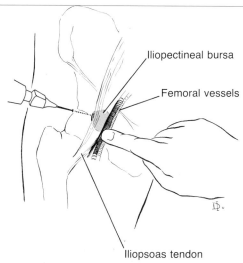

Figure 12–10 Iliopectineal bursa: anterior relationships and injection. The femoral pulse is identified. The needle is inserted as shown, lateral to the femoral pulsation. The tip of the needle is advanced until bone (the ilium) is encountered. This is usually at a depth of 2 inches or less in an average sized person. The needle is from a lateral angle, as illustrated.

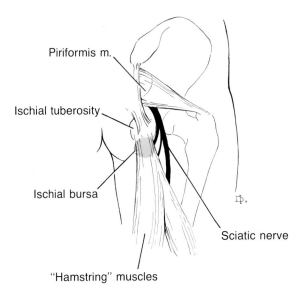

Piriformis m.

Ischial tuberosity

Ischial bursa

Sciatic nerve

"Hamstring" muscles

Figure 12–11 Ischial bursa: posterior view.

Ligamentous Injuries

The application of a valgus or varus stress to the knee joint may result in damage to the collateral ligaments. Severe trauma to the knee usually yields combinations of injuries to the collateral and cruciate ligaments. An isolated cruciate ligament tear is a rare injury and is often not diagnosed.

Medial Collateral Ligament. Most commonly seen are injuries to the medial collateral ligament. The knee is forced into an exaggerated valgus position, usually associated with a twisting component. In the most severe injuries, complete loss of ligamentous continuity occurs, either as a result of avulsion of the ligament from its origin or insertion, or rupture of the ligament in its midportion. Less severe forms of injury result from tearing of fibers of the ligament without evidence of instability.

Examination of the knee should be performed with the patient in the recumbent position (Fig. 12–12). The knee is held in a slightly flexed position with the left hand under the thigh and the right hand grasping the leg under the calf. It is important to be certain that the patient relaxes his quadriceps, as spasm or tension of this mechanism can stabilize the joint. Comparison with the opposite member should be made in determining the presence or extent of instability.

Minor sprains of the medial collateral ligament usually present with pain over the medial joint area. Tenderness can be localized. Little in the way of tissue reaction is seen. The pain is duplicated by acute flexion of the joint. No instability of the joint is noted. A padded dressing covered with an Ace bandage will often afford adequate symptomatic relief and should be used for a ten day period.

Moderate sprains will cause more intense pain. Weight bearing is usually quite painful and no instability is present. There is usually no effusion within the joint. A cylinder cast applied from the upper thigh to the lower leg will afford symptomatic relief and should be worn for a three week period (Fig. 12–13). Weight bearing is allowed and the use of isometric quadriceps exercises is advised during the period of immobilization.

The presence of a complete rupture is usually indicated by the presence of an intra-articular effusion. Instability is often noted by the patient during attempted weight bearing. The application

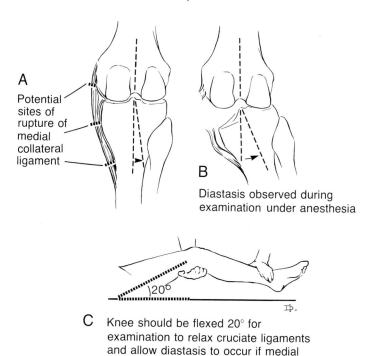

A Potential sites of rupture of medial collateral ligament

B Diastasis observed during examination under anesthesia

C Knee should be flexed 20° for examination to relax cruciate ligaments and allow diastasis to occur if medial collateral ligament is torn

Figure 12–12 Medial collateral ligament injury: technique of examination. *A*. Sites of rupture of the medial collateral ligament are indicated. Rupture occurs due to trauma from the lateral aspect of the knee. *B*. A diastasis is observed, as shown, during examination under anesthesia. *C*. The knee should be flexed approximately 20° during examination for medial collateral ligament injury, to relax the cruciate ligaments.

Figure 12–13 Cylinder cast for medial collateral ligament injury. *A*. A strip of 1 inch adhesive is applied to skin from the upper thigh to the ankle, after skin preparation with Ace adherent spray. An extra few inches of adhesive are left unattached, as shown, and later doubled back as illustrated in inset *(B)*. Sheet wadding is applied next, followed by a circular roll of 6 inch plaster. The distal extra length of tape is incorporated into the plaster wrapping, to prevent downward displacement of the cast when the patient is ambulatory. The cast is molded snugly to conform to the natural contour of the leg *(C)*, and the cast is not bivalved.

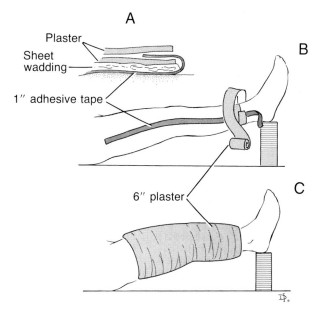

A

Plaster
Sheet wadding
1″ adhesive tape

B

6″ plaster

C

of a valgus stress to the knee will show the presence of instability and will reduplicate the pain. Should there be any question regarding the presence of instability, the extremity should be examined under anesthesia, with subsequent operative repair if instability is verified.

Anterior Cruciate Ligament. As mentioned before, isolated cruciate ligament ruptures are rare (Fig. 12–14). Acute flexion injuries are the most common cause. A bloody effusion within the knee joint associated with a positive "drawer

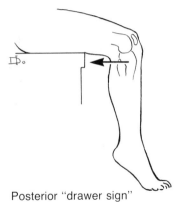

Posterior "drawer sign"

Figure 12–15 Posterior cruciate ligament injury (posterior "drawer sign"). The quadriceps is relaxed by flexing the knee while the patient is seated on a table. Increased posterior mobility of the tibia on the femur simulates closing a drawer, and indicates posterior cruciate ligament disruption.

sign" points to the diagnosis. Operative treatment is usually indicated.

Lateral Collateral Ligament. Injuries to the lateral collateral ligament are rare. Often there is avulsion of a fragment from the head of the fibula, the site of insertion of the ligament. Occasionally there is also an associated stretch injury to the common peroneal nerve, causing foot drop and anesthesia of the dorsum of the foot. Instability requires surgical treatment. Less severe injuries will respond to immobilization in a cylinder cast for a three week period.

Posterior Cruciate Ligament. Isolated injuries to the posterior cruciate ligament are extremely rare (Fig. 12–15). More often the ligamentous injury is a component of other severe ligament damage of the knee joint that requires surgical treatment.

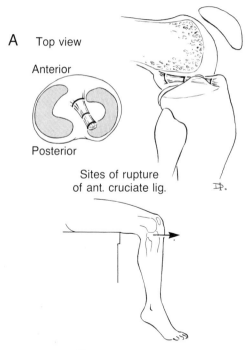

B   Lateral view

A   Top view

Anterior

Posterior

Sites of rupture of ant. cruciate lig.

C   Anterior "drawer sign"

Figure 12–14 Anterior cruciate ligament injury (anterior "drawer sign"). *A* and *B*. Top view and lateral view of knee, showing the sites of rupture of the anterior cruciate ligament. *C*. Test for anterior cruciate ligament injury: the quadriceps is relaxed while the knee is flexed, by having the patient seated on a table. Increased mobility of the tibia on the femur is detected by grasping the calf and pulling the leg forward, toward the examiner. This motion simulates the opening of a drawer.

Meniscal Injuries

The menisci or semilunar cartilages are crescentic segments of fibrocartilage attached to the tibia and are subject to damage with twisting injuries. The medial collateral ligament is contiguous with the medial periphery of the medial meniscus. The lateral meniscus is more mobile and because of this fact is less prone to injury.[8]

Acute Injuries. It is impossible to place too much emphasis on the taking of a thorough history in evaluating the presence of a meniscal injury. The patient usually mentions a twisting injury, most often an inward twisting of the femur with the knee flexed. After the fall, the knee remained in a position of about 20° of flexion. Pain is located over the medial or lateral joint line. The patient may have felt a clicking or popping sensation in the area of pain and tenderness. The knee may have become capable of extension after the initial episode, or it may remain in the "locked" position. The patient who mentions his knee "going out" in the extended rather than the flexed position is usually suffering from an intra-articular disease other than a meniscal injury.

Examination of the joint in the presence of the acute injury will show the presence of an effusion. The knee may be incapable of full extension. An inability to extend the knee fully may be due to intra-articular fluid rather than trapping of the meniscus between the femoral-tibial joint surfaces. Tenderness is present in the joint line over the site of meniscal damage. Rocking of the patella against the femoral surface will usually not produce symptoms. Slight rotation of the tibia on the femur with the knee flexed will often reduplicate the discomfort.

After an x-ray film is taken to rule out the presence of other intra-articular conditions, the joint should be aspirated. The presence of a hemoarthrosis in the absence of ligamentous injury strongly points to the presence of a meniscal injury. If examination of the joint has been difficult up to this point, it may be facilitated by instillation of 5 cc of 1 per cent Xylocaine into the joint.

If the presence of a severe ligamentous injury can be ruled out and the findings point to a meniscal injury, immobilization of the joint in a cylinder cast for a ten day period is indicated. Should there be evidence that suggests that the joint is locked, surgical treatment should be undertaken.

Chronic Injuries. The symptoms as described by the patient are usually less severe than those noted in the original injury. The patient may use the terms "locking" and "giving way." In true locking the joint is caught in a position of flexion, usually about 30°, and requires manipulation by the patient or a companion for relief. The joint may be the site of recurrent effusions arising from a recurrent traumatic synovitis.

The maintenance of quadriceps strength by progressive straight leg weight-lifting is important, but if the diagnosis can be made, surgical treatment is indicated.

Osteochondritis Dissecans

This condition is characterized by sequestration of a portion of the articular surface of the femur. In 85 per cent of cases the disease is localized to the posterolateral portion of the medial femoral condyle. Occasionally the lesion is seen on the lateral condyle. The fragment may not be detached from its site of origin or it may be present as a loose body within the joint.

If the fragment is not detached, the symptoms usually consist of recurrent pain within the joint, sometimes accompanied by effusion. Should the fragment be detached, the presenting symptom is recurrent episodes of locking.

In instances when the lesion is not clearly seen on x-ray films a tunnel view of the femur will clearly show the presence of the lesion.

When the lesion is detected in early adolescence, occasional healing of the fragment will be seen after immobilization for an eight week period in a cylinder cast. Older adolescents and adults usually require surgical treatment.

Osgood-Schlatter's Disease

Also known as osteochondritis of the tibial tubercle, this condition presents as a painful swelling over the tibial tuberosity, made worse by activity and relieved by rest. The condition is commonly first seen in adolescent males and may or may not be related to a traumatic episode. Pain is maximum at the patellar insertion and is accentuated with forced active extension of the knee, or forced passive flexion. Often the lateral radiograph shows irregularity of the patellar tendon insertion.

Treatment is conservative. Acute episodes may be treated with a cylinder plaster cast for two to three weeks, followed by restriction of athletic activity. On such a program the pain usually subsides completely in three to six months.

Chondromalacia Patellae

This disease is characterized pathologically by fibrillation of the articular surface of the patella. The onset may be traumatic from direct blows to the patella but more often results from chronic attritional change. Predisposing factors are recurrent subluxation of the patella and genu valgus.

The clinical syndrome is most commonly seen in adolescents and young adults. Nonlocalized discomfort in the knee joint is the most common symptom and is usually brought on by activity but is felt after the activity is completed. Bending, stooping and forced flexion activities of the knee will ordinarily incite symptoms. A "catching" sensation is often the presenting complaint but is usually differentiated from true mechanical locking of the joint since it occurs in the extended or near extended position. Symptoms are usually intermittent in nature but may become more constant as the disease progresses. Recurrent effusions may be seen in advanced cases.

Quadriceps atrophy may be seen on examination. Retropatellar crepitus and grating can be felt when the patella is manipulated within its femoral bed. Comparison with the opposite knee should be made. The patella may be quite mobile and easily subluxed laterally.

Routine radiographs and a tangential view of the patella may not reveal any abnormality. Occasionally an abnormal lateral facet of the patella with a deficient lateral condyle of the femur will be seen.

Treatment in mild cases should be directed at improving quadriceps strength through the use of resistive straight leg raising exercises. Bent leg raising exercise, knee bends, "yoga" positions and other types of flexed knee exercises should be avoided. Rest from strenuous activity will often help in elimination of symptoms. Failure to improve on this regime should be handled by temporary immobilization of the knee joint in a cylinder plaster cast for two weeks, during which time resistive quadriceps exercises are continued. The oral use of any of the anti-inflammatory agents may also help in alleviating symptoms of the traumatic synovitis of the joint. If effusions are present, aspiration of the synovial fluid and injection of steroid are indicated. The presence of a hemarthrosis should raise the possibility of a meniscal injury; it may, however, be seen with chondromalacia.

Resistant cases may require surgical treatment but the majority of patients may be handled by nonsurgical methods.

Recurrent Dislocation of the Patella

This syndrome is most commonly seen in adolescent females. The patella either displaces laterally over the lateral femoral condyle and remains in this position or merely slips momentarily and returns to its original position. The latter situation is more common and often occurs with mild activity such as walking or dancing. Less commonly, the subluxation occurs with vigorous exercises.

Clinical Syndrome. The patient complains of the knee catching or giving way, often throwing her to the ground. The acute episode is usually followed by an effusion within the joint. The patella will often appear quite mobile and may exhibit considerable retropatellar crepitus. The quadriceps mechanism and especially the vastus medialis exhibits atrophy.

When the knee is examined during an unreduced episode, the obvious lateral position of the patella is seen.

Treatment. If the patient is seen with an acute episode following a traumatic incident, the patella may be easily reduced by applying medial pressure to it with the knee extended and the thigh flexed. X-ray films may show the presence of a fracture, but usually if a fracture is present it may be a disruption of a cartilaginous surface and is not visible radiographically. Aspiration of the hemoarthrosis and immobilization in a cylinder cast for a three week period is indicated and will often result in a cure.

In the more common recurrent subluxation, nonoperative treatment is unsuccessful. When the diagnosis is confirmed, surgical treatment is indicated.

Rupture of Quadriceps Mechanism

A rupture of the quadriceps mechanism may occur without fracture of the patella, through the fibers of the tendon superior to the patella or through the patellar tendon. Often an avulsion of either the superior or inferior pole of the patella may be seen on x-ray films. The injury may follow a forceful contraction of the quadriceps when the body weight is thrust on the extremity or following an acute flexion injury. The diagnosis can be confirmed by the presence of localized tenderness and often a palpable gap is present in the quadriceps, associated with paresis of extension of the knee.

Surgical treatment is indicated.

Bursitis

There are many bursae in the region of the knee joint (Fig. 12–16). They may be the site of infection or inflammation from a variety of causes. Gout and rheu-

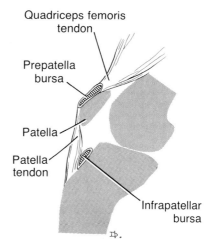

Figure 12–16 Bursae of the knee: prepatellar and infrapatellar. The prepatellar bursa is subcutaneous, and the infrapatellar bursa is located more deeply, posterior to the patellar tendon. Bursitis is treated by injection into the point of maximum tenderness.

matoid involvement are common causes of swelling and local symptoms. Trauma and sepsis are other inciting factors.

Prepatellar Bursitis. This bursa is subcutaneous and lies anterior to the patellar tendon and patella. Inflammations of the bursa result in a visible and palpable swelling which can usually be distinguished from an intra-articular effusion. Work in the kneeling position is the most common cause. Traumatic inflammation of the bursa results in little local tissue response. Gouty and septic involvement of the bursa causes considerable surrounding erythema, local tenderness and heat.

The bursa should be aspirated in traumatic conditions and 1 cc of Hydeltra TBA instilled. Partial immobilization in a padded knee splint for a seven day period is indicated.

If the aspirate is cloudy rather than clear or tinged with blood, the presence of sepsis or gout should be ruled out by smear, culture and examination of the fluid for uric acid crystals. In the absence of sepsis the inflammatory condition resulting from gout and rheumatoid arthritis will often respond to

injection of steroid into the sac as outlined above.

Septic bursitis may be treated by
appropriate parenteral and local use of
antibiotics after the offending organism
is identified. Rest and elevation of the
extremity accompanied by local application of warm moist compresses is
employed.

Infrapatellar Bursitis. This bursa lies
deep to the patellar tendon and anterior
to the upper portion of the tibial tuberosity. It is usually separated from the
synovium of the knee joint.

Pain and local tenderness in the area
of the bursa should be treated by local
injection of steroid in the absence of
sepsis.

Pes Anserinus Bursitis. The bursa lies
adjacent to the tendinous insertions of
the gracilis, semitendinosus and sartorius
muscles on the anterior medial aspect
of the tibia (Fig. 12–17). Traumatic
inflammations of the bursa are treated
by local instillation of a solution of 2 cc
of 1 per cent Xylocaine mixed with
0.5 cc of Hydeltra TBA.

*Semimembranosus Bursitis (Baker's
Cyst).* The popliteal cyst is an enlargement of this bursa which usually communicates with the knee joint posterior
to the medial head of the gastrocnemius.
When enlarged, the bursa presents between the gastrocnemius and the semimembranosus.

The patient often presents with a
painful, palpable mass in the medial
portion of the popliteal space. Recurrent
swelling and subsidence of the mass is
often related by the patient. The presence of inflammation of the bursa may
reflect synovial involvement of the
knee joint secondary to rheumatoid,
gouty and hypertrophic arthritis and
may respond to treatment of these
general conditions. Differential diagnosis includes popliteal artery aneurysm
and synovial sarcoma.

Persistence of the mass requires surgical excision, for which the patient
should be hospitalized.

Ankle and Calf

Sprain

Sprain injury to the ankle often follows
twisting forces. The most common injury follows an inversion and internal
rotation injury in which fibers of the
lateral ligaments of the ankle are torn.
The degree of severity may vary from
tearing of a few fibers to a complete
disruption of continuity.

Injuries to the deltoid ligament usually result from external rotation and
eversion forces. These injuries are accompanied by fractures of either the
fibula or the posterior portion of the tibia.
In fact, an isolated fracture of the posterior "malleolus" of the tibia should suggest the probability of severe damage to
the deltoid ligament.

Acute sprains may be accompanied
by a snapping sound and sensation
noted by the patient. Further attempts at
weight bearing or holding the ankle in a
dependent position cause pain. Swelling and ecchymosis are seen in the region
of the injury. Radiographs of the foot
and ankle should be taken to rule out
the presence of fractures of the malleoli,

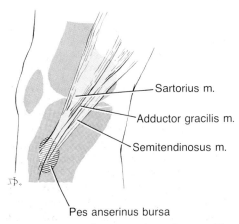

Sartorius m.

Adductor gracilis m.

Semitendinosus m.

Pes anserinus bursa

Figure 12–17 Pes anserinus bursa. The
"goose's foot" bursa is located at the insertion of
the sartorius, semitendinosus and adductor gracilis
muscles in the medial tubercle of the tibia. The
bursa presumably is named for the three separate
tendons which insert at one point.

or avulsion of the malleoli, talus or os calcis. A "sprain fracture" may be treated as a sprain. A tilt of the talus indicates severe damage to the ligamentous structures. Widening of the ankle mortice (secondary to diastasis of the tibiofibular syndesmosis) indicates damage to the tibiofibular and deltoid ligaments and usually requires surgical treatment. The tibiofibular diastasis may occur in the absence of fracture and an unstable joint will result unless it is anatomically reduced.

Treatment. Evaluation of the severity of injury is important in preventing chronic instability of the ankle. In mild cases in which there has been tearing of ligamentous fibers, protection from weight bearing with crutches and the application of a compression bandage with cotton wadding covered with an elastic Ace bandage is indicated. Avoidance of weight bearing for five to seven days followed by gradual institution of active exercises results in return of function after a three week period.

More severe injuries are identified by a greater degree of local tissue reaction. Immobilization is employed in a short leg walking plaster cast for a three week period. Weight bearing per tolerance is allowed.

The presence of a complete rupture may be suspected, either by the presence of a talar tilt noted on an x-ray or by instability detected after instillation of 1 per cent Xylocaine into the area of injury and into the joint. This condition requires immobilization in a short leg walking plaster cast. X-ray films should be taken through plaster to verify that any tilt of the talus has been corrected during application of the plaster. After ten days or following a plaster change necessitated by loosening of the cast, radiographs should be repeated to verify alignment of the mortice. The cast will frequently loosen after reduction of swelling. Weight bearing is permitted after three weeks and plaster is discontinued after six weeks. Unlike other authors, we believe that open treatment of complete sprains of the ankle is not necessary, unless satisfactory alignment of the mortice cannot be obtained.

Chronic Instability of the Ankle

Laxity of the lateral ligaments of the ankle may occur after previous sprains. The patient may suffer from recurrent sprains of the lateral ligaments after even mild activity or walking over uneven ground. A history is given of a previous injury or many minor injuries.

Stress films of the ankle taken in the absence of a recent injury may show a severe degree of talar tilt as compared with the opposite ankle. In this instance, surgical treatment is indicated.

If no talar tilt is demonstrated radiographically, elevation of the lateral aspect of the heel is employed with a $3/16$ inch lateral heel wedge.

Rupture of the Achilles Tendon

This lesion is usually seen in a male aged 35 to 50. The tendon usually ruptures transversely through its narrowest portion. Pain in the region of the rupture followed by swelling and weakness of plantar flexion are noted.

On examination a defect may be seen or palpated in the tendo Achillis when the ankle is dorsiflexed. Local tenderness is present. Retraction of the calf musculature is seen. Some weakness of plantar flexion is present but may be difficult to evaluate because of flexor action of the long toe flexors and posterior tibial muscle.

Operative treatment is indicated.

Tennis Leg

The sudden onset of pain in the posterior aspect of the calf is characteristic of this condition, which occurs commonly in tennis, squash and handball players. The pain feels like a kick in the calf. Dorsiflexion of the ankle is painful.

Although the condition has been ascribed to the rupture of the plantaris tendon, it is most likely that rupture of the fibers of the gastrocnemius along the medial aspect of the musculotendinous junction is the cause.

The use of a ¼ inch heel lift and the wearing of an elastic stocking will help in obtaining symptomatic relief.

Foot

Morton's Neuroma

Intermittent episodes of pain located in the metatarsal region and radiating distally are the presenting features of this condition (Fig. 12–18). The cause is a thickening of the sheath components of the affected plantar nerve. Most commonly affected is the plantar nerve between the third and fourth toes.

The patient complains of pain brought on by prolonged standing or walking. It can sometimes be relieved by removing the shoe.

Compression of the metatarsal arch by the examiner may duplicate the discomfort. Thumb pressure over the dorsum of the involved metatarsal space may also cause pain. Hypesthesia may be present over the plantar aspects of the lateral aspect of the third and medial aspects of the fourth toe.

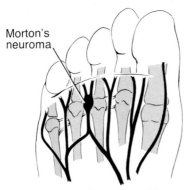

Morton's neuroma

Figure 12–18　Morton's neuroma. Metatarsalgia may occur as a result of a painful condition caused by thickening of the sheath of the plantar nerves. Most commonly affected is the plantar nerve between the third and fourth toes, as illustrated here.

Nonoperative treatment is of little value. When the diagnosis is confirmed, surgical treatment is indicated.

Dissection is performed through a dorsal incision, extending from the web proximally for about 1½ inches. After transection of the transverse metatarsal ligament, pressure on the ball of the foot will usually deliver the neuroma into the wound. Ordinarily the neuroma and the nerve entering and leaving should be removed completely, although occasionally the lesion is simply shelled out. The operation does not involve any major vascular structures, and complications are mainly limited to hematomas or infection. The depth of the incision produces considerable pain in most patients, and two or three days of hospitalization are usually indicated postoperatively. The patient is discharged on crutches, and a cast is not applied.

Plantar Fasciitis

Pain over the medial plantar aspect of the os calcis is characteristic of this condition. The discomfort is brought on by weight bearing, and it can become increasingly more intense. Other than the presence of local tenderness, physical findings are minimal. Radiographs of the area may show the presence of a calcaneal spur. However, in many instances there is no radiographic abnormality. It is felt that the spur, when present, is a contributing factor in the condition, as evidenced by the response to injections and the occasional spontaneous resolution of symptoms.

The use of a felt "doughnut" with the cutout over the painful area is used. Injection of a solution of 1 per cent Xylocaine and 1 cc of Hydeltra TBA is injected into the painful area and angled in several directions into the origin of plantar fascia from the os calcis. Three injections are given at two week intervals and usually result in subsidence of the symptoms.

In resistant cases, operative treatment is indicated.

Spine

One of the problems most frequently encountered by practitioners and emergency room physicians is the patient who presents with pain in the neck or back. Occasionally the pain results from pathological conditions in other organ systems. The history of trauma, however slight, must be documented and evaluated. Onset of pain following a new vocational or recreational activity points to pain of muscular origin. Long-standing discomfort suggests a postural problem. Pain which is worse at night or in the recumbent position may raise suspicion of a neoplasm. The cyclic type of pain in relation to the menses suggests pelvic disease. Pain of skeletal origin is almost always intensified by sitting, standing and activity and any deviation from this pattern should make the examiner suspicious of an extra-skeletal origin of discomfort. Malingering may be difficult to rule out, especially in Industrial Accident Clinics or following automobile accidents.

Discogenic Back Pain

The intervertebral disc is commonly the site of disease resulting in the syndrome of acute or chronic low back pain. The intervertebral discs in the lower portion of the lumbar spine bear the considerable strain of gravity and as a consequence begin to show degenerative changes in the second and third decades. Fissures and tears in the annulus with accompanying dessication of the nucleus pulposus occur with or without accident or trauma. Indeed, disc disease producing back pain seems to occur as commonly in those engaged in sedentary activity as in heavy laborers. Fissures in the annulus usually heal with collagenous tissue. However, loss of fluid content of the nucleus may result in loss of substance, followed by proliferation of osteophytes, a physiological attempt to restore strength to a damaged structure. In other instances, a disc damaged from degenerative change may show no radiographic evidence of narrowing of the height of the disc space or osteophyte formation.

Degeneration of the disc and its inability to withstand stresses cause additional strain on adjacent interspinous ligaments and joint facets and are added factors in the development of chronicity of symptoms.

Degenerative Disc Disease

This syndrome probably accounts for the majority of patients who present with the complaint of acute or chronic back pain.

The patient relates the onset of acute pain in the lumbar region. The pain may have had its onset following trivial activity such as making a bed, bending forward to tie one's shoes, or entering an automobile. A fall or other traumatic incident may be detailed by the patient, such as a lifting episode. The pain is poorly localized by the patient and is often associated with radiation toward the sciatic notch or into the buttock. Standing and sitting increase the discomfort. Lying on the side with the thighs and knees flexed affords some relief. The history almost always reveals that similar episodes occurred previously, following which the patient walked with a pelvic tilt. His symptoms subsequently subsided over a five to ten day period and he was able to engage in all activities again. The intermittent nature of acute symptoms, followed by partial healing of annular tissues, is characteristic of recurring episodes of disc degeneration.

Examination of the patient reveals a pelvic tilt associated with paravertebral muscle spasm. Flexion is present at the hip, with limited mobility of the lumbar segments. Straight leg raising does not usually cause pain referred to the buttock and extremities because of absence of compressive root disease. If straight leg raising is restricted, it is usually equal and bilateral.

Examination of the Back

The patient, wearing a disposable paper gown open in the back, is asked to walk in as nearly normal a fashion as possible. Additional disease, such as deformities in the lower extremities, can then be seen. He is asked to walk, if possible, on heels and toes in sequence, since this allows observation of paresis of the musculature of the lower extremities.

With the examiner seated behind the patient, the patient is asked to stand with both feet flat on the floor. The general posture and the presence of a scoliosis or pelvic tilt is noted.

The patient is asked to flex forward and attempt to touch his toes. More important than measuring the distance from fingertips to floor is observation of how the lumbar segments move in flexion and whether most of the flexion motion is carried out at the hip joints. Flexion may be carried out by veering to the right or left. This maneuver should be repeated during the examination to determine if the patient is feigning disability. The manner in which the patient extends from the flexed position should also be noted by the examiner with special attention to loss of synchronous movement during this effort.

The presence of local tenderness should be explored with evaluation of subjective pain over the sciatic notch and in both gluteal regions along the path of the sciatic nerve. The degree of muscle spasm and symmetry of the muscle masses is evaluated.

With the patient in the recumbent position, with both thighs and knees flexed, the presence of limitation of the hip motion is evaluated (Fig. 12–19). Painful response to internal and external rotation of the hip may point to primary hip disease. The presence of visible atrophy of thigh and calf is investigated. The circumference of the thighs is measured three inches above the superior pole of the patella and the calf is measured around its thickest portion.

Straight leg raising is performed with notation of levels at which pain is produced and areas to which it is referred. In compressive neuropathy pain is referred into the buttock and almost always into the posterior aspect of the extremity. Pain often is referred to this area when the contralateral leg is raised. On the other hand, in acute back conditions without nerve root compression,

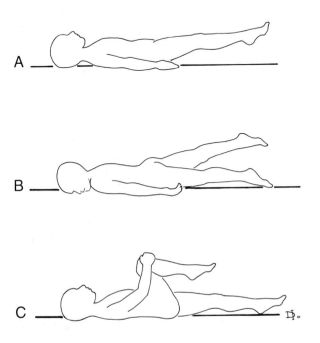

Figure 12–19 Back exercises. Chronic backache is frequently relieved by exercises which improve muscle tone, while not causing increased pain due to aggravation of any organic disease of the spine. Each exercise is repeated ten times daily. These exercises are performed on a firm surface, such as a floor with a soft rug. *A.* The patient is supine, with his heels raised several inches. The thighs are maintained flexed for seven to eight seconds. This exercise strengthens the abdominal musculature. *B.* The extensors of the back are strengthened by extension of the hip while the patient is in the prone position. Each leg is extended alternately and the position is maintained for seven to eight seconds. *C.* The lumbar curve is flattened and lordosis is reduced by a knee-chest exercise which is repeated alternately ten times, for several seconds with each leg.

straight leg raising will often be equally limited, with pain referred into the back region.

The deep tendon reflexes are examined with the patient seated on the side of the examining table. Clonus and plantar reflexes are evaluated. In instances of L5 root compression the posterior tibial reflex may be diminished on the affected side.

Motor power of the lower extremities is tested with special attention to the flexors and extensors of the ankle and toes, where minor differences can easily be appreciated.

Sensory impairment can be screened by alternately using the sharp and blunt ends of a safety pin on the dermatomes of the lower extremities.

X-ray

X-rays of the back should include oblique views of the lumbar spine. Developmental anomalies in the lumbar spine are common but of uncertain significance in relation to back pain. Transitional vertebra formation and spina bifida are frequently seen.

Narrowing of the intervertebral disc spaces is evaluated. The lumbosacral interspace is usually narrower than the L4–5 space, which in turn is wider than more cephalic interspaces. These facts must be kept in mind when evaluating disc space narrowing.

Spondylolysis may be seen on the lateral or anterior-posterior view but its verification may be difficult on the oblique views.

The presence of sacroiliac disease is investigated and special views of the joint should be taken if a suspicion of disease in the area is raised.

Search is made for destructive lesions and degenerative changes in the radiographs.

Films may show narrowing of one or more intervertebral disc spaces with osteophyte formation. Frequently no abnormality is seen on the radiographs.

Treatment. Most important in treatment of the acute painful episode is employment of the recumbent position.

Most often the patient is advised to assume the most comfortable recumbent position, usually lying on either side and flexing both thighs and knees. He is allowed to be upright for meals and allowed bathroom privileges. Pain and muscle relaxant medications are prescribed. The use of local heat helps somewhat in alleviation of pain evolving from muscle spasm.

The importance of bed rest is stressed to the patient. After several days the acute pain has subsided and gradually increasing activity is allowed. Avoidance of bending and stooping is continued for at least a one month period.

In some instances in which the syndrome becomes chronic in nature, a lumbosacral corset is advised. Rectus strengthening and pelvis strengthening exercises are prescribed. Advanced cases with marked disc space narrowing and osteophyte formation frequently respond to the use of Indocin 25 mgm q.i.d. If there are no medical contraindications or harmful side effects, the drug may be used for prolonged periods.

Herniated Disc

The presenting complaint is that of low back pain associated with sciatic radiation. In almost all instances preceding the onset of sciatic radiation there have been several episodes of acute back pain like those described for degenerative disc disease. These previous attacks may have occurred at six month or yearly intervals over a period of several years. It is doubtful if one traumatic incident could result in a herniated disc. The clinical syndrome usually results from many fissures of the annulus, either on a traumatic or a degenerative basis, followed by displacement of the annulus posteriorly. The displaced annulus may cause the disc to bulge posteriorly or it may rupture through the annulus and lie free in the epidural space. Both syndromes cause irritative and compressive neuropathy symptoms.

In the acute syndrome the back pain which was the predominant symptom in previous "attacks" may be secondary to the sciatic symptoms. Sciatic radiation may be experienced into the sacroiliac region, buttock or more distally into the posterior extremity. Paresthesia is almost always present and helps in localization. Weakness of muscle groups is seldom noticed by the patient unless profound.

Chronic syndromes may have been punctuated by recurrent episodes of acute pain followed by partial remissions for several months. These spontaneous remissions may be caused by subsidence of irritative phenomena of the nerve root or possibly diminution of the herniation.

Examination. Loss of mobility of the spine is almost always present, along with incomplete reversal of the lumbar segments in flexion.

Straight leg raising is limited on the affected side, with pain referred into the buttock and along the course of the sciatic nerve. Absence of positive straight leg raising signs in the presence of sciatic symptoms indicates the presence of irritative neuropathy rather than true nerve root compression. L5 root compression due to a herniation at the L4–5 interspace characteristically produces hypesthesia in the great toe associated with weakness of the ankle and toe extensors. The posterior tibial reflex, if obtainable on the opposite side, may be depressed and thus it has clinical significance.

S1 root compression results in hypesthesia over the lateral aspect of the foot and depression of the tendo Achillis reflex. Weakness of the hamstrings and calf musculature may be present. Absence of the patellar tendon reflex may imply L3–4 protrusion or may represent upward displacement of an L4–5 herniation.

X-rays. Radiographs of the lumbar spine quite frequently show no abnormality. Radiographic features of degenerative changes (i.e., disc space narrowing and osteophyte formation) usually do not localize the site of disc herniation. More often the symptomatic disc herniation is at the normal-appearing L4–5 interspace, when there is, for instance, radiographic evidence of degenerative disc

disease at the lumbosacral interspace. In such an instance both discs exhibit evidence of disease, one progressing to chronic degenerative changes and the other evolving into degeneration but with nuclear protrusion.

Myelography may be required to localize the area of disc protrusion. It is usually performed on an inpatient basis immediately prior to surgery.

Treatment. The majority of patients when first seen should be treated with bed rest as described under degenerative disc disease. Many patients with acute symptoms will exhibit improvement with this regimen. Muscle relaxant and pain medications are used along with local heat. Instances have been seen wherein a complete foot drop has improved with nonoperative treatment. Therefore, surgical treatment is employed only for treatment of persistent pain, progressive neurological change or in those instances in which a massive herniation has resulted in cauda equina compression.

Lumbosacral Sprain

Back pain following trauma may be caused by damage to the supporting ligaments of the lumbar spine and to the lumbosacral articulation. The syndrome appears in individuals who have not experienced previous symptoms referable to the lumbar spine. The relationship to a traumatic incident is clear, although it cannot be definitively established that pain has developed from a progressing annular fissure. The inciting force may arise from a twisting movement while carrying a heavy object, or, in the case of two workers carrying a heavy object, one drops his weight and the other suddenly experiences the full thrust of the object. Attempts to lift a heavy object with the spine flexed may cause damage to the ligaments of the lumbar spine as well.

The history of the traumatic incident is taken. Usually the patient reports that the initial pain which occurred after the incident seemed to subside somewhat in the next several hours. On the following day the pain was much more severe and was associated with stiffness and muscle spasm. The patient usually has not previously experienced back difficulties, but if he has, they have usually followed other traumatic incidents. There has been no history of acute back symptoms occurring after trivial motions — the common history of degenerative disc disease. It may nevertheless be difficult to differentiate acute lumbosacral sprain from degenerative disc disease.

Examination reveals flattening of the normal lumbar lordosis and paravertebral muscle spasm. Tenderness is diffuse and difficult to localize. A pelvic tilt may be present. Straight leg raising may be restricted, but is equal in both extremities. The discomfort experienced during the maneuver is localized in the back.

Radiographs may show abnormalities in the lumbar spine which were present prior to the injury. A spine with degenerative changes or a spondylolysis is more subject to injury, but the changes seen on the x-ray films cannot be attributed to the injury.

Treatment of the acute cases consists of bed rest until the severe symptoms have subsided. Ultrasound and massage is helpful after the severe initial phase. Activity is gradually increased. In industrial cases, the length of time before normal duty is resumed can sometimes be reduced by allowing the worker to return to limited or part-time work. This is preferable to returning the individual to full activity before he is ready. The physician often finds himself in a difficult position in this regard but sincere handling of the patient usually minimizes the problem.

If the patient has difficulty with ambulation after the initial acute phase has subsided, a lumbosacral corset is prescribed. During the course of treatment the patient should be seen at frequent intervals for encouragement and reassurance that his injury is not a serious one.

Almost all persons can be expected to return to nearly normal function within several months.

Spondylolisthesis

In this condition one vertebra in the lumbar region slips anteriorly upon the adjacent one. The two major types are those in which there is a defect in the pars-interarticularis and those in which there is no associated defect.[9]

The most commonly seen type is associated with a laminar defect in the pars-interarticularis. This defect is called a spondylolysis, and may or may not result in a forward slipping. The defect is rarely seen before the age of twenty.

The other types of spondylolisthesis are associated with elongation of the lamina, attritional changes of the intervertebral facet joints, or osteomalacia, in which the vertebrae have undergone gradual structural changes.

The patient frequently presents with back pain of long-standing duration. There is often a dragging sensation felt in the buttocks. Symptoms and signs of nerve root compression may be seen in the lower extremities.

When the symptoms are predominantly lumbar the use of a lumbosacral corset is recommended. Often an individual will have periodic and repeated episodes of low back pain and will achieve relief with the intermittent use of his back support.

Surgical treatment is indicated for clinically disabling symptoms and when there is evidence of lumbar nerve root compression.

Cervical Sprain

The rear-end automobile collision is a frequent occurrence on our congested streets and highways. This type of accident has brought the so-called "whiplash injury" into prominence among legal and medical groups and the lay public. The forces and mechanism of this injury have been studied and documented by many authors. Patients who have been subjected to rear-end collisions have been the victims and subjects of both overtreatment and neglect by the medical profession. In addition, these patients have been thoroughly inconvenienced by the other driver.

Mechanism of Injury. If seated in an automobile which is struck in the rear, an individual is propelled forward along with his vehicle and seat. His head and neck, being unsupported, are in effect thrown backward into extension. In addition there is a severe compression force applied to the spine. The opposite effect occurs when the vehicle comes to a halt, causing a forward thrust of the trunk coupled with flexion of the neck. It is probable that the extension and compression of the neck is a major offending force in the cause of whiplash injury.

Symptom Complex. The patient complains of discomfort which begins several hours after the accident. It is not unusual for symptoms to occur in both the anterior and posterior neck musculature. The anterior symptoms are usually evanescent and disappear after several days. Posterior symptoms may increase in severity and be accompanied by headaches, which originate in the cervical region and are accompanied by cephalad and anterior radiation of pain. Pain on rotation of the neck is frequently a presenting complaint. Nonspecific intermittent tingling in the upper extremities usually is caused by scalenus spasm with thoracic outlet obstruction rather than nerve root compression.

Examination. Inspection of the neck may suggest evidence of muscle asymmetry. Paravertebral muscle spasm is frequently noted. Passive motion permitted in flexion, extension, rotation and lateral bending is noted and recorded. Examination of the upper extremities should be included in the examination to rule out nerve root compression.

Radiographic Examination. X-ray films of the cervical spine should be taken to rule out fracture. Flexion and extension views may be necessary in cases of protracted symptomatology but they are usually difficult to obtain in the acute phase of the injury. The presence of degenerative changes may be used as a baseline for comparison with subsequent films, but these changes are common on routine examinations of the adult population.

Treatment. Muscle relaxants and analgesics are used, supplemented by local heat. Symptoms which become bothersome as the day progresses may be helped considerably by a rest of several hours in the afternoon. Severe occipital headaches will be helped by the use of a cervical support. We prefer the plastic adjustable type of so-called "Thomas collar" with padded superior and inferior surfaces. The short-term use of cervical traction may help to relieve bothersome muscle spasm but will often have an adverse effect in the acute phase.

It is thought that the best course for the physician to pursue is to reassure the patient that his symptoms will gradually subside with the passage of time and that frequently this convalescence will be measured in months rather than weeks. The continuing persistent employment of physical therapy modalities over long periods of time is often a deterrent to the patient's convalescence since it may overemphasize to the patient the severity of his injury.

In the majority of instances the patient will gradually improve and be left with no residual effects. Occasionally evidence may be noted on subsequent radiographs of progressive disc space narrowing or new or accelerated degenerative changes which suggest the cause of continuing cervical symptoms.

TUMORS

Bone tumors are a relatively uncommon problem in outpatient orthopedic practice. There is considerable variation in types of tumors, in anatomical distribution and in prognosis.

The most common malignant tumor of bone is metastatic cancer. Metastatic tumors are usually derived from either lung, thyroid, stomach, breast, kidney or prostate. These lesions generally show bone destruction, with or without surrounding sclerosis. Metastatic tumors are seen most commonly in pelvis, spine or proximal long bones. They often present as pathologic fractures. Operative biopsy is indicated for diagnosis.

The most common primary bone tumor is osteogenic sarcoma, usually presenting in patients less than 20 years old. The most frequent site of presentation is around the knee. Prognosis is extremely poor. Differential diagnosis includes infection, Ewing's sarcoma, solitary plasmacytoma, myositis ossificans and eosinophilic granuloma. Open incisional biopsy is indicated, and a pathologic diagnosis by permanent section is desirable before definitive therapy is carried out.

Many benign lesions may be discovered on routine radiographs, taken for fractures or mild skeletal complaints. Cystic lesions result from aneurysmal bone cysts, unicameral bone cysts, nonossifying fibroma, enchondromas, chondroblastomas, and fibrous dysplasia. These lesions usually cause minimal or no complaints by the patient unless they develop a pathologic fracture. Other patients may present with complaints of a mass or growth on an extremity. Giant cell tumor of the tendon sheath, lipoma, ganglion, epithelial inclusion cyst, Dupuytren's fibrosis and pseudosarcomatous fascitis present in the hand and are benign. Excisional biopsy under regional anesthesia is indicated.

One of the most common lesions presenting as a mass is that of an osteochondroma (exostosis). These lesions usually involve metaphyseal areas of long bones, especially about the knee, but may present in the pelvis and scapula. Less than 5 per cent undergo malignant transformation into chondrosarcomas. Excisional biopsy is indicated for complaints of persistent pain secondary to irritation of overlying bursa, interference with joint motion, or suspicion of malignant transformation because of rapid increase in size.

Other soft tissue tumors may present as mass lesions of the upper or lower extremity. Synovial sarcomas commonly occur as soft tissue masses about the knee, hip or shoulder. Rhabdomyosarcomas present as soft tissue enlargement and discomfort within a muscle mass. Any such soft tissue mass requires excisional biopsy, with minimal destruction of normal tissue, followed by study of permanent sections and appropriate radical surgery if indicated.

Other conditions such as multiple myeloma or reticulum cell sarcoma may be discovered in the complete work-up of multiple vertebral compression fractures. Paget's disease may be discovered on routine pelvic or skull films. Hyperparathyroidism may be first discovered on routine hand films. These conditions do not usually require bone biopsy for diagnosis.

Specific treatment of the above conditions is beyond the scope of this text. Generally the malignant lesions require radical excision or amputation, although the ultimate prognosis is still very poor. Amputation is unwarranted until permanent sections have been reviewed by a pathologist expert in evaluating neoplasms of bone, even if a delay of a week or more is necessary after biopsy. Benign lesions usually require simple observation, curettage or local excision. Other malignant lesions such as giant cell tumor, chondrosarcoma and periosteal osteosarcomas are unpredictable in action. They are generally treated with wide local excision, followed by close observation for recurrence.

References

1. Kite, J. H.: Clubfoot. New York, Grune and Stratton, 1964.
2. Lovell, W. W.: Treatment of congenital talipes equinovarus. Clin. Orthop., 70:79–86, 1970.
3. Kite, J. H.: Congenital metatarsus varus. J. Bone Joint Surg., 49A:388–397, 1967.
4. Coleman, S. S., Stelling, F. H., and Jarrett, J.: Pathomechanics and treatment of congenital vertical talus. Clin. Orthop., 70:62–72, 1970.
5. Sharrard, W. J. W.: Paediatric Orthopaedic Fractures. Oxford, 1971.
6. Winter, R. B., Moe, J. H., and Eilers, V. E.: Congenital scoliosis. A study of 234 patients treated and untreated. J. Bone Joint Surg., 50A:1–48, 1968.
7. Phalen, G. S.: Carpal-tunnel syndrome. J. Bone Joint Surg., 48A:211–228, 1966.
8. Smillie, I. S.: Injuries of the knee joint. Baltimore, Williams and Wilkins, 1962.
9. Newman, P. H., and Stone, K. H.: The etiology of spondylolisthesis. J. Bone Joint Surg., 45B:39–59, 1963.

13

The Hand

By PAUL W. BROWN, M.D.

INTRODUCTION

The purpose of this chapter is to make clear what can and cannot be done properly and safely for injured and ailing hands in the Emergency Room and in the Outpatient Clinic. The attending physician should keep always in mind the first dictum of medical practice, "Primum non nocere." Unfortunately, too much is often attempted in the Emergency Room and more hands are harmed by too ambitious attempts at treatment than by too little. When faced with many of the poorer results of too much treatment administered in the interest of "saving time and money for the patient" or for "convenience," the hand surgeon is forced to conclude that the patient would have fared better if he had never seen a physician. When the capabilities and limitations of the Emergency Room and the Outpatient Clinic are honestly assessed, these environments can be properly used to relieve suffering and to treat or prepare the way for treatment of the injured hand. If ignorance or surgical arrogance is fostered in these places, the result will be a steady stream of complications referred to the hand surgeon or to the attorney.

THE ROLE OF THE EMERGENCY ROOM

Evaluation

An assessment of the damage to the hand can be made most thoroughly and adequately if the examining doctor is oriented toward diagnosis rather than therapy. Most injured hands are bleeding and the sight of blood seems to inspire the thought of surgery in many of us rather than an objective analysis of cause and effect. The Emergency Room certainly has great advantages in the treatment of minor trauma, but its highest value is in preparing the patient for proper treatment and in separating what is best handled on the spot from that which requires more extensive treatment.

Control of bleeding is seldom a great problem if one proceeds in a cool and organized manner. If bleeding obscures the wound the logical first step in the assessment of the wound is to stop the flow of blood. A fistful of surgical sponges covered with a mildly compressive elastic bandage will do the job in the majority of cases. I have not known exsanguination from a severed artery in the hand, wrist or forearm to occur, but occasionally it will be necessary to staunch the flow of blood by digital pressure or a tourniquet, a simple procedure which will then allow a full examination of the damage. Such an examination cannot be done well in the presence of a hovering parent or a distraught wife and they should be asked to remain in the waiting room, providing one does not forget to see them later and give them a report of one's findings.

The evaluation itself starts with the history of the injury or complaint. Not only is the nature of the accident or incident important, but also the nature of the environment, the exact time of the accident and the first aid treatment which has been given. The treatment for a laceration of a knuckle incurred by a knife is quite different from that for a laceration inflicted by someone's front teeth, since the contamination factors in the kitchen are quite different from those of the street. The patient's occupation and special requirements for the use of his hand as well as knowledge as to whether he is left-handed or right-handed are occasionally of importance in planning treatment.

The correct position for examination is to have the patient supine with arm outstretched on an armboard or table with a physician seated beside the hand. Good lighting is essential and need not include a glaring light directed into the patient's eyes. Many upright patients tend to faint when an injured hand is examined or manipulated; the supine position obviates this possibility as well as reassuring the patient (Fig. 13-1).

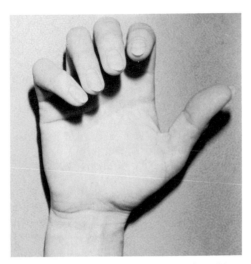

Figure 13-1 Position of examination. Note that the small finger is normally held in more flexion than the ring, the ring more than the middle and the middle more than the index. Also called the position of rest.

Physical and visual examinations are next. Fear and anxiety are the greatest potentiators of pain and if the patient is supine and the physician proceeds in an orderly and confident manner, complaints of pain are seldom severe enough to interfere with the examination. Only rarely will narcotics or sedatives be required; if medication is indicated, diazepam (Valium) will act effectively and safely. An orderly inventory should be taken by tissue system: skin, vessels, nerve, bone and joint, tendon and muscle. Occasionally, the state of a particular structure will not be clear—e.g., the median nerve in a volar laceration of the wrist. In such cases one's curiosity must be curtailed by the admonition "do no further harm." Surgical exploration in the Emergency Room is out of order even in the cause of correct diagnosis. Generally, this will not be necessary and under ordinary circumstances, all damaged structures will be apparent without harming or hurting the patient.

What Can Be Done in the Emergency Room

Most dislocations and many fractures can be reduced in the Emergency Room.

Some wounds can be closed. A spurting artery can be ligated or at least clamped. An occasional extensor tendon can be repaired and a burned hand may be immersed in ice water. Proper splints and dressings can be applied. Ideally, and with few exceptions, that is all! Unfortunately, the ideal is beset with necessary compromises of time, place, economics, bed availability and patient pressures, and we may be forced to extend the Emergency Room beyond its safe limits. For this we will pay a certain price of infection, wound breakdown, scarred-down tendons and other unhappy results. The greater our compromise, the greater the complications, and these will include such misfortunes as reflex sympathetic dystrophies, stiffened fingers and painful hands.

One very important thing the Emergency Room can do is to prepare for proper and prompt management of severe conditions beyond the capabilities of the Emergency Room. When time is important to results, and this is always true where débridement is necessary, the Emergency Room staff can save that time by notifying the attending physician and the operating room and taking care of preoperative and administrative details. The Emergency Room's task is not finished when the decision is reached to treat the patient further in the operating room.

Limitations of the Emergency Room

The limitations of the Emergency Room are implied in the foregoing. Nerves and tendons are not repaired, with certain obvious exceptions which will be dealt with later. Only the most simple skin grafts are undertaken and open reductions of fractures and dislocations are not done at all. Major débridements cannot be done well in the Emergency Room, and only the most obvious superficial burns can be assessed. The hand is terribly unforgiving of poor management and barely tolerant of the moderately good; most of these things can be done better in the operating room than in the Emergency

Room and the damaged hand will insist on proving that time after time.

The Transition to Inpatient Status

The Emergency Room patient should become an inpatient when further care in the operating room is necessary within the next twenty-four hours or when the hand requires constant elevation, frequent observation, dressing changes or skilled nursing care. Cases not requiring immediate surgery but in which there is a reasonable risk of increasing edema should certainly be admitted: included in this category are wringer injuries in children and other crush injuries. Burns of undetermined extent should be admitted as should hand infections which show evidence of progression. Poor treatment in the first 24 hours may cause functional impairment that may take months or years of rehabilitation to correct.

The Outpatient Clinic

The results of treatment of the disabled hand can be facilitated or ruined by the follow-up care given that hand. Every hand surgeon is acutely aware that the postoperative management of the hand is just as important as the operation. Thus the Outpatient Clinic, like the Emergency Room, must have good facilities for examination of the hand. For most patients this is best accomplished with the patient sitting opposite the examiner with the hand resting on a small table of comfortable height. If sutures or wires are to be removed the examination may be painful and it is better to have the patient supine to remove the risk of fainting.

In the Outpatient Clinic dressings can be changed and splints made or adjusted, and a detailed record of the patient's progress in returning function to the hand can be made and kept. As future prescriptions may depend on the rate of progress, it is important that appearance, swelling, coloration, complaints of pain, strength and ranges of motion be carefully recorded. Consistency of nomenclature is necessary if records are to have value. The digits are not numbered, but are named: thumb, index, middle, ring and small. These may be abbreviated Th, I, M, R and S. The joints are metacarpophalangeal (MP), proximal interphalangeal (PIP), and distal interphalangeal (DIP); the thumb has only a single interphalangeal joint (IP). The joints are most commonly agreed to be at zero degrees when extended. If extended beyond this point, it can be recorded as a minus figure. Thus the MP joint of a right small finger which hyperextends ten degrees and flexes to a right angle would be recorded as follows: RtSF MP–10/90. A distinction may have to be made between active and passive ranges of motion (act. ROM and pass. ROM). The usual range of motion of the wrist would be recorded: –60/90; pro. 90, sup. 90.

In the case of nerve injuries careful motor and sensory examination is a necessary part of the record if the rate of regeneration of the nerve is to be assessed. Such recording may play an essential role in future decisions to reexplore a nerve or to intervene with secondary salvage procedures such as tendon transfers.

Most wounds of the hand, surgical and traumatic, are closed with synthetic sutures such as nylon. The simplest and most effective tools for suture removal are iris scissors with two sharp points and a mosquito type hemostat. Wire sutures may also be readily removed with these, although the scissors will not last indefinitely.

Kirschner wires used for internal splinting and for the fixation of fractures and arthrodeses are generally buried just under the skin. Their removal is a simple outpatient procedure requiring the injection of a drop of local anesthetic, a nick in the skin and extraction of the wire with needlenose pliers whose jaws have been filed down to sharp points. Occasionally one cannot find the wire and if its removal is imperative a more effective anesthetic and a more extensive search and a tourniquet are required. Probing for elusive K-wires

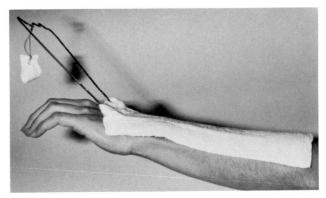

Figure 13–2   An improvised splint of plaster of paris, a bent coat hanger, rubber band and adhesive tape finger sling. When the plaster is set, it is affixed to the forearm with an ace bandage. This particular splint is designed to assist a finger in extension. Slings for each finger can be added.

can be a painful experience for both physician and patient, and it is to be hoped that the former will not prolong the experience when simple measures are not enough.

Proper dressings can certainly be applied in the Outpatient Clinic and some simple splints can be fabricated out of plaster of paris, wire coathangers and rubber bands (Fig. 13–2). Some of the newer thermoplastics such as Orthoplast have some use in this regard. An understanding of what is needed in the way of a splint and some ingenuity are more important for most splints than fancy materials and elaborate equipment.

Equipment

The most essential equipment for dealing with impaired hands in the Emergency Room is an observant pair of eyes. Next most important is plenty of mild soap and water. Helpful but far less necessary are sutures and other surgical paraphernalia. With these priorities clearly in mind the type and extent of proper hand surgery in the Emergency Room can be better defined.

When dealing with wounds of the hand, the examiner or operator should wear a surgical mask. Surgical instruments needed are few and simple, but they should be small and reserved for delicate work. Necessary are a scalpel with expendible No. 15 blades, Adson or tissue fixation forceps, double pointed scissors, mosquito hemostats, a probe, a small bone rongeur, a Bunnell type hand drill and 0.045 inch Kirschner wires. A 4-0 plain catgut suture is adequate for tying off bleeders and 5-0 nylon or polyethylene swaged onto a small curved cutting needle is best for closing wounds of the hand and affixing skin grafts. Simple self-retaining retractors, skin hooks and small rake retractors complete the list. Anything more elaborate than this instrument inventory would indicate that work is being done in the Emergency Room that should best be done in the operating room.

A tourniquet has limited application in the Emergency Room and in the Outpatient Clinic. Simple débridement in the Emergency Room is generally best done without a tourniquet since recognition of devitalized tissue is easier when free bleeding can be seen. When a tourniquet is required, its level of application and duration of use may depend on the type of anesthesia used. A pneumatic blood pressure cuff should be used on the upper arm, a proper pressure for adults being 250 mm of mercury and for children 200 mm. Tourniquets used at wrist and forearm levels may cause nerve damage. A rubber band tourniquet

around the base of the finger is dangerous except for procedures lasting only a
few minutes. Since most patients can
comfortably tolerate a tourniquet on the
arm for about twenty minutes, this can
be useful when carrying out small procedures on the hand under local anesthesia.

Anesthesia

This topic has been dealt with more
thoroughly in Chapter 2, but reference
should be made here to three types of
anesthesia particularly useful to Emergency Room management of the injured
hand. For all of these a solution of 1
per cent aqueous lidocaine is effective
and safe. The first is local infiltration of
the injured area. Producing an intradermal wheal, waiting a few seconds and
then advancing the needle in various
directions while injecting the solution
should be a relatively painless procedure.
A 1½ inch No. 22 hypodermic needle
will suffice for this and the following
methods. For effective use one should
wait approximately ten minutes after
injection before proceeding further.
Solutions with epinephrine should not
be used.

For work on one or two fingers a
block of the digital or common digital
nerve is often useful. The needle is
introduced into the dorsal surface of the
finger web, pointed volarward and toward the metacarpal head, and 2 milli-
liters of lidocaine are injected (Fig.
13–3). This is repeated for the other volar
digital nerve, and if work is to be done
on the dorsum of the proximal or middle
segment of the finger a similar block of
the dorsal nerves may be necessary.
Again it should be emphasized that no
epinephrine should be used.

One of the most satisfactory types of
anesthesia for Emergency Room work
on the hand, wrist and forearm is the
intravenous regional block or the so-
called Bier block. This was described in
Chapter 2, but it can be mentioned here
that this type of anesthesia is easy and

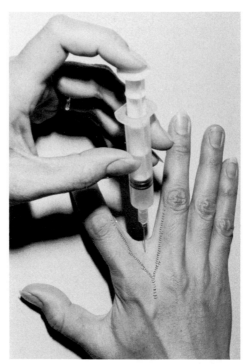

Figure 13–3 Common digital nerve block. The
needle is directed toward the bifurcation of the
nerve. If preceded by an intradermal wheal, the
procedure should be almost painless.

safe to use and is well accepted by
children.

Related to methods of anesthesia are
the safe, simple and analgesic properties of ice water. Ice water immersion
of the painful burned hand is wonderfully
effective in allaying pain and calming the
patient, and is similarly useful for
sprains, fractures and crush injuries. An
ice water bath maintained for up to
twenty minutes not only gives excellent
relief of pain, but if used within an hour
after the injury it may be very effective
in preventing or decreasing the amount
of edema that would otherwise develop.

Dressings and Splints

The hand dressing can be as important
as the surgical treatment itself. Properly
applied it can promote comfort, contribute to healing, and—most important—
help to prevent or decrease edema. Im-

properly applied it can cause pain, contribute to stiffening and in fact irreparably damage a hand. The basic principle should be one of uniform mild compression — the dressing must be firm but not tight. Bunnell's concept of the position of function is still a very useful one in applying hand dressings even though some conditions may call for deviations from this position. These principles state that the hand is best maintained with the wrist in 30 degrees extension with moderate flexion of all MP and IP joints and with the thumb in moderate abduction. In this position both the transverse and longitudinal arches of the hand are preserved.

Wounds, whether sutured or left open, are best covered with fine mesh gauze. Somewhat better are plastic coated dressings such as Telfa or gauze impregnated with bismuth ointment such as Xeroform, since these allow blood to ooze through but do not stick to the wound when removed. Petrolatum fine mesh gauze is also good if the excess grease is scraped free — too much grease tends to cause maceration. Over the gauze are applied several flat gauze sponges; how much of the hand must be incorporated in the dressing is a question to be decided at this time. Any injury of the hand or of a digit causes edema of some degree. Whether this edema will be severe enough to interfere with healing or with return of the hand to normal function depends conjointly on the nature of the injury as well as on the postinjury management of that hand. Though one may hesitate to apply a complete hand dressing for a finger injury, it is safer to do so when there is a question of subsequent edema and pain.

For dressing an individual finger the various sizes of tubular stockinette known as Tubegauz are extremely convenient. Lacking this, a roller bandage gauze can be used, but this must be affixed with strips of adhesive tape. With such circumferential strips, care must be taken not to constrict venous return, and the patient must be cautioned to loosen the strips in the event of increasing swelling.

In dressing the entire hand the fingers should be separated by individual sponges, and the dorsal and volar surfaces of the entire hand, including the wrist, should be overlain with fluffed-up sponges in multiple layers. The dressings are then wrapped snugly with a slightly elastic roll of gauze such as Kling or Kerlex. The goal should be a firm dressing with evenly distributed compression; a compression dressing is definitely not a tight dressing. Material such as sponge rubber foam, polyurethane foam or mechanic's waste may be used in place of the gauze fluffs (Fig. 13–4).

A volar — and occasionally dorsal — plaster splint may sometimes be overlain on the compression dressing where immobilization is needed. A circular plaster cast seldom is needed for injury of the hand until the initial edema has subsided.

Equally important to the compression dressing is continuous elevation of the injured extremity. The duration of elevation is directly proportional to the damage done to the hand. Twenty-four hours will suffice for most injuries, but elevation may be indicated for several days when crushing has been a part of the injuring force. In the case of outpatient treatment, the patient should be instructed to suspend the hand in its dressing from the back of a chair moved next to his bed while he is sleeping. When he is up the forearm can be rested on top of the head or the hand rested on the opposite shoulder. Slings are generally inadvisable as they invite prolonged dependency of the hand and also tend to produce stiff elbows and shoulders.

Static splints for digital fractures are illustrated in Chapter 11. Dynamic splints for uncomplicated problems can readily be fashioned from plaster splints, coathanger wire, rubber bands and safety pins. Such homemade splints may be definitive in some cases or may

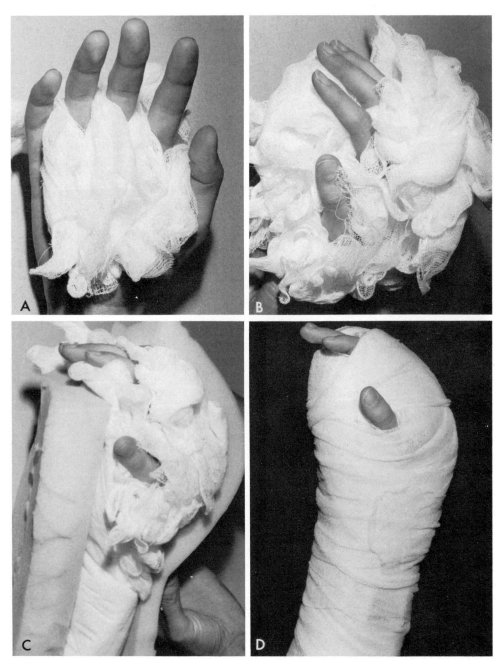

Figure 13-4 Applying the hand compression dressing. *A.* The fingers are lightly separated by surgical sponges. *B.* Many fluffed-up surgical sponges are applied to volar and dorsal surfaces. *C.* ABD pads or strips of polyurethane foam are applied from middle finger joints to just below the elbow. *D.* Firm, but not tight, compression is applied with Kerlix or Kling gauze. Ace bandage may be used but caution is necessary to avoid wrapping too tightly. Note "position of function." Elevation of the extremity should follow.

serve to start treatment until a more
sophisticated brace or splint can be
made by an orthotist.

TRAUMA

Open Wounds

An open wound represents a dual
insult to the hand: first, a break in the
integument with or without other tissue
damage, and second, a factor of contamination. It is the latter which makes the
open wound unique and potentially more
dangerous than the closed injury. Lest
this seem obvious to the point of being
trite, let me point out that many of our
complications and bad results stem from
a lack of understanding of this fundamental. Pasteur's deathbed words are
reputed to have been, "The organism
is nothing, the environment is all." In
dealing with the inherent dangers of
wound contamination, two fundamentals
must be understood: (1) as many of the
contaminating organisms as possible
must be removed from the wound without further damaging tissue, and (2)
the tissue must be managed in such a
way as to discourage multiplication of
organisms. Anything which enhances
such multiplication also enhances the
transition from contamination, a nonpathologic state, to infection, which
definitely is pathologic. The presence
of devitalized tissue, hematoma, foreign
material or edema tends to encourage
infection. Translated into terms of practical action, our task is to remove as
many bacteria as possible by irrigation,
but since complete decontamination
is not possible, we must improve the
environment by débridement and by
proper wound dressing and management.

Débridement. Débridement is the
key to wound healing. It may be as
simple as the housewife holding her cut
finger under running water before applying a Band-aid, or it may be an exacting, time-consuming operation. It implies
the removal of foreign bodies, devitalized or unsalvagable tissue and the
removal of as many bacteria as possible.
Foreign bodies such as splinters or lead
shot may be easily removed, but the
removal of foreign materials injected
under pressure from a grease gun or
paint gun may represent a formidable
challenge. Organic material such as
vegetable matter or bits of clothing must
be removed, but the extraction of metallic bodies such as bullets or pieces thereof is rarely worth the surgical trauma required to find them.

Recognizing and removing devitalized
tissue is the most difficult part of débridement. The hand has little expendable
tissue, and the challenge is to save anything viable which is useful to future
function, yet not to compromise healing
and future function by leaving any dead
or potentially dead tissue within the
hand. Débridement is done without
tourniquet, because bleeding of the
tissues is often the best key to their
viability. Skin which is obviously
avascular should be removed; if in doubt
as to its viability, leave the decision

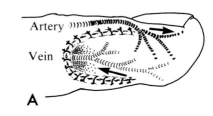

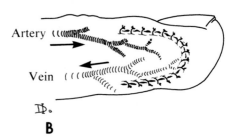

Figure 13–5 Traumatic skin flaps. The major
problem and cause of necrosis in the distally based
flap is inadequate venous drainage.

until two or three days have elapsed (Fig. 13–5). Subcutaneous fat which is dirty or badly traumatized should be removed. Muscle which bleeds freely should be retained; that which does not must be discarded. Bone fragments — even though completely detached from soft tissue — are never removed. If detached and dirty they should be washed off and returned to their place of origin. Nerves and tendons are rarely removed; even though frayed and dirty they may often be salvagable for future function, and therefore the physician should clean them off and leave them in place.

The best aid to the removal of bacteria is copious irrigation with sterile saline. This implies the use of a liter — or in severe cases many liters — of fluid and not a few squirts from a syringe. If the liquid is gravity delivered though a narrow gauge nozzle the stream of fluid can be directed into nooks and crannies and with enough force to flush out bits of contaminants and devitalized tissue as well as a good proportion of the contaminating organisms.

Closure and Nonclosure. There are several conflicting approaches to the management of open wounds. Perhaps the most popular and certainly the most simplistic is to close them all. When this doctrine has been applied to all wounds, disasters such as wound breakdown, gas gangrene, amputation and death have been frequent. To go to the opposite extreme and leave all wounds open is certainly safer but hardly practical for many injuries. The challenge is to recognize those which may be safely closed — or better yet to recognize those wounds which would be benefited from early closure. This determination is often a difficult one: the factors to be considered are the nature and extent of the injury, the degree and type of contamination, the adequacy of decontamination and débridement, and the length of time elapsed from the time of injury. To appraise all of these variables accurately and to apply them to a particular hand calls for objective analysis, knowledge and experience. If there is one simple rule, it must be: "If in doubt, don't close."

Wounds which generally can be safely closed are those which are cleanly incised, those which have been incurred in a relatively "clean" environment, those which have a small degree of soft tissue damage, and those in which less than eight hours have elapsed from the time of injury until the time of closure. A useful distinction between the "tidy" and the "untidy" wound has been made by Rank and Wakefield,[7] but it should be noted that a seemingly tidy wound incurred the day previously does not permit safe closure, as it is no longer clean. Gunshot wounds, crush injuries and wounds incurred in the barnyard are examples of wounds which should not be closed early.

Primary closure means suturing a wound within 24 hours of injury. This is probably the most common method used in the Emergency Room and despite the fact that most wounds so treated heal without complication, we must concern ourselves with those cases which are harmed by such treatment.

Delayed primary closure is done between the second and seventh day and is much safer for most wounds. Such wounds will still heal by primary intention and with fewer complications. The disadvantages for the physician and the patient are the time and inconvenience. A major advantage is that the "second look" at the time of redressing gives one the opportunity to find areas requiring redébridement, an opportunity which is denied by primary closure.

Closure after the sixth or seventh day is called secondary, and is used for more severe, untidy wounds, especially when there is some crushing of soft tissues. Secondary closure of wounds can sometimes be done by wound excision and suturing, but more commonly coverage is obtained with skin grafts or pedicle transfers, and these procedures will seldom be done in the Emergency Room.

With many wounds the doctrine of delayed closure may well be expanded to one of nonclosure. Some open wounds of the hand that are allowed to heal by secondary intention will give end results as good as the same types of wound that have been closed primarily. Transverse wounds of the volar aspect of the palm and fingers do particularly well when dressed properly with relative immobility of the adjoining joints, and will heal as well and as promptly as those which are sutured and with less likelihood of infection and wound breakdown. This doctrine is perhaps a difficult one for both physician and patient to accept, but once the former has seen a few wounds thus treated and has convinced himself of the usefulness of this technique, he will have little difficulty in convincing his patients (Fig. 13–6). For skin flaps which lift up or separate, adhesive tape strips may readily be used instead of sutures. The sterile adhesive Steri-Strips are quicker, cheaper and more comfortable to apply than sutures and they may be effectively used for skin closure as well as affixing skin grafts. Such tape sutures are very useful with a so-called trapdoor laceration, with lacerations of the fingers and on the dorsal surface of the hand.

Fractures and Joint Injuries

Open Fractures. It is widely written and accepted that open fractures of the hand must be closed and also that leaving an open fracture open invites infection. Neither of these dicta is true. If there is any question about the wound healing primarily because of contamination or the nature of the wound, the open fracture will heal better and with fewer complications if the wound is left open than if the wound does not accept closure and breaks down secondarily. The same is true of open joint injuries; contrary to popular teaching an open joint overlain by a dirty wound will do better left open, if active motion of the joint is encouraged. Such joints do not lose their articular cartilage nor do they tend to stiffen appreciably; on the contrary, the joint which becomes infected owing to premature closure often ends up with painful stiffness or ankylosis.

Fractures of the Distal Phalanx. These usually involve the distal tuft and may be remarkably comminuted, but no treatment other than a protective fingertip splint for comfort is necessary.

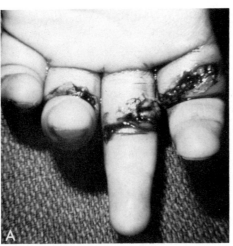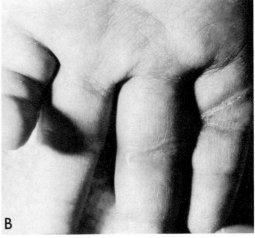

Figure 13–6 Nonclosure technique. Healing by secondary intention. *A*. Volar lacerations with an element of crushing. Underlying flexor tendons divided. Wounds were treated by débridement and copious irrigation, covered with fine mesh gauze and a mild compression hand dressing and suspension. No sutures were used. *B*. Same wounds 40 days later. No edema, no induration. Hand is now ready for reconstructive surgery for the tendons.

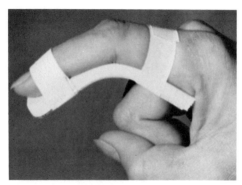

Figure 13–7 Splint for a fracture of the middle phalanx. Splint is aluminum and is padded with sponge rubber. The patient should be instructed to loosen the tape strips if swelling occurs.

This splint is a simple splint of aluminum placed on the volar side of the middle and distal phalanges with the DIP joint flexed fifteen degrees. The end of the splint is curved up to cover the end of the finger to protect it from being painfully bumped.

Fractures of the Middle Phalanx. Shaft fractures of this bone usually result from a crushing injury or from a blow by a heavy object. If undisplaced they should be immobilized for two to three weeks with an aluminum splint taped to all three phalanges with the interphalangeal joints in 15 degrees of flexion (Fig. 13–7). If angulated, the deformity should be corrected before splinting. If reduction cannot be retained by the splint, the fracture should be transfixed with a Kirschner wire drilled in from one side of the finger and left in place for three weeks. A fairly common injury combines a fracture of the volar portion of the phalanx with a dorsal dislocation of the remainder of the phalanx: i.e., a fracture-dislocation of the PIP joint. If not reduced accurately all useful function of this joint will be lost and an open reduction and internal fixation with two Kirschner wires as shown in the illustration is necessary (Fig. 13–8). This is generally a task for the operating room.

Fractures of the Proximal Phalanx. The mechanism of injury of such fractures is usually the same as for the middle phalanx, and volar angulation of the fragments is common (Fig. 13–9). The proper treatment is reduction of the deformity followed by immobilization on a volar splint incorporated into a short arm plaster cast (Fig. 13–10). Placing traction on fingers is not only unnecessary but dangerous. Stiffened fingers may result from traction applied to straight fingers. Sloughs of volar skin and stuck-down flexor tendons may result from traction applied to fingers flexed over a splint. Unstable oblique fractures of the shaft of the proximal phalanx should be internally splinted with a transfixing Kirschner wire as with middle phalangeal fractures.

In reducing fractures of the phalanges or metacarpals care must be taken to

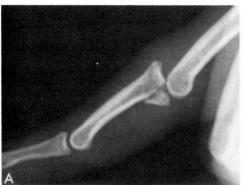
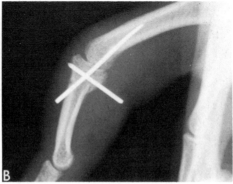

Figure 13–8 Fracture-dislocation of the PIP joint. *A.* Reduction of the dislocation cannot be maintained until the fracture is reduced and stabilized. *B.* This is best done with open reduction and K-wire fixation. The wires are removed in three weeks.

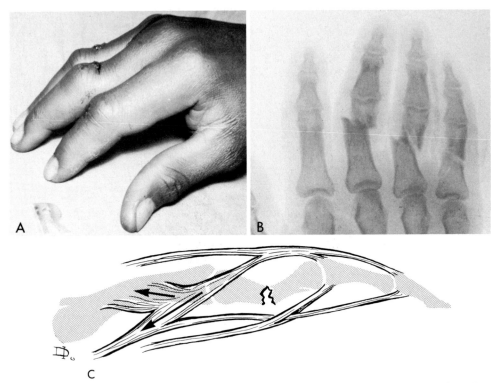

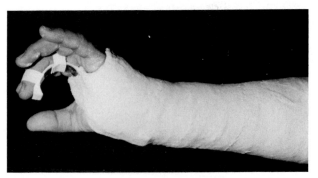

Figure 13–9   Fracture of the proximal phalanx. *A.* Typical deformity of volar angulation. *B.* Comminution, volar and lateral deformity are common. *C.* Volar angulation results from the deforming forces of the intrinsic muscles.

Figure 13–10 Immobilization of the proximal phalanx fracture. A padded aluminum splint is shaped to conform to the moderately flexed finger and the slightly extended wrist and is incorporated into a plaster short arm cast. This splint and cast are also useful for metacarpal fractures.

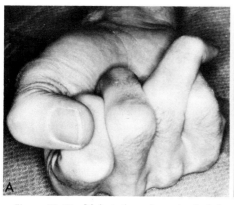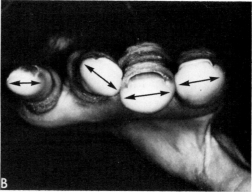

Figure 13–11 Malrotation of proximal phalanx fractures. *A.* This ring finger appeared fairly normal when the fingers were held extended. The deformity quickly became apparent when the fingers were flexed. *B.* Malrotation was apparent when the fingers were viewed end on.

correct rotatory as well as angulatory deformity. Careful inspection of both volar and dorsal surfaces is needed and the fingertips should be looked at end on (Fig. 13–11).

Fractures of the epiphysis of the base of the proximal phalanx in children and adolescents may be corrected by manipulation, but if this is not possible and there are more than 10 or 15 degrees of angulation present, open reduction in the operating room may be necessary to avoid unsightly deformity. Such an injury is most common in the small finger.

Metacarpal Fractures. Most common of these is the neck fracture of the fourth or fifth metacarpals, the so-called boxer's fracture. If loose and easily reduced by manipulation, this fracture can be immobilized with a short arm cast extended over the dorsum of the hand and the involved finger with the finger flexed at the MP joint. Such a splint should leave the middle and distal phalanges free. Most often such fractures are impacted with the metacarpal head and neck flexed 30 to 60 degrees into the palm. In these cases manipulative reduction is usually impossible and they are best treated by accepting the deformity and allowing immediate active use of the hand as soon as symptoms allow, usually a few days. The patient with such an injury must be advised that the "knuckle" of the involved finger will forever remain obscure. The depression of the metacarpal head into the palm may be slightly uncomfortable when tightly grasping an unyielding object, but since metacarpals four and five are quite mobile this will represent only a minor inconvenience for most people. If this is not acceptable to the patient, open reduction and K-wire fixation is the alternative (Fig. 13–12).

Less common but more serious are similar fractures of the neck of metacarpals two and three. As these metacarpals are relatively fixed, prominence of the head in the palm is a deterrent to strong and comfortable grasp. Therefore if closed reduction is not possible, open reduction will be necessary. Two crossed K-wires introduced on either side of the MP joint will stabilize these fractures without the necessity for a cast or splint, and active motion of the MP joints can be allowed immediately. The wires should be removed after three weeks.

Oblique or transverse shaft fractures of the metacarpal which can be reduced can generally be adequately immobilized with a short arm cast which ends at the distal palmar crease, but this plaster dressing must be carefully molded to the transverse metacarpal arch and must be nonpadded. Oblique and unstable meta-

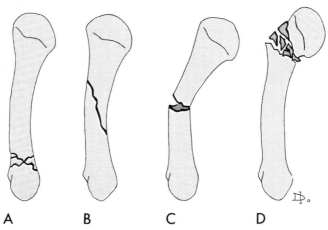

Figure 13–12   Metacarpal fractures. *A.* Comminuted fracture of the metacarpal base—generally stable and requires no splinting. *B.* Oblique fracture of shaft—usually treated with plaster splint or cast. *C.* Transverse fracture of shaft—usually angulates dorsally or displaces—generally best treated with internal fixation. *D.* Boxer's fracture of neck—reduction often impossible.

carpal shaft fractures which tend to telescope require K-wire fixation. Transverse shaft fractures which tend to angulate—and are fairly good risks for nonunion—require open reduction and fixation with crossed K-wires (Fig. 13–13). Intramedullary Kirschner wires introduced through the MP joint tend to give poor fixation and may jeopardize the joint. Fractures of the bases of the metacarpals are of little consequence and may be treated with active motion. Considerable pain and swelling may accompany these, and these symptoms are well handled by ice water immersion if seen within an hour or two of injury.

Fractures of the Thumb and First Metacarpal. Phalangeal fractures of the thumb are treated much the same as those of the fingers, though it is more difficult to shape an aluminum splint to conform to the thumb and thenar eminence, thereby immobilizing the MP joint. Shaft fractures of the first metacarpal are more often comminuted than are fractures of the other metacarpals. They can be readily immobilized by a plaster thumb spica, which is simply a short arm cast extended beyond the interphalangeal joint of the thumb. The thumb should be held in the position of function, i.e., slight flexion and moderate abduction (Fig. 13–14).

Fractures of the Base of the First Metacarpal. Fractures of the base of the thumb metacarpal are generally

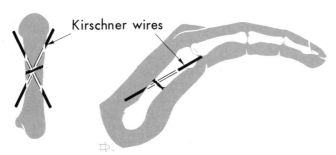

Figure 13–13   K-wire fixation of metacarpal fractures.

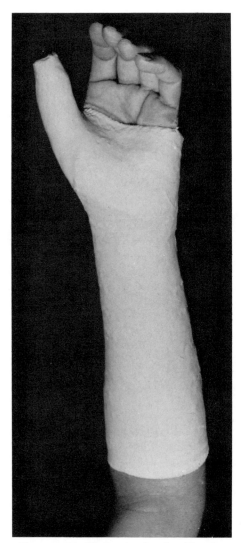

Figure 13-14 Plaster thumb spica. The plaster extends to the end of the thumb and the thumb is in a position of moderate abduction.

extension into the joint are often confused with Bennett's fractures, which, however, are really fracture-dislocations with proximal displacement of the distal fragment and the ulnar base or hook of the metacarpal remaining in place (Fig. 13-15). If the deformity is accepted, disability in the range of motion of the thumb will be moderate, but it is better to treat it by open reduction and Kirschner wire internal fixation. Treatment by skeletal traction is difficult, and often results in failure or complications.

Joint Injuries. Dislocations of the interphalangeal joints, like those of other joints, are emergencies because the functional result following such an injury is in direct proportion to the amount of time elapsed from injury until reduction. Reduction is generally a simple matter of pulling or manipulating the joint into normal position and is often accompanied with a palpable and sometimes audible snap. Ice water immersion for 15 or 20 minutes following reduction will result in decreased swelling and pain. Splinting with an aluminum splint for two weeks may then be followed by careful resumption of active motion.

MP dislocation of the thumb is caused by hyperextension of the proximal phalanx with rupture of the volar capsule and protrusion of the first metacarpal head through the two heads of the flexor pollicis brevis (Fig. 13-16). Reduction is accomplished by manual traction on the thumb while holding the MP joint in flexion to allow relaxation of the flexor pollicis brevis. Occasionally closed reduction will not be possible, in which case open reduction through a transverse incision in the proximal flexion crease of the MP joint is necessary. The same type of dislocation of the index finger MP joint may be seen and reduction is performed in the same manner. Following either open or closed reduction the digit should be immobilized with the MP joint flexed to 45 degrees for three weeks. If reduction is performed within several hours of injury, residual disability should be negligible.

transverse, but they sometimes involve the carpometacarpal joint. The distal, larger segment is angulated in the position of flexion, which is quite compatible with good function. Since these are generally impacted and stable fractures, active motion will give a very acceptable result for most patients. If a patient requires a normal span, as with a pianist, an open reduction and K-wire fixation will be necessary. Base fractures with

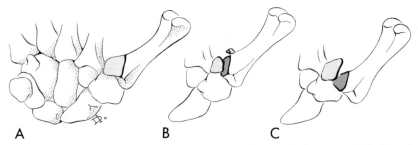

Figure 13–15   Fractures of base of first metacarpal. *A.* Stable—no displacement. *B.* Stable—slight displacement. *C.* Bennett's fracture–dislocation—reduction and fixation usually indicated.

Sprains of the PIP joints of the fingers represent a tear or stretching of the collateral ligaments and capsule. These injuries cause a surprising amount of persistent pain, swelling and stiffness of the joint. The joint should be immobilized for three weeks, and then active but protected motion may be started. Sprains or tears of the ulnar collateral ligament of the thumb MP joint are rarely successfully treated by splinting, and if recognized within two weeks of injury should be surgically repaired. Otherwise a condition of chronic instability called "gamekeeper's thumb" may result.

Carpometacarpal dislocations are uncommon and are difficult to recognize. Both physical deformity—difficult to recognize because of swelling—and a good lateral x-ray help in the diagnosis. They are easy to reduce but usually they promptly resume the position of dislocation when digital pressure is released (Fig. 13–17). They should be reduced manually and one or two K-wires drilled through the dorsum of the hand, transfixing the metacarpal base and the adjoining carpus. This wire should be left in place for three to four weeks.

Burns

Thermal Burns. The most difficult aspect of burn management is recognition of the depth of the burn or the degree of skin destruction. Many burns which at first seem devastating can be well managed on an outpatient basis. The most striking aspect is pain and this

quite often is out of proportion to the depth of the burn. The burn cannot be objectively examined or analyzed until the patient is given relief from the pain and is quieted down, particularly children with burned hands. Ice water immersion is very effective for this and not only gives relief from pain but helps to control subsequent edema. Immersion for 15 minutes or so will soothe the patient and allow careful scrutiny of the burned area. The examiner will want to know the history of the burn and will wish to assess the depth of burn with close attention to the appearance of the wound. Often it is not possible to be sure of either the area or depth of burn, and when in doubt it is important to hospitalize the patient. Superficial burns causing only partial skin loss and leaving adequate elements for normal skin regeneration are called first degree burns (Fig. 13–18). These can be managed in the Emergency Room, though the patient may have to return for regular follow-up examination and dressing changes. A light layer of mafenide acetate (Sulfamylon) cream covered with a regular compressive hand dressing will allow comfort, healing and some motion of the fingers. Dressings should be changed every four or five days until healing is well under way.

Deeper burns which involve the dermis heal slowly by the formation of granulation tissue. Though such granulations will eventually reepithelialize, the quality of this skin is relatively poor and areas greater than one centimeter in diameter

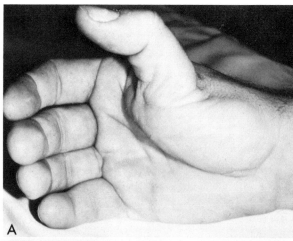

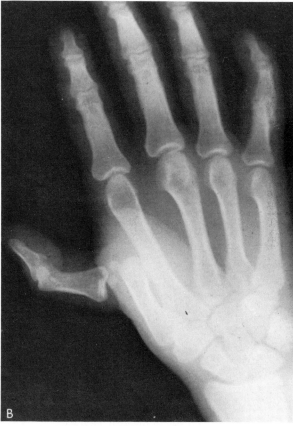

Figure 13–16 MP dislocation of the thumb. *A.* The metacarpal head is prominent on the volar surface. *B.* The proximal phalanx is displaced dorsally and proximally. Note the sesamoid bones.

are best covered with split thickness skin grafts. Such grafts can be laid on the raw areas and then overlain with petrolatum of Xeroform gauze from which most of the grease has been scraped off. The gauze is then covered with the usual bulky dressing. Larger areas of dermal involvement (which some call second degree burns) should be treated on an inpatient basis, since more extensive

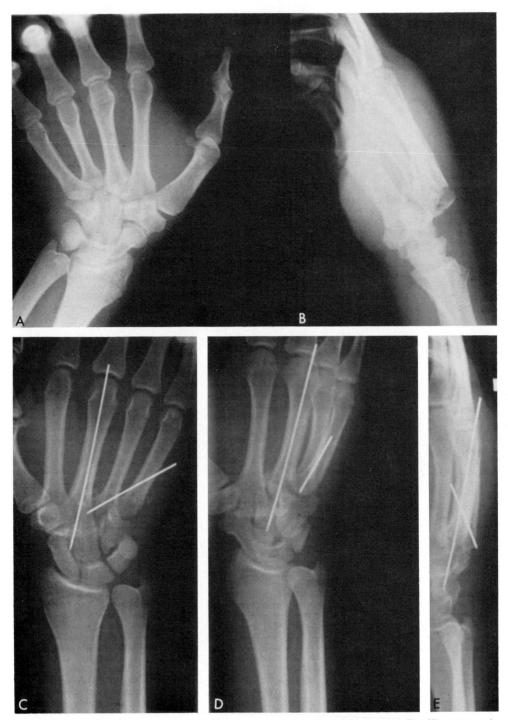

Figure 13–17 Carpometacarpal dislocation. *A*. Not recognized on AP x-ray. *B*. Readily apparent in lateral view. *C, D, E*. Manually reduced and transfixed with two K-wires.

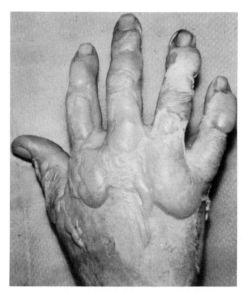

Figure 13–18 Superficial burn of the hand. The bullae are ominous in appearance but portend uneventful recovery with normal function.

grafting as well as daily attention to active motion of the fingers will be necessary.

Deep burns wherein all of the dermis is lost naturally require grafting usually preceded by débridement or escharotomy. Classically such a burned area is said to be anesthetic, but this is only relatively true and early classification of such a burn can be impossible. When in doubt, hospitalize. Electrical burns may appear at first to be small in area, but the apparent burn of the skin may only be the tip of the iceberg and extensive necrotizing damage may underlie it. Proper treatment cannot be planned until the extent of tissue damage is known.

Chemical Burns. Burns from caustic agents such as strong acids or alkalies are fairly common, and the immediate need is for removal or neutralization of the damaging agent. A copious amount of running water is the most effective means for this, but vinegar may be used to neutralize alkalies and chalk or lime water for acid burns. Solid phosphorus is more pernicious in that it is not easily washed free, although its oxidizing ac-

tion will be halted by immersion of the hand in water. The phosphorus particles must be removed manually, and a 5 per cent solution of copper sulfate will neutralize any residual particles.

Cold Injury. Frostbite, though common, is not benign as it represents local freezing of tissues. If extensive, permanent and irreversible damage results. Immediate warming by warm water immersion is the most effective first aid. Remember that frozen or near frozen tissues are damaged tissues and vulnerable to further injury, and thus the water should be warm (37° to 42° C), not hot. Pain may be intense with this type of injury and narcotics and sedatives may be necessary. The degree of damage may not be apparent for several or even many days, and it is often necessary to protect such hands with occlusive dressings. Sympathetic blocks are of little value in this type of injury.

Crush Injury

Crush injuries of the hand are often complex and may combine with fractures, joint damage, skin lacerations or tears, abrasions and injury to vascular structures, nerves and tendons. There is always an element of escape of extracellular fluid into the tissues. Formation of edema and its fixation in the tissues may cause more residual crippling than occurs from damage to any specific tissue or structure. Ice water immersion within an hour of injury will help considerably in preventing and controlling edema. This should be followed by immobilization of fractures, débridement of wounds and control or prevention of infection. A bulky compression dressing and constant elevation of the extremity are extremely important and may have to be continued for many days. The institution of active motion of the fingers within the dressing is also important to help prevent stiffening of joints.

Crush injuries can be deceptive, and the extent of damage may not be revealed until several days have elapsed. If any significant degree of crush has occurred, the patient should be hospitalized.

Wringer injuries of children are still fairly common and many are still mishandled. They may be superficial in degree or severe enough to compromise the entire extremity because of skin loss, severe swelling and the subsequent development of a Volkmann's ischemic contracture. The earlier the injured extremity is seen the more difficult it is to determine the severity of the crush. Even if there is only initial swelling, a few abrasions and moderate pain it is safer to assume the worst and to hospitalize the child, placing a firm compression dressing from fingertip to axilla and keeping the extremity elevated. The surgeon should be particularly attentive to any increasing complaints of pain. If there is obvious increasing swelling of severe proportions, prompt wide fasciotomy in the operating room may be required.

Foreign Bodies

Human beings are continually devising ingenious ways of introducing foreign objects through the skin of the hand. Wooden and bamboo slivers, pencil leads, pins and needles, broken knife points, steel filings and pieces of glass are commonplace. Bullets, often fragmented, shot pellets and the casings of detonating caps blown into the hand as the result of accident, altercation or experiment are also common. Most such objects should be removed, but this will depend on symptoms, size of the object and its location. Shotgun blast injuries at close range are devastating to a hand and a common mistake is to leave the felt or fiber shot shell wad in the depths of the hand because it is not apparent on x-ray films. Glass slivers of astounding size may be introduced through very small wounds. Most glass can be detected by careful scrutiny of x-rays. Children often sustain such injuries by a fall on the outstretched hand, introducing a sliver of broken glass into the palm in the region of the median nerve

and its branches. After the bleeding has been staunched and the pain assuaged there may be no further symptoms. But careful palpation may elicit tenderness, indicating that a piece of glass which should be extracted is present in a dangerous area.

Removal of such foreign bodies in the Emergency Room is usually a practical course and can be done under local anesthesia and tourniquet ischemia when necessary. It is rarely necessary or advisable to close the incision. The foreign body which has been deeply embedded for weeks or months before causing symptoms may not be as easy to locate or remove, and generally such removal should be done in the operating room. Foreign material long embedded may have caused the formation of an inclusion cyst or foreign body granuloma which will also have to be removed.

More important than the foreign body is the risk of infection it entails. After removal it is best to flush the wound thoroughly and to leave it wide open. Tetanus is an ever-present threat with any puncture or penetrating wound, and a booster dose is indicated for those previously immunized.

A barbed fishhook embedded in the finger should be cleansed with soap, the finger anesthetized, the hook passed through the finger, the point and barb clipped off, and the hook then backed out (see p. 1012).

Fingertip Injuries and Amputations

These represent the most common type of hand injuries seen in the Emergency Room and the majority of them can be treated there. Power lawn mowers, automobile radiator fans, power saws, slicing machines and more mundane devices such as knives, handsaws and doors all take their toll of careless or inquisitive digits. As with most hand injuries the physician's goals are to relieve pain and to obtain healing with the best functional result, with appearance as nearly normal as possible. Unfortunately it is not always possible to satisfy both the functional and cosmetic ideal. Female — and some male — patients frequently attribute more importance to the appearance of the hand than they will admit to and will therefore be unsatisfied with an excellent functional result if the appearance is unsightly. Despite some of our surgical pretensions, a cut off finger is a cut off finger, and both patient and physician must recognize that the state of the art is not yet such that the amputated part can be reimplanted and still satisfy the criteria of use, appearance and comfort.

Injuries to the Fingernail and Nailbed. Subungual hematomas usually resulting from a misdirected hammer blow or a carelessly slammed car door are painful, but prompt relief from pain is obtained by burning a hole through the nail directly over the accumulation of blood. This is simply done by straightening a paper clip and heating one end to a red hot temperature over a match or cigarette lighter. The hot end of the paper clip is touched to the nail and as the hematoma wells out, immediate relief from pain is obtained. This is a painless procedure but must be done before the hematoma has clotted.

Partially avulsed nails should be held in place as a temporary dressing by taping them in place with a Band-aid. The loose nail will protect the underlying raw bed until it is sufficiently healed to require no protection. This takes two to three weeks, after which the nail generally is quite loose and can be easily removed. Often the base of the nail is avulsed, leaving one or both sides intact. In such a case the border of the avulsed portion should be trimmed and the nail then held in place with a Band-aid. The base of the nail should not be forced back under the skin or infection may result.

When the nail has been completely avulsed, the bed should be protected by light petrolatum gauze and a dry dressing for about three weeks. Displaced or raised portions of the nailbed should be sutured in place to avoid distortions of the new nail.

If portions of the nailbed have been lost due to slicing or grinding injuries, the lost portion should be replaced by split thickness skin graft, but only after the denuded area has been fully debrided, gently scrubbed and irrigated. The graft should be a thin one and should be sutured in place, leaving the ends of the sutures long so that they may be tied over fine mesh gauze and several thicknesses of surgical sponge. If this stent dressing is then covered with Tubegauz, the finger can be returned to use promptly and the dressing cut free at the end of two weeks.

Injury to the Volar Pad. Most injuries to the volar aspect of the fingertip are caused by lacerating or grinding agents. If reasonably clean or if further surgical cleaning can be done, they may be closed primarily by replacing flaps with sutures or Steri-Strips; if these are absent skin grafts may be used instead. Often such wounds have grease and dirt ground into them and cannot be cleaned satisfactorily. Such wounds should be fully and vigorously cleaned, but not closed. Closure or grafting can be done with more success and fewer complications a few days or even a week or two later. The concept of delayed primary closure is a sound one here and Iselin[4] refers to this as the "delayed emergency."

In those cases where skin has been lost it is often difficult to know if replacement is necessary. It will depend on the digit involved and the width or diameter and the location of the lost skin. Divots or strips of skin loss of approximately one centimeter or less in adult fingers will close satisfactorily by secondary intention. Pieces larger than this should be replaced by split thickness skin grafts, Wolfe grafts (Fig. 13–21), or occasionally by cross finger flaps. If the loss is from the volar pulp of the thumb or index finger or in a child, the loss acceptable without grafting is smaller. Much larger areas of loss will of course heal but may result in hard, irregular or painful volar pads with some distortion or narrowing of the fingertip.

Amputations. The basic rule in the Emergency Room is to save all viable tissue, but this may occasionally need modification. The Emergency Room is not the place for reconstructive surgery of the hand, but prompt action and good judgment here may often make any future reconstructive surgery unnecessary. This is often true in finger amputations because a good job by the first physician may often be the only surgical procedure needed. With any finger amputation the surgeon must satisfy two requirements: to preserve all length possible and to produce a functional digit. Function must take precedence over length unless cosmesis is more important to the patient than use, and it may thus be necessary to shorten the finger to make it more functional. Even more drastic is the injury requiring complete removal of a viable but useless finger in favor of obtaining better overall hand function (see Ring Injuries). Careful judgment is required and sometimes a compromise between the two requirements is necessary, but generally a short nontender finger with good sensation is better than a longer finger whose end is painful or numb. The patient's occupational requirement for the finger (or fingers) may well dictate the proper course.

The thumb is the most important digit for prehension, and preservation of length is most important. Nevertheless, comfort and sensation must also be considered and sometimes shortening is in order. The index finger is next in importance but will function fairly well if a functional portion of the middle segment is preserved. Such an index finger has a suitable key or lateral pinch, but the patient will substitute the middle finger for tip to tip pinch.

There is a distinction between complete and partial amputation (Fig. 13–19). Complete amputation means absolute severance, and reimplantation of severed fingers is beyond our present capabilities, though many patients request that the severed member be "sewn back on." The only purpose that can be served by

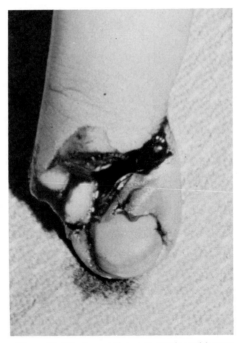

Figure 13–19   Incomplete amputation with comminuted fracture of distal phalanx. Replaced and held in place with a K-wire: no sutures. Excellent result.

a separated digit is as a donation for a skin graft and then only after suitable scrubbing. In partial amputation, there is some soft tissue connection; this is of value only when at least one neurovascular bundle is intact and in such cases careful fixation after cleansing is indicated. The more distal a partial amputation and the younger the patient, the better the chance for survival. In questionable cases the decision should not be made in the Emergency Room; if only one or sometimes two fingers are involved, the repair should be done. If not successful, definitive amputation may be done later in the operating room. In any event, all attempts should be made to preserve the partially amputated finger, though the patient may have to be warned that survival of the finger is in doubt.

Closure of amputation stumps is obtained either by utilization of skin remaining on the stump or by skin graft or transfer. Skin flaps left by the wound

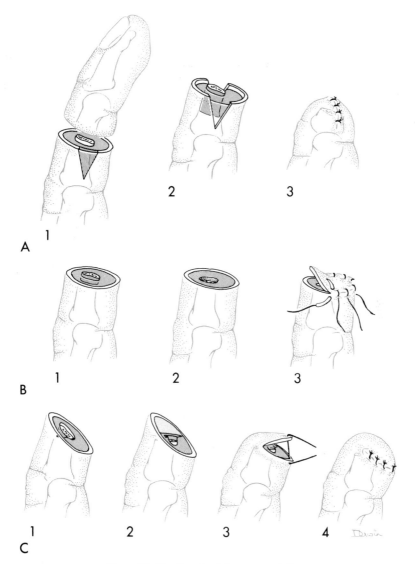

Figure 13-20 Repair of finger amputations.

should be utilized for closure after proper cleansing and removal of fat (Fig. 13-20). If the flap is too short to cover the stump, the phalanx may be shortened slightly, but if shortening is not desirable a combination of flap and graft can be used. Local sliding flaps should be used only by those experienced in their use — they are not generally a suitable method for the Emergency Room. The same is true for pedicle skin transfers, e.g.,

cross finger, thenar, palmar or thoraco-abdominal flaps. These can be used by experts but others may find their disadvantages and complications will be more apparent than their advantages.

If skin must be transferred in the Emergency Room it should be in the form of a free graft and here there is a choice of split thickness or a thin full thickness (Wolfe) skin graft. The technique for these grafts is described in the following section and either of them is useful in closing amputations in the Emergency Room.

Split grafts grow or "take" more readily than full thickness grafts, but the latter result in tougher and more satisfactory coverage. Wolfe grafts are particularly suitable in children but their incidence of survival decreases with increasing age of the patient. Either type of graft should be sutured to the stump end under slight tension with interrupted 5-0 synthetic suture. It is best not to lay them directly on bone and therefore it may be necessary to nibble away enough of the exposed phalanx so that it lies 2 or 3 millimeters below the surrounding soft tissues. Three or four of the sutures should be left long enough to tie over several layers of gauze, forming a stent dressing. Tubegauz over this completes the dressing, which should be removed on day four or five and then replaced for about another week. If injuries to the hand are more extensive than a single finger amputation, a complete compression dressing and elevation of the extremity is required. Multiple amputations and mangled fingers are situations requiring a longer anesthesia and tourniquet time and better surgical conditions than are available in the Emergency Room.

Skin Loss

Loss of skin substance greater than approximately 1 square centimeter generally requires replacement by graft or transfer. This loss is not to be confused with wounds which are gaping but from which no skin has been removed; these will generally close very satisfactorily by suture, by tape or by spontaneous healing. Avulsions of skin are most common on the dorsum of the hand or fingers and can be replaced by split grafts after adequate cleansing. If in doubt about the degree of contamination or the adequacy of débridement, it is far safer to apply a dressing to the wound and to supply skin coverage as a secondary procedure some days later.

Split thickness skin grafts are most satisfactorily obtained with a dermatome, but since these are seldom available in the Emergency Room, grafts no larger than a postage stamp can be taken with a razor blade. The most convenient donor site is the proximal volar aspect of the forearm. The upper anterolateral thigh surface would serve even better, because the donor scar would be seen less frequently. For a graft 2 centimeters square a donor area of approximately 4 centimeters square should be anesthetized using subcutaneous infiltration of approximately 10 cc of 1 per cent aqueous lidocaine introduced with a 2 inch No. 22 needle. It would benefit both surgeon and patient to wait ten minutes after infiltration before cutting the graft, for this should be a painless procedure for both. The aim is to cut as uniform a graft as possible holding the razor blade almost parallel with the skin. The best thickness is 0.014 inch, but such a freehand graft will be quite irregular in both shape and thickness. The donor area of a graft this thick will show multiple punctate bleeding points and no fat. The graft should be transferred immediately to the recipient site and either sutured or taped in place with Steri-Strips. The donor site is covered with a single layer of fine mesh gauze and nothing more. The oozing blood will quickly clot and the patient should allow this gauze to fall off when it is ready to do so—generally in about ten days.

A simple technique is the use of a thin full thickness or Wolfe graft. Though the rate of take of this type of graft is somewhat less than that of split thickness grafts, it is preferable for areas requiring tougher skin, such as palmar surfaces and fingertips. Suitable donor areas are the volar aspect of the upper forearm, the antecubital region and the inguinal crease. The principle is to excise the graft as an ellipse after infiltration with the lidocaine and then to close the donor site as a straight line. After outlining the graft by a full thickness incision one tip of the ellipse is retracted with a skin hook and the graft reflected

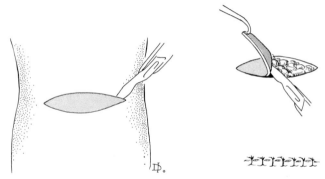

Figure 13–21   The Wolfe or thin full thickness skin graft.

under constant tension; a scalpel is used to cleanly separate the graft from the underlying fat (Fig. 13–21). No fat should remain on the graft. As such grafts tend to curl up they are best sutured in place as with split thickness grafts. On examination after 10 to 12 days such a graft looks terrible, but after another week or two the blackened outer layers will peel off leaving good full thickness skin behind. The graft should be kept dressed until this healing has occurred.

The principal causes of skin graft loss are infection and hematoma. Infection is best prevented by very thorough débridement and irrigation of the recipient site and by a thorough surgical scrub of the donor site as well as careful aseptic technique. Hematoma is avoided by laying the graft on a surface which has ceased to bleed and by maintaining gentle but constant pressure on the graft with a proper dressing. Expressing any delayed hematoma formation from under the graft at three or four days will also help.

Tendon Injury

Flexor Tendons.   Hands with wounds on the volar aspect should be carefully examined for flexor tendon injury. Such injuries are easy to miss if the physician does not specifically watch for them. Sometimes the wound will gape enough to show severed ends of tendons, but frequently what appears to be a severed tendon is a portion of flexor pulley ligament or palmar fascia, and just as frequently a completely severed tendon will be retracted from the wound and not be apparent. The resting position of the hand and fingers is the best guide, especially in young children. A digit with lacerated flexors will demonstrate "hang out" as shown (Figs. 13–22 and 13–23). Intact tendons can be checked by having the patient demonstrate functional flexor digitorum profundus by flexing the distal joint of each finger. The flexor digitorum sublimis is checked by the examiner by holding three fingers in full extension and having the patient actively flex the middle joint of the remaining finger. The flexor pollicis longus is checked by demonstrating active IP flexion of the thumb. Wrist flexors are

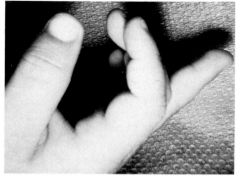

Figure 13–22   "Hangout" due to severed flexor digitorum profundus and sublimus in the middle finger of a child. This position is diagnostic and represents an alteration of the normal stance or position of the rest of the hand.

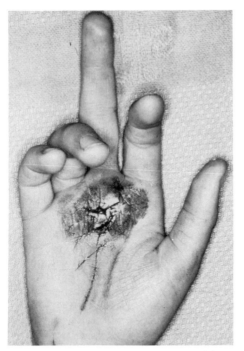

Figure 13–23 Same situation (in an adult) as in Figure 13–22. The palmar wound requires débridement, irrigation and no closure.

easily demonstrated and palpated by active flexion of the wrist, as is the palmaris longus.[1]

The purpose of this examination is to inform the patient of the damage done so that arrangements can be made for flexor tendon repair or grafting in the operating room when the wound is healed. Flexor tendons should not be repaired in the Emergency Room: unfortunately, many are and with uniformly poor results. Flexor tendon repair, either by direct anastomosis or free tendon graft or transfer, requires an experienced surgeon, the best of operating room environments and a sterile field. A transverse laceration of the volar aspect of the wrist may seem to invite primary repair of the underlying severed tendons in the Emergency Room. The temptation should be resisted, thereby avoiding the common complications of suturing the median nerve to severed palmaris or sublimis tendon, suturing tendons together with heavy silk, secondary wound breakdown,

extra scar formation and a complete tenodesis of all the flexors to the digits.

Extensor Tendons. Though it is commonly recognized that primary flexor tendon repairs give poor results, many feel that repairs of extensor tendons are a much simpler matter. This is true for a few specific types and locations of injury, but most of the difficulties encountered in extensor tendon repair and the complications therefrom are so great that the Emergency Room is not the place for them. As with flexors, careful examination is imperative. The patient should demonstrate independent active extension of each of the MP joints and each of the IP joints. The extensor mechanism of the fingers is far more complex than the flexor: MP extension is by action of the extensor digitorum communis for the four fingers, plus the extensor indicis proprius for the index finger and the extensor digiti-quinti for the small finger. The thumb MP joint is extended by the extensor pollicis brevis with an assist from the extensor pollicis longus. The thumb IP joint is extended by the extensor pollicis longus. The PIP joints of the fingers are extended mostly by the intrinsics—the interossei and lumbricals—but with an important contribution from the central slip of the extensor digitorum communis. Repairs of the extremely complex extensor mechanism over the dorsum of the fingers are difficult, and failures are more common than successes; they should be done under the best possible circumstances through a healed wound and in the operating room. With such injuries the proper approach is to thoroughly clean the wound, close it only if relatively clean and then splint the finger and wrist in full extension (i.e., 0°) until wound healing is complete and definitive extensor tendon repair can be carried out.

Lacerations of the extensor hood overlying the MP joint may be repaired if the wound lends itself to primary closure. This very definitely does not include wounds inflicted by human teeth (see later discussion). End-to-end suture with 4-0 to 5-0 wire or synthetic suture can be done and the finger splinted in full extension for four weeks before active motion is allowed. The single buried suture of Bunnell which is widely illustrated and looks very well in drawings is not so easy to use unless one has had considerable experience with it. A simpler technique is illustrated in which two sutures and therefore two knots are used. If the anastomosis is lightly rolled between the fingers the knots will disappear into the anastomotic line and will cause no trouble (Fig. 13–24). With this type of suture the two ends of the tendon can be pulled tightly together with less likelihood of the surgeon breaking the suture and having to rethread it through the tendon, thereby further mangling the tendon ends.

Extensor tendons transected on the dorsum of the hand may be similarly repaired, but only if the wound lends itself to primary closure, and only if both tendon ends are readily accessible

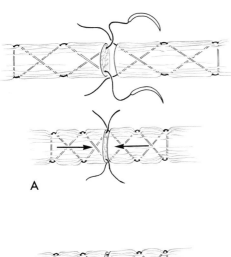

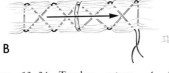

Figure 13–24 Tendon suture. *A.* Simpler method (preferred)—the two knots are buried at the anastomotic line. *B.* Classical Bunnell method —technique more difficult and with little real advantage over the simpler method.

without extending the wound. Following such repair the usual bulky dressing is applied and the finger and wrist are to be immobilized at 0°—i.e., in a straight line—with a short arm volar plaster splint extending to the finger tips for four weeks.

Incipient Boutonniere Deformity. This deformity, a flexion contracture of the PIP joint with hyperextension of the DIP joint, is difficult and often impossible to correct once it has occurred (Fig. 13–25). Prevention is needed, requiring early recognition and treatment. The cause is severance of the central extensor slip over the PIP joint. Such an injury is not very impressive when first seen: usually there is a wound over the PIP joint and an inability to extend this joint actively for the last 20 to 30 degrees, though the joint will have full passive range of motion. Occasionally the wound on the dorsum of the joint will be in the form of a contusion and there will be no break in the skin. Caution is necessary here, for if the central slip is ruptured and the joint is allowed to assume a flexed position, the lateral bands of the extensor mechanism may migrate volarward, starting an insidious chain of events leading to the boutonniere deformity. Primary repair of the central slip is a job for the expert and should not be done in the Emergency Room. It is advisable to treat the wound only and to splint the finger and wrist at 0° with a volar plaster splint for three to four weeks. If the splinting has been constant, satisfactory healing of the central slip will occur in many such cases. If the patient cannot extend the PIP joint fully after removal of the splint, it should be recognized that the tendon has healed with some lengthening, and surgical repair is indicated.

Mallet Finger. Mallet or baseball finger is incurred by avulsion of the insertion of the extensor mechanism at the base of the distal phalanx or by severance of this tendon over the DIP joint. Frequently a fragment of bone will be pulled off the phalanx by the tendon. It is the most common tendon injury

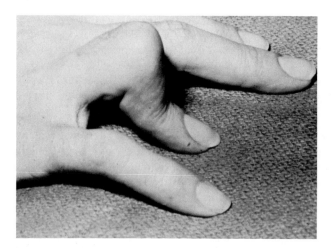

Figure 13-25 Boutonniere deformity. Late result of a rupture of the central slip of the extensor digitorum communis which was missed by the first examining physician. The finger was untreated and the deformity assumed this degree within three months.

and is usually incurred by striking the end of the extended finger and forcing it into flexion against the resisting extensor mechanism. Following this the DIP joint lacks twenty degrees or more of active extension, though full passive extension is possible. It has been widely publicized that treatment must consist of immobilization of the PIP joint in flexion and the DIP joint in hyperextension, and many elaborate splints and modes of internal fixation have been devised for this. They are difficult to apply and more difficult to maintain and are really not necessary at all. If the injury is treated promptly—preferably within a few days of occurrence—by splinting the DIP joint in 5 to 10 degrees of hyperextension, the result will be good, and the patient will be far more comfortable than with more complicated splinting. Three methods are available. The most satisfactory is a so-called safety-pin splint which is available as a stock item from most surgical supply houses (Fig. 13-26). This is a dynamic splint which, properly worn, applies a constant extension force to the DIP joint. It is imperative that it be worn constantly and without exception for a four week period. The patient must have this explained to him and he must cooperate if it is to work. The patient is also given an aluminum "ski tip" splint which he can substitute for the dynamic

splint once or twice a day in order to wash his hands (Fig. 13-27). The patient must be cautioned against flexing the joint while changing splints. A second method is to use only the ski tip splint for the full four weeks. This does not give quite as good a result as the safety-pin splint, as it may leave the DIP joint with a deficit of 10 to 15 degrees of full extension. This deficit is somewhat unsightly but not significantly disabling. The ski tip splint, however, is much simpler and more convenient for the patient to maintain. The third method, which is suitable for children or patients who are unable to cooperate with splinting, is to drill a Kirschner wire the length of the distal phalanx and across the DIP joint while holding

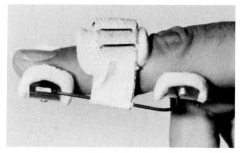

Figure 13-26 The safety-pin splint for mallet finger. When the central band is tightened, the DIP joint will be forced gently into slight hyperextension.

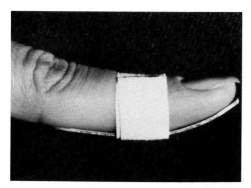

Figure 13-27 The aluminum ski tip splint for mallet finger.

that joint in hyperextension. In placing the K-wire remember that the tuft of the phalanx lies directly beneath the nail and the wire should therefore enter the fingertip about 3 millimeters volar to the nail and not through the volar pad. The tip of the wire may be left protruding, covered with a Band-aid and left in place for four weeks.

Nerve Injury

It is important to recognize nerve injuries in the Emergency Room, but they should be repaired in the operating room. Prompt recognition is important in planning treatment and in advising the patient on aftercare, and it has obvious medico-legal significance. Both motor and sensory examinations must be done before anesthetizing the extremity or any part of it. Obvious perhaps, but a common mistake is to wish one had checked fingertip sensation before the digital block had been done. An elaborate examination is not necessary: gross touch and pin-prick sensations are quickly checked and even in young children the latter should give some idea as to the presence or absence of sensation without the necessity of drawing blood with the examining pin. Radial nerve sensation is of little importance though easily checked over the dorsum of the hand and proximal segments of the thumb, index and middle fingers. Ulnar sensation should be looked

for over the hypothenar eminence, the dorsum of the fifth metacarpal, the dorsal and volar aspects of the small finger, and the ulnar half of the ring finger. Not infrequently the ulnar nerve supplies sensation to all of the ring finger and the adjacent half of the middle finger. The median nerve supplies the rest: the volar aspect of the thumb, index and middle fingers and radial side of the ring finger, as well as the dorsum of the middle and distal segments of these digits.

Transection or damage to the median nerve will result in a thenar palsy with loss of opposition of the thumb. If the thenar eminences of both hands are palpated simultaneously and the patient is directed to abduct and oppose his thumbs the deficit on the injured side is readily apparent. Stab wounds of the proximal palm may transect the median recurrent (motor) branch, leaving the sensory digital branches intact.

Transection of the ulnar nerve gives a motor deficit which is easy to detect. Palpation of the first dorsal interosseous muscle while the patient is attempting to abduct the index finger, or asking the patient to abduct the small finger or to flex the small finger MP joint without bending the PIP or DIP joints will demonstrate paralysis of ulnar innervated intrinsic muscles. A stab wound in the palm may transect the deep ulnar or motor branch, leaving ulnar sensation intact.

In the case of an extremely clean, sharply incised wound occurring within the past hour or so, a primary neurorrhaphy may be indicated, but it should be done in the operating room by a trained and experienced team with proper instruments. In such a case it is the function of the Emergency Room to pave the way for the prompt transition to the operating room. Repair of the ulnar motor trunk or the median recurrent branch is feasible in the operating room. Severed digital nerves of the fingers and common digital nerves of the palm also lend themselves to successful repair when the repair is meticulously done under ideal circumstances, none of which exist in the Emergency Room. In dealing with the wound in the Emergency Room, there is nothing to be gained by the placement of marking or stay sutures in the nerve ends.

Arterial Injury

As with nerve injuries, the role of the Emergency Room is to recognize the injury and to initiate treatment. Transection of both radial and ulnar arteries may or may not cause a bloodless hand. Such an injury should certainly be suspected with a wrist laceration presenting with a blanched, cold hand even though there is little bleeding from the wound, as severed arteries are quick to close up and seldom present in the Emergency Room spouting blood. Such a situation requires a prompt end-to-end arterial anastomosis but it is rare that an Emergency Room will be adequately equipped or manned for such a procedure. If either artery is intact and the other severed, all that need be done is to ligate both ends of the severed artery and the other artery will more than suffice to supply the hand with blood. The same is true for digital arteries; one will do for a finger, but if both are transected the digit will be lost unless prompt repair of one or both is possible.

The Mangled Hand

Industrial and farm accidents cause most of these, though automobiles, home power tools and shotguns make their contribution. The Emergency Room cannot deliver definitive treatment in most such cases, but it can play an absolutely essential role in setting the stage and in expediting such treatment. Assessment of the degree of injury, obtaining x-rays, cutting the red tape employed by hospital administrators, starting initial débridement, starting fluids, controlling shock and premedicating the patient will all serve to get the patient more quickly to the operating theater where complete débridement and repair can be undertaken. The golden period, though an old concept, is not an old-fashioned one, and it states simply that the more time elapsed from injury until proper treatment of the wound, the poorer the prognosis for uneventful healing of that wound.

Degloving and Ring Injuries

Circumferential degloving of a digit is typically incurred by the patient jumping off a truck or platform as the ring on the involved finger catches on an immovable object. The skin is circumcised at the level of the ring and stripped distally by the ring. Usually there is no fracture or dislocation and the extensor and flexor mechanisms are intact, and often the volar digital nerves and arteries as well. After cleansing the denuded digit and the reversed skin, the skin is peeled back onto the finger and the wound will then appear rather innocuous. Despite its good appearance, such a finger is usually fated to extreme functional loss because the subcutaneous veins and lymphatics have been disrupted and are impossible to repair: during the ensuing days the finger becomes markedly swollen, painful and often gangrenous. When first seen in the Emergency Room it is best to warn the patient that he will probably end up with a useless, stiff or painful finger even if the finger does survive. Nevertheless, it is best to attempt to salvage it, and to debride or amputate later on when it is quite apparent to the patient that the finger is a detriment to overall hand function. After proper cleansing and thorough irrigation the skin edges should be approximated loosely with five or six sutures and a complete hand compression dressing applied, followed by continuous elevation for several days.

Degloving of the dorsum of the hand usually results from the hand being jerked out of rollers or similar farm or industrial machines, creating a distally based flap of skin. Circulation to such a flap is often precarious, particularly as regards the venous and lymphatic drainage. Unless it is obvious that vascularity of such a flap is impaired, it should be debrided and lightly sutured in place as above. The patient should be advised that redébridement and possibly skin grafting may be necessary.

Grease and Paint Gun Injuries

Paint or lubricants forcibly injected into a finger from a pressure gun may dissect throughout the finger and hand and even up into the forearm. Such an injury may seem relatively benign for a few hours after the injection, but soon swelling, pain and stiffness become noticeable. Such injuries are surgical emergencies requiring detailed and prolonged dissection and débridement in the operating room under long-acting anesthesia. There are no effective first aid measures, and hot soaks are damaging: the only useful function of the Emergency Room in such an injury is to speed the patient to the operating room for proper and adequate débridement.

A similar injury may be caused by air or gas pressure guns, and the treatment for these is the same. Often the air or gas is a vehicle for abrasives or other foreign material which is forced throughout the tissues of the hand. Since the hand must be opened widely, such injuries carry a high infection risk.

Bites

A bite by human or animal teeth causes bruising and crushing of the skin and underlying tissue as well as laceration. It is an exceedingly dirty and potentially dangerous wound. The treatment consists of meticulous cleansing with soap under anesthesia, copious irrigation and excision of any questionably viable tissue. Such wounds should very definitely not be sutured. Penicillin in heavy doses should be given until it is obvious that infection has not occurred. The open wound should be covered with light petrolatum fine mesh gauze and a dry dressing. Bites from animals of any species pose a risk of rabies, and it is important where possible to impound the animal which inflicted the bite. If there is the slightest possibility that the animal was rabid, immunization of the patient should be started despite the possible complications from this procedure.

Carnivores, particularly cats, carry virulent strains of pasteurella which cause nasty, indolent infections, and these are usually inoculated deep into the tissues of the hand bitten by these animals. Prompt treatment as outlined above followed by antibiotics will decrease the chances of such infection. Human bites are the most common and the most troublesome of all. They are most commonly incurred in fist fights in which the extensor surface of the MP joint is lacerated on the opponent's incisors. Contamination of the MP joint is common, and it is not rare to have such a joint or its extensor mechanism destroyed by the ensuing infection. Closing such a wound may endanger not only the joint but the entire hand or extremity. If the extensor tendon or hood has been severed, it should not be repaired and this should be left for a later procedure after the wound has healed. If the wound is presented several days after the bite, an infection, manifested by pain, erythema, induration and sometimes pus, is already present. The involved area must be widely opened, debrided and left open. Massive doses of an appropriate antibiotic should be used as well as a complete hand dressing, elevation and hospitalization. Such an infection is a serious matter and procrastination or halfway measures will cause serious complications.

Gunshot and High Explosive Wounds

The severity of these wounds depends on the type of structures damaged, the extensiveness of damage and the degree of contamination within the wounds. These factors in turn are dependent on the velocity and mass of the missile, the intensity of the blast and the environment of the hand when wounded. A knowledge of wound ballistics is helpful but not essential if a few basic concepts are understood. The greater the velocity of the missile and the greater its mass, the more energy will be expended in stopping its flight and the greater the mass of tissue that will be damaged by the absorption of that energy. The role of the Emergency Room physician is first to get the facts concerning the injury: the weapon or wounding agent, its caliber and load, the distance of the hand from the weapon, the time of the accident, whether gloves were being worn and what treatment has already been administered. The next task is an assessment of damage. A short but careful examination of the hand, including an x-ray film, should tell if the wound can be handled in the Emergency Room or must go to the operating room for more extensive treatment. In either case the same fundamentals apply: adequate débridement, copious irrigation, nonclosure of the wounds, and a proper hand dressing and splinting followed by elevation and antibiotics and a tetanus booster.

Wounds inflicted by pistols of most calibers and by .22 caliber rifles are classified as low velocity wounds, and damage incurred by them is usually confined to the missile track. The wounds of entrance and exit should be debrided of any damaged tissue and the missile track irrigated generously. A roentgenogram may show that the bullet has fragmented within the hand, and it is usually best to leave these fragments undisturbed unless it is apparent that they are lodged against a vital structure, within a joint or are subcutaneous. Any bullet, particularly those of the larger caliber pistols, may cause a markedly comminuted fracture of a phalanx or metacarpal and occasionally of several bones. The bone fragments should never be removed even if completely detached from soft tissue and blood supply, as they will almost always be incorporated as part of the healing frac-

ture and their removal may result in a serious deficit of bone. The size of the bullet is not a good criterion for the degree of damage: a .45 caliber pistol bullet is a very large missile, but it is quite possible for it to pass through a palm or even a finger with surprisingly little damage.

Far more important than size is the velocity of the bullet. The bullets from most high-powered sporting and military rifles are definitely high velocity. Even though they may pass completely through the hand with little apparent destruction, the energy they expend in the hand is transmitted throughout the entire extremity and may cause great damage a good distance from the missile track. This energy is dissipated in violent shock waves throughout the hand and may cause fractures, nerve damage and other injuries several inches away from the primary wound. Even if no specific structures seem to be harmed, the general disruption of the hand occurring in a few milliseconds may cause extensive edema and microhemorrhage which can permanently cripple the hand. Most such wounds require extensive débridement and intricate internal stabilization of fractures, and this of course should be done in the operating room. The complications and bad results obtained through inadequate débridement and by primary closure of such wounds are innumerable.

Shotgun blasts of the hand vary considerably, depending on the shot load and particularly the distance of the hand from the muzzle. Unfortunately, most such injuries are incurred with the hand directly against the muzzle and the damage sustained may be tremendous. It is not unusual to have several digits or even an entire hand carried away by such a blast. Not only is the force great at close range, but the mass of the shot pellets, wads and burning powder all contribute to blowing a large hole through the hand. Often such hands are gloved and bits of wool, leather and other contaminants are thus distributed throughout the wound. Though plastic wads are supplementing them, wads composed of animal and vegetable fiber and cardboard are still used in many shot shells and are serious sources of tissue destruction and contamination. These are particularly pernicious as they are usually not seen in a roentgenogram and may be easily missed in débriding the wound. The shot pellets themselves are of little consequence and need not be sought unless they are in a joint.

Explosive wounds of the hand in civilians are caused by detonating caps, dynamite, blasting powder, firecrackers, fireworks, and (more *au courant*) tear gas grenades and homemade bombs. Even relatively small charges such as firecrackers may cause extensive wounding if the charge is enclosed within a container or within the grasping hand. Skin loss, multiple lacerations, fractures, amputations and extensive contamination by embedding of foreign material within the hand are seen with these wounds. The débridement and the recognition of salvageable tissue is a complex task and one for the operating room in most cases. Often there are burns associated with these injuries, and phosphorus and other powerful oxidizing agents from fireworks may be embedded in and under the skin.

It bears repeating that no wounds in the above categories should be closed. Delayed primary closure is feasible with many, and the advantages to this are that examination of the wound three or four days after injury offers the opportunity for a second débridement if the first has not proved extensive enough. Many of these wounds are closed secondarily, and in many cases skin grafts and pedicle flaps are necessary.

INFECTION

Most serious infections of the hand start from small beginnings, and bad results stem from treatment which is inadequate or which is started too late. Prevention is best, of course, but once infection has started sharp observation and appropriate early treatment can prevent a progression of the infection into a crippling or loss of the digit or hand. Staphylococci are the most common causative agents, and antibiotics are far less useful than are prompt surgical measures.

Paronychias

Paronychias are infections around the nail. Early in their development swelling, redness and pain occur at the side or the base of the nail. At this stage the infection may often be resolved by warm compresses, but if it has progressed to the point where pus has accumulated around the edge of the nail, the accumulation should be incised with a scalpel passed between the cuticle and the nail. If the infection has progressed to form a subungual abscess, pus will be apparent under the base of the nail, and the proximal half of the nail should be excised. Under digital nerve block the nail is transected distal to the accumulation of pus and the proximal portion of the nail avulsed from its bed. The distal portion of the nail is left in place and the raw bed covered with petrolatum gauze and a small dressing (Fig. 13–28). A Band-aid will suffice for the dressing and should be changed daily for about a week.

Felon

A felon is an infection in the volar pad of a digit which has progressed to abscess formation within the pulp space. Traversing this space are vertical septa running from the periosteum of the volar surface of the distal phalanx to the skin of the volar pad. Increasing pressure within these confined spaces causes severe pain, osteitis and sometimes necrosis of the phalanx. Once recognized, the proper treatment is surgical drainage and the goal is to cut through all the vertical septa and to

Extent of nail removed

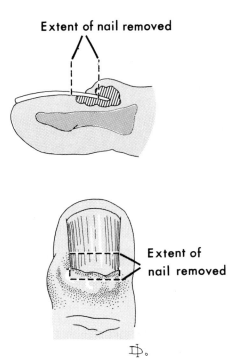

Extent of
nail removed

Figure 13–28   Subungual abscess.

allow free drainage of the entire pulp area. After digital nerve block a straight incision lateral to the nail may do the job, but it is often inadequately made and is therefore not recommended. It is better to extend this lateral incision hockey stick fashion around to the tip of the finger (Fig. 13–29). This distal portion should fall 3 or 4 millimeters volar to the nail bed and should not dip down into the volar skin which forms the tactile pad. Such an extension may result in a painful scar. After the incision is made the knife blade should be passed across the finger, breaking down all of the vertical septa. Pus and areas of necrotic

pulp are removed and the wound lightly packed open with a wick of petrolatum gauze. This wick should not be packed tightly into the wound. A fluffed dressing of the digit and hand is applied and the patient instructed to keep the hand higher than the head. Two days later the dressing should be changed and the gauze wick removed if the induration and erythema are markedly improved. If there is still some swelling and redness, leave the wick in for another two days. It is not necessary to close the incision and it will heal very well by itself as infection subsides.

With severe or neglected felons when the entire terminal digit is inflamed and swollen, a fishmouth incision which extends the above incision around to the other side of the finger is in order. This has been condemned by some, but if care is taken not to run the incision down onto the volar surface or the volar pad, the healed wound will be innocuous. After the incision has been made and the vertical septa transected, the end of the finger should gape open. No attempt should be made to close it, but a folded strip of Xeroform or petrolatum gauze can simply be laid in the wound and treatment proceeds as above.

Tenosynovitis

Infections of the flexor tendon sheaths of a digit usually start from a small puncture wound, but frequently this will be so small and obscure that the point of origin of the infection cannot be detected. These are dangerous infections and prompt recognition and treatment are necessary if a functional digit (or

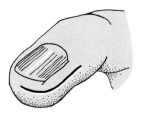
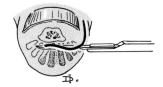

Figure 13–29   Incision for felon.

hand) is to be preserved. In the cases presented early, the patient has a painful finger which may be only slightly swollen but which feels tense to palpation. The finger is held slightly flexed and active flexion of the digit by the patient causes pain along the flexor aspect. Passive straightening of the finger is even more painful. Most such cases will respond to appropriate antibiotics, bedrest, constant elevation of the extremity and a warm, moist, bulky dressing. If, despite these measures, pain, swelling and redness increase and the pain progresses into the palm or wrist, the finger and flexor sheath should be opened through a midlateral incision along the so-called neutral line (Fig. 13–30). This incision should extend the length of the proximal and middle segments of the digit and should be left open, since it will heal spontaneously as the infection subsides. Pus in the sheath may or may not be encountered; if it is extensive, the sheath should also be opened in the palm and free drainage established. Whether to

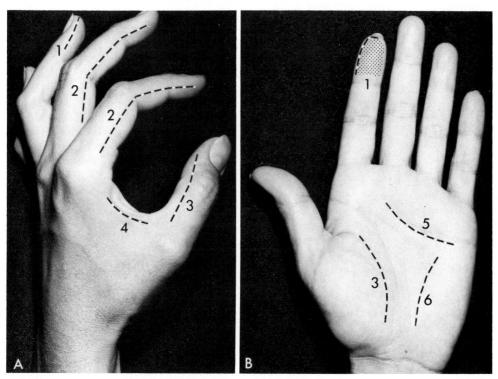

Figure 13–30 A, B. Incisions in the hand for drainage of infection.

1. Felon. This incision falls 3 or 4 millimeters volar to the tip of the nail. The dotted area represents the vertical fascial septa that must be transected by the knife blade. In severe cases this incision may be carried around to the opposite side of the finger forming the "fishmouth" incision.

2. Purulent tenosynovitis. This incision falls in the "neutral" line dorsal to the digital nerve and artery. The "neutral line" intersects the most dorsal portion of the flexion creases of the interphalangeal joints, which are easily determined by acutely flexing the finger.

3. Tenosynovitis of the thumb. The neutral line of the thumb is utilized in most cases, but in severe cases the ulnar border of the thenar eminence may also be opened.

4. Thenar space infection. A curved transverse incision through the dorsum of the thumb web allows direct access to the thenar space.

5. Middle palmar space infection. This incision is made 1 or 2 millimeters proximal to the distal palmar crease and extends from the third to the fifth metacarpal.

6. Hypothenar space infection. The ulnar bursa is approached through an incision on the radial side of the hypothenar eminence.

open the finger or to treat conservatively may be a difficult decision, but in the face of a worsening situation it is better not to procrastinate. An unnecessary incision is better than a finger which has lost function due to sloughed or scarred flexor tendons.

Fascial Space Infections

Several potential fascial spaces exist in the hand and any of them may be infected and become distended with pus. The treatment for all is prompt and adequate surgical drainage followed by treatment as described for tenosynovitis. The *middle palmar space* is most commonly infected. It lies dorsal to the flexor tendons and extends from the carpal tunnel to the distal palm and from the line of the third metacarpal to the hypothenar eminence. In opening this space care must be taken to protect the digital nerves and arteries as well as the flexor tendons and lumbrical muscles. *Thenar space infections* are characterized by marked swelling of the cleft between the first and second metacarpals. Drainage is best obtained through a transverse incision on the dorsum of the distal portion of the thumb web. The *hypothenar space* represents the third palmar space. This is rarely infected, but when it is it points dorsally. The *dorsal subcutaneous space* lies between the skin and the extensor tendons; it is rich in lymphatics and may become very swollen owing to infection in the palm and fingers. The space itself is not commonly infected, but when it is and pus is present, drainage by longitudinal incision is recommended. The same is true for the dorsal *aponeurotic space*, which lies between the extensor tendons and the metacarpals. *Web spaces* are three in number and exist between index and middle fingers, middle and ring fingers and ring and small fingers. When infected they point dorsally and are usually drained by means of a longitudinal incision through the dorsum of the finger web.

Lymphangitis

This generally starts from superficial injury, progresses rapidly and presents as pain, swelling and redness of the hand and sometimes of the forearm. The patient is febrile and toxic and the symptoms rapidly progress up the forearm to above the elbow. There are no findings of tendon sheath or fascial space infections. Subcutaneous abscesses may appear, but usually there are no localizing signs of infection. Surgical drainage is inadvisable except when there is definite localization of pus. The patient should be hospitalized and the entire extremity elevated and kept wrapped in warm, moist compression dressings to the axilla.

Cat Bite Infection

Pasteurella multocida infections from cat bites are treated with antibiotics, drainage where abscess formation has occurred, elevation and heat. These infections generally subside spontaneously in about two weeks.

Erysipeloid Infection

Erysipeloid infections are common in butchers, farmers and veterinarians. These are acute infections which subside spontaneously in about a month. Surgical intervention is inadvisable and penicillin is moderately effective. Wounds incurred while handling raw meat may be infected with Erysipelothrix and these should not be closed primarily, as they will frequently break down and result in more scarring than if left to heal secondarily.

CYSTS AND TUMORS

Ganglion

This is the most common of the extraneous growths of the hand other than warts. Most commonly located on the dorsal aspect of the wrist, ganglia may also be found on the volar side of the wrist and in the palm and fingers. Despite the various methods of injection and needling periodically reported, the best method of treatment for symptomatic or unsightly ganglia is complete surgical excision in a controlled surgical environment. The more complete the excision, the less the incidence of recurrence. The same treatment is indicated for the small ganglia which are found on the proximal flexor pulleys over the metacarpal heads.

Giant Cell Tumor of Tendon Sheath Origin

These are also known as xanthomas and are the second most common tumors of the hand. They are benign but may cause local symptoms or bone erosion. They are usually located in the digits and present as firm, nontender, often irregular nodules. Their proper treatment is excision under tourniquet ischemia. They frequently have extensions around and under the flexor or extensor mechanisms and as their dissection may be complex should properly be done in the operating room.

Epidermoid Cysts

These are also called epithelial inclusion cysts. They develop following injury and are due to the implantation of epithelium into deeper tissues. They develop first as small nodules which are transiently tender and slowly grow to form subcutaneous cysts. Treatment is by surgical excision which can be done easily under digital block if the cyst is in a finger or under local infiltration if it is in the palm.

Mucous Cysts

These are the next most common tumor of the hand. They are present in older persons, usually with degenerative arthritis, and appear as painful cysts on the dorsum of the finger in the region of the DIP joint. Puncturing them produces a clear, gelatinous fluid and this relieves pain temporarily but results in either prompt recurrence or a bothersome ulcerative lesion. More satisfactory treatment is surgical excision of the entire lesion including the overlying skin, replacing the skin with a split thickness skin graft. This can usually be done adequately in either the outpatient clinic or the Emergency Room under digital nerve block and local lidocaine infiltration of a small donor site on the volar aspect of the forearm.

Pyogenic Granulomas and Foreign Body Granulomas

These are of inflammatory origin; the former are external and involve the skin and the latter are deep to the skin and form around a foreign body. The pyogenic granuloma is pedunculated, tender and ulcerated. It can be easily snipped off or excised and the base cauterized with silver nitrate. Foreign body granulomas require careful dissection in a bloodless field and most of them should be excised in the operating room.

Other Tumors of the Hand

Most tumors of the hand are benign and include lipomas, fibromas, enchondromas, hemangiomas, glomus tumors and warts. Warts will generally disappear as mysteriously as they occurred and within a few months. For extensive wart formation, dermatologic consultation is generally indicated.

Squamous cell carcinoma is the most common of the malignancies in the hand. Malignant melanomas occur on the hand and have a particularly poor prognosis in subungual or palmar sites. Early excisional biopsy of palmar nevi is recommended to forestall malignant degeneration.

TENDON CONDITIONS

DeQuervain's Disease

This is also known as stenosing teno-synovitis and is manifested by pain over the radial styloid where crossed by the tendons of the abductor pollicis longus and extensor pollicis brevis. These two tendons share a common compartment covered by the extensor retinaculum. This condition is common in middle-aged females and can cause pain of disabling degree. Palpable tender-ness can be demonstrated over the ten-don compartment on the dorsal radial aspect of the distal radius. The pain is also produced or accentuated by forcible passive flexion of the thumb MP joint. Immobilization of the wrist and thumb in a plaster cast or splint may give re-lief of pain while immobilization per-sists, but the pain usually recurs when normal activity is resumed. Injection of the tendon sheath (not into the tendons themselves) with 2 ml of hydrocortisone gives prompt relief, but the pain usually recurs within a month or so. Repeated injection of the tendon compartment is inadvisable as degeneration and rupture of one or both tendons may occur. The only definitive treatment is surgical release of the compartment, which gives a definite cure in almost all cases. This procedure is best done in the oper-ating room, but if the operator is ex-perienced it may be done on an out-patient basis. Under tourniquet control a longitudinal incision is made directly over the affected tendon compartment. The retinaculum overlying the tendons is slit longitudinally, opening up the entire tunnel. Aberrant tendons and duplication of either of the tendons are common, but excision of these is not necessary. If there is a reactive teno-synovitis, the thickened synovium should be dissected free from the tendons. Some prefer to make a transverse incision, but the longitudinal incision gives almost as good a cosmetic result and has the added advantage that it is easier to avoid the sensory branch of the radial nerve which lies just radial to the tendons. Care should be taken to avoid traumatiz-ing this nerve with either scalpel or retractors as it is often the source of troublesome neuromas. In making the longitudinal incision one should be care-ful to stop short of the transverse ex-tension crease in the skin on the dorsum of the wrist.

Traumatic tenosynovitis can affect any of the flexor or extensor tendons, but is more common over the dorsum of the wrist. It is caused by excessive use of a particular tendon and is bascially an inflammatory response of the teno-synovium to excessive motion. It is manifested by severe pain on motion and tenderness to palpation over the inflamed area. Palpable crepitation is often present when the tendon moves. Although it is similar to deQuervain's disease, surgical intervention is not needed. Splinting the tendon at rest for a couple of weeks will cause subsidence of the symptoms.

Trigger Thumb and Clutched Thumb

Snapping of the thumb when it is flexed is caused by thickening of the annular sheath of the flexor pollicis longus at the level of the MP joint, and it is a condition more common in in-fants than adults. Occasionally there is a concomitant nodule in the tendon it-self. Cure is accomplished simply by longitudinal slitting and excision of the thickened portion of the sheath. This is done by a transverse incision through the flexor crease of the MP joint, care being taken to protect the digital nerves. Occasionally the thumb remains fixed in flexion and cannot be unlocked with-out surgical release. In the newborn, in whom the thumbs are held tightly in the flexed position, the "clutched thumb" condition, the thumbs may sometimes be coaxed into the extended position by steady but gentle manual traction and held thus with plaster casts for several months. If the deformity is associated with con-genital absence of the thumb extensors, reconstructive surgery is necessary.

Trigger Finger

Trigger or snapping finger is usually caused by a constriction in the proximal flexor pulley at the level of the metacarpal head. Often a corresponding nodule or thickening is present on the flexor digitorum profundus or at the bifurcation of the flexor digitorum sublimis. The treatment is release of the constriction by longitudinal slitting of the flexor pulley, which is exposed by a 2 centimeter longitudinal incision through the palmar skin overlying the metacarpal head. A transverse incision is recommended by some, but the longitudinal incision will heal almost as well and allows greater exposure with less danger to the digital nerves and arteries. A trigger finger will sometimes be the first sign of rheumatoid tenosynovitis, in which case a rheumatoid nodule and proliferative tenosynovitis may be found in one of the flexor tendons. An extensive tenosynovectomy may be necessary, and since this is difficult to forecast preoperatively, cases of trigger finger should be operated upon in the operating room.

Ruptured Tendons

Any of the flexor or extensor tendons may rupture as a result of trauma, rheumatoid involvement or other disease process such as tuberculosis. Finding the ruptured ends is not always an easy matter, and when found the severed ends can rarely be satisfactorily anastomosed. A segmental tendon graft or a tendon transfer is therefore frequently required. Such reparative surgery—and this includes avulsion of the flexor digitorum profundus from its insertion—should be done in the operating room.

Metacarpal Boss

The extensor carpi radialis longus and brevis insert on the dorsal bases of the second and third metacarpals respectively. The normal skeleton reveals dorsal bony prominences on each of the metacarpal bases, but in some patients, particularly those whose occupation requires repetitive, forceful wrist extension, a painful swelling and increase in size of this bony prominence may develop. The pain apparently is located in the fibers of insertion of the radial wrist extensors and is relieved by injection of the region with hydrocortisone. Occasionally immobilization of the wrist in extension for about three weeks will be necessary. Surgical shaving of the boss is indicated only when it is very large and persistently troublesome.

ARTHRITIS AND JOINT DISEASE

Rheumatoid Arthritis

Synovectomy, tenosynovectomy, repair of ruptured tendons and other reparative surgery for this disease should be done only in the operating room as well-planned procedures. Steroid injection of rheumatoid joints and tissues is commonly done and may give transient relief of symptoms, but repeated injection may cause such complications as tendon rupture and possibly cyst formation in the subcondylar bone.

Osteoarthritis

Degenerative arthritis of the hand will present in the Emergency Room and Outpatient Clinic either as painful arthritis of the thumb carpometacarpal joint or painful Heberden's nodes overlying the DIP joints of the fingers. The former is treated by arthrodesis or excision of the greater multangular in the operating room. When symptomatic, Heberden's nodes may be quieted by massage with an ice cube for a few minutes. They do not respond well to excision or injection.

Pyogenic Arthritis

Infections of the joints of the hand are usually caused by staphylococci introduced by trauma. Early joint infection is best treated by elevation and moist hot compresses, using antibiotics when appropriate. If these measures don't lead to regression of joint swelling and tenderness in two to three days, the joint should be opened and any debris or inflamed synovium excised. Contrary to some, I believe in leaving the joint wide open and starting active motion immediately. Such joints will heal very well. They will not lose their articular cartilage and will preserve normal or nearly normal ranges of motion.

Villonodular and Chronic Nonspecific Synovitis

A chronically swollen, thickened and moderately tender MP joint may have a hypertrophic proliferative synovitis due to repeated trauma or perhaps a low grade infection. Synovectomy is the prescribed treatment if one intra-articular injection of 25 milligrams of hydrocortisone does not cause subsidence of the findings and symptoms.

NEUROGENIC CONDITIONS

Carpal Tunnel Syndrome

Median nerve entrapment is common in the middle-aged, in the rheumatoid arthritic and following Colles' fracture. It is manifested by tingling and numbness in the median nerve sensory distribution in the hand, usually the thumb, index and middle fingers, but sometimes the tingling is present throughout the entire hand. Pain may be associated with this, and discomfort may involve the entire extremity. It is not rare for the presenting complaint to be pain in the forearm, or in the shoulder, or even in the neck. The patient is often awakened by tingling in the fingers. He may resort to vigorous shaking of the hand or hands to obtain relief. Physical findings may be absent in the early cases but often there is a diminution in median sensation throughout the hand, manifested by a decrease in fine touch and two-point discrimination. There is occasionally thenar atrophy, and paresthesias may occur in the fingertips when the nerve is percussed on the volar aspect of the wrist. The main function of the Emergency Room or outpatient physician is to make a tentative initial diagnosis, so that follow-up studies and further testing can be done. If the diagnosis is confirmed early, surgical release can be done; surgery is very effective in reversing nerve changes. The longer these changes have been present and the older the patient is, the poorer the chance for regaining lost nerve function, particularly if there has been motor loss. An emergency situation exists with the elderly patient who has sustained a fracture of the distal radius which has been reduced and immobilized (usually in the flexed wrist position), and who then complains of pain or numbness in the fingertips. Such an extremity should be elevated and the plaster cast removed. A volar splint should be applied holding the wrist in neutral, even if this means losing the reduction of the fracture.

Reflex Sympathetic Dystrophy

In this category fall several complex conditions such as causalgia, Sudek's post-traumatic atrophy, the shoulder-hand syndrome and others. Such past favorites as scalenus anticus syndrome and cervical rib have now been replaced by the thoracic outlet syndrome, but this too is related to this complicated group. In these there are apparently four components interacting in various combinations: a painful peripheral stimulus, spinal reflex arcs, sympathetic changes and finally interpretation and reaction to these peripheral phenomena by the higher levels of consciousness.

Once such a condition is developed a vicious cycle is established and it tends to be self-perpetuating. Breaking the cycle at any one point is usually not effective and it must be attacked simultaneously at several points. Though it is true that the most "normal" individual may develop a reflex sympathetic dystrophy, more commonly it is seen in the inadequate personality type and in the outright neurotic. The approach then must be to relieve the painful stimulus as well as to deal with the patient's reaction to that stimulus. This is a time-consuming and patience-demanding process, but if the physician persists, often with the aid of a psychiatrist, most of such patients can be improved if not cured. Sympathetic block or stellate ganglionectomy is often tried, but these procedures are rarely effective unless done within the first few weeks of the development of the cycle. The most promising approach is the preventive one which consists of dealing effectively with the painful lesion before a cycle can develop fully. Too often this depressing chain of events is fostered either by neglect of an injury or, even more commonly, by improper treatment, and one of the most common initial events is the tight plaster cast in which the patient's pain is treated by narcotics rather than by the relief of the pressure by bivalving the cast.

Self-Mutilation

Occasionally the Emergency Room or clinic physician will be faced with wounds of the hand which simply refuse to heal despite adequate treatment. These are usually on the dorsum of the hand and may be open or closed. Some patients who prefer to continue with compensation payments rather than return to work will deliberately or sometimes subconsciously keep an open wound of the hand from healing by picking at it or by traumatizing it in other ways.

A simple contusion of the dorsum of the hand may lead to persistent swelling and a painful hand edema which may last for many months. Known as Secretan's disease or peritendinous fibrosis, the condition is seen almost exclusively in insurance or compensation cases. The only treatment is to attempt to get the patient to use the hand as normally as possible and at the same time advise that all litigation be settled.

CONGENITAL DEFECTS

These range from mild syndactyly through innumerable combinations of defects to such severe conditions as congenital amputation of the hand or parts thereof. Few lend themselves to outpatient treatment. One exception to this is the infant who has a supernumerary digit on a small fleshy pedicle. Such a rudimentary finger can be easily snipped off and the small wound covered with a Band-aid. If the pedicle is larger than about 3 millimeters in diameter, there may be a skeletal connection and more elaborate measures may be necessary. Attempts to repair syndactyly, congenital bands, bifid fingers and similar congenital anomalies should not be made on an outpatient basis, as the results obtained therefrom will be unsatisfactory.

DUPUYTREN'S CONTRACTURE

The only definitive treatment for Dupuytren's contracture is palmar fasciectomy, an exacting operation which should be done only in the operating room. In cases where fingers are held contracted into the palm by a single longitudinal fascial band the operation may be simplified by percutaneous fasciotomy which allows a partial release of the fingers. Severance of one or two fascial bands is simple to perform, but care must be taken not to cut too deep or to try for too great a release or the digital nerves, arteries, and flexor tendons may be severed. Under local anesthesia a small bladed scalpel or tenotome is held flat on the palm and sloped transversely through the skin directly overlying the tight band. While applying traction to the contracted finger the knife blade is then turned perpendicular to the band and pushed down through the band. The knife pressure should be released as soon as the band is severed. This is a useful prelude to fasciectomy but is dangerous if one tries to accomplish too much. The small wound need not be sutured but will close spontaneously in about two weeks, after which the more complex operation can be done. During this time gentle but continuous extension splinting of the finger should be used to stretch out the skin and joint capsule.

SNAKE BITE

Time is of the essence in the case of snake bite, and simple first aid measures may greatly decrease the ensuing pain, edema, necrosis and systemic toxicity. If the patient is seen within 30 minutes, incision of the snake bite area and suction can remove a significant amount of venom. The incision should not be the commonly described cruciform type, as a single elliptical incision is preferable. Suction may be applied by mouth if there are no open lesions of the mouth, or by rubber bulb. Appropriate antivenom should be promptly administered, half in the area of the bite and the remainder intramuscularly. If the patient presents himself with a tourniquet on the arm this should be maintained until these immediate measures have been carried out. In no case should the tourniquet be left in place for more than two hours. Since much of the secondary damage may be caused by edema, dependency of the extremity should be avoided. Hypothermia of the hand and forearm with ice packs is quite effective in controlling pain and edema, but numerous cases of great damage from prolonged cold have occurred. Complications of cold injury have been severe enough to cause loss of the extremity above the elbow. Cold should not be used for longer than two or three hours and hospitalization is indicated in all cases.

The median fasciotomy is extremely effective in relieving pain and preventing muscle necrosis in severe bites in which massive swelling is obvious. The skin incision and fasciotomy should be extensive and may extend from fingertip to elbow or higher. These wounds heal very well without closure or they may be subsequently covered with split thickness skin grafts.

References

1. Brown, P. W.: Lacerations of the flexor tendons of the hand. Surg. Clin. N. Amer., 49:1255–1268, 1969.
2. Boyes, J. H. (ed.): Bunnell's Surgery of the Hand. Philadelphia, J. B. Lippincott Co., 1970.
3. Flatt, A. E.: The Care of Minor Hand Injuries. St. Louis, C. V. Mosby Co., 1963.
4. Iselin, M.: Delayed emergency in fresh wounds of the hand. Proc. R. Soc. Med., 51:713–714, 1958.
5. Kanavel, A. B.: Infections of the Hand. Philadelphia, Lea & Febiger, 1939.
6. Milford, L.: The Hand. St. Louis, C. V. Mosby Co., 1971.
7. Rank, B. K., and Wakefield, A. R.: Surgery of Repair as Applied to Hand Injuries. Edinburgh, Livingstone, 1953.

14

The Breast

By JOHN Q. GALLAGHER, M.D.

INTRODUCTION

The female breast has achieved a certain degree of attention by the present generation of the American public. The problems and diseases of this organ deserve an equal amount of attention from the physician—from house officer, family physician and surgeon. Cancer of the breast is the most common cause of death in women between the ages of 40 and 60. In fact, it is generally accepted that carcinoma of the breast is the most common cancer of women in the world today. Diseases of the breast therefore deserve a high degree of consideration in a text such as this which is devoted primarily to the care and treatment of patients not confined to the hospital bed.

During the past hundred years the sheer number of books and papers published on carcinoma of the breast stands in mute testimony to the confusion, controversy and apparent inability of doctors to establish a systematic approach to the treatment of this disease. A course of action that can withstand the vocal and written onslaught of our fellow investigators has yet to be found. The treatment of the patient with carcinoma of the breasts extends over a long period of time. This, in many cases, may encompass a significant number of years in the life of the patient's attending physician. The actual time spent in hospital is relatively small compared with the years of follow-up care and hours spent plotting the best course of action for the individual patient whose free interval is past and who now presents with recurrent disease.

There are problems other than cancer of the female breast, and these, though important to our patients, are proportionally far less complicated and controversial. These will be handled with little trepidation. The purpose of this short chapter, then, is to chart a course of action dealing with problems of the breast from benign to malignant. An attempt will be made to be concise and to summarize the voluminous writings on the subject. The plastic and esthetic properties of the female breast will be avoided and left to those specifically interested in these problems.

443

THE EXAMINATION

Every doctor who as a matter of course in his daily practice examines the female patient would do well to establish a habit of spending three to four minutes teaching the patient to examine her own breasts. He then not only will have conducted a thorough examination, but hopefully will have encouraged his patient to check herself properly and routinely every month. He has then done more than just examine the patient. In the premenopausal woman routine examination of the breast is best done several days after cessation of the last menstrual period because at this time breast enlargement is minimal and a mass is more easily detected. The history is important and discomfort, swelling, skin changes, nipple discharge, as well as time of menopause, hormone therapy, or family history of breast disorders all may prove significant to the patient's problem.

The actual examination should begin with inspection of size and symmetry of the breasts. Skin changes such as erythema or retraction, and any nipple ulceration or retraction are all significant (Fig. 14–1).

Gentle palpation of the entire breast in a systematic fashion should be demonstrated to the patient in both upright and supine positions. This will assure both doctor and patient future familiarity with the texture and consistency of her breasts. Areas of nodularity, old biopsy sites, or abscesses should be accurately mapped out on the patient's chart. Careful palpation of axillary and supraclavicular areas completes the examination. Any change in the future detected by patient or doctor can then be more readily evaluated.

Patients with nodular or cystic breasts as well as those who have been treated for a previous carcinoma can be more accurately followed with routine mammograms (Fig. 14–2). Certainly mam-

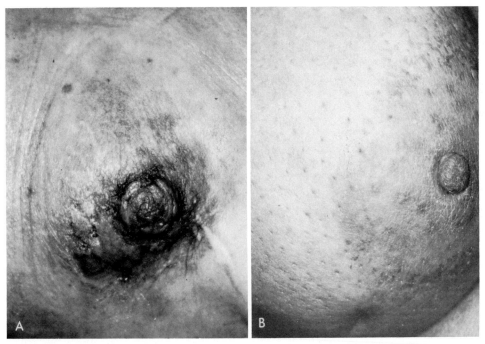

Figure 14–1   Carcinoma of the breast. *A*. Nipple ulceration and retraction in early subareolar carcinoma. *B*. Skin retraction ("peau d'orange") in advanced carcinoma.

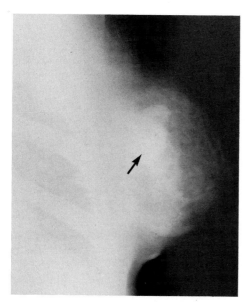

Figure 14–2 Mammogram of patient with carcinoma of the breast. Distortion and irregularity of ducts, increased density and flecks of calcification are the radiographic signs of malignancy in this patient with a mass deep in the breast.

mography is capable of diagnosing and localizing some preclinical cancers, but at present its value is limited to that of a survey procedure. Mammography, xerography and thermography are not substitutes for the history, physical examination, surgical consultation or biopsy. They are valuable aids which must be used with full knowledge of their limitations.

INFLAMMATORY CONDITIONS OF THE BREAST

Inflammatory lesions of the breast, though infrequent, cause considerable morbidity because of their chronic, indolent nature.[7] Engorged breasts in the neonate often become infected but usually respond readily to warm compresses and antibiotics. As always, suppuration is an indication for surgical incision and drainage. Pubertal enlarge-

ment is not really a true mastitis and should be handled conservatively with support and pain medication. The breast abscess as seen in adult women is a complex problem. Mammary duct ectasia, mammary fistulas, and nonspecific inflammation may frequently be confused with carcinoma. The lactating breast is highly susceptible to infection. This condition usually responds quite readily to cessation of breast feeding, antibiotics, and incision and drainage as indicated. Mammary duct ectasia is characterized by dilatation of the large ducts beneath the nipple and areola with periductal inflammation and fibrosis.[1] There may be associated nipple discharge with or without retraction. A painful tumor mass may form, making biopsy mandatory to rule out carcinoma. As the disease progresses, overt abscesses and fistulas may form. In our experience at the University of Colorado we have been singularly impressed by the fact that for any of the chronic inflammatory conditions of the breast—duct ectasia, abscesses or fistulas—simple incision and drainage is not the definitive treatment. The average patient referred to our clinic with a chronic inflammatory condition has previously had one or two incision and drainage procedures. Our approach has been wide excision of the involved area with associated subterminal duct excision, including the entire area beneath the nipple and areola (Fig. 14–3). Because of the chronic infection, delayed primary closure of the skin is suggested. The underlying breast tissue is approximated with catgut or Dexon and three to five days later the skin edges can be pulled together with tape or previously laid sutures. With this approach recurrent disease has not been a problem.

CYSTIC DISEASE OF THE BREAST

In this age of enlightenment women are acutely aware of their susceptibility

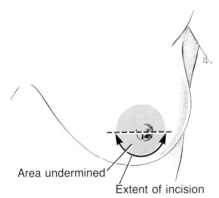

Area undermined

Extent of incision

Figure 14–3 Circumareolar incision for wide excision of diseased duct system. The areola is elevated and the involved area is excised up to the nipple. Deep tissue is then closed, followed by delayed closure of skin in three to five days.

to carcinoma of the breast. No disease of the breast is more common or more confusing than lumpy, tender breasts, usually more pronounced just prior to menstruation. First of all, the patient must be reassured and the normal physiology of the cyclic changes of her breasts explained to her. If there are dominant lumps which are mobile, well-circumscribed and appear fluctuant, the probability of cystic disease increases. Chronic cystic mastopathy (it is not truly a mastitis) is probably the most common breast ailment in premenopausal women. Because of high medical costs, as well as shortage of hospital beds, it appears unnecessary and meddlesome to admit women repeatedly to the hospital and

perform partial mastectomies under general anesthetic.[3] The mental anguish associated with a hospital admission and the possibility of awakening with the loss of a breast is of great significance to the patient. If the patient, when first seen, presents with one or more discrete, fluctuant masses and is in the premenopausal age group, needle aspiration is in order.[10] With the fluid removed and the mass gone the patient can safely receive follow-up care.

Patients who have previously undergone biopsy and have an established diagnosis of fibrocystic mastopathy certainly should have needle aspiration when recurrent masses appear. In the event that no fluid is obtained or if a residual mass is present, the patient should be scheduled for breast biopsy under general or local anesthesia. Cysts that recur within two weeks or those that require multiple aspirations can also be scheduled for elective excision. A high degree of judgment must be used in following a regimen such as this, but it is a safe and conservative approach for the many women who present with this problem. The technique of needle aspiration is simple and relatively painless even without local anesthetic (Fig. 14–4). A syringe of appropriate size with a needle of 22 to 25 gauge is used after thorough cleansing and preparation of the breast. Light finger pressure assists in complete evacuation of the cyst. A common problem is the woman with multiple small cysts throughout both breasts who complains of considerable

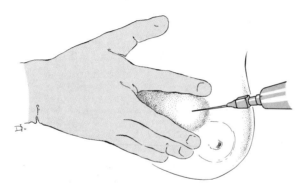

Figure 14–4 Aspiration of breast cyst. The cyst is identified, stabilized and evacuated by light finger pressure while syringe barrel is withdrawn.

pain during the premenstrual period. Reassurance, pain medication, and support with a well-fitted bra will usually suffice. Small doses of diuretics given during the premenstrual period will often be of help. In extreme cases the use of an androgen such as methyltestosterone, 5 mg daily for the first three weeks of the cycle, may relieve the discomfort.

FIBROADENOMA

It is not an uncommon event for the physician to be confronted by a highly concerned young woman in her late teens or twenties who has just noted a firm mass in her breast and wants to be sure that it is not a cancer—right now! These young ladies, frequently accompanied by their distraught mothers, must immediately be assured and placed at ease. They must be told that their age places them in a relatively safe category.[4] To tell these girls that the lump may indeed be a cancer, that they should be admitted to the hospital and given a general anesthetic, and then assure them that if it proves to be a cancer, they will be cured by surgical removal of the breast is an approach that can only be described as barbaric. We have a strict rule at the University of Colorado that women under the age of thirty scheduled for biopsy are positively assured that they will awaken with their lump removed and both breasts present and intact. Permanent sections, consultations with a number of pathologists, and thorough discussion with the patient and her family are in order before any radical surgery is embarked upon in a woman of this age group. Delaying the definitive surgery a number of days to achieve this has not proved harmful. We have, in fact, gone further. The easily accessible, well-circumscribed mass of significant size which presumably is a fibroadenoma is now subjected to biopsy immediately in the office or clinic. This relatively painless procedure can be done with a small amount of local anesthetic, using a disposable biopsy needle* after first incising the skin with a scalpel (Fig. 14–5). When the pathological diagnosis is confirmed the young lady and her physician can then logically and without undue emotion outline the approach for the removal of the benign but worrisome lump. Many superficial, well-circumscribed fibroadenomas can be removed easily, quickly, and less expensively under local anesthesia in the office or hospital outpatient department.

NIPPLE DISCHARGE

The complaint of spontaneous discharge from the nipple is second in frequency only to finding an actual lump in the breast.[8] The resultant worry to the patient is understandable and she must immediately be reassured that this is not necessarily an outward sign of an underlying cancer. Only then should a systematic, logical plan for the approach to this problem be outlined to the patient. First of all, it should be made clear that a nonspontaneous, self-induced discharge is usually harmless and of no pathological significance. The puerperal discharge of lactation is, of course, a normal physiological process. The cloudy, purulent discharge associated with mammary duct ectasia and fistula has been dealt with above. The bloody or serosanguineous discharge which a generation ago was believed to be a sure sign of underlying cancer is of greatest concern to the patient. It is now established that though the underlying cause for this discharge must be determined, it is most likely due to a benign lesion, the most common of which is an intraductal papilloma.

Cytological study, a simple procedure and an additional diagnostic aid, de-

---

*Travenol Laboratories, Inc.

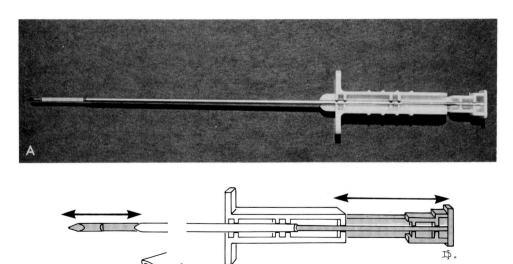

Figure 14–5 Disposable biopsy needle for breast biopsy. *A.* Needle assembled. *B.* Technique of biopsy. The hollow needle and obturator are inserted into the mass with the obturator (shaded portion) withdrawn. The obturator is then advanced by pressure on the plunger. The direction of the needle is then altered slightly, and the obturator is withdrawn, bringing with it a fragment of tissue. Needle and obturator are removed from patient, and tissue is extracted from obturator.

pends wholly on the availability of an interested, diligent and well-trained cytologist. A negative cytological study means nothing. Though we have emphasized the benign nature of these discharges it must be made clear that in patients over the age of 50 years, cancer, not a benign lesion, is the most frequent cause of this discharge.[11] If an associated mass is present there is no problem, as it *must* be excised.

The patient presenting with a discharge and no mass must then be thoroughly examined in an effort to establish the quadrant containing the underlying pathology. This is done by palpating firmly in a radial fashion over the entire breast (Fig. 14–6). If the quadrant which is the source of discharge can be localized, the involved ductal system can then be surgically excised. In an older woman and in patients in whom no preoperative localization can be elicited it is then advisable to completely excise the central duct system. This is done through a circumareolar incision ex-

tending no more than halfway around the areola, as described earlier (Fig. 14–3). The nipple and areola are elevated, the central duct system identified, and a generous underlying wedge of tissue removed, including the contents of the nipple, to assure excision of the entire major duct system. The defect is closed with buried catgut or Dexon and

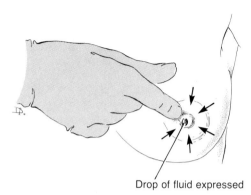

Drop of fluid expressed

Figure 14–6 Radial palpation of duct system to determine source of nipple discharge.

the nipple and areola replaced. The only possible occasion for simple mastectomy would be in the older patient presenting with a significant discharge, no mass, and in whom the previously mentioned excision of the major duct system demonstrated no significant benign lesion to explain the discharge. This decision requires judgment, often aided by consultation with one's colleagues.

CARCINOMA OF THE BREAST

The definitive surgical treatment of carcinoma of the breast has no place in the subject encompassed by this book. The correct surgical approach is and has been under question for the past 80 years.[12] During this time we have seen treatment evolve from conventional radical mastectomy through extended radical mastectomy, and lately to a modified conservative radical operation.[2] This latter approach has been generally accepted in England and is receiving considerable attention in this country. No absolute statement should be made, however, until there is clear-cut evidence from a well-controlled study comparing the various surgical procedures, such as that proposed by the National Adjuvant Breast Project.[5] In order to facilitate and plan the course of primary therapy, including the wishes and desires of the patient, we attempt to establish the exact diagnosis prior to the time of definitive surgery whenever possible. This can be simply done with the use of the disposable biopsy needle in suspicious lesions seen in the office or clinic. A benign diagnosis necessitates performance of an open biopsy if the lesion is at all suspicious. With a diagnosis of carcinoma the situation is clear. When the results of the needle biopsy are known, the course of action can be discussed with the patient and her relatives. Further tests, such as liver functions, bone survey, and so on, may be indicated. It would also seem that there is less chance of tumor seeding with this approach compared to open excisional biopsy at the time of the radical surgery. The operative time saved is obvious.

Postoperative Care

Once the patient has been discharged she again enters that phase in her disease which is relegated to outpatient care. The immediate problems which vex the surgeon or surgical resident assigned to the outpatient clinic concern the skin flaps. Seromas under these flaps require needle aspiration. This must be done carefully under sterile conditions, and a pressure dressing should be applied. Strict instructions must be given to the patient regarding care of the dressing and the importance of returning promptly for a follow-up visit. If a significant amount of fluid reaccumulates after one or more aspirations, a small rubber drain should be inserted for two or three days.

Scattered areas of skin necrosis generally are seen at or near the suture line on the first outpatient visit. These are usually due to faulty technique, such as skin flaps shaved unnecessarily thin or flaps approximated with undue tension, often with large retention sutures. Multiple closely placed skin sutures usually will prevent this problem. Prompt removal of sutures within 10 to 12 days, followed by application of basic principles of wound care should complete this phase. If necessary a skin graft can be performed at the appropriate time. When the wound is clean the graft can be performed on an outpatient basis under local anesthesia.

Physical rehabilitation is an important but frequently neglected factor following radical or modified radical breast surgery. Personal motivation should be stimulated by the surgeon with the help and expertise of the hospital physical therapist. Often this department, so readily available, is grossly neglected postoperatively in the care of the patient who has had a mastectomy. It should be made very clear to the premenopausal patient that she should, under no circumstances, take estrogens in any form, including oral contraceptives (the "pill"). The danger of stimulation of growth of any residual cancer is the reason for this injunction.

Postoperative radiotherapy continues to be a controversial issue. A survey of the literature and the varied statistics leaves one in a state of doubt and confusion. The fact remains, however, that high voltage therapy can, under the proper circumstances, sterilize carcinoma.[6] We recommend postoperative radiotherapy for those patients with one or more positive nodes and for subareolar or medial quadrant lesions.

Is subsequent pregnancy a danger for the premenopausal patient who has undergone treatment for carcinoma of the breast? There is no absolute answer to this question. In the past, carcinoma of the breast in a pregnant woman was thought to be an indication for therapeutic abortion. We no longer believe that this is true. The young patient who has undergone primary treatment for carcinoma of the breast might well consider having a child if she is well apprised of the situation, and is free of disease after two or three years.[4] This question obviously must be carefully and thoughtfully considered according to the needs of the individual — necessitating extremely close rapport between the physician and his patient.

A routine of postoperative follow-up care is mandatory in tumor surgery. The postmastectomy patient should be seen at regular intervals for a thorough examination of the operative sites, areas of lymphatic drainage and particularly the remaining breast. Chest x-rays and mammographic examination of the remaining breast are suggested at yearly intervals. It is well established that at least 7 to 8 per cent of women develop carcinoma in the remaining breast.[11] Any complaints of bone pain, particularly in the back or hips, should be promptly investigated with an appropriate bone survey. These regular examinations reassure both the patient and her physician.

If recurrent disease is found in one of these periodic examinations, the so-called "free-interval" is over. The patient then enters an entirely new phase in the management of her disease. The first and most important consideration is to explain to the patient and her immediate family the full meaning of the presence of recurrent disease. This is best discussed with the closest relatives first.

The explanation possibly may be modified in discussions with the patient on the basis of recommendations from the relatives. A positive approach offers reassurance to the patient. Emphasis should be placed on the many means of therapy at our disposal. The physician should then plan a sequential approach — not offering everything at once, but always having one more additional form of therapy available when the existing one fails. The patient with incurable cancer is often unbelievably optimistic, usually welcoming any form of therapy that may offer a glimmer of hope.

Management of Recurrent Breast Carcinoma

The first treatment of recurrent breast cancer generally lies in the realm of the radiotherapist. He has a success rate of up to 70 per cent in the palliative management of breast cancer. His role is particularly important when the disease involves portions of the bony skeleton within a field which can be treated practically and safely. He can often achieve remarkable results in superficial soft tissue metastasis and not only can alleviate pain but can also prevent pathologic fractures by radiating weight-bearing areas of the skeleton. There are limitations to this form of treatment. It is a local, not a systemic approach, and there is a distinct limit to the amount of radiation which can be given over any period of time. Radiation therapy offers little to the patient with visceral involvement such as metastasis to lung or liver. ^{32}P, a radioactive phosphorous substance, is taken up in areas of bone metastasis and affords significant palliation for patients who have multiple areas of involvement. Pleural effusions due to metastases can be controlled in up to 50 per cent of cases by radioactive gold or colloidal ^{32}P. The skilled radiotherapist can offer much in the way of palliation to the patient with recurrent breast cancer.

The beneficial effects of castration in the female with carcinoma of the breast were first noted by Sir Astley Cooper in 1829. Even today the issue as to who should receive this treatment remains unsettled. From the voluminous writings on this subject it would appear that the patient most likely to respond to oophorectomy is a woman nearing menopause who has soft tissue or osseous metastases and who had a relatively long free interval. Prophylactic castration following mastectomy probably does not add anything when one considers the entire spectrum of the disease. The effect of castration in prolonging survival and the beneficial effects on metastases are likely to be the same whether oophorectomy is performed early or late. We therefore usually wait until the extent or location of metastases makes the need for it obvious. Objective response to oophorectomy then helps to direct the course of further therapy.

As metastatic disease progresses there is usually some throughtful consideration given to further ablative therapy such as adrenalectomy. There have been a number of reports from large referral centers suggesting that adrenalectomy can offer a distinct remission in up to 50 per cent of the cases.[9] This, however, is a procedure which must not be embarked upon lightly. It is an operation of some magnitude, one of the more difficult abdominal procedures. It is performed on a patient with a known fatal disease. Certainly operative mortality figures coming from a large center can be misleading and do not apply to the surgeon who rarely approaches this area.

There are no absolute criteria available to detect the patients who will benefit most from an adrenalectomy. It is generally believed that young patients who have responded to oophorectomy after first experiencing a significant free interval and who now present with primarily bone or skin metastasis stand the best change of receiving significant palliation. Hypophysectomy, too, can produce beneficial results in those patients who satisfy the same criteria as the candidates for adrenalectomy. Postoperative endocrine regulation is not too difficult in the patient of moderate intelligence. Oral cortisone acetate in doses of 50 mg per day and Fluorinef 0.1 mg every other day is generally all that is necessary to control the patient after adrenalectomy.

The beneficial effects of castration in premenopausal women with metastatic breast cancer are similar in many ways to the effects produced by administration of hormones. As experience broadens and data accumulates it is becoming increasingly clear that androgens or their synthetic equivalents have a palliative value in both premenopausal and postmenopausal women with metastatic disease. Androgens are particularly valuable to the younger, premenopausal woman with disseminated disease. Fortunately, it is no longer necessary to submit her to the indignity of visible and aggravating side effects. Fluoxymesterone (Halotestin) and testolactone (Teslac) are oral androgen preparations which are frequently effective with the absence of masculinizing side effects. Estrogens often can offer distinct help to the postmenopausal woman. Since breast cancer in young women can be stimulated by estrogens, they should be used only by postmenopausal women. There can be complications of hormone manipulation. Vaginal bleeding in postmenopausal women may require dilatation and curettage but will usually respond to cessation of therapy. Serum calcium must be followed closely, particularly in patients with osseous metastases. Nausea, vomiting and lethargy progressing to disorientation and coma are signs of hypercalcemia. Treatment includes cessation of hormones, increased fluids, steroids and phosphate.

Significant progression of disease after an adequate trial of hormone manipulation would prompt the physician to change to a new modality of treatment. Administration of corticosteroids offers a high degree of subjective improvement in the patient who is in the latter half of the course of metastatic carcinoma of the breast. There is no hard and fast rule regarding indications and dosages. Oral prednisone in doses of 10 to 30 mg per day is convenient and usually offers a degree of subjective improvement. Once therapy is begun it is generally continued indefinitely.

Chemotherapy can offer hope, and a significant degree of palliation is achieved in selected patients, usually toward the latter stage of their disease. ThioTEPA, 5-Fluorouracil and some of the newer experimental drugs have been used with varying degrees of success. This subject is covered in greater detail in Chapter 25.

SUMMARY

The diseases of the breast have been outlined briefly. Absolute conclusions regarding treatment of breast cancer must be avoided. When we compare the results achieved during the past hundred years with the effort expended on clinical and laboratory research it is evident that the problem is far from solved. The investigators of the next generation can rest assured that this is a fertile field for their interest and efforts. Cancer of the breast is the most common cancer in women and our record in treating this condition is still unsatisfactory.

References

1. Abramson, D. J.: Mammary duct ectasia, mammillary fistula and subareolar sinuses. Ann. Surg., *169*:217–226, 1969.
2. Auchincloss, H.: Modified radical mastectomy: Why not? Amer. J. Surg., *119*:506–509, 1970.
3. Bolton, J. P.: The breast cyst and the hospital bed. Arch. Surg.: *101*:382–383, 1970.
4. Earley, T. K., Gallagher, J. Q., and Chapman, K.: Carcinoma of the breast in women under thirty years of age. Amer. J. Surg., *118*:832–834, 1969.
5. Fisher, B.: The surgical dilemma in the primary therapy of invasive breast cancer: A critical appraisal. Curr. Probl. Surg., Oct.: 1–53, 1970.
6. Gutmann, R. J.: Role of supervoltage irradiation of regional lymph node bearing areas in breast cancer. Amer. J. Roentgenol. Radium Ther. Nucl. Med., 96:560–564, 1966.
7. Handley, R. S.: Benign breast diseases: Surgical aspects. Proc. R. Soc. Med., 62:722–724, 1969.
8. Leis, H. P., Jr., and Pilvich, S.: Nipple discharge. Hosp. Med., November:29–53, 1970.
9. Moore, F. D.: Carcinoma of the Breast. Boston, Little, Brown and Co., 1968.
10. Rosemond, G. P., Maier, W. P., and Brobyn, T. J.: Needle aspiration of breast cysts. Surg. Gynecol. Obstet., *128*:351–354, 1969.
11. Seltzer, M. H., Perloff, L. J., Kelley, R. I., and Fitts, W. T.: The significance of age in patients with nipple discharge. Surg. Gynecol. Obstet., *131*:519–522, 1970.
12. Spratt, J. S., Jr., and Donegan, W. T.: Cancer of the Breast. Philadelphia, W. B. Saunders Co., 1967.

15

The Chest—Thoracic Surgery

453

By MELVIN M. NEWMAN, M.D.

INTRODUCTION— OUTPATIENT EVALUATION AND TREATMENT

Most of the problems in thoracic surgery do not involve primarily outpatient procedures. Diagnostic endoscopy and thoracentesis may be exceptions. The office practice of the thoracic surgeon revolves around questions of diagnosis of tumors, infections or minor trauma. The Emergency Room experience concerns more immediate threats to life which impose urgency upon diagnosis and decision.

History

The office practice of thoracic surgery depends more upon details of the history than do many other specialties. Many patients have had chronic respiratory complaints but the first important question is: Why does the patient present himself *at this time*? Does he have pain, cough, hemoptysis, dyspnea, fatigue or weight loss? How rapidly have symptoms developed?

Physical Examination

Rabin[1] has listed 15 frequently neglected physical findings in four groups:
1. Pulmonary periostopathy and clubbing of digits
   a. Rest pain but no pain on joint motion
   b. Floating or sponginess of nail bed
2. Signs of bronchial obstruction
   a. Bagpipe sign of a partially obstructed bronchus
   b. Pendular motion of trachea toward the side of obstruction or pneumothorax or inspiration and away from the affected side on expiration
   c. The palpable but inaudible rhonchus
3. Specific tracheal signs
   a. Absence of upward laryngeal movement on swallowing (fixation by mediastinal mass)
   b. Deviation of trachea toward right or left sternomastoid muscle
   c. Increased depth of jugular notch (anterior mediastinal tumor)
   d. Fluctuation of trachea on palpation (distension of cervical esophagus)
   e. Respiratory fremitus in tracheal obstruction
   f. Anterior d'Espine's sign (loud tracheal sounds on auscultation over sternum indicate a large anterior mediastinal tumor)
4. Specific signs in the neck
   a. Auscultatory crepitus above the clavicles (mediastinal emphysema)
   b. Ecchymosis at root of neck and over upper thorax (mediastinal hemorrhage)

c. Supraclavicular lymph nodes may become palpable when patient coughs or strains
d. Unilateral loss of bulging on Valsalva maneuver and retraction on Mueller maneuver (carcinoma at apex of lung)

X-ray

The interpretation of roentgenograms is aided by an organized inspection routine.[2] One first looks at the chest wall for symmetry, contraction of interspaces, rib erosion and extrathoracic soft tissue swelling. Next scan the pleura from apex to base for thickening, fluid or air collections, and changes in the leaves of the diaphragm. Next, scan the mediastinum and cardiac shadow for shifts to right or left and abnormal contour. Then look at the lung parenchyma for masses, infiltrates, radiolucencies, or changes in radiodensities between the right and left side or the upper and lower portions of the lung. Compare the vascular patterns right and left. Finally, if infiltrates are present, try to determine if they are alveolar or if they are interstitial (interstitial fibrosis versus Kerley's lines).

Special Techniques

More information about a suspicious area can be obtained by a variety of simple techniques: the apical lordotic projection, oblique projections, the use of coning down and focussed grids to decrease tissue scatter, anteroposterior and lateral tomograms (body section radiography). Since image-intensifying equipment has become generally available, fluoroscopy again has become more popular as a supplement to roentgenograms for assessing mobility of the right and left leaves of the diaphragm, equal ventilation of the right and left lungs, and normal versus abnormal motion of the cardiac silhouette. When supplemented with a few swallows of barium, fluoroscopy may add several dimensions to

our understanding of the x-ray shadows. Finally, there will always be special situations where angiocardiography will be essential for evaluation of superior vena caval obstruction or abnormalities of the heart and the aorta and its branches.

Endoscopy

In these days of increasing hospitalization costs, one tries even harder to complete the diagnostic work-up without hospitalizing the patient. Bronchoscopy and esophagoscopy can be done in the well-equipped office which has all the facilities to cope with emergencies, including untoward drug reactions, hypoxia or cardiac arrest. Bronchograms also can be advantageously done at the same sitting as bronchoscopy if x-ray facilities are available. There has been recent renewed enthusiasm for brush biopsy of smaller bronchi with fluoroscopic control as a means of establishing diagnosis in cases of lung cancer.[3]

Sputum Examination

Sputum studies are useful in proportion to the effort made in securing deep cough specimens. Bacteriologic specimens should be cultured for pyogenic bacteria, mycobacteria and fungi as quickly as possible to avoid overgrowth of saprophytic bacteria. Cytology depends upon rapid fixation to stop autolysis of the desquamated cells. Some cytologists prefer to examine smears fixed in ether-alcohol and others supplement this with study of sections of centrifuged and formalin-fixed sputum. Many cytologists have reported a success rate of 90 per cent in diagnosing bronchogenic cancer from three consecutive sputum smears.[4] The three or four days after bronchoscopy are likely to provide the best sputum specimens for cytology and for culture of bacteria and mycobacteria.

Skin Tests

Skin tests for tuberculosis, histoplasmosis and coccidioidomycosis should be done routinely. We no longer use the blastomycin skin test, which lacks specificity. The Kveim test for sarcoidosis is now of historical interest only, since the antigen appears to be specific not for sarcoidosis but for lymphoid cells.[5]

Lung Biopsy

In many cases the cause of pulmonary infiltration can be determined only from lung biopsy. Modifications of the Vim-Silverman and Menghini needles have been used successfully for biopsies of pleura and lung. A recently developed technique is percutaneous lung biopsy with the high speed, turbine-driven, hollow drill;[6] until we have more experience with this procedure and its complications, it will continue to be done only on inpatients. Diagnoses of carcinoma, tuberculosis, sarcoidosis, pyogenic infection, Pneumocystis carinii infection, and fungus infection have been made in this way. However, an open biopsy of the lung is still frequently necessary in order to obtain adequate material for culture and histological study (Fig. 15–1).

Node Biopsy

When there is palpable lymphadenop-

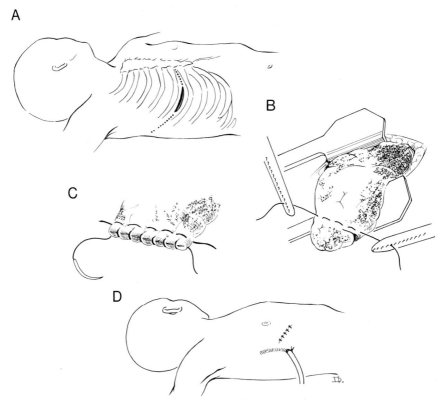

Figure 15–1   Lung biopsy technique. *A.* Lung biopsy can readily be carried out through an anterolateral incision through the right or left fifth or sixth interspace. Bleeding is usually less if one strips the periosteum from the upper edge of the rib, rather than making an incision of the intercostal muscles. The deep portion of the incision is usually somewhat longer than the skin incision. *B.* A continuous basting stitch minimizes blood loss and facilitates suturing. *C.* The over-and-over suture insures hemostasis. *D.* A size 16F to 18F catheter is brought out through a separate stab wound in the midaxillary line and connected to −20 cm suction.

athy, node biopsy or cervical fat pad biopsy under local anesthesia is perfectly feasible as an outpatient procedure.

Mediastinoscopy

When no nodes are palpable, it is preferable to hospitalize the patient for general endotracheal anesthesia and to do a formal mediastinoscopy[7] (Fig. 15–2) and bronchoscopy. Ward has reported success with 100 consecutive mediastinoscopies with local anesthesia.[8]

Indications for Thoracotomy

After preliminary diagnostic studies have been completed, exploratory thoracotomy may be indicated for diagnosis or definitive treatment. Pulmonary resection must have clear justification. The most important question one should ask about any surgical or medical procedure is: What are we trying to accomplish for this patient?

Tuberculosis

Indications for Resection. In the case of tuberculosis there are certain specific indications for resection:

1. A persistent, thick-walled cavity or solid necrotic residual.[9]

2. An area of destroyed lung tissue of limited resistance to secondary infection.

3. The bronchial problems: bronchostenosis, bronchiectasis, bronchopleural fistula.

4. The diagnostic problem of the solid lesion ("coin lesion").

Preoperative Chemotherapy. Surgery is no substitute for rational chemotherapy based on careful *in vitro* studies of sensitivity, followed by the administration of three or more drugs of demonstrated effectiveness for a minimum period of 18 months. Removal of small necrotic foci may lead to a reduction in the relapse rate, but the evidence is meager. If one accepts the basic premise that tuberculosis is a systemic infection, then only prolonged chemotherapy will insure cure, and the place

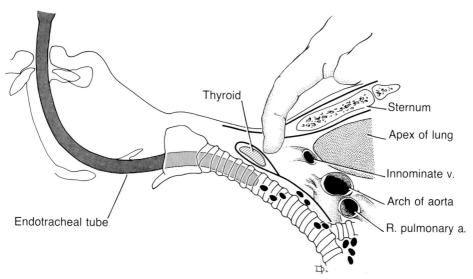

Thyroid

Sternum

Apex of lung

Innominate v.

Arch of aorta

Endotracheal tube

R. pulmonary a.

Figure 15–2 Mediastinoscopy. The neck is entered by a low collar incision which follows the skin creases. Blunt dissection can be carried down along the pretracheal fascia to the bifurcation of the trachea. Nodes can then be selected by inspection through the mediastinoscope and biopsies can be made of them.

of surgery is to cope with localized mechanical problems as listed above.

Selection of Agent. Isoniazid and streptomycin remain the time-tested agents for treatment of tuberculosis due to mycobacteria susceptible to these agents. With new drugs continually coming into the field, it is essential that the surgeon consult updated reviews and recommendations, such as those of the Committee on Therapy of the American Thoracic Society.[10] There are rarely indications today for pulmonary resection in children with pulmonary tuberculosis.[11]

Fungal Infection

Treatment of pulmonary fungal infections parallels that of the treatment of tuberculosis. Agents available for chemotherapy are fewer.[12] Amphotericin B is effective against the widest number of fungi. Penicillin is effective against susceptible strains of actinomycosis and sulfadiazine has been effective against many strains of nocardia. The compound 5-fluorocytosine has been especially promising in cryptococcal infections. Again, the role of surgery is to remove mechanical problems in order to make chemotherapy more effective.

Cancer

Cure. There are certain rules-of-thumb concerning operability in lung cancer. Weight loss still tends to be an ominous sign; it may not preclude resectability of a lesion but it decreases the likelihood for surgical cure. Phrenic or recurrent nerve paralysis does not always preclude resection but again argues against possible cure.

Accumulation of pleural fluid does not necessarily rule out curative resection, providing that the fluid is a result of pulmonary suppuration distal to an area of bronchial obstruction and is not due to seeding of the visceral and parietal pleura by tumor nodules. If the pleural fluid is free of tumor cells, one should not hesitate to perform exploratory thoracotomy.

The popularity of mediastinoscopy (Fig. 15-2) followed studies showing that patients with extensive mediastinal lymph node metastases were not likely to be benefited by pulmonary resection.[13] However, a more recent study has shown a five year survival of 25 per cent of patients who had squamous cell carcinoma with mediastinal metastases who were treated by resection and postoperative radiation to the mediastinum.[14]

Palliation. There are definite indications for palliation by resection: removal of a localized area of suppuration and removal of distressing, intractable hemoptysis. It has been the general experience that, although comfort might be gained from palliative resection, there is no improvement in longevity.

The best results in treatment of lung cancer have been in patients with small asymptomatic lesions discovered by routine roentgenograms.

The Problem of the Solitary Pulmonary Nodule. The extensive chest x-ray surveys done by the U. S. Armed Forces during and after World War II seemed to indicate that in men over the age of 40 the solitary, uncalcified pulmonary nodule might have as high as a 35 per cent chance of being malignant, primary or metastatic. By contrast, Holin et al.[15] found, in a civilian population, 666 solitary nodules in 673,218 films. Only 20 out of the 666 demonstrated malignancy (3 per cent); however, if the group were narrowed down to males over the age of 44 years who had nodules more than 39 mm in greatest diameter, then 8 out of 44 nodules were malignant (35 per cent). In another study McClure et al.[16] did a five year follow-up of 551 patients with solitary nodules obtained from a screening survey in Pittsburgh, Pennsylvania, and found only 13, or 2.4 per cent, developed microscopically proven malignancies. Only 32 out of 551 patients came to surgical diagnosis and 10 out of 32 of these were malignant. There is general agreement that the nodule which shows massive or laminar calcification is probably caused by a granuloma (tuberculosis, atypical mycobacterial infection or fungus infection), whereas scattered flecks of calcium in a nodule are still compatible with cancer. Rigler feels that a notch in the edge of a nodule is strongly suggestive of malignancy.[17] Hamartomas usually have a characteristic pattern of patchy calcification and are readily recognized.

The patients referred to the surgeon represent a selected or skewed sample of the entire group. Overholt and associates[18] reported on 46 patients with asymptomatic tumors discovered by survey films: 26 patients were explored, 23 resected, and 9 (30 per cent) were alive three years later. Wilkins[19] reported 77 patients with asymptomatic nodules of which 33 were carcinomas, 27 being primary and 6 metastatic. There were 50 patients more than age 50 and of these 29 (58 per cent) had cancer microscopically. Davis et al.[20] reported 215 "coin lesions" of which 101 were malignant. Thirty-two patients were without symptoms at the time of operation and had curative resections. Twenty-four of these (75 per cent) survived more than three years. John Steele[21] reported that the asymptomatic patient with a malignant nodule had a 38 per cent chance for surviving 30 months if the lesion were less than 6 cm in diameter and about a 50 per cent chance of survival for lesions of less than 3 cm in diameter.

Results. Once the patient has developed symptoms, most clinics report a survival of only 6 to 8 per cent for the entire group with bronchogenic cancer. Attempts to improve survival of patients with bronchogenic carcinoma have been disappointing. Preoperative supervoltage irradiation was received enthusiastically when it was found that a larger number of tumors were made resectable. However, two carefully randomized series[22,23] have failed to show any improvement in survival. Similarly, chemotherapy has failed to show any benefit in patients in a series from Veterans Administration hospitals[24] or in a university hospital series.[25]

Functional Criteria for Surgery

Pulmonary. One must always ask the question: Is the patient able to afford the loss of any more functioning pulmonary tissue? Many years ago Max Pinner asked the question in a different way: What shall it avail the patient to be "cured" of his tuberculosis if he never again will be able to leave his bed to do a few hours' work or climb one flight of stairs?[26] Often one can gain a useful estimate of the patient's ability to withstand a lobectomy or pneumonectomy by a detailed study of his daily activities. How many flights of steps can he climb? How far can he walk on level ground without distress in either legs or chest? Does he wheeze or become blue with exertion? Can he blow out a match at a distance of two feet with unpursed lips? It is tempting to estimate pulmonary function from the x-ray film, but this is always inferior to actual studies of ventilation and of blood gases. The detailed laboratory values are available in *The Lung* by Comroe[27] and in other textbooks. In general a patient of average size who has at least 2 liters of total vital capacity and who can expel 65 per cent of that in the first second of forceful expiration and who has disease localized to a lobe can probably be tided over an operation. He may have severe difficulty after operation and may require prolonged assistance of ventilation.[28]

Cardiac. Cardiac catheterization has been useful in borderline cases. The normal individual can increase ventilation at least tenfold and can triple his cardiac output with strenuous exercise. Under these circumstances pulmonary artery pressure may rise slightly in the normal individual or may actually fall, whereas the person who has lost more than half of the perfusable pulmonary vascular space will almost always show a rise of 15 to 20 mm of mercury or more in mean pulmonary artery pressure.

Temporary occlusion of the right or left branch of the pulmonary artery with a fluid-filled balloon was first introduced in Sweden by Carlens (1951) and in this country by Paul Nemir (1953); it serves as a "functional pneumonectomy."[29] Arterial blood gas studies at rest and after breathing 100 per cent oxygen for 20 minutes will also tell much about intrapulmonary mixing and the ventilation/perfusion ratios.

Endocrine Abnormalities

Various types of endocrine abnormalities have been associated with malignant tumors of the thymus, of the lung, of the pleura and of the retroperitoneal tissues. These have included paradoxical antidiuretic hormone production, secretion of insulin or insulinlike materials, hypercalcemia from parathormonelike materials, Cushing's syndrome from anomalous ACTH secretion, and secretion of norepinephrine and epinephrine by extra-adrenal pheochromocytomas.[30]

Mediastinal Tumors

Mediastinal tumors are less common than tumors of the lung. One clue to the type of tumor involved is often its position.[31] In the upper anterior mediastinum the substernal goiter can usually be identified easily by fluoroscopy—it is adherent to the trachea and moves upward on swallowing. A little lower in the anterior mediastinum the two most common tumors are thymoma and enlarged lymph nodes involved by lymphoma or Hodgkin's disease. The teratomas, dermoids and embryonal cell carcinomas are all rare. Lymph nodes in the midmediastinum may simulate tumor when they are involved by various granulomas such as tuberculosis, atypical mycobacterial infections, fungal infections, or by involvement by metastatic tumor from lung or esophagus. Posteriorly, the neurofibroma is almost unique.

Thymic tumors have been of special interest because of the association of the thymus with myasthenia gravis, first noted in 1901 by the German pathologist Carl Weigert. On May 26, 1936, Alfred Blalock did the first thymectomy specifically for treatment of myasthenia gravis. His patient, a 19 year old woman who had had symptoms for four years, was well 25 years later.[32] After a lapse from grace for nearly two decades, thymectomy is making a comeback. Current studies by Osserman and associates[33] indicate that thymectomy works as well in men with myasthenia gravis as in women. Duration of symptoms had little prognostic value in their series. Since most patients have either a normal or hyperplastic thymus, it is a waste of time to attempt to demonstrate a tumor in every patient as a justification for thymectomy.

Idiopathic Pleural Effusion

Idiopathic pleural effusion is a different matter (Fig. 15–3). All effusions should be aspirated (Fig. 15–4) and cultured for pyogens, fungi and acid-fast bacilli, and search should always be made for malignant cells by direct smear

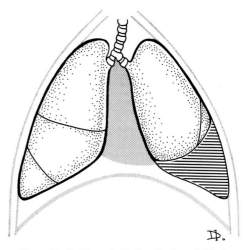

Figure 15–3   Pleural effusion. In pleural effusion, the fluid level curves up along the chest wall. If hydropneumothorax exists, there is an obvious, straight airfluid interface. Hydropneumothorax implies a connection with the bronchial tree.

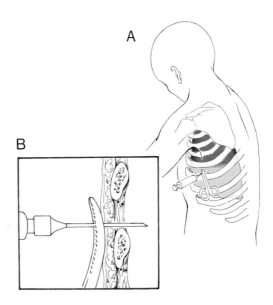

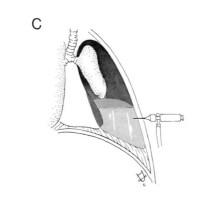

Figure 15–4 Thoracentesis. *A.* Thoracentesis is best done with the patient seated and leaning forward slightly. *B.* An 18 gauge needle with a 45° bevel is introduced just above the top of the rib. A plastic cannula (e.g., Intracath, Longdwel, or Angiocath) works well and is less likely to lacerate the underlying lung than a metal needle. *C.* When large volumes of fluid must be removed, a three-way stopcock between the needle and a 30 to 50 ml syringe permits drainage through a length of rubber or plastic tubing into a collecting bottle.

and in sections of a block of centrifuged sediment. Extensive studies during and since World War II have demonstrated that patients with idiopathic pleural effusion and a positive tuberculin skin test should be considered to have active pulmonary tuberculosis and should be started on chemotherapy.[34] Most experts would prefer to start treatment with streptomycin and isoniazid and para-aminosalicylic acid.

Spontaneous Pneumothorax

Spontaneous pneumothorax used to be considered pathognomonic of pulmonary tuberculosis. Today it usually results from rupture of focal areas of obstructive emphysema which are often in portions of the lung adherent to the apex of the chest from an old infectious process. My own policy is to treat the first or even second episode (Fig. 15–5 *A, B, C*) of spontaneous pneumothorax with catheter drainage of the affected pleural space. However, in individuals who have had episodes on both sides of the chest or more than two episodes on the same side of the chest, the recommendation is for a thoracotomy to excise or oversew areas of blebs (on the surface of the lung) or bullae (originating below the surface of the visceral pleura) and to strip off the parietal pleura to insure a firm symphysis between the surface of the lung and the chest wall. This latter

A

1

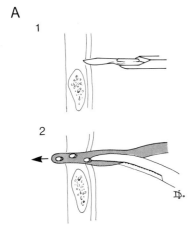

2

Figure 15–5 Closed thoracostomy. Three methods of inserting a chest tube for drainage: *A.* A short horizontal skin incision at the level of the top of the rib permits direct insertion of a drainage catheter supported by hemostat.

procedure does not completely prevent blowouts from the surface of the lung, but it means any such blowout will form a very localized pneumothorax and not be life-threatening.

The former enthusiasm for treatment of emphysema by extensive excision of emphysematous blebs or bullae has been tempered by the increasing evidence that patients with airway obstructive disease have a generalized process affecting the whole lung and that any surgical intervention is likely to have extremely short term benefits. There are a few individuals who have localized giant bullae and minimal evidence of generalized airway obstruction who may still be benefited by judicious local excisions.

Empyema—Resection and Open Drainage

Empyema is still with us despite antibiotics and increased awareness. The diagnosis sometimes can be made by a direct smear of pleural exudate, even though growth of bacteria has been suppressed by antibiotics given prior to consultation. Tube drainage is the first maneuver. If the fluid is very thick or

B

1

2

3

4

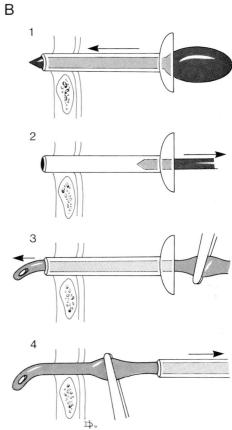

Figure 15–5 (Continued.) *B.* A stab incision in the skin permits insertion of a suitable trocar. The obturator is withdrawn and replaced with a catheter. The sheath is slipped out over the catheter.

C

1

2

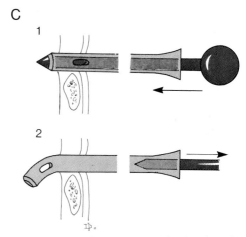

Figure 15–5 (Continued.) *C.* The Argyle catheter comes with a sharp obturator which facilitates insertion through a small skin incision.

the empyema wall quite dense, then we do not hesitate to revert to the old maneuver of rib resection and open drainage.

Each new generation of surgeons (and physicians) must relearn the dictum arrived at by the Empyema Commission of the U. S. Army after World War I:[36] "Empyema is cured only by eliminating the space, either by bringing the lung out to meet the chest wall, or failing this, by bringing the chest wall down to meet the lung (thoracoplasty)."

Chronic Constriction—Decortication

Chronic constriction of the lung by a layer ("peel") of granulation tissue and fibrin is best treated by decortication. There are a few patients with extensive fibrosis of the underlying lung who are not candidates for decortication but who can be treated by chronic open drainage or marsupialization of the empyema cavity to the outside and who remain relatively symptom-free for many years, until they finally succumb to their pulmonary insufficiency. We have not hesitated doing localized Schede full-thickness excisions of the chest wall in order to marsupialize chronic empyema cavities and the patients have been grateful for relief which has often extended for over a decade or more. Fortunately, since few patients are being treated by artificial pneumothorax any more for tuberculosis, the chronic "mixed" empyema (tuberculosis plus pyogens) is almost a museum piece.[37]

Postoperative Problems

Pain

Postoperative care after thoracotomy must not be neglected. Persistent intercostal neuralgia is often troublesome. Light percussion on the chest wall often will locate a "trigger zone." Direct block of this or a block of two intercostal nerves above and below the segment, repeated two or three times, may be all that is needed. Claggett[35] has suggested division of the intercostal nerve above the line of incision prior to opening the rib spreader, since he feels that many cases of intercostal neuralgia in the older patient are the result of excessive traction upon posterior sensory roots in the patient who has already developed considerable stiffening of the thoracic cage. One per cent lidocaine has been an effective blocking agent, as discussed later under rib fracture.

Persistent Air Space

The problem of the persistent air space in the patient who has had recent pneumonia or in the postoperative patient always comes up. One of the most common problems is the pneumatocele which may persist for weeks or months after an episode of staphylococcal pneumonia. This is not a surgical problem. If the patient is asymptomatic and has had adequate antibiotic treatment for his staphylococcal pneumonia, we prefer merely to watch such spaces until they disappear. If there is a fluid level or if the patient has cough, fever or leukocytosis, then we consider this a lung abscess and start with treatment of appropriate antibiotics, based on cultures of sputum or pleural fluid, and this course of antibiotics is usually four to six weeks in duration. Persistent air spaces have also been described in children after pertussis and usually need only careful observation until they disappear.

THE EMERGENCY ROOM

"Chance favors the mind that is prepared."

These words of Louis Pasteur's have been quoted thousands of times but never in a better context than that of the Emergency Room.

Priorities

An ordered system of priorities is essential (a) to save life, (b) to preserve function as far as possible, and (c) to minimize disfigurement.[38] The priorities are:

1. Maintain ventilation
2. Stop obvious external bleeding
3. Replenish the blood volume and insure adequate circulation
4. Treat cardiac wounds
5. Evaluate and treat central nervous system damage
6. Repair the ruptured viscus
7. Stabilize and later reduce and fix fractures

Ventilation

The importance of ventilation can be illustrated by simply holding one's breath. Only a trained athlete such as an experienced underwater swimmer can hold his breath voluntarily for more than 40 to 60 seconds. The accident victim is fortunate if he reaches the Emergency Room within 30 minutes after the catastrophe. Fractures and lacerations about the face with bleeding into the upper airway causes obvious airway obstructions. However, fracture of the larynx must always be suspected when there is laryngeal tenderness, crepitus or stridor, and it may be overlooked until the patient is in serious difficulty. This is one of the few instances when emergency tracheostomy is justified; otherwise it is safer to insert a bronchoscope or endotracheal tube for ventilation and perform a formal tracheostomy sometime in the next 24 hours (see Chapter 10). Tracheostomy is best done over an endotracheal tube in the operating room with adequate equipment, light, and assistance.[39]

Several points cannot be emphasized too often. Instead of "stop, look and listen," the command should be "strip completely, look, feel, and listen." Ventilation can often be observed better by looking at the patient's chest movements from the foot of the bed. Inequality of movement of the right versus the left thorax can often by evaluated by palpation with the fingers on the rib margins and the thumbs laid along the spine. If the patient is awake and cooperative and has an intact glottis, pneumothorax can be detected more quickly by palpation of vocal fremitus than by percussion or auscultation.

Physical Signs and Emergency Treatment

Some physical signs may give clues as to the severity of injury: "splinting" of movements of chest or abdomen, *flail chest* (Fig. 15–6), respiratory distress, ecchymoses at the base of the neck, subcutaneous emphysema, difference in breath sounds between the right and left sides, absence of a point of maximal impulse at the cardiac apex and a change in the percussible liver dullness. *Sucking chest wounds* (Fig. 15–7) can be closed with Vaseline gauze and a bulky dressing held in place by tape. If there is suspicion of a *tension pneumothorax* (Fig. 15–8) do not wait for the x-ray but confirm by thoracentesis (Fig. 15–4) and then insert a thoracostomy tube (Fig. 15–5). Although many textbooks still show insertion of chest tubes in the second interspace in the midclavicular line and the seventh interspace posteriorly, I have come to believe that the patient is much more comfortable if tubes are inserted in the midaxillary line and that they work just as well in this position with less restriction of the patient's movements. As shown in Figure 15–5, the demonstration of free air or blood in the pleural space is followed immediately by insertion of a trocar and a tube. At one time there was enthusiasm for inserting the largest possible chest tube, but again experience has shown that a size 16 catheter is usually more than adequate for the upper tube to remove air and usually adequate for the lower tube to remove blood. Occasionally, one may want to insert a

Figure 15–6 Paradoxical motion—flail chest. *Paradoxical motion* of the chest wall results from multiple fractures of contiguous ribs. Each rib must be fractured anteriorly and posteriorly to cause the chest wall to be pulled in on inspiration and pushed out on expiration. This can markedly decrease alveolar ventilation. Immediate treatment with an endotracheal tube connected to volume-cycled respirator will improve ventilation and bring arterial pO_2 and pCO_2 back toward normal. An elective tracheostomy can safely be done in the operating room at any convenient time in the next 48 hours.

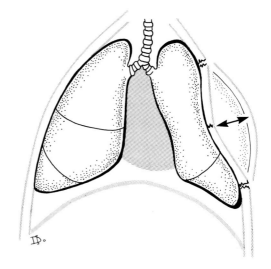

Figure 15–7 Sucking chest wound. A *sucking chest wound* can be occluded by petrolatum (Vaseline) gauze covered by a bulky dressing. If the patient has any evidence of respiratory distress, a thoracostomy tube is inserted in the fifth or sixth interspace in the midaxillary line to remove air and blood and expand the lung.

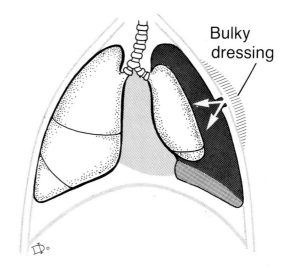

Bulky dressing

Figure 15–8 Tension pneumothorax. *Tension pneumothorax* results from a laceration of the lung which produces a one-way valve effect. During straining or coughing, air is forced into the pleural space under high enough pressure to displace the mediastinum, interfere with ventilation of the other lung and with venous return to the right atrium. Immediate insertion of a chest tube can be lifesaving. Occasionally, tension pneumothorax can result from bronchiolitis, rupture of an emphysematous bulla, or even a necrotizing pneumonia.

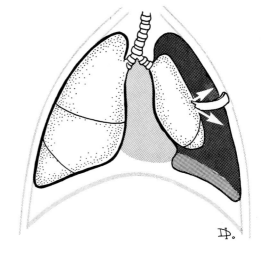

size 24–36 plastic tube by means of direct incision into the pleural space because of rapid bleeding intrapleurally, but bleeding of this magnitude generally requires thoracotomy.[40] The quickest way in general to stop bleeding in the pleural space is to expand the lung expeditiously. This usually requires at least two chest tubes with suction of minus 15 to minus 25 cm of water. If the patient continues to bleed more than 500 ml during the second hour after the tubes have been inserted, this is taken as an indication for immediate thoracotomy. Similarly, if there is an unremitting flow of air from the chest tubes, one has to suspect either a ruptured bronchus or deep lacerations of the lung surface by spicules from fractured ribs, both of which require immediate operation.

Eijgelaar and van der Heide[41] found that x-ray demonstration of air in the deep cervical fascial planes along the trachea and along the large vessels enclosed by the middle cervical fascia was a very strong indication of a ruptured bronchus or trachea.

Subcutaneous emphysema may be annoying but in itself is rarely serious. It can occur from a laceration of the nasopharynx when air is forced beneath the skin, or from mediastinal emphysema from a tracheal laceration, or it may simply represent the end of an involuntary Valsalva maneuver with rupture of alveoli at the periphery of the lung and dissection of the air back along the vascular sheath, as originally described by C. C. Macklin in 1936. When subcutaneous emphysema produces severe discomfort, excess air can often be massaged into a few pockets where it can be aspirated aseptically with an 18 gauge needle.

Stabilization of the Chest

By simple inspection, one can see whether or not there is paradoxical motion of the chest. This implies fractures of several ribs in at least two places, making an unsupported flap of chest wall which is pulled in with inspiration and pushed out with expiration, thus diminishing pulmonary ventilation. Despite recurrent articles in the surgical literature advocating stabilization of the chest wall with towel clips, pericostal stainless steel wire traction sutures, and even Kirschner wire fixation of rib fragments, I remain convinced that internal splinting by artificial ventilation is superior. Blood gases can be maintained in the normal range and the patient requires less narcotics. The original contribution of Moerch and Avery represents the best approach: insert a cuffed endotracheal tube immediately and start artificial ventilation with a volume-cycled respirator. Within 24 to 48 hours the endotracheal tube can be replaced by a cuffed tracheostomy tube. Positive pressure ventilation is then maintained for ten to twenty days, until the chest wall has been stabilized by fibrosis at the fracture sites.[42]

Monitoring of Blood Gases

Cyanosis can be seen only when the patient has more than 5 gm of reduced hemoglobin per 100 ml of blood, and the hypovolemic patient may die before this level is reached. Inadequate ventilation can quickly be demonstrated from an arterial blood sample by a saturation below 90 per cent and a pCO_2 above 50 mm of mercury. Repeated arterial samples are the best guide to the adequacy of ventilation.

Probably the single greatest advance in the treatment of patients with all types of acute pulmonary insufficiency has been monitoring of arterial blood samples. Arterial puncture is easily done by puncture of radial, brachial or femoral arteries with a 20 gauge needle. Currently available equipment for determining arterial oxygen saturation, pH, pO_2 and pCO_2 can give rapid, accurate values as guides to therapy.

Bleeding

External

External bleeding can generally be controlled with finger pressure or pressure dressings initially. Definitive vascular repair or ligation should be done under aseptic conditions in the operating room. More difficult problems arise from lacerations of intercostal arteries or the internal mammary artery and these may require emergency thoracotomy for repair.

Internal

Evaluation of internal bleeding is more difficult. It is important to check pulses and blood pressures in both upper and lower extremities repeatedly for symmetry; this is often a clue to aortic laceration or false aneurysm after blunt trauma. As soon as ventilation and circulating blood volume have been restored to normal, plans should be made for definitive repair (see Chapter 16 on heart wounds).

Treatment of Hypovolemia and Shock

While all the above measures are being taken, other members of the team have begun treatment for hypovolemia and shock. A central venous pressure cannula should be inserted by a convenient route: antecubital vein, jugular vein or subclavian vein (see Chapter 3). At least two plastic cannulas or cut-downs should be inserted. As soon as central venous pressure has been measured accurately, fluid infusion should be begun with lactated Ringer's solution to increase circulating blood volume. Plasmanate can be added as soon as blood has been drawn for typing and cross-match. Up to one liter of low-molecular weight dextran (dextran 40) can be given without interfering with the coagulation mechanism.

Associated Injuries (Diaphragm, Spleen, Liver, Kidney, Brain)

A Foley catheter is inserted in the bladder to monitor urinary output. Cross-match enough blood: most patients subjected to massive injury should have at least six units of blood cross-matched initially. Plan the logical approach to stop any continuing bleeding. Even the least experienced surgeon soon learns that lower thoracic injuries on the left carry a high suspicion of rupture of the spleen, and sometimes laceration of diaphragm and low thoracic injuries on the right may be combined with lacerations of the liver and of the right kidney. Traumatic rupture of the diaphragm (Fig. 15–9) frequently follows a massive, sudden compression of the abdomen and demands immediate surgical repair.

The problem of central nervous system damage is always with us. Few patients subjected to massive injury to the torso and extremities have escaped without a concussion at the minimum. The problem of differentiation between cerebral concussion, contusion and laceration on the one hand and between acute extradural or subdural hematoma on the other is extremely difficult and calls for neurosurgical consultation as early as possible.

Rib Fractures

Uncomplicated rib fractures can cause much discomfort. Analgesics will relieve most patients, but if there are multiple fractures, much more relief can be achieved by intercostal nerve block (Fig. 15–10). Blocks may have to be repeated every six to eight hours for the first few days after injury. The patient is then enabled to ventilate more effectively and to clear the bronchial tree by coughing. In general, strapping of the chest is much less effective in reducing pain and

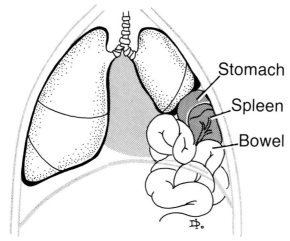

Stomach

Spleen

Bowel

Figure 15–9 Traumatic rupture of diaphragm. Massive blunt trauma to the abdomen can split the diaphragm (usually the left leaf) in the direction of its fibers. The spleen, stomach, splenic flexure of colon, and small bowel may be forced into the pleural space and may markedly interfere with ventilation. Immediate operation is essential. A similar but more slowly developing situation has followed stab wounds (in the left lower chest or left upper abdomen) that lacerate the diaphragm.

is likely to cause blistering of the skin. In a few instances, when one or two lower ribs have been fractured, circumferential restriction of the entire chest by a belt or by tape may give some comfort.

Transportation

Finally, the reader may wonder why the acutely injured patient has not been taken for x-ray studies up to this point. Experience again has shown that the least amount of moving around that need be done in order to accomplish treatment is to the patient's advantage. Plan the evaluation and emergency treatment in a logical fashion so that the patient needs only one trip to the x-ray department, either on the way to the intensive care area or to the operating room. If extremity fractures are splinted before he makes this trip, further blood loss around the fracture sites will be minimized and it will be easier to maneuver the splinted extremity into the best position for x-ray studies.

Summary

In summary, the patient who comes to the Emergency Room after massive trauma must be considered in imminent danger of death. Chest injuries may be involved in more than half of the cases. A logical, preformed plan for diagnosis and decision will save more lives than misguided enthusiasm and technical virtuosity.

ESOPHAGUS

History

Just as with pulmonary disease, it is important to learn why the patient presents with his symptoms at this time. Is there incoordination of swallowing with regurgitation of fluid through the nose, suggestive of neurologic disease? Is there pain in the throat or substernally with swallowing (odynophagia)? Is there difficulty in swallowing (dysphagia), manifested by a vague sensation of soreness or something sticking in the esophagus? Are there symptoms to suggest gastroesophageal reflux,

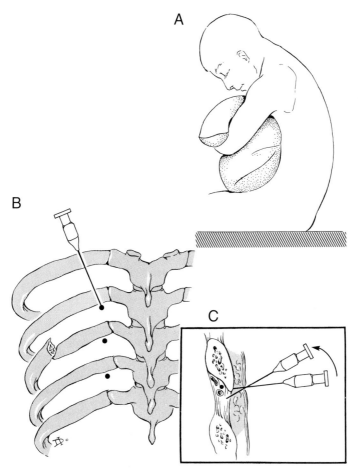

Figure 15–10 Relief of pain from fractured ribs. *A*. The patient is usually more comfortable sitting up with the arms grasping a pillow, thus throwing the scapulae forward. *B*. The sensory fields of the intercostal nerves overlap. In order to relieve the pain of fractured ribs, one must block one nerve above and one below the fractured rib, as well as the nerve adjacent to the fracture. *C*. A 22 gauge needle is inserted through a skin wheal of 1% lidocaine until it touches the lower border of the rib; then it is angled downward to pass just beneath the edge of the rib. It is not necessary to produce paresthesias by contact with the nerve. Five ml of 1% lidocaine injected within a few millimeters of the nerve will diffuse to produce an adequate block. Always get a chest x-ray after the block to be sure no pneumothorax has resulted from inadvertent laceration of the lung during the block.

such as "heart burn," regurgitation when bending over to put on shoes, regurgitation of gastric contents or staining of the pillow during sleep?

Physical Examination

A fairly good index of severity of symptoms is the degree of weight loss. Physical examination begins with a careful evaluation of the mouth and teeth, since symptoms may be related to swallowing large masses of unchewed food. Inspection of the posterior pharynx and base of the tongue with a mirror takes only a few minutes and is often helpful. Only a limited examination of the cervical portion of the esophagus is possible and therefore roentgenography and endoscopy provide much of the relevant information.

X-ray

There have been many excellent descriptions of the x-ray examination of the esophagus; one of the best is by Templeton.[43] A recent concise paper is that by Zboralske and Freedland.[44] The image-intensifying fluoroscope has made the examaination more precise and has stimulated the use of cinefluoroscopic studies. An initial scan using thick barium with the consistency of tooth-paste is often useful in studying motility in the pharynx and the upper esophagus. Thinner barium is more useful for study-ing lower esophagus and reflux. The repeated playback of cinerecords of swallowing and peristalsis gives much more information than can be obtained by the skilled observer with a single observation of the screen. In the case of foreign bodies, the patient can swal-low a piece of soft white bread or absorb-ent cotton saturated with barium sulfate suspension and this will often "hang-up" on the foreign body, which far too often these days is radiolucent. Sometimes esophageal spasm or stricture can be assessed better by observation of the passage of a marshmallow soaked in barium suspension. Special techniques, such as the Trendelenburg position, having the patient stand up and bend at the waist, the Valsalva maneuver, or direct pressure on the abdomen may be useful for demonstrating reflux. Some radiologists use the so-called "water syphon" technique for demonstrating reflux from stomach into the esophagus, but others have felt that this gives too many false positives and may be mis-leading.[45]

Endoscopy

Bronchoscopy and Esophagoscopy

Bronchoscopy and esophagoscopy are often done at the same sitting and will be discussed together here. The history of endoscopy has been concisely reviewed by Richard Meade.[46] The contributions of Chevalier Jackson were remarkable and were largely responsible for the popularization of bronchoscopy and esophagoscopy in this country and in Europe. The classic text of Jackson and Jackson[47] should be more widely read.

Standard Instruments

Many instruments are available for examining the trachea and bronchi. A straightblade laryngoscope of the Jack-son model should be available in infant, child and adult sizes for detailed study of the larynx and pharynx and for the occasional case in which it is difficult to pass the bronchoscope directly. The original tubular Jackson bronchoscope has been modified by Holinger, by Broyles, and by C. L. Jackson (Fig. 15–11). Telescopes (foroblique, retro-grade and right angle) make possible more detailed examination of the mucosa and inspection of segmental orifices. The right angle telescope will serve about 90 per cent of clinical needs. Even if the budget is limited, it is better to purchase two right angle telescopes, since one is often out for repair.

Pediatric Problems

Infants present special problems be-cause the small airway permits passage of only a 3 or 3.5 millimeter tube. Visi-bility has been likened to observing the far wall of a ballroom through a very small key hole. A useful instrument from the urological armamentarium is a size 14 F. panendoscope. The anes-thetist can ventilate the lung intermit-tently through the cystoscope sheath and then a foroblique or right angle telescope can be inserted intermittently for short periods of observation.

Special Instruments and Equipment

Fiberoptic light sources are used on all the newer model endoscopes and are available as replacements for the grain-of-wheat bulbs in older models. Esopha-goscopy can be done with a broncho-

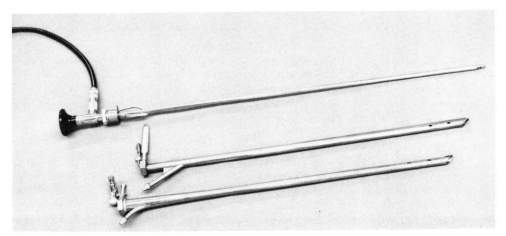

Figure 15–11   Bronchoscopes. *Top.* Right angle telescope with fiberoptic light carrier. *Middle.* Classic Chevalier Jackson tubular design. *Lower.* Modern conical tube found in the Broyles, Holinger and C. L. Jackson instruments.

scope; Jackson's original esophagoscope was a straight tube with a round lip. The Eder-Hufford instrument has a long flexible obturator to facilitate introduction and this is removed as soon as the instrument has passed the cricopharyngeus sphincter; inspection of the mucosa is facilitated by a telescope at the proximal end. I have found an esophagoscope of the Jessberg or Robertson pattern (child and adult sizes) the most useful single instrument (Fig. 15–12). The shape is a transverse oval which gives a wider lumen for inspection with no

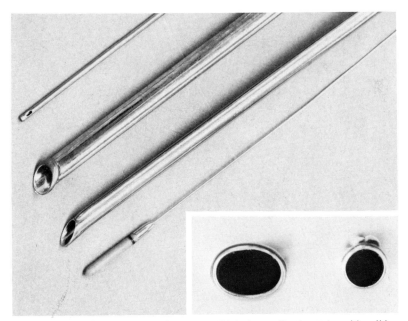

Figure 15–12   Rigid esophagoscopes. *Left upper to Right lower.* Suction tube with solid rounded end and side holes; oval esophagoscope of Robertson or Jessberg type; cylindrical esophagoscope of Chevalier Jackson; soft rubber bougie—"lumen finder." *Inset.* End-on views of Robertson *(left)* and Jackson *(right)* esophasgoscopes to show the marked improvement in working space available with the oval cross-section as compared with the cylindrical tube with the same anteroposterior diameter.

increase in pressure in the anterior-posterior direction over a cylindrical instrument. The end is slightly flared and spatulated, which is of considerable advantage in dealing with esophageal foreign bodies and manipulating biopsy forceps. It is long enough to be passed through the cardia into the stomach conveniently.

In recent years fiberoptic technology has permitted the development of esophagoscopes (Olympus Fiber Esophagoscope, ACMI-LoPresti Gastroesophageal Panendoscope model EF) which permit examination of the esophagus and proximal half of the stomach with somewhat less discomfort to the patient (Fig. 15–13). Despite the fact that these are flexible instruments and are easier to insert than rigid tubes, there have been several reports of esophageal perforations with them. A 5 mm fiber bronchoscope (ACMI-LoPresti Bronchoscope model EB) has the advantage of the capability of being threaded into segmental bronchi. The optical systems give excellent magnified images of the mucosa and permit relatively easy color photography by means of a built-in electronic flash lamp.

In conjunction with the endoscopes, a complete set of suction tips, biopsy forceps, and forceps for removal of foreign bodies is essential (Fig. 15–14).

The Endoscopist

The most important factor in bronchoscopy or esophagoscopy is the endoscopist. An experienced, obviously knowledgeable physician who moves gently but deliberately gives an enormous amount of nonverbal reassurance to the patient.

Premedication

We feel that premedication is essential. Formerly, a short-acting barbiturate such as seconal or amytal was used together with 0.4 to 0.6 mg atropine and a narcotic by intramuscular injection. During the past three years, I have found that diazepam (Valium), 5 to 15

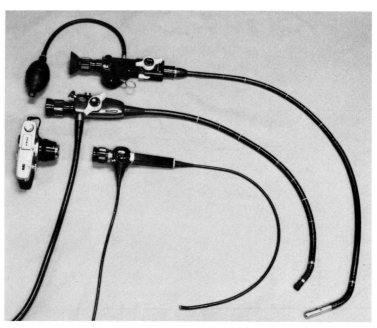

Figure 15–13 Flexible endoscopes. *Top.* Gastroscope. *Middle.* Esophagoscope. *Bottom.* Bronchoscope. The camera at left can be adapted for use with all three instruments.

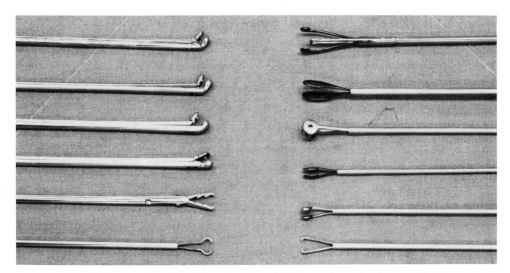

Figure 15–14 Endoscope tips. A variety of endoscopic biting and grasping forceps. The instrument at upper right is a Clerf safety pin closer.

mg orally one hour before the examination, has been superior to a barbiturate in relieving anxiety and producing muscular relaxation. Atropine 0.4 mg is given intramuscularly 30 minutes before the examination to decrease salivation. Depending upon the size of the patient and his previous reaction to narcotics, I have used 5 to 10 mg of methadone orally one hour before the examination, 50 to 100 mg of Demerol (meperidine) intramuscularly or intravenously 5 to 30 minutes before the examination or 5 to 10 mg of morphine intramuscularly. In most patients the combination of diazepam 10 mg and methadone 5 mg by mouth one hour before the examination has been effective for endoscopy and for most minor surgical procedures with local anesthesia.*

---

*Roche Laboratories, the manufacturer of Valium, has the following sentence in the package insert: "Valium (diazepam) is not recommended for bronchoscopy and laryngoscopy because increased cough reflex and laryngospasm have been reported." The manufacturer inserted this because "In early trials with Valium, one investigator reported laryngospasm and coughing in his patient." My personal experience has been that diazepam is an excellent agent for premedication before endoscopy and is not accompanied by any increased incidence of laryngospasm.

An occasional patient may come to the examination quite tense and anxious. Five to 10 mg of Valium given slowly intravenously will produce tranquility, muscular relaxation and amnesia for the procedure.

General Anesthesia

General anesthesia has been used routinely for babies, children and extremely apprehensive adults. Modern techniques for general anesthesia have removed any justification for immobilizing the helpless little patient for endoscopy without premedication or anesthesia, as formerly practiced by Jackson and Jackson and their pupils. Ventilation during anesthesia seems most efficient by the Sanders Venturi attachment which eliminates the need for the cuirasse respirator or other complicated gear.[48] General anesthesia is used routinely in some clinics for esophagoscopy, but our experience has been that most patients tolerate esophagoscopy under topical anesthesia quite well.

Topical Anesthesia

Topical anesthesia was formerly a ritual which involved the use of concentrations of cocaine of from 4 to 10 per cent. Some patients have had severe and even fatal reactions to cocaine, and consequently this was supplanted in many centers by the use of 1 per cent Pontocaine, but reactions continued to occur. In recent years, dyclonine hydrochloride (Dyclone) has been used almost exclusively as our topical anesthetic agent. Our routine is to measure out a total of 20 ml of 0.5 per cent Dyclone in a medicine glass and not to exceed this amount. The pharynx and tongue are sprayed slowly and systematically to eliminate the gag reflex. Since Dyclone has a slower onset of action than Pontocaine or cocaine, this takes about five minutes. The earlier step of placing cotton pledgets saturated with cocaine in the pyriform sinuses has been abandoned, since it is uncomfortable for the patient and adds little to the anesthesia. Instead we have the patient breathe slowly while a mist of Dyclone is sprayed over the glottis. This is followed by three intratracheal instillations of 2 to 3 ml each. The trick here is to have the patient expire completely just before the anesthetic solution is delivered into the glottis through a malleable laryngeal cannula. The patient must take a deep breath and cough and, as a result of the cough reflex, he aspirates the material deep into the bronchial tree. Our patients have had no toxic reactions from Dyclone used in this fashion.

Dyclone shares with Pontocaine and some other topical anesthetic agents the property of inhibiting growth of bacteria, mycobacteria, and fungi. When cultures are of critical importance, lidocaine or even 4 per cent cocaine for topical anesthesia might be preferred. As mentioned previously, positive cultures and positive specimens by cytology are most likely to be obtained from sputum coughed up during the two or three days following bronchoscopy, and these will no longer be affected by the topical anesthetic agent.

In preparation for endotracheal intubation, the anesthesia staff often prefer to use 3 to 5 ml of Xylocaine (lidocaine) injected percutaneously into the trachea. For prolonged endotracheal intubation, percutaneous superior laryngeal nerve blocks with 1 per cent lidocaine have been used, but I feel this technique adds very little to topical anesthesia for a routine bronchoscopy.

An ingenious method for topical anesthesia has been devised by Christoforidis et al.,[79] who have used an ultrasonic nebulizer and cascade impactor to produce a mist of particles of which 80 per cent are less than 10 microns in diameter. Adequate anesthesia can be produced in seven to ten minutes with 4 to 7 ml of 4 per cent lidocaine with no stimulation of cough and virtually no discomfort for the patient. As ultrasonic nebulizers become more available, this method of self-administered topical anesthesia will undoubtedly become increasingly important.

In preparation for esophagoscopy the pharynx and tongue are sprayed with 0.5 per cent Dyclone as for bronchoscopy and in addition, the patient swallows 10 to 15 ml of viscous Xylocaine in small sips, a procedure which gives excellent topical anesthesia of mouth, pharynx and cricopharyngeal area.

Some endoscopists insist upon general anesthesia for all esophagoscopy; however, this does not seem necessary except in children too young to cooperate. There is no good evidence that routine use of general anesthesia will result in a lowered incidence of esophageal perforation.

Position of Patient

In the classic method of Chevalier Jackson the patient was supine for all endoscopy and his head was securely controlled by an assistant. This is still useful when bronchoscopy is performed under general anesthesia, when the assistance of gravity is needed for manipulation and extraction of foreign bodies, and for almost all esophagoscopy. Bronchoscopies at this center are mostly performed with the patient sit-

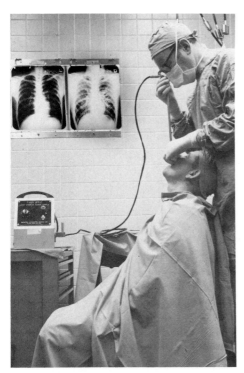

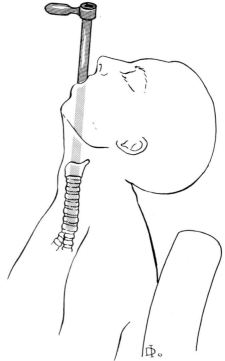

Figure 15–15 Bronchoscopy in the sitting position. *Bronchoscopy in the sitting position* is often more comfortable for the patient. The x-rays are available for continual comparison with the endoscopic findings.

ting in a straight backed chair (Fig. 15–15), or reclining slightly on the operating table or in bed.[49] Patients in this position can breathe more comfortably and have less fear of suffocating. A special assistant is not needed to hold the head.

Foreign Bodies—Technique of Removal with Physiotherapy

Foreign bodies in the air passages may threaten life because of glottic obstruction, and this tends to be a problem more often in elderly or alcoholic patients. The foreign bodies in the lower respiratory tract occur most commonly in children under school age. Jackson and Jackson[47] have presented one of the widest experiences with endoscopic removal of foreign bodies from the bronchi and esophagus. More recently Ernest Cotton and associates[50] have developed a method which uses a bronchodilator by aerosol and postural drainage and coughing,

assisted by the physiotherapist. They have been able to recover more than 80 per cent of inhaled foreign bodies by this method. If the foreign body cannot be coughed up, endoscopy is an important technique that prevents bronchial obstruction and secondary suppuration, which is especially common when vegetable foreign bodies such as peanuts have been aspirated. In the case of the esophagus, the oval cross section of the Jessberg or Robertson type of esophagoscope (Fig. 15–12) is especially useful in manipulating and removing foreign bodies.

Congenital Lesions— Tracheoesophageal Fistula and Atresia of the Esophagus

In *Surgery of the Esophagus* by Sealy and Postlethwait[51] one can find an excellent discussion of congenital anomalies of the esophagus. Commonest is atresia of the midesophagus with tracheoesophageal fistula, which seems to occur about once in 3000 live births. The experienced nurse often makes the diagnosis in the newborn nursery; the clue is excessive production of frothy mucus. Attempts to pass a size 10 to 12 F. soft rubber catheter into the stomach will meet obstruction about 10 cm from the mouth. Occasionally the diagnosis may be missed until the baby has developed considerable respiratory embarrassment from aspiration.

Diagnostic Techniques

Anteroposterior and lateral chest films in the upright postion will show the configuration of the heart and whether or not there is air in the stomach and small bowel; sometimes they will show the gap between the tip of the catheter in the upper segment and the air column in the lower esophageal segment. The severest problem in these babies is aspiration pneumonia; therefore, barium is *never* used to outline the upper esophageal pouch. In most cases, instillation of 1 or 1.5 ml of gastrografin or other water soluble contrast material will give adequate information to plan the operation, the contrast material being aspirated through the inlying soft rubber catheter immediately after exposures have been made. Swenson[52] has used a size 8 F. soft rubber catheter with three holes at the tip which is passed through the nostril into the upper esophageal pouch, on which constant suction is maintained to remove saliva and minimize further aspiration.

Surgical Repair and Results

T. M. Holder et al.[53] collected 1058 cases from 84 pediatric surgeons. Eighty-six percent of the patients fell into group C with a blind upper esophageal pouch and a fistula between trachea and lower esophageal segment. About half

had associated congenital anomalies of heart, gastrointestinal tract, genitourinary system, musculoskeletal system or central nervous system. Imperforate anus was noted 99 times. An extrapleural approach seemed to offer a small but definite advantage in survival over the transpleural approach, because in the event of an anastomotic leak massive empyema did not occur. The Haight type of anastomosis in which mucosa of the upper segment is attached to a full thickness of the lower segment by interrupted fine silk sutures followed by a second layer approximating the muscularis of the upper segment down to the lower segment to cover the inner suture line, seemed to have better survival value but a higher rate of stricture formation, over the end-to-end anastomosis done in one or two layers. Gastrostomy before or after repair did not appear to reduce complications or mortality. The overall survival rate in 431 full term infants with type C malformation who weighed more than 5 pounds was 72 per cent.

Most authors have advised primary repair of the esophagus when the ends of the esophagus can be joined without undue tension. If tension appears excessive at the proposed suture line, then division of the fistula, cervical esophagostomy, gastrostomy, and later reconstruction with transposed colon, will decrease mortality.

Holder, McDonald, and Woolley[54] advocated primary repair except in the critically ill baby or the infant weighing less than $5\frac{1}{2}$ pounds. Various authors have reported that 25 to 40 per cent of infants with tracheoesophageal fistula have been premature. In this group results were remarkably improved by doing a Stamm gastrostomy under local anesthesia as soon as the diagnosis was made to minimize reflux into the trachea. The tracheal fistula was divided by a retropleural approach through the right thorax 18 to 36 hours later. Repair of the esophagus was done 1 to 6 months later, when the infant's condition appeared favorable. By this method they were able to salvage 9 out of 15 patients in a very high risk group.

Carcinoma of Esophagus

Diagnosis

Nearly sixty years have elapsed since Franz Torek of New York City successfully resected a carcinoma of the esophagus transthoracically,[55] yet our salvage rate for patients with this disease has improved but little in the past two decades. Symptoms of mild substernal distress may evolve very gradually into high grade obstruction. Gradual weight loss and nutritional anemia may be ignored initially by patients and physicians. Cancer of the esophagus has often extended considerable distances through the submucosal lymphatics before the patient has disabling symptoms which take him to the physician. Fluoroscopic studies and endoscopy will usually make the diagnosis but some patients are unsuitable for esophagoscopy, especially those who have marked stricture or angulation of the esophagus, patients who have severe cardiovascular disease or airway obstructive disease, or those with severe arthritis of the cervical spine. For patients such as this Fennessy et al.[56] have suggested inserting a catheter down to the level of the lesion under fluoroscopic control and then brushing the surface with nylon and steel brushes to obtain cells and shreds of tissue for microscopic examination.

Treatment

Once the diagnosis is made, one is faced with the decision regarding the feasibility of cure or palliation. X-ray therapy by multiple port or rotational techniques, supplemented by bouginage, has given relief to many patients[57] and a few long-term cures when the tumor is in the lower half of the esophagus. Esophagectomy with reconstruction by transposition of the stomach, colon or jejunum may be feasible if the patient does not have diseases of other systems which would limit his life expectancy. Wilkins and Skinner have reviewed the recent literature.[58] There is general agreement that simple gastrostomy is unlikely to prolong either life or comfort. Intraluminal plastic tubes are occasionally useful in maintaining an open channel through the tumor.

Hemorrhage

Hemorrhage is not a common accompaniment of esophageal disease except for rare catastrophes, such as erosion of an aortic aneurysm into the esophagus. Probably the commonest cause of hematemesis is bleeding from gastric or duodenal ulcer or erosive gastritis.[59] The next commonest is esophageal varices. Finally, there is the Mallory-Weiss syndrome in all its variations, ranging from a simple split of the mucosa of the lower esophagus to intramural hematoma of the esophagus to a full thickness tear into the pleural space, usually on the left. There is almost always a history of excessive intake of food and alcohol and an episode of vomiting immediately preceding the episode of bleeding. Although there is no universal agreement on early use of esophagoscopy, numerous reports indicate that early endoscopy can be valuable in differential diagnosis of bleeding. If frank rupture of the esophagus has occurred, then immediate thoracotomy is indicated.[60] The special problem of esophageal varices will be discussed in Chapter 18 on liver disease.

Hiatal Hernia and Reflux Esophagitis

Diagnosis

Hiatal hernia and gastroesophageal reflux are not necessarily coexistent. By special maneuvers, up to 60 per cent of adults can be shown to have some degree of herniation of the esophageal hiatus. Contrary to earlier studies, the incidence does not increase with age.[61] Stilson et al.[45] examined 1027 patients aged 9 to 90 and found that the Trendelenburg maneuver and straight leg raising were insensitive tests for herniation. A prone or right oblique position detected about 25 per cent of the cases. A block of balsa wood interposed between the abdomen of the prone patient and the examining table revealed approximately 98 per cent of the total hernias discovered and in their hands the water syphon test revealed 93 per cent of the total. Sixty-nine percent of the patients who had a positive water syphon test had a demonstrable hiatal hernia, and 54.5 per cent of the total patients with hiatal hernia had a positive water syphon test. The combination of manometric studies with pH studies in the lower esophagus has been more dependable in diagnosing reflux.[62] This helps to explain some of the failures in preventing reflux after what appeared to be adequate anatomic repair of the hernia.

Sphincter Mechanism—Chalasia and Achalasia

The accumulated experience with cinefluoroscopic and manometric studies has improved our understanding of the lower sphincter mechanism of the esophagus. There is a functional sphincter at the cardia which relaxes in response to peristaltic waves initiated by swallowing. The sphincter works more efficiently when situated below the diaphragm where it is exposed to the positive pressure of the abdomen, than above the diaphragm where it is influenced by the negative intrapulmonary pressure. The acute angle of entry into the fundus of the stomach appears to aid in prevention of reflux. Reflux can occur in the absence of hiatal hernia, as in the series of Hiebert and Belsey,[63] and most patients with hiatal hernia do not have symptoms of regurgitation or

esophagitis. The term "chalasia" (excessive relaxation) has been proposed for the hypotonic cardiac sphincter as the antonym to "achalasia" (failure to relax).

Treatment

Baue and Belsey[64] have emphasized several points in the surgical treatment: (1) adequate mobilization of the lower esophagus and cardia, (2) inversion of the lower esophagus into the fundus of the stomach to maintain the acute angle of entry of the cardia, (3) some type of gastropexy to maintain an appreciable length of esophagus within the abdomen, and (4) adequate approximation of the crurae of the diaphragm to prevent recurrence of the hernia. Urschel and Paulson[65] have reported excellent success with the Belsey repair. Their experience has included a larger number of patients with pulmonary disease secondary to aspiration (50 per cent) than in most other series.

Several authors have reported treating stenosis secondary to peptic esophagitis by effective repair of the hernia followed by bouginage. More severe cases require interposition of a segment of colon or jejunum. Thal[66] has devised an ingenious method for splitting the full thickness of the stricture and filling the defect with a portion of the fundus of the stomach, which then becomes covered by esophageal epithelium. There are still some unsettled problems in the treatment of long-standing peptic esophagitis. Some workers have argued for vagotomy and a drainage operation of the stomach, such as pyloroplasty, while others have felt that vagotomy might predispose to achalasia of the cardia. For reasons not at all apparent, some children with peptic esophagitis develop severe symptoms and a shortened esophagus, while others who are treated symptomatically (antiacids, small meals, sleeping with head of bed elevated on blocks) seem to outgrow symptoms of reflux and an esophageal hiatal hernia can no longer be demonstrated a few years later. The consensus now is that the so-called Barrett's esophagus probably represents areas of peptic esophagitis where the squamous epithelium has been replaced by glandular epithelium from the fundus of the stomach.[67]

Webs and Rings

Webs or rings in the mid or upper esophagus probably represent congenital anomalies resulting from a failure of the formerly solid cord of cells of the embryonic esophagus to canalize completely. The so-called Schatzki ring seems to occur almost always in association with hiatal hernia and seems most of the time to mark the junction of gastric mucosa with esophageal squamous epithelium.[68]

Corrosive Injuries

Chemical Burns—Types

Chemical burns of the esophagus continue to pose some of the most difficult technical problems. Acid burns tend to produce superficial coagulation while alkali burns produce a rapid hydrolytic destruction of protein which may progress through the full thickness of the esophageal wall within a few minutes. Eighty-six percent of the lye burns in the series of Sealy and Postlethwait[69] occurred in children under the age of five years. The series reported by Yudin[70] consisted largely of sulfuric acid burns, because sulfuric acid is commonly used as a dessicant to prevent frosting of storm windows in Russia. By the time the patient reaches the Emergency Room with an alkali burn, attempts at neutralization are of no value, a conclusion borne out by Leape et al.,[71] who in a study of sodium hydroxide burns in animals found that much of the damage was done within the first few seconds after contact. Liquid caustic was worse than granular in their clinical series.

Treatment

Esophagoscopy and Steroids. Previous treatment regimens, such as that published by Salzer in 1920, emphasized avoidance of esophagoscopy for several weeks after the burn. Bouginage was begun three to seven days after the burn and was continued for at least six months. It has been estimated that at least half of the patients did not require this period of extended and uncomfortable treatment. The current approach, as reviewed by Egan,[72] calls for esophagoscopy under general anesthesia within 24 hours after the patient has been admitted to the hospital, since pharyngeal burns are not always accompanied by esophageal damage. If esophagoscopy is stopped at the level of the first evidence of burn of the esophagus, the incidence of perforation will be kept low. If no burns are found in the esophagus or cardia, the patient is kept overnight for observation and then sent home with careful instructions to the parents to watch for any symptoms of interference with swallowing. If there is an esophageal burn, the patient is started on cortisone and an antibiotic. The work of Rosenberg et al.[73] demonstrated the advantages of cortisone in delaying maturation of fibroblasts and inhibiting collagen formation so that the epithelium could regenerate over the burned surface. The addition of antibiotics was especially important in patients who were on cortisone. Yarington and Heatly[74] at the University of Rochester used methylprednisolone sodium succinate (Medrol) intramuscularly in doses of 20 mg every eight hours for children under the age of two and 40 mg every eight hours for older patients. The University of Oregon routine[72] with 60 patients was to use parenteral dexamethasone 1 mg daily or oral prednisone 60 mg daily for three or four days and then a maintenance dose of from 5 to 10 mg of prednisone daily together with ampicillin. The steroids are continued until esophagoscopy, performed at intervals of two to three weeks, demonstrates that the mucosa has healed. Fluoroscopic studies are made six months after steroids are discontinued. Strictures are dilated either with woven dilators (silk or nylon) or with the Hurst type of mercury-filled bougie (Fig. 15–16). More complicated or multiple strictures require a gastrostomy and retrograde dilatation. Ashcraft and Holder found that direct injection of prednisolone into short experimental strictures has aided in their dilation and resolution.[75]

Dilatation. Dilatation therapy can be carried on successfully for many years, as Salzer and many others have demonstrated. When dilatations are done over a previously swallowed string or are carried out over a looped string through a gastrostomy, the incidence of perforation is not great. It is important not to try to proceed too rapidly; Chevalier Jackson's old rule of not increasing the diameter by more than three gradations of bougies at any one sitting is still a good one. Dilatations must be kept up two or three times a week for a pro-

longed period and then from once a week to once a month indefinitely. Some patients learn to swallow a Hurst dilator at home with little difficulty. If a lumen of at least size 30 French through the esophagus can be maintained, the patient can manage baby food. With extensive, long, multiple strictures, either dilatation eventually becomes laborious as maturing collagen continues to contract, or the patient becomes dissatisfied with the multiple dilatations. In such cases esophageal substitution with colon has been helpful. A common technical problem is stenosis of the anastomosis at the level of the cricopharyngeus, since scarring in the area just below the cricopharyngeus is usually very extensive after a lye burn. It is better to err in making the anastomosis directly to the side of the pharynx and a little too high rather than attempt to save the cricopharyngeus sphincter and make the anastomosis through an area of devascularized scar, since this will almost

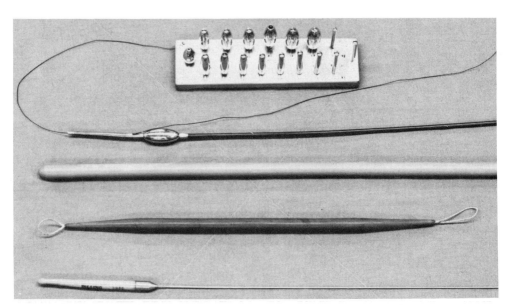

Figure 15–16 Esophageal bougies. *Top* to *Bottom*: The Plummer dilator has a flexible coil spring tip which follows a previously swallowed silk thread. The shaft unscrews and a series of metal olives can be positioned just behind the flexible tip. Next, the Hurst mercury-filled, flexible dilator is probably the easiest for the patient to use at home. The torpedo-shaped Tucker bougies have loops at both ends to facilitate their being drawn antegrade or retrograde in patients with established gastrostomies. The woven nylon Jackson dilators have olive-shaped tips to reduce the likelihood of perforation. Holinger has developed miniature dilators on the same pattern for use in infants with esophageal strictures.

always require a second operation for revision of the stricture. Some surgeons have felt that a second operation for total esophagectomy should be done once the esophagocolostomy has been successfully accomplished, since the incidence of carcinoma in old lye strictures of the esophagus is quite high.

Disorders of Esophageal Motility

Differential Diagnosis

Disorders of motility have already been alluded to. Lindsay[76] has classified these under the headings of muscular disturbances (diffuse scleroderma or generalized systemic sclerosis, dermatomyositis, myasthenia gravis, secondary myasthenia and senility); inervation disturbances (peripheral neuritis, the jugular foramen syndrome, central nervous system lesions of amyotrophic lateral sclerosis, syringomyelia, multiple sclerosis or poliomyelitis, lesions of the medulla from tumor, inflammation or trauma); and psychic disturbances producing the familiar globus hystericus. Some authors have included the pulsion diverticulum which almost always occurs posteriorly between the leaves of the upper and lower portions of the cricopharyngeus sphincter as the result of a postulated asynchrony of the upper and lower constrictor fibers. The Plummer-Vinson syndrome of iron deficiency anemia and dysphagia is well recognized, but the pathogenesis is still unexplained.

Spasm

Spasm of the esophagus can occur alone or may be associated with disordered peristaltic activity of the esophagus. Milder degrees of spasm cause the appearance of the corkscrew esophagus. Diffuse spasm with muscular hypertrophy has also caused dysphagia and in some patients has been associated with pulsion diverticula and hiatal hernia. A long myotomy will relieve symptoms in a majority of patients.[77]

Achalasia

Our knowledge of the lower esophageal sphincter has been increased by the study of patients with reflux and especially by study of patients in whom the sphincter fails to relax, a condition commonly called achalasia. The excellent monograph on achalasia by F. H. Ellis and A. M. Olsen[78] brings together the clinical background and experimental studies. In man there is degeneration of ganglion cells in the lower esophageal segment. In cats failure of the lower esophagus to relax is produced by bilateral cervical vagotomy or destructive lesions in the dorsal motor nucleus of the vagus nerve. The syndrome of achalasia was first described in 1674 by Thomas Willis, who described palliation by bouginage. Plummer in 1906 reintroduced bouginage, and forcible dilatation with a hydrostatic bag remained the method of choice at the Mayo Clinic for many years; however, the safety and even better results following longitudinal myotomy of the lower esophagus (Heller procedure) have tended to displace dilatation in recent years. In the Mayo Clinic experience there was one operative death in 300 cases. Three patients had a postoperative empyema. Ninety-four per cent of 256 patients who could be followed from 1 to $17\frac{1}{2}$ years experienced definite improvement and 83 per cent reported good to excellent results. Eleven per cent had only a fair result, but were still symptomatically improved.

Hydrostatic Dilatation

Because of the simplicity of the procedure, several authors still use some form of hydrostatic dilator. This is definitely not an outpatient procedure since the patient must be observed closely for 24 hours after the dilatation, which is frequently forceful enough to split the mucosa and cause minor bleeding. Perforation has occurred and should be corrected by immediate open operation.

Complications—Esophagitis and Carcinoma

When peptic esophagitis has occurred, it has usually been due to carrying the Heller myotomy too far down on the stomach and completely disrupting the lower esophageal sphincter mechanism or to deranging the phrenicoesophageal support mechanism with subsequent hiatal hernia and gastric reflux. In addition, persistence of dysphagia after a Heller procedure demands further investigation by fluoroscopy and esophagoscopy since there appears to be a markedly increased incidence of carcinoma of the esophagus in patients with achalasia.

SUMMARY

In this short space it has been impossible to cover all aspects of pulmonary and esophageal disease. That work is reserved for textbooks. Whenever possible, attempts have been made to include references to the literature of the past five years, to points of controversy, and to recent reviews in depth. The discipline of thoracic surgery continues to advance rapidly and repeated trips to the current literature will be needed to keep pace with its progress.

References

1. Rabin, C. B.: New or neglected physical signs in diagnosis of chest disease. J.A.M.A., *194*:546–550, 1965.
2. There are many excellent textbooks of roentgenology and not all can be listed here. Three useful texts are:
   (a) Felson, B.: Fundamentals of Chest Roentgenology. Philadelphia, W. B. Saunders Co., 1960.
   (b) Fraser, R. G., and Paré, J. A. P.: Diagnosis of Diseases of the Chest. Philadelphia, W. B. Saunders Co., 1970.
   (c) Medelman, J. P.: Normal Roentgen Anatomy. In C. B. Rabin (ed.): Roentgenology of the Chest. Springfield, Illinois, Charles C Thomas, 1958.
3. (a) Fennessy, J. J.: Transbronchial biopsy of peripheral lung lesions. Radiology, *88*: 878–882, 1967.
   (b) Fennessy, J. J., Fry, W. A., Manalo-Estrella P., and Frias Hidvegi, D. V. S.: The bronchial brushing technique for obtaining cytologic specimens from peripheral lung lesions. Acta Cytol., *14*: 25–30, 1970.
   (c) Willson, J. K. V., and Eskridge, M.: Bronchial brush biopsy with a controllable brush. Amer. J. Roentgenol. Radium Ther. Nucl. Med., *109*:471–477, 1970.
4. (a) Farber, S. M., and Mandel, W.: Diagnosis of bronchogenic carcinoma, cytologic. In D. M. Spain (ed.): Diagnosis and Treatment of Tumors of the Chest. New York, Grune and Stratton, 1960.
   (b) Melamed, M. R., and Cahan, W. G.: Cytology. In W. L. Watson (ed.): Lung Cancer. A Study of 5000 Memorial Hospital Cases. St. Louis, C. V. Mosby Co., 1968.
5. Israel, H. L., and Goldstein, R. A.: Relation of Kveim-antigen reaction to lymphadenopathy. Study of sarcoidosis and other diseases. N. Eng. J. Med., *284*:345–349, 1971.
6. Steel, S. J., and Winstanley, D. P.: Trephine biopsy of the lung and pleura. Thorax, *24*:576–584, 1969.
7. Jepsen, O.: Mediastinoscopy. Copenhagen, Munksgaard, 1966.
8. Ward, P. H.: Mediastinoscopy under local anesthesia. A valuable diagnostic technique. Calif. Med., *112*:15–22, February, 1970.
9. Corpe, R. F., and Blalock, F. A.: A continuing study of patients with "open negative" status at Battey State Hospital. Amer. Rev. Resp. Dis., *98*:954–964, 1968.
10. (a) Treatment of drug-resistant tuberculosis. A statement by the committee on therapy. Amer. Rev. Resp. Dis., *94*:125–127, 1966.
    (b) Fischer, D. A., Lester, W., Dye, W. E., and Moulding, T. S.: Re-treatment of patients with isoniazid-resistant tuberculosis: Analysis and follow-up of 146 cases. Amer. Rev. Resp. Dis., *97*:392–398, 1968.
    (c) Lester, W.: Unclassified mycobacterial disease. Ann. Rev. Med., *17*:351–360, 1966.
    (d) Vall-Spinosa, A., Lester, W., and Moulding, T.: Rifampin in the treatment of drug-resistant *Mycobacterium tuberculosis* infections. N. Eng. J. Med., *283*:616–621, 1970.

11. Newman, M. M.: Surgery for tuberculosis in infancy and childhood. In J. R. Derrick (ed.): Thoracic Surgery in Infancy and Childhood (in Press).

12. (a) Wolstenholme, G. E. W., and Porter, R. (eds.): CIBA Foundation Symposium: Systemic Mycoses. London, J. and A. Churchill Ltd., 1968.

   (b) Treatment of fungal diseases. A statement by the committee on therapy. Amer. Rev. Resp. Dis., *100*:908–910, 1969.

   (c) Drutz, D. J., Spickard, A., Rogers, D. E., and Koenig, M. G.: Treatment of disseminated mycotic infections. A new approach to amphotericin B therapy. Amer. J. Med., *45*:405–418, 1968.

13. Palva, T., Viikari, S., and Inberg, M.: Pulmonary carcinoma. Mediastinoscopic criteria for curative resections. Dis. Chest., *56*:156–158, 1969.

14. Kirsh, M. M. et al.: The effect of histological cell type on the prognosis of patients with bronchogenic carcinoma. Ann. Thorac. Surg., *13*:303–310, 1972.

15. Holin, S. M., Dwork, R. E., Glaser, S., Rikli, A. E., and Stocklen, J. B.: Solitary pulmonary nodules found in a community-wide chest roentgenographic survey. Amer. Rev. Tubercul. Resp. Dis., *79*:427–439, 1959.

16. McClure, C. D., Boucot, K. R., Shipman, G. A., Gilliam, A. G., Milmore, B. K., and Lloyd, J. W.: The solitary pulmonary nodule and primary lung malignancy. Arch. Environ. Health, *3*:127–139, 1961.

17. Rigler, L. G., and Heitzman, E. R.: Planigraphy in the differential diagnosis of the pulmonary nodule; with particular reference to the notch sign of malignancy. Radiology, *65*:692–702, 1955.

18. Overholt, R. H., Bougas, J. A., and Woods, F. M.: Surgical treatment of lung cancer found on x-ray survey. N. Eng. J. Med., *252*:429–432, 1955.

19. Wilkins, E. W.: The asymptomatic isolated pulmonary nodule. N. Eng. J. Med., 252:515–520, 1955.

20. Davis, E. W., Peabody, J. W., and Katz, S.: The solitary pulmonary nodule. A ten-year study based on 215 cases. J. Thorac. Cardiovasc. Surg., *32*:728–770, 1956.

21. (a) Steele, J. D.: The Solitary Pulmonary Nodule. Springfield, Charles C Thomas, 1964.

   (b) Steele, J. D., and Buell, P.: Survival in bronchogenic carcinomas resected as solitary pulmonary nodules. Proc. Nat. Cancer Conf., 6:835–839, 1970.

22. MacMahon, B., et al.: Preoperative irradiation of cancer of the lung. Preliminary report of a therapeutic trial, a collaborative study. Cancer, 23:419–430, 1969.

23. Shields, T. W., Higgins, G. A., Jr., Lawton, R., Heilbrunn, A., and Keehn, R. J.: Preoperative x-ray therapy as an adjuvant in the treatment of bronchogenic carcinoma. J. Thorac. Cardiovasc. Surg., *59*:49–59, 1970.

24. Higgins, G. A., and Wolf, J.: Chemotherapy and lung cancer—Present status. J. Thorac. Cardiovasc. Surg., *51*:449–454, 1966.

25. Slack, N. H.: Bronchogenic carcinoma: Nitrogen mustard as a surgical adjuvant and factors influencing survival. Cancer, *25*:987–1002, 1970.

26. Pinner, Max: Collapse Therapy. In Pulmonary Tuberculosis in the Adult. Springfield, Charles C Thomas, 1945.

27. Comroe, J. H., Forster, R. E., Dubois, A. B., Briscoe, W. A., and Carlsen, E.: The Lung, Clinical Physiology and Pulmonary Function Tests. Chicago, Yearbook Medical Publishers, Inc., 1962.

28. Boushy, S. F., Billig, D. M., North, L. B., and Helgason, A. H.: Clinical course related to preoperative and postoperative pulmonary function in patients with bronchogenic carcinoma. Chest, 59:383–391, 1971.

29. Charms, B. L.: Unilateral pulmonary artery occlusion. In Zimmerman, H. A. (Ed.): Intravascular Catheterization. Springfield, Charles C Thomas, 1966.

30. Lipsett, M. B., Odell, W. D., Rosenberg, L. E., and Waldmann, T. A.: Humoral syndromes associated with nonendocrine tumors. Ann. Intern. Med., *61*:733–756, 1964.

31. Lyons, H. A.: Mediastinal Tumors. In Spain, D. M. (Ed.): Diagnosis and Treatment of Tumors of the Chest. New York, Grune and Stratton, 1960.

32. Viets, H. R., and Schwab, R. S.: Thymectomy for Myasthenia Gravis: A Record of the Experiences at the Massachusetts General Hospital. Springfield, Charles C Thomas, 1960.

33. Papatestas, A. E., Alpert, L. I., Osserman, K. E., Osserman, R. S., and Kark, A. E.: Studies in myasthenia gravis: Effects of thymectomy. Amer. J. Med., *50*:465–474, 1971.

34. Roper, W. H., and Waring, J. J.: Primary serofibrinous pleural effusion in military personnel. Amer. Rev. Tuberc., *71*:616–634, 1955.

35. Claggett, O. T.: Personal communication.

36. Graham, E. A.: Some of Fundamental Considerations in the Treatment of Empyema Thoracis. St. Louis, C. V. Mosby, Co., 1925.

37. Eloesser, L.: Of an operation for tuberculous empyema. Ann. Thorac. Surg., 8:355–357, 1969; Surg. Gynecol. Obstet, 60:1096–1097, 1935.

38. (a) Hewlett, T. H.: Sheft's Initial Management of Thoracic and Thoraco-Abdominal Trauma. Springfield, Charles C Thomas, 1968.

   (b) Hood, R. M.: Management of Thoracic Injury. Springfield, Charles C Thomas, 1969.

(c) Martin, J. D., Jr., Haynes, C. D., Hatcher, C. R., Smith, R. B., and Stone, H. H. (Eds.): Trauma to the Thorax and Abdomen. Springfield, Charles C Thomas, 1969.

(d) Baker, R. J., Boyd, D. R., and Condon, R. E.: Priority of management of patients with multiple injuries. Surg. Clin. N. Amer., *50*:3–11, 1970.

39. Newman, M. M.: Tracheostomy. Surg. Clin. N. Amer., *49*:1365–1372, 1969.

40. Virgilio, R. W.: Intrathoracic wounds in battle casualties. Surg. Gynec. Obstet., *130*:609–615, 1970.

41. Eijgelaar, A., and Homan van der Heide, J. N.: A reliable early symptom of bronchial or tracheal rupture. Thorax, *25*:120–125, 1970.

42. (a) Avery, E. E., Mörch, E. T., and Benson, D. W.: Critically crushed chest. J. Thorac. Cardiovasc. Surg., *32*:291–309, 1956.

(b) Blair, E., and Mills, E.: Rationale of stabilization of the flail chest with intermittent positive pressure breathing. Amer. Surg., *34*:860–868, 1968.

43. Templeton, F. E.: X-ray Examination of the Stomach. Chicago, University of Chicago Press, 1964.

44. Zboralske, F. F., and Friedland, G. W.: Diseases of the esophagus. Present concepts. Calif. Med., *112*:33–51, 1970.

45. Stilson, W. L., Sanders, I., Gardiner, G. A., Gorman, H. C., and Lodge, D. F.: Hiatal hernia and gastroesophageal reflux. A clinicoradiological analysis of more than 1000 cases. Radiology, *93*:1323–1327, 1969.

46. Meade, R. H.: A History of Thoracic Surgery. Springfield, Charles C Thomas, 1961.

47. Jackson, C., and Jackson, C. L.: Bronchoesophagology. Philadelphia, W. B. Saunders Co., 1950.

48. Morales, G. A., Epstein, B. S., Cinco, B., Adkins, P. C., and Coakley, C. S.: Ventilation during general anesthesia for bronchoscopy. Evaluation of a new technique. J. Thorac. Cardiovasc. Surg., *57*:873–878, 1969.

49. Brown, R. K., and Kovarik, J. L.: Bronchoscopy in the sitting position. Surg. Clin. N. Amer., *49*:1421–1424, 1969.

50. Burrington, J. D., and Cotton, E. K.: Removal of foreign bodies from the tracheobronchial tree. J. Ped. Surg., *7*:119–122, 1972.

51. Postlethwait, R. W., and Sealy, W. C.: Surgery of the Esophagus. Springfield, Charles C Thomas, 1961.

52. Swenson, O., Lipman, R., Fisher, J. H., and DeLuca, F. G.: Repair and complications of esophageal atresia and tracheoesophageal fistula. N. Eng. J. Med., *267*:960–963, 1962.

53. (a) Holder, T. M., Cloud, D. T., Lewis, J. E., Jr., and Pilling, G. P.: Esophageal atresia and tracheoesophageal fistula. A survey of its members by the surgical section of the American Academy of Pediatrics. Pediatrics, *34*:542–549, 1964.

(b) Holder, T. M., and Ashcraft, K. W.: Esophageal atresia and tracheoesophageal fistula. Ann. Thorac. Surg., *9*:445–467, 1970.

54. Holder, T. M., McDonald, V. G., and Wooley, M. M.: The premature or critically ill infant with esophageal atresia: Increased success with a staged approach. J. Thorac. Cardiovasc. Surg., *44*:344–355, 1962.

55. Torek, F.: The first successful case of resection of the thoracic portion of the esophagus for carcinoma. Surg. Gynecol. Obstet., *16*:614–617, 1913.

56. Fennessy, J. J., Frias Hidvegi, D. V. S., and Variakojis, D.: Transcatheter biopsy of esophageal lesions. Radiology, *96*:123–126, 1970.

57. Watson, T. A.: Radiation treatment of cancer of the esophagus. Surg. Gynecol. Obstet., *117* 346–354, 1963.

58. Wilkins, E. W., Jr., and Skinner, D. B.: Recent progress in surgery of the esophagus. I: Pathophysiology and gastroesophageal reflux. J. Surg. Res. 8:41–56, 1968. II. Clinical entities. Ibid, 90–104, 1968.

59. Zollinger, R. M., and Nick, W. V.: Upper gastrointestinal tract hemorrhage. J.A.M.A. *212*:2251–2254, 1970.

60. Thompson, N. W., Ernst, C. B., and Fry, W. J.: The spectrum of emetogenic injury to the esophagus and stomach. Amer. J. Surg., *113*:13–26, 1967.

61. Mandelstam, P., and Lieber, A.: Cineradiographic evaluation of the esophagus in normal adults. A study of 146 subjects ranging in age from 21 to 90 years. Gastroenterology, *58*:32–39, 1970.

62. Bombeck, C. T., Helfrich, G. B., and Nyhus, L. M.: Planning surgery for reflux esophagitis and hiatus hernia. Surg. Clin. N. Amer., *50*:29–44, 1970.

63. Hiebert, C. A., and Belsey, R.: Incompetency of the gastric cardia without radiologic evidence of a hiatal hernia. The diagnosis and management of 71 cases. J. Thorac. Cardiovasc. Surg., *42*:352–359, 1961.

64. Baue, A. E., and Belsey, R. H. R.: The treatment of sliding hiatus hernia and reflux esophagitis by the Mark IV technique. Surgery, *62*:396–404, 1967.

65. Urschel, H. C., Jr. and Paulson, D. L.: Gastroesophageal reflux and hiatal hernia. Complications and therapy. J. Thorac. Cardiovasc. Surg., *53*:21–32, 1967.

66. Thal, A. P., Hatafuku, T., and Kurtzman, R.: New operation for distal esophageal stricture. Arch. Surg., *90*:464–471, 1965.

67. Mossberg, S. M.: The columnar-lined esophagus (Barrett Syndrome)—an acquired con-

dition? Gastroenterology, *50*:671–676, 1966.

68. Postlethwait, R. W., and Sealy, W. C.: Experiences with the treatment of 59 patients with lower esophageal web. Ann. Surg., *165*:786–796, 1968.

69. Postlethwait, R. W., and Sealy, W. C.: Chemical burns of the esophagus. In Surgery of the Esophagus. Springfield, Charles C Thomas, 1961.

70. Yudin, S. S.: The surgical construction of 80 cases of artificial esophagus. Surg. Gynecol. Obstet., *78*:561–583, 1944.

71. Leape, L. L., Ashcraft, K. W., Scarpelli, D. G., and Holder, T. M.: Hazard to health—liquid lye. N. Eng. J. Med., *284*:578–581, 1971.

72. Egan, R. S.: Corrosive esophagitis—a review of therapy. Northwest Med., *68*:1007–1009, 1969.

73. Rosenberg, N., Kunderman, P. J., Vroman, L., and Moolten, S. E.: Prevention of experimental lye strictures of the esophagus by Cortisone. Arch. Surg., *63*:147–151, 1951; *Ibid, 66*:593–598, 1953.

74. Yarington, C. T., Jr., and Heatly, C. A.: Steroids, antibiotics and early esophagoscopy in caustic esophageal trauma. N. Y. State J. Med., *63*:2960–2963, 1963.

75. Ashcraft, K. W., and Holder, T. M.: The experimental treatment of esophageal strictures by intralesional steroid injection. J. Thorac. Cardiovasc. Surg., *58*:685–691, *passim*, 1969.

76. Lindsay, J. R.: Functional disturbances of the upper swallowing mechanism. Ann. Otol. Rhinol. Laryngol., *64*:766–776, 1955.

77. Ferguson, T. B., Woodbury, J. D., Roper, C. L., and Burford, T. N.: Giant muscular hypertrophy of the esophagus. Ann. Thorac. Surg., *8*:209–218, 1969.

78. Ellis, F. H., Jr., and Olsen, A. M.: Achalasia of the Esophagus. Philadelphia, W. B. Saunders Co., 1969.

79. Christoforidis, A. J.: Use of ultrasonic nebulizer for the application of oropharyngeal, laryngeal, tracheobronchial anesthesia. Chest, *59*:629–633, 1971.

16

The Heart — Cardiac Surgery

I. PREOPERATIVE EVALUATION
  A. History
    1. Congenital heart disease
       a. Illnesses during pregnancy of mother
       b. Condition at birth
       c. Health since birth
       d. Exercise tolerance
       e. Differential diagnosis
       f. Cyanosis and coagulopathy
    2. Acquired heart disease
       a. Predisposing diseases
       b. What led to diagnosis of heart disease?
       c. Onset of symptoms
       d. Progression of symptoms
       e. Functional disability
       f. Dyspnea
       g. Pain
  B. Physical examination
    1. Inspection
    2. Palpation
    3. Percussion
    4. Auscultation
  C. Radiography
    1. Cardiac chambers
       a. Enlargement
       b. Hypertrophy of walls
       c. Valvular insufficiency
       d. Intracardiac shunt
    2. Great vessels
    3. Chest film
       a. Correct orientation
       b. Bony structure
       c. Cardiac shadow
       d. Lung fields
  D. Electrocardiography
  E. Cardiac catheterization: angiocardiography
    1. Catheterization
    2. Angiocardiography
       a. Site of obstructive lesions
       b. Evidence of valvular insufficiency
       c. Ventricular function
       d. Coronary arteriograms
  F. Laboratory examinations
  G. Drugs

II. ASSESSING THE RISK
  A. Congenital heart disease
    1. Ventricular septal defects
    2. Atrial septal defects
    3. Coarctation of aorta
    4. Patent ductus arteriosus
    5. Mongolism
  B. Acquired heart disease
    1. Tricuspid disease
    2. Mitral disease
    3. Aortic valve disease
    4. Coronary artery disease
  C. Talking to the patient

III. POSTOPERATIVE EVALUATION
  A. Functional progress
  B. Physical findings
    1. Wound
    2. Cardiovascular system
  C. Radiologic evidence
    1. Heart size
    2. Pulmonary vascularity
  D. Electrocardiographic evidence
  E. Laboratory examinations
    1. Blood counts
    2. Biochemical tests
    3. Hemolysis
  F. Drug therapy
    1. Cardiac drugs
       a. Digitalis glycosides
       b. Antiarrhythmic drugs
          (1) Quinidine
          (2) Lidocaine
          (3) Procaine amide
       c. Anticoagulants
          (1) Heparin
          (2) Bishydroxycoumarin (dicumarol)
          (3) Warfarin sodium (Coumadin)
          (4) Platelet inhibitors
          (5) Diuretics
             (a) Thiazides
             (b) Ethacrynic acid: Furosemide
       d. Antibiotics
  G. Special techniques
    1. Phonocardiography
    2. Sound spectroscopy
    3. Ultrasound
       a. Measurement of valve movement
       b. Measurement of left ventricular size and stroke volume

By BRUCE C. PATON, M.R.C.P.(Ed.), F.R.C.S.(Ed.)

Cardiac surgery might not, at first sight, seem a suitable topic for discussion in a text on outpatient surgery. The initial contact between surgeon and patient, however, is likely to be in the outpatient clinic or office, and postoperative visits to the clinic are an essential part of the patient's care. It is in the Outpatient Department, therefore, that the surgeon makes his first assessment of the problem, and it is again in this department that he evaluates, often for many years, the results of the operation.

PREOPERATIVE EVALUATION

The classic approaches of history-taking and physical examination are as important in a complex problem such as the preoperative evaluation of a cardiac patient as in other fields. Even though objective data derived from cardiac catheterization, angiocardiography and pulmonary function tests, and tests of coagulation, renal function and biochemistry combine to fill out and amplify the clinical picture, a surprisingly large proportion of the relevant information can be obtained from the history and examination. In some instances, such as cases of uncomplicated patient ductus arteriosus or secundum atrial septal defect, a history, examination and EKG, chest x-ray or fluoroscopy are all that is needed to make the diagnosis and lay the foundation for advice about operation. Under these circumstances the decision is made neither easier nor more sure by embarking upon more complex and expensive forms of examination. The more complex the problem, however, the greater becomes the need for supporting data to ensure that the right operation is advised at the right time.

History

Certain standard questions are applicable to all types of heart disease. When these questions are asked and the answers to them interpreted with knowledge of the natural history of the disease in question, a full evaluation of the severity of the lesion and the point reached in the natural history of the disease may be obtained. This concept is extremely important, especially in deciding the opportune time for operation. All cardiac diseases have typical life history curves on which the critical points are the origin of the disease, the start of reversible symptoms, the start of irreversible symptoms and death. If these points are mentally plotted along a time base, the patient's individual position on the curve can be fixed and the natural outlook that he faces can be determined.

Congenital Heart Disease

The following questions should be asked:
1. Were there any predisposing illnesses during the mother's pregnancy, such as rubella or other virus diseases, or exposure to toxic drugs? Keeping in mind that the heart and cardiovascular system are completely formed by the tenth week of intrauterine life, most of the factors likely to cause defects should presumably affect the fetus within this period. The rubella syndrome can develop in mothers exposed during the second trimester, but cardiac defects are not as common as defects of other systems when exposure is that late.
2. What was the condition of the child during and immediately after delivery? Was cyanosis present? Was a murmur heard? Was there respiratory difficulty?

3. What has been the health of the child since birth? Specific questions should be asked about:
    a. Rate of growth and development
    b. Exercise tolerance
    c. Frequency of respiratory infections
    d. Changes in color of skin and mucous membranes with exercise or crying
    3. Petechial hemorrhages or difficulties with coagulation
    f. Fainting spells or blackouts
    g. Feeding problems, especially dysphagia

It is sometimes difficult to assess with accuracy the exercise tolerance of a child. Obviously, if the child is not yet crawling or walking this may be difficult, but the general levels of activity may be an indication. In older children other factors may obscure the true state of affairs. Often the exhortations of parents, school authorities and doctors may result in the child becoming relatively inactive and giving up sports which he previously played without difficulty. If the question is then asked, "Well, what do you do after school when no one is there to stop you?" a more honest appraisal may be reached. The child may say that he plays football, throws baskets or plays baseball without difficulty. How well does he keep up with his brothers or schoolmates? Don't just accept a protective mother's answer that "Oh no, Jimmy can't play baseball!" Jimmy may be able to do a lot of things that his mother never knew, and the mother may have to be out of the room before the doctor receives a truthful reply.

The differential diagnosis between congestive heart failure and pneumonia is difficult to make in small infants. If, for instance, parents say that a six month old child was in hospital on several occasions during the first three months of life with "pneumonia," the correct interpretation may be that the infant was in congestive failure. Dysphagia and respiratory problems within the first few weeks of life may suggest a vascular ring. Many children with left-to-right shunts have an increased frequency of upper respiratory infections. This frequency, however, is not necessarily related to the severity of the lesion, the size of the shunt or the presence of pulmonary hypertension.

If cyanosis has been prolonged and severe, important coagulation defects are present which must be recognized and treated before operation (see page 537). Questioning about bleeding and bruising may not disclose the problem, but if the answers to such questions are positive, tests of coagulation should be made. Syncope occurs with lesions such as aortic stenosis but other cardiovascular and neurologic causes must be sought.

Acquired Heart Disease

Most patients with acquired heart disease are adult by the time symptoms become severe enough for operation to be considered. The origin of the disease, however, may have started in youth and questions about early health are not inappropriate. For instance:

1. Were there obvious predisposing diseases? Rheumatic fever, acute pericarditis, or history of a murmur during childhood?

2. At what time and under what circumstances was a diagnosis of cardiac disease first made? Was the diagnosis made because symptoms led to an examination or was an examination made for routine purposes of insurance or employment and the diagnosis made then?

3. If the patient was asymptomatic when the diagnosis was first made, when did symptoms first develop and what were the symptoms?

4. What has been the progression of symptoms since they first developed?

5. To what extent is the patient now functionally disabled? As with children, extensive and detailed questioning is often necessary to arrive at a true picture of disability. The reply to such a question as "How well do you manage stairs?" may be deceptive unless it is then determined that in the normal course of daily life the patient never encounters stairs. A comparison of the patient's capabilities with that of his spouse may be useful. A patient may admit that his wife now seems to walk too fast, or that during the lunch interval his business associates walk too quickly. What was the patient able to do 12 or 6 months ago that he can no longer do?

All these questions are directed toward discovering the nature, severity and progression of symptoms. Merely to note in the chart that a patient has "two-block D.O.E." (dyspnea on exertion) seldom tells the whole story.

Dyspnea is the commonest symptom of cardiac disease and signifies pulmonary congestion. Although it is evidence of left-sided failure, it also occurs with pulmonary hypertension or increased pulmonary blood flow. Patients with pulmonary venous hypertension and incipient left-sided failure often start coughing with exertion, as well as becoming dyspneic.

Nocturnal dyspnea is a significant symptom when present. "Two-pillow orthopnea," however, is a meaningless description. Many normal people sleep with two pillows and patients with genuine nocturnal dyspnea find that two pillows provide insufficient elevation and support.

Medical purists have long taught that leading questions should not be asked. If this pedantic role is strictly adhered to as though there were a legal sanction upon asking such questions, much useful historical information remains unacquired. If a patient is asked a straight question such as "Do you ever become so short of breath at night that you have to sit up on the side of the bed?" both patient and doctor are likely to have the same concept of the severity of the symptom. The answer is usually a plain "yes" or "no."

Of all symptoms of acquired disease none is more difficult to elucidate than pain. Ryle (1928) described a sequence of questions to ask about pain which has not yet been improved upon:

1. Character
2. Severity
3. Location—chest, abdomen, superficial or deep, for example
4. Extent—covered by a hand or a fingertip
5. Radiation
6. Time of onset of first attack
7. Length of each attack
8. Time between attacks
9. Precipitating factors
10. Relieving factors
11. Associated symptoms—vomiting, sweating and faintness, among others

In most instances answers to these questions will provide a clear picture not only of the symptom but also of the etiology.

Physical Examination

Inspection

A systematic approach to examination of the heart starts not with the application of a stethoscope to the chest but with general observation of the patient and an examination of the periphery. Examination begins as soon as the patient walks into the office. Is he young or old, fat or thin, emaciated or short of breath? Does he move around easily and with assurance or slowly and cautiously as though expecting the onset of pain, or is he incapacitated by shortness of breath? What is his color? Is there generalized cyanosis, or the cyanosis of peripheral stasis? And, perhaps the most important distinction of all, does he look ill or well?

The patient should be stripped to the waist at about 45° elevation and seated in a good, slightly side-directed light. Note pulsations in the neck. Are they arterial or venous? If venous, estimate roughly the venous pressure and the presence and magnitude of an accentuated V-wave. If arterial pulsation is obvious, is it normally located in the carotids, or is it suprasternal as is characteristic with coarctation of the aorta? Does the pulse pressure seem to be abnormally wide? Inspection of the precordium is directed toward determining the cardiac apex, any obvious asymmetry of the chest, pulsations and signs of cardiac activity. The weight, size and configuration of the patient must be taken into account in interpretation of all these findings.

Palpation

Palpation starts at the periphery with examination of the pulses. Are pulses present or absent? What is their volume, timing, rate and rhythm? What is the blood pressure and are there inequalities of pressure between limbs?

Feel over the precordium and neck for thrills, which should be timed against the cardiac cycle. When the ventricles become hypertrophied, their activity is transmitted to the precordium as distinctive impulses. Right ventricular hypertrophy is best felt along the left sternal border as a rather sharp tapping impulse, while left ventricular hypertrophy is transmitted as a strong rolling, heaving apical impulse. During systole the hypertrophied right ventricular outflow tract travels directly anteriorly during contraction, but the left ventricle, in contracting, pushes the whole heart forward in a somewhat rotatory manner, imparting a much broader, more widely distributed thrust to the precordium.

Percussion

In the classic sequence of physical examination, percussion follows palpation, but it contributes little to examination of the heart per se. It is very useful in detecting pleural effusions and large pneumothoraces. But percussing out the cardiac apex is not of much help except perhaps when a pericardial effusion dampens the precordial manifestations of cardiac action.

Auscultation

Because auscultation is instinctively regarded as the most important facet of cardiac examination, it is worthwhile to reconsider the information that may already have been acquired by this stage of the examination before a stethoscope is used. The presence or absence of cyanosis of cardiac origin immediately separates patients with right-to-left shunts from all others. The peripheral pulse wave can be diagnostic of coarctation, aortic stenosis and insufficiency, and it suggests a patent ductus. Artrial fibrillation points to mitral disease, especially stenosis, arteriosclerotic disease or thyrotoxicosis. Tricuspid insufficiency may be diagnosed from the venous pulsation. Visible wide arterial pulses reconfirm an impression of aortic insufficiency. The precordial impulse indicates left or right ventricular hypertrophy and, if pulmonary valve closure is palpable, pulmonary hypertension. The presence, location and timing of thrills are pointers to a diagnosis of patent ductus, valvular stenosis or insufficiency, ventricular septal defects, tetralogy of Fallot and unusual shunts such as rupture of a sinus of Valsalva. By the time, therefore, that auscultation is started the diagnosis has often been made and the stethoscope merely confirms what has already been found.

For the finer points of auscultatory diagnosis any standard textbook of cardiology should be consulted. It is important, however, that the surgeon have a system for listening to the heart. Each area—aortic, pulmonary, tricuspid and mitral—should be listened to in order. By timing against the pulse or precordial impulse the first and second sounds can be confirmed. Then listen to the sounds individually. Are two or more sounds present? Are they of normal volume? If they are split is this a constant finding during all phases of respiration? Next listen to the systolic and diastolic intervals. Murmurs are usually graded in intensity on a basis of I to VI, I being the softest and VI so loud that it can be heard without direct application of the stethoscope to the skin. Murmurs should be analyzed for the location of maximum intensity and radiation, magnitude, character, precise timing within systole or diastole and impingement upon the opening and closing sounds.

Aortic murmurs are accentuated by making the patient sit up, lean forward and exhale. Similarly, low-intensity mitral diastolic rumbles are best heard when the patient is tilted over to the left side. If the patient is made to sit up and down in bed a couple of times and then listened to while he is lying on his left side, some hard-to-hear murmurs of mitral stenosis may become audible.

Not all murmurs signify cardiac disease, and it is obviously important to try to distinguish as simply as possible between significant and insignificant murmurs. This problem arises most often in children, and the commonest insignificant or "functional" murmurs are: (a) A low-frequency musical or grunting murmur best heard between the left sternal border and the apex. (b) A soft, blowing, early systolic murmur heard over the pulmonary area, associated with normal splitting of the second pulmonary sound. The chest x-ray and EKG should also be normal. (c) Venous hum: this high-pitched hum is usually heard on the right side over the superior cava, but occasionally it may be heard in the left intraclavicular region and is confused with the continuous murmur of a patent ductus arteriosus. The hum changes with alterations in the position of the neck and may be obliterated by compressing the jugular veins.

Most innocent murmurs are of low-grade intensity, and they are never associated with other abnormalities such as thrills or cardiomegaly, or with changes in the chest x-ray or EKG.

After auscultation is complete, determine if the patient is or is not in congestive failure. Venous pulsations have already been noted. Examine the lungs for rales and pleural effusions and palpate the liver for enlargement, tenderness and pulsation. Gross ascites is usually found without difficulty, but a small volume of ascites may be impossible to detect. Ankles and legs are examined for edema. If there is any doubt about the patient's functional capacity have him walk up the hallway or some stairs or "mark time" in the office and observe for yourself the effects of exercise.

When the history and physical examination are completed, an anatomical diagnosis has usually been reached. The functional capacity of the patient has been assessed from both history and examination. In most cases, therefore, ancillary tests such as radiography and cardiac catheterization are used to confirm a diagnosis already made and to provide objective data of its severity.

Radiography

A full "cardiac series" should be taken on all patients at the first visit. This includes plain PA and lateral views of the chest, and PA, right and left oblique views after a barium swallow. Oblique views are not worth taking in children under two years of age. At subsequent visits a PA view may be all that is necessary to determine if the size of the heart has changed and to view both lung fields.

In order to interpret the cardiac findings in a chest x-ray, knowledge of normal anatomy is required (Fig. 16–1). Alteration in configuration of the cardiac shadow can then be interpreted with knowledge of the chamber involved. Some principles which influence the enlargement of cardiac chambers and the great vessels are important.

Cardiac Chambers

1. Enlargement is more likely to be caused by increased intracameral volume than by increased pressure. The increase in volume may be due to addi-

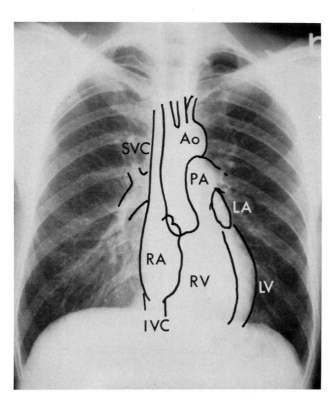

Figure 16–1 Normal AP chest film, with cardiac chambers outlined. SVC, superior vena cava. RA, right atrium. IVC, inferior vena cava. AO, aorta. PA, pulmonary artery. RV, right ventricle. LA, left atrium. LV, left ventricle.

tional flow derived from an intracardiac shunt, retrograde flow secondary to valvular insufficiency, or dilatation due to myocardial disease or failure.

2. Hypertrophy of the walls may be considerable before the external dimensions of the heart are noticeably enlarged. Stenotic lesions, therefore, are not associated with great cardiac enlargement until failure induces ventricular dilatation.

3. When valvular insufficiency is present the chamber immediately upstream is enlarged the most. If the insufficiency is of an atrioventricular valve, both upstream and downstream chambers are enlarged.

4. When an intracardiac shunt is present, enlargement involves the downstream chamber and great vessel.

Great Vessels

The pulmonary vessels and aorta increase in size for three reasons: (1) increased intravascular volume (flow or congestion), (2) poststenotic dilatation, and (3) intrinsic disease of the vessel walls. Pulmonary vessels may also be increased in number.

The size of a vessel is closely related to the flow within it. Because increased flow usually affects one or another of the cardiac chambers, isolated enlargement of the pulmonary artery or aorta is more likely to be due to poststenotic dilatation or localized disease than to increased flow. An increase in flow also enlarges distal vessels, such as the peripheral pulmonary vasculature.

Looking at a Chest Film

A good working system for looking at chest films is the assessment of the following factors in the order listed:[3]

1. Check that the film is correctly viewed. Left stomach bubble and left cardiac apex—normal; right stomach bubble and right cardiac apex—situs inversus (dextrocardia); left stomach bubble and right cardiac apex—dextroversion.

2. Survey the bony structure, looking for defects due to noncardiac disease as well as those associated with cardiovascular disease such as rib-notching.

3. The overall size and localized enlargements of the cardiac shadow should be noted and interpreted according to their anatomical sites. A knowledge of the best view for evaluating enlargement of each chamber is important, because enlargement apparent in one view may be confirmed or refuted by appearances in another view (Table 16–1).

4. The lung fields. Examine lung parenchyma, vascular patterns and extrapulmonary lesions such as effusions. The lung fields are best divided into upper, middle and lower thirds for comparison between both sides.

Evaluation of the pulmonary vessels should distinguish between vascularity (the number of vessels), perfusion (increased or decreased flow) and congestion (with associated signs of decompensation). Differences between central and peripheral vascular patterns are also important. Severe pulmonary hypertension, for instance, may be associated with large hilar vascular shadows but with attenuated, sparse peripheral

TABLE 16–1 Optimum Views for Cardiac X-ray

Target	Best Viewing Angle
Right Auricle	AP
Right Ventricle	RAO
	Lateral
Pulmonary Artery	AP
	Lateral
Left Auricle	AP (with barium)
	LAO (with ba)
	Lateral (with ba)
Left Ventricle	LAO
Aorta	
ascending	AP; LAO
arch	LAO
descending	LAO

LAO—left anterior oblique
RAO—right anterior oblique
AP—anteroposterior

shadows. In high flow, left to right shunts, however, enlargement of the vessels extends to the periphery.

Some changes are more obvious in upper than lower zones or vice versa. The "upturned mustache" effect, in which hilar vessels turn toward the upper lobes, is characteristic of mitral stenosis, but a large main pulmonary artery without peripheral enlargement suggests pulmonary valve stenosis.

Engorged lymphatics in the basal lobes are the basis for the so-called Kerley lines associated with pulmonary venous hypertension and failure.

Serial observations are essential. In the long-term followup of cardiac patients changes in the x-ray appearances may tell a story more graphically than the patient's words.

Electrocardiography

Few surgeons become expert at electrocardiographic interpretation and in most instances this is fortunately not necessary.

In the diagnosis and follow-up of operable heart disease the features of the electrocardiogram most important to the surgeon are: (1) the rhythm, (2) the heart rate, (3) major defects in conduction, (4) evidence of ventricular hypertrophy, (5) evidence of acute ischemia, (6) changes associated with drugs such as digitalis, and (7) evidence of electrolyte imbalance (Fig. 16–2).

Especially in congenital defects specific electrocardiographic changes are associated with certain lesions. Because left axis deviation is so unusual in young children, it is a finding of great significance. A severely cyanosed infant with left axis deviation almost certainly has tricuspid atresia. An older child with left axis deviation and evidence of a left-to-right shunt at the atrial level has an endocardial cushion defect of some variety unless other evidence proves differently.

Evidence of ventricular hypertrophy is not usually of significant help because other clinical signs of these changes have usually been elicited by the time the electrocardiogram is read. If, however, the electrocardiographic evidence does not fit with other clinical evidence a re-evaluation of the situation is obviously necessary. In patients with multiple valvular lesions in whom it is difficult to assess the relative importance of defects, the electrocardiogram may give valuable evidence of ventricular preponderance.

Cardiac Catheterization: Angiocardiography

Although few surgeons carry out cardiac catheterization on their patients it is important that the cardiac surgeon be totally familiar with all normal values, with methods for calculating cardiac output, and vascular resistances with interpretation of data (Tables 16–2 and 16–3).

Catheterization

The following information is obtainable by cardiac catheterization:
1. The presence, anatomic location, magnitude and direction of shunts.
2. The presence, location and severity of valvular obstructive lesions.
3. The presence, location and severity of valvular regurgitation.
4. Cardiac output, vascular resistances, and responses to stimuli such as exercise, hypoxia, or drugs.

Angiocardiography

Cardiac catheterization determines changes in physiology, but angiocardiography outlines the changes in anatomy, and it is the anatomy that the surgeon has to change in order to alter the physiology. Angiocardiography provides the following information:
1. Evidence of the exact site of intra-

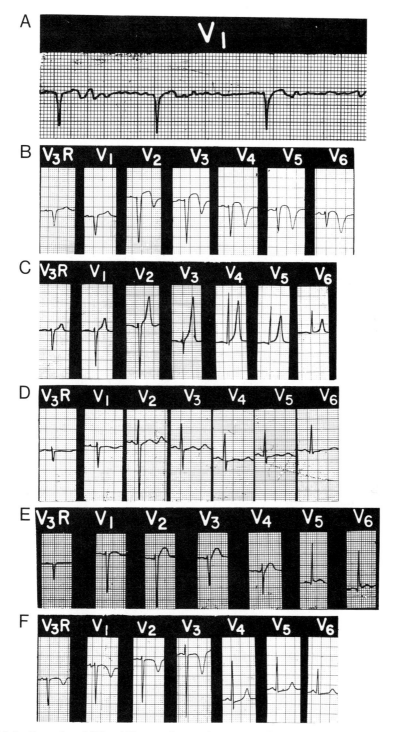

Figure 16–2 Examples of ST and T wave changes due to several causes. *A.* Digitalis effect with atrial fibrillation. *B.* Acute ischemia and infarction. *C.* Hyperkalemia. *D.* Hypokalemia. *E.* Hypercalcemia. *F.* Hypocalcemia.

TABLE 16–2 NORMAL VALUES FOR INTRACARDIAC PRESSURES

| | PRESSURE (mmHg) | | |
	Systolic	Diastolic	Mean
Right atrium	3–7	−2 to +2	2–7
Right ventricle	15–30	0–7	
Pulmonary artery	15–30	5–15	10–20
Pulmonary wedge			5–12
Left atrium			4–12
Left ventricle	100–140	4–12	
Aorta	100–140	65–90	70–90

ventricular obstructive lesions. Although catheterization may accurately locate an infundibular obstruction in the outflow tract of the right ventricular, only angiocardiography delineates the exact location, length and severity of the obstruction. It is from the angiocardiographic appearances and not from the pressure data that the surgeon can determine the technical difficulties involved in the operation.

2. Evidence of valvular insufficiency. The assessment of mitral and tricuspid insufficiency from pressure tracings alone is not very accurate. A left or right ventricular injection of dye, however, may indicate 'the severity of the lesion.

Aortic insufficiency can similarly be evaluated, but because measurement of aortic diastolic pressure is such a good test for determining the degree of insufficiency, angiocardiography is not essential merely to diagnose this lesion.

3. Ventricular function and contractility can be accurately assessed from cineangiocardiograms. Knowledge of ventricular function is of great importance in cases of valvular disease and when dyskinetic or akinetic areas are suspected in patients with coronary disease and postinfarction scars.

4. Coronary arteriograms should probably be made in all patients in the "coronary age group," i.e., males above 35 and females above 45, regardless of the lesion for which they are being investigated. Obviously in patients being evaluated for coronary disease, good bilateral cineangiograms are a *sine qua non*. In other patients, however, it may be of great importance to know whether

TABLE 16–3 FORMULAE FOR CALCULATING COMMON PARAMETERS

Cardiac output (Fick method):

$$CO = \frac{O_2 \text{ consumption (ml/min)}}{\text{Systemic A–V } O_2 \text{ difference (vols. \%)}}$$

$$\text{Vascular resistance (R)} = \frac{\text{Pressure gradient}}{\text{Flow}}$$

$$\text{Pulmonary vascular resistance} = \frac{\text{Mean PA pressure–Mean LA pressure} \times 80}{\text{Pulmonary blood flow}}$$

(Normal: under 3 units, or 240 dynes-sec/cm⁵)

$$\text{Systemic vascular resistance} = \frac{\text{Mean arterial pressure (mmHg)}}{\text{Cardiac output (L/min)}}$$

(Normal: under 20 units, or 1600 dynes-sec/cm⁵)

the coronary vessels are normal. If a patient with severe aortic valvular stenosis has angina he may also have coronary disease and might be better off with both valve replacement and coronary bypass than with valve replacement alone. Before the advent of successful direct operations upon the coronary arteries, knowledge of the state of the coronary vessels was important only in assessing the risks involved in an operation. But indications for coronary angiography in patients with primarily noncoronary lesions have now been widened, because if coronary lesions are discovered it may be possible to incorporate their treatment into the overall management of the patient.

Laboratory Examinations

The following tests should be made routinely on all cardiac patients: CBC, electrolytes, BUN, creatinine and urinalysis. Liver function tests are indicated if there has been clinical suspicion of abnormal hepatic function.

Tests of coagulation are not normally necessary unless the patient has been receiving anticoagulants, or if there has been a history of abnormal bleeding. Patients with severe cyanotic heart disease commonly have a variety of coagulation defects and should be appropriately investigated. The older the patient and the more severe the cyanosis, the greater the likelihood of a severe defect of coagulation (see page 541). If left uncorrected these defects may lead to severe and uncontrollable small vessel hemorrhage during the course of the operation, and excessive and even fatal hemorrhage in the postoperative phase.[19]

Drugs

Most patients with acquired heart disease who require operation are already receiving one or more drugs by the time they are seen by the surgeon. Drugs most commonly given are digitalis, diuretics, potassium supplements, tranquilizers and anticoagulants. It is important that these drugs and their doses be noted.

It is sometimes advantageous to change the digitalis preparation that is being given. Digitoxin, for instance, is a long-acting preparation which is only slowly excreted. Experience has shown that it is advisable to stop all digitalis administration at least 48 hours before operation to prevent digitalis toxicity during and after operation. If the patient is receiving digitoxin there will be only a minimal reduction in digitalis action in this interval. If, however, the patient has been receiving digoxin, which is much more rapidly excreted, then the digitalis level will be much lower by the time of operation and the danger of digitalis toxicity will be greatly reduced. Chronic use of digitalis and diuretics can induce severe and critical reductions in total body potassium. If a patient is receiving digitalis and diuretics the physician should ensure that supplemental potassium is also given; the preadmission serum potassium level should be between 3.8 and 4.5 mEq/L.

Anticoagulants are often given to patients with atrial fibrillation who may or may not have already suffered from peripheral emboli. There is no need to restore the prothrombin level to normal before operation, and too sudden a cessation of Coumadin anticoagulation may induce rebound hypercoagulability. Arrange the dosage so that the patient is admitted to hospital with a prothrombin time of 30 to 40 per cent of normal. Bleeding complications are rare if the prothrombin time is at this level.

There is no need to start antibiotic treatment before the patient is admitted to the hospital. Note any allergy to antibiotics so that appropriate agents can be chosen which will not induce reactions.

If the patient has focal infections of the urinary tract or oropharynx, time is saved by treating these appropriately on an outpatient basis before admission.

ASSESSING THE RISK

One of the most important decisions the cardiologist and cardiac surgeon have to make is the determination of the point reached by the patient on the natural history curve of his defect. The diagnosis is often simple to make. No unique skill is required to diagnose aortic insufficiency, but great judgment may be necessary to decide upon the correct time for operation. Numerous factors must be taken into account in assessing the risk in each case.

Congenital Heart Disease

Different factors are important at different stages of childhood. But, in general, children either require operation in infancy because the severity of the defect is causing crippling and life-threatening hemodynamic difficulty, or operation can be safely delayed for several years until the child is older.

In small infants, the following factors increase the risk of operation: pulmonary hypertension, severe cyanosis, prematurity, superimposed respiratory complications and additional severe congenital defects.

Obviously the risk is greater with a severe than with a less severe defect. But even patients with severe defects can be operated upon with an acceptable risk if operation results in a radical improvement in hemodynamics. An infant in congestive failure with a large patent ductus arteriosus may be transformed almost immediately by closing the ductus. The operation, in this instance, results in rapid, total hemodynamic cure. On the other hand, an infant with preductal coarctation of the aorta, a patent ductus and pulmonary hypertension may be minimally improved by correction of the defects because severe pulmonary hypertension secondary to pulmonary vascular changes will persist and may result in death of the patient.

Complete correction of a defect does not always carry with it a smaller risk than a palliative operation. Total correction of tetralogy of Fallot or of large ventricular septal defects in small infants has proved to carry a high risk. Whereas a palliative shunt or banding of the pulmonary artery can usually be done with a small risk and considerable improvement in the child.

The principle to be followed in choosing the correct operation for a small infant, therefore, is to make the least possible change that will produce significant hemodynamic improvement. Total correction can usually be deferred until a later date.

In older children many factors applicable in infancy still apply. But the child, by living, has demonstrated to some extent his ability to tolerate his lesion. The complexity of the defect, congestive failure, pulmonary hypertension and severe cyanosis adversely affect the outlook. Of these, pulmonary hypertension is the most important.

It is helpful to determine preoperatively whether pulmonary hypertension is "fixed" or "reactive." During cardiac catheterization the response to 100 per cent oxygen, hypoxia (10 per cent oxygen), vasodilators (Priscoline) and exercise should be determined. If pulmonary hypertension is fixed there will be no reduction in response to 100 per cent oxygen and vasodilators, but hypertension may become more severe if the patient breathes only 10 per cent oxygen. Severe fixed pulmonary hypertension carries a grave prognosis because surgical correction of the underlying defect will not favorably affect the basic pulmonary vascular pathology. If, however, pulmonary vascular resistance falls and pulmonary hypertension is reduced by oxygen and vasodilators, then it can be assumed that correction of the defect and diminution in pulmonary blood flow and pressure will result in improvement of the pulmonary pathology. Pulmonary hypertension does not always revert completely to normal, depending upon the severity of the original lesion, the totality of correction and, possibly, the age at which operation is done. The longer and more established the pulmonary hypertention, the less likely it is to disappear after operation.

Congestive failure is not necessarily a bad prognostic factor, provided that the failure is not due to myocarditis, endocardial fibrosis or irreversible pulmonary hypertension. When failure is secondary to a mechanical problem such as a stenotic valve which can be restored to normal function by an operation, the outlook is good. In young patients with multiple rheumatic valvular lesions, assessment of the relative importance of myocardial and mechanical valvular factors is very difficult. Measurement of pressures such as the left ventricular end-diastolic indicates at best only the current functional capacity of the left ventricle. These measurements do not indicate the ability of the ventricle to recover once the valvular lesion has been repaired. At the moment no such method is available. In young patients, fortunately, if a severe valvular lesion exists some improvement can be expected after repair even if myocardial disease also exists.

Congenital heart disease is also encountered, with less frequency, in adults. Sometimes the lesion has been recognized but left untouched for many years. At times a palliative operation has already been carried out and a definitive operation is contemplated. Correction of tetralogy of Fallot in the older teenager or adult has been thought by some to carry with it a very high risk. But others, such as Beach (1971), have demonstrated that total correction can be carried out without excessive risk. Most patients in this age group with tetralogy have already had a palliative operation. Many return for definitive operation when cyanosis is severe and disability is increasing. Coagulation defects are extremely common in such patients and should be corrected preoperatively. Correction involves multiple 500 cc exchange transfusions with removal of the patient's blood and immediate replacement by fresh plasma. If this is done every two days until coagulation returns to normal, these patients can be operated upon without risk of severe hemorrhage. The theory behind this technique is that these patients are deficient in certain clotting factors and also have active clotting inhibitors in their plasma. By exchange transfusion the deficiencies are restored and active inhibitors removed. The replacement of the blood withdrawn by normal fresh plasma is an essential part of the technique. The mere reduction of hematocrit as advocated many years ago does little to restore clotting to normal.

Complete anatomical analysis of the lesion by cardioangiography is essential. If the pulmonary arteries and pulmonary valve annulus are of adequate size and if stensois exists only at the infundibular level, no great surgical problem is present. If, however, an extensive reconstruction of the infundibulum, pulmonary valve annulus and pulmonary arteries is necessary, the complexity of the operation is increased and the possibility of a less than perfect result is proportionately enhanced. Operative mortality after repair of the uncomplicated defect is 10 per cent or less and a good result with restoration of functional normality may be anticipated in about 80 per cent of survivors.[10]

Ventricular septal defects are rarely found in adults. The critical factor in assessing the surgical problem is whether or not the patient has pulmonary hypertension. If fixed severe pulmonary hypertension exists with only a small left-to-right shunt then a poor result may be anticipated, and the risks involved may not be worth the small gain in function. If, however, a large left-to-right shunt is still present, closure should be advised, the risk of operation should not exceed 5 per cent and the improvement to be gained should be considerable.

Atrial septal defects are not uncommonly found in adults and there are numerous instances of people living into their seventies with a secundum atrial defect. Once again, the presence and severity of pulmonary hypertension are critical factors. Pulmonary hypertension has been found by some to revert to normal after closure of the defect, but others have not found this to be true. In general, asymptomatic adults in their forties and fifties with secundum defects can be operated upon with very little risk if they do not have severe pulmonary hypertension. The risks of operation increase in proportion to the severity of symptoms and the magnitude of pulmonary hypertension. If pulmonary hypertension is severe, it does not regress after operation. The need for operation is based upon balancing the patient's symptoms and their progression against the anticipation of the possibility of improving the pulmonary hypertension by closing the defect.

Coarctation of the aorta is technically more difficult to deal with in adults than in children. The aorta is less flexible, and atherosclerotic disease may exist in the proximal segment. In pregnant women acute dissection of the proximal aorta has often been reported. For this reason resection and repair in females should always be advised at an age before pregnancy is likely. The older the patient the greater and more fixed is systemic hypertension, and the greater the technical risks associated with operation.

Patent ductus arteriosus is very uncommon today in adults because of the ease with which the diagnosis is made in children and the good results from closure during childhood. Pulmonary hypertension may be present, but if a left-to-right shunt exists, closure should be advised. The ductus and associated great vessels may be brittle and technical problems should be anticipated. If an aneurysm of the ductus is present, the risks increase considerably but partial bypass may make the technical problems of closure easier.

Mongolism and other forms of mental deficiency are not uncommonly associated with congenital heart disease. The decision as to whether or not operation should be carried out in such children involves an assessment of the incapacity due to the mental deficiency, the severity of the cardiac defect, the risks involved and the overall improvement anticipated in the child's condition and ability to look after himself, enjoy life and benefit from remedial training. The wishes of the parents are paramount. The author's personal opinion is that few children with mental deficiency should be denied operation, especially if the risks involved are reasonably low. If the quality of the child's life might be improved by increasing his physical capabilities, then operation would seem to be entirely justified.

Acquired Heart Disease

Several factors are common to the assessment of patients with acquired heart disease, among them the relative importance of valvular malfunction and myocardial disease. If the primary problem is a mechanically poor valve and the myocardium seems to be strong, then a good result can be anticipated and the mortality rate should not be high (Table 16–4). If several valves are involved the risk increases, mainly because of associated myocardial disease with chronic congestive failure, complicated drug therapy, and coexisting pulmonary problems.

Patients with stenotic lesions are often more improved by operation than those

TABLE 16–4 MORTALITY AFTER OPERATION*

Aortic valve replacement	5–12%
Mitral valve replacement	8–15%
Multiple valve replacement	8–25%
Open mitral commissurotomy	1–2%
Closed mitral commissurotomy	1–2%
Coronary bypass:	
1 vessel	5%
2 to 4 vessels	8–40%

*Rates based upon published figures.

with valvular insufficiency. The reasons for this are not entirely clear. The heart is usually smaller in patients with valvular stenosis than in those with regurgitation. Increased volume loads due to regurgitation may result in greater myocardial stretching and subsequent fibrosis than in pressure loads. Resection of the papillary muscles during replacement of the mitral valve has been blamed as a cause of impairment of left ventricular function. Most surgeons, however, still resect these muscles in order to make an adequate cavity for the prosthetic valve. Regardless of the causes, heart size in patients with regurgitation will decrease neither as rapidly nor as completely as in those with valvular stenosis.

The New York Heart, Association classification of functional severity is a useful index by which to select patients to be operated upon, but is not necessarily a prognostic indication of how patients will fare after operation. Patients in Class I should probably never be operated upon. Patients in Class II may be operated upon under some circumstances, and those in Classes III and IV are almost by definition candidates for operation. Some of the most dramatic results are obtained in patients in Class IV, perhaps because they have the greatest reasons for improvement.

Very few patients should now be regarded as inoperable. Severe congestive failure per se is not a contraindication. Massive cardiomegaly with clear-cut evidence of mild valvular disease but severe myocardial dysfunction or very severe renal, hepatic or pulmonary disease may suggest that the lesion is inoperable. But every surgeon can point to individual patients in whom these conditions existed and who were helped by operation. The prospect for such patients without operation is universally grim.

Renal function should always be assessed preoperatively. If the BUN is normal and urinalysis does not indicate infection or proteinuria, no further investigation is necessary. If the BUN and creatinine are elevated and creatinine clearance is depressed, the risk of renal dysfunction postoperatively is increased. If these changes seem to be on the basis of chronic congestion rather than primary renal parenchymal disease, the prospect for improvement after operation is good. Primary renal disease cannot be expected to improve and may impose a significant risk during the immediate postoperative phase. Once the initial recovery phase has been reached the period of risk has usually passed.

Hepatic function is sometimes depressed by chronic congestive failure. Improvement of congestive failure after operation may result in a similar improvement in hepatic function. During the postoperative period, when the products of hemolysis secondary to perfusion must be effectively handled by the reticuloendothelial system, pre-existing diminution of hepatic function may contribute to temporary postoperative jaundice.

In patients with suspected hepatic dysfunction, defects of coagulation should be sought and can, if found, be corrected preoperatively.

Respiratory disease often accompanies cardiac disease and in most cases is secondary to it. Patients with independent chronic obstructive respiratory disease must be very carefully evaluated by pulmonary function tests. Even severe respiratory disease may be tolerated during the postoperative phase with the aid of respirators, and correction of cardiac defects, especially those contributing to pulmonary congestion or hypertension, may greatly improve the overall respiratory state. But severe obstructive respiratory disease considerably increases the risks of operation and should be recognized as a deleterious factor.

Previous embolic episodes may be both an indication for operation and a source of added risk. About 50 per cent of patients with previous emboli are found at operation to have an intra-atrial clot which can be the origin of intraoperative emboli, or if inadequately removed, the propagating point for later emboli. Recognition of this danger also decreases it because intraoperative techniques should prevent dissemination of emboli.

If a patient is hemiplegic there is a slightly increased risk of postoperative pulmonary complications because the cough of these patients is not as strong as is normal. Aphasia may present some nursing problems and the details of pre- and postoperative care should be explained in great detail to aphasic patients since their disability isolates them from those who attend them.

Neurologic problems should be carefully noted before operation because neurologic complications of open cardiac surgery are not unknown, and if the preoperative state is not carefully noted, postoperative problems may be difficult to evaluate.

Other associated diseases are occasionally encountered. Diabetes of moderate severity does not impose any great problem. Severe diabetes associated with diminished renal function obviously adds to the risks, but under these circumstances the real question is whether cardiac disease or diabetes imposes the greater threat to the patient's life.

Gout is not uncommon in association with valvular disease. The commonest complication of this association is an acute flare-up after operation, and the patient should be warned that this may occur.

Marie-Strümpell's ankylosing spondylitis is sometimes associated with valvular disease. The patient with a rigid spinal column and no movement of the thoracic cage is particularly liable to pulmonary complications. The ribs, however, can be retracted without difficulty through a midline sternotomy.

Hematologic diseases such as thrombocytopenia or chronic leukemia present special problems. Any hematologic disease which might affect coagulation must be fully investigated and, if possible, corrected before a cardiac operation is contemplated. Chronic leukemia is not a contraindication to operation, but platelet dysfunction is common in these patients and their ability to clot properly must be assured.

Tricuspid Disease. Of all valvular lesions this is perhaps the most difficult to assess. Clinical examination is helpful if there is obvious venous pulsation in the neck, distinct murmurs, hepatomegaly and peripheral edema. Starr (1969)[16] found that in approximately one-third of patients who required tricuspid valve replacement there was no preoperative evidence of significant disease.

Hemodynamic measurements made at cardiac catheterization are often undiagnostic. Cardioangiography with injection of dye into the right ventricle will confirm the presence of tricuspid regurgitation. But because the catheter must pass through the tricuspid valve, false positives are not uncommon. Isolated tricuspid disease is uncommon and the overwhelming clinical picture may be that of the associated aortic or mitral disease. The surgeon's finger at the time of operation probably remains the best means for evaluating tricuspid function.

Severe tricuspid disease may cause persistent hepatic dysfunction, ascites and peripheral edema. If the operation is postponed until these have been fully compensated, there may be unnecessary delay. A reasonable period of bed rest and preoperative therapy is advisable, but as soon as improvement has reached a recognizable plateau, operation should be carried out.

It is not possible at this point (1973) to present an overwhelmingly enthusiastic picture to the patient of the results of tricuspid valve surgery. Annuloplasty seems to afford temporary improvement but breakdown of the repair is common. Prosthetic replacement, especially by ball valves, is associated with a high rate of valve dysfunction due to thrombosis and impingement of the cage upon the septum. Fascia lata valves have been found to have a distressing tendency to shrivel up in this locus, and too few homografts have been used for any definite conclusions to be drawn. In most series the operative mortality rate is higher when the tricuspid valve has had to be replaced than when tricuspid disease has not been present, an increase which is probably not due to any intrinsic problem with replacement of the tricuspid valve, but rather reflects the severity of cardiac disease in these patients.[17]

Mitral Disease. More surgical experience has been gained with the treatment of mitral stenosis than with any other valvular disease. During the past decade there have been changes both in the surgical approach to this problem and also in the nature of the problem itself. Whereas the early experience with mitral stenosis was with closed commissurotomy in young patients, present experience is with open operations on older patients.

Patients in Class I do not require operation. They will usually live for many years without disability. As soon as symptoms develop and the patient moves into Class II, operation should be seriously considered. One of the genuine tragedies of medicine is the young woman with mitral stenosis who suddenly develops atrial fibrillation, cerebral embolism and hemiplegia. Recognition, therefore, is necessary not only of the diagnosis but of the phases of danger. As the patient approaches 40, atrial fibrillation with attendant dangers of embolism becomes more likely. Once atrial fibrillation is established, embolism is a constant danger which can be ameliorated by relief of the stenosis.

Most patients in Classes III and IV should be operated upon. The type of operation depends upon the experience and inclinations of the surgeon. Closed commissurotomy has produced excellent results in many patients, but blind operations on so vital a structure as the mitral valve would seem to contravene good surgical principles. The operation can, however, be carried out with a mortality rate of about 1 to 2 per cent and with excellent functional results. The operation, however, has certain intrinsic limitations. It should not be carried out when there is calcification or associated insufficiency of the valve, nor when there has been preoperative embolism. It is no longer a satisfactory approach to re-operation, and, because there is always a danger of inducing mitral regurgitation, it should never be carried out in a hospital where facilities do not exist for the immediate use of cardiopulmonary bypass.

Open commissurotomy does not have a significantly greater mortality rate than the closed operation. The long-term results (ten years) in large numbers of patients have still to be evaluated. But this operation, like all others on the mitral valve, should be regarded as palliative. If open operation can obtain a better functional result with more valve mobility and more normal function than a closed operation, it might be anticipated that the long-term results would be good.

Valve replacement is reserved for those patients with accompanying insufficiency, calcified valves or extreme degrees of fibrosis and subvalvular contraction of chordae and papillary muscles. The choice of valve is still a matter for individual preference because no single technique has been shown to be unequivocally superior to all others. Operative mortality for isolated mitral replacement is 5 to 8 per cent in many centers, although higher and lower figures are also quoted. The postoperative embolic rate has been reduced to less than 5 per cent with recent prosthetic valves. This major reduction in embolic rates in the past few years has been due to changes in valve design, especially the development of totally cloth-covered prosthetic rings and struts. Because embolic episodes are no longer such a major complication, the real issue in the choice between a synthetic prosthetic valve and a tissue valve now revolves around the relative stability and longevity of the different types of valve.

Valvuloplasty for mitral insufficiency

can be a very effective operation when the valve is not calcified and is still mobile. Valve replacement is necessary in all other cases of mitral insufficiency.

Although functional results as measured by improvement in symptoms are good after mitral valve replacement, objective data obtained at postoperative catheterization often show residual gradients across the prosthetic valves which increase with exercise.[18] Pulmonary hypertension and vascular resistance decrease so that at rest they are at approximately the upper limit of normal, but with exercise both pressure and resistance increase. There is often no correlation between improvement in symptoms and objective data, and patients with persistent severe pulmonary hypertension are sometimes dramatically improved and able to resume activities long since given up. The scientist worries about the objective data, but let us not forget that the patient is more concerned with his symptoms.

Aortic Valve Disease. Of all acquired valvular defects aortic stenosis is perhaps the most satisfactory to treat. Patients with severe symptoms and congestive failure preoperatively improve rapidly after operation: heart size comes down even before the patient leaves the hospital and exercise capabilities are restored even to patients in their late sixties and seventies.

How severe should aortic stenosis be before operation is warranted? Several factors must be considered: symptoms such as angina or syncope make operation a fairly urgent necessity. If shortness of breath without failure is the major symptom the gradient across the valve should be measured. Operation should be advised if the gradient is greater than 50 mmHg at rest and rises with exercise. If the cardiac index is much below normal a lesser gradient may be significant. But in most instances valves with a gradient of about 30 mmHg have remarkably few pathologic changes except for some thickening of the cusps and a few millimeters of fusion at the commissures. Although this fusion can

be relieved it is not worth subjecting a patient to a major operation to do so little. If this grade of aortic stenosis coexists with another valvular lesion which demands operation it is worthwhile to look at the aortic valve at the same time and relieve whatever stenosis exists.

Left ventricular end diastolic pressure (LVEDP) is an important index of ventricular function and if elevated above 15 mmHg suggests myocardial dysfunction. If the LVEDP is very high, the cardiac index low and the gradient moderate, myocardial fibrosis may be severe. The risk of operation is increased and the final result may be poor. Electrocardiographic evidence of left ventricular strain or peri-infarction block is also a bad prognostic sign. The presence of these electrocardiographic changes has been held to be a contraindication to operation because of the high mortality rate that is associated. This has not been our experience, but postoperative difficulties, arrhythmias and failure may be expected more frequently in these patients than in those with more normal electrocardiograms.

After a patient with aortic stenosis becomes symptomatic, death ensues in three to five years. Therefore, the onset of symptoms is a pressing indication that operation should be carried out with reasonable urgency. Although sudden death has often been thought to be a major feature of aortic stenosis, congestive failure is more commonly the terminal event.

All patients with aortic stenosis should have selective coronary arteriograms before operation to distinguish between angina due to the valvular disease and that due to coronary arterial disease. If both diseases are present they may both be treated at the same operation with valve replacement and saphenous vein bypass of the stenotic coronary artery.

Patients with aortic insufficiency have a different natural history pattern from those with aortic stenosis. Whereas those with stenosis are usually in their fifties before symptoms develop, patients with insufficiency are commonly in their thirties when dyspnea on exertion, nocturnal dyspnea and congestive failure become manifest.

The optimal moment for operation is more difficult to decide in patients with aortic insufficiency than in those with stenosis. Some patients with aortic insufficiency and huge hearts with a wide-open valve are capable of considerable physical exertion, to an extent quite beyond the usual expectation. After symptoms develop, about five to seven years elapse before death.[15] Therefore, although the development of symptoms is an ominous sign, there is no extreme urgency in advising operation. It is presumed that ventricular fibrosis is likely to develop progressively in patients with large hearts and, since it is irreversible, it diminishes the result of the operation. For this reason operation is usually advised soon after patients become symptomatic. Age should be taken into consideration, for an asymptomatic patient in his twenties with free insufficiency probably has almost a decade before him without symptoms. A man in his early forties is likely to develop symptoms within a short span of time.

Diastolic pressure measured by a sphygmomanometer is as good an indication as any of the severity of insufficiency. If the diastolic pressure is greater than 60 mmHg, insufficiency is mild; between 50 and 60 mmHg it is moderate; and below 50 mmHg it is severe. It is important to notice the heart rate when diastolic pressure is measured. If the rate is rapid, the diastolic pressure will not be as low as when the rate is slow, and the severity of the insufficiency will be minimized.

Heart size, left ventricular end diastolic pressure, cardiac index, evidence of pulmonary congestion and severity of symptoms must be taken into consideration in deciding about operation.

Coronary Artery Disease. There are four results of coronary atherosclerosis for which operation may be necessary:

(a) occlusion, partial or total, of one or more coronary vessels; (b) postinfarction scars and left ventricular aneurysm; (c) postinfarction intracardiac defects such as ventricular septal defect or papillary muscle dysfunction and mitral insufficiency; and (d) conduction defects requiring insertion of a pacemaker.

With the development of saphenous vein bypass of coronary lesions a wide new field of surgical treatment has opened up. Localized endarterectomy and patch grafting is of limited usefulness because the number of patients with localized lesions suitable for this type of correction is small. Saphenous vein bypass, however, has wide application in patients with severe single or multiple vessel disease.

The indications for operation in patients with coronary artery disease have not yet been fully worked out. The attitudes of different cardiologists vary greatly. At one end of the spectrum of enthusiasm are those physicians who believe that everyone with angina should have coronary arteriograms and that perhaps one or two out of every five patients may require operation. At the other end are those physicians who believe that only young patients with angina severe enough to cripple should be investigated, and that only patients with multiple vessel disease should be operated upon. The disparity in these viewpoints probably arises because we still don't know the precise natural history of coronary disease. While statistical evidence is extensive in some respects and permits an overall prognostication of longevity of people with angina or after infarcts, there is no good data which includes angiographic studies of patients with and without operation with figures comparing longevity, incidence of reinfarction and so forth, in groups of patients with comparable symptoms and anatomical lesions. Nor are there sufficient long-term studies on patients after saphenous vein bypass to permit a good analysis of long-term longevity and complications. A moderate approach between these two extremes would comprise the following: Coronary arteriography should be advised in all young patients with angina of any degree and in all patients below 65 years old with severe or disabling angina. If a man can live a reasonable life, continue to work and indulge in other activities, albeit with medication, then some physicians would not advise arteriography. But if a patient cannot work, has to change his job because of symptoms, or becomes severely restricted in his social and family life, arteriography is strongly indicated. Angina increasing in intensity and frequency is also an indication.

All patients with unusual chest pain which could be angina should also have arteriograms. Angina does not always present itself in the classical severe form and may be manifest by relatively mild pain, or pain in the jaws or arm without chest pain. But some such patients have significant lesions.

If dyspnea in addition to angina is an important symptom, cardiac catheterization should be carried out and left ventricular function assessed both by pressures and by angiography. Evidence is accumulating that poor left ventricular function may be a contraindication to operation, although a successful bypass graft can result in immediate improvement of ventricular dynamics.

Age must be considered, both chronological and physiological. A well-preserved 70 year old man with angina of recent onset would probably be a candidate for operation. But a sick man of the same age with two previous infarcts and severe angina would probably not be considered suitable, but might be considered a candidate for carotid sinus stimulation.

Involvement of several vessels is not a contraindication to operation. Total obstruction of a vessel, as seen on the arteriogram, does not mean that the vessel distal to the obstruction is completely occluded, this is especially true of the right coronary artery in which good vessels can almost always be found distal to an area of total obstruction. Operative mortality for saphenous vein bypass

varies between 5 and 25 per cent, depending upon the type of lesion, the number of grafts that must be inserted and the state of the myocardium. If the patient has only obstruction of the right coronary with no failure, the risk is low, but if there is triple vessel disease requiring three grafts, poor distal runoff and failure, the risks are obviously much greater.[4]

In patients with postinfarction scars and ventricular aneurysm the most important indication for operation is congestive failure. Cardiac catheterization and left ventricular angiography should be used to confirm the diagnosis and to demonstrate the extent of dynamic impairment. Failure of an aneurysm to fill with dye may be due to clot. A large area of paradoxical expansion is always associated with reduced cardiac output. Coronary angiograms should be made because vein bypass may be necessary to improve function of the healing left ventricle. An occasional patient may require operation because of repeated peripheral embolism arising from clot within an aneurysm.

Similar indications obtain in patients with postinfarction ventricular septal defects or papillary muscle dysfunction. The extent of failure and all other hemodynamic data must be fully assessed. Operation is indicated solely to cure the physiologic disability and not to deal with the anatomical lesion alone.

Talking to the Patient

It is essential both morally and legally that the surgeon talk with the patient and explain what is advised, why it is advised and what may be expected. Many cardiac operations on children are prophylactic—closure of a secundum atrial septal defect or a small ventricular septal defect, for example—and parents are entitled to a frank discussion of the need for an operation. It would be easy to tell a parent that the child has a "hole in the heart" and *must* have an operation. In many instances a defect may be present, but there is no urgency about operation, and operation should be arranged when financial, social and other factors are convenient.

Questions that patients ask fall into several categories. First, they want to know what is wrong with them, why an operation is necessary and what the risks are. The answers should be forthright and as complete as the background of the patient will permit. Second, they want to know what to expect, where the incision will be, how long the operation will take, how long they will be in hospital, how long the convalescence will be, and the details of postoperative diet, drugs and activities. Some patients have strange ideas about the technical aspects of cardiac surgery, and it is surprising how many patients believe that the heart is totally removed from the body, repaired, and returned to its original site. Third, the patient will want to know about the financial cost. Crippled Children's Services and other agencies pay for the care of many patients, but it is advisable to have someone in the admissions office who is conversant with the costs of cardiac surgery and the helping agencies available to plan with the patient how best to deal with these problems.

Except for details of postoperative convalescent care all these questions should be answered before the patient is admitted. For several years, all cardiac surgical patients admitted to the University of Colorado Medical Center have received an explanatory booklet which also serves as notice of admission. Similar explanatory booklets or sheets are easily made up to answer local needs.

POSTOPERATIVE EVALUATION

Details of postoperative follow-up vary with each patient and each lesion. But certain principles can be followed in assessing how well a patient is recovering from the operation.

Functional Progress

By the time the patient leaves hospital he is on his feet most of the day and capable of looking after all personal needs. Thereafter, progress depends upon his own efforts as well as physiologic recovery. It is impossible to detail exactly what every patient may or may not do. Recovery from a cardiac operation is similar to retraining an athlete— progressive, acceptable and tolerable activity is desirable. Whatever the patient can do without undue tiredness, pain or shortness of breath is acceptable. Between four to six weeks after operation the patient should be back to full activity. Patients with prosthetic valves should be warned against undue activity for three months in order that complete healing and fixation of the valve may take place before it is subjected to the tachycardia and increased blood pressure of exertion.

Few patients discuss the resumption of sexual activity. But provided that reasonable exercise capability has been achieved there is no reason why sex should not be resumed.

The patient's achievement in resuming and improving upon preoperative exercise tolerance is probably the best single sign of satisfactory progress. If the patient has been asymptomatic before operation total resumption of activity must be aimed at. The greater the disablement before operation the greater the possible improvement. Questioning of patients must be detailed and as objective as possible to evaluate improvement in exercise tolerance. Patients sometimes feel that they should always report improvement so as not to disappoint their doctor. This otherwise priaseworthy attitude should not deceive the physician. Return of symptoms and a decrease in exercise tolerance after a period of improvement should always be regarded as an ominous sign. If operation has involved closure of a shunt, it should be determined whether the shunt has reopened; if a prosthetic valve has been used, other signs of valve dysfunction should be looked for.*

Physical Findings

During routine postoperative examination the following points should be noted:

Wound

The wound should be well healed, without infection or keloid formation, and painless. The midline sternotomy wound is notorious for poor healing with a broad scar or the development of keloids. Midline epigastric herniae occasionally develop at the lower end of a midline sternotomy where the linea alba has been divided. Wire sutures may become prominent and painful, especially in thin patients. If sufficient time has elapsed for the sternum to heal and a wire suture causes discomfort, it should be removed.

Cardiovascular System

Examination should be carried out in the routine manner and is a comparison between pre- and postoperative features. After a successful operation, congestive failure should have disappeared or diminished, cardiac action should be quieter and palpable evidence of ventricular hypertrophy should decrease. Changes in murmurs must be correlated with what is anticipated. After relief of pulmonary valvular stenosis, for instance, the murmur is always still present, although often of a more vibratory character. Patients with prosthetic aortic valves all have a short systolic murmur. However, in addition to listen-

*See page 524, Syndromes of prosthetic valve failure.

ing for the expected, listen also for the unexpected, the signs that tell of trouble. Redevelopment of murmurs which had previously disappeared, the appearance of new murmurs or changes in character or intensity of murmurs which have been long present should always arouse suspicion. The disappearance of a murmur caused by a surgically induced shunt is equally important. If fever is present the important question is whether or not the patient has endocarditis. Malaise, anemia, petechial hemorrhages, splenomegaly, changing murmurs and newly developed congestive failure point to infectious endocarditis. But a sense of reasonable well-being in spite of the fever, pericardial rub or pleural effusion, lymphocytosis and splenomegaly suggest that the patient has a postcardiotomy syndrome.

Radiologic Evidence

Heart Size

Reduction in heart size should be anticipated after most operations (Fig. 16-3). The few exceptions include cases in which heart size has been normal to start with, and in a few lesions such as tetralogy of Fallot in which heart size increases after operation. After operation for stenotic lesions heart size tends to come down more rapidly and completely than after operation upon regurgitant lesions.

After a left-to-right shunt has been closed, heart size should decrease within a few weeks. Persistence of cardiomegaly should suggest that closure of the defect has been incomplete.

Pulmonary Vascularity

When pulmonary vascularity has been increased before operation and the cause has been completely eliminated by operation, vascular patterns should return to normal within three months. Although flow through the lungs is acutely restored to normal by the operation the

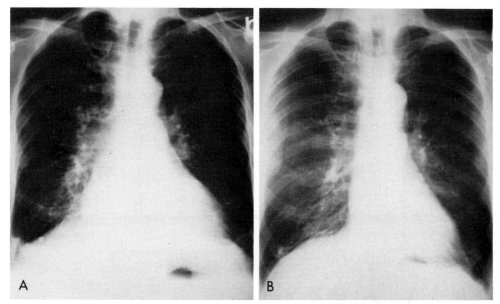

Figure 16–3 Preoperative *(A)* and postoperative *(B)* chest x-rays of a patient with aortic stenosis. A gradient of 167 mmHg was present across the aortic valve before replacement by a ball valve. Film *B* was taken four months after operation.

vessels still remain large and it takes time for them to respond to the diminished flow by a decrease in size. Persistently increased vascularity for more than three months after operation should be regarded as evidence of incomplete closure or reopening of the defect. If vascularity increases after a period of diminution, reopening of the defect should be suspected.

In those defects in which diminished pulmonary vascularity is present preoperatively, an increase in vascular patterns is apparent immediately after operation and should remain unchanged. An excessive increase in vascularity should raise the suspicion that a right-to-left shunt has been converted into a left-to-right shunt by breakdown of the repair.

Electrocardiographic Evidence

After a successful operation electrocardiographic evidence of ventricular hypertrophy should recede (Fig. 16–4).

The interval during which recession may be anticipated varies with the degree of hypertrophy. But after successful replacement of the aortic valve for aortic stenosis signs of left ventricular hypertrophy may begin to diminish within two weeks of operation.

Conduction defects of the right bundle are constantly present after right ventriculotomy and are related to incision of the anterior wall of the right ventricle. This abnormality does not alter the prognosis.

Other arrhythmias and conduction defects commonly seen are atrial fibrillation and flutter, nodal rhythms, premature ventricular contractions and, occasionally, complete heart block.

The arrhythmia is most often related to the underlying pathology. But electrolyte abnormalities or digitalis toxicity should be sought.

Complete heart block is almost invariably iatrogenic and is present from the moment of operation. In rare cases, complete heart block can revert to normal sinus rhythm many years after oper-

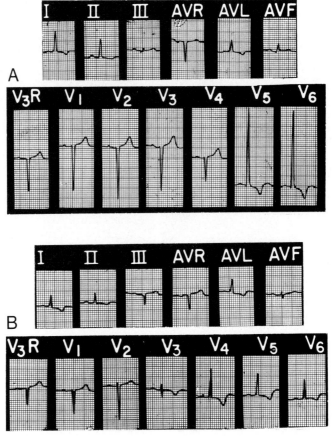

Figure 16–4   Electrocardiographic evidence of regression of left ventricular hypertrophy within eight months of replacement of a stenotic aortic valve. *A.* Before operation. *B.* Eight months after operation.

ation. This is a happy exception to the rule that if complete heart block is present when the patient leaves hospital it should be regarded as permanent and treated accordingly.

Laboratory Examinations

Blood Counts

Routine blood counts should be made at the first two or three postoperative visits, and subsequently thereafter if there are indications such as fever or anemia.

During the first week to ten days after an operation involving extracorporeal circulation the hematocrit falls to 30 to 32 per cent because the generation of cells circulated through the pump has a shorter life span than normal. Within a month after operation the hematocrit should be back to normal. If the hematocrit is not normal by this time a source of bleeding or hemolysis should be sought.

The development of anemia months or years after operation should always be a source of concern. If the patient has a prosthetic valve, hemolysis should be suspected (see page 524). A combination of fever with anemia raises the possibility of bacterial endocarditis. An iron deficiency anemia is probably due to chronic blood loss; therefore, it should be remembered that patients with prosthetic cardiac valves are not immune to carcinoma of the colon. Look for the usual causes of anemia.

Biochemical Tests

Routine electrolyte examinations should rarely be necessary as part of the follow-up examination. By the time a patient leaves the hospital he should be in electrolyte balance. If prolonged treatment with digitalis and diuretics is necessary, periodic measurement of serum potassium is important to ensure that potassium supplementation is adequate.

In some patients with preoperative impaired renal function the BUN becomes elevated after operation. Renal function may take several weeks to return completely to normal and an elevation of BUN a month after operation is not necessarily a sign of permanent renal damage.

If liver function has been depressed before or after operation, standard tests of function are necessary to confirm that improvement has occurred.

Hemolysis

Hemolysis is a possibility in several situations after cardiac surgery. Any situation in which a leak may occur around or through a valve or intracardiac patch may give rise to hemolysis. Mild jaundice and anemia are the clues. A falling hematocrit not responding to iron or transfusion, and an elevated bilirubin provide objective data. Plasma hemoglobin and haptoglobin levels, an elevated reticulocyte count and a shortened red cell life confirm the clinical diagnosis.

Drug Therapy

Cardiac Drugs

Digitalis Glycosides. The most important function of these is their positive inotropic action. Systolic contractile force and cardiac output are increased and the Starling curve relating left ventricular stroke work to left atrial filling pressure moves upwards and to the left (Fig. 16–5). Stroke volume is increased and elevated ventricular end-diastolic pressure is restored to normal. The heart rate is slowed, especially in patients with congestive failure. This slowing in rate may be not so much a primary action of the drug as a secondary effect of the increase in cardiac output. If there is atrial fibrillation, the frequency of signals from the atrium to the A-V node is so great that many impulses are extinguished within the node. The frequency of ventricular response depends upon the refractory period of the A-V node. Digitalis prolongs the refractory period so that a greater number of atrial signals fail to pass through the A-V node, and the ventricular response becomes slower. Vagal activity is increased, slowing ventricular response.

Digitalis also has important peripheral actions. In normal subjects digitalis induces arteriolar and venous constriction. In patients with congestive failure the opposite occurs and there is an indirect vasodilator action. There is also

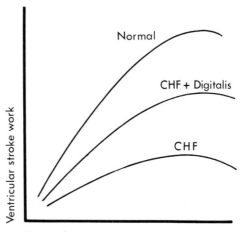

Figure 16–5   The effect of digitalis on the Starling curve is shown. Cardiac function, depressed in congestive failure, is improved by digitalis, but is not restored to normal.

a shift in pooled blood from the portal to the systemic venous bed.

Salutary effects are produced by digitalis in patients with heart disease but without failure. The stress of a chronic pressure load is withstood better by a digitalized myocardium, and with improvement in contractile force the necessity for increased sympathetic tone is reduced. Systemic and pulmonary venous pressures are reduced and symptoms are proportionately alleviated.

The effect of digitalis is in proportion to the dosage. A small effect is achieved by a small dose, and maximal effect is obtained by the maximum tolerable dose.

The effects of digitalis are influenced by several factors, including electrolyte levels (especially potassium), endocrine hormonal actions and other drugs. High serum potassium levels diminish the inotropic effect of digitalis but also reduce the incidence of toxic arrhythmias. Low potassium levels do not affect the inotropism of digitalis, but a low serum potassium, by itself, increases myocardial contractile force.

The electrocardiographic effects of digitalis are characteristic. The earliest effect is a sagging depression of the S–T segment. As digitalis action increases, S–T depression becomes more marked, heart rate slows, and the P–R interval is prolonged. If toxicity develops, multiple ventricular extrasystoles, pulsus bigeminus and various degrees of heart block may appear.

The cardiac glycosides are all toxic and the margin between therapeutic effect and toxicity is quite narrow. If a rapidly metabolized agent such as digoxin is used, toxic manifestations should disappear within 12 hours of the last administration of the drug, but if a long-acting agent such as digitoxin is used, toxic effects will persist.

The common symptoms of toxicity are:

Gastrointestinal—anorexia, nausea, vomiting, abdominal discomfort, diarrhea. Anorexia and nausea usually appear first, and early digitalis toxicity should be suspected in any patient receiving a maintenance dosage who suddenly loses appetite and becomes nauseated.

Cardiac—changes in rate, rhythm and conduction. Ventricular extrasystoles, pulsus bigeminus, paroxysmal tachycardia, bradycardia and, in extreme cases, ventricular tachycardia and fibrillation. Any of these changes should be taken as an indication of toxicity and treated accordingly.

Miscellaneous systemic effects—headache, visual disturbances, skin rashes, and eosinophilia have all been reported. With the exception of headache these symptoms are uncommon.

When a patient develops signs and symptoms of digitalis toxicity three steps must be taken: (a) stop all further doses, (b) measure serum electrolytes, and (c) obtain a new EKG trace. If the potassium concentration is low, supplementary potassium should be given. If the primary manifestation of toxicity is a cardiac arrhythmia, extra potassium may have to be given intravenously. A dose of 3.0–5.0 mEq given slowly IV may immediately stop a bigeminal rhythm or multiple extrasystoles. Even if the serum potassium concentration seems to be within normal limits, intracellular levels may be low, and a small dose of potassium given intravenously may be very beneficial without changing the plasma concentration to a measurable extent.

Antiarrhythmic drugs, quinidine, procaine amide, lidocaine and propanolol may be used when severe digitalis toxicity leads to dangerous supraventricular and ventricular arrhythmias. Great care must be taken in their use because of their propensity to lower cardiac output. Diphenylhydantoin is useful in the conversion of digitalis-induced supraventricular and ventricular arrhythmias to normal sinus rhythm with very little concomitant reduction in cardiac output.

Patients treated chronically with digitalis and diuretics should receive potassium supplements (15 mEq one to three times a day). Potassium should not be given to patients with seriously impaired renal function.

Digitalis Preparations. There are many different preparations available. The commonest in use are:

Digoxin for oral, IM or IV use. Loading dose is 1.0–1.5 mg in divided doses over 24 hours; maintenance dose by mouth is 0.25–0.50 mg per day. Digoxin begins to act within one hour of intravenous administration and within a few hours of an oral dose. Excretion is quite rapid and most of its effectiveness disappears within 48 hours of stopping administration.

Digitoxin (U.S.P.). This is a very potent, slow-acting preparation. The dose is 0.6 mg IV, followed by 0.2–0.4 mg every 4 to 6 hours for a total dose of 1.2 mg. Oral dosage to 0.6 mg twice at 12–hour intervals, then 0.1–0.2 mg per day. After intravenous administration 6 to 10 hours are necessary before its effect begins. After stopping chronic usage, 2 to 3 weeks may elapse before complete regression of action and disappearance of blood levels.

Antiarrhythmic Drugs. Several drugs are used specifically for their antiarrhythmic actions. Other drugs such as potassium have isolated usefulness in the treatment of specialized arrhythmia. The most commonly used antiarrhythmic drugs are described below.

Quinidine. Like many arrhythmic drugs, quinidine increases the refractory period of cardiac muscle, decreases excitability and slows conduction. The drug is absorbed rapidly by mouth. About 15 per cent is excreted and the rest is metabolized. Use of quinidine is indicated by the conversion of atrial fibrillation or flutter, ventricular and nodal tachycardias to normal rhythm. It is useful in the suppression of frequent premature beats. A test dose of 100–200 mgm should be given before regular dosage of 200 mgm every four to six hours. The dose is increased daily to 400 mgm and then to 600 mgm every six hours, to a maximum of 600 mgm every two hours for five doses. Toxic effects (cinchonism) include vertigo,

headache, and tinnitus. Hypotension with widening of the QRS complex occurs sometimes and typical drug rashes are not uncommon.

Lidocaine. Although lidocaine is absorbed after intramuscular administration it is given intravenously in the treatment of arrhythmias. The usefulness of lidocaine is greatest in the emergency treatment of ventricular arrhythmias. Onset of action is almost immediate, and it has an effective half-life of 15 to 20 minutes. Metabolism takes place almost entirely within the liver. The initial dose is 1 mg per Kg which can be repeated after five minutes, or a continuous infusion can be used in a dose of 1 to 2 mg per minute. A convenient dose is 1.0 gm in 500 ml of saline given by microdrip infusion. Toxic side effects are primarily related to the central nervous system. Large doses may cause drowsiness, convulsions or collapse. One of the advantages of this drug is that doses up to 5 mg per Kg do not depress myocardial contractility.

Procaine amide. Absorption of procaine amide from the gastrointestinal tract is effective within 60 to 90 minutes of oral administration. The effect of a single dose lasts 5 to 10 hours. Procaine amide is eliminated unchanged via the kidneys.

Although procaine amide is most effective in the treatment of ventricular arrhythmias it is also useful in the treatment of atrial premature contractions and atrial tachycardia, and is moderately successful in the prevention of recurrent atrial fibrillation. About 90 per cent of patients with ventricular premature contractions respond to this drug.

Daily divided doses of 1.0 to 6.0 gm are used to start treatment. A stable therapeutic level should be obtained within three days. More even levels are obtained by smaller doses every four hours than by larger doses every six hours. Procaine amide can be given intravenously, 100 mg every five minutes, for emergency treatment. Blood pressure should be carefully monitored during such treatment.

Toxic effects, especially after intravenous use, include hypotension, widening of the QRS complex and myocardial depression. Nausea, vomiting and skin rashes may occur. A syndrome similar to systemic lupus erythematosus has also been reported after prolonged oral administration. If the drug is stopped the symptoms slowly disappear.

Anticoagulants. Anticoagulants are given preoperatively to patients with valvular disease, especially mitral disease, atrial fibrillation and a history of peripheral embolism. Some patients may have been receiving anticoagulants for a long time before being seen by the surgeon. It is not necessary to stop therapy completely before operation. If the prothrombin time is greater than 30 per cent of normal at the time of operation unusual bleeding is not usually encountered.

In many such patients anticoagulation is restarted again after operation even if a prosthetic valve has not been inserted. It is difficult to know how long anticoagulation should continue. There is some evidence that stopping anticoagulation leads to a rebound phenomenon with hypercoagulability and an increased likelihood of embolism. But it is also clear that the incidence of embolism after, for instance, a good mitral commissurotomy is much less than that before operation and that the increased flow rate through the valve diminishes the chances of subsequent episodes. No hard and fast rules can be given.

After insertion of a prosthetic valve, anticoagulation is usually started as soon as chest tubes are removed. In spite of conflicting evidence and the hope that a prosthetic valve might be designed which is without embolic complications, most surgeons still anticoagulate patients with prosthetic valves. Most embolic episodes occur within the first year after operation but there is no period beyond which immunity from embolism is assured. If contraindications to anticoagulation (such as peptic ulceration) develop more than a year after insertion of a prosthesis, it is probably safe to stop treatment.

The anticoagulants most commonly used are heparin, bishydroxycoumarin (dicumarol) and sodium warfarin (Coumadin).

Heparin. Heparin inhibits the clotting of blood and acts on all three stages of coagulation. The clotting time is prolonged in proportion to dosage. It is not effective when given by mouth, but is effective after subcutaneous, intramuscular, or intravenous injection. Heparin is metabolized by the liver and has a relatively short half-life; some is excreted in the urine.

Administration for immediate effect is by intermittent intravenous injection. A dose of 1.0 mg per Kg is therapeutically effective and prolongs the clotting time two to two and a half times normal for four to eight hours. When treatment is being initiated, clotting time should be measured prior to injection of the dose and approximately 30 minutes later. This enables the physician to assess the peaks and troughs of therapeutic effectiveness.

Continuous IV administration (200 mg heparin in 500 ml of 5 per cent dextrose in water) gives a more continuous therapeutic benefit but is more difficult to control.

For long-term use the subcutaneous route is necessary. A very fine needle (No. 25 or 27) should be used and injections should not be given repeatedly in the same site. An initial dose of 30,000 to 40,000 units is given and, thereafter, about 20,000 units every 12 to 24 hours. The clotting time should be measured a few times about midway between each dose to try to establish a satisfactory therapeutic level.

Heparin is counteracted by protamine sulfate in an intravenous dose of one to one and a half times the dose of heparin. Antagonistic effects are rapid and clotting time should be normal within seven to ten minutes of administration.

Protamine can itself act as an anticoagulant if given in too large a dose. It can also result in temporary pulmonary hypertension and a reduction in cardiac output if given too rapidly. For these

reasons the appropriate dose of protamine should be diluted in 100 to 150
ml of 5 per cent dextrose and given over
a 10 to 20 minute period.

Bishydroxycoumarin (dicumarol). The
effects of this agent are very similar to
those of warfarin sodium (Coumadin).
The most important action of these drugs
is to depress the prothrombin complex,
but other clotting factors are also
affected. Administration is oral and there
is a latent period of 12 to 24 hours before
an effect is obtained. It is important that
this latent period be taken into account
when treatment is being started and
when the dosage schedule is being
worked out. If the drug is taken in the
afternoon the effect of that dose will not
be measureable until the following day.
(The latent period is longer with warfarin sodium.)

Numerous factors affect the action of
this and similar drugs; among them are
the following. (a) Diet: a change in fat
intake by changing vitamin K absorption
may influence the response. (b) Liver
function: depression of hepatic function,
from whatever cause, increases the patient's susceptibility to the drug. The
development of postoperative serum
hepatitis, for instance, should be an immediate indication for a drastic reduction
in the dosage. (c) Intercurrent diseases:
during minor intercurrent diseases such
as flu, the dosage should be reviewed and
prothrombin times measured more frequently than usual to make sure that
desirable therapeutic levels are maintained. (d) Drugs: sulfonamides, quinine, quinidine steroids and salicylates
in excess of 1.0 gm per day increase
sensitivity to these drugs. These drugs
should either be avoided or increased
vigilance should be maintained if their
use is essential.

The most important complication of
anticoagulant treatment is hemorrhage.
If the prothrombin time is kept between
two to two and a half times the control
time or 20 to 25 per cent of normal,
hemorrhagic complication should be
rare. If the prothrombin time falls below
15 per cent of normal, spontaneous

hemorrhage—retroperitoneal, intracranial, nasopharyngeal, gastrointestinal
or into the urinary tract -- is increasingly
likely. Some hemorrhagic complications
such as bleeding gums may be relatively
trivial, but severe gastrointestinal bleeding may be catastrophic. When bleeding
occurs treatment with the drug should
be stopped. If hemorrhage is not severe
this alone may be adequate. But vitamin
K (2.5 to 5.0 mg by mouth) may have to
be given. In severe cases the dose of
vitamin K may have to be increased to
10 mg parenterally. For immediate effect
transfusions of fresh blood or fresh
frozen plasma will restore coagulation
to normal.

Warfarin sodium (Coumadin). The
initial dose is 20 to 30 mg by mouth followed by a dialy maintenance dose of
2.5 to 10 mg depending upon sensitivity
of the patient to the drug. The latent
period between ingestion and response
is 24 to 36 hours and the effect of a
single dose may last for four to five days.
This delayed action is extremely important in calculating doses and in determining why a dose may seem to be too
small or too great. The prothrombin time
you measure today reflects the dose of
the day before yesterday. The complications and antidotes necessary are the
same as with dicumarol therapy.

Platelet inhibitors. The initiating
feature in the development of a thrombus
is the aggregation of platelets. If this
process could be prevented the subsequent deposition of thrombus could be
avoided. Two functions of platelets can
be measured: (1) platelet aggregation,
which is the tendency of platelets to
stick to each other, and (2) platelet adhesiveness, which is the tendency of
platelets to adhere to foreign surfaces.
Induced diminution in either of these
activities could be beneficial in preventing the development of thrombi
upon prosthetic valves.

Several nonsteroidal anti-inflammatory agents such as aspirin, sodium
salicylate, and sulfinpyrazone have
been found to inhibit ADP-induced
platelet aggregation and to prolong

platelet life. This both explains some of the complications of treatment with these drugs and also raises the possibility of preventing thrombus formation by the administration of these or similar drugs. Patients with prosthetic valves have been given these drugs with inconclusive results, but it seems likely that within the next few years potent agents will be developed to prevent platelet aggregation and thrombus formation.

Diuretics. *Thiazides.* These drugs are effective orally and are useful in the treatment of congestive failure and hypertension. They induce loss of both sodium and potassium, and dietary supplementation with potassium, 1.0 gm three to four times per day, is necessary during prolonged administration. Thiazide drugs are contraindicated if there is renal failure. Eight or nine different drugs in this group are available, all of roughly equal potency. Dosage depends upon the drug used. Toxic effects include skin rashes, gastrointestinal disturbances, hyperglycemia and even diabetes. In susceptible patients a flare-up of gout may occur.

Ethacrynic acid: Furosemide. These are very potent agents which induce a profound diuresis within 30 to 60 minutes of ingestion. Diuresis of both sodium and potassium is greater than with thiazides. Because of the potency of these agents they should not be used unless congestive failure is severe, and even then should be given in small doses, 20 to 50 mg, to see what effect is obtained. These drugs can be given safely when renal function has been impaired.

Antibiotics. The general principles which govern the use of antibiotics obtain in cardiac surgery. Most surgeons give antibiotics prophylactically to cover the period of operation, and the evidence is that infections are thereby reduced. By the time a patient leaves hospital antibiotic administration has usually been stopped.

Antibiotic coverage should be given to all patients with congenital or valvular disease, or after prosthetic replacement, dental work, urologic manipulations, operations for noncardiac disease or intercurrent infections which are more than trivial. Young patients with rheumatic heart disease should continue to take penicillin prophylactically until the age of 35.

Special Techniques

Phonocardiography

Phonocardiograms are not made routinely in the followup of all types of cardiac patient, but they are useful when following patients with prosthetic heart valves. One of the earliest signs of mechanical malfunction of a prosthetic valve is a change in the heart sounds. In following a large group of patients it is impossible to recall precisely the exact nature of the heart sounds from visit to visit. The phonocardiogram therefore makes a good documentary record of the sounds and provides measurable objective data of changes.

The first sound of a normally functioning aortic prosthesis is louder than the second, and the magnitude of aortic opening sound to aortic closing sound (AO/AC) should be greater than 0.7 — a ratio of 0.5 to 0.7 is borderline and a ratio smaller than 0.5 is presumptive evidence of aortic ball variance.

Sound Spectrography

By recording heartsounds on tape and then transmitting recorded sounds through a sound spectrograph, a contoured representation of sound intensity can be obtained. This has been used to document aortic ball valve sounds. An aortic opening sound of 19,000 to 14,000 cycles per sec. is satisfactory, but an opening sound of less than 13,000 cycles per sec. is suspicious of ball variance.[6]

Ultrasound

Echocardiography, the use of ultrasound waves to determine certain intra-

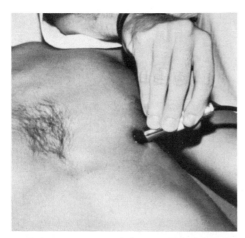

Figure 16–6 The technique of taking an echocardiogram. The crystal is placed on the precordium and directed toward the valve to be examined (the mitral valve, in this instance).

cardiac functions, has developed in the past few years to a state of useful precision. A crystal from which sound waves emanate in the ultrasound frequencies is placed against the chest wall (Fig. 16–6). The waves penetrate the thorax and return as echoes to be picked up and translated on an oscilloscope into discernible patterns. The technique is useful in that an immediate answer is obtained, there is no discomfort to the patient, and an objective measurable record is obtained. Two functions can be measured by this technique that are useful in the follow-up of postoperative patients.

1. Measurement of Valve Movement. The movement of valves, both natural and prosthetic, can be measured with precision.[8] It is easier to examine movements of the mitral and tricuspid valves than of the aortic. To examine the mitral valve, the crystal is placed at the cardiac apex and directed upward toward the right shoulder tip along the axis of the mitral valve. The tricuspid valve is examined with the crystal in the right fourth interspace to the right of the sternum pointing slightly downward and to the left. The aortic valve is examined with the crystal in the right supraclavicular fossa close to the attachment of the sternomastoid muscle. The beam is directed downward and to the left along the axis of the first part of the ascending aorta and through the aortic valve.

Natural valves reflect the sound waves in characteristic patterns. The movement of the cusp can be measured on the tracing in mm, and the restricted movements of a stenotic valve or excessive motion of a prolapsing cusp are also measurable (Fig. 16–7). A prosthetic valve reflects sound waves from its component parts, cage or struts, ball or disc, and suture ring. Echoes from the cage and suture ring remain relatively stationary while the echo from the ball moves more extensively. The physical nature of the moving ball or disc is important in correct interpretation of the waves. Sound waves, for instance, pass more slowly through silastic rubber than through normal tissue. Waves that pass through a silastic ball, therefore, take longer to return than those which pass through tissue, and the object may be interpreted as being further away from the crystal than it actually is.

The movement of a mitral prosthesis can be measured to within 0.1 cm. This degree of accuracy is sufficient to determine a significant reduction in motion due to the buildup of clot or sticking of the poppet.

The technique is probably not of sufficient accuracy to determine small changes in the diameter of silastic ball poppets in aortic valves, but gross changes in movement can be determined.

2. Measurements of Left Ventricular Size and Stroke Volume. Measurements of left ventricular size and stroke volume can be derived from relatively simple measurements of the distance between echoes from the anterior and posterior walls of the ventricle, and movement of the annulus of the mitral valve. This method provides a noninvasive method for measuring these parameters continuously, for preoperative and postoperative evaluation.

3. Pericardial Effusion. Echocardiog-

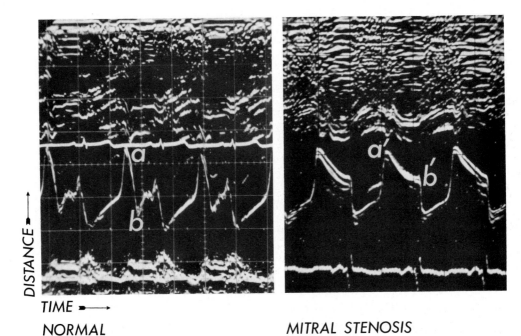

DISTANCE ➡

TIME ➡

NORMAL

MITRAL STENOSIS

Figure 16–7   Echocardiograms of normal and stenotic mitral valves. Because the tracing is a function of both distance and time the slopes of ab and a'b' depend upon the distance moved by the mitral cusp and the speed with which the cusp moves. In *A*, ab has a steep slope indicating rapid extensive movement. In *B*, the slope is shallower because the stiff stenotic valve moves neither as far nor as fast as normal.

raphy is a useful and accurate method for determining the presence of pericardial effusions. Echoes are received from the anterior and posterior pericardium and ventricular walls. The distance between the pericardial and ventricular echoes is a measure of the size of the effusion.

Scanning

Detection of a pericardial effusion is sometimes difficult. The patient presents with radiologically discernible cardiomegaly. If the heart has previously been small and congestive failure has not developed, the increase in heart size is almost always due to fluid, but if the heart has previously been large the detection of intrapericardial fluid may not be easy.

A radionuclide such as ^{131}I or ^{99m}Tc is injected intravenously and a scan made of the thorax. This scan can then be superimposed upon an AP chest film. Normally very little distance separates the cardiac from the pulmonary and hepatic blood pools and the cardiac scan can be almost exactly superimposed upon the cardiac shadow. If the scan is less than 80 per cent of the cardiac shadow or if there is an appreciable distance between the cardiac and pulmonary scans, the inference is that the pericardium is greatly thickened or there is a pericardial effusion (Fig. 16–8). The smallest effusion detectable by this means is 200 ml.

COMPLICATIONS

Complications Common to All Operations

1. Postcardiotomy Syndromes

The various syndromes have been comprehensively reviewed by Kirsh

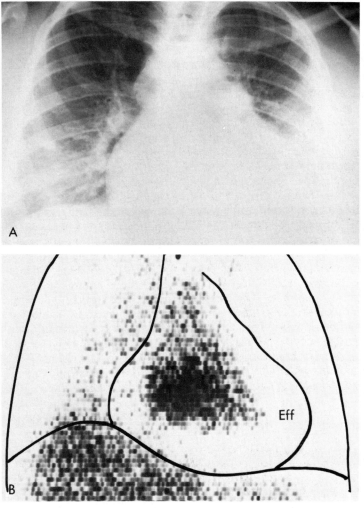

Figure 16–8 AP film and radioactive scan of a patient with a large pericardial effusion. The cardiac shadow, radiologically, is large *(A)*. The scan *(B)* demonstrates a small central blood-filled cardiac shadow (dark area) surrounded by a wide light area of effusion (Eff) which does not pick up the radionuclide.

(1970). Three have been recognized, but as the etiology of none is known the relationship between them is also obscure.

The *postpericardiotomy syndrome* is characterized by pericarditis and pleuro-pericardial involvement with fever, chest pain and friction rubs. It usually develops two to three weeks after operation. A fever of 101° to 104° F. is common. The patient feels generally unwell with sweats, chills and myalgia. The white cell count is elevated with a normal lymphocyte count. Improvement takes one to four weeks. Activities should be restricted: aspirin, 10 gr q.i.d., may be sufficient to alleviate symptoms. Steroids are rarely necessary. If the patient is receiving anticoagulants and salicylates are contraindicated, acetaminophen is a useful substitute.

The *postperfusion syndrome* is not as common as the postpericardiotomy syndrome and occurs in only about 5 per cent of patients after operations in which extracorporeal circulation has been used. Fever, lymphocytosis and splenomegaly are the distinguishing features. Atypical lymphocytes, constituting 25 to 80 per cent of the white count, appear in the blood soon after the development of fever and persist for as long as three months. The syndrome usually starts within the first six weeks after operation and lasts for two to four weeks. The course is benign. Pleuropericardial complications are not a feature. Treatment consists of aspirin or other antipyretics. There is strongly suggestive evidence that this syndrome may be caused by a cytomegalic virus transmitted by blood transfusion.

A *biphasic postcardiotomy syndrome* has also been described by Kahn (1967). The first phase starts a few days after operation with fever, tachycardia and a vesicular periorbital rash. The second phase starts three to six weeks later with similar fever, perioral lesions and pleuropericardial manifestations. Atypical lymphocytes are found in the blood smear but not in such high proportion as in the postperfusion syndrome.

2. Infection

Infection may appear in the late postoperative period in two ways: (a) as a wound infection, or (b) as bacterial endocarditis or septicemia.

Wound infection becomes apparent with all the classic local signs of calor, dolor, rubor and tumor. If an infected stitch is the source of trouble it must be removed. If infection involves the sternal stitches a decision must be made about the stability of the sternum, the possibility of deep mediastinal infection and even the possibility of sternal osteomyelitis. A superficial wound incision may be a minor complication, and a mediastinal infection with sternal dehiscence is potentially catastrophic. If an infected sinus grows along the tract of an infected suture the patient may have to be readmitted to hospital for curettage of the tract.

Bacterial endocarditis is a potential hazard in all patients with intracardiac defects before or after operation. After valve replacement infection develops in a small percentage of patients, with perhaps slightly greater frequency after graft replacement than after prosthetic replacement.

The patient with infection presents with some signs and symptoms similar to those of the postcardiotomy syndromes. Fever, elevated white count and splenomegaly are found. But perhaps the most important immediately distinguishing feature is the obvious illness of the patient with septicemia and endocarditis, whereas most patients with postcardiotomy syndromes maintain a good appetite and feel reasonably well in spite of fever. Changing murmurs, petechiae, emboli and splinter hemorrhages may be found. Numerous blood cultures must be made as soon as the diagnosis is suspected and before antibiotic treatment is started. Although the prognosis is grave if infection develops on a replaced valve, recovery is possible, sometimes after prolonged antibiotic treatment and sometimes after removal and replacement of the infected valve.

3. Congestive Failure

Congestive failure must not be taken as a satisfactory diagnosis, per se. The physician must always look beyond the immediate situation to determine the underlying cause. Postoperatively, congestive failure may be due to a continuation of the cardiac problem for which the operation was performed or it may be due to the development of a new complication.

If the patient was in chronic failure before operation, weeks or months may elapse before failure disappears in spite of a hemodynamically excellent result. Severe myocardial fibrosis or coronary disease may slow down or prevent total recovery.

Congestive failure occurs after operations for congenital as well as acquired disease. After total correction of the tetralogy of Fallot many patients are left with persistent right ventricular hypertension, a closed interventricular septum, and a right ventricle recovering from a large incision. Congestive failure is common, but almost always responds satisfactorily to standard management with digitalis and diuretics.

The most ominous onset of failure is that which occurs after a period, perhaps a long period, of well-being. The first suspicion must always be that something has gone awry with the technical result of the operation. A patch on a septal defect may partially dehisce, a previously opened valve may have slowly restenosed, or a prosthetic valve may no longer be functioning adequately. Technical problems are usually fairly easy to pinpoint. Recatheterization may be necessary to confirm and measure a reopened shunt, the development of a new murmur being the warning clue. Only after it is certain that the result of the operation is still technically intact should other sources of trouble be invoked. Myocardial disease, coronary disease, or systemic hypertension may be responsible. Myocardial factors are most difficult to diagnose and are often established only by elimination of other causes, including findings of decreased myocardial contractility or elevated end diastolic pressures.

The treatment of congestive failure in the postoperative patient is no different from that prescribed in other circumstances. Immediate recourse to increased diuretics and salt restriction is not always necessary. The patient's activities, diet and habits should be reviewed; he may have been indulging, soon after operation, in activities which are too strenuous, and sometimes a short period of bed rest is all that is necessary to restore compensation. If failure is severe and a technical problem exists, the patient must first be admitted to hospital; failure is then treated and the hemodynamic situation and the necessity for reoperation is reassessed after failure has abated.

4. Wound Problems

Disruption. If a thoracotomy wound disrupts at all, it almost always does so before the patient leaves hospital. Infection is the commonest cause of late disruption and must be treated accordingly. Not all disruptions of sternotomy wounds must undergo reoperation. If there is no infection, the skin is intact and the wound is stable from a ventilatory point of view, the final endpoint may be firm fibrous union. Minor degrees of sternal movement and clicking may be annoying to the patient but may be preferable to another operation and the risk of introducing infection where none already exists.

The midline sternotomy is the most frequently used incision for cardiac operations. Cosmetically it leaves much to be desired. It protrudes above a fashionable level in girls and often heals as a wide scar, occasionally as a true keloid or hypertrophic scar. Painful keloidal healing is difficult to deal with. Excision and resuture may result in an acceptable scar, and local injections of hydrocortisone may also relieve symptoms and diminish scar formation.

In children a pigeon-breast deformity may develop after midline sternotomy. This can, in part, be avoided by taking good periosteal sutures as part of the closure. These stitches tend to prevent eversion of the sternal edges in the flexible juvenile chest.

5. Rhythm Problems

Arrhythmias and conduction problems are common. Some begin during the operation and persist; others start postoperatively and may be intermittent or permanent.

Atrial Fibrillation. This is probably the most frequent arrhythmia. Provided the rate of ventricular response is adequately controlled with digitalis, the patient will probably tolerate the irregularity. Cardiac output can, however, be increased by restoring normal sinus rhythm. If an attempt is made at electrical conversion within the first two weeks after operation normal rhythm may be achieved but seldom persists. If there is a delay of four to six weeks the likelihood of permanent conversion is greater. At the time of electrical conversion the patient should be fully digitalized and should receive quinidine after conversion. Patients with atrial fibrillation also tend to have a slightly higher incidence of peripheral emboli after valve replacement than patients in sinus rhythm.

Atrial Flutter. Atrial flutter sometimes develops after operations which involve the right atrium such as closure of an atrial septal defect. The arrhythmia is sometimes resistant to therapy and sinus rhythm cannot be restored. The usual treatment is full digitalization followed by a course of quinidine. Electrical conversion is rarely of value in restoring sinus rhythm.

Nodal Rhythm. Nodal rhythms do not seem to be as persistent as atrial arrhythmias. A nodal rhythm is quite common at the end of operation but usually disappears within a few days. An occasional patient develops chronic nodal bradycardia. This may reduce cardiac output to the point of disability; if the rate remains constantly below 55 per minute, thought should be given to the need for a permanent transvenous pacemaker.

Heart Block. Most instances of complete heart block after cardiac operations are iatrogenic. Patients with endocardial cushion defects, large ventricular septal defects and tetralogy of Fallot run a small (5 per cent) risk of induced heart block. With detailed anatomical knowledge of the course of the conduction bundle and satisfactory surgical techniques for placing sutures without injuring the bundle, the risk should be small. Complete block may develop during aortic valve replacement and, very rarely, with mitral valve replacement. In some cases, the block is temporary, but if block persists for four weeks after inception a permanent pacemaker should be inserted. Two drugs are

of limited usefulness in complete block — isoproterenol hydrochloride and ephedrine. Steroids appear to be of benefit in patients with postinfarction block.

Isoproterenol may be used intravenously in an emergency — 0.05 to 0.1 mg, or 1 to 2 mg in 500 ml of 5 per cent dextrose in water. Sublingual absorption (10 to 15 mg) is sometimes helpful. Ephedrine 15 to 60 mg by mouth, has a beneficial effect in some patients. Prednisone 10 to 15 mg per day may be tried if there are no other contraindications and especially if myocardial ischemia rather than direct mechanical damage to the bundle is suspected.

There is some evidence that prolonged iatrogenic heart block in children may not have as serious a prognosis as was once thought. But with increasing reliability of pacemakers the risks of a fatal standstill would not seem to be worth taking, and insertion of a pacemaker is advisable.

6. Respiratory Complications

By the time the patient leaves the hospital most complications have been successfully treated. A few complications may become chronic and require continued management.

Tracheal or Subglottic Stenosis. After prolonged ventilation by a respirator with a cuffed endotracheal tube, there is some mucosal damage in almost every patient. Minor degrees of noncritical stenosis may occur unnoticed in many patients. If severe stenosis occurs it may not become manifest for several weeks until the patient returns with respiratory distress and stridor.

If ventilation has been through an oro- or nasotracheal tube the commonest site for stenosis is subglottic. On laryngoscopy subglottic swelling with a slit-like orifice can be seen. If ventilation has been via a tracheostomy the site of obstruction may be at the healed tracheostoma or lower down, at the level of the cuff or tip of the endotracheal tube.

When the patient is first seen he may be in acute and potentially lethal respiratory distress. If the obstruction is subglottic a tracheostomy below the obstruction will afford relief, or it may be possible to pass an endotracheal tube through the narrow passage. If the obstruction is secondary to a previous tracheostomy, obtaining a good airway may be difficult. In the case of stenosis at an old tracheostomy, reopening the wound may permit the passage of a tube into the distal trachea.

Stenotic areas lower down pose the greatest problem. It is difficult to dilate these areas via the larynx through a bronchoscope. But bronchoscopy may be necessary initially in order to determine the site of obstruction. Reopening the tracheostomy provides better and closer access to the stenosis. Depending upon the site of obstruction, an uncuffed tracheostomy tube or a longer endotracheal tube may be passed through the narrow part.

Subglottic obstruction is due to granulation tissue and swelling. Radiotherapy has been used successfully in reducing the size of these masses. Most of the more distal obstructions are due to contracting scar tissue although there may be superimposed edema. Tracheograms should be made to delineate the problem.

There are two long-term solutions — first, repeated dilatation; second, resection and repair. Through a tracheostomy the distal areas of obstruction can be dilated with Hegar dilators. Topical anesthesia is necessary. At first dilatation may be necessary every 48 hours. Eventually a permanent lumen of adequate caliber may be achieved. If dilatation is not successful, definitive repair is the only solution.

Pleural Effusion: Hemothorax. Small effusions may collect because of congestive failure, and in most instances there is no need to tap them. If respiratory distress is due to excessive accumulation of fluid, thoracentesis* may be necessary.

The management of hemothorax is a source of discussion. If a patient acquires a sizeable hemothorax, should or should it not be evacuated surgically and a decortication carried out? Much of the information about the management of these cases comes from military sources and from observing the course of events in traumatic cases. This information may not be directly applicable.

If the hemothorax is small or moderate and does not contribute to respiratory distress, and if there is no evidence of infection within it, it should be left alone. Aspiration is not necessary and may introduce infection, and it is inadvisable if the patient is receiving anticoagulants. Hemothoraces of this magnitude will be absorbed quickly without residual constrictive fibrothorax. In children even quite large collections will be absorbed if given time. If the hemothorax is large or seems to be infected, tube thoracotomy,† followed possibly by decortication, may be necessary.

7. Complications of Valve Replacement

Embolism. Peripheral embolism as a major complication of valve replacement became apparent soon after the first prosthetic valves were inserted. During the first few years of experience with valve replacement, the incidence of embolism was very high — 10 to 15 per cent after aortic replacement and 30 to 50 per cent after mitral valve replacement. Research indicated that the emboli arise from junctional areas between cloth and metal. Fibrin and pseudoendothelium adhere to the cloth but break away from the metal. By covering metallic parts with cloth this problem can be significantly reduced. With most valves used in the past three years the incidence of embolism after valve replacement of all sorts has been reduced to 3 to 5 per cent.

Embolism after homograft replacement is not unknown, although it is less than that after prosthetic replacement.

---

*Thoracentesis is discussed in Chapter 15.

†Chest tube is discussed in Chapter 15.

Some authors, Gonzalez-Lavin and Ross (1970),[5] and Barratt-Boyes and Roche (1969)[1] have reported large series without embolism, but Wallace et al. (1971)[20] reported a 2.5 per cent incidence.

It is important to realize that only a small proportion (about 1.5 per cent) of embolic episodes are fatal, and about an equal percentage result in residual damage. Most episodes are transient and without sequelae.

The value of long-term anticoagulation has not been clearly established, although in some reported series there have been large differences in embolic rates between anticoagulated and non-anticoagulated patients. Most surgeons feel that carefully controlled anticoagulation significantly reduces the incidence of emboli and should be started unless strong contraindications exist.

Hemolysis. After valve replacement, hemolysis is usually an indication of valve malfunction. Hemolysis has been reported in patients with a Beall disc mitral valve without mechanical malfunction. Perivalvular leaks, ball variance, and clots on the suture ring causing leakage through the valve can hemolyze cells.

If hemolysis is mild the hematocrit can be maintained with iron therapy. If, however, the hematocrit continues to fall, blood transfusion may be necessary. When hemolysis is severe, even transfusion at regular intervals is inadequate, and reoperation is then mandatory.

Other factors must be considered. Prosthetic valves with silastic poppets may develop ball variance, and the hemolysis is then a sign of variance. If other evidence of variance coexists, reoperation becomes a matter of some urgency. If the prosthetic valve is of a type (e.g., metal ball) in which variance is not possible, other causes for hemolysis must be considered.

Syndromes of Prosthetic Valve Failure. Increasing long-term experience with valve replacement has made it abundantly clear that no type of valve—prosthetic, homograft or heterograft—is devoid of problems. Although some of these difficulties have been referred to elsewhere in this chapter the subject is of such importance that the various syndromes should be collectively described. Although the clinical manifestations are those of congestive failure, embolism, hemolysis and arrhythmias, it is perhaps easiest to look separately at the difficulties with aortic and mitral valves.[7]

Aortic valve failure. When faced by a patient with probable valve failure it is very important to know precisely what type of valve has been used. Ball variance, for instance, has only been reported in valves with silastic balls. Not all valves with silastic poppets have a high incidence of variance, whereas some, such as the Starr-Edwards model 1000 aortic valve (no longer used), had a high incidence of variance. Disc valves (Kay-Shiley), free-floating valves, or tilting valves (Bjork-Shiley, Wada) are subject to cocking and fixed tilting of the disc. Homografts and heterografts are liable to cusp rupture and retraction and, occasionally, massive calcification.

Loss of the opening valve sound is pathognomonic of ball variance, but this sign is found in only about 25 per cent of patients with variance. If still present, but diminished in intensity so that the opening sound is less than half the intensity of the closing sound, variance is likely. Sound spectrograms can detect loss of high frequency components better than phonocardiography.

The late appearance of hemolysis, failure, emboli, arrhythmias and new murmurs should all be taken as evidence of a mechanical problem. Palpitation, dizzy spells, syncope and angina may also be warning signs. When these symptoms are associated with jaundice or anemia the diagnosis should be assumed unless there is overwhelming evidence to the contrary. Prosthetic aortic stenosis is due to a clot that prevents normal movement of the poppet, either as a collar on the suture ring or a thickening around the struts or apex of the cage. Aortic insufficiency, however, is most likely to be due to uneven accumulation of a clot, permitting leakage around the poppet, or a leak around the fixation ring.

Aortic insufficiency, ranging between minor and severe, is a common complication of homograft valve replacement. The late appearance of an aortic diastolic murmur may signify development of a tear in a cusp and the patient's progress must be watched very carefully in case insufficiency increases to produce hemodynamic difficulty. A diastolic murmur without a change in diastolic pressure is not of hemodynamic importance, but may presage impending difficulties.

Mitral valve failure. As with aortic valves the single most important warning indication is the development of symptoms after a good result without trouble.

Mechanical problems with mitral prostheses are most frequently associated with clinical evidence of pulmonary congestion and left-sided failure. If the signs and symptoms are persistent, a "steady-state" problem such as a valve leak is probably the cause. If paroxysmal episodes predominate, an intermittent cause such as acute tilting or sticking of a ball or disc is probably present. Progressive evidence of mitral stenosis indicates a buildup of clot on the valve that restricts motion but preserves competence, whereas evidence of insufficiency indicates that some process is preventing proper closure of the poppet, or that there is perivalvular leakage.

Variance has been uncommonly found in mitral ball valves. Disc valves may wear at the edges and become notched.[12] When this happens free movement is impaired. Usually the initiating force is an accumulation of fibrin between the disc and the ventricular wall which pushes the disc against the opposing struts. A metal disc may prevent notching but does not prevent cocking and tilting. As soon as one of these syndromes is suspected every possible means must be used to confirm or deny the diagnosis. Auscultation, phonocardi-ography, spectrography, ultrasound, radiology (including fluoroscopy and angiocardiography), and laboratory data should all be used in evaluation.

If the evidence points definitively or strongly to a diagnosis of mechanical malfunction, whether of the aortic or the mitral valve, reoperation should be planned for an early date. The mortality rate for emergency reoperation is 60 to 80 per cent, but for a semi-elective reoperation the mortality rate is only 10 to 15 per cent.

8. Congestive Failure

If a patient develops left ventricular failure after valve replacement, two questions must be answered. Is there some problem with the replaced valve? Is failure due to myocardial or coronary disease? Clinical examination may or may not provide the answer. If there is a new murmur or a louder murmur than before, or if valve sounds have changed, a valve defect must be suspected. If failure supervenes without these changes endocardial or myocardial fibrosis may be the cause. When failure begins soon after operation it may be due to too early activity, inadequate digitalization, or improper adjustment of diet or diuretics. When, however, failure starts after a period of improvement and well-being, other causes must be sought. Assessment must first be made of valve function, using radiologic, ultrasound, phonocardiographic and other necessary methods. Cardiac catheterization and angiocardiography may be necessary to demonstrate perivalvular leaks because not all of these are clinically audible.

Management depends upon the findings. Late left ventricular endocardial fibrosis has been described after ball valve replacement of the mitral valve and occurs to some extent after all types of prosthetic mitral replacement. The lesion is a response to turbulence and the impingement of (Fig. 16–9) ventricular filling jets on the endocardium. Clinically, patients with this problem present

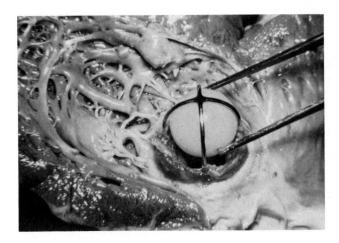

Figure 16–9 Left ventricular endocardial fibrosis one year after insertion of a prosthetic mitral valve. Fibrosis of this type is due to the effects of turbulent flow emitting through the valve and striking the ventricular wall.

with congestive failure; management is difficult because a precise diagnosis is not possible, nor is there specific treatment.

Coronary disease should be treated according to the usual indications. Coronary ostial stenosis due to a jet lesion from an aortic prosthesis has been successfully treated, and this lesion and more distal occlusions could be treated by saphenous vein bypass.

PACEMAKERS

The necessity for a pacemaker may be either temporary or permanent.

Temporary pacing may be required (a) after cardiac operations, (b) after myocardial infarction, (c) when permanent pacing fails and before permanent pacing is re-established, and (d) before placement of a permanent pacemaker.

The indications for use of a permanent pacemaker are: (1) complete heart block in an adult with a rate less than 50 per minute and with Stokes Adams syncopal attacks, congestive failure, or functional disability because of low cardiac output; (2) failure to respond to medical treatment by establishment of an adequate heart rate; (3) symptomatic bradycardia without complete heart block; and (4) iatrogenic complete

heart block which has persisted for longer than six weeks.

Pacemakers may be classified as *fixed rate* in which the rate is present at the factory; *variable fixed rate* in which there is a possibility of changing the rate, but which always delivers a regular signal to the heart, regardless of intrinsic cardiac rhythm; *synchronous* in which the atrial impulse is picked up by a special electrode and used to trigger delivery of an impulse to the ventricular; and *demand* in which the R-wave is used either to stimulate or to inhibit the impulse generated by the power source. Demand pacemakers are most useful in patients with intermittent conduction problems.

Temporary pacing is established by passing a transvenous electrode percutaneously via a subclavian vein into the right ventricle. If it is not possible to enter the subclavian vein percutaneously a cut-down is made of an external jugular or cephalic vein and the lead passed into the vein under direct vision. The external end of the lead is attached to a battery-operated power source which can be arranged in a sling to enable the patient to be mobile.

Insertion of Endocardial Leads

Temporary. Temporary pacemaker leads are inserted using a technique similar to that for subclavian vein cannulation.* Under local anesthesia in the fluoroscopy room a large No. 14g needle is inserted into the subclavian vein. A No. 5 temporary pacing electrode is passed easily through this and the needle withdrawn. Positioning of the electrode in the right ventricle is done under fluoroscopic control. The lead is firmly attached to the skin by a stitch.

Permanent. There are several techniques for installing a permanent pacemaker, but only one will be described in detail (Fig. 16-10). The type of anesthesia depends upon whether or not the patient already has a temporary pacemaker lead. If temporary pacing is controlling the heart rate, general anesthesia is safe and may be desirable. If the rate is not being controlled, local anesthesia is safer.

The patient is positioned on his back with the left arm outstretched. Drapes are arranged to expose the area from the midline to the midaxillary line and from the level of the xiphoid to the line of the jaw and trapezius muscle. Two incisions are possible and depend upon the individual potential for subcutaneous pockets. If a battery pocket would best be made under the pectoral fold (e.g., in someone who has plenty of subcutaneous fat and space), a one and one half inch incision is made over the deltopectoral groove parallel to the clavicle. A second incision is made later, below and lateral to the first, parallel to the pectoral fold. In a thinner patient a longer incision is made, through which a pocket can be made under the pectoralis major muscle. Through the first incision the cephalic vein is exposed and traced to its entrance into the subclavian vein. Two ligatures are placed around the vein and the distal one is tied. A small incision is made in the vein and the lead passed medially and positioned under fluoroscopic control. The tip of the lead should be wedged in the apex of the right ventricle. When a good position has been achieved, a "jumper" cable with alligator clips is attached to the outer end of the endocardial lead and taken to an external power source. Pacing is tested through the newly placed lead. If pacing is satisfactory the stylet wires are removed and the position of the lead is re-examined and pacing retested.

If a single large incision has been made the leads can now be attached to the power source, while any temporary pacing system is disconnected. The power source is then buried under the pectoral muscle in a pocket of suitable size.

When only a small incision has been made for exposure of the cephalic vein, a second incision is made parallel to the pectoral fold. A subcutaneous pocket is developed, and a tunnel made from the pocket to the first incision with a long clamp. A clamp is then passed through the tunnel from above downward and a chest tube, or similar tube is drawn upward through the tunnel. The ends of the leads are pushed firmly into the open end of the tube, which is then withdrawn downward, pulling the leads through the tunnel. The ability to pace should again be tested in case the manipulation might have displaced the lead tip. The lead is fixed in the power source which is buried within the pocket. A small rubber drain is brought out from the pocket through a dependent exit. Before the patient leaves hospital an EKG and chest x-ray and x-rays of the batteries should be made for future reference.

Changing of Pacemaker Battery

For elective changing of a pacemaker battery the patient is admitted to hospital one day before the operation, and can usually be discharged 24 hours following operation after satisfactory function of the new battery has been confirmed.

The patient is positioned on the table with the battery location suitably exposed. Electrocardiogram leads are

---

*Subclavian vein cannulation—see discussion in Chapter 3.

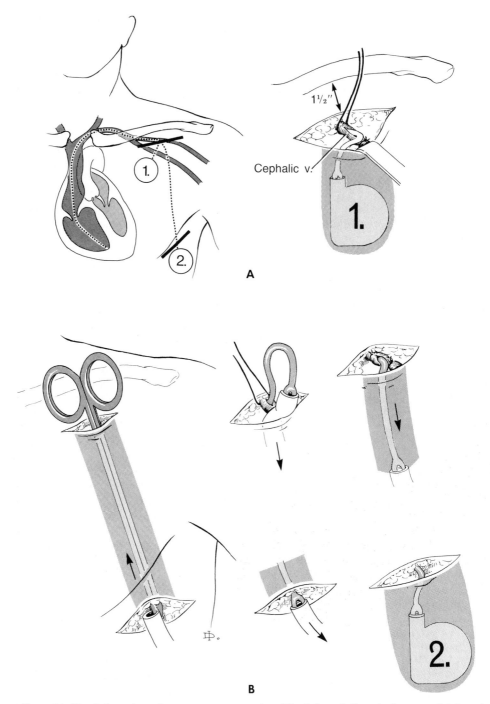

Figure 16–10 A. Insertion of transvenous pacemaker. The left cephalic vein is exposed below the clavicle and the lead passed into the right ventricle. The same incision may be made large enough to make a subcutaneous or submuscular pocket for the generator. *B.* Insertion of transvenous pacemaker. A pocket for the generator may be made subcutaneously below the pectoral fold. The pacemaker leads are easily drawn downward through a tunnel after temporarily inserting them within the open end of a chest tube.

attached for continuous monitoring. Under local anesthesia (1 per cent Xylocaine, without epinephrine) an incision is made over the battery, usually by reopening the old wound. The smooth endothelialized pocket around the battery is opened widely enough to permit exteriorization of the battery. Depending upon the system for attachment of the endocardial leads to the battery, the appropriate connections are loosened. An alligator clip lead is made ready and led off the table to an external battery source. With a minimum of delay the battery is detached from the leads and the alligator clips immediately fastened to the bare ends of the endocardial leads. Cessation of pacing can thereby be reduced to a few seconds.

The external power source should be provided with a variable input so that the threshold required to pace the heart can be measured and noted for future reference. The new battery is brought into proximity to the lead ends, the alligator clips are removed and the connection made between leads and new battery with minimal delay. If any problems of manipulation arise, the leads are immediately withdrawn and reconnected to the external power source, which should not be turned off until reconnection to the new battery has been safely accomplished.

The battery is replaced in its pocket. A quarter inch rubber drain is brought via a small stabwound to the exterior and the pocket is liberally irrigated with bacitracin before resuturing of the wound in layers.

The drain can be removed within 24 hours and stitches may be removed after seven days.

Assessment of Pacemaker Failure

The causes of failure to pace are (1) battery failure, (2) breakage of lead, (3) dislodgement of endocardial lead, (4) failure of electrical component other than battery, (4) perforation of endocardial lead through myocardium into pericardium, and (6) fibrosis around lead resulting in increased electrical resistance.

With these causes in mind the following tests should be made when a patient presents with pacemaker failure:

1. Is the pacemaker pacing but the patient not picking up the impulse? Examine the EKG. The pacemaker spikes should be visible if the batteries are still working.

2. Is the impulse strong enough to cause pacing? Measurement of the pacemaker artifact on the EKG is deceptive, but it may be of help if the measurement can be compared with a similar previous tracing. X-ray examination of the batteries can determine if they have become seriously rundown. The time since implantation of the batteries will also be a valuable clue. Most batteries should last 24 to 30 months.

3. Is the impulse getting to the heart? Take x-rays to examine for fractured leads. Several views should be taken from different angles. X-rays will also demonstrate a change in position of a lead or apparent perforation of the myocardium. If a specific cause such as a lead fracture or worn-out batteries can be determined, appropriate steps can be taken to remedy the situation. If a cause cannot be determined, exteriorize the battery under local anesthesia, remove the leads from the battery and attach them by jumper cable to an external power source. The threshold for pacing can then be determined. If the threshold is normal, the power source should be renewed, but if it is excessive, the old lead may have to be removed and replaced by another. If no pacing can be achieved, the electrode is probably fractured and must be replaced.

Transvenous leads may become fixed by fibrosis to the tricuspid valve or the right ventricular endocardium. Attempting to pull out such a fixed lead by force is hazardous. If the lead does not come out easily the safest course is to insert a second lead by an alternative route.

PERICARDIAL PROBLEMS

Pericardial Effusion

The clinical manifestations of pericardial effusion depend upon the nature of the underlying disease and the hemodynamic changes due to the effusion. Trauma, uremia, infections, neoplasms and collagen diseases are among the many possible causes. In some instances the primary cause is obvious, in others a detailed search must be made for the cause, and open pericardial and myocardial biopsy may be a necessary part of the investigation.

Fatigue, dyspnea, orthopnea, abdominal swelling and peripheral edema are the presenting features. Venous pressure is elevated and engorged neck veins are easily seen. Precordial activity is diminished, but there is evidence by palpation and percussion of an enlarged heart. Radiologically a large globular heart shadow is seen, with elimination of the usual indentations along the cardiac borders.

Special diagnostic investigations include cardiac catheterization with angiography, scanning with radioactive isotopes and echocardiography. The diagnostic intracardiac pressures are a raised venous pressure, and elevated end-diastolic pressure in both ventricles. Systemic pressure and cardiac output are both reduced. If the right atrium is filled with radiopaque dye the distance between the atrial wall and the edge of the cardiac shadow can be measured and represents the depth of effusion. When severe tamponade supervenes, the patient is clinically in shock. He is cool, peripherally cyanosed, with a small, thready, rapid pulse; cardiac output is diminished acutely in spite of high venous pressure.

The intrapericardial volume necessary to induce tamponade is variable and depends, in part, upon the rapidity of accumulation of fluid. Pericardium does not stretch acutely and, therefore, even 150 ml of effusion accumulated rapidly in a previously normal sac may elevate intrapericardial pressure sufficiently to reduce venous return and impede diastolic filling. If, however, the development of effusion is slower, the pericardium may have time to stretch and several hundred ml may accumulate without tamponade.

In either circumstance removal of a relatively small (25 to 50 ml) volume may reduce intrapericardial pressure sufficiently to improve cardiac function.

Never decide, therefore, that there cannot be tamponade because the volume of pericardial fluid seems to be too small. Nor should a conclusion be reached that a large effusion should automatically result in tamponade.

Pericardiocentesis

Before embarking upon elective pericardiocentesis examine the scanning and radiologic evidence carefully to determine if the effusion is loculated and to assess the size of effusion.

There are three routes of entrance into the pericardium: (a) through the angle between the xiphoid process and the left costal margin, (b) at the cardiac apex, and (c) through the left fourth or fifth interspace just lateral to the sternum. The preferred route is (a) because there is the least chance of damaging neighboring structures—lung, internal mammary artery, left anterior descending coronary artery—via this route.

The patient is positioned in a sitting position elevated to about 45°, and the lower chest and upper abdomen are thoroughly prepared and draped (Fig. 16–11). Under local anesthesia a long 20g needle is inserted in the angle between the left costal margin and the xiphoid process in an upward and posterior direction. The needle is inserted with a 20 ml syringe attached and the operator aspirates while advancing the needle. An alligator clip lead attached to the needle acts as one lead of an EKG which is monitored continuously while the needle is inserted. A change is noted if the myocardium is entered.

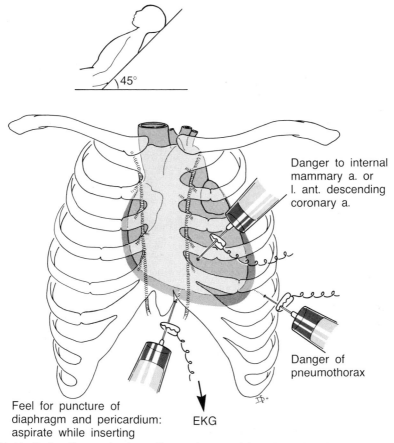

45°

Danger to internal
mammary a. or
l. ant. descending
coronary a.

Danger of
pneumothorax

Feel for puncture of
diaphragm and pericardium:
aspirate while inserting

EKG

Figure 16–11 Pericardiocentesis. A needle may be passed into the pericardium via the three routes indicated. Each route has some disadvantages. An EKG lead is clipped to the needle to monitor contact between needle and myocardium.

It is usually possible to feel the needle puncture the central tendon of the diaphragm and pericardium and immediately thereafter fluid may be aspirated into the syringe. If movement of the heart is felt against the needle tip, the needle is withdrawn slightly. If a large volume of chronic effusion must be drained, a small plastic tube can be introduced into the pericardial sac through the lumen of a large-bore needle and left in position, draining into a container.

Pericardial Drainage

If pericardiocentesis is not successful a simple method of pericardial drainage has been described by Schlein (1970).[14] Under local anesthesia a five inch vertical incision is made in the midline over the xiphoid process. Dissection is carried down through the linea alba to the diaphragm. The xiphoid process is raised superiorly, the fibers of the diaphragm are divided and the pericardium exposed and entered. Ample drainage is obtained and, if necessary, a tube can be left within the pericardial sac for prolonged drainage.

Constrictive Pericarditis

In constrictive pericarditis the heart becomes entrapped by a thick encircling fibrous scar which obliterates the pericardial sac and may become calcified. Venous return is reduced by contracted scars around the caval orifices, and diastolic filling is impeded by constricting pericardial scar.

Venous congestion, hepatic enlargement, ascites and peripheral edema highlight the clinical picture. Peripheral cyanosis and cool extremities reflect a low cardiac output.

The techniques of radiology, scanning and ultrasound used to demonstrate a pericardial effusion can also be used to determine the presence and thickness of pericardium. Pericardial calcification is sometimes easily seen on a plain film, but the mere presence of calcification does not by itself denote constriction.

The treatment of constrictive pericarditis is widespread pericardiectomy, from phrenic nerve to phrenic nerve, with release of scar around the caval openings.

CARDIAC TRAUMA

Closed Injury

Evaluation of the integrity of heart and great vessels should be part of the investigation of every patient who has sustained a crushing or deceleration injury of the thorax. Attention should be directed along two lines.

1. Is there damage to the heart? There may be myocardial contusion of every degree from a mild bruise to infarction readily discernible by electrocardiography. Atrial and ventricular walls, including the septum, may rupture, giving rise to a hemopericardium or a large intracardiac shunt. Disruption of the papillary muscles can cause mitral insufficiency.

Accumulation of a pericardial effusion may result in tamponade, and development of a shunt or valvular dysfunction may cause congestive cardiac failure.

Myocardial contusion may cause the symptoms and effects of myocardial infarction and is probably commoner than most statistics would indicate.

2. Have the great vessels been damaged? Severe deceleration injuries may rupture the aorta. The commonest site for this is at the ligamentum arteriosum, but it may also occur in the ascending aorta, intra- or extrapericardially, and at the roots of the main branches of the aortic arch. A widened mediastinal shadow, seen by x-ray, should immediately arouse suspicion of aortic injury. If subsequent pictures indicate that widening is progressive, aortography is essential to demonstrate the lesion. The *treatment* of closed injuries depends upon their nature. Contusions should be treated like myocardial infarctions of comparable severity. Rupture of a chamber into the pericardium may first require pericardiocentesis for relief of tamponade before definitive repair. Intracardiac shunts require open operation, but if congestive failure can first be controlled medically risks may be decreased.

Penetrating Injuries

Stab and gunshot wounds in and around the heart demand rapid evaluation and action if lives are to be saved. Two questions have to be answered immediately:

1. Is the patient bleeding to death?
2. Is there acute tamponade, and an equal but different threat to life?

Massive free bleeding into pleura and pericardium leads to acute hypovolemic shock. The most important distinguishing feature between hemorrhage and tamponade is the presence of high venous pressure in the latter. If, however, there is a combination of massive hemorrhage and tamponade the intrapericardial pressure necessary to induce tamponade is not as great as in a patient with a normal blood volume. Venous pressure may not then be elevated.

Penetrating thoracic wounds which injure the heart alone are uncommon, except after stab wounds. Gunshot wounds are likely to involve lung, esophagus, trachea and great vessels and these possibilities must be constantly kept in mind.

Cardiac tamponade is more likely after stab than gunshot wounds. Out of 547 patients with thoracic gunshot wounds treated in Vietnam only 7 presented with tamponade.

The outcome after cardiac injuries depends upon the size of the wound and the interval between injury and treatment. Small wounds, less than 1 cm in length, may seal themselves quite rapidly, especially if the wound is a clean stab of a ventricle. Atrial wounds are less likely to seal spontaneously. Large wounds may cause death due to blood loss before treatment can be started. But if the patient reaches the Emergency Room alive, he has, by definition, demonstrated that the wound is temporarily compatible with life.

Treatment

Immediate evaluation includes: (a) assessment of shock, (b) search for signs of tamponade, (c) examination of entrance and exit wounds and a determination of organs which may have been injured, and (d) chest x-ray for signs of hemopericardium, hemo- and pneumothorax.

Immediate treatment includes: (a) assurance of airway and ventilation, (b) insertion of catheters for measurement of venous pressure and infusion of blood and fluids, (c) insertion of chest tubes for drainage of hemothorax and pneumothorax, and (d) pericardiocentesis, if there is direct evidence of, or strong suspicion of, tamponade.

Indications for immediate operation are: (a) evidence of massive continuing hemorrhage, (b) immediate evacuation of 1000 ml to 1500 ml of blood by tube thoracostomy, followed by 500 ml blood loss in the first subsequent hour, (c) redevelopment of tamponade after one successful pericardiocentesis, and (d) evidence of injury to esophagus, trachea or great vessels.

THE FUGITIVE CATHETER

The use of plastic catheters for intravenous infusions has become so widespread in the past few years that needles have become almost passé. An unpleasant dividend of this technique is the loss of a catheter into the cardiovascular system. There are two common causes of this complication. Either the catheter is improperly secured to the skin, so that it becomes disconnected and slips intravenously, or the end of the needle previously inserted into the vein for passage of the catheter severs the catheter, and the free segment is carried away by the circulation.

If loss of the catheter is recognized at the moment of occurrence, rapid application of circumferential pressure high and proximal on the same limb may catch the catheter. Palpation is extremely deceptive, especially around the elbow. Don't cut down on what is presumed to be a catheter without radiological proof of its presence.

Take x-rays of the limb and thorax. If the catheter is radiopaque it will be spotted in the limb, right side of the heart or pulmonary artery. Because radiopaque catheters are now available, no catheter which is not radiopaque should ever be put into the cardiovascular system. Searching for a nonopaque catheter is frustrating and unfruitful.

If the catheter is lodged in the limb, a tourniquet is applied to prevent migration and it is removed under local anesthesia. Special instruments such as the Dormia basket catheter and the Ross snare are needed for removal of a catheter from the heart.

There is still some controversy over the best therapeutic approach to this problem. Many patients are now walking around harboring within them a piece of plastic catheter without any symptoms. In most instances there are no sequelae. There have been occasional reports of septic emboli and hemorrhage and removal of all fugitive catheters has been advised.

A middle-of-the-road course seems acceptable. All catheters still in the limb should be removed. An attempt should be made to extract, by cardiac catheterization, all catheters within the heart. If the catheter is in the distal pulmonary arteries, leave it alone.

Antibiotics should be given for about one week after the incident. Anticoagulants do not seem warranted (any more than with endocardial pacemaker electrodes). At any sign of further complications, the catheter should be surgically removed.

References

1. Barratt-Boyes, B. G., and Roche, A. H. G.: A review of aortic valve homografts over a six and one half year period. Ann. Surg., *170*:483–490, 1969.
2. Beach, P. M., Bowman, F. O., Kaiser, G. A., and Malm, J. R.: Total correction of tetralogy of Fallot in adolescents and adults. Circulation, *43*, Suppl. I:37–43, 1971.
3. Daves, M. L.: Skiagraphing the mediastinal moguls. New Physician, *19*:48–54, 1970.
4. Favaloro, R. G.: Surgical Treatment of Coronary Arteriosclerosis. Baltimore, Williams and Wilkins Co., 1970.
5. Gonzalez-Lavin, L., and Ross, D.: Homograft aortic valve replacement: A five year experience at the National Heart Hospital, London. J. Thorac. Cardiovasc. Surg., *60*:1–12, 1970.
6. Hylen, J. C., Kloster, F. E., Starr, A., and Griswold, H. E.: Aortic ball variance: Diagnosis and treatment. Ann. Intern. Med., *72*:1–8, 1970.
7. Hylen, J. C.: Durability of prosthetic heart valves. Amer. J. Heart, *81*:299–303, 1971.
8. Johnson, M. L., Paton, B. C., and Holmes, J. H.: Ultrasonic evaluation of prosthetic valve motion. Circulation, *42*, Suppl. II: 3–7, 1970.
9. Kahn, D. R., Ertel, P. Y., Murphy, W. H., Kirsh, M. M., Vathayanon, S., Stern, A. M., and Sloan, H.: Pathogenesis of the postcardiotomy syndrome. J. Thorac. Cardiovasc. Surg., *54*:682–687, 1967.
10. Kirklin, J. W.: The Tetralogy of Fallot from a Surgical Viewpoint. Philadelphia, W. B. Saunders Co., 1970.
11. Kirsh, M. M., McIntosh, K., Kahn, D. R., and Sloan, H.: Postcardiotomy syndromes. Ann. Thorac. Surg., *9*:158–179, 1970.
12. Paton, B. C.: Reoperation for fibrinous stenosis of disc mitral valve prosthesis. J. Thorac. Cardiovasc. Surg., *57*:726–731, 1969.
13. Ryle, J. A.: The clinical study of pain: With special reference to the pains of visceral disease. Br. Med. J., *1*:537–540, 1928.
14. Schlein, E. M., Bartley, T. D., Spooner, G. R., and Cade, R.: A simplified approach to therapy of uremic pericarditis with tamponade. Ann. Thorac. Surg., *10*:548–551, 1970.
15. Segal, J., Harvey, W. P., and Hufnagel, D.: A clinical study of one hundred cases of severe aortic insufficiency. Amer. J. Med., *21*:200–210, 1956.
16. Starr, A.: Acquired disease of the tricuspid valve. In Gibbon, J. H., Sabiston, D. C., and Spencer, F. C. (eds.): Surgery of the Chest. Philadelphia, W. B. Saunders Co., 1969.
17. Vander Veer, J. B., Rhyneer, G. S., Hodam, R. P., and Kloster, F. E.: Obstruction of triscuspid ball valve prostheses. Circulation, *43*, Suppl. I:62–67, 1971.
18. Vogel, J. H. K., Paton, B. C., Overy, H. R., Pappas, G., Davies, D. H., and Blount, S. G., Jr.: Advantages of Beall valve prosthesis. Chest, *59*:249–253, 1971.
19. Von Kaulla, K. N., Paton, B. C., Rosenkrantz, J. G., Von Kaulla, E., and Wasantapruek, S.: Preoperative correction of coagulation in tetralogy of Fallot. Arch. Surg., *94*:107–111, 1967.
20. Wallace, R. B., Giuliani, E. R., and Titus, J. L.: Use of aortic valve homografts for aortic valve replacement. Circulation, *43*:365–373, 1971.

17

Peripheral Blood Vessels—
Vascular Surgery

By J. CUTHBERT OWENS, M.D.

INTRODUCTION

This chapter is devoted to the identification of conditions which require hospital admission, conditions which can be cared for on an ambulatory basis, and conditions which warrant little or no treatment other than a thorough education of the patient. Over 80 per cent of patients seen on an outpatient basis with peripheral vascular disease require neither hospital admission nor surgery. However, the vascular system is interrelated with all systems of the body. The clinician must therefore be alert to all possible diagnoses and therapeutic methods available, since the vascular problem may be either caused by or influenced by associated disease entities. Failure to accept this broad approach leads only to confusion regarding the method of therapy which will result in the most beneficial outcome. Although a completely successful outcome is not possible for all patients, reasonable success should be expected in the vast majority of patients suffering from peripheral vascular disease. Success requires a clear understanding of the various conditions that comprise this common group of disorders. Success also requires early recognition of the early stages of disease and an adequate differential analysis of the method of treatment best suited for the individual patient.

THE CLOTTING PROCESS

The literature dealing with clinical problems of blood coagulation abounds with information concerning bleeding disorders. Most of the clotting tests are structured to investigate hypocoagulability; however, many more people die from intravascular thrombosis than from clotting deficiencies. Intravascular thrombosis is not only the most frequent cause of death but is also a significant factor in the daily disability of a large percentage of the population. Conceivably, there is a balanced relationship between factors which increase the activity of clotting and naturally occurring clotting inhibitors which have a reduced activity and intravascular clotting. Fibrinolytic activity may be involved and may be spontaneous, reduced or absent. It is difficult but not impossible to measure hypercoagulability in clinical situations. Several clotting parameters must be checked simultaneously. Once there were more tests for investigating clotting factors for bleeding problems than for clotting; now hypercoagulability interests both the clinical and research fields. Areas of interest include studies to explain the reasons for anticoagulant failure; screening for potential "clotters"; means to identify doubtful cases of intravascular clotting; hypercoagulability potential of certain drugs (e.g., oral contraceptives), and many others.

The coagulation of blood is the result of an enzymatic chain reaction in which activators, precursors, activated enzymes and inhibitors, and additional components such as calcium participate.

Basic Steps in the Coagulation Process

The three phases of clotting are: Phase I, initiating events and formation of thromboplastin; Phase II, conversion of prothrombin to thrombin; Phase III, conversion of fibrinogen to fibrin, followed by stabilization and polymerization of fibrin.

Clotting Factors

To help classify the complex mechanisms of blood coagulation, Von Kaulla has classified the factors of the clotting system into three major groups:

1. Origin

Factors Present in Blood Before Clotting	Clotting Factor*	Factors Formed During Clotting
fibrinogen	I	fibrin
prothrombin	II	thrombin (active for short period, then neutralized by antithrombins)
calcium	IV	
proaccelerin	V	
proconvertin	VII	
antihemophilic globulin, AHG	VIII	These clotting factors are "activated"
plasma thromboplastin component, PTC	IX	
Stuart-Prower factor	X	
plasma thromboplastin antecedent, PTA	XI	
Hageman factor	XII	platelet factor 3* (released)
fibrin stabilizing factor	XIII	blood thromboplastin, III
platelets		activated factor X + factor V + phospholipids + Ca^{++} complex)

*The clotting factors have Roman numerals; platelet factors have Arabic numbers.

2. Fate

Factors Consumed During Clotting	vs. Clotting Factor	Factors Not Consumed During Clotting	
(relatively little present in serum)		(serum relatively rich in these factors)	
antihemophilic globulin (antihemophilic factor, AHF)	VIII	proconvertin	VII
		plasma thromboplastin component	IX
proaccelerin	V	Stuart-Prower factor	X
prothrombin	II		
fibrinogen	I		

Origin of Clotting Factors. The liver manufactures several factors. The origin of most of the others is presently unknown. Presently, investigators are attempting to determine the organ or organs which synthesize antihemophilic globulin. If such an organ is identified, transplantation of this organ into a hemophiliac patient may cure his disease.

Fate of Clotting Factors. The fate of clotting factors circulating in human blood is essentially unknown. It has been established that the liver clears plasminogen activator and possibly activated factor X, the Stuart-Prower factor. Some clearing occurs in the reticuloendothelial system and some of the clotting factors can enter the extravascular space.

Stability of Clotting Factors. Two aspects of the stability of the clotting factors which are important for therapy are (1) the "shelf" life and (2) the biological half-life.

"Shelf" life is the term given to the duration of stability of clotting factors in shed blood and in isolated factors derived from shed blood. Shelf life can be modified by storage conditions. An example is factor VIII, antihemophilic globulin. This highly unstable factor can be stabilized for more than one year by proper treatment.

Biological half-life of a clotting factor is determined on the basis of serial blood specimens drawn from a patient who has received a transfusion of blood or a blood fraction. Biological half-life is the

3. Stability.

Factors Stable in Shed Blood	vs.	Factors Unstable in Shed Blood (unless certain techniques of conservation are used)	

Important for selection of blood or blood product: fresh blood or fresh frozen plasma vs. "bank blood" or blood products; platelet concentrates and factor VIII preparations

		Platelets (loss of viability) antihemophilic globulin	VIII
plasma thromboplastin component, PTC	IX		
plasma thromboplastin antecedent, PTA	XI		
Stuart-Prower factor	X	prothrombin	II
proconvertin	VII	proaccelerin	V
fibrinogen	I		
plasminogen (fibrinolytic enzyme system)		free plasminogen activator	

length of time until the immediate post-transfusion value has decreased 50 per cent. Biological half-lives vary for each factor, from a few hours to several days.

Dynamic Relationship Between Clotting Factors and Clotting Inhibitors. The clotting factors have a relationship to each other as well as to the naturally occurring clotting inhibitors. The relationship is dynamic and the activity or concentration of one or more of them may change very rapidly under physiological or pathological stimuli. Examples include:

(1) *physiological changes*—physical stress may cause an increase of factor VIII and fibrinolytic activity; and
(2) *pathological changes*—
  1. Premature separation of the placenta in which there is release of tissue thromboplastin into the maternal circulation
  2. An increase in fibrinolytic activity or the appearance of clotting inhibitors may appear in thoracic surgery
  3. Fibrinolytic activity may increase in surgery on the liver
  4. A release of partial thromboplastin from the hemolysis of erythrocytes in a mismatched transfusion
  5. Consumption coagulopathy may occur during an acute rejection crisis of transplanted organs

These changes are dramatic when they occur abruptly and are noted chiefly in hospitalized patients. However, there are many examples of changes in the clotting mechanism which develop slowly, over a period of weeks or months. Patients with these conditions are often seen on an outpatient basis. It is therefore essential that they be identified early in the process of change. Examples include:
  1. Liver disease, with a reduction of components of the prothrombin complex
  2. Kidney disease, in which there may be disturbances of platelet function

  3. Collagen disease, in which there is an appearance of clotting inhibitors
  4. Cancer of the prostate, which may show an increase of fibrinolytic activity and thrombocytopenia
  5. Release of tissue thromboplastin in many malignancies

Septicemia may induce intravascular clotting, which may develop slowly or within a period of hours, resulting in severe consumption coagulopathy.

Phase I. Initiating Events and Thromboplastin Formation

Initiating events. Two events initiate extravascular hemostasis and pathological intravascular blood coagulation. Of *primary importance* is the contact of blood with rough wettable surfaces. This event plays a prominent role in the initiation of normal blood coagulation and hemostasis, and also may induce pathological intravascular clotting. When the smooth nonwettable surface of the vascular endothelial lining is damaged, the collagen-containing basement membrane is exposed. This exposed membrane initiates the clotting mechanism by activating factor XII, triggering release of platelet 3 factor from the platelets. It may also activate erythrocyte erythroplastin, which is a partial thromboplastin. Of *secondary importance* is the admixture of tissue thromboplastin. Thromboplastin is a lipoprotein found in almost all human tissues which plays an auxiliary role in normal hemostasis and an important role in some instances of diffuse intravascular clotting. Tissue thromboplastin will produce an erroneous result in studies of coagulation *in vitro* if it contaminates the blood specimen. This is particularly true when a question of hypercoagulability is involved.

Blood thromboplastin formation is the result of the first phase of coagulation. Thromboplastin formation has a lag period of several minutes from initiation to completion. The reaction is initiated when Hageman factor XII is activated by contact with rough surfaces. This factor interacts with factor XI, in a chain reaction which eventually results in the formation of blood (intrinsic) thromboplastin. Other factors which participate in formation of blood thromboplastin are plasma thromboplastin antecedent (XI), plasma thromboplastin component (IX), antihemophilic globulin (VIII), Stuart-Prower (factor X) and proaccelerin (V). For this chain reaction to follow its proper course, calcium ions are required and phospholipids are released from platelets as platelet factor 3.

All components of the normal "intrinsic" process of blood clotting are derived from blood, except the rough wettable surfaces which are primary initiating factors in coagulation. The constituents derived from blood include "blood thromboplastin," which evolves during the process and which converts prothrombin into thrombin. It is presently thought to be a complex made up of activated factor X, factor V, phospholipids from platelets, and Ca^{++}. The exact sequence of interaction of these clotting factors is not clearly established and is subject to some controversy.

The "extrinsic" pathway of blood coagulation occurs when extravascular or extrinsic material ("tissue thromboplastin") is mixed with blood. The extrinsic clotting chain reaction which follows is shorter than the intrinsic pathway, because factors XII, XI, IX, and VIII are bypassed. In addition, platelets are not required, since tissue thromboplastin contains the necessary phospholipids. Tissue thromboplastin probably forms a complex with factor VII and Ca^{++}. Factor VII is not required for the "intrinsic" pathway. Calcium ions activate factor V, which acts with factor X in converting prothrombin into thrombin.

Phase II. Thrombin Formation

Thrombin formation is the second basic step in the coagulation process. Thrombin is formed by conversion of prothrombin into thrombin by thromboplastin. This requires about ten seconds. Generation of blood (intrinsic) thromboplastin does not require the presence of proconvertin VII for full activity. The combined kinetics of the first and second phases of clotting are measured in the thrombin generation test, which measures the amount of thrombin formed. It is a useful method to discover hypercoagulability. The extrinsic clotting system contributes to formation of thrombin formation in extravasated blood, and consequently it is important in hemostasis. Prothrombin was the first member of the so-called prothrombin complex to be discovered. All factors of the prothrombin complex are related to prothrombin conversion into thrombin and are synthesized by the liver. Clotting factors which are synthesized by the liver drop to low levels in the presence of severe liver disease. In addition to the prothrombin complex, fibrinogen I and antithrombin III levels decrease in liver disease.

Vitamin K is required for biosynthesis in four of the five factors of the prothrombin complex: prothrombin II, proconvertin VII, Christmas factor IX and Stuart-Prower factor X. Each of these are reduced by prothrombin-reducing agents such as coumarin drugs (Coumadin, dicumarol, among others). Prothrombin II and proconvertin VII are also reduced in patients with liver disease. Proaccelerin (factor V) is not reduced by prothrombin depressing agents but is reduced by severe liver disease. Hemorrhagic diathesis is produced by severe isolated or combined deficiency of the factors of the prothrombin complex. Bile must be present in order for vitamin K to be absorbed from the intestinal tract. Prolongation in prothrombin time is caused by absence of nonabsorption of vitamin K, or the congenital or acquired absence of any of the factors of the prothrombin complex.

Phase III. Fibrin Formation

Fibrin formation is the third and final step in blood coagulation. It depends primarily on thrombin concentration. Thrombin is a proteolytic enzyme which hydrolyzes peptide bonds in the fibrinogen molecule, permitting them to form the fibrin monomer. Fibrin monomers combine to form fibrin polymers, from which the fibrin network is produced. In some pathological conditions, fibrin monomers can be found in the circulating blood. This situation indicates that the patient is a potential candidate for intravascular clotting.

Fibrin stabilizing factor is required in the formation of a firm and physiologically useful clot. Fibrin stabilizing factor is probably a transaminase, requiring calcium and thrombin for its activity. This factor is totally missing in rare congenital cases and is markedly reduced in some diseases. A weak clot is then formed which does not become well organized. Poor wound healing results and bleeding may occur within a few hours to days after any type of trauma. All clotting tests are normal in these patients, except for fibrin stabilizing factor XIII.

A normal clot consists of a fibrin network which incorporates proteins, erythrocytes, leucocytes and platelets, *Clot retraction* occurs when the fibrin fibers slowly draw together, a process termed syneresis. Clot retraction depends in part on the presence of normal platelets. Poor or absent clot retraction *in vitro* is an indication of a low platelet count or an abnormal platelet function. Clot is organized *in vivo* by the ingrowth of fibroblasts within a few days unless a pathological condition results in fibrinolysis. Normal hemostasis requires passage of time for development, in a clot, of firmness and adherence to tissue and wound surfaces. A good firm clot may not develop in the presence of a low fibrinogen level, deficiency of fibrin stabilizing factor, fibrinolysis, a reduced platelet count, or poor platelet function.

In summary, the three phases of clotting are: formation of blood thromboplastin (Phase I); conversion of prothrombin to thrombin (Phase II); and conversion of fibrinogen to fibrin, followed by stabilization of fibrin (Phase III). Calcium is required for each of these phases, and removal of calcium results in uncoagulability of the blood. Tests are available for each phase: prothrombin consumption test for Phase I; prothrombin time for Phase II; thrombin generation test for Phases I and II; and thrombin time for Phase III.

Endogenous Inhibition of Clotting

Studies indicate that some intravascular fibrin formation proceeds slowly on a continuous basis. This process is controlled by endogenous clotting inhibitors and by the fibrinolytic enzyme system. Clotting inhibitors are theoretically necessary to prevent the clotting process from spreading beyond the area where it is required. However, if endogenous clotting inhibitors increase, a more or less pronounced hemorrhagic diathesis may develop. When the activity of endogenous clotting inhibitors is reduced beyond a certain point, there is increasing evidence that a potential danger of intravascular clotting exists. The key factor in this phenomenon may be antithrombin III.

Endogenous clotting inhibitors are known as antithrombins and antithromboplastins. The *antithrombins* are: antithrombin I—the fibrin clot which absorbs thrombin; antithrombin II—the thrombin inhibitor which immediately neutralizes thrombin; antithrombin III—a serum antithrombin which progressively neutralizes thrombin; (antithrombin IV is no longer recognized as a specific entity); antithrombin V—pathological macroglobulins which interfere with fibrin polymerization; and antithrombin VI—a pathological mixture of fibrinolytic breakdown products derived from fibrinogen or fibrin, which may interfere with fibrin polymerization. Markedly reduced antithrombin III activity has been reported in association with intravascular clotting. Low levels have been found in families with hereditary thrombophilia. Another natural inhibitor is heparin, which is present in very small amounts in blood. This inhibitor needs a cofactor for its anti-coagulant activity, which is probably antithrombin III. Blood normally contains antiheparin activity known as platelet factor 4 or antiheparin platelet factor, which is derived from the throm-bocytes. Heparin inhibits thrombin and also probably interferes with the activation of factor IX by factor XI.

Antithromboplastins include those which are considered to be "normal," and also pathological inhibitors which interfere with blood thromboplastins. The latter are found primarily in the gamma-globulin fraction. They are generally specific inhibitors of factor VIII.

Endogenous clotting inhibitors are generally called "circulating anticoagulants."

Predisposing Factors

The clinician's interest in the etiology of venous thrombosis begins with prevention of this disease. An account of "clotting very quickly" may occasionally be extracted from the patient's history. Examples include a history of trivial trauma which has been accompanied by clots or an erythematous area on the skin suggestive of phlebitis. A past history of one or more bouts of minor or major thrombophlebitis may be elicited. An additional aspect is a family history of clotting tendency. These patients should be considered for special laboratory studies. The most common predisposing factor is the patient's presenting disease.

Associated diseases which commonly accompany venous thrombosis include pneumonia, typhoid fever, septicemia, chronic ulcerative colitis, carcinoma, lymphoma, localized and generalized cardiovascular disease. Other associated conditions are seen in a wide variety of obstetrical and surgical illnesses. A high incidence of venous thrombosis is noted in various forms of trauma, including venipuncture or prolonged intra-venous cannulation, advancing age, prolonged debilitating illness, and rapid changes in the hemodynamics of the body during shock or dehydration. The predisposing factors also include drug abuse and contraceptive medications. Surgery was formerly followed by a high incidence of venous thrombosis. The incidence is now lower, probably as a result of improved preoperative, intra-operative and postoperative hemodynamics. Other factors contributing to decreased incidence of thrombosis include passive exercises of the lower extremities performed at frequent intervals postoperatively until the patient is completely awake. Early postoperative ambulation is important. Particular attention should be directed toward any condition which leads to venous stasis due to immobility of the lower limbs, especially with advancing age, bed rest and prolonged sitting.

Hypercoagulability. Identification of Individuals Who Have a Tendency to Intravascular Clotting

Patients with evidence of repeated thromboembolism have previously been studied by various individual coagulation tests. Most of these tests failed to detect "chronic clotters," and "clotters" were therefore usually best identified by their history alone. Recently, however, there has been renewed interest in these tests because of the thromboembolic events which have occurred in association with use of oral contraceptive drugs. Clinicians should realize that it is naive to attempt to use a single test for the evaluation of hypercoagulability of the blood. Widely different triggering events and resulting alterations occur in the clotting process which predispose to intravascular thrombosis. Entirely different coagulation procedures are required to reveal the danger of intravascular clotting in amaurosis fugax, which may be due solely to an increased spontaneous aggregation of platelets, as compared to a disseminated carcinoma, in which necrosing cells may cause massive penetration of thromboplastic material into the circulation. Appropriate therapy may be determined after identifying the abnormal clotting parameters. In these two examples aspirin would prevent the platelet aggregation in amaurosis fugax, while thromboembolic complications of disseminated carcinoma would necessitate adequate levels of heparin. Endogenous clotting factors have received little attention until recently, when it was found that a normal level of antithrombin III activity is important to prevent thromboembolism. It is believed that many other endogenous factors are important in preventing thromboembolism.

Even if the laboratory detects the existence of hypercoagulability *in vitro*, it should not be stated that the patient will develop intravascular thrombosis. It does, however, warn the clinician of the patient's propensity to clot. The predisposing events or factors are the catalysts which convert a clotting tendency into an actual thromboembolism. A combination of tests identified as the *hypercoagulability panel* is required to screen the various parameters of the coagulation system to produce meaningful results for the clinician. These tests include: (1) *thrombin generation test,* (2) *thromboelastography,* (3) *euglobulin lysis test* (increased in primary fibrinolysis), (4) *platelet aggregation* (may be increased in amaurosis fugax, transient ischemic attacks and recurrent vertigo), (5) *platelet count* (high count reveals clotting tendency while a low count may indicate hypercoagulability, diffuse intravascular coagulation, or both), (6) *circulating soluble fibrin monomers* (their presence indicates a preliminary stage of clotting), (7) *fibrinogen* (if high, hypercoagulability is enhanced; if low, disseminated intravascular coagulation is suggested), (8) *fibrin degradation (split) products* (presence is due to fibrinolysis and is indirect evidence of clotting; if high, strong evidence is present for disseminated intravascular coagulation), and (9) *antithrombin III activity* (in which a low level indicates reduced pro-

tection against clotting. All oral contraceptives cause the level to be low, so other tests are required. Antithrombin III activity is deficient in hereditary "clotters"; high in infants and children, decreasing to normal by early twenties; if subnormal or normal in coumarin-treated patients, then subcutaneous heparin is the drug of choice. In liver disease it may be low or absent.)

Any patient receiving oral contraceptives or who has any other predisposing condition and a personal or family history of clotting, migraine headaches, vascular catheterization, angiography, elective surgery, corticosteroids or prolonged bed rest should be treated cautiously. In iatrogenic hypercoagulability from the "pill," it is necessary to stop the drug at least three weeks before elective surgery. Mass laboratory screening of patients for hypercoagulability is not practical and is not advised. Clinical screening is essential for all patients but specific conditions warrant further study by the laboratory.

VENOUS DISEASE

Thromboembolic Disease

Venous thrombosis and its complications are among the most common diseases seen on an outpatient basis. These diseases occur both as acute processes and as chronic conditions.

Definition and Classification

Venous thrombosis may be defined as a partial or complete occlusion of a vein by a thrombus. An antecedent or secondary inflammatory reaction is present in the wall of the vein. Its importance lies in its frequent occurrence and its serious, sometimes fatal, sequelae.

Venous inflammatory processes are associated with local thromboses which invariably evoke secondary inflammatory reaction. The two processes of thrombosis and inflammation cannot be separated from each other. Variation in the degree of inflammatory reaction has led to a classical division of venous disease into two categories — phlebothrombosis and thrombophlebitis. This categorization is not universally accepted. Barker states that there is always some inflammatory reaction present in every case and therefore all cases should be included under the one term of thrombophlebitis.

Differing philosophies regarding the specific diagnosis of phlebothrombosis or thrombophlebitis seem unrealistic since all states of thrombus formation are directly related to the time elapsed and the clinical signs which are present. The clot may vary from initial sludging to formation of an organized clot. Thrombophlebitis theoretically has an organized clot and phlebothrombosis an unorganized clot. Phlebothrombosis as a specific diagnostic term should be assigned only after objective histopathological examination of the specimen. Thrombophlebitis is the more appropriate term to use unless the thrombus has been examined microscopically, since all stages of clot formation are present until treatment is instituted. Such a philosophy frees the clinician from emotional attitudes toward treatment.

Thrombophlebitis may affect any vein. It may occur at the confluence with venous tributaries, in a patchy or scattered fashion, or it may be localized. It may be fulminant or it may develop insidiously. The most common location is in the veins of the lower extremity. The incidence of thrombophlebitis of the upper limb is increasing in frequency because of the increased use of indwelling catheters and the awareness of the syndrome of "effort vein thrombosis." This is a thrombosis of the subclavian vein resulting from venous entrapment in the thoracic outlet. Venous clotting in the lower extremities may be categorized by its location — in the superficial veins, the deep veins, or both. Iliofemoral thrombophlebitis was previously called *phlegmasia alba dolens* or "milk leg." The diagnosis was usually made when a severe inflammation of a lower extremity occurred postpartum. The popular term used today for extensive iliofemoral thrombophlebitis is *phlegmasia cerulea dolens*. However, this term should be used only to identify a venous thrombosis of the lower extremity which is so extensive that gangrene is considered a potential complication. Diagnosis should preferably include only the anatomical site and severity of the venous thrombosis. Complications such as sepsis, ischemia, or pulmonary emboli are recognized when they occur during the course of the disorder. Veins of the intestine, liver, kidney, lungs, brain, pelvis, breast, and chest wall may also be involved. Clotting in these areas may accompany or complicate thromboembolic lesions of the peripheral veins in the extremities.

Etiology and Pathogenesis

Intravascular thrombosis is not yet completely understood. The common denominators leading to the development of thrombosis, irrespective of the primary disease or operative procedure, are: (1) primary endothelial lesions of the vein wall with subsequent inflammation and thrombosis; (2) slowing and eddying of the blood flow with sludging and inflammatory reaction in the wall of the vein; and (3) physical and chemical changes in the blood itself, producing hypercoagulability. Thrombophlebitis is the end result of an imbalance in the physiochemical forces which maintain the vein endothelium undisrupted and the blood in a fluid state.

When blood coagulates, the final result is the formation of fibrin which is the stroma of the "clot." This white fibrin matrix produces the network which catches the thrombocytes, leucocytes and erythrocytes. This process may be normal, decreased (hemorrhagic diathesis), or increased (abnormal thrombosis).

When the clotting process is enhanced, the contributing or triggering factor may be localized and result in a thrombosis. A thrombus may produce an embolus, or it may be diffuse, causing obstruction of small vessels in various organs such as the kidney. When the diffuse process is extensive, a marked consumption of clotting factors occurs which is termed *consumption coagulopathy*.

Endothelial Lesions. The early phases of thrombus formation are basically the same as those of hemostasis. The process begins on a damaged intravascular endothelial lining where circulating platelets stick to the collagen.

Changes in the clotting mechanism resulting from aberrant electrical potentials on the vein wall are also reported as a possible etiology. As the charges decrease, the repulsion of platelets is reduced and this ionic potential permits platelets to adhere to the intima of the vein. This results in the formation of thromboplastin, which then induces fibrin formation. With successive increments of coagulum, the thrombus formation is propagated. The local clotting process is potentiated when stasis or a hypercoagulable state of the blood is present. Much investigation is being carried out to measure *platelet adhesiveness*, which is the tendency of platelets to adhere to surfaces, and *platelet aggregation*, which is the tendency of platelets to stick to each other. When these two parameters are reduced or increased in activity, patients have a tendency either to hemorrhage or to develop intravascular thrombosis. By using a drug such as aspirin, which reduces both platelet adhesiveness and aggregation, intravascular thrombosis and emboli may be lessened or prevented in arterial clotting disorders. However, these drugs do not prevent thromboplastin from being released from damaged tissue. Reduced platelet adhesiveness may play a role in hemorrhagic diathesis. Aspirin or aspirin-containing drugs should therefore never be administered to a patient with even a slight bleeding tendency.

The common sites of involvement by thrombophlebitis are the veins of the extremities—the femoral, popliteal and tibial veins, the subclavian, axillary and iliac veins, and the superior and inferior vena cava. Venous thrombosis may be localized or it may be confluent, with several venous tributaries involved. It may also occur in a patchy or scattered fashion. The disease may be either fulminating or insidious in onset. Although thrombophlebitis characteristically presents in one lower extremity, phlebography and autopsy studies have demonstrated similar lesions in the asymptomatic limb. Since numerous nonthrombotic disorders may present similar clinical features, it is not uncommon to question the reliability of signs and symptoms of venous thrombosis when they are based previously on a clinical impression. However, in the majority of patients the manifestations of the disease process are clear-cut and diagnosis is ordinarily simple. In some patients the manifestations may be so bizarre and erratic that a diagnosis can be made only by exclusion.

Thrombophlebitis

Clinical Features

The cardinal findings in thrombophlebitis are those of inflammation: Celsus' classical quartet of dolor, calor, tumor and rubor. Redness may be present disproportionately and may occur concurrently with other symptoms and signs. The following clinical patterns refer mainly to thrombophlebitis of the lower extremity, but analogous manifestations can be expected elsewhere.

Local Manifestations. 1. *Subjective pain* in varying degrees is often sensed as "soreness" or "pins and needles" in the involved area, and the extremity may feel heavy. It is accentuated by motion or dependency, and relief is obtained by inactivity and elevation. Muscle cramps usually indicate deep vein thrombophlebitis. Severe low back or groin pain may accompany iliofemoral thrombophlebitis. Causalgia is a burning type of pain which is sometimes present when there is evidence of decreased arterial supply to the foot. A common complaint in superficial veins is the burning pain localized to the course of the greater or lesser saphenous vein.

2. *Objective pain* may be elicited by indirect compression on the vein. This maneuver is recommended only as a rapid screening method. The well-known Homan's sign is deep pain evoked in the upper posterior calf on dorsiflexion of the foot with the knee extended. Grasping the entire muscle mass of the calf also causes pain. The misleading aspect of this sign is that it is positive in a large number of nonthrombotic disorders, particularly those which involve the muscles or nerves of the calf. It has no significance when the venous thrombosis is situated above the knee.

Another misleading test is Lowenberg's sign which elicits pain in the calf when a blood pressure cuff is applied to the region of the knee and inflated to 100 to 120 mm mercury. A modification of this test is the Ramirez sign in which the blood pressure cuff is placed on the leg and inflated to 40 mm mercury. Pain may be produced in the region of the thrombotic calf vein, and should disappear promptly with release of the pressure. Another test is the Perthes' test which is positive if the patient develops pain upon walking with a tight elastic bandage on the leg, or a tourniquet on the thigh produces pain. This test was popularized as a method to determine deep vein obstruction in patients having varicose veins. However, when the Perthes' test is positive, treatment is required for venous thrombosis, not varicose veins. These tests also may be misleading when specific nonthrombotic disorders are present.

3. *Tenderness* of a mild, moderate, or marked nature is provoked by direct digital pressure along the course of the involved vein. This simple test is probably the most accurate method of diagnosing thrombophlebitis, for it locates the most inflamed site. This test can be used to rule out nonthrombotic disorders as well as to follow the response to therapy. Since it requires a detailed anatomical examination of the extremity, this type of examination should differentiate between deep vein thrombosis and such common entities as superficial thrombophlebitis, gastrocnemius muscle injury, sciatic nerve neuritis or entrapment syndromes as well as the less common nonthrombotic leg disorders. Tenderness of the deep veins is diffuse or radiating over the course of the vessel and is usually confined to sections where the veins can be easily delineated, as in the inguinal region, Scarpa's (femoral) triangle, Hunter's (adductor) canal, or popliteal fossa. A positive Bancroft's sign is tenderness induced by firm, steady pressure in the midportion of the calf, anteriorly toward the tibia. This is a far better method of examination than Homan's, Lowenberg's, Ramirez' or Perthes' tests. Tenderness may also be elicited by pressure over the malleoli or plantar surfaces.

4. *Color changes* usually present as red linear streaks corresponding to the path of the superficial vein, and the involved extremity has an inflamed appearance. Dusky cyanosis may occur distal to the occlusion of a large vein. Occasionally, a pale blue or white appearance of the extremity may follow spasm of an artery which rests against an inflamed vein. The red lines are warm to the touch; the pale areas are cool or cold. When a significant amount of deep vein obstruction results in a bluish foot and leg, elevation of the extremity does not produce much of a decrease in the blue color. The same results are noted when subclavian or axillary vein thrombosis obstructs the venous outflow of the upper extremity.

5. *Local swelling* or *induration* of the red streaks and tissues immediately adjacent to either of the saphenous veins or their tributaries produces cordlike prominences which may remain for several weeks after anti-inflammatory therapy has eliminated the red streaks and pain.

6. *Edema* results from congestion of

the venous, lymphatic and capillary beds beyond the thrombophlebitic obstruction. Gross edema from distal blockage of larger veins causes disproportion and a doughy feel to the limb. Swelling is not characteristic of superficial thrombophlebitis since the saphenous system conveys no more than 20 per cent of the venous circulation from a normal limb. Ambulatory patients are more likely to have edema than bed patients since gravity influences the location of swelling. The more cephalad the venous occlusion, the more likely it is that the patient will have discomfort from the swelling and the higher the incidence of venous thrombosis as verified by phlebography. Edema and a waxy, pale discoloration accounts for the typical appearance of *phlegmasia alba dolens* (milk leg). In the early stages the skin may be cool. Later, when reflex vasospasm is relieved by the inflammatory reaction, the leg becomes warm. Occasionally, there may be marbleization (cutis marmorata) or "cobweb" mottling of the skin (harlequin skin).

7. *Enlarged or dilated veins* may appear and be diagnostic of the presence of a deep vein obstruction due to the increased load of venous return through venous collaterals. The veins of the involved foot and leg may become quite prominent. As many as three sentinel veins may appear over the tibia on the upper third of the leg (veins of Pratt). The superficial venous tributaries in the groin may become prominent with iliac vein thrombosis, or with bilateral prominence of these vessels when the inferior vena cava is involved. With subclavian, innominate, or superior vena cava venous occlusions, prominent veins are noted in the shoulder area.

Systemic Manifestations. 1. *Fever* may be slight or absent, depending on the amount of perivenous inflammatory reaction and the presence or absence of infection. Fever is usually limited to the early stages of the disease and subsides within a few days. An unaccountable, transient subnormal temperature is sometimes one of the earliest signs of thrombophlebitis (Michaelis' sign).

2. The *pulse rate* increases in a step-ladder fashion. Tachycardia may occur when a significant amount of inflammation and edema develops.

3. The *erythrocyte-sedimentation rate* tends to parallel the degree of fever. Although it is nonspecific, this test is used as an index of resolution or progression of the disease.

These systemic signs become extremely important when thrombophlebitis is being considered in patients with paralysis of the lower extremities. The legs are invariably swollen in these patients, and incapable of producing pain.

Typical Clinical Patterns

The general clinical patterns are fairly consistent in thrombophlebitis but the symptoms and signs may vary. The atypical or rare forms are less easily identified and the condition may be recognized only at autopsy.

Deep Thrombophlebitis (Thrombophlebitis of the Femoral Veins and Veins of the Muscles of the Calf)

The most common location of thrombophlebitis is in the veins of the calf, or in the superficial, deep and common femoral vein, or both. The symptoms and signs are variable, and may include none or all of the clinical manifestations described in the preceding section. Common presenting symptoms include:

1. Calf pain, especially with contraction of gastrocnemius and soleus muscles
2. Pain in the thigh
3. Edema in calf or thigh
4. Pulmonary embolus from a silent thrombosis of calf or femoral veins

An uncommon presenting symptom is a paradoxical embolus to the arterial system, in a patient with a patent atrial or ventricular septal defect.

Superficial phlebitis, which occurs in the saphenous system, may progress into deep phlebitis by extension through perforating veins or by extension across the saphenofemoral junction at the fossa ovalis. Deep thrombophlebitis of the common femoral vein may progress to involve the iliac vein and inferior vena cava. When iliofemoral thrombophlebitis occurs, the thigh almost invariably becomes swollen. Deep thrombophlebitis may be life-endangering because of the production of pulmonary emboli or because of the consequences of massive venous occlusion, with hypovolemia and gangrene (see later discussion). Deep thrombophlebitis may later subside completely or may produce the postphlebitic syndrome, characterized by chronic edema, pain and ulcerations of the lower legs, particularly at the malleoli.

Superficial Thrombophlebitis (Thrombophlebitis of the Saphenous Veins)

Although this is a common condition occurring with or without varicose veins, it may be associated with more serious problems. Its symptoms are pain, local tenderness, reddish-blue discoloration and usually the formation of a palpable cord localized to lesser or greater saphenous veins or their tributaries. Since deep venous thrombosis may also be present, the outcome may depend on its detection and the type of therapy instituted. The saphenous vein carries only a small amount of the venous return from the extremity. Therefore generalized swelling of the leg and foot should not occur unless deep vein thrombophlebitis is present, or unless the patient has a history of the postphlebitic syndrome. Propagation of the thrombus to the saphenofemoral junction may be the source for a pulmonary embolus. Therefore, it is essential that patients with superficial thrombophlebitis be followed by frequent examinations to evaluate the extent of the local tenderness and vein changes from the thrombosis.

Silent Thrombosis (Unorganized Clot)

The presence of a silent thrombosis should be considered in questionable thromboembolic states, especially when predisposing factors are present. Silent thrombosis is the term used to identify an unorganized clot; it may be unsuspected until a pulmonary embolus has occurred and death is imminent, or in other cases, there may be varying degrees of apprehension, malaise, chest pain, cough, fever, tachycardia, cyanosis, dyspnea, pallor, hypotension, and sweating. In pulmonary embolization, a pleural rub or rales may lead the observer to conclude that an embolus is the cause of shock, and a thorough search for the source of the embolus in the lower extremities or pelvic vein is sometimes rewarding. Hemoptysis is absent or is a late manifestation. Electrocardiographic tracings are equivocal or may be mistaken for coronary occlusion, and the roentgenographic opaque triangle of pulmonary infarction is rarely seen. A small primary embolus which has been overlooked may be followed in a week or ten days by a fatal secondary embolization. When the histories of a majority of patients with fatal emboli are carefully reviewed, a primary embolus is usually noted. This impression has recently been supported by reports regarding patients who have undergone a pulmonary embolectomy. Roentgenological changes or a pleural rub are usually not evident until two or three days after embolization has recurred.

Massive Venous Occlusion

This uncommon disease of the limb is actually an accentuation of iliofemoral thrombophlebitis. It can be classified into three venous thrombotic entities according to the severity of signs and symptoms. Iliofemoral thrombophlebitis per se is the mildest of the three (see discussion of deep thrombophlebitis earlier). The two severe forms are *phlegmasia alba dolens* (milk leg) and *phlegmasia cerulea dolens* (blue phlebitis).

Phlegmasia Alba Dolens. This is a syndrome caused by severe iliofemoral thrombophlebitis. Historically it was called "milk leg" because of its occurrence in the postpartum period. In the majority of patients it occurs on the left side, supposedly due to inherent abnormalities of the iliac vein such as an internal web or compression from the right iliac artery as it crosses over the left common iliac vein. Clinical findings are caused by severe venous thrombosis as well as by some degree of lymphatic obstruction. The onset of edema is sudden and is accompanied by severe pain. Swelling of the thigh is a characteristic feature and local tenderness can be elicited in the groin over the femoral triangle and possibly above, in the iliac fossa. The superficial collateral veins in the inguinal area become dilated and are usually prominent. The foot is cool early and later becomes warm. Pedal pulses are palpable although difficult to feel when foot and ankle edema is marked. However, capillary flow is good and ischemia is not a problem. Fluid loss into the extremity may be significant and hypovolemia may become a problem.

Phlegmasia Cerulea Dolens. This syndrome is the most severe of those associated with iliofemoral thrombophlebitis. Gangrene of the leg is strongly considered as a possible complication. The onset is usually violent with agonizing pain. The extremity is cold, tender, cyanotic, sometimes swollen, and suffused with a violescent discoloration. It finally becomes shiny, livid, markedly edematous and develops blisters on the toes and foot. Vasospasm is severe and gangrene may ensue because of arterial deficiency. To differentiate this entity from acute arterial occlusion, one should remember that arterial occlusion alone never results in edema. Also, the absence of a history of intermittent claudication should exclude chronic arterial disease as a contributing factor. If arteriospasm is complete or sustained, the gangrene is "dry" and well demarcated; otherwise, the gangrene is the "wet" or venous type. The progression is usually swift and the outcome may be death from shock or pulmonary embolization. In almost all cases, it is associated with an underlying condition. Arterial deficiency in deep-vein thrombosis ranges from no decrease to complete absence of the arterial flow. Since a large amount of blood and fluid is sequestered in the thrombotic limb, hypovolemia is a potential hazard and may require treatment.

Thrombophlebitis of the Superficial Veins of the Breast and Chest Wall

This is a rare variant of superficial thrombophlebitis which occurs in both men and women. It has been called "vestigial mastitis" because of its predilection for "the milkline," "sclerosing periangiitis," or more recently "Mondor's disease." Initial manifestations are pain, local tenderness, a confined local reddening of the skin, and the appearance of a subcutaneous fibrous ridge. If the arm is raised, the firm ridge or cord is converted to a shallow cutaneous groove. Histologically, the lesion is a sclerosing endophlebitis. The condition usually is self-limiting and subsides spontaneously without complications. It may be mistaken for lymphatic permeation from an occult mammary cancer but no relation to cancer is known to exist.

Thrombophlebitis of the Subclavian or Axillary Vein

This is a relatively benign variety of thrombophlebitis which may be misinterpreted as arising from cancer. The manifestations are indistinguishable from thrombophlebitis elsewhere. The arm is swollen due to venous obstruction and prominent veins are usually noted over the pectoral area. Raising the arm during examination fails to relieve the blueness or venous engorgement of the extremity. Because this condition sometimes follows sudden abduction of the arm, it has been called "effort thrombosis" or "straphanger arm." Usually the patient has a history of a thoracic outlet syndrome which traps the subclavian vein between the clavicle and the first rib. Details of the thoracic outlet syndrome will be discussed later in the chapter.

Migratory Thrombophlebitis

This condition appears as isolated, red, painful areas, usually involving superficial veins in separate parts of the body. It has been associated with cancer, thromboangiitis obliterans, nonbacterial endocarditis, collagen disease, drugs and familial traits toward clotting. Underlying disorders should be searched for and the patient's clotting profile should be studied.

Pelvic Thrombophlebitis

Pelvic vein thrombosis may be difficult to diagnose unless evidence of the predisposing gynecologic and obstetrical conditions are noted on pelvic examination. Systemic manifestations may raise suspicion of venous thrombosis in the pelvis. Occasionally, when the hypogastric vein is thrombosed, perivenous inflammation may involve the obturator nerve which passes beneath the vessel. Discomfort may then be referred to the adductor muscles of the thigh or to the knee.

Inferior Vena Cava Thrombosis

Occlusion of the inferior vena cava by an isolated thrombus is rare because of the large volume of blood flowing through the vessel. Occasionally vena caval occlusion occurs from extension of iliac vein thrombophlebitis. When an isolated thrombosis does occur, associated disorders causing the condition include tumors such as lymphoma or hepatoma, trauma, retroperitoneal fibrosis, scleral obstruction of the hepatic veins, and massive infection in children who develop severe dehydration and ·blood dyscrasias. Swelling and congestion may appear in the lower extremities and dilation may appear in the superficial veins on the anterior abdominal wall. Venous flow occurs from the groin toward the umbilicus in the superficial

epigastric veins, instead of in the opposite direction as is normal. Other than the occurrence of pulmonary emboli, the most serious complication is extension of the venous thrombosis into the renal veins, causing the nephrotic syndrome.

Superior Vena Caval Thrombosis

Many diseases may cause this disorder, such as tumors, aortic aneurysms, mediastinitis and histoplasmosis. The head—particularly the conjunctiva—becomes edematous and cyanotic; the arms and chest swell and dilated veins appear on the neck, arms, and upper trunk. The patient may develop vertigo and syncope with exercise.

Septic Thrombophlebitis

Most cases are sequelae of infected sites of venous catheters or are seen in conjunction with burns of the extremities, or following obstetrical and gynecologic manipulations. There are the usual local manifestations of thrombophlebitis plus cellulitis, abscess formation, and accentuated systemic reactions. Cavernous sinus thrombosis from jugular venous dissemination may appear long after chronic mastoiditis has subsided. Neonatal omphalitis may give rise to portal vein thrombosis several months later. Other types of septic thrombophlebitis include pylephlebitis, renal vein thrombosis, vena caval thrombophlebitis, mesenteric vein thrombosis, acute cor pulmonale due to thrombotic occlusion of the pulmonary arteries, and pelvic phlebitis.

Pulmonary Embolism

The diagnosis of pulmonary embolism can be very difficult to make. Most competent clinicians lean toward diagnosis and treatment of pulmonary emboli on suspicion alone because of the difficulties in establishing a firm diagnosis, and because of the risk of death and disability when it goes undiagnosed.

Any major hospital should recognize

the importance of immediate procedures to establish the diagnosis of a pulmonary embolus. Sudden death is admittedly uncommon in patients who die as the result of pulmonary embolism. However, these patients are often received from smaller institutions in precarious condition, and further delay in establishing diagnosis may result in a fatal outcome. Errors in diagnosis are reduced when an expert team is available to perform the necessary diagnostic procedures. Centralization of equipment, personnel and facilities is therefore essential. Pulmonary emboli may arbitrarily be divided into massive, moderate and minor; or massive pulmonary embolism, branch embolism and peripheral embolism. Variables relating to preexisting pulmonary or cardiac disease, acute right heart failure, tachypnea, and cyanosis are the hallmarks of massive or critical embolus.

A plain chest film is initially taken to differentiate embolism from other diseases such as pneumothorax, aneurysm of the aorta and acute cardiac conditions. Decreased vascular markings lead to the suspicion of an embolism or pulmonary infarction. A normal film does not exclude a pulmonary embolus. Angiography is essential if embolism is suspected.

Radioactive lung-scanning should precede angiography, since a normal scan excludes a massive or branch embolus. Lung-scanning is currently performed with I^{131}-labeled albumin administered intravenously and inhalation of radioactive xenon.

Differential Diagnosis

The more common disease entities which may be confused with thrombophlebitis are listed in Table 17–1.

The superficial veins of the lower extremities are frequently a source of "false phlebitis." Many women, particularly women with varicose veins, develop pain and tenderness on the medial aspect of one or both limbs just

TABLE 17–1 DIFFERENTIAL DIAGNOSIS OF DEEP THROMBOPHLEBITIS
"False phlebitis" ("hormonal phlebitis")—pain in saphenous veins immediately prior to menstrual periods and during pregnancy
"Epidemic phlebodynia"—painful cords in the legs during cyclical periods of water retention in women
Cellulitis
Lymphangitis
Superficial (saphenous) thrombophlebitis
Muscle strain
Muscle rupture—gastrocnemius or plantaris
Sciatic neuritis
Posterior tibial neuritis
Entrapment neuritis
Spontaneous night cramps
Arterial insufficiency
"Restless" or "crazy" legs
Lymphedema, congenital and acquired

prior to menstrual periods. The pain is frequently described as burning in nature, and the complaint is localized to the saphenous veins and is termed "hormonal phlebitis." When the extremity is elevated, the vein collapses (an event which does not occur in thrombophlebitis). Pain subsides following menstrual flow. During pregnancy and when anovulatory hormones are used, a similar discomfort may occur, and the patient also notices fluid retention and increased prominence of the limbs. A detailed history and examination plus elevation of the limbs should exclude venous occlusion. Discontinuance of the anovulatory hormones usually relieves symptoms. Another entity known as "epidemic phlebodynia" has been described in young women who develop palpable cordlike structures in the legs. This is thought to be a variant of water retention. Elevation of the limbs allows the superficial veins to collapse. Ballottement or percussion of the saphenous system should demonstrate venous patency. No specific treatment is of benefit because the condition eventually subsides spontaneously.

Congenital and acquired lymphedema may simulate the chronic postphlebitic syndrome, but can be distinguished in most patients by history and physical examination. Patients with lymphedema should be treated initially with pneumatic compression applications, elevation of the extremities, diuretics and elastic stockings. Surgery should be utilized only for refractory or grotesque cases, such as elephantiasis. Pelvic venography is now utilized to identify patients with iliac vein entrapment by the common iliac artery, since this appears to be a cause of unilateral lymphedema in some patients (Fig 17–1).

Cellulitis, with or without lymphangitis, may also be difficult to differentiate from venous thrombosis. However, in most instances of cellulitis the fever is high, which is unlikely in thrombophlebitis unless it is septic. Leucocytosis or a shaking chill also differentiates cellulitis from thrombophlebitis. Antibiotics

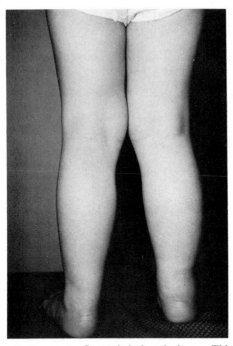

Figure 17–1 Congenital lymphedema. This child with bilateral mild edema was treated with the Jobst pneumatic pressure machine at weekly intervals. Her condition was stable and did not require surgery. Currently, pelvic venography is utilized in such patients to look for entrapment of the iliac vein.

would exclude the possibility of differentiation.

Superficial thrombophlebitis of the saphenous veins in the thigh or calf presents a disturbing problem, since these veins overlie the course of the deep venous system in these two areas. Palpation of a tender cordlike structure, erythema localized to the saphenous vein, or establishment of patency of the vein by elevation or ballottement, and percussion and comparison of the measurement of each extremity's circumference will assist in establishing the diagnosis. When in doubt the patient should be assumed to have deep vein thrombosis also and should be treated accordingly.

Muscular complaints in the leg may easily simulate deep vein thrombophlebitis. Mention has been made previously of the signs which may mimic the presence of thrombophlebitis. These are positive Homan's, Lowenberg's or Ramirez' signs which may be elicited in numerous muscular as well as sciatic nerve disorders. Moreover, all of these conditions may coexist. Muscle strain or rupture of the gastrocnemius or plantaris muscle after direct trauma or following unaccustomed sudden or strenuous exercise in middle-aged men or women can cause severe discomfort in the calf of the leg with swelling, tenderness and a "diagnostic" dorsiflexion sign. A history of diffuse tenderness located medial or lateral to the midline of the calf, swelling over the muscle rupture area, and the presence of ecchymosis at the ankle or lower third of the leg establishes the diagnosis of a ruptured muscle. Plantaris muscle rupture may be present, with tenderness which is usually high in the calf and in the popliteal space, but occasionally in the midcalf. Leg soreness may occur following spontaneous night cramps. Treatment with quinine, benadryl or chloroquine should result in relief for the majority of patients. Included in the differential diagnosis is a strange syndrome identified as "restless or crazy legs." The history of its presence periodically during or after a stressful situation, fatigue or hormonal changes, and the presence of minimal physical findings other than tender muscles in the extremities should help establish this diagnosis. Following femoral-popliteal bypass, swelling of the thigh and leg may occur owing to disturbance of lymphatic channels and increased flow of arterial blood. If calf discomfort occurs, this is strongly suspicious of thrombophlebitis. Most often, this occurs in an extremity which was severely ischemic from recent acute arterial occlusion. The leg pain develops within 48 hours after reconstruction and tenderness is usually localized to each of the compartments of the leg. Tenderness is present in the lateral, posterior or anterior areas of the leg. These findings usually exclude venous thrombosis unless it is demonstrated on phlebography.

Another difficult diagnostic problem is the differentiation of thrombophlebitis from sciatic nerve irritation due to entrapment neuritis. Tenderness over the sciatic nerve on the posterior aspect of the thigh and absence of adductor canal tenderness or tenderness in the calf and the posterior aspect of the thigh will exclude the diagnosis of thrombophlebitis. The possibility of both conditions being present may need to be considered. Peripheral neuritis may be localized to one extremity but usually is more generalized. Nerve tenderness is frequently bilateral.

Supplemental Diagnostic Aids

A number of clinical observations can be utilized to establish the diagnosis of acute venous thrombosis, chronic venous insufficiency, and varicose veins. The two latter disorders do not warrant immediate further study. However, because thromboembolism may have serious and often fatal complications, supplemental diagnostic aids may be necessary. Ancillary diagnostic measures are being employed with increasing frequency in three types of patients with suspected venous disease: those with *silent thrombosis*, when thrombophle-

bitis is suspected but signs and symptoms are minimal or nonexistent; those in whom *pulmonary embolism* is suspected or established but no peripheral evidence of thrombophlebitis is displayed on examination; and patients who are believed to have diseases which are considered in the *differential diagnosis* of thrombophlebitis. The following diagnostic procedures have been proposed in the group of disorders which have a high incidence of deep vein thrombosis.

Phlebography

The importance of phlebography is now reemphasized for both acute and chronic venous disease. Three methods of study may be used: ascending phlebography from the foot, in which the superficial and deep veins of the extremity are studied; direct femoral vein puncture, in which venous pressure and the iliac portion of the venous system are investigated; and osseous phlebography, which is used when venipuncture cannot be performed. The os calcis, malleoli, femoral condyle or greater trochanter can be used, depending upon which segment needs to be evaluated.

Phlebography is indicated to confirm or deny a diagnosis of acute or chronic venous thrombosis and also to locate the source of pulmonary emboli when thrombophlebitis is not observed clinically. It may help to identify the location of venous pathology and follow the course of therapy. It may reveal whether a segment of deep vein is patent and available for a venous graft to an unobstructed normal deep vein. Phlebography can be used to identify perforating veins or venous "lakes" in varicose veins, and in the postphlebitic syndrome with ulceration of the lower extremities. This technique is also used to establish the presence of extra- or intra-iliac vein occlusion in venous or lymphatic disorders. The technique for performing phlebography is extremely important to reduce false readings. Phlebography should be reserved for patients on whom additional information is necessary to assist the clinician in the course of management and therapy.

Doppler-Effect Flowmeter

This is a convenient method of demonstrating blood flow in the superficial and deep veins by means of ultrasound. Some clinicians believe it is more accurate than a physical examination. It is useful in detecting patency of the major veins of an extremity, but it is of no value in demonstrating pathology in their branches or for venous thrombosis when the vein is unobstructed and the venous flow is not affected. It can be a screening technique for patients with a questionable diagnosis.

Impedance Plethysmography

This is another noninvasive screening technique used for occult deep vein thrombosis. The technique is subject to less error than the Doppler technique since probe placement is not critical in measuring the electrical impedance of the extremity. The procedure is based on the observation that impedance varies with blood volume. The normal changes in venous hemodynamics which occur with respiration are greatly reduced or abolished in the presence of partial or complete venous obstruction. These patterns in blood flow can be assessed indirectly by measurement of changes in the electrical impedance of the extremity. The simplicity of the technique permits it to be used at the bedside. Both lower and upper extremities can be evaluated simultaneously. Probably the most important use of this technique is the detection of deep vein thrombosis in asymptomatic patients.

Venous Pressure

This is a valuable procedure which has been used for some time to evaluate varicose veins and chronic deep vein obstruction or insufficiency. Measurements are now usually taken only when phlebograms are being performed. It has been observed that, in foot veins, venous pressure is elevated when there is a proximal venous obstruction. In both iliac thrombophlebitis and lymphedema, comparison of pressures in the femoral veins may reveal the source of the disorder. Iliac thrombophlebitis is four times more common on the left than on the right because of external compression by the right iliac artery or the presence of an intraluminal web. A difference of 2 mm Hg between the two sides indicates iliac vein obstruction. Confirmation is made by exercise when there is an increase of 3 mm Hg or more in venous pressure. When phlebography is contraindicated, venous pressures may be useful in supporting other findings.

Isotope Tests

Several labeled isotopes have been used to localize venous thrombosis in lower extremities. The most commonly accepted method is I^{125}-fibrinogen localization, which is injected into the saphenous vein to provide direct evidence of venous thrombosis in the lower extremities. The use of ^{113m}Indium has recently been reported by Rutherford et al. as a means of providing a quantitative measure of the functional status of leg veins. This procedure appears to be a useful method to appraise the effectiveness of both medical and surgical therapy in venous disease, especially for patients with the postphlebitic syndrome.

Thermography

The clinical use of thermography or infrared photography has had limited acceptance as a screening device for venous disorders. This is probably due to the high cost of the apparatus and the availability of other simpler methods which record information of more importance than temperature alone.

Complications and Sequelae of Thrombophlebitis

The outcome of thrombophlebitis in any particular case is unpredictable since the course of the disease does not always appear to be governed by the usual natural history. It is often controlled with little or no treatment, only to recur weeks, months or years later in the same vein or in another one. Sometimes it shows a stubborn progression, cannot be contained, and leads to death or chronic incapacitation.

Complications begin when the thrombus extends by continuity; it then shrinks and becomes firmer or more adherent, and finally it may fill the entire lumen or float beyond its site of attachment and block other veins. A severe perivenous inflammation may occur, with constitutional symptoms present. Suppuration of the affected vein may ensue and remain localized or result in bacteremia and septic emboli. Even when infection does not occur, the thrombus may detach and become a pulmonary embolus and infarction, which sometimes is fatal. Restoration of vein function may occur, or contraction and permanent obliteration of the vein may develop.

The fate of the thrombus depends upon the degree of derangement of the vessel or the blood. If the involvement is minimal, the entire process can undergo rapid resolution. Significant inflammation or disease prolongs the abnormality. Disturbances in circulation or changes in coagulation aggravate the condition. Gangrene may occur from thrombosis of large venous trunks and collateral veins, and marked spasm of the distal arterial tree.

The main pathophysiological manifestation of thrombophlebitis is obstruction to venous blood flow. The degree of venous impairment varies according to the vessels involved, the extent of the process, the presence of aggravating factors and the availability of collateral circulation.

"Postphlebitic syndrome" is the result of severe derangement of the venous vasculature and adjacent tissues in an extremity, and manifests itself as dermatitis, cellulitis, pigment deposition and infection. Cutaneous ulcers are typically located about the medial and lateral

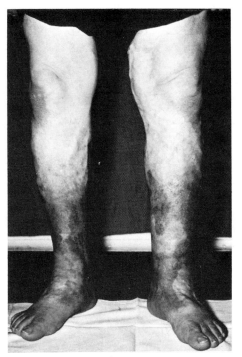

Figure 17–2 Superficial varicose veins secondary to chronic deep thrombophlebitis. Ligation and excision of varicose veins is contraindicated and treatment consists of the standard therapy for the postphlebitic syndrome, as described in the text.

malleoli and are rarely found on the upper portion of the leg. Because some collateral circulation is available, the extremity generally does not become gangrenous. Varicose veins may develop on a secondary basis (Figs. 17–2 and 17–3).

Treatment of Thrombophlebitis

When treating thrombophlebitis, it is important to do no harm. No single therapeutic agent or specific is known at present which will either prevent or cure all types of thrombophlebitis. A disease with such a varied pathogenesis and clinical course as thrombophlebitis can be expected to respond capriciously to therapy. It is essential that a working plan be followed which is based on the appreciation of both the initial manifes-

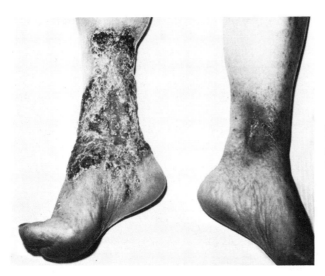

Figure 17-3 Squamous carcinoma arising in chronic postphlebitic ulcer. Ulceration present for many years at the ankle; finally underwent malignant degeneration.

tations and the potential complications of the disease.

The objectives of therapy are:

1. To recognize all predisposing and contributing factors and to eliminate them whenever possible.
2. To neutralize any forerunners of the disease, some of which may be dormant or masked.
3. To provide protection to the vessel walls.
4. To aid embarrassed venous return and enhance circulation.
5. To reduce the clotting potential of the blood.
6. To decrease established phlebitis.
7. To encourage dissolution of clots and prevent propagation of thrombi.
8. To combat incidental or superimposed infection.
9. To support the patient's own resources for mitigating the disease and its complications.

Prophylaxis. Prevention begins with history-taking and identification of the factors which predispose to thrombophlebitis. The patient is asked about allergies and tendencies to bruise or bleed easily; he should also be questioned about quick clotting and erythematous reactions in superficial veins adjoining the site of an injury. A history of previous thrombophlebitis may be elicited by discussing varicosities. The presence of polycythemia, arteriosclerosis, or congestive heart failure will indicate a predilection to thrombophlebitis.

The physical examination is often contributory. Obesity, cardiac dysrhythmias, or impingement on the veins from pregnancy, garters, girdles, or fractures should be noted. Multiple old scars and bruises, especially of the ankles and legs, should lead to careful evaluation of the venous system. Deep venous incompetence, which is particularly significant in geriatric patients, may be identified by a few simple maneuvers. Probably the best determining factor of deep vein incompetence is a history of swelling in one extremity before noon every day.

To aid the physician in detecting patients most susceptible to thrombophlebitis, a clotting profile should be obtained for those patients who have a history of venous thrombosis. Clotting profiles should also be obtained for patients who are presently on, or have recently used, medication which has a known incidence of thromboembolic complications, and for patients who have specific disorders which may predispose to thrombophlebitis. A simple approach is the use of a clinical scoring table like that shown in Table 17-2, which is a modification of a

TABLE 17–2 SCORING SYSTEM FOR RISK
OF THROMBOEMBOLISM*

FACTOR	POINTS
Age 50 or more	3
Major abdominal or pelvic surgery	3
Presence of cancer	2
Serious postoperative complications	2
Prolonged operation (three hours or more)	2
Obesity	1
Varicose veins	1
Abdominal distension	1
Infection, particularly intra-abdominal or retroperitoneal	1
Prolonged immobilization (ten days or more)	1
Heart disease	1
Shock during or after operation—systolic pressure below 80, with pallor and tachycardia for 30 minutes or more	1
Blood dyscrasia or anemia (Hb. 10 gm or less)	1
Previous thromboembolic disease	1
Dehydration	1

*A total score of 6 or more indicates susceptibility to thrombophlebitis.

table devised by Farmer and Smithwick. Any patient whose total score reaches 6 during hospitalization is considered susceptible to thrombophlebitis.

Other criteria, such as the presence of ulcerative colitis, soft tissue trauma and fractures may be added.

The reversal of some conditions which predispose to thrombophlebitis may be impossible at short notice in surgical patients. Nevertheless, useful prophylactic measures can be instituted at the time of hospital admission. When surgery is elective and one can temporize, the risk of thrombophlebitis may be lessened in several ways:

1. Overweight individuals are placed on dietary control.
2. Smoking is forbidden.
3. Varicosities are treated when possible.
4. Physiological imbalances are rectified as much as possible. Patients with reduced pulmonary function are started on breathing exercises; fluid and electrolyte deficits are replaced; anemia is corrected and lagging nutritional states are stimulated by anabolic agents; diabetes is meticulously regulated; hypertension, congestive heart failure and cardiac arrhythmias are controlled within limits. In patients with osteoporosis, the reconstitution of nitrogenous and mineral deficiencies may require months of therapy.
5. Dermatologic disorders such as eczema and epidermophytosis are treated.
6. Chronic infections, such as those occurring in the bronchi or urinary tract, are noted. Antibiotics and anti-inflammatory agents are used as indicated.
7. The tone and architecture of the blood vessels must be sustained. Sympatholytic drugs or sympathetic nerve blocks may be indicated. Elastic compression bandages are often recommended preoperatively. The benefits of an oscillating bed have been demonstrated in various centers, but oscillating beds are generally considered impractical.
8. Rest and preparation of the body is recommended for the stress of surgery. Rest means repose; it is not synonymous with total inactivity.
9. Common sense and proper surgical technique are the best precautions against postoperative complications. Proper positioning of the patient on the operating table is vital.

Modern anesthetic techniques permit fairly rapid recovery but the physician should be alert for signs of hypotension, excessive blood loss, laryngeal edema, gastric regurgitation or dilatation, or cardiac irregularities. All patients should be kept in the recovery room until they are fully reactive. Sedation should be kept to a minimum to facilitate hourly deep breathing.

Some of the programs instituted preoperatively may need to be continued during and immediately after surgery. Some surgeons recommend that all patients who were ambulatory before surgery receive dorsiflexion several times at the termination of the operative procedure to increase the flow within an already lethargic venous circulation. Active and passive use of leg muscles is beneficial immediately after operation unless contraindicated. Early ambulation must be individualized. Elastic stockings or elastic bandages are rarely applied above the knee because they exert a tourniquet effect at the knee. Above the knee bandages are actually unable to compress the thigh. They are uncomfortable to keep in place, and the extra cost is not justified. Venous catheters

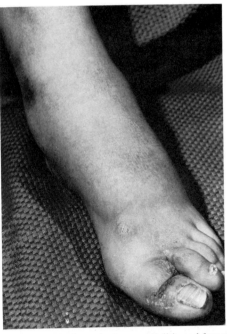

Figure 17–5 Lymphedema, cellulitis and fungal infection of the foot superimposed on chronic thrombophlebitis. Treatment is given as in the postphlebitic syndrome, and in addition potassium permanganate immersion is prescribed for 30 minutes, three times per day for three days. The potassium permanganate solution is 1:1000 (120 mg in 1 quart of water.) Systemic antibiotics are also administered.

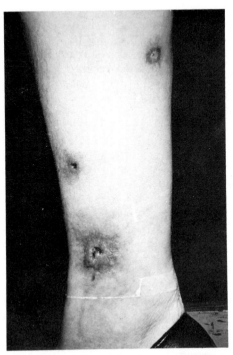

Figure 17–4 Chronic leg ulcers resulting from vasculitis. Often mistaken as postphlebitic ulcerations.

should be inspected frequently and discontinued as soon as possible. Cutdowns should be confined to the upper extremity unless they are life-saving, and should be used no more than 24 hours.

If immobilization is prolonged, passive and active exercises should be started early with the help of a trained physiotherapist. Stasis may be the precursor of sludging and clotting of the blood, but active exercise must be limited by the patient's endurance.

Treatment of the Postphlebitic Syndrome. Patients with this syndrome require education and support on a long-term basis. Patients in our clinic are given the following instructions:

Instructions for Patients With Postphlebitic Syndrome

Your condition is known as the postphlebitic syndrome. It is important that you thoroughly understand this plan of treatment. The condition which you have may lead to complications which will be severely incapacitating, but *with your cooperation* we may control your present disability and gradually restore you to comfort and useful activity.

What Is the Postphlebitic Syndrome?

The postphlebitic syndrome refers to the condition which frequently follows inflammation of the deep veins of the lower extremity. It may range in severity from mild painless swelling of the feet and legs to tremendous enlargement of the entire extremity, accompanied by varicose veins, deep leg ulcers, and even *dangerous* infection. Either one or both legs may be involved.

The process begins with inflammation and clotting of the blood in the veins of the feet and legs. At this stage, there is tenderness in the calf muscles, usually accompanied by swelling of the legs and fever; this is called "phlebitis." Most cases of phlebitis subside without further trouble. However, two things may occur during the phlebitis which lead to the postphlebitic syndrome:

First, the vessels which carry blood from the legs back to the heart, called veins, become plugged. This blocks the drainage of blood from the legs, and the resulting back pressure may cause swelling.

Second, another network of smaller vessels which accompany the veins carries tissue juices from the legs back to the heart; these, too, are called lymphatic vessels. They, too, may become inflamed and obstructed, particularly if there is any infection in the foot or leg. This blocks the lymph (tissue juice) drainage from the legs, and will also cause swelling of the legs and feet which your doctor calls *edema.*

Both the veins and the lymphatic vessels contain one-way valves, which assist in the return of fluid to the heart with movement of the muscles. These valves act the same as the handle of a water-pump, which removes water from a well. When these valves are damaged, the fluid may move in both directions when the vessels are compressed by the muscles. This, plus plugging of these damaged vessels, results in increased back pressure and a more sluggish circulation. Therefore, any smaller vessels which are able to take over by detouring around the obstruction are also blocked by the swelling. Now a vicious circle has developed, in which swelling of the legs and obstruction of the damaged vessels with the loss of the valves aggravate one another.

This last point is extremely important, for the plan of treatment aims to break up the vicious circle by removing a key link in the cycle, namely, by *keeping the swelling out of your legs.* In addition, infection which is present should be cleared by your doctor, and good foot care should be instituted to prevent any future occurrence or recurrence of infection.

No matter how advanced your postphlebitic syndrome may be, proper treatment will result in marked and encouraging improvement, but your full cooperation is absolutely essential. From the beginning, your attention should be directed toward keeping the swelling out of your legs. This will prevent further damage to the remaining drainage vessels and allow new ones to develop and take over the work of those which have been damaged. Special problems, such as varicose veins and leg ulcers, will be handled at the proper time—AFTER THE LEG SWELLING IS UNDER CONTROL.

Plan of Treatment

Two methods are used to remove and prevent a recurrence of swelling in your legs:
(1) Elevation of the legs on at least two pillows;
(2) Elastic stockings, applied whenever you are erect, and occasionally necessary in some patients when the legs are elevated.

Elevation removes the fluid from the legs by means of gravity. When the legs hang down, gravity works against the drainage vessels, and swelling prevails.

The elastic stocking gives the drainage vessels support, and milks fluid from the legs. Seldom is an elastic stocking necessary above the knee since it is more difficult to put on and to keep in place, does not compress the thigh as well as the leg and may produce a garter effect at the knee and intermittently prevent drainage from the leg.

Powder the legs before applying the stocking, especially during the summer. In most cases, the stocking may be left off the extremity while it is elevated in bed—but be sure to put the stocking back on before arising in the morning.

The Postphlebitic Routine

(1) The first step in your treatment is to get *all* of the swelling out of your legs by

means of elevation. This may be accomplished during one night's rest. However, in a few cases, it may take days. Your doctor may prescribe "water pills" to assist the removal of the excess fluid in your legs.

(2) Once you have removed *all* of the swelling, you are ready to start a gradual increase in walking. Remember that you regulate your walking so that you *never allow swelling to return in your legs*. Observe that a *full feeling* beneath the stocking warns you that swelling has just begun to appear. Stop walking or allowing your legs to be down when this fullness appears. They need to be elevated above the level of your body immediately. This fullness may develop in 15 minutes, 2 hours, or even more or less. Don't be discouraged, for improvement will soon begin.

When the time for this fullness has been noted, your next period of walking will be just short of this time. For example, if the fullness appears in 90 minutes, elevate your legs at 60 minutes after arising for 15 minutes, then walk or have them dependent for only 60 minutes (30 minutes less than the fullness period) and elevate them again above the level of your body. This time routine is continued for the remainder of the day. The same routine is continued for a few days and then the dependency period increased to the previous time of fullness. If no fullness occurs then walk or have the legs dependent until fullness does occur. When it does reappear then repeat the routine of elevation, starting again 30 minutes prior to the new noted time of fullness. Now you are walking more than before. In this manner, you will increase the time you are up, in accordance with your findings. Some people will quickly increase their walking time and in a few weeks return to full activity, without swelling in their legs; others will have to go very slowly, being up for only short intervals each day for a week or more, until new drainage vessels develop which will allow longer walking periods without swelling of the legs.

During the period of increasing activity, there are three rules to follow:

(1) Always reapply your elastic stockings *before lowering your legs from bed in the morning or during the day.*

(2) When you are up, *walk*, for walking helps fluid drain from the leg by muscular milking action on the vessels. When you are not actually walking, elevate your legs, either in bed or on a chair. Be an executive; put your feet on the desk!

(a) Do not *sit* with your legs hanging down.

(b) Do not *stand* in one position when you could be sitting with your legs elevated.

If it is imperative that you return to work, you may do so if the swelling does not occur for at least two hours after standing. However, frequent rest periods should be taken at work, and if possible the legs should be elevated on a chair so that progress will continue. When you are able to be on your feet the entire morning without swelling, the time is approaching when you will be free of swelling the entire day with elastic stockings.

Three things retard this program:

(1) Failure to cooperate—routine has not been followed.

(2) Obesity—reduction in weight will be ordered by your doctor, and will be most helpful.

(3) Infection—failure to remove this hinders your efforts in the program. In addition, poor foot care delays the possibility of a successful outcome.

Keep your feet as clean as your face!

Even though you have returned to normal activity, and no swelling appears in your legs with or without elastic stockings during the entire day, there is always the possibility that at some future date you may have a return of this swelling, and it will be necessary for you to repeat the routine. If you discontinue the use of elastic stockings when you are free of swelling it is suggested that you wear them when you are required to sit or stand for long periods.

Conclusion

You must remember that no matter how slow your progress may seem to you now, the *quickest* way for you to return to useful and normal activity is to follow this postphlebitic routine religiously. So when you feel your legs getting heavy and tight under the elastic stocking—take warning, and *elevate your legs.*

Remember—KEEP THE SWELLING OUT OF YOUR LEGS!!!!

Varicose Veins

Abnormally enlarged veins are termed varices or varicose veins. Varicosities usually occur in the lower extremities. They are important clinically because they predispose to venous thrombosis and venous insufficiency. Generally they are dilated, elongated and tortuous. However, a significant number of patients have a long saphenous vein which is straight, thick-walled and apparently normal in appearance, but which shows free reflux of blood into tributaries which are obviously varicose. A normal variant which may be misleading is *venous ectasia*. This is a condition, usually occurring in men, who have leg veins which are prominent but neither tortuous nor thick-walled. These patients usually have similarly enlarged veins in their upper extremities. The valves in these veins are competent and the condition is asymptomatic.

Varicose veins may be classified as *primary* when they are the result of congenital or acquired incompetence of valves or weakness of the wall of the veins. *Secondary* varicose veins are the superficial collateral tributaries which develop following venous occlusion from thrombosis. The differentiation can be very difficult unless an adequate history is obtained and the state of the patient's venous return is carefully evaluated.

Etiology

Varicosities are caused by the presence of one or more of the following: increased intraluminal pressure, destruction of the venous valves, deterioration of the vein wall, or a lack of support of the veins by the surrounding tissues. Once varices occur they usually become self-perpetuating, with increasing dilatation and incompetence. The examining physician frequently finds it difficult to determine whether the varicosities are congenital, familial or acquired. Congenital or familial origin is generally considered a factor in at least 65 per cent of the cases. Acquired varicosities are caused by repeated trauma to the lower extremities, pregnancy, thrombosis in the deep veins, occupations requiring long periods of standing, obesity, under-

garments which constrict the thighs, and chronic infections requiring prolonged rest. Each of these factors should be carefully scrutinized in taking the history, for the cause of the disease often has a bearing on the type of treatment.

The *congenital* varicose veins are seen in patients who present with venous insufficiency soon after puberty. These patients often develop small arteriovenous fistulae with or without cutaneous hemangiomas. They usually have a hereditary history of varicosities and form large varicosities during pregnancy. They frequently present markedly incompetent superficial veins without a history of trauma, deep vein thrombosis or infection.

Varicosities which develop after *trauma* are fairly common, although a history of superficial or deep vein thrombophlebitis occurring after injury may be difficult to obtain. Incompetent veins do not develop until weeks or months after the trauma and do not necessarily show enlargement of the entire saphenous system. Physical findings demonstrate that the varicosities are due to incompetent valves in the perforating veins which connect the superficial veins with the deep veins below the saphenofemoral area. Varicose veins per se do not produce morning swelling of the leg or ankle unless obvious arteriovenous fistula or lymphedema is present. Therefore, any patient presenting with a history of past or present leg edema should be carefully studied, since the cause of lower extremity complaints for the problem may not be due to the obvious varicose veins. Cardiac, hepatic or renal disease may be the cause of edema. No patient should have surgery for varicose veins when leg edema is present. If there is a past history of leg edema in the morning, the cause should be treated and under control before surgery is undertaken. Varicose veins which develop in the postphlebitic syndrome should rarely be ligated or removed since they constitute a small but important pathway for venous return.

Another intriguing aspect of congenital

varices is the presence of macroscopic arteriovenous connections. These can be noted at surgery by opening the saphenous vein and viewing the minute arterial connections under magnification. These A–V connections become prominent during pregnancy and in cirrhotic patients.

Pregnancy is probably the most common acquired cause of varicose veins. Varices do not usually form until the second or third pregnancy. Increased abdominal pressure is a major factor, but hormonal factors are also believed to play a large part in the etiology. Treatment is preferred in the first trimester and no later than the seventh month. Most patients should avoid surgery for varicosities which develop during pregnancy since the majority lessen or disappear following delivery. Surgery can be scheduled in the immediate postpartum period or during an elective period. Labial varices are seldom treated unless they fail to regress after delivery. Labial varices suggest the presence of pelvic varices, especially in the broad ligament. Many obstetricians fear the possibility of hemorrhage from labial varices during an episiotomy and may therefore advise a caesarean section. If noted during pregnancy, labial varices should be operated upon on a prophylactic basis between pregnancies. When surgery must be performed for labial varices during pregnancy, it should be performed as early as possible to lessen the possibility of infection of the labia occurring as a complication and creating a serious problem during and after delivery. Surgery is definitely not advised during the third trimester.

One entity not relieved by varicose vein surgery is a *"restless leg syndrome."* The most common cause of this complaint in women is the stress produced from career commitments or the seemingly endless responsibilities of caring for a number of aggressive children. Due to the tension of the environment the patient experiences fatigue in her legs and finds they are uncomfortable during the evening. She frequently describes them as "crazy legs" and finds comfort only in rest, sedation or walking on a cold floor.

A word is in order regarding the commonly used term, *varicose vein ulcers.* This term should be abandoned, for it implies that the ulcer is due to varicose veins. There is no such entity unless a significant arteriovenous fistula is present. Incompetent veins feeding the area may be a contributory factor but the main source of the disability is disorder in the deep venous system. These patients should not be informed that excision of the incompetent superficial veins can cure the ulcer. On occasion the ulcer may heal but healing is short-lived, since the problem involves the deep venous system. Ninety per cent of the lower extremity blood returns to the systemic circulation via the deep venous system.

Anatomy

The lower extremity has two systems of venous outflow, the deep and the superficial. The deep system is represented by the posterior tibial, the anterior tibial, and the peroneal veins which drain to the popliteal vein and then into the superficial femoral vein at the adductor canal. The superficial vein forms the common femoral vein after receiving the profunda femoris vein at the inferior portion of the fossa ovalis in Scarpa's triangle. This is just below the saphenofemoral junction. The superficial venous system, represented by the long (greater) and short (lesser) saphenous veins, is the site of varicose veins. The two systems are connected by communicating veins which pierce the deep fascia of the extremity. There are usually two or three communicating veins in the thigh and approximately six in the leg. The long saphenous vein drains the medial aspect of the foot, crosses anterior to the medial malleolus, continues up the inner aspect of the leg, going behind the condyles of the tibia and femur. It progresses in an oblique line to the fossa ovalis where it enters the common femoral vein just inferior to the inguinal ligament. Besides the numerous penetrators which join the long saphenous vein with the deep system, there is occasionally a communication with the short saphenous vein which drains into the popliteal vein. In many instances, two long saphenous veins pass the medial area of the knee and join at the lower third of the thigh or continue to the saphenofemoral junction. Three to five tributaries are present near the saphenofemoral junction. Some of these may join the common femoral rather than the long saphenous vein. As mentioned earlier, an accessory saphenous vein may be noted at the saphenofemoral junction joining directly with the femoral vein or connecting with the saphenous vein just below the saphenofemoral junction. Valves are present in both the long saphenous and the perforator veins. Those in the long saphenous vein open superiorly, while the perforator valves open toward the deep system. The saphenous nerve closely accompanies the vein from the medial malleolus to the lower third of the thigh where it enters the adductor canal and continues cephalad as the femoral nerve.

The short saphenous vein begins on the lateral aspect of the foot and runs 1 cm posterior to the external malleolus. It drains the lateral aspect of the leg. It usually ascends to the tendon of Achilles and then progresses up the posterior midportion of the calf to enter the popliteal space. In some cases it penetrates the deep fascia and joins the popliteal vein, usually at the mid-upper third of the leg between the heads of the gastrocnemius muscle. This vein also has several perforators connecting with the deep veins of the leg. The short saphenous vein is accompanied by the sural nerve from the medial malleolus to the upper portion of the calf, where the nerve continues on to join the sciatic nerve in the area of the popliteal fossa.

Anomalies of both the long and short saphenous veins are common and should be searched for during the examination and at operation. Failure to recognize anomalies is the most common cause of development of so-called "recurrences."

The deep veins are in a fascial compartment, surrounded by muscle. The deep veins are the chief component of the "venous heart" which is responsible for the major part of the venous drainage from the lower extremity. In contrast, the superficial veins lie in the subcutaneous fatty tissue and have relatively little support from surrounding tissue. The superficial system of saphenous veins contributes only a small portion of the total venous return from the lower extremity. The deep veins have bicuspid valves which maintain the flow of blood upward. They do not permit backflow unless they are incompetent. Blood flow is propelled upward by contracting muscles beneath the fascia, assisted by a combination of other forces such as capillary pressure and cardiothoracic aspiration produced by respiratory movements. Fluctuations in venous flow are demonstrated by impedance plethysmography. The role of muscle contraction can be demonstrated in varicose veins when their content is decreased during ambulation. Here muscle contraction directs the blood from the superficial system toward the deep system via the communicating veins which are supplied by one-way bicuspid valves.

Symptoms

Symptoms of varicosities vary among patients. However, careful questioning almost always reveals some symptomatology when prominent veins are evident. In every case, the examining physician should completely examine the lower extremity, including the arterial system, to exclude any other basis for the patient's complaints. Disfigurement of the extremities is obviously an indication for operation but it is very much overemphasized. The true reason for evaluating the patient for surgery is frequently not listed.

There may be an increased tendency to fatigue of the muscles of the leg, and a sensation of fullness, congestion and soreness in the region of the veins after standing for a variable period of time. The actual course of the long or short saphenous veins may be traced by the patient as the bothersome site for the patient's complaints, especially during the period of two or three days just prior to menstrual flow at which time the veins appear larger. There may be burning pain and itching in the area overlying the varices. Muscular cramps occasionally occur, particularly at night. The patient's symptoms often seem disproportionate to the amount of actual pathology observed; nevertheless, they almost invariably clear up on removal or obliteration of the involved veins. Swelling when present is minimal and localized around the ankle after the patient has been on his feet all day. Swelling occurs in the evening and disappears during the night.

Primary varicosities seldom show skin changes. Secondary varicosities frequently show skin changes, and symptoms which pertain both to the varicosities and to the underlying venous disorder. Itching, dermatitis, morning edema, fibrosis and ulceration in the region of the ankle are usually the result of deep vein incompetency or trauma.

Little can be done for telangiectatic veins unless bleeding, following minor trauma, occurs.

A few minor varices should not be blamed for all of the patient's leg symptoms.

Examination

Inspection of the lower extremities is conducted with the patient standing on a foot stool. Distended veins may be related to the long or short saphenous system. Spiderlike intracutaneous venules may be separate or related to obvious large vein varicosities. Similar small venular dilatations occurring at the ankle or foot suggest deep venous insufficiency, long-standing varicosities with a history of repeated pregnancies or a strong history for congenital varices. This small group of patients, termed

"vein formers," are the patients who may develop recurrent varicosities following adequate varicose vein surgery.

A number of tests are available for examination of varicosities. Some should be abandoned, others used only when indicated, and a few should be conducted regularly on all patients. Varicosities below the knee are almost always plainly visible to the examiner; however, frequently the long saphenous vein in the thigh with its connecting tributaries from the leg and occasionally the short saphenous vein are not obvious due to a large amount of subcutaneous fat. This prevents proper mapping of the venous pattern. Accurate determination of the size of the vein being examined is difficult to assess, and areas where incompetent perforators are present may be obscure. Tourniquet tests are usually valueless in these patients, for the flow pattern seldom can be demonstrated. This problem is far more evident in females than in males. The following tests are advised:

Percussion or ballottement test (Schwartz-Heyerdale) is utilized to identify the course of the long and short saphenous veins. This test augments the information obtained from visualization and simple palpation. It also demonstrates variables such as the presence of more than one long saphenous vein, or a variable course of the short saphenous vein. The short saphenous vein should be traced into the popliteal vein or into the long saphenous below the knee or in the thigh. It may also have connections to the popliteal and long saphenous veins. In addition, when there is a marked enlargement of the long saphenous vein in the thigh, an incompetent perforator may be looked for at this point. Patients are permitted to feel the size of the enlarged incompetent main vein in the thigh during percussion. The percussion is extended around the medial aspect of the thigh to determine if additional accessory saphenous veins are present, and to determine where a tributary enters the saphenous system. Percussion may also demonstrate that a soft bulge on the leg is actually muscle herniating through a small fascial defect. This can be confirmed by its appearance and disappearance during dorsiflexion on the foot. No pulse wave is transmitted from one of these bulging areas.

To perform the percussion or ballottement test, the examiner's hand is placed at the level of the lower third of the medial aspect of the thigh with the fingertips on the area where the vein is expected to be present. The other hand is used for percussion or ballottement of the vein below this level. By moving both hands along the vein, it is possible to map the vessel and its branches completely. Experience with this method allows the examiner to determine the size of the vessels, their course, the amount of scarring in the vein wall, and the number of incompetent perforators. The latter may be observed at points of bulging of the vein at the thigh or along the leg medial to the tibia. The percussion test does not establish competence of the venous channel or the direction of flow.

Tourniquet tests (Brodie-Trendelenburg) are used mainly for patients who have questionable varices or to rule out any connection between the short and the long saphenous vein in the thigh. It is difficult to determine the vein causing reflux in the short saphenous vein—that is, whether the reflux comes from the popliteal vein, or the long saphenous vein, or a perforating vein. Control of the reflux with digital pressure at these sites separately or in combination will clarify the direction of flow.

The tourniquet walking test (Perthes' test) has often been suggested as a means for demonstrating deep vein incompetency. In this test, which involves placing a tourniquet on the thigh and instructing the patient to walk, if the veins empty below the tourniquet it is concluded that the deep veins are incompetent. A modification is the use of an elastic support to the knee. In this case, if discomfort develops shortly after ambulation, the deep venous system is considered occluded. The presence of edema during the morning or early afternoon hours is a more reliable means of evaluating the efficiency of the deep venous system. Until proved otherwise, the deep venous system is considered functionally adequate if morning or early afternoon edema does not occur. No patient should have a total saphenous system excision or stripping until edema which occurs early in the day is controlled for several months. Venography or supplemental procedures may be performed to confirm the adequacy of the deep venous system but they are not essential when an adequate history and physical examination do not disclose the presence of edema. The examiner must understand the stages of venous insufficiency which result from progressive involvement of the valves. The Trendelenburg test is frequently used, in which the patient is told to lie supine on the examining table with his lower extremity raised above the level of the body until all superficial veins are collapsed. Thumb pressure is applied over the fossa ovalis or a tourniquet applied lightly at midthigh or the upper leg. Specific sites may be controlled by thumb pressure in the calf during the time the tourniquet is in place. The patient is then allowed to stand erect and the following observations are made: (1) retrograde filling of an incompetent vein to the tourniquet, with the vein below this area remaining empty; (2) rapid filling of the saphenous vein from the deep system below the tourniquet, demonstrating perforator incompetence; (3) sudden retrograde filling of the vein approximately 15 seconds after the tourniquet is released, denoting total vein incompetence; and (4) sudden filling of the vein below the tourniquet before it is released, demonstrating incompetence of the short saphenous vein or the perforating veins. The tourniquet may be applied at any point along the lower extremity.

These methods of examination determine the incompetence of the long or short saphenous vein or both, and allow the examiner to recommend the type of surgery necessary to remove the veins. These tests have limited usefulness since most patients with varicose veins are women, generally with moderately obese thighs, in whom the long saphenous vein flow pattern cannot be determined with these test maneuvers.

Treatment

Surgeons vary widely in their initial treatment of varicose veins. A thorough understanding of normal and abnormal anatomy, pathology and physiology of these vascular channels is necessary. Without such an understanding various complications such as deep vein thrombosis, nonhealing ulcers, uncontrolled edema, lymphorrhea, causalgia and even loss of the leg are possible following surgery.

When there is indecision regarding the benefits which may be obtained from surgery because the patient's complaints are indecisive or the varicosities are borderline, nonoperative treatment is advisable. Elastic stockings from toe to knee are prescribed and supplemented with intermittent elevation of the lower extremities above body level for short periods daily. Long periods of sitting or standing are to be avoided, especially in women prior to menstrual periods. Panty girdles and other constricting garments and the varied use of high heeled and flat soled shoes are inadvisable. Mild exercise is suggested on a regular basis. Anxiety from stress of career or homelife is investigated, for such stress may cause muscle tension resulting in fatigue in extremities, called "restless" or "crazy" legs (see above). Frequently this entity is misdiagnosed as being due to varicose veins, even when the veins are not significant in appearance and unlikely to be the cause of the patient's discomfort.

Operative Treatment

Indications for surgery may be listed as: (1) symptoms localized to superficial veins or the entire extremity; (2) superficial thrombophlebitis of less than 24 hours duration, with no evidence of deep vein involvement; (3) appearance — cosmetic; (4) prophylaxis against deep venous thrombosis and its complications; and (5) "recurrent" varicosities.

Unnecessary surgery should be avoided; when in doubt, nonoperative measures should be instituted at least for a trial period. Isolated vein surgery or slcerosing is discouraged. A cardinal rule in vascular surgery holds that in order to interrupt vascular flow permanently, a vessel needs to be ligated and partially excised or recanalization and bridging will occur. This is nature's method of recovery.

Surgery for varicose veins does not always necessitate hospital admission. The following procedures can be performed on an outpatient basis in the operating room with no more risk than occurs with admission.

1. *High Ligation of the Long Saphenous Vein with Excision of a Segment.* This procedure is adequate if incompetence is present only at the saphenofemoral junction. However, frequently the segment is not obliterated due to incompetent perforators. Objections to this operation brought forth the second procedure:

2. *High Ligation of the Long Saphenous Vein and its Tributaries with Excision of a Segment.* Dissection and partial excision of the tributaries are absolutely necessary for examination of anatomical variations which may be present at or near the saphenofemoral junction. However, the objection to this treatment alone is the same as (1).

3. *High and Low Excision and Ligation of the Long Saphenous Vein.* Whether or not the tributaries have been dissected back and excised in the high ligation, this method still does not remove the varicose segment. Recurrences occur due to a bifid or dual saphenous vein. In addition, a communicating vessel may develop as a result of an incompetent perforator.

4. *High Ligation and Excision Followed by Retrograde Sclerosing Therapy.* This

procedure probably has the highest incidence of complications since sclerosing therapy has been added to a surgical procedure; these complications are listed below.

5. *High and Low Ligation with Retrograde Sclerosing Therapy at Both Sites* (see No. 4).

6. *Isolated Injection of Small Varicose Segments.* This procedure has the disadvantages listed for sclerosing therapy and should be used only when the major component has been ligated and excised. Too frequently these isolated varices are connected and are the result of an incompetent major system (the long or short saphenous). The procedure merely leads to recanalization with further damage to the vessel.

7. *High Ligation and Excision of the Long Saphenous Vein with its Tributaries, Followed by Segmental Ligations and Partial Excision of the Vein.* Even with an extremely thorough examination before operation, perforators and communicating veins could easily be missed. This procedure is designed to locate and ligate the perforators and communicating veins.

8. *High Ligation of the Long Saphenous Vein and its Tributaries Followed by Stripping of the Entire Long Saphenous Vein, Utilizing the Intraluminal (Babcock, Meyers, Emmerson, Zollinger), or Extraluminal (Mayo) Stripper.* By performing this segmentally, the vein in the thigh can be inspected in its entirety, and any variables present may be observed and surgically excised. One modification of this technique is to make two incisions, at the groin and at the ankle, and to strip between the two points. This latter procedure is probably the most common method presently performed in most hospitals. However, its use should be discouraged, since it is a crude, blind technique which misses variables and allows "recurrences." It also necessitates a full-length elastic bandage which is objectionable due to limitation of flexion postoperatively and discomfort at the knee. The potential of deep vein thrombosis in the extremity is increased as a result of the trauma of surgery and the subsequent postoperative splinting. Sludging can be demonstrated by phlebography or one of the flow tests.

9. *High Ligation of the Long Saphenous and Tributaries with Stripping to an Area Just Below the Knee, Followed by Complete Excision of the Lower Segment Along with Scar Tissue and Fascia.* This procedure is more radical than is required.

The short saphenous vein may be treated by the same forms of therapy tabulated above.

A few patients may not be completely cured during the initial operation. They may have to return for further treatment, at which time an isolated segment may be ligated and excised. Excision is preferred to sclerosing therapy for obliteration of an isolated segment after operation. Therefore, enough operating time should be allowed to clear a patient's varicosities so that there will be a minimal chance of recurrent varices. Admittedly, the procedure is more lengthy than other approaches but it assures the patient of complete extirpation of the offending viens with few exceptions. Only one extremity is operated upon at a time.

We recommend high ligation and excision of the long saphenous vein and its tributaries, followed by segmental excision or stripping technique (techniques 7 or 8). The short saphenous vein is treated similarly either at the same time or at a later date.

Anesthesia

The anesthetic should allow ambulation as soon as possible following surgery. Epidural is preferable, although light general or local may be employed. Spinal anesthesia is not desirable because of the possibility of long motor paralysis and spinal headache. Epidural anesthesia may occasionally produce spinal headache when the dura has been entered. Properly applied local anesthesia can also be very satisfactory.

Virtually all patients are ambulatory within two or four hours after operation and are instructed to walk a few steps or move every hour during the day. Ambulation is gradually increased until the patient is able to walk well. If general or spinal anesthesia is used, passive exercises should be carried out immediately after operation and for several minutes of every hour until the patient is capable of ambulation.

Local or epidural anesthesia has been used in all but 8 of 456 cases in which we have performed the excision and stripping technique. Excluding the 8, these patients were discharged after a few hours under observation without being admitted to the hospital. We do not mean to imply that excision and stripping of varicose veins is a simple operation or that it could be an office procedure. The operations were closely supervised, and in no instance have we or the patients felt that postoperative care was neglected. The few possible complications could easily have developed even if the patient had been admitted to the hospital. All patients received medication for sleep and pain, plus thorough instructions before leaving the hospital.

Reasons for discharging these patients immediately after surgery are: (1) vacant beds in hospitals are often limited and should be available for patients who need admission; (2) postoperative therapy in the hospital offers very little which cannot be provided at home; and (3) financial saving to the patient and "third party" programs is considerable.

The procedure most often performed is high ligation and excision at the saphenofemoral junction with wide excision of the tributaries followed by complete stripping of the long and sometimes the short saphenous veins. When this method of extirpation of the saphenous vein is performed, it is probably hazardous to discharge the patient, especially if a pressure dressing is applied to the entire extremity. We advocate stripping only below the knee following complete excision of the varicosities in the thigh.

Preoperative Preparation

Morning swelling and ulcers are allowed to clear before surgery is performed; treatment of the sequelae of the postphlebitic syndrome is discussed below. Occasionally varices are marked on the skin before surgery, although the surgical procedure excises the incompetent segments causing the varices. When they are marked, this is done the day before surgery on veins which do not follow the usual course or have a bizarre pattern. An ordinary pen is used. The areas are scratched with a needle beside the marking before skin preparation is started and while anesthesia is being instituted.

Operation (Fig. 17–6)

We prefer a high longitudinal or slightly oblique incision from 3 to 5 inches long. This incision has specific advantages: (1) The incision is in line with the vessel which has been percussed and palpated and also with the femoral vein and artery so that it allows better visualization of these vessels should control be necessary. (2) Transverse incisions have a greater probability of cutting lymphatic vessels and traumatizing lymph nodes, sometimes resulting in lymphedema and lymphorrhea. We believe that the ankle swelling which may appear after operation is not necessarily an indication of deep vein thrombosis but is more characteristic of lymphedema. (3) Excision of a large segment under direct vision is readily possible by this type of incision. In addition, more of the wound is utilized since it is in line with and not transverse to the axis of the vessel.

The remainder of the incisions are also longitudinal along the course of the vessel except the one used in the popliteal space for the short saphenous vein. We have found that this incision has a better cosmetic appearance on the extremity, particularly in females, since the lines of a woman's stocking run longitudinally rather than transversely.

Care and Method of Ligation. After the incision has been made up to the inguinal crease, the long saphenous vein is dissected to the saphenofemoral junction, with careful ligation of all tributaries, dissection of each tributary back as far as possible, and wide excision of each segment. From three to five tributaries may be expected. Because there may be a direct connection between the femoral vein and one of these tributaries or an accessory saphenous vein, the femoral vein is gently exposed and inspected on both the medial and lateral aspects to obviate recurrent varicosities originating from this area. Any blunt dissection against the axis of the vein is avoided to obviate puncture of the vessel. The saphenofemoral junction is then doubly ligated flush with the femoral vein, with the distal ligature being a transfixion suture. Dissection should be cautious because of the presence of the small external pudendal artery which traverses the inferior portion of the fossa ovale. This artery may have its course over or beneath the long saphenous vein at this point. If it is damaged, it should be carefully ligated, since it is notorious as a site of postoperative bleeding.

Method of Segmental Stripping. The inferior segment of the saphenous vein is dissected under direct vision and an attempt is made to localize the highest perforator, which is usually just inferior to the groin incision. Any communicating or perforating vessel is directly visualized, clamped, and ligated. The superior dissection also locates any accessory saphenous vein which may be present. The inferior segment of the long saphenous is utilized to locate the mid-thigh point of incision. A large majority of the incompetent perforators occur at this site. The superior wound is not closed until the segment between the two incisions has been dissected or stripped out. Here one end of the vessel is converted into the other wound and the perforator is ligated when present. In most cases the entire segment is removed under direct vision by gently pulling up (rather than back) on retractors. After the segment has been removed, the first incision is closed with interrupted sutures, carefully obliterating any pockets where serum may collect. The operation is then continued inferiorly in the same manner, with the third incision approximately four inches above the knee, avoiding the flexion crease. This third incision is important in looking for a perforator or a bifid saphenous vein; when the latter is present both segments are stripped to the ankle. The next incision is just below the knee. When two saphenous veins are present in this area the incision is made at a point midway between the two vessels. The dissection of the saphenous vein in the thigh is done under direct vision to minimize the possibility of recurrences and the incidence of postoperative hematoma. Close observation is made for a communication with the short saphenous vein at any point along the long saphenous vein in the thigh even though it was not found on preoperative examination. In such cases the short saphenous vein is excised or stripped at the same operation.

Occasionally no incision is made below the knee if the operator is confident that the long saphenous is a single segment which goes directly to the ankle. In such a case, the next incision is made over the internal malleolus in a longitudinal direction, and the stripper is placed into the lumen of the vein at this site. However, the procedure is much easier to perform if a fourth incision is made inferior to the knee. When the stripper is passed, care is taken that the first attempt allows easy passage of the stripper, since occasionally the vessel may go into spasm and make the second passage difficult. Perforation of the vein wall may occur. When the operator is not sure of the specific course taken by one of the vessels observed, they can easily be traced by passage of the instrument.

Many types of intraluminal strippers are available—some have filiform tips, others have olive or acorn ends and some allow injection of saline to distend

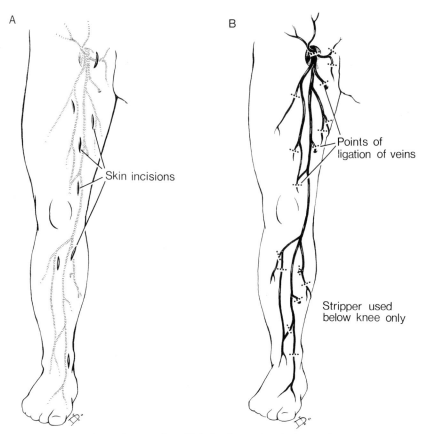

Figure 17-6 Surgery for varicose veins. High ligation and stripping of the greater saphenous vein is performed as described in the text. This operation can be performed on an outpatient basis when suitable anesthesia and postoperative recovery facilities are available.

the vessel so that the stripper may be passed through a tortuous vein. The only type of stripper necessary is one which is sufficiently flexible and has small olive or acorn tips which are interchangeable.

The short saphenous vein is stripped and excised in approximately one out of ten cases. A transverse incision is made at the popliteal space and longitudinal incisions are placed at the mid-calf and 1 cm posterior to the external malleolus. It should be noted that a longitudinal incision is not made across the popliteal space.

Four anatomical variations of the short saphenous vein are possible. In 57 per cent of cases, the short saphenous vein goes directly into the popliteal vein through the popliteal space; in 21 per cent, the same connection with the popliteal vein is present but a tributary is evident coursing up the posterior aspect of the thigh and going into the deep system at a higher point; in 12 per cent, the short saphenous vein does not enter the popliteal vein but connects with the long saphenous vein near the saphenofemoral junction; and in 10 per cent, the saphenous vein enters the deep fascia below the popliteal space, coursing between the two heads of the gastrocnemius to join up with the popliteal vein. The stripper is introduced from the ankle to aid in identifying variables.

Only one lower extremity is operated upon at a time.

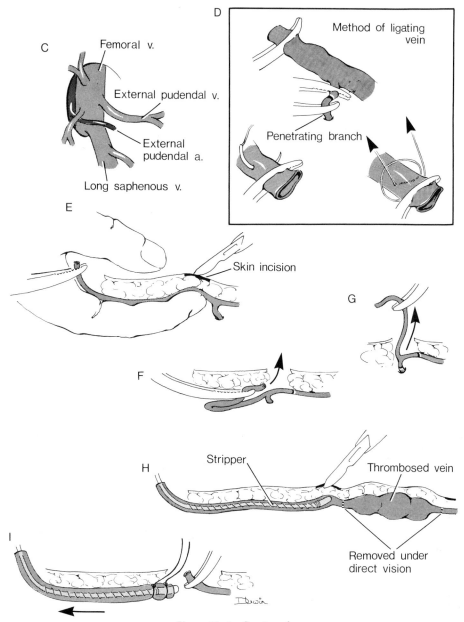

Figure 17–6 Continued.

The incidence of recurrence has been less than 5 per cent, and half of these were vessels which had been missed at operation and therefore should not be considered recurrences.

Postoperative Care

The extremity is wrapped with an elastic bandage from the toe to the knee. Instructions are given to walk a few minutes of every waking hour and to elevate the extremity between ambulatory periods and at night. Mild sedation is given for pain and discomfort. Antibiotics are not indicated. Most patients return to their occupations within five or six days. On the seventh day, the wounds are inspected and the sutures generally removed.

Sclerosing Therapy

Sclerosing injections are not used at our institution because recanalization is common following this method of treatment. When varicosities do recanalize (usually within two years) they are worse than when originally seen. It has been our experience that the most bizarre patterns of varicose veins have been in those patients who have had repeated sclerosing therapy.

Causes for Recurrences

Excluding recurrences which follow other procedures, the majority of recurrences are the result of missing or subsequent opening of incompetent veins connecting the saphenous and deep venous circulation. Three explanations for missed varicosities are (1) failure to ligate and excise points of communication with the deep penetrator; (2) failure to ligate and excise all tributaries at the saphenofemoral junction including an accessory saphenous vein; (3) failure to make sure that both sides of the femoral vein are under direct vision; and (4) failure to recognize the occasional long saphenous vein which is bifid just above the knee.

Incompetency of the saphenous vein from the saphenofemoral junction is the same as incompetency from a deep penetrator connecting the saphenous vein at the superficial femoral vein.

Varicose Veins with the Postphlebitic Syndrome

Varicosities occur in two out of three patients with the postphlebitic syndrome. They invariably have morning swelling, whereas the patient with varicose veins alone has ankle swelling only late in the afternoon. Treatment of varicosities in the presence of the postphlebitic syndrome is not undertaken until a minimum of six months' therapy has been successfully accomplished. The swelling should be controlled until it occurs only late in the afternoon. Therapy regarding postphlebitic syndrome has been discussed earlier.

Varicose Veins with Acute Superficial Thrombophlebitis

Extremities of patients with acute superficial thrombophlebitis are closely examined for deep vein involvement. If no such evidence exists, they may receive high ligation and excision with stripping regardless of the presence or absence of varicose veins. This procedure was very frequently performed a decade ago but due to the successful use of anti-inflammatory drugs, few now require surgery.

ARTERIAL DISEASES

Peripheral arterial diseases are manifested most frequently in the lower extremities, but they are not clinically limited to these areas. Any acute or insidious pathological change occurring in an arterial vessel distal to the heart is considered as peripheral arterial disease.

Vasospastic Disorders

The three most common vasospastic disorders are Raynaud's phenomenon, acrocyanosis and livedo reticularis. Each of these conditions may occur as a primary disorder, as a secondary condition due to an underlying systemic disease, or as an entity resulting from some mechanical irritation to a major artery proximal to the symptomatic area.

Raynaud's Phenomenon

Raynaud's phenomenon is the most common vasospastic condition. A typical case involves first the tip of one or more fingers and later may progress to include the entire digit and even the hand. Usually the disorder begins unilaterally and later becomes bilateral. The toes and feet may be included in the symptomatology but never without the presence of upper extremity findings. Symptoms and signs are characterized first by intermittent pallor or a cyanosis and finally by reactive hyperemia. Numbness initially occurs in the digit(s), and "burning" paresthesias may develop later during the erythematous phase. Swelling of the involved fingers often occurs. Even though gangrene of the part is frequently feared by the patient, nutritional lesions are absent or limited to the skin, usually of the fingertips alone. These lesions vary from petechial spots and spontaneous subungual hematomas to frank ulceration. The condition is most often noted in young females and is initiated by exposure to cold, trauma or emotional stress.

Any patient with Raynaud's phenomenon needs further study to determine the underlying basis for the condition. Three possibilities are presently considered: (1) the rare primary group, termed "Raynaud's disease," which includes patients in whom an underlying cause is not established within two years; (2) the secondary group includes Raynaud's phenomenon due to associated conditions such as collagen diseases, metabolic occlusive arterial disease, neurogenic lesions, drug and heavy metal intoxication, and blood dyscrasias; and, (3) Raynaud's phenomenon related to repeated mechanical trauma to the shoulders, hands and fingers. Occasionally in these patients there is clinical evidence of the thoracic outlet syndrome. In this group of patients there is continuous or intermittent irritation of the subclavian artery or vein or brachial plexus.

The studies required to determine the underlying basis for the Raynaud's phenomenon begin with a blood clotting profile and digital capillary examination. Plethysmography may be used to document the arteriolar blood flow. Laboratory procedures should be ordered cautiously when the only complaint is that of color changes in the extremity. Elaborate studies costing the patient hundreds of dollars are unjustly ordered when no other sign or symptom is evident from history or physical examination. "Artful procrastination" is advised when considering these studies,

yet close attention is paid toward treatment of the symptomatology.

Treatment of Raynaud's phenomenon is generally concentrated on protection from exposure to cold, trauma and emotional stress.

Medical Treatment. 1. The patient is thoroughly educated as to the nature of the condition and reassured that extensive gangrene will not occur. Known factors which precipitate vasoconstrictive episodes and occasional ischemic changes on the fingertips such as cold, emotional upset, trauma, cigarette smoking and infection are included in the discussion. During winter weather, warm clothing is advised including heavy stockings and gloves and protection of the head. Special heating devices for hands and feet may be suggested. Summer weather does not exclude additional protection, for it may be necessary in drafts or low evening temperatures. A change of climate may be advised, though it is rarely necessary.

2. Psychiatric evaluation is suggested only when it is needed to prevent or reduce significant manifestations of emotional instability.

3. The use of tobacco is strongly discouraged. Evidence of its effect is easily identifiable by finger symptomatology, gross evidence of sweating or vasoconstrictive activity demonstrated by plethysmography during a period of smoking.

4. Prophylactic care of hands and feet is mandatory. Any surgical procedure on digits is ill-advised and should be discouraged since minor trauma may precipitate vasospasm and ischemia. When digital surgery is necessary, local anesthesia to the digit should never be used. Many of these patients are excellent candidates for causalgic pain syndromes. They are therefore warned of the hyperesthesia which may follow trauma or infection to their hands or feet, and informed that pain can be treated by medical or surgical sympathetic denervation.

5. Even though empirical ordering of laboratory procedures is not advised, underlying diseases or physical causes are constantly considered concurrently

with treatment of Raynaud's phenomenon.

6. Several approaches to therapy may be initiated.

a. Mechanical entrapment causing arterial or neurological irritation in the shoulder area from a thoracic outlet syndrome may require some method of medical sympathetic denervation. Irritation may occur when shoulder exercises are advised before considering surgery, or following excision of the first rib in which an upper thoracic sympathectomy has not been performed (Fig. 17–7).

b. If an underlying systemic disease, such as one of the collagen diseases, is present and if ulcerations are present, the use of subcutaneous heparin is prescribed on a long-term basis. Sympatholytic drugs are also used to relieve superficial pain and to attempt to maintain a more normal digital color pattern. A third approach to drug therapy is the use of reserpine or methyl dopa.

None of the treatments for Raynaud's disease and Raynaud's phenomenon are entirely satisfactory. Oral administration of sympatholytic drugs, sublingual use of nitroglycerine, and intramuscular injection of estrogens have been used with varying results. These drugs have not produced sustained changes in signs and symptoms. The role of sympathectomy is also inconsistent. Almost all patients will show improvement for the first six months following operation, but half of the patients will subsequently develop a recurrence of symptoms and signs. The greatest improvement occurs in patients with digital-artery thrombosis and in those individuals who have been classified as primary Raynaud's phenomenon. The outcome is poor in patients with scleroderma and other connective tissue diseases in which sympathectomy is contraindicated. These disorders are difficult to diagnose in their early stages, and the prognosis with any treatment may therefore be difficult.

c. The following therapy is advised in patients with Raynaud's phenomenon:

The most promising drug presently being used is reserpine, a drug with a potentially dangerous central depressant action. This effect is seen with oral therapy, in which doses should be about 0.25 mg daily. The preferred method of administration is intra-arterial, using 0.5 mg into the brachial artery. Some reports maintain that relief of pain and ulceration may be present for as long as six months. In addition, the patient may again become responsive to therapy, such as sympatholytic drugs, to which he had become resistant.

Oral or intramuscular injections of reserpine are prescribed as tolerated from 0.25 to 1 mg. The blood pressure is regularly monitored on each visit to avoid the discomforts and hazards

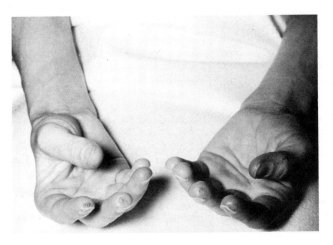

Figure 17–7 Raynaud's phenomenon due to entrapment in thoracic outlet. Note fingertip necrosis. Treatment: first rib resection and simultaneous extrapleural thoracic sympathectomy.

which may occur if it is significantly lowered. The side effects of reserpine are described in the instructions given to the patient. Reserpine administration has been reported to deplete catecholamines with or without depletion in serotonin. Response to reserpine has been very gratifying in patients with Raynaud's phenomenon, but further studies are necessary to determine the safety and long-term benefits of this form of therapy.

Methyl dopa is another promising drug for treatment of Raynaud's phenomenon. This drug is preferred initially in patients who have moderately severe signs and symptoms; patients with minor complaints should not be treated with methyl dopa. Dosage ranges from 1 to 2 gm per day, and side effects normally are minimal. The mechanism of action may depend on a relatively biologically inert metabolite of the drug-binding alpha receptors (Ahlquist's protein) on cutaneous blood vessel walls. The strongly vasoconstricting catechol, norepinephrine, is thereby displaced.

Six sympatholytic drugs are prescribed separately for a few days to one week at a time to determine their effects on pain, temperature, skin color and the function of involved digits. These drugs are azapetine phosphate (Ilidar) 25 to 100 mg; dihydro ergot alkaloids (Hydergine), 0.5 to 1 mg orally or sublingually; phenoxybenzamine hydrochloride (Dibenzyline) 15 mg; tolazoline hydrochloride (Priscoline), 25 to 50 mg; nylidrin hydrochloride (Arlidin), 6 to 12 mg; or cyclandelate (Cyclospasmal), 100 to 200 mg when necessary three times a day and at bedtime. Since the response to each of these drugs may vary, a record of the benefits and side effects observed will determine which drug or combination of drugs will be most beneficial. Medication should be used when symptoms are expected. Medication is therefore taken prior to exposure to an adverse environment, rather than on a specified time schedule. However, when vasospasm, pain or ischemic ulcerations are continuously present, regular administration of medications is indicated. Because of recent success obtained by reserpine therapy, sympatholytic drugs have lost much of their popularity. Their use is now reserved to cases in which reserpine produces little if any benefit or is contraindicated. Sympatholytic drugs are also indicated when sympathectomy is being considered. When sympatholytic drugs produce a good response, relief of symptoms should be expected following sympathectomy.

Surgical Treatment. Surgical measures may be indicated when medical therapy fails to control digital complications, such as pain, subungual hematoma, recurrent ulcerations, paronychia, atrophy of soft tissue and osteoporosis. The strongest indication for surgery is the presence of the thoracic outlet syndrome and the traumatization of subclavian vessels. This is rarely seen. We treat the thoracic outlet syndrome by removal of the first rib via the axilla or the posterior thoracic area. Shoulder exercises are often prescribed for at least three months before surgery is undertaken. The patient is advised to elevate both shoulders and bring them forward during the day on a frequent schedule. The shoulder exercises should also be performed at other times, as when passing through a doorway and when stopping for a red light while driving. The objective is to correct a sagging shoulder posture, relieving the scissors effect on the soft tissues of the thoracic outlet caused by two "bony blades," namely, the clavicle and the first rib. Many patients will have very dramatic relief of symptoms while most, when properly diagnosed, will receive some amelioration of symptoms by exercise alone. When cervical ribs are demonstrated by x-ray, both the cervical rib and first rib are excised. When the clavicle or first rib is abnormal, or when the subclavian artery is already occluded, definitive vascular surgery and first rib removal via the clavicular bed are required. Shoulder exercises are contraindicated in these patients.

An upper thoracic sympathectomy is almost always performed when the first rib is removed for Raynaud's phenomenon. When thoracic sympathectomy is indicated, excision of the second and third ganglia are essential for ablation of sympathetic activity from the upper extremity. However, to lessen the possibility of an inadequate sympathetic denervation because of the possible presence of anatomic variables, T_4, T_3, T_2, and the inferior half of T_1, are excised. The preganglionic fibers entering T_1 (which fuses with the inferior cervical ganglion) are avoided so that a Horner's syndrome will not develop. When sympathectomy alone is performed, benefit is frequently less than optimum, although most patients do obtain some relief. Lumbar sympathectomy for lower extremity involvement requires ablation of L_2 and L_3 but a wider excision including L_1, L_2, L_3 and L_4 is usually performed. In males, L_1 is not included in the excision on one side to avoid possible impotence postoperatively. Good results should be expected from this procedure in most patients. When Raynaud's phenomenon is present in all four extremities, sympathectomy is performed at six-month intervals or only three extremities are denervated, to avoid the hazard of orthostatic hypotension and the nuisance of excessive perspiration in the undenervated areas of the trunk. Spacing the procedures allows time for readjustment of sympathetic tone in the proximal areas of each involved extremity. There is no indication for sympathectomy when scleroderma is accompanied by Raynaud's phenomenon, for the results have not been found to be worthwhile. Treatment for this condition is directed toward the underlying disease.

Acrocyanosis

Acrocyanosis is a benign vasospastic disorder in which bluish color, coldness and moistness of the hands and feet are usually persistent rather than transient. The cyanotic appearance becomes more intense in a cold and stressful environment. These changes are not accompanied by pain, and complications rarely occur. Patients obviously appear to have a dysfunction of the sympathetic nervous system and are classified as "sympathetic reactors." Other patients with similar problems include those in whom color changes are not predominant but whose hands and feet are constantly cold and clammy: the "wet fish" hand. In acrocyanosis, the volar aspect of the hands and feet are very moist while the dorsal aspect is usually dry. Interestingly, the cyanotic appearance disappears on elevation and during sleep. The underlying cause for this disorder may be due to some circulating hormonal agent or to a high intrinsic tone in the muscular media of the vessels.

The only therapy which is usually required is assurance of the patient that the cause of the intense blueness of the hands is merely the patient's embarrassment in public. All patients should also be warned to avoid an extremely cold environment, trauma and infection, for they are excellent candidates for the bizarre sympathetic disorders which occur in patients who are "sympathetic reactors."

Sympatholytic drugs may occasionally be prescribed. Sympathectomy is unwarranted, for the disease is almost always uncomplicated except for the signs previously described. These signs usually are less evident in later life.

Livedo Reticularis

Livedo reticularis, unlike acrocyanosis and Raynaud's phenomenon, is not localized to the digits, hands and feet but characterized by a purplish "fish net" mottling of the skin of the legs, thighs, forearms, arms or trunk. Superficial ulcerations, when present, are situated proximal to the hands and feet. Treatment is symptomatic. Rarely is a sympathectomy justified unless the ulcerations become progressively larger and fail to heal in spite of appropriate débridement, antifungal drugs and antibiotics. Sympatholytic drugs, reserpine or methyl dopa may be tried. A search for an underlying collagen disease or blood dyscrasia is advisable. As with Raynaud's phenomenon and acrocyanosis, education of the patient is essential. The patient should particularly avoid cold temperatures and emotional stresses.

Acute Arterial Spasm

Acute arterial spasm has often been blamed but never proved as the primary cause of ischemia of tissue. Therefore, it should be considered, diagnosed and treated as a contributory factor to the ischemic findings.

Acute arterial spasm has a significant role in the outcome of iliofemoral thrombophlebitis or phlegmasia cerulea dolens and arterial injury. In addition, certain patients during examination and at surgery demonstrate a marked tendency toward arterial spasm which often cannot be satisfactorily explained. Other conditions should be considered, such as vasculitis, hypercoagulability, high levels of circulatory catecholamines, hypovolemia, hypertensive disorders and other physiopathologic states. These patients usually have a rapid progression of their disease and frequently are poor candidates for surgery.

Acute Peripheral Arterial Occlusion

Acute occlusions of peripheral arteries necessitate early and accurate diagnosis followed by emergency medical and surgical procedures. Signs and symptoms relate to the occluded site, the extent to which the vessel(s) is occluded, the extension of the associated embolus or thrombus, and the promptness with which appropriate therapy is instituted. Embolization is the most likely cause when pallor, pain, decrease or loss of sensation and function occur with a decrease or absence of distal pulse(s). Thrombosis, although often acute with similar findings, is usually insidious in its development and preceded with prodromal complaints.

Embolism, thrombosis or trauma with or without laceration may cause arterial occlusion. Embolectomy provides a much higher success rate than a thrombectomy since an occluding thrombus encompasses a longer segment of an artery which almost always has extensive vascular disease.

Extremities and Aortic Bifurcation

Aortic, femoral and popliteal artery bifurcations are the usual sites of lodgement of arterial emboli, since the vessel narrows at the point of its division. The axillary and brachial artery bifurcations are the usual sites for occlusion of the upper extremity arteries. Seldom do occlusions of upper extremity arteries cause a loss of the part, even without treatment. However, the hazard of losing the extremity does exist and the possibility of morbid changes such as contracture, pain, and forearm claudication is significantly high; therefore, an embolectomy is indicated to assure maximum restoration of function in the great majority of cases. Aortic, iliac, and lower extremity embolectomies are always indicated, especially when the embolus is lodged at the aortic bifurcation, for not only may the patient lose both lower extremities but also his life, when surgery is inordinately delayed. When any degree of abdominal pain accompanies the signs and symptoms of an aortic bifurcation embolus, a mesenteric artery occlusion should be considered until proved otherwise. The presence of multiple emboli should be considered as a common occurrence.

Origin of the Emboli

Most emboli originate in the heart from an auricular thrombus due to fibrillation, vegetative disease of the aortic or mital valve, or from a mural thrombosis following myocardial infarction. Other sources are atherosclerotic plaques from the wall of the aorta or major artery, platelet aggregate material in an atherosclerotic ulcer, a clot within an aneurysm, pulmonary vein thrombosis or a thrombus in an injured artery. Other causes for embolization include missiles, tumor particles, paradoxical emboli through a right to left shunt in the heart, air, amniotic fluid and fat. However, all except fat are so rare that unless the history is reinforced by clinical findings, they are not considered. Fat emboli are fairly common following trauma.

Fewer large arterial emboli are noted today due to improved therapy for cardiac lesions. Cardiac and peripheral vascular surgeons routinely check for unexpected emboli peripherally following surgery.

Diagnosis

The classical signs and symptoms of acute arterial occlusion of an extremity usually result in the proper diagnosis. However, the classical signs and symptoms are not present in all patients. Therefore, the examining physician needs an "index of suspicion" to lessen the hazard of an increase of mortality or morbidity. Accompanying the suspicion of the presence of an acute arterial occlusion must be an aggressive attempt to utilize supplemental diagnostic procedures.

Arterial occlusion should be considered in a patient who presents with sudden or insidious complaints referrable to an extremity which, without injury or infection, demonstrates pallor when the extremity is in a horizontal position and becomes worse on elevation. Pain per se is not important initially in more than half of the cases. However, when the discomfort of paresthesia or numbness is listed as pain the percentage is much greater. Decrease or loss of sensation and function is related to the site of and extent of the occlusive segment in addition to previously present vascular disease. On the skin the lines of demarcation of sensation and temperature changes seldom coincide, and the occlusive site is frequently proximal to the area of symptomatic changes. A decrease in distal pulse amplitude is synonymous with an absent pulse in a patient with blood pressure which is normal or above normal.

Supplemental diagnostic aids such as arteriograms, the use of a Doppler flowmeter, oscillometric readings or plethosmography may confirm the suspicion of arterial occlusion. Arteriogram studies are beneficial, not only to confirm the site of occlusion, but also to determine the patency of the distal arterial system. Due to the potential of multiple sites of occlusion in one or both lower extremities, arteriograms should be performed preoperatively and also following removal of the embolus, thrombus, or repair of the injured vessel.

Left atrial enlargement, atrial fibrillation, recent myocardial infarction or a history of intermittent claudication are clinical findings which may indicate presence of an embolus or thrombus in the extremity. In approximately 10 per cent of patients no source of embolus is demonstrated. Calf or forearm tenderness is usually present in more than one compartment in patients with arterial embolism. In patients with venous thrombosis, however, only the posterior compartment of the leg is tender and this usually occurs only in the midline of the calf.

Objectives of Treatment

(1) Relieve arterial spasm by intra-arterial tolazoline hydrochloride (Priscoline) 25 mg, paravertebral sympathetic blocks, continuous epidural or spinal anesthesia, or sciatic or median nerve infiltration. Caution must be exercised in diagnosis and treatment if the patient is in shock or has a lowered blood volume. (2) Do not allow extremes of temperature to the ischemic part. (3) Protect extremity from trauma with cotton wadding or foam rubber and board to the foot of the bed. The extremity is placed in a de-

pendent position by elevating the head of the bed on blocks to increase available blood flow by gravity and to attempt to relieve discomfort. (4) Administer anticoagulants immediately, utilizing heparin, 7500 to 10,000 units intravenously. When heparin is used, the treatment for arterial spasm should be limited to an intra-arterial sympatholytic agent, or a sciatic or median nerve perineural infiltration. Anticoagulant therapy lessens the likelihood of further emboli, slows the progression of a preexisting arterial thrombus and retards development of venous thrombosis and sludging in the distal arterial tree. Its use may save the patient from arterial occlusion elsewhere and may also save the occluded part when surgery is delayed or not undertaken. When surgery is not performed, heparin is administered subcutaneously 15,000 to 20,000 units every 12 hours, keeping the clotting time around 15 minutes, or three times normal just prior to the subsequent injection.

(5) Surgery may have to be postponed if acute arterial occlusion occurs in a community which does not have personnel or facilities to perform definitive vascular surgery or if operating room space or specialized personnel are unavailable, or for other reasons including the patient's condition. Regardless of the reason for postponement, the aforementioned procedures plus the administration of antibiotics should be instituted prior to transfer to another hospital or to surgery. Acute arterial occlusion is an urgent-emergent condition; it is not critical except when acute mesenteric vascular occlusion is suspected. (6) The optimal period for surgery is within ten hours of occurrence for an extremity arterial occlusion, but immediately for a major mesenteric vascular occlusion. Later exploration is justified for the extremity only if patency of the distal major major vessel can be clinically demonstrated. An arteriogram is warranted in most cases; it should always be performed prior to completion of the surgery. Operation is definitely indicated for patients with an embolus to the bi-

furcation of the aorta or the common iliac artery. Unless contraindicated, patients with arterial emboli or thrombi are continued on half of the prescribed therapeutic dosage of heparin and 5 gr of aspirin orally twice daily after operation to minimize the danger of a second embolus or thrombus. If the patient is on heparin during hospitalization he is usually converted to oral Coumadin or aspirin for long-standing prophylactic therapy. Some patients may need fasciotomies because of (1) the inordinate delay of the procedure, (2) relief of the obstruction permits a high arterial pressure to flow into a markedly dilated and atonic arterial tree, (3) a compartment may have been penetrated and bleeding may occur in a confined space, or (4) deep pain occurs in a compartment area postoperatively after relief of the acute occlusive site. Fasciotomies are not performed unless definitive arterial surgery has also been attempted. The exceptions are listed under the next section, *Arterial Injuries.* When multiple compartment fasciotomies fail to relieve the deep pain and arterial circulation has not been adequately reestablished, amputation may be warranted. Superficial pain is relieved by sympathetic denervation.

In either medical or surgical treatment, consider the cause. In arterial injury, occlusion is due to local factors alone; return of circulation is highly possible and should always be sought regardless of the time element. However, in embolus or thrombosis, inherent diseases are already present and time is of the essence. Before undertaking any procedure, the body as a whole should be considered. Anticoagulants, sympatholytic drugs, sympathetic blocks, sympathectomy, and definitive vascular surgery all have their uses. Treatment should be for function; viability does not necessarily mean return to function.

Arterial Injuries

The conservative or non-operative approach to arterial injuries is no longer an acceptable means of treatment. To prevent crippling, loss of limb or organ, or loss of life, both military and civilian surgeons have demonstrated that an aggressive and confident application of current surgical procedures is mandatory. Injury to a major artery is not unusual in a hospital emergency department, nor is overt trauma the chief cause of the injury. There is a significant incidence of vascular injuries which occur during diagnostic procedures, at operation, and during therapeutic cardiopulmonary bypass. Occasionally these occur as late occlusions and do not present for diagnosis until the patient returns for a followup examination with symptomatology of vascular insufficiency.

Diagnosis

Diagnosis of an arterial injury is not always obvious. The classical sign is a significant bright red bleeding with the ischemic extremity appearing pale, cadaverous or mottled, cold to touch, with collapsed veins and absence of pulses. Recognition of arterial injury is usually not difficult in a nonobtunded patient who complains of pain in a nonbleeding extremity with characteristic diagnostic signs. However, the signs may be misleading in the presence of arteriosclerosis, shock or arterial spasm. It is not necessary to confirm diagnosis by the absence of a peripheral pulse. The conclusion that a decreased distal pulse is due to spasm should not be entertained for a prolonged period, for spasm alone does not cause loss of tissue. As stated previously, a decreased distal pulse should be considered synonymous to an absent distal pulse until proved otherwise. With a normal, or even with a decreased distal pulse, a definitive diagnosis sometimes cannot be made until débridement of the wound reveals a vascular injury. All injuries above the wrist or ankle should be explored if a peripheral pulse is diminished or absent, provided the patient is not in shock. This aggressive approach should be taken to increase the possibility of a successful outcome and to combat the high incidence of vascular injuries without laceration following blunt trauma. In blunt trauma there may be no penetration of the skin but the distal arterial pulse is decreased or absent due to an intimal tear, perivascular hematoma, soft tissue edema or entrapment of the artery between fragments of bone. Following a fracture, dislocation of a joint, snake bite, or prolonged use of an improperly placed tourniquet, an interesting index of major vascular injury is the presence of "fracture blisters" in the distal portion of the extremity. In these patients, compartment fasciotomies are performed routinely after the injured artery is repaired. The deep fascia is unable to expand under pressure of muscle edema which may occur preoperatively from a snake bite (usually only one compartment is involved) or shortly after repair of the artery when diapedesis occurs. An expanding hematoma may be present in only one compartment. Both the muscle edema and the expanding hematoma may thereby further occlude the arterial circulation when arterial injury is present or they may obstruct the artery by their resultant pressure. As previously mentioned, a fasciotomy is never performed without arterial repair unless definite evidence of muscle edema or an expanding hematoma has been demonstrated as the cause of the arterial insufficiency to the extremity. Penetrating wounds are frequently an indication of vascular injury and may constitute an immediate threat to life from exsanguination. Late sequelae of secondary hemorrhage, false aneurysm and arteriovenous fistulas may be equally hazardous and are further reasons for an aggressive operative policy. Additional criteria demanding operation are: a pulsating or expanding hematoma and a penetrating wound over the course of a large vascular bundle such as the neck, axilla, brachium, antecubital space, femoral-inguinal area, popliteal space, and the forearm and leg areas. A patient presenting with a penetrating wound in these areas should be admitted to the hospital either for exploration of the involved compartment(s), or for observation for a decrease in muscle or nerve function or arterial supply to the distal part. These patients are observed for a minimum of 24 hours. Wounds which penetrate the fascia in these areas should not be considered minor because the potential of an avoidable amputation is too great. Occasionally a fasciotomy may be required following muscle rupture below the elbow or knee when the rupture is accompanied by bleeding and no major artery is involved.

Treatment

Treatment must follow certain guidelines both at the emergency site and en route to the hospital via ambulance as well as within the hospital Emergency Department. The following protocol is not intended to suggest that the techniques and concepts are original but to identify procedures that are expected to give satisfactory results for ambulance attendants trained as emergency medical technicians, Emergency Department personnel, and surgeons who perform the definitive arterial repair.

Emergency care begins by pressure directly to the wound to control bleeding. When this is unsuccessful in stopping hemorrhage a tourniquet may be employed. The tourniquet should not be loosened until a pressure dressing has been applied and blood or plasma expanders are available to treat or prevent shock. If hemorrhage is excessive when the tourniquet is released, bleeding may be controlled by pressure over the major artery proximal to the site of injury. Clamping a vessel blindly with hemostats must be avoided, since this may lead to damage of veins and nerves and may crush a portion of the artery. Airway obstruction, cardiac arrest and monitoring of shock have priority over hemorrhage. Sterile technique should be utilized at the hospital to prevent infection. Arteriography, although not always essential, may be necessary to determine the presence of a preexisting arterial lesion, the type of vascular injury which has occurred, or a more exact localization of the site of arterial injury.

Definitive treatment of arterial injuries requires special facilities. Every general surgeon has been trained to do definitive vascular surgery, but the equipment necessary for quality care of a patient with an arterial injury may not be available. When these prerequisites are not present, immediate treatment of the injury should be limited to hemostasis, wound care and stabilization of the patient so he can be safely transferred to a hospital having the required special facilities. Details are essential for successful arterial surgery. Eighty per cent of all arterial injuries should have a successful outcome, and compromise does not serve the patient's interest and increases the possibility of an unsuccessful result.

Preoperative measures include continuation of emergency procedures plus the following: (1) A central venous pressure catheter is placed through the brachial or jugular vein or directly into the subclavian vein. If indicated, transfusion or plasma expanders are started. Vascular surgery is ordinarily contraindicated on hypotensive patients, but occasionally control of hemorrhage and revascularization of tissue is a prerequisite for control of shock. (2) Antibiotics, preferably penicillin and streptomycin, are begun in heavy doses. (3) Tetanus toxoid or human antitoxin is administered. (4) If the patient is normovolemic following shock therapy, spinal or brachial block anesthesia is advised according to the location of the injury. If shock is predictable, general anesthesia is preferred. Occasionally, intra-arterial sympatholytic drugs such as tolazoline hydrochloride (Priscoline), 25 mg, or dihydro ergot alkaloids (Hydergine), 0.5 mg, or epidural, spinal or paravertebral sympathetic blocks are used in an attempt to obtain return of pulsations in a vessel injured without laceration; if pulsations do not return, operation is immediately scheduled. Sympatholytic drugs and sympathetic blocks are contraindicated when there is arterial laceration or shock.

Failures in arterial repair result from: (1) poor vascular surgery technique including too much tension on the anastomosis; undue operative trauma or injudicious débridement of the vessel; improper application of sutures with reliance on external thrombosis rather than internal fibrin seal; or stenosis of the vessel at the anastomotic site resulting from a continuous suture being placed too tightly. Use of interrupted sutures may prevent a stenosis. (2) Incomplete total wound management, especially inadequate débridement and failure to eliminate dead space. (3) Failure to perform distal clean-out of the thrombus followed by operative arteriographic proof of total vessel patency. Occasionally an arterial injury may occur following a diagnostic arteriography due to underlying disease and hypercoagulability. Platelet aggregation may be noted at the injured site within the vessel. These patients require the administration of heparin or aspirin during operation to prevent a recurrence of the occlusive process. (4) Inadequate measures to control arterial spasm. (5) Failure to utilize the technique of fasciotomy to control complications of muscle edema and hematoma. (6) Inadequate measures to prevent or eliminate shock; incomplete control of total body hemodynamics before, during and after operation. (7) Failure in management of massive and multiple injuries, particularly in elderly patients with pre-existing disease.

Infection, hemorrhage and reocclusion are the most frequent complications postoperatively and following discharge from the hospital.

Chronic Occlusive Arterial Disease

Chronic occlusive arterial disease has previously been regarded as a degenerative vascular disease which chiefly affects elderly males and people who have diabetes mellitus, both men and women. More elderly persons with chronic occlusive arterial disorders are seen now than in the past because the average life span is increasing. This condition is now being diagnosed with increasing frequency in younger, nondiabetic patients.

The clinician is increasingly apt to assess the circulatory reserve of the body's organs and extremities before making any conclusions regarding the choice of definitive medical or surgical treatment. Earlier and more accurate diagnosis has been made possible by various mechanical, electronic and laboratory facilities which were previously used only on an experimental basis. Nevertheless, confusion continues to exist regarding the complexities of possible diagnoses and therapeutic methods available in chronic occlusive disease.

Diagnosis

Arteriosclerosis obliterans is the most common peripheral chronic occlusive arterial disease. Symptoms are usually manifested in the lower extremities. Vasospastic conditions and vasculitis must be considered in the differential diagnosis. Any of these disorders may be complicated by infection, thromboses or embolism. It is not uncommon for a patient to have multiple arterial occlusions, either partial or complete. They may occur in the symptomatic area as well as in the opposite lower extremity, of the carotid, renal, coronary, subclavian and mesenteric arteries. These possibilities have a significant bearing on the diagnosis, prognosis and future course of treatment. It is important to note if there is a family history of vascular disease: coronary disease or cerebral arterial disease, hypertension, diabetes, gangrene of an extremity or a hypercoagulable state. Other important aspects in the patient's history are age, sex, occupation, race, smoking habits, hobbies and the presence of cardiac disease, diabetes mellitus or anemia. Prior injury to any area of the body may also be pertinent. Neurological complaints and intestinal complaints must be included, even though they may seem bizarre. Inquiry should be made of a history of ulceration or frostbite of the extremities. A reduction in exercise tolerance must be described, including the character, location, period of onset and duration, and aggravating conditions relating to the pain. Loss of sexual function in the male is an important indication of aorto-iliac occlusive disease (Leriche's syndrome).

Pathology

Although the histopathologic picture of chronic occlusive arterial disease may vary, the changes may be classified as follows:

Segmental, involving short distances of the aorta, iliac, femoral, popliteal, carotid, vertebral, subclavian, celiac, mesenteric and renal arteries. Treatment for these lesions is chiefly surgical. The etiology is primarily arteriosclerosis, but may occasionally be due to a previous injury, a localized arteritis of unknown origin or mechanical entrapment.

Diffuse, involving arteries throughout most or all of their length. Treatment may be surgical or medical depending on adequate distal arterial patency. The etiology is also chiefly due to arteriosclerosis, with an occasional case caused by a more extensive arteritis.

Small vessel disease associated with metabolic, allergic and hematalogic disorders. The diseases include diabetes mellitus (Figs. 17–8 and 17–9), collagen diseases, polycythemia vera, dysproteinemia and other conditions. Treatment for these conditions is chiefly medical.

The Lower Extremities

Arteriosclerosis obliterans is the commonest disease of the lower extremities.

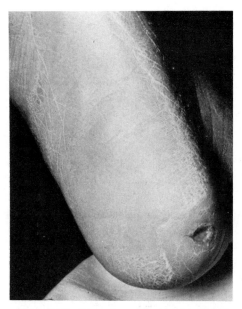

Figure 17–8 Ulceration of the heel in a diabetic patient. Although the ulceration is small and relatively painless, osteomyelitis is present and the patient required hospitalization for extensive débridement. Small vessel arterial disease in these patients frequently leads to the loss of the digits or parts of the foot, even when pedal pulses are present.

The symptoms of arteriosclerosis obliterans are entirely the result of ischemia of tissues. The symptoms are increased in relation to the proximity of the occluded artery, the extent of obstruction in the potential collaterals, and the time involved in the development of the occlusion. The appearance of symptoms may be gradual and unnoticed, or it may be misinterpreted due to the slow progression of occlusion. Symptoms may also be sudden in onset when a thrombus obliterates a relatively short segment of the artery. Sudden occlusion may not be interpreted as an acute process if excellent collateral channels are present. The disability period may be so short that the patient at first believes the symptoms will ultimately disappear. Symptoms may, however, stabilize to that noted in the slow process of arterial obliteration. A third pattern is observed when the occluded segment involves such a short area of the artery that the

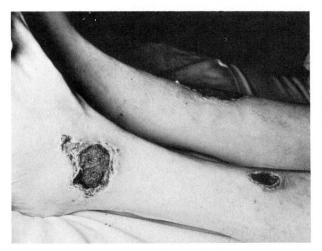

Figure 17–9 Ulcerations of the lower extremities in a diabetic patient complicated by proximal arterial occlusions and small vessel arterial disease. Successful "take" of skin grafts occurred on the fifth attempt but not until definitive arterial surgery and bilateral lumbar sympathectomies had been performed.

symptoms are mild or absent. The previously mentioned abrupt episodes may occur in sequence, with partial subsidence after each episode. However, the extremity becomes more symptomatic each time this occurs.

Location of the Occlusion

Location of the occlusion will frequently determine the site and extent of the signs and symptoms. The sites may be situated in the distal aorta, iliac, femoral or popliteal arteries. When high and low occlusions are present, high occlusion decreases the arterial flow to a certain degree and low occlusion further diminishes the blood flow. In isolated occlusions the prognosis is worse with the more distal occlusions. In aortoiliac artery occlusion the early course of the disease consists of an incomplete occlusion of one of the common iliac arteries (Fig. 17–10). This area later becomes completely occluded by thrombosis or dissection of blood beneath the atherosclerotic plaque. The process ultimately involves the other iliac artery and propagates upward toward the renal arteries. Occasionally only the terminal portion of the aorta is involved. The most common entity noted today is not the syndrome of bilateral aortic occlusion, first described by Leriche in 1923, but a unilateral common iliac artery occlusion with early encroachment on the opposite common iliac vessel. This type of occlusion process is most commonly noted in men in the fifth and sixth decades of life. When both common iliacs or the abdominal aorta is occluded, impotence is common and the Leriche syndrome is present. Impotence may also occur with bilateral occlusion of both hypogastric arteries alone.

The most common site of occlusion is in the superficial femoral artery, beginning in Hunter's canal just proximal to the origin of the superior geniculate artery. Occlusion extends proximally by thrombosis until the process reaches the area of the profunda femoris artery, which is the major collateral to the superior geniculate artery and the distal vessels. Primary occlusion of the popliteal artery is seen more often in women and young men, and is more frequently noted in the upper half of the vessel below its beginning at the exit of Hunter's canal. Popliteal occlusion may stop just proximal to the origin of the anterior tibial artery or it may extend further to the tibioperoneal bifurcation. More extensive involvement may result in a diffuse, segmental disease involving the anterior tibial, posterior tibial and peroneal arteries. Multiple segmental occlusions occur far more commonly when the primary occlusion

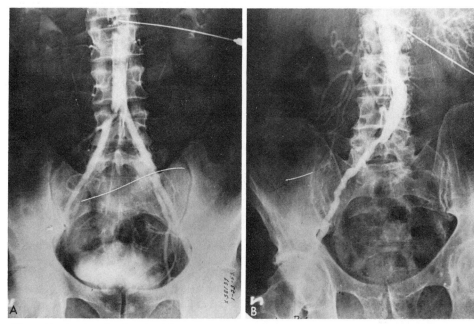

Figure 17–10 Arteriosclerosis obliterans. *A*. Localized occlusion of the right common iliac artery was treated with endarterectomy. *B*. Diffuse disease in this patient extended from the aorta down the left iliac artery, which was completely occluded, and was also extensive in the right iliofemoral system. Surgery was not performed because of the diffuse nature of the disease.

occurs below the inguinal ligament. This distribution is probably due to the slow flow rate present with distal occlusions, compared to the high flow rate which is present through collaterals which are available with an aortoiliac occlusion.

About one third of superficial femoral artery occlusions will be bilateral within five years. However, one extremity does not necessarily mirror the severity of the other.

Symptoms

Pain is the most significant early symptom which brings the patient to a physician. This symptom may be of four types: intermittent claudication, night cramps, superficial foot pain and ischemic or deep neuritic pain. The latter two types are often grouped together as rest pain.

Intermittent claudication is derived from the Latin word *claudicare,* which means "to limp." It is the most common and usually the earliest symptom of chronic occlusive arterial disease. The term has evolved to mean intermittent discomfort due to arterial insufficiency in any area, whether it be in the abdomen or the lower or upper extremity. This symptom is a classic sign of muscle ischemia and accumulation of toxic metabolites. The site of the pain will establish the site of occlusion, which is proximal to the area of discomfort except in diffuse small vessel occlusion. Claudication may be described as a pain, ache, cramp, numbness or sense of fatigue in certain muscles during exercise. Rest relieves the distress quickly. It may be the only subjective complaint elicited by the patient for years while other symptoms develop slowly. A patient may have a short segmental occlusion with good collateral circulation and a pedal pulse, yet complain of intermittent claudication. The most common area of the claudication complaint is in the calf, and other diagnoses are often entertained when the pain is in other areas.

Foot claudication may be vague when

tibial vessels alone are occluded. Since some patients are poor observers of their symptoms it may be necessary to educate them as to the types of discomfort they may note when walking.

Another type of claudication is the "pudendal syndrome" in which pain develops in the thighs and buttocks during intercourse. These patients have been described as having aortoiliac occlusive disease.

Occasionally venous congestion may be interpreted as claudication when the leg has the discomfort of heaviness or a "bursting" sensation. No relief occurs when the patient stops walking unless the extremity is elevated. In contrast, in arterial occlusion the claudication disappears within minutes after stopping, or even sooner, and elevation increases the pain. The past history and a physical examination should confirm the presence of deep venous obliterative disease.

Night cramps or nocturnal claudication is a calf pain which occurs only at rest and usually during the night, awakening the patient. The pain is not specific for arterial occlusive disease, for night cramps also occur in venous insufficiency, pregnant women, vitamin D deficiency patients, and hypoparathyroidism when the arterial circulation is normal. Night cramps due to arterial disease also occur in diabetic patients. In these cases, pain is related to a disturbance in muscle metabolism.

Superficial foot pain (causalgic type) varies in description and location on the toes, foot or the lower portion of the leg, but it is best characterized as a superficial burning pain with hyperesthesia and is sometimes severe enough to be disabling. This variable type of pain is usually grouped with ischemic neuritis and possibly nocturnal claudication and labeled rest pain. It may influence the method of treatment as well as the prognosis. It is similar to nocturnal claudication (night cramps), but is classified here as an entity separate from rest pain or ischemic neuritis. The examining physician may thus understand the types of pain which occur from occlusive arterial

disease. Though an ischemic neuropathy is present, causalgic pain is identified as being a complaint related more to the sympathetic nervous system than the somatic root pathways. Besides numbness, there may be tingling or prickling paresthesia. In spite of normal skin temperature the patient may complain of burning or coldness and hyperesthesia of the toes or part of the foot. This may persist even though necrosis or gangrene does not evolve. It is most often seen in patients with diabetes mellitus, in whom hyperesthesia may be disproportionate to the amount of arterial insufficiency. Its presence may result in injury, ulceration, and infection without the patient's knowledge that these complications are occurring. The numbness and hyperesthesia seen in diabetic patients is considered more of a manifestation of diabetes than ischemic neuropathy. The same pain pattern may occur from certain types of injury and infection and are not specific for arterial insufficiency. Those patients with arteriosclerosis obliterans who manifest this type of pain say that its presence is noted when the bed sheets contact the toes or foot and often complain that walking elicits the discomfort with each step. The latter discourages ambulation and thereby leads to further deterioration of the extremity, both by shortening the time of intermittent claudication and by the more rapid appearance of trophic changes due to disuse. Means of separating this causalgic type of pain from deep ischemic pain will be discussed later under treatment.

Ischemic neuritis is a disabling deep foot or leg pain that frequently requires hospitalization. It may follow the pathway of one or more peripheral nerve trunks. Gangrene or ulceration need not be present. It is frequently severe and difficult to relieve. Occlusive disease is usually extensive. Patients most often receive some relief by hanging their legs over the side of the bed or by sleeping in a chair to aid circulation by gravity. This often produces edema of the foot and ankle, thereby causing additional

pneumatic cuff is inflated to a point midway between systolic and diastolic pressure, and fluctuations in pressure are recorded in millimeters of mercury, or as one to four plus. Oscillometric records should be made in midthigh and midcalf, on both legs.

Doppler Flowmeter. This new, noninvasive technique for measurement of blood flow is increasingly accepted as a useful method. The special equipment required will be a valuable asset to any peripheral vascular clinic.

Arteriography. In most cases final decision regarding the advisability and type of surgery will be based on a study of arteriograms. These examinations are now usually performed by the radiology department in most hospitals, though surgeons should be familiar with the techniques and the complications. When arteriography is performed in the operating room, it is usually performed by the surgeon, with consultation from the radiology staff. In these cases, a single injection is usually made and a single film is taken. In most cases, however, a plastic catheter is inserted in the radiology department, allowing multiple injections and rapid-sequence radiography with high-speed bi-plane cassette changers and image intensifying fluoroscopy.

Arteriography should be performed to evaulate areas of the circulatory system outside of the region in which pathology is suspected and surgery is being considered. For example, arch aortography with visualization of both carotids and vertebral arteries is indicated in patients who are being considered for carotid artery reconstruction — e.g., in amaurosis fugax and recurrent small strokes. Abdominal aortography is indicated in patients who are under consideration for renal artery reconstruction for hypertension. The distal aorta as well as both iliacs and femoral arteries should be visualized in patients with claudication, even if it seems that the major pathology exists in only one femoral artery.

Arteriography can be performed by the Seldinger technique, which makes it possible to perform selective injections into several arteries, or by the translumbar needle approach. As was mentioned above, a needle or short catheter can also be introduced directly above the area which is under investigation, and this is the technique commonly used in the operating room. Overnight hospitalization is suggested if a translumbar aortogram is performed, or if selective arteriography is performed with a long catheter. Translumbar aortography should not be performed in hypertensive patients, or if the patient has any tendency toward bleeding.

Treatment

The indications for medical and surgical treatment vary, depending on the area of the body in which arterial occlusive disease is present. Indications also depend on the patient's general medical status, the extent of arterial disease elsewhere, and on the patient's symptoms.

The patient must be evaluated regarding cerebral, renal and cardiac status before any major elective vascular reconstructive procedure is recommended. The extent of disease in these three systems has considerable bearing on the risk of surgery and on the patient's life expectancy.

Elective vascular reconstruction may be recommended for relatively minor symptoms related to the carotid arteries, whereas elective reconstruction for claudication may be deferred if the patient can assume a more sedentary occupation. Repeated embolization from ulcerated plaques is an indication for "prophylactic" surgery in the carotid, iliac or femoral system. Abdominal angina may be sufficient indication for celiac or superior mesenteric artery reconstruction. Rest pain and impending ulceration of the digits is an indication for reconstructive surgery if a reconstruction can be performed.

The nature of the operation also varies, depending on the patient's disease and the materials available. Saphenous vein interposition or bypass has been more satisfactory for femoral–popliteal surgery than either endarterectomy or prosthetic grafts. If the patient has a good saphenous vein, reconstructive surgery can be recommended more forcefully than if previous phlebitis or surgery has eliminated the availability of the greater saphenous vein. A saphenous graft is considered nearly essential if the proposed graft would be anastomosed to a small popliteal artery or would cross the inguinal crease.

The indications for sympathectomy vary, but this procedure may be the only available means of increasing blood supply to the skin, and it has been a useful means to relieve rest pain in some patients who have poor "run off" from the popliteal artery, with only one or two branches of the popliteal artery patent. Sympathectomy is commonly performed as an adjunct to aortoiliac reconstruction, and can usually be counted on to produce a warm foot immediately after operation. The possibility that sympathectomy can produce a "steal" syndrome is still debated, and it appears to be possible that a unilateral sympathectomy could worsen the flow to one extremity, by increasing the cutaneous blood flow on the sympathectomized side.

In questionable cases, or those in which surgery would not be beneficial, nonoperative (medical) management is indicated. The patient is educated to the long-term management of his extremities, using the guidelines set forth below:

Instructions to Patients with Arterial Insufficiency

You have a condition which is going to require you to live carefully to prevent serious complications and to enable you to be comfortable. The name of the disease is arteriosclerosis obliterans. It means simply that the blood vessels carrying blood to your tissues are choked by an aging process also known as "hardening of the arteries." This is similar to the plumbing in a house which has become clogged with lime deposits over the years. The water will not flow as freely as it did when the pipes were new. Patience is required.

Unlike the pipes in your home, the vessels cannot be totally replaced. You must live with what you have. It is possible to live comfortably, provided that you are careful and follow certain simple rules. Details are of the utmost importance and must be followed. What would be a minor injury to someone else may well mean the loss of a leg for you.

1. Care of Other Diseases

If you have any other diseases be sure that they are under control. Diseases such as heart disease, diabetes, or skin diseases are most important. Be sure to see your physician about these periodically.

2. Exercise

Walk at least two miles a day. The more you walk the more you will be able to walk. This does not mean two miles at a stretch, but interrupted by periods of rest prior to extremity fatigue or pain. Do not walk until the pain occurs and then stop for rest. You must exercise like an athlete with rest before you develop extremity discomfort. Walking keeps the muscles in condition. A period of inactivity allows the muscles to waste away and they will not return to their former condition. If you follow this routine you should in a few weeks be capable of walking further distances before finding it necessary to stop for rest.

3. Guard Against Injury

When the circulation is good, small scratches heal promptly; when the circulation is not good a small scratch may become a large ulcer that will not heal in spite of good treatment. If you note anything wrong, see your doctor immediately; do not wait until it looks serious.

You may have noticed that the sensation in your legs and feet is not as good as it was previously. This may allow you to injure yourself without knowing it has occurred. One of the more common offenders is heat. Burns caused by heating pads, lamps, and hot water bottles are serious; none of these should be used at any time. In addition, pressure areas from shoes and socks may not be noted due to this loss of sensation. A brief, thorough inspection after your daily foot bath is indicated.

4. *Keep Yourself Warm*

In cold weather keep yourself warm. Cold causes further constriction (spasm) of the blood vessels. This means that you must not only keep your feet and ankles warm but all of your body. Long underwear is excellent. One thing that is often forgotten is the head; your head exposes many vessels to cold, which may cause vessel constriction elsewhere in the body. Warm, dry, clean, well-fitting socks are most important and should be considered as medicine.

5. *Infection and Self-Treatment*

There are only five things which should touch your feet and legs in the way of medicines. These are mild soap, water, 70 per cent alcohol, powder, and PLAIN lanolin. You should NOT use anything else unless your doctor specifically orders it. "Put nothing on your feet that you wouldn't put in your eyes," excluding soap, alcohol and powder.

Infection occurs easily in legs and feet and must be guarded against at all times. A daily foot bath is imperative. The skin of your face is in good condition and you wash it every day. The skin of your feet and legs is not in good condition and you must wash your extremities every day—preferably twice daily. IF YOU WASH YOUR FACE, WASH YOUR FEET. Inspect them thoroughly after washing. If you see anything suspicious, such as itching between the toes, cracks between the toes, corns or callouses, see your doctor. DO NOT TRY TO TREAT THEM YOURSELF.

6. *Care of the Feet*

a. *Shoes* should extend a half inch beyond the toes and be wide enough to allow all the toes to move. There should be no seams or other projections inside. They should be examined inside with your hand for small stones, nails, and creases before putting them on each time. A torn lining should be removed or repaired. If possible two pairs of shoes should be used, to be worn on alternate days and allow them to dry and be aired before putting them on again.

b. *Socks* should be of ample size but should not bunch or wrinkle, thereby causing points of pressure. They should provide some cushioning of the sole and top of the foot against the shoe.

c. As mentioned before, a daily inspection of the feet should be made and anything suspicious such as itching or cracks between the toes should be reported to your doctor.

d. Again, a daily foot bath is a necessity. Using warm, but not hot, water and a mild soap, a thorough washing should be done, paying particular attention to the areas between the toes and around the nails. The feet should be thoroughly dried. A light oiling with lanolin at night and a dusting with a mild antifungal powder in the morning are important.

e. A word about corns and callouses, which are due to poorly fitting shoes. They should never be removed by you at home; it is absolutely necessary that they be taken care of by a trained person. Once they are removed, their recurrence should be prevented by properly fitted shoes. Therefore, if you have a corn or a callous have it examined by your doctor; do not cut it or treat it yourself.

f. *Toenails* must be properly cut and trimmed. Do not cut them yourself, especially if you have poor eyesight. To do so you must sit at an awkward angle. Your doctor or foot specialist is trained to see that they are properly managed. A small cut by the pressure of a toenail is just as important to you as a cut by any other means. If you find it necessary to trim your own toenails and you have good eyesight and no loss of sensation on your toes they should always be trimmed straight across using a toenail clipper, never a razor blade or scissors.

7. *General Instructions*

The above things you must do yourself. If you have any questions after reading this, be sure to ask your physician to clear up anything you do not understand. He will ask you questions to be certain that you do understand these instructions. They are important.

There are times when he will vary these instructions, give other medications, or recommend other procedures. Follow his instructions to the letter. Remember that the attention you pay to details in the care of your feet may save them.

Arteritis

Inflammatory diseases of the arteries which are referred to as arteritis are difficult to classify. As a group, they occur more frequently than is generally realized and are often associated with underlying conditions such as the collagen diseases, thromboangiitis obliterans, and allergies to proteins, toxins, antigens and some medications. Any area of the vascular system may be involved but the inflammation usually involves small and medium-sized vessels. Diagnosis should be considered when medium-sized arteries are painful upon palpation. However, muscle biopsy including a small artery is frequently necessary for diagnosis except when arteritis is localized to major arteries.

Thromboangiitis Obliterans

Thromboangiitis obliterans is the most controversial disorder in the group. This disease has recently become much less common, probably because of a better understanding of arteriosclerosis obliterans. Numerous factors have been considered as the etiology of the disease. It occurs in patients with hypercoagulability and local arteritis due to a mechanical entrapment of the popliteal artery and vein in the adductor canal, or the gastrocnemius muscle, or the subclavian artery and vein in the thoracic outlet area. It may also be caused by generalized vasculitis, resulting in peripheral gangrene. The exact cause is unknown and its identification as a specific disease is questioned by many clinicians. However, when the signs and symptoms of chronic arterial occlusion occur and thromboangiitis obliterans is considered, tobacco smoking is found to be closely related to the development of the disease. There is no doubt that smoking has an aggravating influence on its progress. Another unusual feature is its predilection for white males. It occurs primarily between the ages of 20 and 40 years and is manifested by intense inflammation of the arteries and veins primarily and the nerves secondarily. Thrombosis of the small and medium-sized arteries and veins progresses ultimately to larger

vessels. Any or all of the arteries in the body may be involved, but the condition is predominately localized to the lower extremities.

Diagnosis. Thromboangiitis obliterans is considered in a patient who has objective evidence of arterial occlusion in peripheral arteries, is a young male and an habitual smoker. Frequently there is a history or evidence of superficial thrombophlebitis and the arterial occlusive process is progressive in each of the lower extremities and may also involve the upper extremities. Vasospasm often accompanies the condition and Raynaud's phenomenon, with blanching, cyanosis or mottling of the skin of the part as well as excessive sweating, may be noted. The major difficulty in differential diagnosis is to determine whether chronic arterial occlusive disease is thromboangiitis obliterans or arteriosclerosis obliterans, especially in patients in their fifth decade.

Arteriograms are an essential diagnostic procedure to rule out arteriosclerotic segmental occlusion of the iliac or femoral arteries. A hypercoagulation panel is ordered on all patients, especially those who presently have or have had superficial thrombophlebitis and those with a family history of arterial occlusion in a young male relative.

Treatment. Since the etiology of this condition is undetermined, treatment is directed toward symptomatic relief rather than specific therapy. It should be recognized that patients with thromboangiitis obliterans go through remissions and exacerbations.

Acute stage. Abstinence from *tobacco* is most important, and the clinician must try to persuade the patient to stop smoking. Sedatives and tranquilizing agents are of little benefit. Whiskey, 1 ounce four or five times a day may be beneficial, but is never administered when tranquilizers have been prescribed.

Pain is relieved in a manner similar to that used for arteriosclerosis obliterans patients.

Edema usually indicates an advanced degree of ischemia and its presence increases the amount of pain. Therefore movement of the foot is encouraged and an oral diuretic is administered daily.

Treatment of infection is similar to the method described in the previous section on arteriosclerosis obliterans.

Anticoagulants, namely heparin, are prescribed subcutaneously in doses ranging from 10,000 to 20,000 units twice daily. Coagulation times are determined periodically to keep below 20 minutes just prior to the subsequent injection. Hypercoagulation studies should be done on all patients prior to the use of heparin or any drugs, especially Butazolidin which may be prescribed for its anti-inflammatory characteristics.

Additional medical therapy should include routines similar to those described for arteriosclerosis obliterans, such as progressive ambulation, foot care and elevation of the head of the bed.

Surgery is not performed in the acute stage. However, if there is hyperesthesia and burning pain over the involved foot and medical sympathetic denervation does not produce prolonged relief, sympathectomy is indicated. Amputation is avoided in the acute stage. Prognosis is determined by the temperature of the foot and the trophic changes; if the foot is cool while appearing inflamed, the prognosis is poor. Diagnostic biopsy of a peripheral artery is contraindicated. In the past this disease responded poorly to all forms of treatment; present methods of care of the extremities have reduced the amputation rate.

Chronic Stage. Thromboangiitis obliterans is primarily due to arterial occlusion, but it is frequently associated with and aggravated by vasospasm which reduces collateral circulation to the part. Vascular flow improves and symptoms are usually relieved when the vasospastic component is released by a lumbar sympathectomy. The effects of sympathectomy may be more striking than in arteriosclerosis obliterans. Sympathectomy is done when the acute stage subsides and the foot improves; blanching on elevation diminishes and previously absent pulses may return.

Reconstructive procedures are rarely performed; however, arteriography should be routinely undertaken for proper evaluation of the disorder.

Collagen Diseases

Three collagen diseases may be considered when symptoms of peripheral chronic arterial occlusions occur and arteriosclerosis obliterans and thromboangiitis obliterans have been excluded. These diseases are periarteritis nodosa, disseminated lupus erythematosus and scleroderma. Diagnosis of periarteritis nodosa is difficult and often requires an arterial biopsy. Raynaud's phenomenon may accompany the symptoms. Disseminated lupus erythematosus may also be difficult to diagnose unless the characteristic "butterfly" skin eruption of erythema across the bridge of the nose and malar region is present. Biopsy of the involved area may be required to confirm the clinical diagnosis. A few patients may have symptoms and signs of Raynaud's phenomenon. Unlike periarteritis nodosa and thromboangiitis obliterans, alteration of peripheral pulses is uncommon and gangrenous changes are rare. Scleroderma is not usually difficult to diagnose especially when it is characterized by a diffuse induration of the skin and associated with vasomotor disturbances and visceral involvement. Raynaud's phenomenon frequently precedes the skin induration and trophic changes of the toes and fingers. Ulceration and even gangrene may occur at the tips of the digits. Peripheral pulses may be difficult to palpate because of vasospasm and the leathery and nonpliable character of the skin overlying the vessels. Occasionally calcinosis occurs as painful focal lesions over the joints of the extremities.

Other Forms of Arteritis

Other forms of arteritis are temporal arteritis, erythema nodosum, erythema induration of nodular vasculitis, steroid vasculitis and nonspecific arteritis.

Temporal arteritis and steroid vasculitis are especially important to a surgeon. Temporal arteritis may be diagnosed by the pain and tenderness which occur over the temporal arteries and is accompanied by diffuse headaches, fever, malaise and weakness. There may be redness and induration over the temporal artery as well as disappearance of the pulsations. The condition should not be taken lightly for intracranial involvement may cause blindness. Biopsy of the temporal artery is frequently requested to confirm the diagnosis; dramatic relief of pain usually occurs. Steroid vasculitis may develop in patients who have been on cortisone or prednisone for several years. Leg ulcers may develop as a complication of the vasculitis.

Another group of arteritides includes those due to anatomic factors or direct trauma such as crutch arteritis, adductor canal arteritis or thrombosis; and to thoracic outlet syndromes resulting in arteritis and thrombosis.

Treatment for generalized arteritis is basically symptomatic and is directed toward removal of sensitizing factors. Steroid therapy should be avoided until all other therapy fails or an acute episode develops. In acute episodes, cortisone, 200 to 300 mg daily, or prednisone, 40 to 50 mg daily, is prescribed until symptomatic relief occurs; then the dosage is reduced until maintenance is established. The maintenance dose should be the smallest possible to achieve comfort and rehabilitation. Ultimate withdrawal of medication should be sought. Temporal and cranial arteritis should be treated with steroid therapy early lest blindness ensue. Leg ulcers which are caused by steroid arteritis are treated by subcutaneous heparin 10,000 to 15,000 units twice daily. In a few patients with periarteritis nodosa, sympathectomy may be necessary for relief of hyperesthesia, and superficial pain as well as any vasospasm in the ischemic part. Sympathectomy is not performed for any patients with scleroderma in spite of the belief that it may benefit the patient. Most surgeons who have performed a fairly representative number of sympathectomies on these patients agree that their results have not been beneficial.

Treatment of localized arteritis consists of removal of the anatomic cause of trauma and definitive therapy toward the specific artery involved.

Aneurysms

Abdominal Aortic Aneurysm

One of the most impressive achievements of medical progress in recent years has been the effective surgical treatment of abdominal aortic aneurysms. With the availability of aortic homografts and later synthetic cloth prostheses, the general consensus among the medical profession is that few individuals with abdominal aortic aneurysms should fail to have surgery for this potentially lethal lesion. Although the surgical mortality is reported to have been reduced to an acceptable level for both symptomatic and asymptomatic aneurysms, there is some doubt that this level of mortality has been achieved on a nationwide basis. Candidates for surgery are invariably advanced in years and always have systemic atherosclerosis. These individuals represent some of the poorest risks for a surgeon, especially when the surgery entails such an extensive operative assault as removal and replacement of an abdominal aortic aneurysm. The problem is compounded when the expanding and ruptured aortic aneurysm demands immediate surgery and does not permit case selection. Every surgeon therefore must consider the general status of the patient in assessing operative risk and be qualified to understand the many problems of diagnosis and treatment which must be solved before operation is undertaken in the individual instance.

Clinical manifestations of abdominal aortic aneurysms are often difficult to separate from other symptoms which frequently appear in the sixth, seventh and eighth decades of life. The mean age of the occurrence of abdominal aortic aneurysms is 65 to 75 years of age.

Most of the lesions are asymptomatic when first diagnosed; however, some patients demonstrate a rapidly expanding or ruptured aortic aneurysm. Between these two extremes is a group of individuals who complain of vague abdominal symptoms. These are usually gastrointestinal in nature and are related to duodenal displacement by the aneurysm or to a change in bowel habits occurring from occlusion of the inferior mesenteric artery included in the aneurysmal dilatation. Back pain is common and is difficult to distinguish from symptoms of hypertrophic arthritis which may accompany the lesion.

An abdominal aortic aneurysm may be detected by palpation of a pulsatile mass anywhere in the abdomen but usually located to the left of the midline of the epigastrium and several centimeters below the umbilicus where the normal aorta bifurcates. Occasionally a significant pulsation can be transmitted through an abdominal mass or the aorta may be easily palpated owing to marked curvature of the spinal column. A false impression of the presence of an aneurysm may occur in the hypertensive female patient in whom the aorta "buckles" from elongation and seems widened because of its tortuosity. Many aneurysms are first detected by radiologists when they review abdominal films obtained for other reasons. Calcification in the wall of the aneurysm is observed in the AP abdominal x-ray and may be more frequently found on a slightly over-exposed lateral film. Aortography is not ordered except (1) when a diagnosis of tortuous aorta is considered; (2) additional surgery for correction of a renal hypertension is contemplated; and (3) severe distal chronic occlusive arterial disease is present and adequate patency beyond the occlusive area(s) may be a problem during and immediately following abdominal aorta surgery. Aortography is not routinely performed because the majority of abdominal aorta aneurysms are localized

below the renal arteries and even very large aneurysms may have an axial blood flow which appears normal on aortography. An ultrasound device has recently been used to diagnose abdominal aortic aneurysm as well as to follow the size of the lesion. However, this apparatus is not widely available.

Palpation of the pulsatile mass may elicit mild tenderness. When rapid expansion or rupture has already begun, tenderness is always present and severe rigidity of the abdominal musculature may develop, preventing detection of the underlying pulsatile abdominal mass.

Symptoms of rapid expansion or rupture may range from severe abdominal pain and immediate death to almost any symptom listed for acute abdominal conditions. A history of a past myocardial infarction is common and symptoms of chronic occlusive disease of the lower extremities may be present in at least half of the patients. Unlike peripheral arterial aneurysms, abdominal aortic aneurysms are rarely the source of arterial emboli to the lower extremities.

Aneurysms may be *classified* as: (1) asymptomatic, when they are dormant and may enlarge to tremendous proportions without any significant complaints; (2) expanding, when they are potentially lethal; or (3) ruptured, when death is inevitable without surgical correction.

The expanding aneurysm produces symptoms ranging from mild back, flank, hip and abdominal pain to severe pain related to the enlarging mass. No hemodynamic changes occur. Upon rupture, blood escapes from the aortic wall and may go (1) through the anterior wall into the peritoneal cavity; (2) into the retroperitoneal space or the mesentery; and (3) into a hollow viscus such as the intestine or inferior vena cava.

Time of rupture prior to hospital admission is significant. Half of the patients presenting with a ruptured abdominal aneurysm survive for 24 hours and a third have had symptoms of rupture for over 96 hours. Symptoms of expansion precede or accompany the rupture in about 60 per cent of patients, and these—together with symptoms of "double rupture"—have been described as characteristic of aneurysms. Diagnosis of a ruptured abdominal aortic aneurysm may be made by three findings: (1) presence of a palpable, pulsatile, midabdominal mass; (2) pain in the abdomen and back with radiation to the groin, genitalia, hip or thigh; and (3) hemodynamic signs of continuous blood loss. With these findings, only a hematocrit, urinalysis and blood cross-matching should be obtained, for delay of surgical treatment by consultation on special studies may be fatal to the patient.

Selection of patients for operation is not always so clear-cut; an aneurysm should be considered as a malignant lesion and surgery should not be delayed. However, many patients with abdominal aortic aneurysms may have severe pulmonary disease as well as generalized atherosclerosis involving coronary, cerebral, mesenteric or renal arteries. Any of these conditions may lead to death or morbidity before the aneurysm ruptures, and elective removal of the aneurysm only assures the patient that he will not have a ruptured aneurysm.

Several questions should be answered before patients are electively selected for operation:

Is an abdominal aortic aneurysm significantly lethal to warrant surgery in all but a few patients? Even though the number of patients studied has been small and some reports are retrospective, there has been a fairly universal acceptance that an aneurysm will enlarge and rupture in a majority of patients within three years. All patients have a progression of their atherosclerosis, especially those who have symptomatic aneurysms, and a third have an even chance of dying from atherosclerotic disease or a ruptured aneurysm. The risk for surgery increases significantly in patients over 70 years of age and also depends upon the experience and capability of the surgeon performing the procedure.

Does aneurysmectomy restore to the patient the life expectancy he would have *had without risking a potentially lethal lesion?* Excluding surgery for ruptured aneurysms which are obviously survival procedures, most experienced surgeons agree that life expectancy is as much as doubled for a 5-year period.

What size abdominal aortic aneurysm is hazardous? The incidence of rupture increases in relation to its size. In lesions which are less than 7 cm in size the incidence of rupture is 4 per cent; the incidence of rupture rises to 82 per cent if the aneurysm is larger than 7 cm in diameter. The smallest measurable size for an aneurysm is 4.5 cm. Operative mortality rates for elective aneurysms range from 5 to 18 per cent while 34 to 85 per cent of those which are ruptured have a fatal outcome.

What are the criteria for operation? These can be listed as: (1) symptoms of pain or tenderness, suggesting impending rupture; (2) evidence of expansion; (3) associated iliac artery occlusive disease; (4) an aneurysm which is greater than 7 cm in size; (5) the occurrence of peripheral emboli; (6) patients who are less than 70 years of age; and (7) aneurysms which have ruptured. Contrary to general belief, only a small percentage of patients expire immediately from exsanguination when an abdominal aorta ruptures. Obviously the ultimate outcome of the lesion varies with the location and rapidity of the hemorrhage. The majority of patients with a ruptured abdominal aorta leak into their retroperitoneal or mesentary attachment areas for hours or even days. The average period between the onset of symptoms of rupture and death has been reported as ten hours. This is more than adequate time to hospitalize the patient and implement emergency surgery. In view of this common pattern, the high risk patient with an asymptomatic aneurysm may only be examined every two to three months. At each visit the size of the pulsatile mass is determined by measuring its distance from the umbilicus. A two-way scout film of the abdomen may be taken and the calcification in the wall noted. An ultrasound device may also be valuable for denoting any change in the size of the lesion. The patient is informed that he should contact his surgeon and make himself immediately available at the hospital if he experiences severe abdominal pain. This approach has been very successful for the few patients in this category in our clinic.

Improvement in monitoring, surgical technique and supportive therapy should result in a high incidence of survivors. Patients with symptomatic aneurysms should be operated upon; patients with asymptomatic aneurysms should have excision and replacement of the lesion according to the aforementioned guidelines. Otherwise, if they are included in a high risk group, they should be examined at regular intervals and should be counseled on importance of abdominal systems.

Late complications following discharge include: (1) constipation frequently due to ischemic changes of the left colon; (2) occlusive distal arterial disease; (3) the development of a false or true aneurysm at the proximal suture line; and (4) postsymptomatic pain in the thighs on the tenth postoperative day if a lumbar sympathectomy was performed as an additional procedure. A patient with a diagnosis of anuria following abdominal aorta surgery should be evaluated for iatrogenic ureteral artery obstruction due to the close relationship of these excretory ducts to the aneurysm. Ureteral compression is so frequent preoperatively that a routine intravenous pyelogram is advised prior to surgery whenever possible.

Iliac Artery Aneurysm

Isolated aneurysms of the iliac arteries are rare; therefore intelligent and successful management depends upon a knowledge of their natural history. Aneurysms of the iliac arteries are an arteriosclerotic disease occurring most often in elderly males. They are generally extensions of an aneurysm of the lower abdominal aorta. Occasionally mycotic types occur; rarely they appear during or after pregnancy and a few cases have been reported in children from a congenital weakness in the arterial wall. Their onset is insidious and their occult location in the pelvis may obscure the diagnosis. Rectal and vaginal examinations are often more informative than abdominal palpation. Most patients are asymptomatic when the aneurysm is diagnosed, for it may be found during examination for an unrelated condition. When symptoms are present the complaints usually are of abdominal and back pain. As with aneurysms elsewhere iliac artery aneurysms continue to enlarge and elongate, and the enlargement continues until it impinges upon surrounding viscera or it ruptures into the bowel or retroperitoneal area. When an asymptomatic aneurysm is diagnosed, operation may be elective unless there are specific contraindications. When aneurysms rupture, surgical intervention is mandatory.

Lower Extremity Aneurysms

Aneurysms of the lower extremities are much less common than abdominal aortic aneurysms. They are most frequently due to arteriosclerosis, especially in patients over fifty years of age. Additional causes are trauma, mycotic arteritis and necrotizing arteritis. Popliteal aneurysms occur more frequently than femoral aneurysms and are often bilateral (Fig. 17–11). Multiple aneurysms are frequently noted in the abdominal aorta, iliac and femoral arteries when the cause is arteriosclerosis and especially when a popliteal aneurysm is present. Occasionally multiple aneurysms of the superficial femoral artery may be observed which are described as "rosary bead" aneurysms. It is interesting that both the femoral and popliteal aneurysms occur at sites where muscles do not cover the vessel completely and where frequent flexion of the thigh and leg may weaken a diseased vessel. It has been postulated that the terminal portion of the superficial

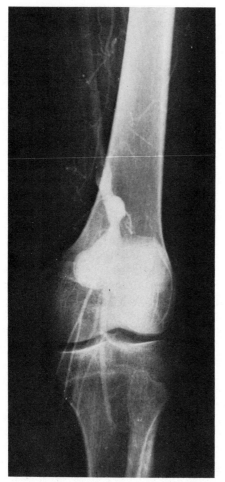

Figure 17–11 Popliteal artery aneurysm, as revealed by arteriography. These aneurysms frequently cause ischemic lesions of the digits because of embolization of fragments of thrombus. Treatment recommended is exclusion by proximal and distal ligation and use of an autologous saphenous vein bypass graft.

of the artery. A normal pulsation may be transmitted through a mass of lymph nodes, tumor or abscess and should be considered in the differential diagnosis. If a pulsatile mass is thought to be an abscess it should not be incised until aneurysm has been excluded from the diagnosis.

When an aneurysm lies beneath a muscle mass such as the adductor magnus on the medial aspect of the thigh, the lesion(s) have been misdiagnosed as muscle ruptures. Elastic compression to the site may cause thrombosis of the aneurysm or distal emboli.

Pressure of an aneurysm on neighboring nerves may result in a characteristic radiation of pain. The first symptom of a popliteal aneurysm may be pain in the heel from pressure on the popliteal nerve. Both femoral and popliteal aneurysms may retard or obstruct adjacent venous return. Auscultation over the aneurysm may reveal a short systolic bruit; however, the majority of aneurysms do not have murmurs unless arterial stenosis with turbulence is present. If the murmur is a continuous to and fro machine-like bruit, an arteriovenous fistula must be present. Arteriography should be performed routinely for all peripheral arterial aneurysms to confirm the diagnosis and to establish the exact site and extent, the possible presence of more than one aneurysm, and the patency of the arterial system distal to the abnormally enlarged vessel.

Complications of lower extremity aneurysms are not uncommon and may result in loss of the limb or loss of life.

Femoral and popliteal aneurysms are usually asymptomatic until complications occur. Rupture of either is not common but a distal embolism or a sudden thrombotic occlusion which may cause irreversible gangrene of the extremity is always a possibility. Therefore, elective treatment by excision and graft or an exclusion bypass procedure is strongly recommended once the diagnosis is established. Multiple aneurysms in the vessels pose a problem in priorities and management; an abdominal

femoral artery is intermittently compressed by the tendinous hiatus of the adductor magnus muscle as it emerges from Hunter's canal to become the popliteal artery. This compression contributes to the development of a poststenotic dilatation which later develops into a popliteal aneurysm. A similar compression may be caused by the arcuate ligament behind the knee.

Diagnosis of femoral and popliteal aneurysms is usually made by palpation of a pulsatile swelling along the course aortic aneurysm should be approached surgically prior to the correction of lower extremity aneurysms.

The femoral artery aneurysm is more apt to be diagnosed early since it is easily observed by the patient as a pulsatile mass in the groin. Popliteal aneurysms frequently go undiagnosed unless a complication occurs, since the popliteal artery is behind the knee and is not routinely palpated during the average physical examination. Its presence should be considered when a patient develops an ischemic toe or an ischemic spot on a toe with good pedal pulses and no origin for emboli can be determined by history or physical examination.

Any patient who develops an acute thrombosis of a popliteal or femoral artery aneurysm has a poor prognosis for limb salvage unless distal thrombotic material is immediately removed at surgery and viability of the limb is maintained by a patent distal arterial bed proven by arteriography. Results depend upon the time of recognition, the time surgical intervention is undertaken, and the condition of the distal arterial vasculature. If good viability of the extremity is present and continues to be maintained, the operation may be scheduled as an elective procedure while the patient is maintained on subcutaneous heparin.

Visceral Arteries

Visceral arterial aneurysms are presently diagnosed much more frequently than in the past because of increased awareness of these lesions, the widespread use of aortography and improved vascular surgical techniques.

Any visceral vessel may develop an aneurysm. Although the three most common sites are the splenic, renal and hepatic arteries, aneurysms of the superior mesenteric, inferior mesenteric, pancreatic, pancreaticoduodenal, gastroduodenal, right gastroepiploic, celiac and cystic arteries have been reported.

Etiologically, visceral aneurysms have been listed as arteriosclerotic, congenital, mycotic, traumatic, dissecting, false aneurysm secondary to focal arteritis and to periarteritis nodosa. Multiple congenital visceral aneurysms are known to occur in the presence of polycystic disease of the kidneys, liver and other viscera.

Visceral aneurysms are usually asymptomatic until complications occur. Intraabdominal rupture is a major complication which may be fatal if undiagnosed.

Splenic Artery. Aneurysm of the splenic artery is probably not as rare as was once thought. It is one of the most frequently occurring intra-abdominal aneurysms and is the only aneurysm that is found in more women than men. In the past, the overwhelming majority of cases were identified at operation or autopsy and as a result aneurysm of the splenic artery was associated with an extremely high mortality. In recent years opinions regarding the prognosis of splenic artery aneurysms have been encouraging. Although splenic artery aneurysm is not often seen, its importance should not be underestimated for the alert physician may recognize it by its clinical pattern. Surgical intervention is indicated as an elective or life-saving measure.

The precise cause of aneurysm of the splenic artery is unknown. The majority are atherosclerotic in origin, but a significant and interesting finding of localization of the arteriosclerosis to the splenic artery alone has been reported. The second most common cause is a congenital defect. A peculiar relationship may exist between the third trimester of pregnancy and the development of rupture of a pre-existing aneurysm of the splenic artery. Any pregnant or recently postpartum woman who develops upper abdominal pain, especially in the left upper quadrant, that is associated with signs of intraperitoneal bleeding, should be considered as a possible instance of splenic artery aneurysm. Surgical intervention is immediately indicated. There may also be some unexplained relationship to its occasional presence in patients with portal hypertension.

Several clinical features are sufficiently

characteristic to suggest the presence of this lesion. The symptoms produced are of two types: those occurring before rupture and those occurring after rupture. The most common symptom before perforation is pain in the epigastrium or the left upper quadrant. Associated with this pain are a host of other symptoms, most of which are referable to the gastrointestinal tract. Most patients are asymptomatic, especially those in whom the aneurysm has been noted as an incidental finding during aortography, a routine film of the abdomen or surgery. Physical examination may reveal little besides tenderness in the upper abdomen. Other findings may be splenomegaly, a pulsatile tumor or a systolic murmur in the upper abdomen.

The most common clinical manifestation of splenic artery aneurysm is the typical calcification in roentgenograms of the abdomen. The calcified aneurysm appears as a round or oval shadow of increased density in the left upper quadrant or epigastrium. The periphery of this shadow is sharply delineated and the central portion presents a mottled appearance. If the patient is not asymptomatic, he should receive a translumbar aortogram to establish the diagnosis. Once the diagnosis is proved, surgical therapy is recommended.

The major complication is rupture which commonly occurs in two stages—the so-called "double rupture," a common occurrence for all ruptured aneurysms. Following the first leak, the patient may improve clinically and in this brief interlude the diagnosis and surgical treatment is life-saving. Some time after the primary rupture, a secondary hemorrhage occurs into the greater peritoneal cavity, stomach or colon. Even with immediate surgery the mortality rate is exceedingly great.

Renal Artery. Aneurysms of the renal artery must be managed surgically because of the complications they may cause within the kidney and their frequent association with hypertension. Unlike their splenic artery counterpart, renal artery aneurysms do not often rupture except during the third trimester of pregnancy or early postpartum period. They are most commonly due to atherosclerosis, although some have a congenital origin. Multiple aneurysms may develop in the presence of fibromuscular hyperplasia. It is not uncommon for renal artery aneurysms to be found bilaterally. They rarely enlarge enough to be palpable and although signet ring calcification does occur, it is unusual.

As with aneurysms elsewhere in the body, many patients with renal artery aneurysm are asymptomatic until complications develop. Since the aneurysms are usually saccular, a mural thrombus contained within the aneurysm may produce embolic infarctions in the kidney parenchyma. Another complication is the formation of a dissecting hematoma distal to the aneurysm. A majority of patients have hypertension as well as pain in the flank, lumbar region, lower back or upper abdomen, and hematuria ranging from a few cells to a massive hemorrhage. Renal artery aneurysms caused by trauma may either rupture or form an arteriovenous fistula. The latter may be iatrogenic following mass ligation of both artery and vein during a nephrectomy.

Renal artery aneurysms are diagnosed much more frequently since translumbar aortograms have become routine for occlusive peripheral vascular disease and for many patients with hypertension. Radiographic studies should include excretory urography and nephrotomography. Once the diagnosis is made, immediate surgery is indicated. Previously, nephrectomy was the procedure of choice, but current techniques of vascular surgery can usually preserve renal function.

Hepatic Artery. Hepatic artery aneurysms, like those of the splenic and renal arteries, have characteristic features which may lead to a definite diagnosis.

As in other aneurysms, the most common cause of hepatic artery aneurysm is arteriosclerosis. A variety of causes other than congenital have been implicated, including direct extension by an inflamed gallbladder, infected emboli, trauma from a previous biliary operation or an external penetrating injury.

The most frequent finding which leads to suspicion of the existence of a hepatic artery aneurysm includes a triad of symptoms of jaundice, abdominal pain and gastrointestinal hemorrhage. Roentgenologically there may be a calcification of the aneurysmal wall, a filling defect of the duodenum and narrowed duodenum cap. Occasionally a murmur may be present, and if the aneurysm enlarges sufficiently a pulsatile mass is found in the right upper quadrant. Any of these findings may suggest the need for aortography to establish the diagnosis.

The major complication is rupture either into the peritoneal cavity or gastrointestinal tract. Several instances of rupture into the portal vein have been reported at operation or postmortem as a hepatic artery–portal vein fistula.

In view of the potential complications, surgery is advised. Collateral blood supply to the liver may be sufficient to allow resection of the artery without a graft replacement although its use is recommended.

Mycotic Aneurysms

The term "mycotic" is used to identify those aneurysms which originate from inflammatory destruction of the arterial wall, especially the internal elastic lamina. The most common source of infection is of *intravascular origin*. These lesions may develop from: (1) infected emboli from endocarditis which lodge in the vessel lumen or in the vasa vasorum; (2) microorganisms deposited directly on the intima of the vessel or in the vasa vasorum; and (3) extension of infection from aortic or pulmonary valves to the proximal portion of the aorta or pulmonary artery. When the causative infection extends to the vessel from a contiguous or neighboring inflammatory

process, the source is classified as of *extravascular origin*. Very rarely, the lesion may result from a distant extravascular source of infection and is termed a "primary mycotic aneurysm." These lesions are not associated with any demonstrable intravascular inflammatory process or with any infection from surrounding tissues; but during the course of bacteremia, an intimal defect caused by arteriosclerosis may permit the infection to obtain a foothold. Bacteremia may also cause secondary infection in congenital, traumatic and arteriosclerotic aneurysms and may result in aneurysmal rupture.

The course of the lesion depends on the virulence of the bacterial agent causing it. If it is highly virulent, the vessel wall is destroyed and rupture may occur before an aneurysm forms. This may happen less than two weeks after symptoms begin; however, symptoms are usually present for several weeks before the aneurysm ruptures, if it ruptures at all. Unfortunately most of the aneurysms are located in visceral and cerebral arteries and the aorta rather than peripherally. Circulatory impairment may be noted distally but gangrene is uncommon. Diagnosis is therefore determined by the presence of infection, chiefly bacterial endocarditis, and the rapid development of an inflamed painful pulsatile mass.

Treatment requires heavy doses of antibiotics, ligation of the artery if necessary to prevent exsanguination, or excision and restoration of vascular continuity if the infection is under control. It may be necessary to sacrifice the arterial supply to the involved part to save the patient's life. Due to the widespread use of antibiotics very few mycotic aneurysms may be encountered in afebrile patients in which the bacterial endocarditis has been at least temporarily arrested. Conversely a mycotic aneurysm may be the focus for a fever of unknown origin. Excision of a mycotic aneurysm has been reported to have cured a bacteremia.

Extracranial and Aortic Arch Occlusive Disease

Numerous descriptive terms are employed to identify the less common occlusive lesions of the great vessels arising from the aortic arch. The terms include nonspecific arteritis of Takayasu or pulseless disease, Martonell's syndrome, thrombotic obliteration of the aortic arch branches, and the aortic arch syndrome. Among the more common disorders are occlusion, stenosis or atherosclerotic ulceration of the extracranial and vertebral arteries. Each of these lesions may be present singularly or in combination with lesions of the aortic arch branches. The most common cause of partial or complete occlusion of the great vessels is arteriosclerosis. Less frequent causes are fibromuscular hyperplasia, arteritis, embolism and dissecting aneurysm.

Arteriosclerotic lesions usually occur at the origins and bifurcations of the brachiocephalic arteries. Usually these sites of atherosclerotic changes have progressed to a stenosis or occlusion in the first one or two centimeters of the great vessels, the first centimeter of the vertebral arteries, and the first centimeter of the internal carotids at the common carotid bifurcations before they are detected. Recently clinicians have realized that many mild intermittent cerebral ischemic symptoms are the result of small emboli originating from friable thrombotic material within atherosclerotic ulcerations which have not advanced to the point of stenosis or occlusion of the vessel.

As with atherosclerotic lesions found elsewhere in the body, males are predominant and the usual age of occurrence is over 50 years. Younger males occasionally develop atherosclerotic lesions in a frequency similar to that which occurs in other sites of the arterial system. When symptoms occur in young women, however, the primary pathologic change is usually due to arteritis and usually occurs at the origins of the great trunks arising from the aortic arch.

Fibromuscular hyperplasia occurs infrequently and is usually present in the internal carotid artery. It has a corrugated or "string of beads" appearance on arteriography because of the irregular muscular hyperplasia and intervening pseudoaneurysms present in the vessel.

Dissecting aneurysm should be considered when clinical evidence of cerebral arterial insufficiency is present. An embolism lodged at the innominate or carotid bifurcation is an uncommon cause for cerebral ischemia and when it occurs immediate surgery is required; otherwise irreversible brain damage ensues rapidly in many patients.

Any patient with symptoms and signs of cerebral insufficiency should be evaluated for lesions of the extracranial arteries as well as the arteries originating from the aortic arch. Surgery for these lesions may be corrective as well as prophylactic, especially in patients with transient localized cerebral ischemia and in individuals who have an initial or recurrent stroke. Early diagnosis is essential, especially in a completed major stroke; some patients may be amenable to definitive surgical treatment if diagnosis and therapy are accomplished within a few hours after the symptoms occur.

Indications for surgery are:
1. Transient focal cerebral ischemia in which patients have a correctable lesion of the carotid and vertebral arteries;
2. Aortic arch syndrome.

Questionable indications for surgery are:
1. An occasional patient with a completed stroke;
2. Extracranial embolic obstruction;
3. Asymptomatic stenosis of extracranial carotid artery, unless surgery is performed for another lesion.

Contraindications for surgery are:
1. A progressing or acute completed stroke;

2. Arteriographic evidence of both intracranial and extracranial stenosis or occlusion of the internal carotid and basilar arteries;
3. Complete occlusion of the internal carotid artery both intra- and extra-cranially.

Transient Ischemic Attacks

Lesions which cause transient ischemic attacks occur in the area of the bifurcation of the common carotid and involve the internal carotid artery, the vertebral artery and occasionally the proximal segments of the branches of the aortic arch.

Approximately 50 per cent of the cases of cerebrovascular insufficiency result from extracranial lesions. A small number of these are due to a decrease in the blood flow resulting from a stenosis or occlusion of the internal carotid artery. However, the majority of the transient cerebral ischemic attacks or "little strokes" are due to small emboli arising from an atherosclerotic ulcer with or without the presence of internal carotid stenosis. Stenosis may occur from bleeding beneath an atherosclerotic plaque. A significantly high proportion of patients who have a stroke present a history of intermittent cerebral ischemic symptoms prior to the catastrophic neurologic episode.

Diagnosis. The identification of transient ischemic attacks is usually not difficult when the symptoms are considered as prodromal evidence that a stroke may develop at a later date. A variety of symptoms may occur, such as brief episodes of light headedness and vertigo, blurring of vision or blindness, headaches, diplopia and short periods of paresthesia and paresis or incoordination of the extremities, especially on one side. These symptoms should not be ignored for they may be the only clue that a lesion is present in the extra-cranial or aortic arch vessels.

Upon physical examination the area of stensois may be located by a palpable decrease or absence of carotid pulsations and the presence of a bruit over the site. However, the finding of a bruit does not determine the severity of the stenosis nor does the absence of sound exclude the presence of a pathologic change in the vessel wall. A bruit is not noted with an atherosclerotic ulcer unless stenosis is also present. A stenosis may progress to complete occlusion and the bruit disappears. Although the bruit frequently is systolic in phase, it may be continuous when the area of stenosis is extremely small. Bruits in the neck must be distinguished from the systolic murmur of an aortic valve disorder and from venous hum, both of which have characteristic locations of intensity and sounds. The use of a Doppler flowmeter may be used to screen these sounds heard by auscultation. Occasionally a thrill may be palpated over the bifurcation of the carotid artery. The firm mass of an atheroma also may be noted on palpation.

Ophthalmodynamometry is useful as a method of comparing the diastolic pressures of the retinal arteries of the two sides. It supplements clinical findings and other methods of diagnosis, especially carotid arteriography.

Cerebral angiography is the most useful diagnostic procedure, since it determines the presence, location, number and severity of the lesions in the great vessels of the aortic arch, carotid and vertebrobasilar arterial systems. Angiography should be performed in patients with symptoms of transient ischemic attacks in whom surgery is contemplated. However, angiography is indicated for stroke patients only when the benefits from surgery are uncertain.

Treatment. Treatment of intermittent cerebral ischemic episodes must be individualized because the identification of the site and type of underlying pathology is more often important for the prevention of a future stroke than for the treatment of the existing one. The possibility of intracranial hemorrhage or tumor must always be kept in mind whenever the patient with a stroke or intermittent ischemia is evaluated.

A useful approach is to divide the

development of a stroke into three phases: Phase I includes the patient who recovers rapidly from transient ischemic attacks. A Phase I patient warrants thorough study to determine if surgery is indicated. Here the location, severity and accessibility of the vessel or vessels involved determines the procedure. If surgery is not advised, the hypercoagulability of the blood is inhibited with Coumadin or platelet antiadhesive drugs. Phase II describes the patient who experiences an advancing stroke in which the localized neurological changes progress but the brain tissue remains viable temporarily. A rapid recovery demonstrates that the brain tissue is viable. Treatment requires immediate lowering of blood viscosity with low molecular weight dextran or heparin, or a platelet antiadhesive drug such as aspirin. Many clinicians are reluctant to use heparin since it may cause hemorrhage into the infarcted area. For the same reason some clinicians are against surgery to relieve the obstructed extracranial vessel. Others believe that either method of therapy is beneficial only if the procedure is undertaken early enough to precede cerebral infarction. Phase III identifies the patient who has a progressive or acute completed stroke. In this individual a brain infarct has occurred and no method of treatment will restore blood flow to the damaged area.

Briefly, surgery is indicated principally for Phase I patients who are characterized by transient ischemic attacks. In Phase II patients, who have had a stroke with recovery, surgery is indicated if an infarction probably has not occurred. The procedure should usually be delayed for four to six weeks. Surgery is contraindicated in Phase III patients, in whom brain infarction is almost a certainty.

Aortic Arch Syndrome

Reduction in flow in the innominate, left carotid or left subclavian artery may be due to either of two mechanisms. The first mechanism is diminution or elimination of flow through these arteries as the result of pathologic reduction in the vascular lumen. The second mechanism is termed the "vertebral-subclavian steal syndrome." Because the results of surgery in these patients is usually excellent, operation is indicated.

Diagnosis. When pathologic changes occur in the proximal portion of the innominate, left carotid and left subclavian arteries, blood supply may be decreased to the extracranial tissues, the intracranial tissues and/or the upper extremities. Symptoms are similar to transient ischemic attacks. Syncope and convulsions may occur when the patient is placed in an upright position. Other findings are intermittent "claudication" of the forearm, decrease or absence of pulsations in the cervical carotid artery or in the upper extremity of the involved side, facial atrophy, optic atrophy and presenile cataracts.

The "steal" syndrome occurs in patients with stenosis or occlusion in the proximal left subclavian or innominate arteries. In this syndrome, the patient is usually unaware of any problems in his upper limbs but has symptoms of cerebral vascular insufficiency, including lightheadedness or a feeling of "blacking out" after using the involved extremity above his head or when standing up quickly. The symptoms occur when pressure in the distal subclavian artery is less than that of the vertebral artery. In these patients, blood may flow in a reverse direction from the vertebral to the subclavian artery during exercise, which causes an increased demand for blood in the tissues and an increased flow through the vessel with the least resistance. The syndrome does not usually occur when significant occlusive lesions are present in all three of the great vessels of the aortic arch. Neurological changes are usually not present.

If a single arch vessel is occluded, it is usually the left subclavian. Occlusion of the innominate artery produces an additional possibility for "steal" from the cerebral circulation since both the vertebral and the right common carotid arteries would have reversed flow to the right subclavian artery.

Besides diagnostic arteriography, supplementary findings include a discrepancy in the pulses and blood pressures between the two upper extremities, and a bruit heard over the anterior chest, the supraclavicular fossa, and over the proximal course of the arch vessels involved. The bruit is heard with stenosis rather than occlusion.

A Doppler flowmeter may also be used to locate the area of stenosis or claudication. A "steal" syndrome may be confirmed by the use of two oscillometers. Recordings are made above the elbow of each limb while the carotid artery is compressed on the involved side. Plethysmography may be used as an alternate method.

Treatment. Treatment for the subclavian steal syndrome is surgical, anastomosing the distal subclavian-vertebral area to the carotid through a cervical incision. Bypass procedures are performed for occlusions of the carotid or innominate arteries. Results are good for patients with arteriosclerosis but the long-term result for patients with arteritis is usually poor due to the generalized nature of the disease.

Vertebral Basilar Arterial Insufficiency

Vertebral artery disease can be divided into three categories: (1) patients with disease at the proximal orifice of the vessel who have no carotid artery disease; (2) patients with stenosis in both the vertebral and carotid arteries; and (3) patients with a normal vertebral artery with a proximal subclavian artery obstruction resulting in a "steal" syndrome.

Cerebral symptoms from vertebral artery occlusion are rare but occur, and may require surgery. However, when carotid artery occlusion or stenosis is present simultaneously, surgery for the carotid artery disease is usually performed.

Fibromuscular Hyperplasia

Fibromuscular hyperplasia is generally considered to be a disease of the renal arteries and is one of the causes of renovascular hypertension. However, it may also occur in the internal carotid artery as a separate condition, or in both the renal and carotid arteries. It is characterized by a systolic bruit over the involved artery. When the internal carotid artery is affected, intermittent symptoms of cerebral dysfunction may occur, without progression to a stroke. It is confirmed upon angiography by the "string of beads" appearance of the internal carotid artery. There is stenosis of the lumen between each of the small dilated segments. Since the entire internal carotid vessel is often involved, definitive vascular surgery is difficult. It may be impossible to insert a bypass graft, but dilatation has been reported to be successful.

Kinked Internal Carotid Artery

A kinked or buckled carotid artery occurs most frequently on the right side and is often unjustly diagnosed as a carotid aneurysm because of the prominent pulse in the neck. The extracranial portion of the internal carotid artery may be obstructed owing to the high position of the aortic arch or elongation with resulting "volvulus," "buckling" or "kinking" of an artery which is fixed at either end. Some observers have reported that the entity causes cerebral insufficiency. The first case of definitive surgery on the carotid artery for cerebral ischemia performed by this author (1953) was for a Phase II type of stroke which was found to be caused by a kinked internal carotid artery.

Diagnosis is made by symptoms of cerebral insufficiency, a prominent pulsation in the neck, production or aggravation of symptoms by a change in position of head and neck, and evidence of kinking confirmed by angiography. Generally the condition is considered benign. However, if an actual obstruction is demonstrated by arteriogram and no other cause for the symptomatology is noted, surgery is indicated.

Emergency Carotid Artery Surgery

Embolectomy is indicated only when immediate surgery can be performed. Otherwise, revascularization of an already infarcted brain may occur, resulting in a hemorrhagic infarct. The surgeon is rarely consulted early, so few operations are advised. There is also controversy regarding immediate surgery on a patient who has developed an acute neurologic deficit which progresses or fails to recover. Most clinicians try to avoid surgery and manage the patient with a method similar to that for a completed stroke. At present there is no secure means of identifying which patient has an infarct and which has a simple ischemic area of the brain.

Emergency surgery is advised for patients with transient ischemic attacks whose arteriograms show a very small amount of flow through the stenotic area of the internal carotid artery. Emergency surgery is also indicated for patients whose bruit disappears after arteriography and those in whom arteriographic contrast medium shows extremely narrow or obstructed carotid artery lumen.

Asymptomatic Stenosis of Extracranial Carotid Artery

In the past, asymptomatic patients with a bruit over the bifurcation of the carotid artery or the first part of the subclavian artery were closely followed. However, a more aggressive approach has recently been employed, in which nonstenotic lesions associated with atherosclerotic ulcers and transient ischemic attacks are removed. Surgery is also indicated for the asymptomatic patient with a stenotic carotid lesion. A more aggressive policy of prophylactic surgery is now recommended by many, to lessen the likelihood of thrombosis and a resulting stroke. Patients who demonstrate early senile mental changes confirmed by relatives are classified as symptomatic. The totally asymptomatic lesion is still controversial and needs further study as to the benefits derived from prophylactic drugs versus definitive surgery. Since these studies will not solve the problem soon, individualization is necessary for each patient before a policy is established.

MISCELLANEOUS DISEASES

Celiac Axis and Mesenteric Vascular Disease

Ischemic gastrointestinal disease may involve both the arterial and venous systems of the stomach and intestines. It may or may not be occlusive. Until recently experience with mesenteric vascular disease was confined to the advanced state of massive midgut necrosis which necessitated extensive resection of small intestine and variable amounts of colon. This resulted in death or crippling gastrointestinal symptoms for most patients. Today, several ischemic bowel syndromes are considered, diagnosed and treated successfully.

Etiology and Pathogenesis

The clinical syndrome of chronic mesenteric arterial insufficiency is not common despite the high incidence of atherosclerosis in the vessels which supply the stomach and intestines. The acute occlusive process usually occurs in the orifice of the origin of the artery or in the proximal 1 to 2 cm of the artery, and may be caused by an embolism, thrombosis or trauma. A nonocclusive type may also occur with infarction, but this is usually the result of extremely poor perfusion of the intestine secondary to shock.

Fibromuscular dysplasia may occur in the celiac, superior mesenteric and inferior mesenteric arterial systems similar to that noted in renal and carotid artery stenosis. Aortic dissection may extend to or originate in the mesenteric vessels. Even though the celiac axis and the superior mesenteric arteries are the common sites for occlusion, the inferior mesenteric artery is most frequently reported to be occluded in aortic atherosclerosis or aneurysm. When the inferior mesenteric artery is not occluded, it may provide collateral circulation with the superior mesenteric artery and the branches of the hypogastric artery. Therefore it may be the primary collateral vessel to the intestinal tract as well as to the extremities. This pattern of collateral arterial circulation should be recognized during aortography prior to abdominal aorta resection.

Other causes for mesenteric vascular occlusion are extrinsic compression of the celiac artery by the crus of the diaphragm or from the celiac ganglion. Occlusive lesions resulting from drugs such as methysergide maleate therapy and oral contraceptives are presently being reported with more frequency. Intestinal parasites have been reported as etiological agents, and patients with vasculitis from periarteritis nodosa and thromboangiitis obliterans may develop intestinal ischemia. All patients with mesenteric vascular occlusion due to arterial or venous thrombosis should have hypercoagulability studies similar to those advised for thromboembolism.

Necrosis of the intestine following sequential lumbar sympathectomy and ileofemoral bypass graft has been described when a marginal mesenteric arterial circulation was present. The phenomenon has been called the "aortoiliac steal" syndrome. Another postoperative mesenteric vascular syndrome which may result in bowel necrosis is the vasculitis which occasionally occurs following repair of a coarctation of the aorta.

An understanding of the *anatomical patterns* of the normal abdominal visceral circulation and its variations is essential in order to relate the possible syndromes of occlusive arterial diseases to the patients' signs and symptoms. There are three primary sources of blood supply to the stomach and intestines: the celiac axis, the superior and inferior mesenteric arteries and the two hypogastric arteries.

The superior mesenteric artery, which originates 1.5 cm below the celiac axis, supplies the gastrointestinal tract from the duodenum to the transverse colon and is involved in 90 per cent of clinically significant vascular disorders. Unlike the celiac axis, which forms a right angle with the aorta, the superior mesenteric artery has an obtuse angle course downward. This may have some bearing on its higher incidence for vascular disease, especially embolization. Its major collateral to the inferior mesenteric artery is via the middle colic artery through the marginal artery to the left colic artery branch of the inferior mesenteric artery.

The inferior mesenteric artery, which arises below the renal arteries and proximal to the aortic bifurcation, terminates as the superior hemorrhoidal artery, which joins the middle hemorrhoidal artery—a branch of the hypogastric artery. Chronic occlusion of any one of these three systems does not usually initiate symptoms because collateral flow is plentiful; usually occlusions of two or three of the major vessels or a combination of stenotic and occlusive lesions are necessary to produce clinical manifestations. Bowel necrosis is not inevitable even when occlusion occurs in all three systems. Symptoms are almost always present in chronic gastrointestinal ischemia due to stenosis or occlusion of the celiac axis or the superior mesenteric artery; however, these symptoms are uncommon when stenosis or occlusive lesions involve only the inferior mesenteric and hypogastric arteries. The inconsistency of symptoms is due to the marked variations in the functional capacity of the arterial collateral network.

Occlusion of the celiac artery by an embolus of atherosclerotic thrombotic disease does not ordinarily produce symptoms and is often discovered unexpectedly at surgery or necropsy. It has been postulated as a possible cause for acute peptic hemorrhagic necrosis and ulceration. Recurrence is unlikely due to the short length of the celiac vessels and extensive collateral circulation. Rarely the celiac axis may be absent; variations in its three branches, the left gastric, the hepatic and the splenic arteries are very common. The major collateral circulation between the celiac axis and the superior mesenteric artery occurs through the gastroduodenal artery, which carries blood from the hepatic artery to the superior pancreaticoduodenal artery. The latter vessel joins the inferior pancreaticoduodenal artery, which is a branch of the superior mesenteric artery. There are also other means for collateral circulation between the celiac and superior mesenteric arteries.

Acute Mesenteric Ischemia

There are three distinct syndromes of acute mesenteric ischemia: acute mesenteric artery thrombosis, mesenteric ischemia without vascular occlusion and superior mesenteric artery embolus.

Acute Mesenteric Artery Thrombosis. This, like other acute atherosclerotic occlusive lesions of the peripheral vascular system, is commonly preceded by signs and symptoms of ischemic episodes. Many patients have a history of weight loss, postprandial pain, diarrhea, malabsorption with occult blood in the stool, and the presence of an abdominal bruit prior to the episode when the abdominal pain becomes steady or colicky. This stage is followed by the classical signs of an intra-abdominal catastrophe and symptoms of bowel necrosis develop with abdominal distention, vomiting and bloody diarrhea. Fever, a marked leucocytosis and radiological evidence of dilated bowel loops are present in the late stages. The patient usually appears more ill than noted on physical examination. However, the abdominal pain is often so severe that narcotics do not bring significant relief.

There have been reports of successful revascularization without bowel resection even on patients with generalized peritonitis for over 24 hours. Perhaps a good therapeutic result can be obtained with this method but the outlook previously was bleak.

Patients who have survived massive small bowel resections for acute mesenteric vascular occlusion generally have malabsorption, steatorrhea and negative nitrogen balance. To improve the fat absorption in such patients, isocaloric substitution of medium-chain for long-chain dietary triglycerides has been found advantageous. Periodic hospitalization for hyperalimentation infusions has been advised. Recent attempts to use the formula for home infusions via an established permanent infusion tract are promising.

Acute Embolic Occlusion. Acute embolic occlusion of mesenteric arteries should be suspected when there is a sudden onset of severe abdominal pain followed by a forceful evacuation of the bowel, with or without melena, plus a history of heart disease, dysrhythmias and evidence of peripheral embolization elsewhere. Acute mesenteric artery thrombosis is frequently fatal due to the delay in diagnosis and treatment; the outcome of acute embolic occlusion to mesenteric arteries is potentially more favorable.

Other signs and symptoms of an embolic episode include vomiting, appearance of being severely ill out of proportion to physical findings, leucocytosis and an abdominal roentgenogram which shows absence of intestinal gas. Later signs simulate the symptoms of acute mesenteric artery thrombosis.

Since the embolus is usually lodged in the region of the midcolic artery, the first part of the jejunum appears normal at operation. On the other hand, mesenteric thrombosis causes ischemia of the entire small intestine from the origin of the jejunum to the midtransverse colon. An embolus is relatively easy to remove from the midcolic artery; a thrombus is more difficult to extract when it lies at the origin of the superior mesenteric artery in the retroperitoneal area.

Acute Mesenteric Nonocclusive Ischemia. This is very difficult to differentiate from acute occlusive mesenteric vascular disease except by arteriography, absence of prodromal symptoms and the presence of a hemodynamic crisis resulting in a severe reduction in intestinal blood flow. The latter is caused by hypovolemic shock, prolonged use of vasopressor therapy, low cardiac output conditions and congestive heart failure. Severe atherosclerotic stenosis of the mesenteric arterial vessel may or may not be present, but when present it contributes to the results. Therapy is directed toward improving the low cardiac output state and not toward any surgical procedure. Mesenteric vascular dilatation by continuous epidural anesthesia should be initiated as well as local infiltration of an anesthetic at the base of the mesentery. Intra-arterial vasodilatation and anticoagulants are used to prevent blood sequestration.

Acute Inferior Mesenteric Artery Occlusion. This condition is much less common than superior mesenteric vascular ischemia. Occlusion of the inferior mesenteric artery may produce two syndromes of acute colorectal ischemia: spontaneous thrombosis and iatrogenic ischemia due to ligation of the artery during resection of the abdominal aorta for occlusive disease or an aneurysm.

Spontaneous thrombosis usually occurs in an elderly patient who has advanced generalized atherosclerotic disease. The patient complains of diarrhea and left lower quadrant pain of short duration. Leucocytosis is usually present. Proctoscopy reveals an edematous, pale or cyanotic friable rectal mucosa. Abdominal distension, shock, ileus and peritonitis occur as the ischemic process progresses. Immediate laparotomy is indicated.

Signs and symptoms of postoperative colorectal ischemia are identical to those of spontaneous thrombosis but are obscured during the postoperative period. Roentgenologic findings are marked spasms and irritability with narrowing of the colon. A "thumb printing" appearance occurs from the thickened and irregular mucosal folds and scalloping of the mucosal pattern. The mucosa may slough, and ulceration is noted. Treatment is identical to that advised for spontaneous thrombosis. However, some patients may develop a minor degree of ischemia resulting in edema and bleeding or sloughing of the mucous membrane only. Fibrosis and segmental strictures may form later with constipation and a roentgenologic picture of a pipestem or fibrotic left colon. The surgeon may prevent this condition by reconstituting the blood supply to the rectosigmoid colon following aortic resection.

Acute Mesenteric Venous Thrombosis. This occurs in 15 to 25 per cent of all mesenteric vascular occlusions. It may occur simultaneously with venous thrombosis elsewhere in the body, such as portal vein thrombosis with cirrhosis of the liver, a hepatoma, intra-abdominal infection or injury to mesenteric veins. A hypercoagulable state may be present in any of these patients.

The signs and symptoms of this entity are similar to those of acute mesenteric venous occlusion except that the progression of symptoms is slower. At operation, arterial occlusion presents a pale-appearing bowel, whereas venous occlusion presents an engorged, bluish, edematous bowel. Both sides of the circulation are occluded ultimately. Prognosis for venous thrombosis is generally better than for intestinal infarction resulting from arterial thrombosis. Treatment involves resection of the necrotic bowel followed by anticoagulation.

Chronic Intestinal Ischemia

Chronic visceral ischemia is known by many terms such as abdominal angina, splanchnic ischemia, intestinal angina, abdominal intermittent claudication, and chronic occlusion syndrome of the mesenteric arteries. The classical symptoms are postprandial pain and weight loss. The diagnosis is often obscure, partly because the main intestinal arteries may become stenotic or almost completely occluded without occurrence of any physiologic change. The slow progression of atheromatous disease permits the progressive development of a profuse collateral circulation between the celiac and superior mesenteric arteries and the superior and inferior mesenteric arteries. At least two and frequently all three mesenteric artery systems usually must have severe occlusive disease in order to produce the abdominal angina syndrome. Stenosis of the celiac artery alone may produce severe symptoms in one individual while another who has occlusion of both the celiac and superior artery may have no abdominal complaints.

Diagnosis is first suspected when the patient complains of postprandial pain accompanied by weight loss. Postprandial pain results from intermittent gastrointestinal ischemia and is frequently severely cramping in character. It may occur immediately after eating, or be delayed for over thirty minutes. It may last for more than an hour with radiation from the periumbilical region or the midepigastrium to the back. The severity of the pain often can be related to the size of the meal. The patient may restrict his food intake to lessen the pain. Weight loss may thus range from moderate to severe over a period of several months. Malabsorption may be a contributory factor to the weight loss. Flatulance, abdominal distension and a change in bowel habits may occur. Physical examination usually reveals an abdominal bruit and evidence of atherosclerosis in other areas of the body. The bruit is not diagnostic since other abdominal atherosclerotic lesions may be present.

Diagnosis rests mainly on a clear arteriographic delineation of the major stenosis or occlusion in the mesenteric arteries. Lateral views are usually necessary to demonstrate the lesions in the proximal superior mesenteric and proximal celiac arteries. Collateral circulation patterns are a helpful finding for diagnosis especially when the inferior mesenteric artery is tortuous and markedly dilated.

Almost all of the chronic visceral ischemic diseases exhibit external compression of the celiac axis by the crus of the diaphragm or the celiac ganglion, and atherosclerosis of the celiac axis and superior mesenteric arteries.

Treatment is primarily surgical and usually involves thromboendarterectomy, a prosthetic or autogenous vessel bypass, or reimplantation of the diseased vessel into the aorta. Surgical treatment may also require transection of the median arcuate ligament of the diaphragm or celiac ganglion as it courses over the celiac artery.

Cold Injuries

Cold injuries produce peripheral vascular changes which cause characteristic symptoms and lesions. Concepts of the effect of cold have been influenced by old remedies, misinterpretation of signs and symptoms, and incorrect evaluation of research. Some modes of therapy have proved to be of unquestioned value, some are controversial, and some have proved useful in the laboratory but have not yet had adequate clinical trial.

Recent studies have clarified the pathogenesis of cold injury and provided a basis for new approaches to the management of these injuries. Management begins before hospital admission and continues with treatment of sequelae which occur after hospital discharge. Many basic questions have been answered, particularly those concerning the frequency of ice crystal formation within the cells and the role of vascular changes in the pathogenesis of the lesions. Evidence is available that cold per se, acting by an unknown mechanism, may be an important factor in producing trauma.

A reasonable estimate of prognosis can be obtained after consideration of the conditions of exposure. The degree of injury from cold is the result of four factors in the environmental situation: temperature, moisture, wind, and duration of exposure. Temperature and moisture determine the type of lesions which will develop, and the wind and duration of exposure determine how rapidly and how severe the lesion will appear. Cold injury may develop from prolonged exposure to relatively mild degrees of cold. Therefore, in cold injury, specific terms such as chilblain, trench foot, immersion foot and frostbite are not necessarily a means of classifying the degree of injury but a way of identifying the different modes of development.

Chilblains

The mildest form of cold injury is known as chilblain. It occurs after prolonged exposure of uncovered areas of the body in a climate which is moderately cold (60° F. to freezing) and extremely humid. It is usually seen on the dorsal aspect of the hands of outdoor workers, and on the anterior tibial surface of the lower extremities of young women. It is said to be common in the bare knees and cheeks of British school boys. Acute and chronic states are recognized. The chronic form, which is caused by repeated episodes of exposure, is termed pernio, Bazin's disease or erythrocyanosis. The local lesions are swollen and have a deep, reddish purple discoloration. They form blisters which may ulcerate and produce pigmented scars after healing very slowly. The acute form has a bluish red color. It is swollen, hot, and associated with itching and tenderness. Occasionally, it may cause a burning pain. Treatment is symptomatic and includes advice that the patient dress warmly and prevent continued exposure. Anti-inflammatory and sympatholytic agents may be indicated to reduce pain and swelling.

Immersion or Trench Foot

Immersion or trench foot is seldom seen in civilian life. Its presence has been most frequently reported in sailors or soldiers who have wet feet for prolonged periods in temperature ranging from 68° F. to freezing. Dependency or immobility of the extremity and constriction by clothing or shoes are predisposing factors. Chilling and anoxia of the extremity accompanied by general body cooling and venous stasis results in nerve, muscle and blood vessel changes. As in patients with frostbite, it is not uncommon to observe that the patient has a previous history of personality instability, a labile peripheral vascular system, and a marked tendency to perspire on his hands and feet. These individuals are characterized as sympathetic reactors and are often noted as problem cases in peripheral vascular clinics.

On first examination, the clinical manifestations include an ischemic, cold, swollen appearance of the feet and legs. Subjectively, there is a numb, tingling, itching and cramping pain and a mottled discoloration of the skin. Unlike frostbite the tissues are resilient to palpation. The skin is soft and often very friable. This first stage is termed the prehyperemic phase. It may last for a few hours to several days, and is followed by a hyperemic phase of several weeks. In this stage the pain may be severe; the feet are red, swollen and hot. Blisters appear, and ulcers and gangrene may occur. The third, or posthyperemic phase, is characterized by residual edema and deep pain. Superficial burning pain, hyperhidrosis and cold sensitivity are also present. This phase may continue for months or years.

Prevention requires education of the patient, chiefly those individuals who may experience a cold, wet environment. Rubber footwear should not be worn if possible since it causes an extremely humid environment within the shoes. It is necessary to keep the feet dry at all times. Spare socks should be carried by persons who are prone to wet feet or are in an environment where feet may easily become wet. Periodic elevation, massage and air drying are suggested, and constrictive clothing should be avoided.

Treatment is similar to frostbite except that thawing is not necessary.

Frostbite

Frostbite is the severest form of local cold injury. The injured area initially becomes white. Upon thawing, the sequence of response has three phases: (1) local skin erythema, (2) a wheal at the site of injury, and (3) a flare in the marginal tissues.

Classification. Some clinicians prefer to classify frostbite into two types: *superficial*, which results in superficial dry freezing, and *deep freezing*, which is deep frostbite. This means of identification delineates what should and what should not be thawed before the patient arrives at the hospital. Superficially frozen tissue should be thawed as soon as possible and deeply frozen tissue should be thawed only after arrival in the hospital. Since it is customary to classify frostbite according to the extent of tissue damage, the commonly accepted gradients of thermal tissue injury are preferred (Figs. 17–12, 17–13, 17–14 and 17–15). First degree: erythema, swelling, burning, and tingling without the formation blisters. Second degree: blister or bleb formation, edema, anesthesia, and paresthesia which is marked by hyperemia on rewarming. Third degree: full thickness injury with early edema, early necrosis and gangrene but without loss of a part. Fourth degree: complete necrosis and loss of a part.

First and second degree frostbitten skin is cold and crisp. It may be moved freely over bony surfaces before it is thawed. Third and fourth degree frostbitten skin is not pliable over bony prominences and feels solid or wooden to palpation. On the other hand, all four

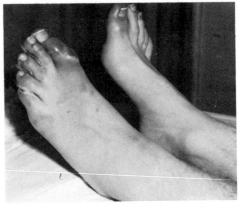

Figure 17–12   Frostbite: first and second degree at twenty-four hours. Following rewarming, second degree frostbite exhibits blister formation and first degree frostbite is erythematous. Sensation is preserved.

types of cold injury may be similar on palpation after they are thawed.

Prevention. (1) *Predisposing or suceptibility factors.* Through the ages, beginning with Hippocrates' writings "on air, waters and places," certain types of people have been observed to have an increased susceptibility to frostbite. As mentioned above in the section on Immersion or Trench Foot, the responses of these individuals (who are

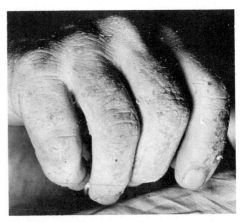

Figure 17–13   Frostbite: fourth degree, fourteen hours after rewarming. Absence of edema is an ominous sign, and it was predicted that the fingers would be lost eventually because of total absence of sensation.

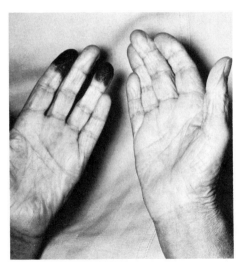

Figure 17–14 Frostbite: second degree, three weeks after injury. The blue skin eschar present subsequently peeled off, leaving normal tissue underneath. While it is true that the ischemia appears superficial in this patient, the point is made that surgical débridement of frostbite should not be aggressive unless wet gangrene appears.

called sympathetic reactors) have verified the role of psychic and personality factors in frostbite. Members of the Armed Forces who have developed frostbite after exposure to a cold environment have had an increased incidence of neurasthenia, poor adjustment,

poor motivation and excessive sweating. Persons with similar physiological and personality traits have been noted in civilian studies on frostbite. Since these people are inclined to place themselves in danger, it is essential that the Armed Forces and industry identify them and not assign them to duty or work in severely cold climates. They are readily recognized by their nonconforming habits and evidence of sweating on hands and feet. This does not imply that all patients with frostbite fit into this group; there are many cases in which exposure was quite unavoidable. Another group exists which is not particularly susceptible but is apparently uninformed: the dedicated outdoor sports enthusiasts. This group has increased in number with the popularity of winter sports.

Racial susceptibility has not been clarified although certain individuals such as Eskimos and arctic fishermen appear to have greater resistance to cold. They are thought to have developed a cold acclimatization at the cellular level. Studies on adaptation to cold by animals appear quite convincing but similar human response have been inconclusive.

Environmental Factors. The depth of cold penetration into the tissues and the duration of exposure of the affected part

Figure 17–15 Frostbite: fourth degree, several weeks after injury. The dessicated necrotic digits eventually underwent autoamputation, which is the preferred method of treatment whenever possible. This method allows preservation of maximum length, since the deep tissues occasionally are viable for a greater distance than the epithelium. Skin grafting can be performed when necessary following autoamputation.

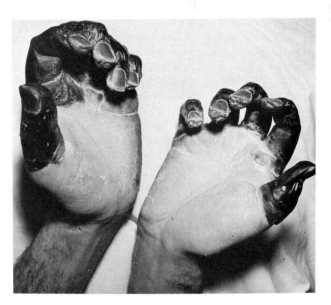

to the cold environment are the final determinants of the severity of frostbite. This conclusion is based on inquiries from weather stations in the area where the exposure occurred. Inquiries must be made regarding the ambient temperature and other environmental factors which increase heat loss by either conduction or convection. A temperature of 22°F. or below apparently produces the highest incidence of frostbite (Table 8–1).

The type of clothing worn is obviously important. Studies have shown that wool cloth beneath an outer garment of closely woven windproof fabric makes excellent use of the insulating properties of still air.

Proper headgear and footwear are extremely important. Gloves should be worm at all times, especially when hands must come in contact with metallic objects.

A sound educational public health program should be continually stressed for individuals who live in or are transients in cold regions. The neglect to cover properly some specific area of the body often determines the pattern of injury.

Early Treatment. Superficial frostbite should be thawed immediately to reduce the total time of cold exposure and lessen the potential of a freezing injury.

Simple methods are often effective: to thaw the face, place a warm hand over the area until it becomes painful; fingers are best treated by placing the hand in the opposite axilla; and feet are warmed by placing them on the abdomen of a companion beneath the clothing. When hot objects are used, extreme caution should be taken to avoid burning of the insensitive cold part. Rubbing or application of snow or slush is absolutely contraindicated.

When deep frostbite has occurred the core body temperature should first be raised. Constricting clothing or boots should be loosened to avoid circulatory loss. Rapid rewarming is not recommended unitl the patient reaches a medical facility. This avoids the possibility of a frozen part being thawed and then refrozen, which is likely to cause the loss of some of the part.

After arrival at the hospital immediate measures are taken in the emergency department to raise the body temperature to normal. Monitoring for shock is instituted, along with its treatment if present.

Rapid thawing is accomplished by immersion in whirlpool, if available, of the injured part or parts for two or more hours at 104° to 107.5°F. (40 to 42°C.) until the distal vascular bed shows flushing. The prognosis is favorable if there is prompt return of sensitivity in the skin and large pink blisters appear extending to the digit tips. Unfavorable prognostic signs are additional trauma to the cold injured part(s), ruptured blebs, purple or reddish-blue blebs, cold and cyanotic digits distal to the blebs, and complete absence of edema after severe injury. Thawing is painful. Rewarming may require the use of analgesics, or intra-arterial or intravenous injection of 25 mg of tolazaline hydrochloride (Priscoline) or 0.6 mg of dihydro ergot alkaloids (Hydergine). These may be used at the physician's discretion.

Patients who show evidence of hypothermia of the legs or the entire body should be hospitalized with bed rest until body temperature has returned to normal, edema subsides, and the blebs dry. Cold injury which does not result in a lowering of the body temperature and frostbite which is localized only to the hands, ears or nose does not require more than a short hospital admission or treatment in the Emergency Department. In these patients the same procedures are instituted at home or on an outpatient basis as for patients admitted to the hospital.

The frozen areas are cleansed with antiseptic soap and water if the extremity was already thawed when first seen. Aseptic precautions are taken in the hospital, using sterile sheets, footboard, cotton between the toes and reverse isolation until the blebs are dry. Frost-bitten fingers are covered with sterile dressings with cotton between the digits. Blebs should not be ruptured. Tetanus prophylaxis is administered either by a toxoid booster or human antitoxin. The injured parts are immersed in a whirlpool at body temperature with antiseptic soap for 20 minutes twice a day and the patient is encouraged to move every joint of every part not only while in the whirlpool but also during the intervening waking hours.

Débridement or amputation is not instituted until the skin begins to separate. If digital circulation appears to be impaired and digital motion is limited by the constricting black eschar, lateral escharotomy is undertaken during the second or third week.

Antibiotics are administered if superimposed infection develops.

Summary. Since most patients with superficial or deep frostbite have been warmed before medical treatment is sought, physicians working in the Emergency Department should accept the responsibility of educating the lay public and ambulance and rescue personnel. All individuals engaged in pre-hospital emergency care should be trained in the technique of rapid re-warming. If the geographical site of cold injury is far enough away from the hospital to delay treatment significantly, emergency health personnel should begin rapid thawing procedures. If refreezing may occur or adequate warming equipment is unavailable, thawing should not be done until the patient arrives at the hospital. Dry heat should never be used for thawing, for the already injured tissues may easily be burned.

Reimplantation of an Extremity

In an Emergency Department which receives a large number of traumatized patients, patients occasionally are referred for reimplantation of a dismembered extremity. It is rare to have both the patient and the dismembered part meet the criteria for reimplantation. Before an Emergency Department physician alerts a speciality service, he must recognize that the procedure of reimplantation of a limb is still under investigation and certain guidelines must be reviewed before this treatment is initiated.

General Criteria

Only an upper extremity should be considered for reimplantation. At present, lower extremity reimplantation is confined to the experimental laboratory.

When a severed part does not accompany the patient, transportation personnel are advised to obtain any tissue left at the scene of the accident. If the tissue is not used for reimplantation, the skin on the part may be available for grafting at the amputated site or elsewhere on the body.

The dismembered extremity must have the potential of viability; that is, the extremity must reach the hospital within six hours after injury.

Tissue destruction of the dismembered part and of the patient's amputated stump must not be extensive.

The candidate must be young.

The patient must have been in good general health prior to the accident.

The plan must be explained thoroughly to the patient and his relatives and they must agree to every aspect of the undertaking.

Team A (responsible for patient) and Team B (responsible for severed extremity) are designated and necessary liaison between the two teams is established. The teams should include a general and vascular surgeon, a neurosurgeon and an orthopedic surgeon.

After team assignments are made in the Emergency Department, both the patient and the severed extremity are transported to the operating room.

Only those hospitals designated as Category I and Category II (see p. 8) should undertake a limb reimplantation. All other hospitals should arrange for transfer of the patient and the limb to a hospital in one of these categories.

Team Responsible for the Patient

Team A, which is responsible for the patient, should:

Establish the monitoring procedures required for patient.

Establish hemostasis, avoiding the use of nonvascular hemostats on major vessels.

Insure that the patient's condition is stabilized.

Draw blood and send it to the laboratory for type and cross-match, with a standby request for whole blood.

Administer tetanus immunization and antibiotics to the patient.

Begin copious irrigation of the patient's wound. No resective débridement of the patient's wound should be performed in the emergency department.

Identify all structures to anticipate and lessen problems upon arrival in the operating room.

Team Responsible for the Severed Extremity

Team B, which is responsible for severed extremity, should:

Place the severed extremity in iced water.

Identify all structures.

Perfuse the artery with iced Ringer's lactate, low molecular weight dextran or a heparin solution of 100 units per kilogram of extremity weight in normal saline.

Add 2 million units of penicillin to the perfusate solution.

Irrigate the open wound copiously. As with the patient's wound, no resective débridement of the severed extremity should be performed in the Emergency Department.

Anatomical Order

The anatomical order of the reimplantation in the operating room may vary slightly among surgeons but in general the following order is used: bone approximation, establishment of circulation, nerve anastomosis, approximation of muscle and tendons, skin suture, and fasciotomy in the forearm.

Postreimplantation management begins with continuous control of the arterial circulation, regulation of the patient's fluid hemodynamics, maintenance of satisfactory urine output, continuation of antibiotic administration, daily use of low molecular weight dextran and treatment of edema of the extremity.

After discharge, physiotherapy is scheduled regularly. Further repair may be required to accomplish a maximal outcome.

Thoracic Outlet Syndrome

Much of the confusion regarding the diagnosis and treatment of shoulder girdle compression syndromes has abated since 1962 when Falconer and Li and Claggett reported their experience with first rib resection for severe thoracic outlet syndrome. This syndrome grouped together all of the possible causes for neurovascular signs and symptoms of the upper extremities including scalenus anticus, costoclavicular, cervical rib, hyperabduction, shoulder-hand, fractured clavicle, effort vein thrombosis or pneumatic hammer syndromes. The authors advised that the first rib be resected in patients who were unresponsive to physiotherapy, traction, collars and even scalenotomies. Their studies and reports of other workers have shown that all shoulder girdle compression syndromes have one problem in common—compression of the brachial plexus and the subclavian artery and vein, usually between the clavicle and the first rib (Fig. 17–16). Therefore, the thoracic outlet syndrome should be considered in all neurologic and vascular complaints of the upper extremities.

Resection of the first rib for thoracic outlet syndrome was cautiously accepted

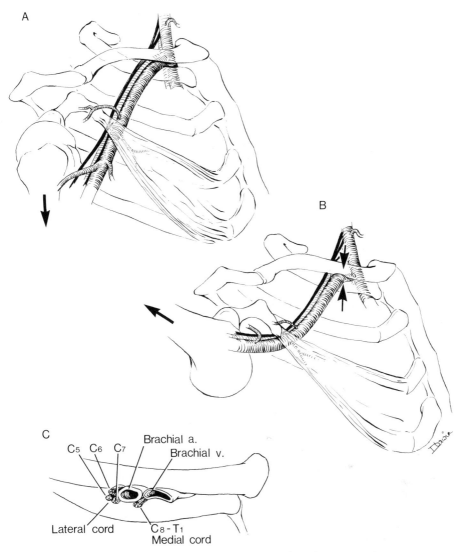

A

B

C

C5 C6 C7   Brachial a.
                Brachial v.

Lateral cord   C8 - T1
                Medial cord

Figure 17–16   Pathological anatomy in thoracic outlet compression.

at first because the two surgical approaches available at the time, namely the supraclavicular and the parascapular, were complicated, traumatic, somewhat hazardous and provided limited exposure. However, since the introduction of the relatively simple transaxillary approach by Roos in 1966, first rib resection has been used almost to excess. The author agrees that approximately only one patient out of five with shoulder girdle complaints should be considered for surgery. The remainder either respond to physiotherapy or their symptoms are so mild that surgery is not indicated. In the ten year period prior to the introduction of the first rib resection concept we performed only one scalenotomy and one claviculectomy, and approximately 30 upper thoracic sympathectomies. Therefore, when the new procedure was introduced we had a large backlog of classical thoracic outlet syndrome patients in whom first rib resection was indicated. Our surgical success rate has been high because of careful screening.

Symptoms

Symptoms may be grouped into neurologic and vascular complaints. The most common neurologic symptom is aching pain in the side or back of the neck, extending across the shoulder and down the arm into the forearm and hand. The pain may radiate in all directions from the point of compression. Numbness and tingling are frequently experienced in the hand, usually localized to a C_8–T_1 distribution, and fine coordination may be affected. Any sustained upper extremity activity aggravates the pain and causes paresthesias and weakness. These activities include combing hair, painting, throwing a baseball or football or other use of the hands above shoulder level, reaching, using a typewriter, holding a newspaper, a telephone or a steering wheel. The pain is usually not noticed until after the arm is used. It may be particularly troublesome at night, often causing the patient to awaken.

Vascular complaints may be divided into arterial and venous symptoms. Arterial symptoms range from coolness, cold sensitivity and pallor of the hand on elevation to a Raynaud's phenomenon or occlusion of the subclavian artery. Venous symptoms vary from edema, stiffness of the fingers, and venous engorgement in certain elevated arm positions or shoulder depression when carrying heavy objects to acute thrombophlebitis of the subclavian or axillary vein (Fig. 17–17).

The onset of symptoms may be either spontaneous or post-traumatic. Most patients with spontaneous symptoms are thin females in their twenties or thirties, while male patients usually have a muscular body build. The post-traumatic group may include anyone who has re-

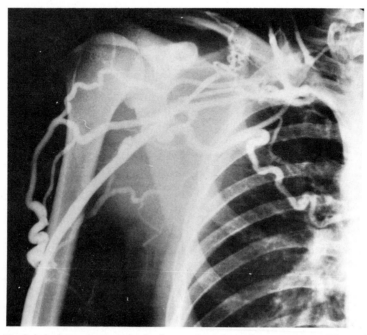

Figure 17–17 Subclavian vein thrombosis due to thoracic outlet entrapment. The patient also had hypercoagulability causing priapism. Treatment was given with heparin followed by first rib resection.

ceived an injury to the shoulder, clavicle or neck. Any severe jerking injury to the shoulder or neck such as the so-called "whiplash" auto injury may precipitate the outlet syndrome. The appearance of arm symptoms may be delayed for several days, weeks or even months after the injury, and the symptoms tend to respond poorly to physical therapy. Other examples of traumatic etiology of the syndrome are brachial plexus palsy following arm abduction and long-term exposure to vibrating tools.

Patients may represent mild, moderate or severe forms of the syndrome. The mild complaints include occasional numbness and tingling of the extremity, especially at night and most often on patients who sleep with their arms above shoulder level. They do not seek or need medical attention. The moderate group has pain in the neck, shoulder, arm and hand for which they seek diagnosis and care. The severe form has limitation of ordinary activities, pain and loss of sleep. Complications such as Raynaud's phenomenon, emboli, thrombophlebitis or muscle atrophy may also occur in the severe category.

Many of the symptoms described by patients are so similar that a diagnosis can often be considered from the history alone. However, confirmation must be made by physical examination.

Signs

Signs may be divided into vascular and neurological changes. The compression of the brachial plexus and subclavian vessels is demonstrated with the arm in a 90 degree, abduction–external–rotation (AER) position, without shoulder elevation. With this maneuver the clavicle swings posteriorly and inferiorly from its fixed fulcrum at the sternoclavicular joint, creating a scissorlike entrapment of the plexus and subclavian vessels against the first rib and producing a decreased or absent radial pulse, a blood pressure fall of 15 mm Hg or greater, and a bruit of the subclavian artery either above or below the clavicle. With both arms elevated in the 90 degree AER position and the subclavian artery partially occluded, the fingers are flexed rapidly to demonstrate the "claudication test." Forearm pain and finger paresthesias occur within a few seconds in an extremity with an outlet syndrome, and the arm will soon collapse from fatigue and discomfort. An extremity without arterial compression may be exercised for over a minute with little or no distress. Positive findings with these manuevers do not necessarily identify the patient as having a thoracic outlet syndrome. However, these tests assist in confirming the diagnosis in individuals whose pulse is obliterated at less than 90 degree abduction and who identify the level of abduction as the position at which their complaints are reproduced, or in patients who have neurological complaints without vascular signs. It is possible to produce pulse obliteration or murmurs in the subclavian artery in various positions of the head and arm in many normal individuals, especially young women. This suggests that even in the normal adult the thoracic outlet is limited to little more than enough space to permit the passage of the subclavian vessels and the brachial plexus. A change in posture such as an abnormal descent of the shoulder girdle in adults, a fractured clavicle, hypertrophy of the scalene muscles, a large scalene tubercle on the first rib, a cervical rib or any other condition which may compromise the reserve space available predisposes to a thoracic outlet syndrome.

Neurologic signs include reproduction of the symptoms by thumb pressure in the supraclavicular fossa over the subclavian artery and brachial plexus, tenderness to tapping in the same site, pinprick hyperesthesia in the hand (most often in the C_8–T_1 (ulnar) dermatome), weakness of the interosseous muscles of the hand innervated by the ulnar nerve, and weakness of the biceps and triceps muscles and the hand grip. Normal tendon reflexes are usually present and nerve conduction times of the ulnar and median nerves are almost always normal. The ulnar nerve is more often involved than the radial and medial nerves because it is formed from the C_8–T_1 cervical roots, the lowest cord of the brachial plexus. This portion of the cord lies directly on the first rib and therefore may receive the greatest compression in the bony "scissor blade" of the clavicle against the rib.

Differential Diagnosis

Differential diagnosis includes herniated cervical disc, cervical spondylosis, carpal tunnel syndrome, bursitis, capsulitis, tendonitis, shoulder or wrist arteritis, myositis, angina pectoris, multiple sclerosis and carcinoma involving the brachial plexus. Each entity may be confused with a thoracic outlet syndrome. Appropriate studies including x-rays must be used to differentiate these disorders. However, none of these conditions present the symptoms and signs of both a neurologic and vascular nature.

Treatment

Treatment first considered is a means to enlarge the thoracic outlet by improving posture and exercises to strengthen shoulder suspensory muscles. The patient should be told about the anatomical reason for the complaints, that is, the scissors effect of the clavicle and first rib upon the neurovascular structures in the outlet area. To relieve this, the patient is instructed to elevate both shoulders and push them forward when passing through a doorway or when stopped for a traffic light when in an automobile. Soon the patient unconsciously reverses the abnormal descent of the shoulder girdle and symptoms lessen or disappear. Additional measures for relief of symptoms are traction, heat, ultrasonic treatments and rest from all activities. These measures are beneficial

to most patients in mild to moderate groups.

When conservative measures fail, surgery may be considered but usually only after nonoperative means of treatment have been used for at least three months. Surgery requires the removal of the first rib. This allows the plexus and vessels to drop slightly and the clavicle has no hard surface against which to trap these structures. The preferred approach for rib removal is via the axillary route. If definitive vascular surgery is necessary, the clavicular approach may be incorporated as a separate incision.

Complications may be an occasional wound infection, a brachial plexus injury from retraction, or residual hyperesthesia when the upper thoracic sympathetic ganglia have not been removed. Other complications include residual neck pain because the entire posterior portion of the rib (and the cervical rib when present) was not included in the resection, and postsympathectomy neuralgia over the anterior superior portion of the chest and shoulder on approximately the tenth postoperative day. The latter may be relieved by sympatholytic drugs as reported elsewhere in this chapter.

Arteriovenous Fistulas

An arteriovenous fistula is a direct communication between an artery and a vein that permits the blood to bypass the capillary circulation. William Hunter first demonstrated the true nature of arteriovenous fistulas in 1757 when he observed an iatrogenic fistula which developed following a surgical puncture of the brachial artery and vein. Since this historic observation many clinicians and physiologists have studied these lesions, but not until 1968, when Holman published the results of his experimental studies, was there clarification of the physiologic changes which may occur from abnormal arteriovenous communications. He listed changes as follows:

Physiologic Changes

a. *Immediate Effects*
  (1) Both stystolic and diastolic blood pressures are decreased.
  (2) The pulse rate increases.
  (3) The venous pressure increases distally as well as proximally to the fistula.
  (4) The cardiac output increases in proportion to the size and location of the fistula.
  (5) The heart and the proximal artery temporarily decrease in size due to the diversion of blood from a high pressure system (arterial) to a low pressure system (venous), as seen in massive hemorrhage.
b. *Remote Effects*
  (1) Part of the normal capillary bed is bypassed permanently because of the fistula.
  (2) Total blood volume gradually increases in relation to the amount of flow through the fistula.
  (3) Proximal vasculature, namely, the heart, artery and vein, dilate gradually because of increased volume of blood traversing the fistula into a low resistance system (venous).
  (4) Extensive collateral circulation develops because the fistula has a low resistance to flow and the artery proximal to fistula constricts. The constricted artery contributes to an increased collateral circulation which in turn, because of the volume delivered, results in the artery dilating distal to the fistula.
  (5) Heart musculature hypertrophies slightly due to dilatation, overdistension and increased work load caused by an increased volume of flow.
  (6) Pulse pressure widens when the lowered blood pressure recovers. The systolic pressure returns to its prefistula level or higher and the diastolic pressure falls.

Physiological changes depend upon the size of the fistula, its location in the arterial tree, and the patency of the vein proximal to the fistula. Variations therefore depend entirely upon the quantity of blood diverted through the fistula.

Closure of the Fistula

Closure of the fistula by compression of definitive repair produces the following changes:
a. *Immediate Effects*
  (1) Both the systolic and diastolic blood pressures rise and then fall to readings above prefistula levels because the previously low peripheral resistance is eliminated, but the increased blood volume remains in the newly intact vascular system.
  (2) Pulse rate and cardiac activity decrease.
  (3) Venous pressure decreases proximal to the fistula.
  (4) Cardiac output decreases markedly.
  (5) Heart size increases for a short period due to overdistension from the continued presence of an increased blood volume in the newly intact vascular system.
b. *Remote Effects*
  (1) Blood pressure gradually returns to prefistula levels.
  (2) Total blood volume gradually decreases to normal.
  (3) Pulse rate gradually lowers to normal range.
  (4) Dilatation in the vasculature proximal to the closed fistula, namely, the heart, artery, and vein, gradually subsides but cardiac hypertrophy may be irreversible when the fistula is of a long duration.

Etiology

Arteriovenous fistulas may be congenital or acquired. The congenital type is the most frequently encountered.

Congenital arteriovenous fistulas may occur in any area of the body but are most often noted peripherally. Peripheral fistulas may be classified as: (1) hemangioma; (2) microfistulous arteriovenous aneurysm; (3) macrofistulous arteriovenous aneurysm; and (4) anomalous mature vascular channels. These classifications are based on the alterations which occur during the development of certain mesenchymal cells into mature blood vessels. Since both arteries and veins differentiate from a common capillary plexus one vessel may function as the other in certain areas of the embryo and during specific stages of embryologic life. In addition, it is always possible that any of the infinite number of communications which existed initially between arteries and veins may persist after birth, resulting in congenital arteriovenous fistulas.

Acquired arteriovenous fistulas most frequently result from penetrating wounds such as those from gunshot, stab wounds, flying sharp objects or fragments of bone. A second cause is the spontaneous rupture of an arterial wall into the accompanying vein, as when a mycotic aneurysm ruptures into its neighboring vein. Iatrogenic arteriovenous fistulas may be produced inadvertently during surgery or diagnostic procedures involving major arteries or veins.

Sites of Arteriovenous Fistulas

Extremities. Congenital arteriovenous fistulas are most often noted in the extremities, mainly the legs. Any part of the limbs may be involved, including the bones. Usually the lesion has multiple channels which are diffuse or extensive. Even when multiple communications exist, the lesion may appear to be discrete or confined to a relatively small area.

Diagnostic features of congenital arteriovenous fistulas of the lower limbs include the presence of varicose veins. When varices are unilateral, in an unusual location, and present early in life for no apparent reason, one should suspect a congenital arteriovenous fistula. Further suspicion should be aroused when ulcerations develop on the distal parts of the foot, a site where venous ulcers do not occur, and when elongation of the limb is noted. The communications may be so large that the varicosities pulsate. Increased warmth over the fistula may be expected. Pain localized to the site of the lesion usually indicates that thrombosis is occurring and may be considered a good prognostic sign. Bruits or thrills are usually not present, and the bradycardiac sign seldom can be demonstrated. The congenital fistula usually is not associated with cardiac effects except in infants. Some lesions become progressively larger at puberty or increase their arteriovenous components following minor trauma or exercise.

When surgery is being considered arteriograms should be ordered routinely to determine the extent of the lesion. Frequently the presence of an arteriovenous fistula is demonstrated only by the early appearance of the venous phase of the arteriogram. Oxygen saturation samples may be taken from the vein proximal to the fistula and compared with a sample from a similar vein on the opposite limb. A Doppler flowmeter may be used to assist in the diagnosis and to delineate the limits of the lesion.

Treatment for congenital arteriovenous fistulas is often unsatisfactory. Surgery is discouraged unless the lesion can be demonstrated as discrete or localized, for the lesion is frequently found to be more extensive than contemplated and complete excision is impossible. An approach which is too aggressive may result in the loss of a limb. Serious hemorrhage, extensive ulceration or infection may develop from extensive congenital arteriovenous fistula of an extremity. An amputation may be advisable in some patients with this type of lesion. One promising approach is the use of cryotherapy followed by a pressure dressing. This method of therapy initiates thrombosis within the vascular sinusoids and is not likely to cause permanent damage to tendons and nerves. The procedure is especially advised for hemangiomas of the hand, and although a permanent cure does not result often, it may be used as a palliative procedure every few years. Sclerosing solutions and irradiation therapy are useless methods of therapy in the opinion of this writer.

Acquired arteriovenous fistulas are also most often noted in the extremities and are due almost invariably to trauma. The appearance of a fistula may be delayed for several days because of a hematoma at the site of communication between two vessels. The factors determining the volume flow through the fistula are the size of the opening, its location in the main arterial tree, the absence of fibrosis around the fistula and the duration of the fistula. These factors may be extensive enough to cause an increased blood volume, cardiac enlargement, cardiac failure and thrills localized to the fistula. Hemihypertrophy may be present if a fistula occurs at an early age before the epiphysis closes. Elevated venous pressure produces varicose veins which may pulsate, edema and skin pigmentation about the ankle, and chronic induration similar to that seen in a postphlebitic syndrome. Distal ischemic changes, including gangrene, may occur when the fistula is large and collateral circulation is inadequate.

The skin is warmer in the area of the fistula than the skin of the opposite limb. However, the skin distally may be cooler than that of the companion extremity.

A machinelike murmur accentuated during systole is audible over the fistula and a systolic thrill is palpable. Both are eliminated by pressure over the vein proximal to the fistula. Temporary closure of the fistula by compression causes the heart rate to slow and the diastolic pressure to increase—a positive Branham's sign. Other techniques used to locate the site of fistula are venous pressure (increased), oxygen saturation of the venous blood, thermography, flowmeter studies and arteriography.

Treatment involves some method of definitive repair. Excision of the fistula and reestablishment of the normal arterial and venous flow is preferred as early as possible. When minor vessels are involved, quadruple ligation and excision alone can be performed.

Aorto-inferior Vena Caval Fistulas. These may be spontaneous due to rupture of an abdominal aortic aneurysm into the inferior vena cava, or trauma caused by a penetrating wound, including iatrogenic fistulas from lumbar disc operations.

Aorto-inferior vena caval fistulas require early diagnosis and repair. If they go unrecognized, the early fatality rate is high owing to their size and proximity to the heart. The physiological changes occur in an extreme degree with possible additional findings such as massive swelling of the lower limbs and trunk and bleeding from the rectum and urinary tract.

If a patient undergoing surgical removal of an intervertebral disc has an unexplained drop in blood pressure or develops congestive heart failure postoperatively, he should be examined for the presence of an aorto-inferior vena caval or iliac arteriovenous fistula. An audible machinelike bruit in the lower abdomen is diagnostic. Emergency repair is advised in almost all patients.

Pulmonary Arteriovenous Fistulas. These may be congenital due to persistence of embryologic arteriovenous connections or they may be acquired during pulmonary venous or arterial hypertension, specific types of obstructive lung disease, hepatic cirrhosis and certain infections such as *Schistosoma cercariae.*

Pulmonary arteriovenous fistulas may be separated into two groups—those with a pulmonary arterial blood supply, which are the most frequent, and those with a systemic blood supply.

The lesion with a pulmonary *arterial blood supply* causes a certain amount of the pulmonary circulation to bypass oxygenation in the lungs and flow directly into the left side of the heart and into the general circulation. This abnormal pulmonary blood flow pattern results in chronic arterial hypoxia which produces symptoms of cyanosis, dyspnea, polycythemia and clubbing of the digits. The lesions may be single or multiple, and the majority occur superficially in the lower lobes of the lungs. Hereditary telangiectasis is a common finding. A continuous bruit with systolic accentuation at the time of deep inspiration is a diagnostic sign. The chest roentgenogram will usually show one or more well-circumscribed, noncalcified nodules with vessels connecting them to the hilum, and an angiogram confirms the diagnosis.

The pulmonary arteriovenous fistula with a *systemic blood supply* is very rare. The connecting vessel may be a bronchial, internal mammary, or intercostal artery, or the aorta. Collateral circulation may be so extensive that rib notching may develop. The signs and symptoms are those of a left-to-right shunt. The common complaint is dyspnea and easy fatigability. Diagnosis is confirmed by chest roentgenogram and angiograms.

The fistulas may be localized to the lung or they may have associated abnormalities of hereditary telangiectasis of the skin, mucous membranes and other organs. The arterial supply is often multiple and may be bilateral. Surgery is advised if the fistulas are single, show localization when multiple, or cause symptoms or progressive enlargement. However, surgery is not advised unless changes occur when the fistulas are multiple and diffuse, or single and asymptomatic.

Renal Arteriovenous Fistulas. These may occur with or without a functioning kidney distal to the fistula.

Fistulas associated with a functioning kidney may develop from a congenital, acquired or idiopathic origin. Congenital lesions are angiomatous or cersoid in appearance and have multiple arteriovenous connections. Acquired fistulas result from hypernephroma, trauma, atherosclerosis or inflammation. The hypernephromous lesions are due either to tumor invasion of the large vessels of the kidney or to the neoplasm becoming necrotic and forming arteriovenous communications within the tumor mass. Traumatic renal arteriovenous fistulas are caused by penetrating wounds and iatrogenic wounds following pyelolithotomy or percutaneous renal biopsy. Lesions from subacute bacterial endocarditis and other types of infection are rarely noted today.

Diagnosis is based on the findings of a continuous machine-like bruit localized to the renal area, diastolic hypertension, congestive heart failure and hematuria. Renal ischemia may occur from an infarct distal to the arteriovenous communication(s). An excretory urogram may be used as a screening procedure prior to the detailed renal arteriogram study which precedes surgery. Preservation of the kidney is desirable but is seldom accomplished due to the extent of the lesion or the presence of renal infarcts.

Renal arteriovenous fistulas have been reported following nephrectomy and frequently have been blamed on mass ligation of both renal artery and vein during surgery. However, since all of the patients reported did not have mass ligation of the vessels, it is thought that other factors contribute to renal arteriovenous fistulas. These factors include the formation of a hematoma or infection in the area of the pedicle, or transfixion of the vessels without simple ligation.

Diagnosis is based on the presence of the characteristic bruit, signs and symptoms of congestive heart failure and the usual elevated systolic pressure and lowered diastolic pressure resulting in a widened pulse pressure. Aortography is necessary to confirm the diagnosis and demonstrate the character of the lesion.

Portal Circulation Arteriovenous Fistulas. These are rare, but should be considered whenever a patient is studied for portal hypertension. Congenital lesions frequently are associated with hereditary telangiectasis and are localized either within the liver parenchyma or extrahepatic vessels. Gastrointestinal bleeding may occur because of rupture of the lesions in the submucosa. Acquired arteriovenous fistula may result from spontaneous rupture of a visceral abdominal artery aneurysm into the portal circulation, or it may be iatrogenic following mass ligation of an artery and vein during splenectomy, gastrectomy or other intra-abdominal surgery in which the vein accompanying the artery is part of the portal circulation. Penetrating or blunt trauma is also an etiological factor as with arteriovenous fistulas in other sites.

Clinical manifestations of portal hypertension occur, such as esophageal varices, ascites and splenomegaly. The diagnosis is suspected in the presence of the usual continuous bruit and confirmed by selective arteriography.

Surgery is indicated. Extrahepatic lesions require excision; revascularization of the vessels depends upon the site of the fistulas. Intrahepatic fistula usually necessitates a hepatic lobectomy.

Arteriovenous Fistulas of the Neck and Face. These have become rare due to the early aggressive surgical approach toward repair of traumatic injuries to vessels in this area of the body. Congenital arteriovenous fistulas are less common than acquired lesions. Vessels involved in acquired lesions are the common carotid artery and internal jugular vein, and the thyroid, vertebral and subclavian arteries and veins. Penetrating wounds are the common cause, whether they result from violence or iatrogenically following surgery or a diagnostic procedure.

The usual history demonstrates evidence of a penetrating wound or surgery to the neck or face followed by a hema-

toma which ultimately becomes pulsatile and presents an audible continuous bruit and palpable thrill. Neurological signs of cerebral ischemia may occur and the patient complains of pain and a continuous disturbing sound in his head or neck. With a carotid artery and internal jugular vein communication it is common for the patient to develop a unilateral exophthalmus (Fig. 17–18). Occlusion of the carotid artery proximally abolishes the bruit and decreases the pulse, but the procedure may cause siphoning the distal intracranial bed through the "thirsty" fistula and syncope may occur. However, when the maneuver is carefully performed it helps to locate the precise site of the fistula. Arteriography is indicated to confirm the diagnosis and character of the lesion.

Surgery is advised since the morbidity from these lesions is high. Excision with

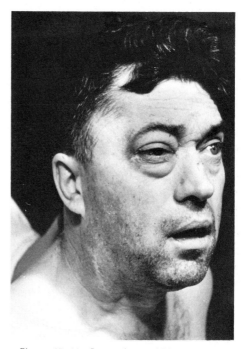

Figure 17–18 Internal carotid-internal jugular arteriovenous fistula causing unilateral exophthalmos. The fistula was created previously at another hospital in an attempt to improve cerebral ischemia. The fistula was divided and the vessels repaired with a satisfactory result.

revascularization of the involved structures is indicated for carotid-jugular and subclavian lesions while vertebral and isolated neck vessels with arteriovenous fistulas may be excised and ligated only.

Congenital arteriovenous fistulas of the head and neck are almost invariably multiple and often involve the underlying bone. The most frequent complaint is of a cosmetic nature but hemorrhage or sudden enlargement with pain may occur. Surgery is frequently unsuccessful unless a radical resection is accomplished. Therefore the lesion is studied thoroughly prior to any surgical decision, and the patient is completely instructed as to the problems involved with and without operation.

Pelvic Arteriovenous Fistulas. Like other fistulas, these are divided into those which are congenital and those which are acquired. Congenital fistulas have multiple arteriovenous connections with the branches of the internal iliac vessels and seldom cause hemodynamic changes in the systemic circulation. Symptomatology usually occurs just prior to menstruation or during pregnancy. When the uterus is involved vaginal bleeding may occur at any time. Diagnosis is made by the presence of a pulsatile mass noted on pelvic examination and a continuous bruit over the lower abdomen. Arteriography should be performed to assist in establishing the site and size of the lesion before surgery is undertaken. If the patient is asymptomatic, surgery is not always suggested since complete excision of the lesion may require extensive surgery.

Acquired arteriovenous fistulas result from penetrating trauma including instances which occasionally develop following hysterectomy. They are thought to be caused by ligation of both artery and vein by transfixion without prior simple ligation. These fistulas usually enlarge and produce hemodynamic changes. As with congenital arteriovenous lesions the presence of a pelvic pulsatile mass and a continuous bruit is diagnostic. Arteriography is advised prior to surgery, which should be performed as soon as possible after diagnosis is made.

Sympathetic Disorders

The diagnosis and treatment of disorders of the sympathetic nervous system has had a colorful and interesting history for more than a century. The first classic description of pain related to the sympathetic nervous system was made in 1864 by Mitchell, Morehouse and Keen, who reported burning pain in soldiers with gunshot wounds of peripheral nerves, an entity which Mitchell eight years later termed causalgia. Sympathetic ablation as therapy for specific disorders was advocated by Jennisco in 1897 and by Jaboulay two years later. They advised periarterial sympathectomy as a method of treatment for epilepsy, glaucoma, migraine and ulceration of the feet. Following their reports, the leading advocate for the diagnosis and treatment of sympathetic disorders was René Leriche, who published many articles on the subject beginning in 1913. Sympathectomy achieved widespread popularity for peripheral vascular diseases about thirty years ago, but this popularity was lost when ganglionic blocks were introduced and reconstructive vascular surgery was developed a decade later.

Diagnosis

Diagnosis of sympathetic disorders is based on careful clinical evaluation of vascular and neurological changes due to congenital or familial conditions, vascular diseases, trauma, metabolic abnormalities, infections and combinations of these lesions.

There are *four primary reasons* for treating conditions which are related to overactivity or underactivity of the sympathetic nervous system: (1) the presence of vasospasm; (2) the need for small collateral channels when there is obstruction of a major arterial vessel;

(3) the relief of causalgic type pain; and (4) the elimination of hyperhidrosis.

Clinicians frequently have widely divergent opinions about the value of therapy involving the sympathetic nervous system because some patients fail to achieve the expected results from treatment. Therapy involving the sympathetic nervous system has much to offer patients when the *limitations* are clearly understood and properly ordered. A sound knowledge of the variations in anatomy of the sympathetic nervous system and the pathophysiology of the patient's condition is essential before treatment can be advised. The results of treatment may be influenced by improper choice of drug, inappropriate technique used in blocking sympathetic ganglia, improperly performed sympathectomy, and the failure to appriase clinical results by objective measurements.

Relief of pain is one of the most interesting and dramatic responses to medical or surgical sympathetic therapy, specifically in patients who have causalgia or causalgic type pain which is burning, hypersensitive, numb and superficial in nature. No relief of deep pain of somatic root origin should be expected.

The beneficial effects of sympathectomy are not always permanent in vasospastic and occlusive arterial disease. Another problem is that sympathectomy may produce unexpected bizarre pain syndromes postoperatively in patients with causalgia.

Sympathectomy for vasospastic conditions such as Raynaud's phenomenon consistently fails to have the same lasting effect in the upper extremities that it has in the lower extremities. Sympathectomy may produce dramatic improvement in the initial postoperative period when performed for Raynaud's phenomenon, which is secondary to other diseases. However, its effect is generally so short-lived that the procedure is considered of little value, especially when scleroderma is present. For the primary type of Raynaud's disease, sympathectomy is valuable for relief of pain but is not necessarily useful for the abnormal color changes which frequently recur postoperatively.

The dependent rubor in severe occlusive disease is due to paralytic vasodilatation or chronic hyperemia in the small peripheral vessels and therefore sympathectomy is not indicated. However, the procedure may be warranted for causalgic type pain in patients with chronic arterial occlusive disease. An intra-arterial sympatholytic drug such as Priscoline may identify the type of pain which may be relieved by surgery.

Since arteriosclerosis obliterans is a progressive disease, the development of a rich collateral bed does not change the possibility of further thrombosis of the vessel. Any patient with rapid progression of disease usually has the poorest effect from a sympathectomy.

The means by which sympathetic tone returns is obscure. It has been suggested that "intrinsic tone" or increased sensitivity to circulatory catecholamines develops. Reserpine has been found to reduce the catecholamine content of the tissues.

There also has been much published about *regeneration* of sympathetic nerve fibers postoperatively. There are several proposed theories as to why autonomic activity returns following sympathectomy. Regeneration has been classified as early (within one year) or late (after a year or more). Theories for early return of sympathetic activity are: (1) the sympathectomy was not adequate; (2) an anatomically complete sympathectomy cannot be performed, since the sympathetic trunks frequently have anatomical variations; and (3) the sympathetic pathways readjust when fibers cross over from the contralateral side. One theory for late regeneration is that the remaining intact fibers of the sympathetic nervous system respond to a stimulus produced by nearby degenerating fibers. Fine branches develop from these fibers and contact the adventitial cells of remaining axons to reach the degenerated structures. Theories to explain early or late regeneration are: (1) the disease for which the sympathectomy was performed may progress and the resulting reduction in blood flow may be considered erroneously to be caused by a regeneration of a sectioned sympathetic chain; and (2) the vessels are hypersensitive to circulatory catecholamines, the amino-oxidase content of the arterial wall is lowered, and the normal synthesis of acetylcholine in the arterial wall is eliminated.

"Regeneration" is most often noted, and is considered more significant, in patients under forty who underwent sympathectomy two or more years prior to the return of sympathetic tone. The earlier the return of symptoms, the more likely that an inadequate sympathectomy was performed; reoperation is indicated for these patients.

Occasionally one hears of a patient who was relieved of *intermittent claudication* following a lumbar sympathectomy. However, there is overwhelming evidence that sympathectomy is not useful for uncomplicated intermittent claudication. Any improvement results indirectly from the relief of foot symptoms as well as the manner in which the patient ambulates.

Sympathectomy should not be advised for patients who have no chance for revascularization of the extremity or for those whose bizarre pain patterns *might* be relieved by sympathectomy. The *"hope for improvement"* is not a logical reason for performing a sympathectomy, especially in a patient whose extremity is doomed to amputation. On the other hand, sympathectomy should not be performed when definitive vascular surgery is indicated.

Indications for Sympathetic Denervation

These can be divided into three groups of disorders: vascular, neurological or both. Selection of patients is therefore based on careful clinical evaluation of these systems.

Vascular Disorders. These are evaluated first as to the presence and degree of peripheral arterial flow by palpation, oscillometry, plethysmography, Doppler flowmeter technique and arteriography. Collateral circulation is determined by the degree of blanching on elevation, the extent of cutaneous congestion on dependency, and the time of venous filling in the toes and foot. Blanching of the toes and forefoot should not occur in less than 120 seconds; upon dependency, flushing time should be 20 seconds or less in the same area and venous filling should be 30 seconds or less. A constant red or purplish-red color on a dependent foot denotes poor collateral circulation and sympathectomy to improve vascular flow is contraindicated.

The presence or absence of vasospasm should be recorded. The simplest method is to block the posterior tibial nerve inferior to the medial malleolus. An increase in toe temperature and improvement in its cutaneous circulation denotes a probably successful result following sympathectomy. A plethesmograph provides additional methods of evaluating an active vasoconstrictor mechanism. This instrument measures the pulsatile blood flow to a digit by recording the character of the pulse deflection and pulse waves. One reliable method is to record toe readings in a warm environment. If, when the patient is exposed to a cold atmosphere, the plethesmographic reading does not go below 50 per cent, the patient is considered to have a collateral circulation adequate to warrant sympathectomy.

Sympathetic blocks may be used to select patients for sympathectomy—the stellate ganglionic block for the upper extremity or the lumbar sympathetic block for the lower limb. Both procedures are unreliable if the block is technically incomplete. The validity of the test depends on the expertise of the clinician performing the block, the absence of anatomical variables in the sympathetic ganglia, and the use of instruments and tests which identify specific physiologic changes in the extremity following the procedure. A Horner's syndrome occurs after a successful block of the sympathetic impulses to the cervical chain. However, a Horner's syndrome does not prove that the post-ganglionic sympathetic fibers supplying the involved upper limb were anesthetized. This needs to be verified by demonstrating the absence of sudomotor activity with a skin resistor or evaluating the digital blood flow with a plethesmograph or recording temperature changes with a thermocouple in a temperature controlled room. Tests for the accuracy of the procedure are also required when a lumbar sympathetic block is performed. When digital temperature or blood flow decreases, a sympathectomy is not advised. Neither spinal nor epidural anesthesia should be utilized to evaluate pain problems related to the sympathetic nervous system, since somatic root and sympathetic type pain patterns cannot be differentiated.

Unless a definite positive response is obtained by one test, multiple tests for patient selection should be performed. The optimum test is the one which is the simplest and most frequently utilized by a clinician who thoroughly understands the patient's problem and the limitations of the diagnostic procedure.

Causalgia. Causalgia or causalgic type pain may develop from injury, infection, venous or arterial disorders or peripheral nerve conditions. Although the pain has many interesting aspects, it is most often characterized as a superficial burning pain with hyperesthesia localized to the involved site or part. It may occur on any surface of the body but is most often localized to an extremity. Therefore, clinicians who treat vascular diseases see it in patients with vascular disorders and in patients referred for consultation for pain of possible vascular etiology. Relief for these patients rests on an accurate diagnosis and adequate medical or surgical sympathetic denervation.

Various names are used to identify "causalgia." The common names are acute atrophy of bone, Sudeck's atrophy, traumatic angiospasm, reflex nervous dystrophy, post-traumatic osteoporosis, minor causalgia, neurovasospastic phenomenon, and chronic traumatic edema.

The pain may be totally related to the sympathetic nervous system or to a combination of somatic root pain and sympathetic pain. Similar types of pain are seen in vascular disorders such as Raynaud's phenomenon, thoracic outlet syndrome, postsympathetic neuralgia, pain of arterial or venous etiology associated with rest pain and postphlebitic ulcers, frostbite, and so on. In some of these conditions the vascular signs may be of minor importance; the pain is the major complaint for which the patient is requesting relief. Proper therapy depends upon consideration of the vascular changes as well as the character of the pain preoperatively and postoperatively. Many patients are "sympathetic reactors" who are prone to develop causalgic type pain following any disorder, whether it results from trauma, a circulatory condition, an infection or a metabolic abnormality.

The most outstanding *symptom* of causalgia or causalgic pain is *burning type of superficial pain*. The superficial aspect is emphasized to differentiate it from deep pain which has a somatic root origin, e.g., traumatic neuritis, abscess, ischemic neuritis, neuromas, and so forth. Other descriptions of causalgia are "throbbing," or "viselike."

The pain may occur instantaneously but most often it is delayed for days or weeks. On the extremity, the pain referral is distal and occupies chiefly the palm of the hand, the fingers, toes or plantar surface of the foot.

Hyperesthesia is the second most conspicuous complaint and may be localized to a sensory nerve. Frequently there is an area of numbness closely related to the area of hyperesthesia.

Increased sweating of the involved hand or foot may be very marked in traumatic or vasospastic disorders. Often a past history of sweating can be obtained.

Vasomotor changes may vary from vasoconstriction to vasodilatation. The involved part may be warm and erythematous initially and may later manifest vasoconstriction, being pale, cool and wet. Patients with arteriosclerosis obliterans commonly show a shiny, scaling, dry foot.

Additional signs may include stiffness of joints, swelling and roentgenologic evidence of spotty osteoporosis.

Diagnosis is based on a history of an overactive sympathetic nervous system, with superficial burning pain exceeding the expected amount, and hyperesthesia localized to a sensory nerve.

Diagnosis may be readily established by injecting Priscoline, 25 mg, or Hydergine, 0.6 mg, intravenously or into the proximal artery. Prior to the injection, the patient is told to classify his pain as 100 per cent, and after several minutes he will be requested to determine what percentage of the original pain remains. The pain is evaluated by stroking the area of complaint before and after the injection. If over 50 per cent relief is obtained for 30 minutes or more, one can conclude that at least part of the pain is related to the sympathetic nervous system. A similar method may be used to monitor the results following oral intake of sympatholytic drugs or a sympathetic block. Any residual pain may or may not be related to the somatic root.

Hyperhidrosis. This is a rare pathological condition of excessive perspiration limited to the palmar surfaces of the hands, the feet and the axilla. Patients are invariably young, nervous individuals with serious psychological and social problems. The sweating may be extremely annoying, embarrassing and even incapacitating in certain occupations. When the patient is under a nervous strain, water may literally drip from his fingers and cause him to avoid handshaking, piano playing, typewriting or touching objects such as delicate materials. When the patient's feet are involved, his socks and shoes are so wet that they become foul-smelling and the skin easily becomes macerated and subject to fungus infections.

Relief seldom is obtained by either medical treatment or psychotherapy; however, when these approaches have failed, surgical removal of the sympathetic nerve pathways is indicated and produces relief. When all four extremities are involved and more than two extremity sympathectomies are being considered, they should be staged at six month intervals to allow readjustment of thigh and arm sudomotor activity. No more than three extremities should be denervated.

Phantom Limb Pain. This pain often is described as causalgic in type. When pain is localized to the distal portion of the phantom limb and is described as burning and superficial in character, the same approach to diagnosis and treatment as described previously for causalgia is taken. Stump pain is not related to the sympathetic nervous system.

Additional Conditions. Additional conditions for which some method of sympathetic denervation may be considered are herpetic neuralgia, postparalytic pain and rheumatoid arthritis.

Treatment

Prompt diagnosis and treatment lessens the likelihood of fixed patterns of pain, which causes dysfunction and atrophy of the part.

The nature of the disease, the physiologic basis for the pain, and the possibility of therapeutic relief are explained to the patient in an attempt to obtain his cooperation. This patient-doctor understanding is best obtained by injecting one of the sympatholytic drugs in the manner previously described. Following a favorable response to an intra-arterial or intravenous sympatholytic drug the physician prescribes an oral sympatholytic drug such as Ilidar, 25 to 150 mg three times a day; Hydergine, 0.5 to 1.5 mg four to six times a day; or Dibenzyline, 10 mg three times a day. Each medication is adjusted to patient response and usually is advised just prior to bedtime when the pain is often most severe.

A paravertebral sympathetic block is indicated when previously described diagnostic methods are short-lived, the pain does not lessen, the medications cause too many side effects or permanent relief from pain does not seem to be forthcoming. The block is routinely checked for adequacy by confirming the absence of sweating by gross evaluation or a skin resistance apparatus.

When pain relief occurs for four or more hours following any of these methods, the treatment is repeated as often as is feasible.

A sympathectomy is indicated when drug therapy or intermittent paravertebral sympathetic blocks fail to elicit progressive improvement in a few weeks, when the pain is so severe that other methods of therapy seem unwarranted, or when additional indications for sympathectomy are present. These include diffuse small vessel involvement, ischemic slow-healing superficial ulcers, the need for development of small collateral channels or vasospasm. Occasionally a sympathectomy may be justified to relieve the pain in a patient with dependent rubor. However, the procedure is contraindicated unless the major portion of intolerable pain is demonstrably sympathetic in origin.

Postsympathectomy Pain Syndromes

Unexpected postoperative pain patterns may develop in patients who have had a sympathectomy. These pain patterns may be separated into five types according to the time of occurrence and site of origin.

Type 1. Type 1 is the recurrence of the preoperative pain approximately six days after an apparently adequate sympathectomy and during the period when the temperature of the foot lessens. It seems to occur only in patients with severe ischemia who have disabling rest pain and dependent rubor. Sympathectomy is ordinarily contraindicated in such patients to improve circulation but may on occasion have been done for pain. Possible explanations for the pain are: hypersensitivity of the vessels to circulatory catecholamines or an unknown hormone, or to an intrinsic change in the smooth muscle. Injection of Priscoline, 25 mg, into the proximal femoral artery is effective treatment for this type of pain.

Type 2. Type 2 is the reappearance of the preoperative pain within three months after supposedly adequate sympathectomy. Possible reasons for the recurrence are: a readjustment of the sympathetic pathways, a less than adequate sympathectomy or similar causes as listed above in Type 1. A more extensive sympathectomy unilaterally or bilaterally is required for relief.

Type 3. Type 3 is the reappearance of the preoperative pain one year or more after an adequate sympathectomy. This type probably is due to "regeneration" or the readjustment of the sympathetic pathways. Treatment is the same as was advised preoperatively for the pain and may require a higher sympathetic block, a contralateral sympathectomy if the block relieved the pain, or a more extensive sympathectomy.

Type 4. Type 4 is the most common syndrome and is identified as postsympathectomy neuralgia. The pain usually occurs about ten days postoperatively, proximal to the preoperative site of pain. It manifests itself as a causalgic type of pain and is localized chiefly to the lateral, anterior or medial areas of the thigh. It often includes the buttocks, with a deep pain in the sacroiliac area of the involved side. It is possibly due to irritation of the preganglionic fibers on the anterior spinal nerve during surgery. The pain is usually limited to a period of three months. Sympatholytic drugs may be used orally, intravenously or intra-arterially on the involved side to relieve the complaints.

Type 5. Type 5 is the appearance of pain in the operative site months following surgery. The pain is localized to a sensory nerve which was traumatized during operation and is termed postsympathectomy causalgia. Relief is obtained by the methods previously described for medical sympathetic denervation.

If the clinician following the patient

postoperatively does not understand these pain patterns, he may unjustly consider the sympathectomy as a failure or the sequelae too severe and frequent to advise sympathectomy for other patients. One very intriguing aspect of these pain syndromes is that their incidence is extremely high in patients undergoing sympathectomy for causalgic type pain.

Chronic Leg Ulcers

Chronic leg ulcers have concerned clinicians since early times because of their common occurrence and the difficulty of their cure. Chronic ulcers of the extremities are almost always a symptom or complication of another illness. Although most leg ulcers are secondary to venous or arterial disease, some result from insufficient innervation of tissues, ulcerating neoplasms, blood disorders, endocrine disturbances or other local and systemic diseases. Careful analysis of these various etiologies may help to establish a rational system of treatment. Sometimes the diagnosis is obvious. More often, the history needs to be more detailed and the examination may necessitate specific laboratory procedures such as biopsy, culture, angiography and other means to uncover a systemic disease. The location of the ulcer, its appearance, the degree of pain and the number of lesions present are important aspects in distinguishing one type of ulcer from another. Some characteristic features of several types of chronic ulcers are listed here to assist the clinician in determining the correct diagnosis and factors which influence healing of the ulcer.

Venous Ulcers

In 1868 John Gay wrote that "ulceration is not a direct consequence of varicosity but of other conditions of the venous system of which varicosity is not infrequently a complication." Over one hundred years later some clinicians continue to believe that postphlebitic leg ulcers require that varices be injected, ligated or excised. However, many individuals with severe varices do not suffer from ulceration, and patients with chronic venous insufficiency and ulceration of the legs often do not have varicose veins. There is no noticeable difference between ulcers with or without varicose veins. There are a few venous leg ulcers which have a "venous lake" beneath the lesion, and a few with an identifiable vein "feeding" the ulcer through a nearby perforator. There are also those which can be termed "varicose vein ulcer" due to trauma, infection or localized minute arteriovenous connections. But attention must be directed to the essential problem of hydraulics, namely the leg muscle pump. This leg pump is an efficient system in normal people but it has such little reserve that standing for long periods in one position will cause edema of the ankles. Venous return may be impaired by arterial insufficiency, arterial venous fistula, defects in the relay pumping mechanism, and venous obstruction due to structural defects, functional changes or both. Chronic venous insufficiency, therefore, may occur from thrombosis in the deep veins with or without recanalization; incompetency of the deep, perforating and superficial vein valves; failure of muscle contraction due to knee or ankle joint changes from arthritis; prolonged dependency and immobility of the lower limb, or a combination of these causes as well as arterial insufficiency affecting the capillary flow.

Rarely does a postphlebitic ulcer appear earlier than two years following deep vein thrombophlebitis. The mean period is usually seven years. The appearance of a venous ulcer is preceded by edema, induration and reddened pigmentation of the skin in the medial malleolar region, accompanied by a sensation of distention and severe itching. This may progress to pain upon walking or bathing. Ultimately a superficial single ulcer develops over a thrombosed vein.

Complications occur when the ulcer is permitted to remain open and develop repeated infections. Further induration and scarring occurs, producing the chronically edematous leg, reducing the possibility of early healing. This chronic tissue inflammation often leads to calcific changes in the surrounding tissues and the foot is drawn into equinus.

Hemorrhage seldom occurs in a large ulcer but is frequent in smaller lesions.

Chronic venous ulcers rarely become malignant unless they have failed to heal in fifteen or more years.

Patients with a history of repeated episodes of thrombophlebitis and patients with recurrent ulcers should be investigated for hypercoagulability.

Treatment of chronic venous ulcers has been discussed previously in this chapter. Two surgical approaches which are increasingly less popular are lumbar sympathectomy and skin grafting of the ulcer. Indications for sympathectomy have previously been discussed. Causalgic type pain not controlled by medical means and the additional presence of small vessel disease are usually the only reasons for performing a sympathectomy. Grafting should not be considered as a means of curing the ulcer, but only as a method of covering an infected and chronically indurated area.

Arteriovenous Fistula Ulcer

Leg ulcers may occur from arteriovenous fistula. This vascular short circuit bypasses the capillary system and delivers a higher pressure to the veins. Venous hypertension causes ulcers as well as skin pigmentation, induration and varicosities.

Diagnosis of traumatic arteriovenous fistula is not usually difficult. It is based on a history of trauma, the presence of a thrill and continuous murmur at the site of the scar, dilatation of the superficial veins, an increased oscillometric index above the fistula and a decreased index beneath it. Treatment is localized to correction of the arteriovenous fistula following arteriographic studies.

Ulcers due to congenital arteriovenous fistula are quite different. The fistulae are multiple and small. The surrounding area may have the appearance of a large singular hemangioma or many small ones.

Diagnosis is suggested by added length of the extremity, presence of angiomas or vascular nevi, varicosities (usually appearing in infancy or adolescence), inability to collapse the varices by elevation, elevated oscillometric index and rarely, a thrill or continuous murmur. Arteriograms will determine the site and extent of the lesion.

Treatment ideally is directed toward excision of the arteriovenous fistula. However, unless the fistula is well localized and is not diffuse in character, patients seldom benefit from surgery. Supportive treatment is the best approach for the majority of patients.

Dependency and Immobility Ulcers

Ulcers of dependency and immobility occur in the aged arthritic, in persons with chronic congestive heart failure and in patients with any other condition which results in limited ambulation.

Immobility and dependency of the limbs in patients with severe arthritis may cause edema complicated by ulcers, which are usually located in the lower third of the legs, often in the region of the malleoli.

Patients with chronic heart failure and respiratory difficulties may be obliged to remain seated both day and night with their legs dependent. This dependency and immobility results in venous hypertension of the limbs which causes ulcers of the legs, when combined with excessive leg edema, hypoproteinemia, distention and skin fissures. These ulcers tend to weep copiously and become infected.

Therapy includes elevation of the leg to lessen edema, cardiac medication, diuretics and application of Unna boots even after the ulcers have healed.

Traumatic Ulcers

Traumatic ulcers of the legs are common and may be factitious or neurotropic in origin.

Pain may be of diagnostic importance in an ulcer related to trauma. Ischemic ulcers are the most painful, especially hypertensive ischemic ulcers. Dependency decreases the pain of an ischemic ulcer. Venous ulcers and most of the other ulcers mentioned here are usually only mildly painful. Neurotropic ulcers are easily identifiable by their lack of pain. Wound care includes débridement, moist soaks and antibiotics. Unna paste boots which are changed periodically may be of therapeutic value.

Arteriosclerotic Ulcers

Arteriosclerosis obliterans of the lower extremities may produce a spontaneous, isolated ischemic ulcer. However, the ulcer is usually initiated by trauma. The ulcers are localized most frequently in the digits, occasionally in the foot, and more rarely in the leg. They are almost always unilateral on the extremity, which is pulseless and cool. There is usually a prior history of intermittent claudication. Pain is often lessened by dependency and the ulcer has a pale gray base.

So-called "senile ulcers" are ischemic lesions due to arteriosclerosis of the small vessels in the skin. There is neither obliteration of the pedal pulses nor a history of intermittent claudication. The most important factor in their appearance is some insignificant trauma. They occur most often in people in the eighth or ninth decade of life.

Treatment is the same as that described in the section on arterial diseases. A senile ulcer may not heal until a lumbar sympathectomy is performed. Unna paste boots are also recommended for senile ulcers.

Hypertensive Ulcers

Hypertensive ischemic ulcers occur as the result of obliterative lesions of the small arterioles. They begin with the appearance of a pigmented or purpuric spot of variable extent or a reddened spot which becomes cyanotic in a few days. An ischemic superficial necrosis then occurs from which an ulcer with a grayish base is formed. Frequently the ulcer is bilateral and symmetrical and located on the anterior lateral or posterolateral aspect of the leg near the junction of the middle and lower thirds. The ulcer may be very painful and resistant to treatment. No visible circulatory changes are present and there is seldom any edema. Lumbar sympathectomy relieves the pain and promotes healing. Treatment of the hypertension is indicated.

Diabetic Ulcers

In diabetic individuals arteriosclerotic ulcers are not uncommon and ulcerated plaques *(necrobiosis lipoidica)* may occasionally be seen. Small vessel disease is often present in diabetics. These patients may develop one or more isolated areas of ischemia on the leg, presenting a chronic black eschar with little or no inflammation. Pedal pulses are usually present and there is no history of intermittent claudication.

The recommended treatment is a lumbar sympathectomy. Attempts to excise and graft the ischemic lesion invariably fail unless a healthy bed for grafting can be identified during surgery.

Corticosteroid Ulcers

Patients may present with necrotic, punched-out ulcerations on an extremity after receiving corticosteroids for arthritis for fifteen or more years. These lesions are seldom painful except in the base of the ulcer. Treatment requires débridement, application of wound-stimulating ointments, and heparin injected twice daily into the subcutaneous tissue of the abdominal wall. Most of these ulcers ultimately heal with this regimen. The lesion is caused by an obliterative arteritis.

Neurotropic Ulcers

These ulcers develop from repeated trauma to the extremities of patients with myelopathies and neuropathies such as syringomyelia, transverse myelitis, tumors or injuries of the spinal cord. Ulcers also occur from peripheral nerve disturbances such as neuritis, leprosy, injuries or tumors of nerves. The ulcers develop as plantar lesions on the toes, or over bony prominences on the leg, ankle or foot. They are usually single, indolent, deep and infected.

Routine wound care and antibiotics are advised.

Vasculitis Ulcers

There are a number of systemic diseases which are characterized by generalized vasculitis. Among these conditions are lupus erythematosus, necrotizing angiitis, periarteritis nodosa, rheumatoid arthritis, and allergic vasculitis. Proliferative and degenerative inflammation of the capillaries and arterioles occasionally develops in one or more areas of the leg, resulting in necrosis and ulceration. Scleroderma ulcers are found on the toes, feet and bony prominences. Leg ulcers from vasculitis are frequently localized in the lower third of the leg but occasionally may present at a higher level. They may be single but are usually multiple; they are small in size with bluish-purple, indurated edges and are mildly painful. Treatment is directed toward the specific disease and usually requires corticosteroids. Subcutaneous heparin, administered in the abdominal wall, is prescribed for healing the ulcers.

Hematologic Ulcers

The most common hematologic ulcers derive from sickle cell disease. They may occur on the foot, ankle or leg, and are caused by ischemia secondary to thrombosis of small arterioles. Treatment is difficult and may require skin grafting.

Other hematologic conditions which may cause leg ulcers are spherocytic anemia, thalassemia, polycythemia vera, leukemia and dysproteinemias such as macroglobulinemia and cryoglobulinemia.

Treatment is directed toward the underlying disease and the ulcer is handled in a manner similar to that described for a postphlebitic ulcer. Antibiotics are usually indicated.

Frostbite Ulcers

Ulceration from frostbite occurs on the digits and feet. However, leg ulcers (chilblains) may occasionally develop, most frequently in young female children or adolescents. They are usually localized to the posterior anterior aspect of the lower third of the leg. Chilblains are more prevalent in humid climates with low but not necessarily freezing temperatures. Patients often are sensitive to cold and the lesions which develop on the legs during cold weather improve spontaneously in the summer. Pain can be severe during the period preceding the ulceration. Treatment has been discussed in the frostbite section earlier in this chapter.

Miscellaneous Ulcers

A number of systemic or nonvascular diseases may cause leg ulcerations. Among these are reactions to drugs such as bromides, ergot and methotrexate; infections, including fungus, syphilis, tuberculosis and other bacterial organisms; metabolic conditions such as pyoderma gangrenosa (associated with chronic ulcerative colitis), Gaucher's disease, gout and porphyria cutanea tarda; tumors such as basal cell epithelioma, Kaposi's hemorrhagic sarcoma, lymphoma, hemangio-lymphangioma and malignant melanoma; and many other isolated conditions.

General Measures of Treatment

Excluding the treatment required for the underlying disease most leg ulcers require a variety of approaches, each related to specific findings noted on examination of the lesion and the limb. The number of dyes, antiseptics, ointments and other materials used for local treatment is endless. Generally the simplest and least expensive form of therapy is the most successful. Antibiotics are seldom used in leg ulcers unless cellulitis, diabetes, ischemia or a blood dyscrasia is present. Antifungal drugs are frequently used, since most leg ulcers contain fungi which are synergistic with the bacterial organisms inhabiting the ulcer.

All predisposing factors must be investigated and eliminated when possible. Diabetes must be controlled, arterial circulation reestablished when considered to have a reasonable chance of being successful, anemia corrected, hypercoagulability averted, and so on.

The application of heat from any source to an ulcerated extremity is absolutely contraindicated. Moist soaks which utilize body heat are less hazardous and more logical.

Chronic or indolent ulcers should be cleansed frequently with saline soaks and exposed for a couple of hours daily to prevent maceration. When circulation is adequate and edema is present, the affected extremity should be elevated above body level until the edema subsides. If enzymatic ointments are used for chemical débridement, mechanical débridement must not be abandoned. Ointments which stimulate the growth of healthy granulations are advised for nonischemic limb ulcers. However, the ointment should produce no harm to surrounding tissues, or "daughter" ulcers may appear. A fungicide soak such as potassium permanganate (1:10,000) applied for thirty minutes three times a day for three days should routinely be used prior to the application of an Unna paste boot.

Ischemic ulcers should be kept dry to discourage bacterial growth. Aqueous solutions of mercurochrome or tannic acid are good drying agents. A logical policy is to keep moist ulcers moist and dry ulcers dry when gross infection is not evident and there is some doubt regarding the cause of the ulcer.

When the patient is ambulatory and there is adequate arterial circulation to the limb, elastic support stockings represent a practical approach. This treatment should be accompanied by leg elevation for short periods prior to the development of swelling. Unna paste boots may be substituted for elastic stockings. Diuretics may help the patient to keep the limb free of swelling. Subcutaneous heparin is frequently prescribed for patients who have vascular ulcers which are refractory to other forms of palliative treatment. Anti-inflammatory agents or sympatholytic drugs are prescribed for pain. See the section on sympathetic nervous system disorders.

Surgical procedures are usually discouraged. However, skin grafts may be applied to large chronic venous ulcers, and lumbar sympathectomy may be utilized for small vessel disease and causalgic type pain. Arterial revascularization is utilized for proximal occlusions of large arteries, and Achilles tendon lengthening is recommended for equinus deformity which limits the use of the leg pump. Palliative measures should be utilized on an outpatient basis before surgery is considered.

The time required to heal chronic leg ulcers varies according to the size of the ulcer, the local condition of the tissues, the nature of the underlying disease, and the general physical condition of the patient. Few ulcers are totally refractory to treatment.

Lymphedema

Lymphedema refers to the collection of lymph in the skin and subcutaneous tissues due to an abnormality of the lymphatic system. It may be classified into primary and secondary types, both of which include several clinical symptoms. Primary lymphedema is thought to be caused by an inherent lymphatic disorder while secondary lymphedema has an obstructive or akinetic cause. Early changes in the patient with classical lymphedema consist of dilatations of the lymphatics and widening of the tissue spaces owing to edema. Later the connective tissue proliferates and may show stages of inflammatory cell infiltration, pigmentation and scarring of the enlarged lymphatics.

The skin in lymphedema is normal or has a pale appearance. Edema does not occur in the skeletal muscle; it occurs only in the fascial planes and in the skin and subcutaneous tissue.

Normal lymphatics have the capacity to drain away free interstitial fluid. When protein-bound dye is injected into the subcutaneous tissue of an edematous leg, it passes very rapidly via the lymphatic channels toward the groin. Therefore, although fluid is rapidly entering the subcutaneous tissues, the lymphatics normally limit the amount of edema by returning the transudate to the circulation. The protein concentration of this normal edema fluid is low. The main characteristic of lymphedema fluid, however, is its very high protein content. This high protein content is responsible for the organization and fibrosis in the cutaneous and subcutaneous tissues, usually not seen in other cases of edema.

Etiology and Classification

In primary lymphedema lymphangiography demonstrates a developmental anatomical variation of the lymphatics. The lymphatic vessels are narrowed and few in number. Hyperplasia with dilated and tortuous lymphatic vessels is observed less frequently. Complete agenesis of the lymphatics and lymph glands is very rare. Females are more frequently affected than men (three to one) and no race is immune.

The predominant feature of secondary lymphedema is obstruction of the normal lymphatic flow, most commonly resulting from inflammation due to infection, but often due to neoplastic disease and other causes.

Classification of Lymphedema

a. Primary
  1. Congenital—at birth
  2. Lymphedema praecox—onset prior to 35 years
  3. Lymphedema tarda—after 35 years
b. Secondary
  1. Obstructive
    (a) Lymphatic
      (1) Chronic infections—bacterial, parasitic, fungal
      (2) Malignant disease
      (3) Surgical resection of lymph glands
      (4) Injury
      (5) Irradiation—x-ray, radium
    (b) Venous
      (1) Normal or enlarged lymphatics
      (2) Hypoplastic or obstructed lymphatics
  2. Akinetic insufficiency
    (a) Causalgia
    (b) Paralysis

Primary Lymphedema

Congenital Lymphedema. Congenital lymphedema may be divided into two types: simple and hereditary. Simple lymphedema occurs at birth or shortly thereafter and involves only one member of a family. The hereditary type affects several members of a family and has become known as Milroy's disease, although both the simple and the hereditary type are often identified with this term.

The condition is mildly progressive until puberty when it frequently becomes worse and may affect part or all of the upper or lower extremities, or both. Ulceration of the skin does not occur. There is an absence of pain, and recurrent attacks of infection seldom occur. Because the skin remains in good condition, the problem is cosmetic rather than functional. Kinmonth's lymphography studies demonstrated hypoplasia of lymph channels in all three types of primary lymphedema, but complete aplasia and severe lymphangiectasia was much more frequent in the congenital group than in the other two types.

Patients with hypoplasia of the lymphatic channels show no other congenital changes in the lymphatic system. Congenital nonhereditary lymphedema is often combined with ovarian dysgenesis in which it is often bilateral and, unlike other forms of lymphedema, prone to regress spontaneously. The finding of other congenital anomalies is not unusual in patients with congenital lymphedema.

Lymphedema Praecox. The most common type of lymphedema, it characteristically occurs at puberty and has no familial history. It predominately affects females and is usually limited to the left lower extremity. The swelling begins spontaneously, usually with swelling of the foot or ankle, and spreads upward; increasing during prolonged standing, just prior to menstruation and during warm weather. It is frequently temporary at first. Elevation of the extremity produces temporary decrease of the edema but not disappearance. The amount and extent of the edema are determined by the degree of inherent lymphatic dysfunction present. In time the soft pitting edema progresses to pitting edema with fibrosis; ultimately the extremity becomes unsightly and uncomfortable. Pain and ulceration do not occur and infection is infrequent.

Varicose veins rarely are noted in patients with lymphedema praecox.

Although the pathological basis of the disease is unknown, it is considered to be an inborn error, not only in the development of the lymphatics but in other organs of the body as well.

Lymphedema Tarda. Lymphedema tarda is the occurrence of primary lymphedema in patients over 35 years of age. This is probably no more than a delayed appearance of lymphedema praecox in patients who have a defective lymphatic system but are more resistant to precipitating factors such as venous entrapment by the common iliac artery. The influence of this factor in lymphedema tarda as well as in the other two types of primary lymphedema needs investigation to determine its incidence,

relationship to clinical findings, and whether or not this group of patients needs to be reclassified as the secondary type.

Edema in lymphedema tarda is usually less extensive and occasionally may be limited to the genitalia and thighs.

Differential Diagnosis. Edema due to renal or cardiac conditions or to hypoproteinemia must be excluded before primary lymphedema can be considered. However, any of these conditions may be a precipitating factor when abnormal lymphatics are present.

Premenstrual edema, pregnancy and prolonged standing, especially in women, causes fluid to accumulate in the lower limbs. This type of edema disappears rapidly with elevation as well as diuretics, and fibrosis does not occur. Malignant tumors of the abdomen, genitalia and kidney should be suspected in middle aged or older patients who have lymphedema.

Postphlebitic syndrome edema is differentiated by a history of deep vein thrombosis and pain, skin discoloration and ulceration.

Lipedema, when it occurs, is always present in women; it is bilateral and painful and the feet are not involved. Abnormal deposits of fat are present in the lower part of the body and in the lower limbs. Pitting is not present, the skin is soft and pliable, and edema disappears at rest.

Other conditions include pretibial edema from myxedema, arteriovenous fistula, Klippel-Trenaunay's syndrome in which there is elongation of bones, hemangiomas of the skin and swelling of the leg, and edema due to certain drugs such as corticosteroids and progestin which subsides when the drugs are discontinued.

Diagnostic Studies. Lymphangiography, the intradermal injection of a blue dye or radiopaque contrast media into a lymph tract, demonstrates the lymphatic pathways. In primary lymphedema there may be hypoplasia, hyperplasia or agenesis. Secondary lymphedema is identified by the presence of multiple collateral channels, dermal backflow and changes in the regional lymph glands. When tumor involves lymph glands, it may completely replace the lymph node(s).

Phlebography of the lower extremities establishes the presence of a venous etiology for edema but is useless for patients who are thought to have primary lymphedema. On occasion the determination of the protein concentration of the edema fluid may help to establish a diagnosis. Controversy prevails as to the benefits of radioactive protein studies.

Complications. The chief complication of lymphedema is erysipelas. The slightest abrasion or laceration may introduce bacteria. Recurrent infections destroy additional lymphatics and the lymphedema progresses. Antibiotics should be prescribed and foot hygiene stressed.

Occasionally a lymph fistula may develop from a skin vesicle and drain for weeks, making ligation of the proximal lymph channels necessary.

Secondary Lymphedema

Secondary lymphedema is caused by obstruction of the lymphatic or venous systems or from an akinetic insufficiency of the extremity.

Lymphedema resulting from neoplastic invasion of lymph pathways is found in patients with malignant disease of the breast, uterine cervix, uterus, vulva, bladder, prostate gland, skin or bones. The clinical signs and symptoms of the primary malignant lesion may not precede the appearance of lymphedema. Therefore, a neoplasm must be ruled out if unexpected swelling of an extremity occurs, especially when the lymphedema develops after forty years of age. Other malignant conditions which may cause secondary lymphedema are Hodgkin's disease, lymphosarcoma and Kaposi's sarcoma. Many of these lesions may be complicated by simultaneous venous occlusion of the femoral or iliac veins.

Surgical removal of lymph nodes and lymph vessels for malignant disease of an extremity or following a radical mastectomy with a block dissection of the axillary lymph nodes may predispose to secondary lymphedema. Occasionally the upper extremity becomes edematous immediately after the operation and gradually progresses into a severely edematous limb termed *elephantiasis chirurgica*. However, in other patients there may be a delay of months or years before the extremity becomes edematous. Several explanations can be given for the discrepancy in the time before lymphedema occurs. Lymphedema which occurs immediately after surgery is probably caused by a complete excision of the lymphatic pathways. An axillary venous thrombosis can be a major contributory factor to the swelling. The later occurrence of swelling may be caused by lymphangitis and secondary obstruction of the remaining lymphatic channels due to a minor accident. A thoracic outlet syndrome prior to, shortly after or some time after surgery may be a contributory factor. The author has noted the presence of this entity in a mild to moderate degree in several patients with postmastectomy lymphedema. Shoulder exercises and avoidance of prolonged periods of abduction help to lessen or eliminate edema from the extremity. Recurrence of tumor at a higher level or lymphangiosarcoma should be considered as additional causes of late edema.

Radium and roentgen rays are often mentioned in the literature as provoking a fibrous reaction in the tissues within the area of treatment and producing further obliteration of lymphatic channels, thus aggravating or causing edema. As mentioned previously we have not been able to prove conclusively that irradiation has been a primary contributor to edema. If it does participate significantly in the process all other possibilities should be excluded before this mode of therapy is blamed.

Venous entrapment of the left common iliac vein by the right common iliac artery has been discussed. It probably should be listed under secondary lymphedema even though it could be a contributory factor to lymphedema praecox or lymphedema tarda.

Obstructive lymphedema, which is more common than primary lymphedema, is caused by inflammation from infection more often than by malignant tumors or iatrogenic causes. Chronic or recurrent inflammation leads to occlusion of lymph channels by thrombosis, which in turn causes lymph stasis and results in fibrosis. With each successive infection the edema increases. The common offending organism is the streptococcus. However, fungus infection of the feet may contribute to recurrent attacks of infection, although edema from this cause is usually limited to the foot and ankle.

Parasitic invasion of lymphatic tracts is frequently seen in the Middle or Far East. The most common organism is filaria; the eggs and larvae provoke an inflammation in the lymph glands and vessels with ensuing fibrosis and obstruction of the normal flow of lymph. This type of lymphedema, referred to as elephantiasis, often involves the external genitalia and lower extremities with the development of a markedly deformed limb. In patients with *elephantiasis,* multiple projections identified as *lymphostatic verrucosis* may occur on the toes.

Patients with intolerable pain in an extremity, such as causalgia, or individuals with motor paralysis of a limb may develop secondary lymphedema because of immobility. These conditions cause an akinetic insufficiency within the lymph pathways owing to the accumulation of tissue fluid within the extremity. Without active movement of the limb, the lymph vessels have to transport a volume of fluid much higher than they are capable of handling. The lymph channels enlarge in a manner similar to that seen in lymphedema when the lymphatic pathways are obstructed. Consequently, the valves fail to close and valvular insufficiency of lymph circulation develops. In patients with prolonged lymphatic obstruction the vessels may disappear, either by lymphatic thrombosis or by perilymphatic fibrosis and contracture. The most serious complication of lymphedema is lymphangiosarcoma, which may develop in these obstructed lymphatics.

Any kind of burden on the lymphatics may upset the delicate balance between lymph formation and transport, whether it is due to venous stenosis from scars or arterial entrapment, thrombophlebitis causing a rise in capillary blood pressure, increased capillary permeability due to bacterial invasion, burns, or other injuries, occlusion of lymph channels by malignancies, block excision of lymph glands, or lymphangitis.

Differential diagnosis of secondary lymphedema is made by lumphangiography, pelvic phlebography and determination of the protein concentration of the edema fluid after a detailed history and an evaluation of the clinical state of the patient is obtained. The possibility that the lymphedema is due to a malignant lesion must always be considered.

Treatment for Primary and Secondary Lymphedema

Lymphedema can usually be controlled medically by a combination of simple measures. Most patients do not have a major functional deformity and therefore surgery is usually unjustified. The cause of the lymphedema must first be established by the history, clinical assessment and specific examinations such as lymphograms, pelvic phlebograms and biopsy of the edematous tissue before therapy can begin.

Medical treatment must be instituted before fibrosis develops. Control of the edema is begun by using high daily doses of oral diuretics such as chlorothiazide and B-complex vitamins for a few days or a week or on a daily basis.

The lymphedematous extremity should be elevated whenever possible. The patient should use a portable pneumatic compression device for at least an hour each day until optimum results have been obtained. The edema can usually be reduced significantly; however, tissue hypertrophy will not be affected. Tailored elastic stockings or leotards should be ordered when edema has been reduced to its least amount. A pure rubber bandage may be used over a cotton stocking until the elastic stocking is available. The same bandage may also be applied over the elastic stocking for those patients whose edema is more difficult to control.

Patients with postmastectomy lymphedema should support the limb in a sling during the day and exercise it as well as elevate it on pillows during the night. Bandages and a gauntlet elastic support should be applied during the day. The intermittent pneumatic compression machine should be used energetically each day. Diuretics may be prescribed with the usual precautions taken to avoid hypokalemia and electrolyte disturbance. However, the use of diuretics has been somewhat disappointing.

Regular swimming exercises may be of benefit. The patient should avoid standing or sitting for long periods since limb movements propel the lymph. Encouragement of short intervals of elevation should be emphasized repeatedly.

Patients should be evaluated as to treatment response. Occasionally patients who have been under treatment for some time should stop using diuretics or elastic supports to determine if withdrawal of therapy is possible. For patients with advanced lymphedema in which fibrosis is present, treatment usually must be continued indefinitely.

Patients with an advanced type of lymphedema or an identifying cause such as venous entrapment should be considered for surgical therapy.

Traditional operations, such as the excision of all peripheral lymph-bearing subcutaneous tissue, have not met with prolonged success. These procedures are based on the theory that the lymph vessels below the muscle fascia are patent and subcutaneous fluid may be drained by these channels. These procedures are done in stages, one half of the leg at a time. Following surgery, the reduction of edema should be maintained by the same procedures mentioned in the nonsurgical management. More often than not the limb returns to its former size in a few years. Modifications of traditional surgical procedures have been performed, such as excising the skin with the subcutaneous tissue and muscle fascia and covering the defect with split thickness skin grafts.

Other operations include the implanting of nylon or silk threads in the subcutaneous tissue to provide new extralymphatic drainage channels, burying a shaved skin pedicle flap to enhance lymph drainage by transferring subcutaneous lymphatics into the deep compartment of the limb, implanting lymph vessels into lymph nodes by microsurgical technique, creating lymphaticovenous anastomosis and transposing omental tissue into the subcutaneous tissue. None of these procedures have been widely accepted.

When the common iliac vein is entrapped by the right common iliac artery and there is elevation of the venous pressure inferior to the occlusion, a silastic bridge is placed beneath the artery, after intimal adhesions within the vein lumen are excised. Trimble et al. have attained successful results in the majority of patients operated upon.

Indications for surgery in primary and secondary lymphedema are: (1) failure to reduce the limb size in spite of adequate medical management; (2) functional impairment; (3) significant skin changes; (4) recurrent infections; (5) presence of a malignant lesion obstructing the lymphatics; (6) evidence of venous entrapment of the common iliac vein(s) and resulting elevated venous pressure; (7) unsightly appearance; and (8) emotional problems related to the deformed limb.

Following excisional surgery, the limb must receive elastic support and supplementary diuretics. If an aggressive postoperative program is not contemplated this type of surgery is ill-advised, for even with such a plan, excisional operation for lymphedema leaves much to be desired. However, patients who undergo the procedure have fewer incidences of infection than untreated patients.

Patients who have recurrent lymphangiitis, cellulitis or a minor open wound should receive vigorous antibiotic therapy routinely.

Lymph Collections in Wounds

Lymph collections in wounds, often identified as a seroma, serum collection, or lymphocele when chronic in nature, is a surgical complication which is of concern, especially if it occurs in the areas of the axilla, groin or adductor canal. The incidence is higher when transverse incisions have been performed or local venous occlusion is present. Repeated aspiration of the loculated amber-colored lymph fluid accompanied by a pressure dressing occasionally fails to eliminate the problem. In these patients the lymphocele requires excision and transfixion suture of the patent lymphatic vessel(s). The same may be necessary when a persistent lymph fistula is present; however, a pressure dressing often causes the lymphatic duct to clot and lymph drainage ceases. Invariably lymphedema is present in these patients postoperatively and usually requires additional therapy.

References

1. Baker, A. G., Jr. and Roberts, B.: Long-term survival following abdominal aortic aneurysmectomy. J.A.M.A., *212*:445–450, 1970.
2. Barker, W. G.: Surgical Treatment of Peripheral Vascular Disease. New York, Blakiston Division McGraw-Hill Book Co., 1962.
3. Fairbairn, J. F., II, Juergens, J. L., and Spittell, J. A., Jr. (eds.): *Allen-Barker-Hines* Peripheral Vascular Diseases. Fourth edition. Philadelphia, W. B. Saunders Co., 1972.
4. Haimovici, H.: Thromboangitis obliterans: a nosologic reappraisal. J. Cardiovas. Surg., *4*:83–86, 1963.
5. Hedblom, E. E.: Disturbances due to cold. *In* Conn, H. F. (ed.): Current Therapy. Philadelphia, W. B. Saunders Co., 1971.
6. Hermann, G., Schechter, D. C., Owens, J. C., Starzl, T. E.: The problem of frostbite in civilian medical practice. Surg. Clin. N. Amer., *43*:519–536, 1963.
7. Holman, E.: Abnormal Arteriovenous Communications: Peripheral and Intracardiac; Acquired and Congenital. Second edition. Springfield, Ill., Charles C Thomas, 1968.
8. Homans, J.: Exploration and division of the femoral and iliac veins in the treatment of thrombophlebitis of the leg. New Eng. J. Med., *224*:179–186, 1941.
9. Kinmonth, J. B., Taylor, G. W., Tracy, G. D., and Marsh, J. D.: Primary lymphoedema: clinical and lymphangiographic studies of a series of 107 patients in which the lower limbs were affected. Brit. J. Surg., *45*:1–10, 1957.
10. Knize, D. M., Weatherley-White, R. C. A., Paton, B. C., and Owens, J. C.: Prognostic factors in the management of frostbite. J. Trauma, *9*:749–759, 1969.
11. Markowitz, A. M., and Norman, J. C.: Aneurysms of the iliac artery. Ann. Surg., *154*:777–787, 1961.
12. Milroy, W. F.: Chronic hereditary edema: Milroy's disease. J.A.M.A., *91*:1172–1175, 1928.
13. Owens, J. C., and Coffey, R. J.: Collective review: aneurysm of splenic artery, including a report of six additional cases. Int. Abst. Surg., *97*:313–335, 1953.
14. Owens, J. C.: Indications for lumbar sympathectomy, *In* Dale, W. A. (ed.): Management of Arterial Occlusive Disease. Chicago, Year Book Medical Publishers, 1971.
15. Roos, D. B.: Transaxillary approach for first rib resection to relieve thoracic outlet syndrome. Ann. Surg., *163*:354–358, 1966.
16. Rutherford, R. B., Reddy, C. M. K., Walker, A. G., and Wagner, H. N.: A new quantitative method of assessing the functional status of the leg veins. Amer. J. Surg., *122*:594–602, 1971.
17. Trimble, C., Bernstein, E. F., Pomerantz, M., and Eiseman, B.: A prosthetic bridging device to relieve iliac venous compression. Surg. Forum, *23*:249–251, 1972.

18

The Abdomen—
Gastrointestinal Tract

By GEORGE J. HILL, II, M.D.

INTRODUCTION

The abdomen is a demanding, hidden region containing a multitude of organs which are highly active in the physiology and metabolism of the body. The general surgeon is charged with responsibility for surgical diseases of abdominal viscera, including the gastrointestinal tract, mesentery and peritoneum. In addition, many of the retroperitoneal organs and systems challenge the surgeon's diagnostic judgment and therapeutic skill. Symptoms and signs mimicking gastrointestinal disease arise in major vascular structures, urogenital organs, the spine, musculature, spinal cord and peripheral nerves, and the lymphoreticular system. An appropriately wide differential diagnosis must be kept in mind when dealing with an abdominal complaint. The wise surgeon should request consultation when he suspects that disease has entered viscera which are outside his field of expertise.

The outpatient who presents an abdominal problem must be viewed in the spectrum of priorities ranging from those who will require immediate surgery to those for whom surgery may not be necessary at all.[5] Immediate operation is obviously indicated for the patient with an aortic aneurysm who comes to the door in shock with a brief history of severe pain in the back and abdomen.

Yet severe back pain may also be a complaint of the malingerer. So the surgeon must have the courage and skill to decide correctly on either immediate action, or firm reassurance for nonoperative management.

A careful history should be taken and thorough physical examination completed before elective surgery is performed. However, an urgent need for surgery or the presence of several simultaneous emergencies may restrict the surgeon in his goal of completeness. No matter how busy he is, however, he should always review the pertinent details of the history and he should *personally* confirm the important aspects of the physical examination. There is little justification for planning to spend several hours in the operating room without first performing a careful review of the case prior to surgery. If the surgeon is unwary, he will be unprepared when he encounters an unexpected carcinoma, a fallopian tube abscess or a ureteral calculus. A subsequent review of the history will often reveal the details which were overlooked when the patient was hustled off to surgery. Appropriate laboratory tests must also be considered and used as guides in determining the diagnosis and the necessity for surgery.

Surgery is frequently the most appropriate and least complicated diagnostic test for the study of puzzling abdominal complaints. In patients who present a relatively good risk for surgery, laparotomy should not be the last test considered to solve a diagnostic dilemma. It is unwise to allow a patient to wait for weeks while a long series of x-rays, laboratory tests and consultations are performed and then finally, grudgingly, consider exploratory laparotomy. Laparotomy is also indicated as a "staging" procedure in patients who are being considered for resection of carcinoma of the lung,[2] and in current experimental studies of the staging for chemotherapy and radiation therapy of Hodgkins' disease[51] (Prosnitz, 1972) and non-Hodgkins' lymphomas.[27]

Intra-abdominal pathology can usually be found in patients with severe chronic illness of undetermined origin, who have definite findings referable to the abdomen. Operation may be of benefit by correction of the lesion, or it may be the only means by which medical therapy can be initiated on a scientific basis.

A sick patient with abdominal complaints should be carefully supervised during his initial period in the hospital. Regardless of the duration of his illness, close professional observation is indicated until definitive treatment is instituted and he has shown definite improvement.

Patients are often separated from their relatives or friends for several hours as they are pushed to unfamiliar rooms or corridors, waiting for the next step in their "work-up." The elderly patient with chronic small bowel obstruction due to carcinoma of the cecum may vomit and aspirate while undergoing a simple x-ray of the abdomen in the Outpatient Department. The patient with toxic megacolon may go into shock while waiting in line at the outpatient laboratory to have a venipuncture. The surgeon in the Outpatient Department must be aware of these possibilities. A nasogastric tube may be unpleasant for a sick, distended patient to swallow. But if the surgeon inserts the tube before his patient leaves for the x-ray department, he may be rewarded by having the gastrointestinal contents drained into a basin instead of into the patient's bronchial tree.

SYMPTOMS AND SIGNS

Symptoms of illness may be observations which are narrated in the history or extracted by questioning the patient. Although some symptoms are so specific that the diagnosis is clear or the necessity for surgery is obvious, most are relatively nonspecific. Symptoms must therefore be judged in the context of the entire history and physical examination in order to arrive at an appropriate decision.[12]

A careful record should be made of *pain*. Inquiry should be made into the acute, chronic or relapsing nature of pain, and the duration of episodes if recurrent. Acute pain is perhaps more likely to be an urgent surgical problem than chronic pain, but a patient with a myocardial infarction should not be operated upon with the mistaken opinion that he has acute cholecystitis. "Mild" pain must be viewed in the light of the individual who describes it; if he is concerned about cancer he may minimize the symptoms; if he is obese he may have a localized infection well protected by fat; and if he is stoic he may inadvertently mask the seriousness of his pathology. Radiation of pain is frequently a helpful sign,[37] since subdiaphragmatic pathology radiates to the shoulder, pancreatic lesions radiate to the back, and ureteral colic may radiate to the testicle. A past history of related abdominal pain may be important, even though the patient is unaware of its significance. The patient with gallstone ileus may have suffered from indigestion and biliary colic for years, but may not reveal it except on direct questioning.

The patient may be aware of a *mass*, and if so the physician can usually confirm this on examination. However, even in the absence of a palpable mass, this history may provide an important clue. The mass is usually frustratingly evanescent in patients with intermittent intussusception due to cecal tumors, and patients with hernias also may give a history of an intermittent mass which appears only after vigorous exercise or a long period of time spent in the erect position. In some cases, the patient is better able to define the mass than the physician because of tenderness at its edges; this is an especially common finding in large tumors. A mass in the mesentery, greater omentum or of the intestines may be apparent to the patient but not palpable when he later visits the physician, the mass having shifted on its mobile mesentery. The history of a definite intra-abdominal mass should be taken seriously when narrated by a stable, intelligent patient or parent of a child. A series of visits should be arranged for sequential examinations, until it is clear that the mass did not reappear or a diagnosis has finally been made.

Weight loss is not, by itself, a condition which warrants surgery, but it may be an ominous indication of serious illness. Cancer is perhaps the most common serious illness associated with weight loss, but the surgeon and patient may be gratified to discover that chronic peptic ulcer, chronic appendiceal abscess, or some such benign disease is the cause of loss of appetite and weight. The loss in weight may be more apparent to the patient than to the doctor, as when a heavy patient begins to find it easy to maintain an "ideal" weight, without calorie-counting. Yet any history of loss in weight should be taken seriously, especially when associated with specific abdominal symptoms and signs.

Diarrhea and *constipation* are rarely obvious indications of surgical disease, although a change in bowel habits often seems clear in retrospect when a diagnosis of cancer of the colon has been made. In practice, constipation and diarrhea are usually problems for the internist or the pediatrician, and the surgeon is not consulted until surgical disease is finally apparent or suspected. Diarrhea with surgical implications may be the florid bloody mucus of pregangrenous ulcerative colitis or explosive hyperperistalsis due to chronic incomplete ileal obstruction. It may be seen in gastrojejunal-colic fistula and in hypersecretion produced by stimulation from the islet cell tumors of the pancreas described by Zollinger and Ellison (1955).[72] It may be the result of protein, water, electrolyte or mucus loss from Menetrier's disease of the stomach or villous adenoma of the rectum. It may be due to massive gastrointestinal bleeding—"diarrhea" being the complaint of the patient just prior to fainting from blood loss. Constipation may be so subtle that only the patient is aware of a change—having a stool every two days is abnormal, if he formerly had two bowel movements per day. It may be complete—obstipation—but of such recent onset that the physician is lulled into complacency until the cecum explodes. Cecal distention is a dangerous complication of colonic obstruction, which occurs in patients with *competent* ileocecal valves. Constipation is a common complaint of aging patients, related to decreased roughage in the diet, decreased exercise, and more subtle histopathological aspects of aging. The problem may be compounded by diverticulosis, which in itself is a disease of aging, and which (to prevent diverticulitis) is frequently treated with stool softeners and elimination of dietary roughage. The most common surgical diseases causing constipation are diverticulitis and carcinoma of the rectosigmoid. Other diseases which are commonly associated with constipation are gastric ulcer, painful hemorrhoids and intermittent volvulus of the sigmoid colon.

Complaints of intestinal *"gas"* are nonspecific, but may be troublesome enough to warrant gastrointestinal x-rays, especially if persistent or associated with other symptoms. The patient may describe belching, flatulence, borborygmi, cramps or "indigestion." In the majority of these patients the symptoms are due to relatively benign pathologic conditions, or to anxiety and aerophagia. However, carcinoma of the gastrointestinal tract may also cause chronic distention and hyperperistalsis. Pancreatic enzyme secretion may be blocked by obstruction from carcinoma of the pancreas, thus interfering with digestion in the small bowel. The consequences include steatorrhea, diarrhea, excessive intestinal gas and alterations in bacterial flora of the gut. "Indigestion" or "heartburn" is thoroughly nonspecific but is often the presenting symptom in surgical conditions such as peptic ulcer, hiatus hernia, chronic cholecystitis, hepatoma and other cancers of upper abdominal viscera.

Tenderness may be mentioned by the patient and should be carefully considered by the surgeon. Abdominal pain is too common a problem to bring each case to a surgeon's attention. But a history of well-localized tenderness is a significant consideration for surgeons, and the point of maximum tenderness may give an important clue to the organ in which pathology is located.[5] Especially significant is tenderness at the right costal margin (gallbladder), right lower quadrant (appendix) and left lower quadrant (sigmoid colon). Epigastric tenderness is usually less ominous, especially when of several days duration and associated with the other signs and symptoms of benign peptic ulcer. Flank tenderness is sometimes a serious indication of penetrating intra-abdominal disease (appendicitis, carcinoma, diverticulitis), but it usually is a sign of illness in the genitourinary or musculoskeletal system. Bilateral lower abdominal tenderness is common in acute pelvic inflammatory disease, which usually can be confirmed by the presence of normal peristalsis, and characteristic findings of tenderness or a tubal mass on pelvic examination.

Abnormal stools may be significant to surgeons, especially if associated with weight loss and change in frequency of bowel movements. Small, hard stools are often described by patients with lesions of the descending and sigmoid colon, and may be explosively passed into the abdomen by patients with diverticulosis. Narrow stools streaked with blood or mucus are the hallmark of carcinoma of the rectum, but all too often are ascribed initially to hemorrhoids. Watery bowel movements may be described by patients with ulcerative colitis, regional enteritis, granulomatous colitis and a host of other conditions which are not primarily surgical diseases. The presence of blood and mucus increases a surgeon's interest, but a thorough diagnostic evaluation, sigmoidoscopy and barium studies are indicated to establish the diagnosis. In general, inflammatory and autoimmune diseases of the gastrointestinal tract are treated medically, except for obvious complications such as abscess, obstruction and bleeding. Foul-smelling bowel movements may be due to blood ("tarry" stools), pancreatic insufficiency, or the change in intestinal flora associated with a "blind loop" syndrome. The history of passage of worms may lead to suspicion of ascariasis in a child with biliary or small bowel obstruction and may thereby suggest a trial of medical therapy instead of laparotomy. On the other hand, a history of pinworms (*Enterobius vermicularis*) may lead to laparotomy in a child with chronic abdominal pain, since pinworm infestation of the appendix may necessitate appendectomy if the pain does not subside after treatment with piperazine.

Increased girth is a common problem in our affluent society and may be a sign of cirrhosis as well as obesity. But several surgical conditions often begin with such a history, including ascites from metastatic cancer, distention from chronic distal small bowel obstruction, and a mass of nonobstructing intra-abdominal or retroperitoneal tumor. The lean, athletic, previously healthy young person who notices an inappropriate increase in girth should be examined with great care, and consideration should be given to an exploratory laparotomy.

Lymphosarcomas and carcinoma of the ovary or testis will occasionally be discovered in these patients.

Fatigue is the most nonspecific of complaints, but may be the indication for surgery in the presence of other unresolved problems when there are symptoms or signs referable to the abdomen. *Fever*, like fatigue, is relatively nonspecific, but if documented and apparently not factitious, it may be due to pathology which can be uncovered at laparotomy.[3] Diseases range from lymphoma and tuberculosis to appendicitis and retroperitoneal abscess. In many cases, surgery may not only be diagnostic but also therapeutic.

Vomiting should always be viewed by a surgeon as a potentially serious symptom. Even if the cause is a nonsurgical lesion (acute alcoholism, gastroenteritis), persistent vomiting may cause gastroesophageal ulceration or rupture. And if prolonged vomiting occurs from obstruction, the patient may develop serious electrolyte disturbances which must be corrected appropriately. Hypokalemic hypochloremic *alkalosis* occurs from peptic ulcers which obstruct the pylorus or first portion of the duodenum. And metabolic *acidosis* is the result of chronic loss of small bowel contents from vomiting.

When vomiting is constant, the likelihood of a surgical lesion is increased. But nonsurgical lesions should still be considered, including myocardial infarction, uremia and drug toxicity. And if vomiting is present without nausea, increased intracranial pressure from primary or metastatic brain tumor should be suspected. The appearance and odor of vomitus is of great importance. "Kelly green" vomitus from an infant is usually the sign of an acute surgical abdomen. The presence of massive bloody vomitus should be an obvious indication for prompt surgical consultation. Fecal odor or appearance is usually associated with a surgical lesion, whereas watery vomitus containing free acid (Topfer's positive) is usually less ominous. Vomiting of blood in elderly patients is less likely to be resolved without surgery than a similar situation in young people. Hematemesis in cirrhotics should receive vigorous attention, a Sengstaken-Blakemore tube, and prompt surgical consultation. Inadequate treatment of the bleeding cirrhotic may lead to hepatic coma.

The surgeon's response to vomiting should be a desire to quantify, characterize and alleviate the problem. He may thereby prevent development of a complication which *necessitates* surgery or of complications following the *necessary corrective* surgery.

Signs of disease are revealed on physical examination. The surgeon's skills must include the ability to perform a complete examination of all areas of the body, but in practice he may frequently limit his examination to the abdomen and pelvis, lower gastrointestinal tract and other areas which he believes are most pertinent to the patient at hand. If the patient does not have a competent referring physician, it is obvious that the surgeon is responsible for performing and recording a complete examination. This is the situation in most large charity surgical clinics. However, in many instances, the patient may have recently undergone a complete evaluation by an internist and has been referred to the surgeon for a specific question regarding the abdomen. If this is the case, it is neither tactful nor economically feasible for the surgeon to repeat all aspects of the examination and to reinterrogate the patient about all aspects of the past history and systems review.

If major surgery is contemplated, or if a minor problem is raised which has a complex differential diagnosis, the surgeon should not restrict himself to an examination of the abdomen. He should perform a thoughtful, though possibly limited, examination of the rest of the patient. He will observe the temperature, pulse and respiration. Like Sherlock Holmes surveying his clients and his antagonists, he will study the eyes for proptosis, anisocoria and oculomotor palsy, listen to the voice, and study the skin for signs of malnutrition or cancer. He will examine the oral cavity and neck,—the latter especially for thyroid masses or lymph nodes—the breasts and the peripheral pulses. He will listen to heart and lungs, the former for rhythm and murmurs and the latter for wheezes and rhonchi. The chest film may disclose cardiomegaly and many types of pulmonary lesions, but only auscultation will reveal rhonchi and rales. These signs of pulmonary pathology may alter the risk of surgery and indicate steps necessary in preoperative preparation. The patient should be asked to cough, and then observed for involuntary repetition of coughing and production of sputum. The genitalia, groins and gait of patients take little time to evaluate. The surgeon is usually better equipped by training and interest than the internist to assess abnormalities in these areas.

The *examination* of the abdomen should ordinarily be systematic, thorough and unhurried, although the approach may be altered in the presence of localized tenderness or obvious urgency. It should include—in this order—the conventional aspects of inspection, auscultation, percussion and palpation. It should conclude with a digital pelvic and rectal examination. Visual examination of the female genitalia should be performed with a speculum. The rectosigmoid should be studied by proctoscopy when possible, especially during evaluation of gastrointestinal bleeding, diarrhea, anal or rectal pain, and in the general examination of men and women over age 35. A stool specimen should be tested for occult blood if possible, and its color and consistency noted. Inspection will reveal abnormality in abdominal contour, or the presence of localized masses and hyperperistalsis. Auscultation is most effective if performed in the quiet period before the intestines are displaced by palpation. The quality, quantity and pitch of peristalsis is recorded. In patients suspected of having tumors or vascular lesions, a careful ear is tuned to listen for bruit. Percussion is useful to outline solid masses, such as the liver edge or tumors. Tympany may reveal the pathology of air obliterating the liver

edge in perforated ulcer, or the distended stomach obstructed at the pylorus. Air-fluid levels may be detected when obstruction is present further along the gastrointestinal tract and in patients with ascites. Percussion is also useful as a gentle form of palpation, to localize areas of tenderness, especially in apprehensive patients. Palpation may be done with one hand or two, using either the fingertips or the palms, depending on the organ being evaluated and the preference of the examiner. The succussion splash of a chronically distended stomach is best elicited with two hands, whereas one hand lying on the other is frequently the best method for ballottement of deep masses. Experienced surgeons frequently "walk" gently around the abdomen with their fingertips in the examination of patients with localized tenderness. Abdominal tenderness is sometimes described as "rebound," which is a relatively useless term unless *referred* rebound tenderness is specified. This term is restricted to tenderness which is "referred" from the palpated site to another point within the abdomen.

A useful maneuver to distinguish anxiety and hypochondriasis from true abdominal tenderness is to use the stethoscope for palpation of the abdomen. The surgeon should appear to listen through the stethoscope and the patient will then attempt to remain quiet and relaxed as pressure is applied. If the patient truly has abdominal tenderness, he will promptly clarify the situation, but the hypochondriac will often let the surgeon press deeply into his abdomen with the stethoscope.

Palpation of the abdomen usually begins in the right upper quadrant. Keeping in mind the structures normally present in each area and the potential pathology in each organ, the surgeon next systematically examines the epigastrium, the left upper quadrant, the mid-abdomen, and the lower abdomen from right to left. The groins are examined for hernias, lymph nodes and quality of vascular pulsations. The examination concludes with a rectal and pelvic examination. Although the surgeon may

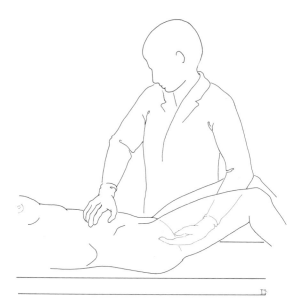

Figure 18–1 Bimanual examination of pelvis and abdomen. Patient is supine, in the position for usual pelvic examination. Surgeon has left hand on abdomen, right hand in pelvis (vagina or rectum), and is standing at the patient's side.

utilize all of the approaches and techniques described in Chapters 20 and 21 (female genitalia and proctology), he is most likely to utilize the pelvic and rectal examinations for the bimanual assistance which they provide in assessing the abdomen. He will, therefore, most likely keep the patient in the supine position, with the patient's knees flexed and the hips flexed and rotated laterally. This type of examination is most effective if the surgeon is standing at the patient's side, rather than at the foot of the bed (Fig. 18–1).

The usual pattern of palpation is modified when the patient is known to have a tender or painful area in the abdomen. In this situation, the most tender area is usually examined last, to avoid disturbing the patient prematurely.

The patient with acute cholecystitis may be unable to inspire deeply when the surgeon is pressing at the right costal margin, a phenomenon known as "Murphy's sign." Costovertebral angle tenderness frequently indicates the presence of pyelonephritis. Involuntary contraction ("spasm") of the abdominal musculature may be present over inflammatory pathology, whereas guarding (voluntary contraction of muscle) may be either the response to a factitious complaint or a protective mechanism to avoid pain during examination.

ORGANS AND SYSTEMS

Although it is true that pain may be referred to a distant region, the location of the symptom or sign is the most useful single guide to identification of a diseased organ.

Unfortunately, general agreement has not been reached regarding the terms which are used to describe the surface area and regions of the abdomen. The classic definitions of the anatomists (Fig. 18–2 *A*) have been modified greatly in practice in the United States, and precise definitions of the regions of the abdomen are now rarely given by surgeons in practice. Variations in body habitus produce considerable variation in the surface features of anatomy, and the underlying organs are also relatively inconstant. From a practical point of view, I refer to the regions shown in Table 18–1 and Figure 18–2 *B* and *C*.

Referred Pain

Pain may be referred out of the abdomen from many diseases of abdominal organs. Common examples are:

Right shoulder—Liver, diaphragm, duodenum

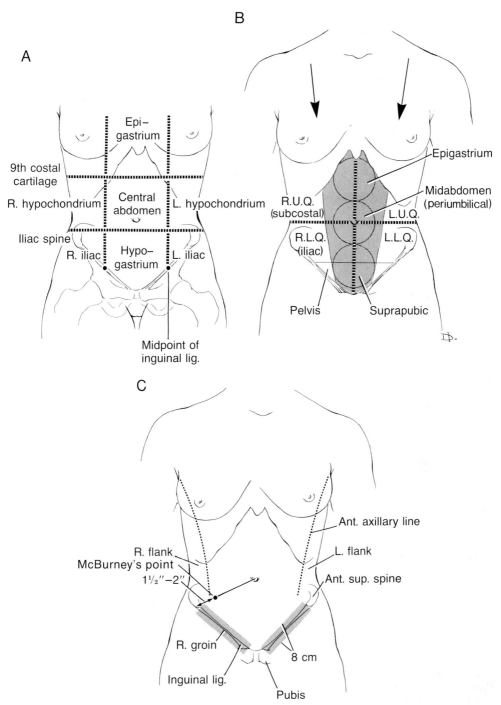

Figure 18–2 Regional surface anatomy of the abdomen. *A.* Classical anatomy (From Cope, 1968). *B.* Practical surface anatomy (from Botsford and Wilson, 1969). *C.* Flanks, groins and McBurney's point. Flanks extend posteriorly to lateral margin of sacrospinalis muscle.

TABLE 18–1   REGIONAL ANATOMY OF THE ABDOMEN FROM A
PRACTICAL POINT OF VIEW

REGION	LANDMARKS	CONTENTS AND ORGANS FROM WHICH SYMPTOMS ARE REFERRED
Right upper quadrant (right subcostal; RUQ)	Superior to umbilicus and right to midline	Liver Gallbladder Bile ducts Duodenum (1st and 2nd parts) Lesser sac Pylorus Right kidney Right adrenal gland Right colon and hepatic flexure Head of pancreas
Epigastrium (subxiphoid)	Upper third of area between midclavicular lines	Stomach; duodenum (3rd and 4th parts) Distal esophagus Celiac artery Pancreas, body Transverse colon
Left upper quadrant (left subcostal; LUQ)	Superior to umbilicus and left of midline	Spleen Splenic flexure and upper left colon Left adrenal gland Left kidney Tail of pancreas
Periumbilical (midabdomen)	Middle third of area between midclavicular lines	Pancreas, body Transverse colon Duodenum (3rd and 4th parts) Superior mesenteric artery Greater omentum Abdominal aorta Small bowel (Appendicitis symptoms appear here)
Right lower quadrant (right iliac; RLQ)	Inferior to umbilicus and right of midline	Appendix Cecum Right ureter Right Fallopian tube and ovary Right iliac lymph nodes Right iliac artery
Suprapubic	Lower third of area between midclavicular lines	Bladder Uterus Appendix (occasionally) Right or left ovary and Fallopian tube Transverse colon, omentum and small bowel (occasionally)
Left lower quadrant (left iliac; LLQ)	Inferior to umbilicus and left of midline	Sigmoid colon and rectosigmoid junction Left ureter Left Fallopian tube and ovary Left iliac lymph nodes Left iliac artery

Table 18–1 *continued on opposite page.*

TABLE 18–1   Regional Anatomy of the Abdomen from a
Practical Point of View (*Continued*)

Region	Landmarks	Contents and Organs from which Symptoms are Referred
Other regions of the abdomen are:		
Groins	Approximately 4 cm superior and inferior to Poupart's (inguinal) ligament	Inguinal and femoral hernias Lymph nodes Femoral nerve (entrapment) Common femoral artery and vein Iliopsoas muscle
Flanks	Superior to iliac crest and lateral to anterior axillary line	Kidneys Ureters Adrenals Iliopsoas muscle Retroperitoneal appendix Retroperitoneal sigmoid colon Tail of pancreas (left)

Left shoulder — Spleen, diaphragm
Back — Pancreas, kidneys
Groin — Ureter, tubes and ovaries, appendix
Legs — Intervertebral disc, nerve root, lumbar abscess, obturator hernia

SURGICAL DISEASES OF SPECIFIC ORGANS

The differential diagnosis of abdominal disorders can be greatly simplified by the laboratory procedures and tests which are now available on an outpatient basis. These studies are summarized in Table 18–2.

Abdominal Wall

Trauma, in general, warrants a period of close observation in a holding area, such as the "overnight ward" described in Chapter 1. If penetrating trauma occurred, exploratory laparotomy is the safest approach and should usually be performed if the wound was larger than that resulting from an ice pick. Major injuries to the abdominal wall from knives, bullets and other large missiles almost always require laparotomy.

It should be remembered that a high velocity gunshot wound can produce extensive necrosis for several centimeters around the tract of the missile. Intra-abdominal damage can therefore occur with tangential bullet wounds which do not even traverse the peritoneal cavity. Blunt trauma produces the greatest problems in management, for it is often difficult to assess the likelihood of intra-abdominal damage. It is necessary to remember that the amount of force, the duration of the period of injury, and the nature of the trauma may give clues to the likelihood of intra-abdominal lesions.[9, 53] A deep abdominal abrasion from a seat belt after an auto crash at high speed is a sign of sufficient trauma to rupture viscera in the abdomen.[69] Paracentesis may indicate a need for prompt surgery, but a "negative" tap in such a patient does not rule out the possibility of significant injury. Blast injury commonly causes ruptured viscera. The problem is to assess the severity of the blast and the proximity of the patient to it. Fractured ribs may be a sign of trauma severe enough to rupture spleen, liver or other organs—especially in children, whose ribs are less liable to fracture than the brittle ribs of adults.

Infections of the abdominal wall can

TABLE 18-2 OUTPATIENT PROCEDURES
AND TESTS — ABDOMEN AND
GASTROINTESTINAL TRACT

Barium contrast x-rays
  Esophagram (including Trendelenburg position
  and Valsalva maneuver)
  Gastrointestinal series (GI series), (including
  cross table lateral for visualization of the
  retrogastric area)
  Small bowel followthrough, with films every
  one-half to one hour until barium is in the
  colon, thus measuring transit time and residual barium in stomach
  Barium enema. Should precede GI series if
  there is a question of a colonic lesion. Lateral
  film usually required to show a rectal lesion.
  Postevacuation and air contrast films are best
  for delineation of polyps
  Barium must be removed with cathartics or
  enemas. The surgeon must assure himself
  that the patient is adequately instructed in
  elimination of barium

Gastrografin (Meglumine diazotrite) x-rays
  Studies are similar to those performed with
  barium, producing a poorer delineation of
  masses, but safer if there is a question of GI
  tract perforation. Gastrografin is satisfactory
  for outlining the point of bowel obstructions

Needle biopsy
  Vim-Silverman or Menghini liver biopsy, or
  Vim-Silverman biopsy of a large, superficial,
  and well-circumscribed tumor

Paracentesis
  Four-quadrant tap (20 ml syringe and a No. 18
  or 20 needle) for diagnosis of blood, pus, chyle,
  ascites, urine or other fluid
  Peritoneal irrigation for diagnosis of hemoperitoneum. If four-quadrant tap is negative use
  peritoneal dialysis catheter or large plastic
  catheter such as EZ cath or Intracath
  Paracentesis, therapeutic, with trochar, or peritoneal dialysis catheter, or large Intracath or
  EZ cath. May instill chemotherapeutic agent
  when a nearly complete removal of fluid has
  been achieved

Blood tests
  Hematocrit
  White blood cell count
  Differential
  Platelet count
  Liver function tests: lactic dehydrogenase, serum
  glutamic oxalacetic transaminase, serum pro-
  teins and protein electrophoresis, cephalin
  floculation, cholesterol, prothrombin time,
  alpha-fetoglobulin
  Amylase

Stool tests
  Fat, blood, mucus, muscle fibers

Gastric analysis

Blood, free acid, acid-fast bacilli, and response
  to stimulation (histalog or histamine)

Intestinal absorption studies
  Schilling test (radioactive vitamin B–12)
  D-xylose

Cholangiogram
  Intravenous
  T-tube

Cholecystogram, oral
  One day or three day test
  Intravenous pyelogram

Plain x-rays
  Flat ("kidneys, ureters and bladder"—KUB)
  Upright (to look for air fluid levels)
  Chest film (shows diaphragms best)
  Lateral decubitus (if patient is unable to stand
  up)
  Spot films (to look for air bubbles, calcification,
  fecalith, among others)
  Repeat films (to look for movement or lack of
  movement in air bubbles and densities)

Sigmoidoscopy, anoscopy, proctoscopy

Papanicolaou test
  Peritoneal fluid, gastric aspirate, colonic irrigation

Esophagoscopy⎫ Fiberoptic 'oscopy is safest for
Gastroscopy ⎬ outpatient use. Records can be
            ⎭ color film with Gastrocamera

Esophageal pressure and pH recording for hiatal
hernia and reflux

Tests on abdominal fluid
  Blood count (after fluid has been heparinized)
  Bacteriologic tests: Gram stain, Ziehl-Neelsen
  stain, culture (routine, anaerobic, TB and fungal) and sensitivities
  Enzymes: LDH, amylase (also place fluid on
  unexposed x-ray film, and if emulsion is di-
  gested, amylase is shown to be present)
  Miscellaneous: Ether extraction—to differentiate pus from chyle. (The upper—ether—
  layer becomes turbid when mixed with chyle,
  which contains fat, but turbidity remains in
  the lower layer if the fluid is pus.)
Fistula studies
  X-ray: Sinogram (with Hypaque injected);
  barium administered in 'ostomy by enema
  or by mouth
  Charcoal or Carmine red: by mouth, to prove
  presence of GI fistula and to show transit
  time to fistula
  PSP–IV to show urinary tract fistula; must alkalinize fistula drainage and voided urine every
  15 minutes to look for dark red color of PSP
  dye

usually be managed on an outpatient basis by incision and drainage as described in Chapter 4. However, an abdominal wall infection associated with crepitation requires immediate hospitalization for treatment. In this case, the tissues are infiltrated with gas produced by gram negative (e.g., coliform or Bacteroides) or gram positive (e.g., Clostridium) organisms.

Tumors of the abdominal wall must be histologically categorized and may then be treated appropriately on an inpatient or an outpatient basis, as described in Chapter 5. In general, however, even benign tumors are best treated by sufficiently deep anesthesia to warrant hospitalization. Calcification is no certain indication if benignity, for it may occur in malignant as well as benign tumors (Fig. 18–3). Congenital defects and hernias almost always require hospitalization for definitive repair. Useful preparation in the outpatient clinic includes instruction for reduction in weight, evaluation of cough, a search for prostatic hypertrophy, and investigation regarding constipation, if any of these predisposing causes for hernia are present. It is not necessary to perform a test for residual urine and a barium enema

on all men prior to herniorraphy. Nevertheless, it is important to evaluate the urinalysis and urological history, and to perform a sigmoidoscopy on men over age 40 who have recently developed hernias.

Inguinal hernia[41,47] may be "indirect" (a congenital weakness of the internal inguinal ring) or "direct" (an acquired weakness of the floor of the inguinal canal). Distinction can frequently be made on the basis of the age of the patient or the location of the hernia. Direct hernias are uncommon in young men and usually do not descend into the scrotum. The weakness of the floor of the inguinal canal in a direct hernia is medial and may be adjacent to the pubic tubercule. It is, however, of little practical importance to distinguish between these two types of hernias preoperatively. The distinction can be made at the time of surgery on the basis of location in reference to the deep inferior epigastric vessels. Indirect hernias arise lateral to the epigastric vessels and direct hernias occur medial to the vessels. Hesselbach's triangle, the classic site of direct hernias, is bounded by the epigastric vessels, Poupart's ligament, and the lateral border of the rectus abdominus muscle.

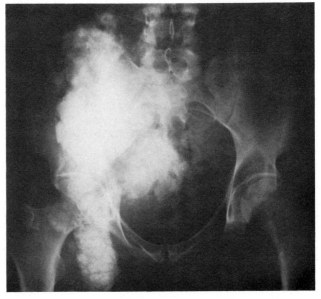

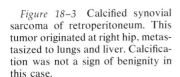

Figure 18–3 Calcified synovial sarcoma of retroperitoneum. This tumor originated at right hip, metastasized to lungs and liver. Calcification was not a sign of benignity in this case.

The repair of an inguinal hernia must, in either case, include closure of the defect and establishment of a secure floor of the inguinal canal.[68] Inguinal hernia also occurs in women, in whom it is called hernia of the canal of Nuck. Recurrent inguinal hernias nearly always begin as a defect adjacent to the pubic tubercule (in the "direct" area). Inguinal hernias may be operated upon under light general anesthesia or local anesthesia, and would therefore, be suitable for an outpatient operating room. However, if a femoral hernia is unexpectedly encountered, a deeper dissection should be performed and Cooper's ligament used for the repair.[41] This may present an awkward problem for a surgeon who is operating with relatively little assistance available. In general, therefore, inguinal hernia repair in the Outpatient Department should be reserved for healthy young men who have a strong probability of a congenital, indirect hernia (for technique see Chapter 23).

Femoral hernia may present in the groin, simulating an inguinal hernia, but it usually produces a relatively lower (inferior) bulge. It is more common in women than men, and is rarely seen in young people. Femoral hernias frequently become incarcerated, even when small. A small, hard tender groin mass which appears to be a lymph node should immediately raise the question of an incarcerated femoral hernia, especially if the patient has become ill. Incarceration of one wall of the bowel (Richter's hernia), with strangulation and perforation is not uncommon. A Richter's type of hernia requires immediate hospitalization and surgery, with preoperative antibiotics as expectant treatment for peritonitis.

Umbilical hernia is relatively uncommon in adults, although it is a significant cosmetic and psychological problem in children (see Chapter 23). In adults, incarceration and strangulation may occur, especially in debilitated, obese, or cirrhotic patients. Hospitalization is recommended for repair in adults, since the likelihood of complications is greatly increased by associated medical conditions. Frequently, only greater omentum or properitoneal fat will be found in the hernia, but it may be unexpectedly troublesome to achieve hemostasis in adults. Postoperative bleeding usually consists of hidden intraperitoneal bleeding and is not easily visible in the wound.

Other types of abdominal wall hernias are relatively uncommon. Paraspinal (lumbar) hernias occur in the triangle of Petit.[50] Spigelian hernias occur along the lateral border of the rectus muscle. Obturator canal hernias may present with discomfort in the buttocks. Ventral hernias are common complications of partial or complete postoperative wound disruption, in which case they are termed incisional hernias. They also occur occasionally in the linea alba on a congenital basis. All of these hernias should be recognizable to the outpatient surgeon, but should be treated only on an inpatient basis.

Intercostal nerve entrapment may occasionally produce pain and a small tender mass which simulates a Spigelian hernia at the lateral margin of the rectus sheath. A test for this diagnosis is local infiltration with anesthetic, which can be performed in the Outpatient Clinic. If the symptoms recede temporarily, and then return, exploration of the area should be carried out. The nerve should be freed up from the entrapment, or resected if a neuroma has developed.

Peritoneum

If the surgeon is consulted because of a diagnosis of peritonitis, he will undoubtedly hospitalize the patient and initiate therapy leading to surgery with appropriate drainage, resection or repair. Occasionally a patient may be extremely ill and the diagnosis is unclear, the possibilities including stroke, pneumonia, peritonitis and intraperitoneal hemorrhage. Paracentesis may then provide an immediate answer, revealing any of several types of fluid: blood, pus, gastric guice, small bowel contents, feces, bile or pancreatic juice. Each of these

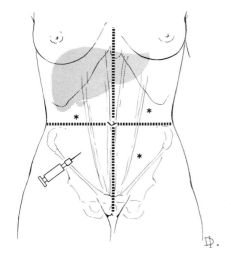

Figure 18–4 "Four quadrant tap"—diagnostic abdominal paracentesis. Abdomen is prepared with surgical prep solution. Needle is advanced carefully, just inside the peritoneum. All four quadrants may be tapped. Color or odor may be diagnostic immediately. See Table 18–2 for lab tests performed on fluid.

types of fluid can be identified tentatively by appearance and odor and should be examined histologically and bacteriologically as well. Four-quadrant tap (Fig. 18–4) provides the quickest and safest means of aspirating fluid for a diagnostic test. If only a small amount of fluid is present, peritoneal irrigation may be necessary to obtain a diagnosis (Fig. 3–4). Intraperitoneal fluid may be a chronic, recurring problem, and therapeutic paracentesis (Fig. 18–5) may provide useful palliation. Recurrent ascites may be a complication of hepatic vein thrombosis, cirrhosis, metastatic cancer or miliary tuberculosis. These forms of ascites can usually be distinguished easily from chylous ascites and pseudomyxoma peritonei, each of which may be more suitably treated by exploratory laparotomy to attempt correction of the primary problem.

Liver

The patient with surgical disease of the liver will usually present with either a right upper quadrant mass, jaundice, pain or fever, or various combinations of these problems.

The problem of a right upper quadrant mass can rarely be solved without a tissue diagnosis. It may be due to hepatomegaly, an enlarged gallbladder, a tumor of or adjacent to the liver, or a host of less common conditions. Occasionally the liver may be made more easily palpable as the result of pulmonary emphysema and flattening of the diaphragm, but this will rarely produce symptoms of right upper quadrant discomfort. The liver may be enlarged as the result of venous distention, heart disease, hepatic vein thrombosis or cirrhosis. Diffuse disease such as hepatitis or cholangitis may cause enlargement, pain, tenderness, jaundice and fever. Liver abscess may also present with a right upper quadrant mass.

If the liver is grossly nodular and the patient is cachectic, a careful search for distant metastases should be made before liver biopsy is undertaken. But if the patient is otherwise well, it may be most expeditious simply to biopsy the liver. Needle biopsy is frequently sufficient, and may be performed in the Outpatient Department. A significant degree of jaundice or abnormal clotting parameters are contraindications to needle biopsy. The patient *must* be closely observed for several hours afterward. The Menghini (1959)[42] needle is the easiest and safest to use, although the specimen obtained is smaller than that obtained with the Vim-Silverman needle. If the patient has a solitary tumor, hospitalization for an open liver biopsy in the operating room is recommended. Occasionally an enlarged or displaced liver lobe may be discovered and may lead to concern. Riedel's lobe is a classic trap for the unwary. We have also seen one patient with apparent hepatomegaly which was actually a congenital rotation of the liver associated with omphalocoele that had been repaired in infancy.

Liver scan will occasionally be very helpful in defining the size and location of lesions (Fig. 18–6), but it is expensive,

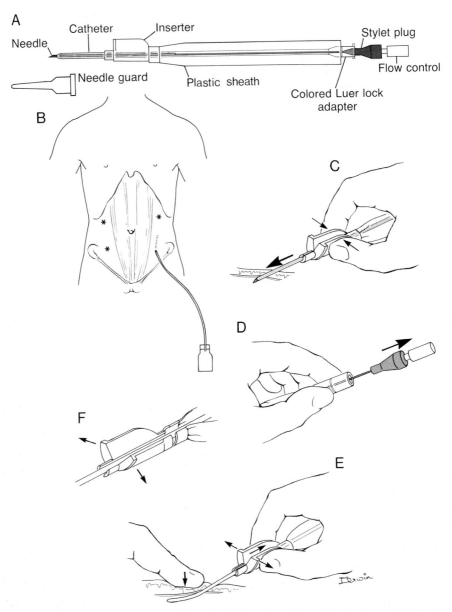

Figure 18–5 Therapeutic paracentesis. Sterile radiopaque Teflon catheter is inserted percutaneously into one of the four abdominal quadrants, following percussion of abdomen to identify and avoid gas-filled viscera. We prefer a catheter and needle unit in which needle is *inside* the catheter. The needle can safely be withdrawn after insertion into the abdomen. Suitable catheters are: Deseret E-Z Cath, 16 ga., 12 inches, Cat. No. 2254; and Deseret Angiocath, 16 ga., 5¼ inches, Cat. No. 2854.

and, of course, does not usually reveal the precise nature of the disease. Selective arteriography is also helpful in identifying the number and size of hepatic lesions. Transfemoral celiac and mesen-teric arteriograms (Fig. 18–7) may be performed on an outpatient basis, if the patient is observed for signs of intestinal ischemia or bleeding for a few hours after the study.

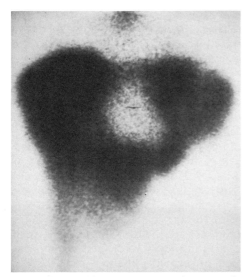

Figure 18-6 Liver scan. 14 cm hepatoma in medial segment of the left lobe, seen preoperatively with Tc[99] scan.

In the series of major liver tumors reported by Malt (1970),[39] 26 out of 63 were found to be benign, and excision was curative. The most common benign

tumors are hamartomas and hemangiomas. Malignant tumors include metastatic tumors, and solitary or multicentric hepatomas.

Jaundice raises questions of hepatitis, cirrhosis, hepatoma, cholangitis, common duct stones, carcinoma of the pancreas, metastatic carcinoma and toxic drug reactions. It is rarely suitable to study and treat the patient with jaundice of unknown etiology on an outpatient basis, so the work-up of this condition involves prompt hospitalization. The patient should be followed closely by a surgeon, but hospitalization under the care of an internist is usually preferred. In any case, a full set of liver function tests should be obtained when the patient is first seen, and stool and needle precautions should ordinarily be instituted.

If the patient has previously undergone biliary tract surgery, the presence of common duct stones or stricture is a likely possibility, and the operations required are formidable procedures.[65] The mortality in reoperation is approximately ten times higher than the mor-

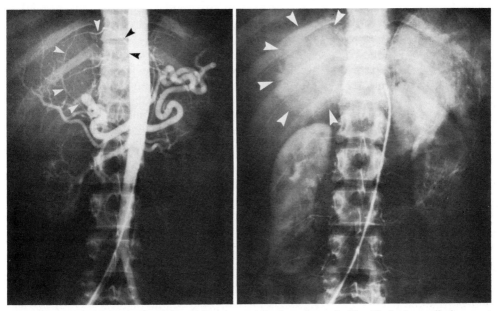

Figure 18-7 Hepatic arteriography. Celiac artery injection of case in Fig. 18–6, shows displacement (arrows) of arterial branches in early phase, and venous tumor "blush" (arrows) in late phase. Patient is now free of disease 12 months following left lobectomy.

tality in first operations on the biliary tract (Glenn, 1965).[22]

Right upper quadrant pain is more commonly due to disease of the gallbladder than to liver disease. However, all of the lesions which produce hepatomegaly can also present with pain, and some conditions produce pain with little or no enlargement in the liver. Hematobilia is one such condition. Although it usually occurs as a complication of injury to the liver, it may occur from a benign or malignant tumor. The presentation may be in the form of intermittent gastrointestinal bleeding of unknown origin, and the presence of pain due to distention of the biliary tree may be the only clue to the site of bleeding. Arteriography will usually reveal a lesion if it is performed when bleeding is active or if a mass is present within the liver. Post-traumatic hematobilia usually requires hepatic resection, although healing has been reported without surgery.[28] Hematobilia also occurs as a rare, usually end-stage complication of carcinoma of the gallbladder, bile ducts or pancreas.

Fever of unknown origin may be the result of diffuse or localized infection of the liver or its surrounding tissues. Many of these patients will also have pain, tenderness, a mass or jaundice or all of these. But any patient with a fever of unknown origin should have a careful study of liver function, and should be considered for a liver scan and possible arteriography. If there is any reason to suspect liver abscess, spot films or tomograms of the liver may show the telltale gas bubbles or air fluid levels which localize the abscess.

Liver abscess may occur as a result of cholangitis, amoebae, or echinococcus cysts; by metastatic spread from elsewhere in the body (especially the portal system or pelvis); or on a primarily idiopathic basis. Drainage is a major surgical procedure, but the condition must often be recognized in obscure and confusing manifestations in outpatients.[25] Elevation of alkaline phosphatase and a solitary defect on liver scan may provide the essential clues to diagnosis. Amoebic abscess is rare in the United States, except in those who have lived or traveled in Mexico or the tropics. The treatment is usually medical, Flagyl being the preferred drug at the present time (Chapter 4), since it is equally effective and less toxic than Emetine. Echinococcus cysts are encountered in specific geographical regions where the cycle of the dog tapeworm has been established. These lesions are not uncommon in Alaskan Eskimos and Indians. The patients should ordinarily be hospitalized for drainage.

Increasing numbers of gonococcal infections are being seen in outpatient clinics in recent years, and a manifestation of this infection in the perihepatic tissues may mimic hepatitis or acute cholecystitis. This disease is known as the Curtis-Fitzhugh syndrome, and was recently reviewed by Trimble (1970).[63]

The evaluation of the patient with possible liver disease should be done with the differential diagnosis in mind, so that appropriate questions, examinations and tests are requested and performed. The patient should be questioned regarding his exposure to hepatic toxins, alcohol, jaundiced persons and needles. He should be asked if he is known to have had gallstones or has had fatty food intolerance or dark urine, or clay-colored stools. A careful record should be made of the size of the liver on physical examination, indicating its edge in relationship to the costal margin and umbilicus, and an estimation of its size in centimeters (not finger-breadths) from the costal margin at specific points (e.g., xiphoid line, midclavicular line, anterior axillary line). The presence or absence of tenderness, irregularity, firmness and mobility should be recorded. The patient should be observed for palmar erythema, asterixis and spider angiomata of the skin. Masses or tenderness in other areas of the body may be a definite clue to the origin of the liver disease, especially if a rectal cancer or supraclavicular nodes are palpated. Intravenous cholangiograms can be performed on an outpatient basis, but they usually contribute little in patients with clinically obvious jaundice. An oral cholecystogram or cholangiography does not visualize the biliary tract if the bilirubin is greater than 4.0 mg per cent. Intravenous cholangiography also has definite hazards, including idiosyncratic anaphlaxis and severe fever. T–tube cholangiogram is useful in patients who happen to have jaundice postoperatively, and in whom a T–tube is still in place. In these patients the need for additional surgery may be clarified by an out-patient x-ray which reveals retained stones or a biliary tract stricture.

Diaphragm

Hiatus hernia is the most common surgical disease of the diaphragm. Sliding hiatus hernia is observed in up to 10 per cent of GI series in which it is looked for. Paraesophageal hiatus hernia is less common but is more likely to produce symptoms or incarceration than a sliding hernia. Sliding hernia should be treated medically until it is obvious that symptoms ("heartburn," regurgitation, dysphagia) or complications (aspiration pneumonia, esophagitis) will not subside without surgery. Esophagitis may progress to stricture, which usually requires surgery, though dilations by bougie may provide long-term success is cases where stricture is mild. The decision to recommend hiatus herniorraphy should be based not only on symtoms and intractability, but also on documentation of acid reflux in esophageal motility studies (Chapter 15), which can be performed on an outpatient basis. Hiatus hernia may be relatively asymptomatic and discovered only incidentally in the course of a GI workup for gallstones or sigmoid diverticulitis ("Saint's triad"). If hiatus hernia is present, a repair can usually be performed at the time of cholecystectomy with little additional morbidity.[4]

Rupture of the central tendon of the diaphragm may occur as the result of trauma, and can be followed by incarceration of stomach or colon within the chest.[19] Symptoms of intrathoracic borborygmi and "heartburn" during defecation may be bizarre consequences of this lesion which should be corrected by surgery. Diaphragmatic rupture is more common on the left side than on the right. However, intrathoracic displacement of the liver through a ruptured right diaphragm may cause acute embarrassment of hepatic or pulmonary function if unrecognized. Rupture of the right diaphragm may be erroneously diagnosed as a hemothorax, in which case an attempt may inadvertently be made to insert a chest tube into the intrathoracic liver.

Subdiaphragmatic infection is usually the consequence of previous surgery or trauma, and may become apparent only after the patient has been discharged from the hospital (Fig. 18–8). The diagnosis should be suspected in a patient with low grade intermittent fever, recurrent pleural effusion, and leukocytosis. Other signs include subcostal or costovertebral ache and tenderness, a paralyzed or sluggish motion of the diaphragm, displacement of liver or spleen, a defect on liver-spleen scan, or a subphrenic accumulation of air. Displacement of the stomach may be apparent on abdominal x-ray or GI series. When the diagnosis is strongly suspected, the patient should be admitted for final preoperative studies and surgical drainage.

Fenestration of the diaphragm is the result of a congenital weakness which causes a bulge in the center of one of the hemidiaphragms, but it usually is of no functional significance.

Tumors of the diaphragm are rare, but sarcomas may occur in this organ. More common, however, are metastatic tumors, or local invasion from cancer in adjacent organs. The prognosis is very poor. The diagnosis of a neoplasm involving the diaphragm can frequently be suspected from inspection of the chest film.

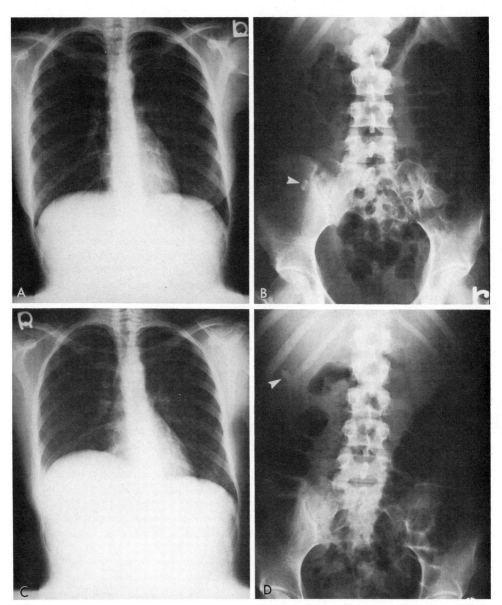

Figure 18–8   Subphrenic abscess. Subphrenic abscess caused by an unrecognized fecalith of the appendix. *A*. Normal chest x-ray when admitted with acute appendicitis in January 1971. *B*. Abdominal x-ray showing fecalith (arrow) in appendiceal abscess, January 1971. Fecalith was not seen at this time and was not removed. *C*. Elevated right diaphragm, June 1971. *D*. Abdominal x-ray, June 1971. Laminated fecalith is now visible in RUQ (arrow).

(*Figure continued on following page.*)

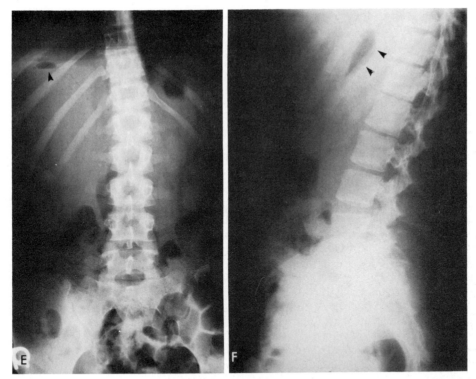

Figure 18–8 (Continued).   E. Upright film shows subphrenic air-fluid level (arrow). *F.* Lateral film shows location of subphrenic abscess (arrow). Patient recovered promptly following rib resection, drainage and removal of fecalith.

Biliary Tract

Gallstones represent the major surgical problem in the biliary tract, producing complications of acute and chronic infection, septicemia, gallstone ileus, biliary cirrhosis, pancreatitis and death. Gallstone disease is also associated with typhoid carrier states and carcinoma of the gallbladder. Acute cholecystitis has a particularly high mortality in the aged population, diabetics and patients with leukemia. It occurs with increased frequency in families with congenital spherocytic anemia, and in patients with collagen diseases such as systemic lupus erythematosus, where it may occur as acalculous cholecystitis. Vagotomy and gastric resections are followed by an increased production of gallstones, probably as the result of poor emptying of the gallbladder.

Gallstones should be suspected in patients who have intolerance to fried or fatty foods, or who describe "bloating," or dyspepsia after ingestion of cabbage, cucumbers, cauliflower or onions. Many patients will have a long history of mild complaints, while others will have only one or two severe episodes of pain before seeking medical attention. The disease may first present as an episode of acute cholecystitis with fever and right upper quadrant pain. Most of these patients will improve with hospitalization and treatment with intravenous fluids, nasogastric tube, antibiotics and sedatives. Morphine should not be administered since it produces spasm of the sphincter of Oddi. Intermittent biliary colic may occur without fever or tenderness and is probably the result of passage of small calculi through the sphincter. Occasionally patients will have jaundice intermittently or temporarily during an episode of acute cholecystitis, and yet be found not to have common duct stones when surgery is performed.

The presence of gallstones is a sufficient indication for cholecystectomy in patients who are otherwise well, since the complications of gallstones are usually more hazardous than the risk of surgery. Common duct exploration should be added to the operation if there are clear signs of common duct stones, stricture, or obstruction, or if jaundice is present. If there is a significant past history consistent with obstruction, operative cholangiography should be performed, and if the duct system is not completely normal, exploration is carried out. The risk of the operation is increased very little by common duct exploration, although if stones are present in the duct, the overall morbidity and mortality are increased somewhat. Multiple small stones are more hazardous than a single large calculus, since small stones are more likely to escape and become lodged in the common duct. This fact is taken into consideration in deciding whether to recommend surgery in patients who are poor operative risks.

The overall mortality for cholecystectomy is approximately 1 to 2 per cent, but should be less than 0.5 per cent in elective operations in otherwise healthy individuals. The mortality in 1090 consecutive cholecystectomies reported by Seltzer (1970)[58] was 1.6 per cent. The mortality for all operations on the biliary tract in 2358 patients reported by Glenn and McSherry (1963)[21] was 1.7 per cent. Glenn, McSherry and Dineen (1968)[23] also reported an overall nonfatal complication rate of 6.9 per cent in 3217 patients with biliary tract operations for nonmalignant disease.

The diagnosis of gallstone disease is made in most cases by oral cholecystography. The reliability of this test is most impressive when it is positive; that is, when gallstones are seen. The stones may be so small that they can be seen only when dye has coated them and they layer out on an upright film. Very few false positives are seen—that is, those in which gallstones are believed to be visualized on x-ray but are not found at the time of surgery. On the other hand, failure to visualize the gallbladder does not prove that the organ is diseased, and

it may concentrate the dye properly if the test tablets are administered for two or three more days. Temporary failure to function occurs during episodes of acute illness, such as with an active peptic ulcer. The reverse situation may also be true, and a "normal" oral cholecystogram may be present in a patient who actually has gallstones. If the patient has a good history for recurrent biliary colic, exploration and even cholecystectomy may be indicated, since very small stones may not even be palpable intraoperatively and will be revealed only when the gallbladder is opened. In cases of acute cholecystitis or jaundice, the oral cholecystogram is of little or no help, since the gallbladder will not be visualized. Occasionally, an intravenous cholangiogram is helpful in such patients, but usually the decision regarding diagnosis and surgery must be made on clinical grounds and other laboratory evidence. We routinely obtain an alkaline phosphatase and prothrombin time in patients suspected of having gallstone disease, since mild or transient obstruction of the common duct will cause elevation in alkaline phosphatase, and impairment of liver function may cause serious derangement in the production of the essential clotting factor, prothrombin. Bilirubin and bilirubin fractions should also be obtained since subclinical jaundice may occur, and these would be an indication for further study of the common duct. Amylase is also an important laboratory test, since—like the bilirubin—if it is elevated, the surgeon is alerted to a more complicated situation.

Other diseases of the biliary tract frequently present a dilemma for the surgeon, especially if they are completely asymptomatic, or if the patient is a poor operative risk. Occasionally, oral cholecystogram demonstrates a small, immobile radiolucent defect in the fundus. This frequently represents a polyp, or rarely, an adenoma. It should be possible to rule out the presence of a gallstone by repositioning the patient and obtaining another x-ray. These patients usually should be operated on simply to rule out the presence of carcinoma, since virtually the only cases of cancer of the gallbladder which are cured occur in patients in whom a small, localized, asymptomatic cancer is present and is removed completely with a cholecystectomy. The annual mortality for cancer of the gallbaldder is actually as high as the mortality for benign disease of the gallbladder, in spite of the rarity of this tumor. Calcification in the wall of the gallbladder (Fig. 18–9) is another uncommon condition, which should probably be operated upon in otherwise healthy patients, but which does not

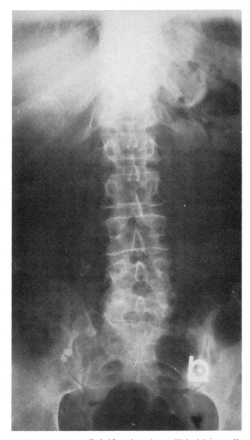

Figure 18–9 Calcification in gallbladder wall. Seventy-four year old woman with recurrent myocardial infarctions and chronic obstructive pulmonary disease. Abdominal x-ray obtained when calcification was accidentally observed during chest fluoroscopy. No symptoms related to gallbladder. Operation was not advised.

present the risk of biliary tract obstruction which is present in patients with small gallstones.

The elderly patient with asymptomatic or nearly asymptomatic chronic cholecystitis presents a philosophical problem for the surgeon and internist. In properly selected elderly patients, the mortality for elective cholecystectomy is only slightly higher than that for the population at large. Ibach (1968)[36] reported a 2.3 per cent mortality in elective cholecystectomies in 151 patients over age 60, but the mortality was increased to 16.7 per cent for emergency operations. If surgery is contemplated in the very elderly patient, the work-up must be meticulous and must include assessment of renal, cardiac and cerebral function.

Unusual manifestations of primary or secondary disease of the gallbladder include painless hydrops (in which the gallbladder may become massively distended with "white bile" as the result of complete occlusion of the cystic duct), emphysematous cholecystitis (clostridium infection of the gallbladder, with gas production in the lumen and wall) and Courvosier's sign (distended gallbladder in a jaundiced patient—the classical sign of carcinoma of the distal common duct or head of the pancreas). The classic sign of gallbladder enteric fistula is a patient with small bowel obstruction who has air in the biliary tree. The gallbladder or common bile duct may develop pressure necrosis as the result of gallstones,[31] with subsequent perforation and bile peritonitis. Likewise, gangrene of the gallbladder may occur, especially in the elderly diabetic patient.

Trauma to the gallbladder or common duct may rupture the biliary tract and cause acute bile peritonitis. This condition is increasingly common as the result of seat belt injuries in high speed automobile accidents. Stab wounds and gunshot wounds may lacerate the biliary tract, and any patient who has bile-stained retroperitoneal tissues or free bile observed at laparotomy must have the source of the bile determined, or disaster will usually result in the post-operative period. The gallbladder may be entered inadvertently by a needle during liver biopsy, and the resulting bile peritonitis will usually require exploration within a few hours.

Stricture of the common bile duct or hepatic ducts may occur from trauma or carcinoma, or on a congenital basis, but most of these cases are the result of prior surgical damage to the biliary tree. Reconstructive surgery for correction or palliation is usually a complex matter, but the end results may be extremely gratifying.

Postcholecystectomy syndrome is a condition which plagues the surgeon and the patient. The cause is unknown, but the symptoms may be the same as those for which cholecystectomy was performed initially. A proper work-up of such patients should include cardiac, neurologic, pancreatic, gastric, colonic, renal and psychiatric studies. Occasionally such patients are found to have new or retained stones in the common duct or T–tubes. Some have had incomplete cholecystectomies. Some have a long residual cystic duct stump which forms and releases stones. Ideally, these patients should be identified by intravenous cholangiograms, careful review of outside hospital records and operative notes, and liver function tests. But occasionally exploratory reoperation on the biliary tract may be necessary,[22] unless non-operative treatment is successful.[66] In patients who no longer have gallstones, occasionally a tight, stenotic ampulla of Vater will be found during operative cholangiography or common duct exploration. Transduodenal sphincterotomy is indictated in such patients and will frequently relieve their symptoms completely.

Stomach and Duodenum

Peptic ulcer disease is the cause of most of the surgical problems related to the stomach and duodenum. Duodenal ulcers, benign gastric ulcers, gastritis, esophagitis, and a multitide of complications provide a steady series of challenges for the outpatient surgeon. In addition, cancer, trauma, congenital and developmental abnormalities are seen in these organs.

Peptic ulcer disease is still incompletely understood, in spite of the efforts of laboratory scientists and clinicians. The parietal and chief cells of the fundus of the stomach secrete hydrochloric acid and pepsin, respectively, in response to stimulation both by the hormone gastrin and by the vagus nerves. Gastrin is released from the gastric antrum when the antrum is distended by food or liquid, or is bathed in an alkaline medium. The vagal response is triggered by the sensation of hunger, and may therefore be initiated by endogenous or exogenous insulin. We believe that gastric mucus probably plays a role in protecting the gastric mucosa from the digestive effects of acid and pepsin in the stomach, and that alkaline secretions of bile, pancreatic juice and Brunner's glands normally protect the duodenum from acid digestion. Acid output is increased by physical or psychological stress, and the mechanism of ulceration has been postulated as due to a decrease in secretion of gastric mucus which occurs from adrenal cortical steroid activity.

Men have higher gastric acid production than women, and peptic ulcer disease is more frequent in men than in women. In general, patients with duodenal ulcers have higher gastric acid output then patients with benign gastric ulcers, and patients with benign gastric ulcers have relatively higher acid output than patients with carcinoma of the stomach. Gastric acid production decreases in the last few decades of life, but complications from previously active peptic ulcers may occur after acidity has decreased to low levels. The most common complications of peptic ulcers are bleeding, pain, obstruction and perforation, and these are the most common indications for operation. Gastric ulcers on the greater curvature have a higher incidence of malignancy than those on the lesser curvature, and are therefore subject to greater scrutiny and earlier operation than ulcers on the lesser curvature.

Duodenal ulcers most commonly occur in the first and second portions of the duodenum. Anterior ulcers are complicated by perforation whereas posterior ulcers penetrate into the pancreas, eroding into the gastroduodenal artery and causing bleeding and pancreatitis. Typically, the symptoms of duodenal ulcers are intermittent epigastric pain and tenderness, especially aggravated by anxiety and hunger, and relieved with rest, food and antacids. Frequently, a predisposing stimulus can be found, such as a family problem or other psychological conflicts. The symptoms are usually aggravated by alcohol or tobacco, although this may not be recognized by the patient. Occasionally, drug ingestion may be the inciting cause. Aspirin, indomethacin and phenylbutazone are the most common offenders at the present time.

Benign gastric ulcers frequently have a history similar to that of duodenal ulcers, but in many instances there is no clear history of pain related to hunger and anxiety and relieved by food and antacids. Giant benign gastric ulcers sometimes occur in the presence of only moderate amounts of gastric acidity. Occasionally, patients with duodenal ulcers will develop duodenal and pyloric obstruction, and simultaneous channel ulcerations in the gastric antrum. Reflux esophagitis and gastroesophageal stricture may later develop in these patients. It is apparent that some gastric ulcers are similar in etiology to duodenal ulcers, while others appear to be caused by some other factor as yet undetermined.

Investigation of the patient with presumed peptic ulcer disease involves obtaining a careful history and physical examination, followed by the necessary laboratory tests to document and confirm the diagnosis. In most cases the history will be characteristic, although in older patients the problem may be mainly related to obstruction from previous scarring, and the question of pyloric carcinoma may thus be raised. Physical examination frequently reveals only mild to moderate tenderness in the patient with an acute peptic ulcer and nothing else. If obstruction is present at the pylorus or duodenum, a succussion splash may be present, and vomiting will have occurred intermittently. The stool and vomitus should be examined for gross and occult blood.

Laboratory tests which are useful include the gastrointestinal x-ray series, in which the esophagus, cardia, stomach and duodenum should be evaluated. Fluoroscopy will often be more useful than the plain films in revealing spasm and irritability of the duodenum. The fiberoptic gastroscope can be used in the Outpatient Department and a record of the appearance of the ulcer obtained on color film. If there is any question of malignancy, gastric washings can be obtained and Papanicolaou's stain performed (Fig. 18–10).

Gastric analysis with histalog stimulation is recommended for assessment of gastric secretion. The techniques and results in 1249 normal subjects, 1261 patients with peptic ulcer and 169 patients with gastric cancer were presented by Grossman (1963).[26] Grossman's technique is as follows:

The patient is fasted overnight. The stomach is intubated, the residual content removed and continuous suction applied for four 15-minute periods (basal secretion). Histolog is given subcutaneously in a dose of 0.5 mg per kg body weight. Aspirations are continued for four additional 15-minute periods. The concentration of free HCl is determined by titration with 0.1 N NaOH to pH of 3.5 with Topfer's indicator or a pH meter. The output of free HCl is expressed in mEq/hr in the basal and posthistalog collection periods.

Values in normal subjects and patients are summarized in Table 18–3. Additional data from histalog stimulation tests are presented in Wormsley and Grossman (1965).[70]

Another test in common usage is the augmented histamine test of Kay, in which maximum acid output (MAO) is measured following a dose of 0.04 mg per kg subcutaneously of histamine

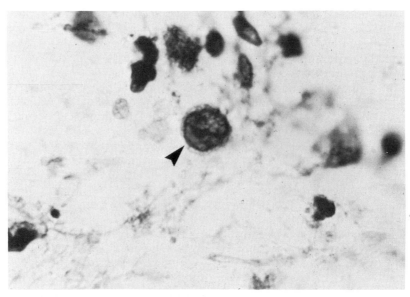

Figure 18-10 Cytologic diagnosis of gastric malignancy. Cancer was positively diagnosed on the basis of the Papanicolaou smear shown here of gastric wastings. Patient had previously had gastric ulcer which had healed slowly, but epigastric distress persisted and washings were therefore obtained. At exploration, reticulum cell sarcoma was found and patient has remained well 18 months following total gastrectomy.

phosphate. These patients should be premedicated with 50 mg mepyramine maleate 20 minutes before histamine is administered. Correlation of MAO with density of parietal cells per unit area was shown by Myren (1968).[45] In 84 patients with duodenal ulcer, he found a mean MAO of 32 mEq/hr (range 10–70). In 19 patients with gastric ulcer, MAO was 15 mEq/hr, and in 12 patients with gastric cancer, MAO was 6.5 mEq/hr.

The medical management of peptic ulcer disease has changed relatively

TABLE 18-3   GASTRIC SECRETION OF FREE ACID (mEq/hr)*

	BASAL MEAN	UPPER LIMIT OF NORMAL (ULN)	HISTALOG (0.5 mg/kg) MEAN	UPPER LIMIT OF NORMAL (ULN)
CONTROL SUBJECTS				
Men	2.44	6.6	11.64	24.3
Women	1.33	4.1	7.53	15.9
DUODENAL ULCER		% above ULN		% above ULN
Men	5.29	28	19.91	36
Women	2.87	25	13.42	31
GASTRIC ULCER		% above ULN		% above ULN
Men	1.45	5	9.68	7
Women	1.00	5	6.95	12
GASTRIC CANCER		% above ULN		% above ULN
Men	0.45	1	3.25	0
Women	0.16	0	1.46	0

*Adapted from tables in Grossman (1963)

little in the past two decades. The basic elements are: antacids, anticholinergics and sedatives; bland diet with frequent feedings; elimination of tobacco and alcohol; and correction of underlying psychological stress, if it can be identified. I prefer Maalox or Gelusil for antacid (30 ml four times daily, between meals); Maalox causes loose bowel movements, whereas Gelusil is slightly constipating. Tincture of belladonna provides a useful means of titrating anticholinergic activity. It is begun with a dose of eight drops three times daily, one-half hour before meals. The dose is increased by two drops every two days until blurring of vision or dryness of the mouth indicate that the maximum tolerable dose has been reached. Phenobarbital, 15 mg three or four times daily, is a safe and inexpensive sedative. Many patients prefer Donnatal, as a combination of barbiturate and anticholingergic. A convenient bland diet of six equal feedings for outpatient use is shown below:

Surgery for peptic ulcer disease has been recommended for relatively liberal indications during the past decade or two, since the operations have become less radical and the results of surgery have been generally satisfactory. Subtotal gastrectomy produces excellent control of peptic ulcer disease but frequently causes weight loss and other untoward symptoms, particularly the "dumping syndrome." On the other hand, vagotomy and a drainage procedure will produce a satisfactory result in approximately 90 per cent of patients, and the mortality and morbidity are more acceptable than that resulting from subtotal gastrectomy. The results of vagotomy and drainage in 436 patients reported by Whittaker (1967)[67] are typical of many large series. He reported an operative mortality of 2.2 per cent, a recurrent ulcer rate of 5 per cent, reoperations in 1.1 per cent, and a satisfactory result in 91 per cent of patients.

The operation performed is selected

*Six Meal Bland Diet**

Six meals of equal size are eaten during the day, as follows:

Breakfast
  Bananas and cream
  Soft boiled egg (1)
  Toast, butter and jelly (1 piece)
  Coffee (4 oz) with cream and sugar

Midmorning
  Cream of wheat with sugar and cream
  Custard
  Milk (8 oz)

Noon
  Cream soup
  Chicken
  Baked potato with butter
  Ice cream
  Milk (4 oz)

Midafternoon
  Egg nog (8 oz)
  Jello with cream (total 4 oz)
  Cookies (4)

Supper
  Hamburger (¼ lb)
  Baked potato
  Buttered peas
  Milk (4 oz)
  Canned peach half

Evening
  Cream soup (4 oz)
  Milkshake (8 oz)
  Sandwich: cream cheese and jelly

Substitution for variety: eggs may be poached, scrambled or served as omelet; other tender, lean meats may be used; other refined cereals are permitted such as rice, noodles, macaroni, spaghetti, melba toast, rusk and zweiback; well-cooked vegetables such as carrots, beets, squash; also ripe bananas, cooked pears, applesauce, junket, tapioca, plain cake and milk toast.

Vitamin supplement must be taken daily. This diet is deficient in vitamin C.

Alcohol, coffee and tea are prohibited on this diet.

*Adapted from Moore, F. D.: *Metabolic Care of the Surgical Patient*. Philadelphia, W. B. Saunders Co., 1959, p. 933.

by the surgeon on the basis of his experience and the findings present at surgery. It appears that vagotomy and pyloroplasty is the easiest and least hazardous operation, but the recurrence rate following this operation is probably somewhat higher than that following vagotomy and antrectomy. Antrectomy as performed in most institutions is simply a distal 30 to 50 per cent gastrectomy. Although techniques are available to identify the antrum by pH measurements, they are rarely used in clinical practice. The alternative operation of vagotomy and gastroenterostomy is rarely used in the United States because of the relatively high incidence of stomal ulcer. Gastroenterostomy alone does have an important role in the treatment of the elderly patient with a chronically obstructed gastric outlet from previous peptic ulcer disease, who has low gastric acidity. The surgeon must be certain that gastric carcinoma has not developed, however, before he performs the gastroenterostomy.

There seems to be little indication for subjecting a patient to several years of antacids and multiple frequent meals, and there now is little reason to insist that a patient suffer two or three serious complications before ulcer surgery is undertaken. Indeed, it is now appropriate to offer pyloroplasty and vagotomy as treatment for many patients at the time of their first major complication (Fig. 18–11), especially if they have had a definite history of ulcer disease for several months or years, and have been unable to control the symptoms on reasonable medical management.

The evaluation of a patient who presents with acute pain can be complex, and occasionally it is impossible to determine preoperatively whether or not the patient has a perforated ulcer. The rigid, "boardlike" abdomen and absent peristalsis are sometimes present from diseases such as pulmonary embolism (Fig. 18–12), while on the other hand, perforated ulcer does not always produce free air in the subdiaphragmatic areas (Fig. 18–13).

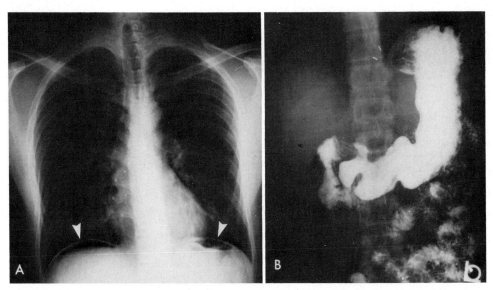

Figure 18–11   Perforated duodenal ulcer with free air. Thirty-two year old transient laborer. Ulcer symptoms for many years. Acute onset of abdominal pain, rigid abdomen, no peristalsis. Upright chest film *(A)* taken three hours after onset of pain shows free air under left and right diaphragm (arrows). Small gas bubble in stomach is inferior and medial to subdiaphragmatic collection. Patient underwent immediate operation (pyloroplasty and vagotomy) and had an uneventful course. GI series seven weeks later *(B)* shows normal gastric emptying, and typical cloverleaf post-pyloroplasty deformity of antrum and pylorus.

Figure 18–12 Pulmonary embolus causing "acute abdomen." Forty-six year old man with past history of active duodenal ulcer one year previously and fracture of patella three months previously. Acute onset of severe abdominal pain, rigidity and mild dyspnea. No peristalsis. Upright chest x-ray normal *(A)*. After some debate among attending physicians, patient was not operated upon. Symptoms persisted, rales developed, and right basilar infiltrate appeared in 48 hours *(B)*. Pulmonary angiogram *(C)* at 1.75 seconds demonstrated major occlusion in right main pulmonary artery and distal occlusions in branches of left pulmonary artery. Inferior vena cava plication was performed. Abdominal symptoms and signs slowly subsided.

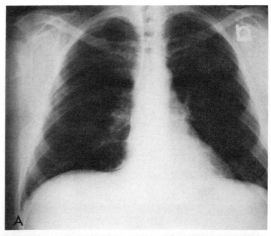

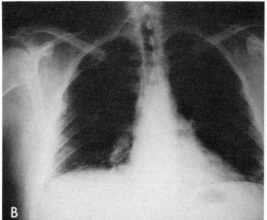
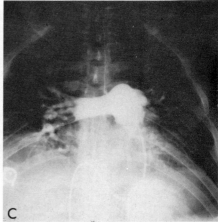

Acute upper gastrointestinal bleeding is likewise not necessarily due to a peptic ulcer, even in patients with a long history of a peptic ulcer. Erosive gastritis, esophageal varices or a Mallory-Weiss ulcer may be present, and the surgeon must be thoughtful as he prepares his patient for operation. Ideally, the patient should be tested with a Sengstaken tube and undergo gastroesophagoscopy and an upper gastrointestinal x-ray series before he has an emergency laparotomy. The surgeon must be prepared to deal with these and other, less common, causes of acute upper gastrointestinal hemorrhage. Yet delay is sometimes fatal, since irreversible shock, transfusion reactions, hepatic or renal decompensation may be the result. And it

should be remembered that steady bleeding in the patient over age 60 is unlikely to stop without surgery. A good rule for emergency operation is that after the deficit is replaced, if more than 500 ml of blood is required every eight hours to maintain stability, surgery is indicated.

The virulent ulcer diathesis caused by Zollinger-Ellison tumors may be suspected on the basis of repeated episodes of ulceration and high acid outputs. These patients should be prepared for total gastrectomy, since this is the operation which will be necessary unless the primary tumor is found and all tumor can be completely resected. Surgical exploration of the pancreas will usually reveal the primary tumor, but metastases

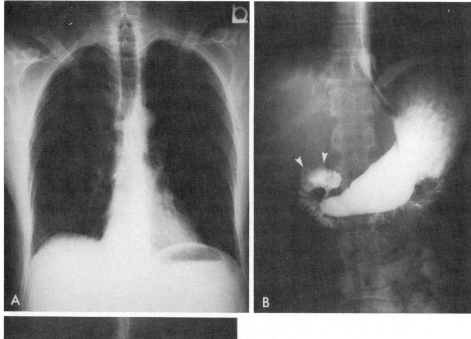

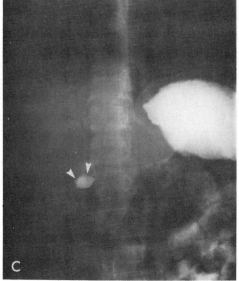

Figure 18–13 Perforated duodenal ulcer—no free air. Fifty-two year old businessman with well-documented past history of peptic ulcer disease and previous myocardial infarctions. Developed acute epigastric pain, hypotension, arrhythmia. Upright chest film showed no free air on two occasions *(A)*. EKG's showed changes consistent with new infarction. After 12 hours, blood pressure was declining and pain was worse. Upper GI series with Gastrografin showed apparent leak (arrow) from duodenum *(B)*, confirmed on film taken 30 minutes later *(C)* (arrow). He underwent immediate laparotomy, plication of perforation into lesser sac, and had an uneventful postoperative course.

or multiple tumors may be present when the patient is first seen.[10]

Gastritis may occur as a mild irritative lesion of the gastric mucosa, or it may be ulcerative, with bleeding or even perforation. The causes appear to be similar to the causes of peptic ulceration, but an underlying event or medication is usually involved as well. Com-mon presentations in the Outpatient Department include pain (similar to that of acute duodenal ulcer), or bleeding, which may be mild to massive. Among the commonest inciting causes are ingestion of alcohol, other drugs, severe stress, major burns and increased intracerebral pressure. Gastritis may appear as a consequence of acute, excessive ingestion of alcohol or in chronic intemperate usage of alcohol—the mechanism postulated being diminished conjugation of endogenous histamine by the intoxicated or cirrhotic liver, leading to locally increased concentrations of this gastric secretagogue. The four other common toxic compounds which at present are significant causes of gastritis are: corticosteroids, aspirin, phenylbutazone (Butazolidin), and indomethacin (Indocin). Acute hemorrhagic gastric ulcerations due to burns (Curling's ulcer) or cerebral pressure (Cusing's ulcer) are not commonly seen in outpatients. The treatment for acute hemorrhagic gastritis is not completely satisfactory. Hospitalization is required, and iced saline lavage is usually tried initially. Most severe cases are operated upon because bleeding fails to cease, and procedures utilized include vagotomy with pyloroplasty or antrectomy, subtotal gastrectomy, or total gastrectomy. In most cases the diagnosis is made at surgery performed for massive bleeding—after negative gastrointestinal series and unsatisfactory gastroscopy have been obtained. In mild or self-limited cases, the diagnosis is made at gastroscopy, and the gastrointestinal series is normal. No patients have survived total gastrectomy for acute hemorrhagic gastritis at Colorado General Hospital, so our preferred surgical treatment at the present time is vagotomy with a drainage procedure.

Adenocarcinoma of the stomach is declining in frequency in the United States, but it is still a major concern in every patient who has a gastric ulcer which does not heal promptly and completely by medical therapy, and in patients who have low gastric acidity. Patients with pernicious anemia commonly have anacidity and a high incidence of carcinoma of the stomach. Other cancers of the stomach include lymphocytic lymphosarcoma, reticulum cell sarcoma, leiomyosarcoma and carcinoid tumors. The most common benign tumor is leiomyoma, which may be grossly and microscopically identical to leiomyosarcoma, except that the malignant variant is larger and metastasizes. All cancers of the stomach may present in the same way, with bleeding, dyspepsia, weight loss, perforation, obstruction, or by signs of metastases in distant locations. Although many patients with adenocarcinoma of the stomach present with advanced disease, guarded optimism is appropriate for specific categories of patients.[24] Favorable indications include: symptoms for more than three years, gross resectability, tumor less than 4.0 cm in diameter, and negative lymph nodes. "Curative" resections have a 25 per cent five-year survival and even "palliative" resections for carcinoma of the stomach have a 5 per cent five-year survival. Occasionally a small gastric carcinoma may be overlooked in a patient with large "Krukenberg" metastases to the ovaries. Therefore, bilateral ovarian adenocarcinoma should stimulate a search for a primary tumor in the upper gastrointestinal tract.

Giant hypertrophic "gastritis" (Menetrier's disease) may simulate tumor in its presentation. This condition is one in which large folds of gastric mucosa develop, secreting mucus and causing symptoms of partial or intermittent gastric obstruction. The x-ray is similar to that for lymphosarcoma of the stomach, but a skilled gastroscopist will recognize the lesion without difficulty. The patient may be depleted by loss of water, protein and electrolytes from the hypertrophic mucosa. The treatment is surgical, usually with a sleeve resection of the involved portion of the stomach.

Bezoars may cause obstruction and discomfort or perforation. Foreign bodies may be ingested accidentally or deliberately by children and may occasionally need to be removed surgically (Chapter 23). Psychotic patients will often swallow large masses of objects, and dozens are sometimes removed by gastrotomy. Fruit pulp bezoars are seen in raw citrus fruit eaters who have undergone a gastrojejunostomy or pyloroplasty; and obstruction, perforation and death have been recorded in such patients.

Other duodenal diseases which are amenable to surgical correction include adenocarcinoma and sarcoma — both of which are rare — annular or ectopic pancreas, malrotation, benign tumors, superior mesenteric artery compression (Wilkie's disease), and post-traumatic or postoperative fistula. Duodenal diverticulum is a relatively common condition, but rarely produces complications which require operation.

Duodenal trauma is a common sequela of severe blunt trauma, especially from automobile accidents. Retroperitoneal rupture must be considered in all such patients, even when peristalsis remains present. The presence of blood in the stomach or air in the retroperitoneal tissues should lead to strong suspicion of this lesion. The temptation is to assume that the blood was due to facial trauma and was swallowed by the patient, and that the little air bubbles present on x-ray really aren't extraluminal. However, when the question has seriously been raised, it is best simply to perform an exploratory laparotomy and inspect the entire retroperitoneal duodenum.[9,53] Gastric trauma is easier to diagnose, since the stomach is usually injured only by violent force or penetrating injury, in which case exploratory operation is obviously indicated. The injury to the stomach is usually visible, since the stomach is anteriorly located and not retroperitoneal like the duodenum.

Preparation for elective surgery of the stomach and duodenum is ordinarily performed as an inpatient. It should be remembered that large fungating gastric cancers may be infected with clostridium and other anaerobes. If cancer is suspected in a patient with achlorhydria, preoperative oral antibiotics or dilute hydrochloric acid solutions are indicated. The elderly patient with a chronic obstructing ulcer and a distended stomach should not be expected to "open up," and thereby avoid the need for surgery. This kind of patient should be intubated for the few days required for preoperative preparation. Intubation serves to decompress the stomach, reducing the danger of aspiration and allowing the stomach to regain some of its normal tone. Preparation is mainly directed at restoration of a normal metabolic state, correcting the hypochloremic, hypokalemic alkalosis which is usually present. When proper metabolic balance is restored, a simple gastroenterostomy is often all that is required.

Syndromes following surgery of the stomach and duodenum may be challenging for the outpatient surgeon, since the technical details of the operation and the psychological characteristics of the patient often play an intermingling role in the illness. Occasionally the problem may be solved by a gastrointestinal series, which may demonstrate partial stomal obstruction or a twisted afferent or efferent loop. But it should be remembered that stomal (marginal) ulcer may be difficult to visualize on GI series, and may be recognized only by its side effects such as pain, bleeding, or — rarely — perforation and abscess, or gastrojejuno colic fistula. It may be necessary to re-explore the patient if a significant question regarding marginal ulcer arises, since these ulcers cannot necessarily be seen even with fiberoptic gastroscopy. Bile reflux gastritis is a recognized complication of gastrectomy or pyloroplasty, and if significant enough, corrective surgery may be required.

Evaluation of postvagotomy symptoms should include a Hollander test, which is the insulin stimulatory test for vagal function. In the presence of an intact vagal nerve, administration of insulin will stimulate release of gastric acid. The test requires that adequate hypoglycemia be obtained and that the patient be able to form gastric acid, since an *increase* in acid is measured in the test. The Hollander test is the best test for an intact cephalic phase of digestion and can be performed in the Outpatient Department if trained personnel are available to watch for symptoms of hypoglycemia, so that glucose can be given promptly to reverse the symptoms. Hollander's test (1946) is performed as follows:

A light diet is given the previous day. The patient is fasted overnight. A Levin tube is swallowed without water. Regular insulin (15 units) is administered intravenously after aspiration of the stomach for basal sample and collection of basal blood sugar specimen. Stomach is aspirated every 15 minutes and blood sugar specimen is obtained every 30 minutes for 2 hours. Specimens are analyzed for free (pH less than 3.5) and total (pH less than 7.0) acid. A *positive* test is a well-defined rise in free acid, in a patient who is capable of making free acid. The blood sugar must fall to 50 mg per cent or less in order to constitute an adequate stimulus for the cephalic phase of digestion.

In Hollander's series, 84 per cent of all duodenal ulcer patients studied had positive tests prior to surgery. Ninety-eight per cent of duodenal ulcer patients who had free acid *and* an adequate fall in blood sugar had a positive test preoperatively. Fifty-two per cent of patients who had bilateral vagotomy were negative two weeks postoperatively, and most of the other vagotomized patients had equivocal tests (inadequate fall in blood sugar or no free acid, and so on).

The "dumping syndrome" is a complication of gastric or duodenal surgery which is characterized by varying degrees of nausea, warmth, light headedness, bloating and diarrhea. Some patients may describe syncope, vertigo, headache, tachycardia or palpitations, sweating, flushing or pallor, and abdominal cramps. The syndrome occurs to a mild degree in about 10 per cent of patients who have been operated upon for peptic ulcers. In about 75 per cent of these patients the symptoms can be controlled with diet alone, and only 1 per cent will require additional corrective surgery.[29] Severe dumping is rarely a complication of vagotomy and pyloroplasty, and is more commonly a complication of gastrectomy after a Billroth II anastomosis than after a Billroth I anastomosis. It occurs with increasing frequency in patients with extensive gastric resection and in those with large anastomotic stomas.

The etiology appears to be due to rapid transit of undigested, hyperosmotic food into the small bowel, where it rapidly draws fluid into the intestinal lumen, lowering blood volume 5 to 10 per cent and raising intraluminal pressures. The condition is exacerbated by large meals, carbohydrates and liquid taken with meals. Milk and candy may be very badly tolerated by these patients. Reactive hypoglycemia has been implicated in some patients as the cause of late postprandial symptoms. Recently, deficiency in intestinal lactase activity has been described as the cause of dumping due to ingestion of milk.

Dietary treatment consists of frequent feedings of small, dry meals with high protein intake, and carbohydrates of 100 gm or less initially. Fluids are not to be ingested for one hour after eating, and patients are encouraged to lie down for a half hour or so after meals. In more difficult cases, tranquilizers, barbiturates, anticholenergic drugs and serotonin antagonists may be indicated (e.g., chlorpromazine, phenobarbital, belladonna, and cyproheptadine, respectively). Narcotics should be avoided, although Lomotil may be used on a temporary basis until control is achieved with diet and other drugs, or until the patient is being prepared for operation.

Surgical correction usually consists of revision of the stoma, conversion from Billroth II to Billroth I or vice versa, or interposition of an antiperistaltic segment of jejunum. The patient should not be allowed to become physically and emotionally crippled before reoperation is undertaken.

Spleen

Splenectomy is performed for a number of reasons and is virtually the only operation performed on the spleen. Few patients are subjected to long-term evaluation by surgeons prior to splenectomy, for elective splenectomy is usually recommended only after a thorough evaluation by a competent hematologist. The surgeon's major responsibility is to assess the risks and determine that the patient is in optimum condition for the operation. The four major indications for splenectomy at present are: hypersplenism, diagnostic evaluation, pain and trauma.

Hypersplenism is produced by any disease which causes enlargement of the spleen, including lymphosarcoma and storage diseases. If the disease is a transient one, such as malaria or mononucleosis, splenectomy is usually not indicated. But if hypersplenism becomes a major continuing problem, splenectomy may be indicated even if the spleen is not enlarged on physical examination. Hypersplenism is recognized by increased rate of hemolysis of red cells, leukopenia and thrombocytopenia. Patients with idiopathic thrombocytopenic purpura are greatly improved or cured by splenectomy in up to 50 per cent of cases. Splenectomy cures the anemia and symptoms of hereditary spherocytosis, although the underlying abnormality in the red cell membrane is unchanged. Hypersplenism in rheumatoid arthritis (Felty's syndrome) is a well-established indication for operation.[49,56]

Pain or discomfort is usually not the major indication for splenectomy, but it frequently is the deciding factor for this operation in patients with gigantic splenomegaly, as in lymphoma. And it may be the clue to splenic injury which leads to operation. Pain may be in the area of the spleen, or—when bleeding has occurred—it will be referred to the left shoulder.

Splenectomy for diagnostic purposes has recently been utilized in the staging of lymphomas and Hodgkin's disease. The efficacy of the procedure in clarifying the stage cannot be questioned seriously, but the safety and ultimate benefit to the patient must still be regarded as under investigation.[17] Occasionally, long-term remissions have been reported following splenectomy for lymphosarcoma.[35]

Trauma is the indication for most emergency splenectomies. The spleen is easily injured, and even a small laceration of the capsule or tear at the splenic pedicle will usually be treated better by splenectomy than by sutures or pressure in the faint hope that bleeding will stop. Patients who have blood loss from abdominal injuries should have the spleen examined carefully regardless of the nature and location of the injury, since force is so easily transmitted to this delicate organ. One of the most common indications for splenectomy is, sadly, a small laceration in the splenic capsule or short gastric vessels during the performance of hiatus herniorraphy or vagotomy.[48]

Other indications for splenectomy or procedures on the spleen include its resection during radical surgery on the stomach, left kidney and adrenal, and colon. It is removed in the course of a distal or total pancreatectomy, and as a part of the classic splenorenal shunt for portal hypertension. The spleen is removed in preparation for renal transplantation in some hospitals, and splenic homotransplantation has been attempted in a few patients in treatment of hemophilia, since factor VIII (antihemophiliac globulin) is apparently manufactured in the spleen. The usefulness of splenic transplantation is still unproved, since all of these patients are believed to have died in the early postoperative course.

Splenic needle biopsy and splenoportography have frequently been performed in some hospitals, and would technically be possible on an outpatient basis. But the operating room and a surgical team should be prepared for the possibility of bleeding and should be ready for an emergency splenectomy in every instance.

Diagnostic dilemmas include the left upper quadrant discomfort of patients with rapidly enlarging spleens in malaria and infectious mononucleosis, and the possibility of delayed rupture of the spleen following trauma. While it is true that accidental rupture of the spleen during trivial trauma has been reported in these conditions, the incidence is apparently very low. For this reason, left upper quadrant discomfort in such patients is not an indication for immediate splenectomy. The problem of "delayed post-traumatic rupture" of the spleen is a troublesome one which may require considerable judgment to anticipate. Furious bleeding may occur from a spleen 10 to 14 days after injury, but in most cases there has been premonitory evidence of injury through a fall in hematocrit and evidence of hemoperitoneum or fractured ribs.

The late sequelae of splenectomy are relatively minor in most cases. Failure to clear the aging blood cells can be recognized in the peripheral smear of otherwise normal patients who have undergone splenectomy. Transient elevation in platelet count may produce alarm when the count exceeds 1 million per cm, and such patients should usually be anticoagulated for a few weeks, initially with heparin, followed by warfarin. These are often the same patients who are observed after splenectomy for late complications of subphrenic abscess, pulmonary embolus or splenic vein thrombosis. The outpatient surgeon must be aware of these ominous complications and assure himself that the patient is in good health before final release from follow-up. Among children with storage diseases who have undergone splenectomy for hypersplenism, there is an increased incidence of untimely death from septicemia. Recently, several medical centers have also suggested that significant morbidity and mortality from infection may be a problem after "staging" laparotomy for Hodgkin's disease.

Pancreas

Pancreatic disease most commonly is manifested to the surgeon in the form of pain—epigastric, periumbilical or back pain in most cases. Pancreatitis (acute or chronic), traumatic injury to the pancreas, adenocarcinoma of the pancreas, abscess and pseudocyst are the most common surgical conditions of the pancreas in adults. Other conditions, less commonly seen, are ectopic pancreas, islet cell adenoma and pancreatic exocrine insufficiency following pancreatectomy. Diabetes mellitus is a disease of the pancreas that has considerable medical significance, but the surgeon is ordinarily involved with its manifestations in other organs. Recently, however, pancreatic homotransplantation has been tried and may be of benefit in the future for patients with severe complications of diabetes (see Chapter 24).

Acute edematous pancreatitis may mimic almost any other disease of the upper abdomen, but classically it presents with midabdominal pain and tenderness, fever, elevation in the serum amylase and cessation of peristalsis. Predisposing causes include gallstones, alcohol ingestion, mumps, penetrating peptic ulcer (Fig. 18–14), or a large meal.[40] In Howard's series (1960) of 371 patients, 50 per cent of pancreatitis was due to gallstones, 25 per cent to alcoholism, 5 per cent was secondary to surgical operations, and the etiology was undetermined in 20 per cent of cases. The disease is also seen with increased frequency in patients with chronic renal disease, in cases of homotransplantation, and in patients on high doses of corticosteroids. In these conditions, diagnosis may be more difficult because serum amylase may be elevated by decreased renal clearance. Regardless of the apparent benignity of the illness, acute pancreatitis should be considered an insidious, potentially fatal illness, and immediate hospitalization is imperative. The initial treatment should begin in the outpatient area with insertion of a nasogastric tube and institution of intravenous fluids. The loss of plasma into the abdomen may be exceedingly rapid, and untreated patients may show signs of hypotension or dehydration within only a few hours. The diagnosis is rarely certain until recovery has begun— usually within four to seven days, and during this period of time other abdominal catastrophies are still possible in the differential diagnosis—even in the

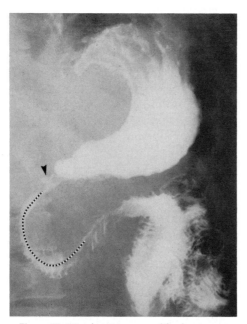

Figure 18–14 Acute pancreatitis due to penetrating duodenal ulcer. Patient presented with acute epigastric pain, nausea, jaundice and silent abdomen. Developed fever, required colloid and electrolytes solutions to maintain blood pressure. GI series showed penetrating ulcer (arrow) and wide "C" loop of 1st, 2nd and 3rd portions of duodenum (dotted line). Amylase 71, bilirubin 11.1. At laparotomy, extensive peripancreatic inflammation and fat necrosis was present, and presence of ulcer was confirmed. Drains were placed along pancreas and T-tube in common duct. He gradually improved and recovered completely.

presence of an elevation in serum amylase. The role of early diagnostic laparotomy has been increasingly emphasized in recent years because the mortality rate from pancreatitis has not been increased by exploratory laparotomy,[18] and other causes of the acute abdomen may thereby be diagnosed and treated appropriately. The overall mortality from acute edematous pancreatitis is approximately 5 per cent.

Acute hemorrhagic pancreatitis is a more serious manifestation of acute pancreatitis. It may be rapidly fatal, or it may have a protracted course leading to slough of the pancreas and delayed recovery, or death from retroperitoneal abscess and hemorrhage. The mortality rates reported range from 50 to 100 per

cent. The antecedent causes and treatment are the same as for acute edematous pancreatitis, although surgical intervention is usually justified to confirm the diagnosis and to remove the necrotic organ.[18] The amylase may or may not be elevated, but hemorrhagic ascites and shock are common.

Chronic relapsing pancreatitis may occur after one or more episodes of acute pancreatitis in some unfortunate individuals, who develop recurrent episodes of abdominal pain similar to acute pancreatitis, but without alterations in fluids and electrolytes and without signs of life-threatening illness. Many of these patients are alcoholics and chronic users of tranquilizing and narcotic drugs; the cause and effect relationships are unclear, but it is believed that alcoholism predisposes to this type of pancreatitis. Amylase elevation may occur with episodes of pain. Stippled pancreatic calcification becomes apparent through deposits of calcium soaps on the surface of the pancreas and stones in the pancreatic ducts. It is the responsibility of the outpatient surgeon to recognize this disease and identify the patients, usually with x-rays of the abdomen that are examined carefully for pancreatic calcification. Preoperative work-up includes a GI series and small bowel follow-through, with cross-table lateral films to search for pseudocyst. The patients should also have an oral cholecystogram (and possibly an IV cholangiogram) so a search can be made for biliary tract calculi or postinflammatory obstruction of the sphincter of Oddi and ampulla of Vater. After these studies have been obtained, it is appropriate to admit the patient for definitive pancreatic exploration, operative duct sialography, and appropriate surgical repair or pancreatectomy.

Traumatic pancreatitis may occur with blunt or penetrating trauma, and the force required is usually sufficient to lead to suspicion of severe intra-abdominal trauma. Hospitalization is indicated. However, the late sequelae of abscess and pseudocyst may be apparent only following discharge, and they present a difficult problem in the clinic. Early operation for abscess is important, for a small duodenal leak may be the cause of this lesion. Pancreatic pseudocyst is best operated upon after it has fully matured, and delay is indicated if the patient's condition will tolerate postponement. If the diagnosis is uncertain, hospitalization for close observation is indicated.

Adenocarcinoma of the pancreas is an increasingly common and highly fatal malignancy. Only 1 to 2 per cent of patients with carcinoma of the pancreas survive for five years. Early carcinomas of the ampulla of Vater, which present with jaundice and occult bleeding, are said to have a 33 per cent cure rate from radical pancreaticoduodenectomy (Whipple operation). Adenocarcinomas of the head, body and tail of the pancreas have a dismal prognosis in spite of partial or total pancreatectomy. The mortality for the radical operation is high, and metastases may become apparent soon after surgery, so the ideal therapy has not yet been determined. Nevertheless, the patient suspected of carcinoma of the pancreas should be admitted for thorough evaluation. A needle biopsy of the liver will frequently demonstrate incurability, and no further operation is then required unless biliary or gastric obstruction develops. Appropriate studies include evaluation of the C–loop of the duodenum (first, second and third portions) on GI series, liver function tests, and stool fat assays. Conflicting opinions regarding radical versus conservative operations have been expressed by Crile (1970)[14] and Hicks and Brooks (1971).[30] Crile cites a longer survival rate for patients undergoing a bypass operation than for those undergoing a standard Whipple operation. Hicks and Brooks emphasize the importance of total, rather than subtotal, pancreatectomy in order to remove intrapancreatic metastases.

Hormone-producing tumors of the pancreas include islet cell adenomas (insulin or glucagon), Zollinger-Ellison tumors (gastrin), and carcinoids (serotonin). The diagnosis of these neoplasms is usually made because of their peripheral symptoms, which may be of long-standing duration prior to surgery. The presence of Whipple's triad (hypoglycemia, symptoms of hypoglycemia when the blood sugar is low, and correction of the symptoms by raising the blood sugar) should lead to a study for islet cell tumor. The study should include selective arteriography, which has been increasingly useful in identifying these tumors and may be an important guide to resection of all suspicious areas of the pancreas. In the presence of recurring episodes of hypoglycemia with syncope or psychosis, exploration of the pancreas may be indicated, even in the absence of a positive tumor blush on arteriography.

Zollinger-Ellison tumors should be suspected in every patient with a virulent ulcer diathesis or recurrent ulcers with high acid production. Unfortunately, many of these patients present such urgent situations that proper acid and arteriography studies are precluded. It is therefore a responsibility of the outpatient surgeon to think of the problem and request the appropriate studies when seeing a patient with a severe or recurrent peptic ulcer. Glucagon-secreting adenomas are unusual, but should be suspected in patients with diabetes mellitus which is unresponsive to therapy. Carcinoid tumors of the pancreas may present all of the manifestations of other carcinoids. All of the functioning pancreatic adenomas may be relatively slow-growing, and repeated resection of metastases may be indicated to control symptoms on a palliative basis.

Postoperative management of the pancreatectomized patient presents relatively little difficulty in insulin regulation, even if total pancreatectomy has been performed. The patients can usually be managed as mild diabetics, with 30 to 50 units of regular and NPH insulin per day, administered by test with observation of urine sugars. They are usually well-regulated by the time they leave the hospital, but should be rechecked at clinic visits. The exocrine management of the patient with ductal obstruction from pancreatic carcinoma or with a total pancreatectomy is sometimes a greater problem, and requires considerable patience to manage. Several preparations of pancreatic extract are available, including pork pancrelipase ("Cotazym") and beef pancreatin ("Viokase"). Some patients will be better managed with either one or the other. Tablets are taken in large amounts— up to 40 to 50 per day, and may be spaced as desired by the patients (2 to 10 with each meal, or 2 to 4 every hour when awake). The control of steatorrhea is an easily recognizable guide to the dosage.

Esophagus

The terminal, intra-abdominal portion of the esophagus is of concern in the differential diagnosis of abdominal complaints, for it may be the seat of a variety of conditions presenting as pain, dysphagia, bleeding or shock. These and other aspects of esophageal problems are also discussed in Chapter 15.

The most common problems of the distal esophagus are caused by hiatus hernia. Regurgitation of acid and interference with normal peristalsis may cause ulceration and fibrosis. The initial symptoms may be substernal discomfort and "waterbrash" regurgitation, although the patient may present with weakness from anemia and occult GI bleeding may be found. Later, persistent "burning" discomfort may be noted, followed by inability to pass solid food into the stomach. Occasionally a startling presentation occurs when a patient has swallowed a large piece of meat which completely fails to pass the cardio-esophageal junction. The diagnosis should then be confirmed by barium esophagram. The obstruction may be relieved with ingestion of a teaspoon of papain paste (prepared from proteinase from Carica papaya), or household meat

tenderizer mixed in water, taken every hour for four to six hours. Proteolytic treatment should only be used if the obstructing bolus is known to be meat alone, without bone. Impacted meat containing bone fragments should be removed carefully through the esophagoscope. Esophagoscopy should later be performed in all cases to rule out carcinoma. Medical therapy for hiatus hernia may preclude surgery, if it is instituted before irreversible stricture has occurred. The treatment consists of elevation of the head of the bed on 6-inch blocks of wood, a bland diet, and antacids. Esophageal dilatation may restore a narrow esophagus to a satisfactory lumen, and may be attempted before scheduling elective esophageal reconstruction. Bougies are also useful in postoperative treatment, if a too-snug hiatus herniorraphy has been performed. The Hurst (mercury-filled) bougies are generally the safest and most useful for outpatient treatment.

Other problems which present with symptoms similar to hiatus hernia include the following conditions, which can usually be distinguished on a barium esophagram: megaesophagus and achalasia (failure of the cardioesophageal junction to open properly during swallowing); chalasia (a congenital defect producing free gastroesophageal reflux); scleroderma (a leathery ineffective esophagus, associated with other aspects of this collagen disease); and chronic stricture from lye ingestion. The indications for surgery and the results of operations in these conditions have been reviewed in Chapter 15 and additional information can be obtained from Rees, 1970.[52]

Bleeding from the esophagus may range from massive to minimal, even when due to varicose veins of portal hypertension. But every clinic surgeon should have at hand an esophageal balloon such as the Sengstaken tube. This tube should be *immediately* inserted, filled and positioned as both a diagnostic aid and a therapeutic maneuver when a patient appears vomiting massive amounts of blood.

Rupture of the esophagus may be either insidious or obvious. The most common cause is endoscopic instrumentation or dilatation, and for this reason it should be a particular concern of the outpatient surgeon. In these cases it is frequently a localized perforation which initially causes only discomfort and a low grade fever. The diagnosis should be confirmed by esophagram with a water soluble contrast medium (e.g., Gastrografin). Free perforation is usually a devastating event and should lead to immediate hospitalization. Rupture may be caused by strenuous vomiting (Mallory-Weiss laceration), blunt or penetrating trauma to the chest or upper abdomen, carcinoma (which may be either adenocarcinoma of the stomach or squamous carcinoma of the distal esophagus), or it may be idiopathic. A localized mediastinal abscess which occurs after perforation during esophageal dilatation may not require immediate surgery, but *must* be observed in the hospital. Free perforation into the chest or mediastinum obviously requires immediate drainage, and usually a resection or repair.

Small Intestine

Disease of the small intestine must be suspected or recognized by the surgeon, but there is little which he can do on a definitive basis for it in the Outpatient Clinic. Some conditions require immediate or urgent surgery—these are usually obvious, in cases where complete obstruction, volvulus, perforation or peritonitis are apparent. The elderly patient may have a lethal disease of the small bowel but display relatively few abdominal findings or complaints until terminal. Mesenteric vascular disease is apt to, be insidious in many cases, except in the classic situation of rheumatic heart disease, arterial fibrillation, sudden onset of abdominal pain, and melena—the result of an embolus to the superior mesenteric artery.

Obstruction can usually be suspected in cases of distention, hyperperistalsis, crampy pain and failure to pass flatus. Vomiting may occur late in cases of low ileal obstruction, or it may occur early in jejunal obstruction, in which case distention may be absent and the abdominal plain x-ray will be of less help than a Gastrografin swallow. Jejunal obstructions are most difficult to diagnose on clinical grounds, but should be suspected in postgastrectomy patients who suddenly begin to vomit unexpectedly, or in patients with small upper abdominal hernias. A common cause of small bowel obstruction in men is an incarcerated inguinal hernia. An immediate, careful examination of the groin is indicated in all patients with distention and vomiting. In patients who have had previous abdominal surgery, intestinal adhesions are a frequent late cause of bowel obstruction. Such patients must be operated on promptly, following the useful general rule that "the sun shouldn't rise on an unoperated bowel obstruction." In-hospital management without surgery is occasionally appropriate for patients with multiple previous laparotomies for obstruction, for patients with recent surgery and incomplete obstruction, and for patients with extensive intra-abdominal tumor. These patients should have a nasogastric tube inserted without delay, and an intestinal decompressing tube (Miller-Abbot, Cantor, etc.) should be inserted later when the patient has been admitted to the hospital.

Bleeding from the GI tract may be a troublesome problem, especially if slow and intermittent. If immediate placement of a nasogastric tube rules out gastric bleeding, the insertion of a small bowel tube may be performed in the clinic. The progress and contents of the long tube should be assessed during the period of preoperative preparation. All too frequently, GI bleeding from the small bowel may cease prior to surgery, and the bleeding site may then be difficult or impossible to locate without the help of ancillary studies such as an arteriogram, or a positive aspirate from the tube. In the work-up of patients with chronic anemia of unknown etiology, with or without demonstration of occult blood in the stools, small bowel bleeding should be considered. Causes may include benign or malignant tumors (especially adenocarcinoma), or vascular malformations such as hemangioma and arteriovenous malformation.[11] In these cases, fluorescein may localize the bleeding site. The patient should be given a soft string to swallow, tied to a small washer, which is allowed to advance through the bowel until the washer is in the colon. When bleeding again occurs, 5 ml of fluorescein solution is injected intravenously. The string is then withdrawn and examined under ultraviolet light (the Woods' lamp of the dermatologist) for fluorescence. If rapid GI bleeding is occurring from an unknown source, hospitalization is obviously indicated, and a selective mesenteric arteriogram should be performed as soon as possible. We have been able to identify the source of intestinal bleeding with arteriography prior to surgery in three patients in the past 16 months (duodenal ulcer, small bowel hemangioma and sigmoid diverticulum).

Chronic disease of the small bowel may utilize surgery for diagnosis or management of complications. The most common indication for this type of surgery is regional enteritis, which should rarely require surgery for diagnosis, except when its presentation occurs during its first complication. In general, regional enteritis is a disease of slow onset and progression, in which granulomatous changes begin in the musculature, serosa and mesentery of the ileum (regional ileitis, Crohn's disease). As the disease progresses, the mucosa becomes involved with ulcerations and strictures, and manifestations may appear in the colon and proximal small bowel or stomach. Occasionally the disease first presents as either an inflammatory lesion of the colon (granulomatous colitis) or proximal gastrointestinal tract. It may also present as "burned out" disease, such as that which occurred in President Dwight Eisenhower.[34] "Skip" areas are common, so conservative surgery is indicated when operations must be performed. Approximately one third of patients who are operated upon will require no further treatment; approximately one third will continue to have intermittent symptoms, and one third will eventually develop another complication which requires surgery. The diagnosis is made by barium follow-through examination of the small bowel in patients who have crampy episodes of pain, low grade fever, weight loss and intermittent diarrhea (Fig. 18–15). If surgery is utilized for regional enteritis it should be reserved for complications resistant to medical management, including obstruction, perforation, bleeding and intractable pain associated with a palpable mass.

Other chronic diseases of the small bowel may be diagnosed by laparotomy; these include Whipple's disease, sprue and lymphosarcoma. The increased effectiveness and safety of transoral small bowel biopsy with a tube has rendered many of these operations unnecessary. Enzyme determinations have clarified the nature of many illnesses, especially chronic milk "allergy" in adults, associated with mucosal lactase deficiency.

Pneumatosis intestinalis is a condition in which air is present in the wall of the bowel. In adults it is frequently asymptomatic and is discovered incidentally during abdominal radiography performed for a variety of reasons. It is frequently associated with peptic ulcer, carcinoma of the stomach and rupture of pulmonary blebs. In children, however, it is usually caused by severe enterocolitis, which requires emergency surgery.[60]

Congenital abnormalities of the small intestine are not commonly encountered in adults. Meckel's diverticulum may be a cause of bleeding, and ectopic gastric mucosa may cause bleeding or perforation. Malrotation may present for the first time in adults, although the diag-

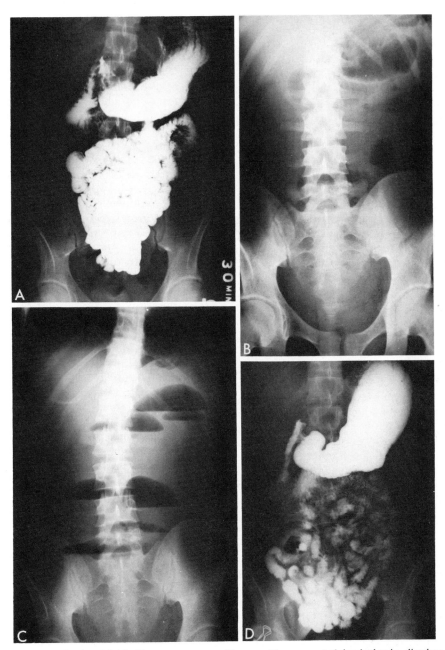

Figure 18–15   Regional ileitis. Twenty-one year old man with recurrent abdominal pain, diarrhea, and gastrointestinal x-rays characteristic of extensive regional ileitis. The typical features seen are *(A)* entrapment of the small bowel in a mass of inflammatory tissue with shortened mesentery and abnormal mucosal pattern. Small bowel transit is rapid, but entry into colon is greatly delayed. In the next five months he had several episodes of partial small bowel obstruction and finally appeared with distention and vomiting. Flat film showed only enlarged gas-filled loops of intestine *(B)*, but upright film showed the air fluid "stepladder" which is characteristic of complete small bowel obstruction *(C)*. He underwent lysis of adhesions, resection of the distal ileum, construction of an end ileostomy. He has subsequently gained weight and had only mild symptoms, which have not required hospitalization. Vitamin B-12 absorption is normal, indicating adequate function of residual ileum. Small bowel x-ray nine months postoperatively *(D)* shows increased mobility in small bowel, improved mucosal pattern, and normal transit time.

nosis can usually be suspected by the presence of other anomalies.

Recent developments in pharmacology have produced new chronic and acute diseases which must be remembered in patients with abdominal pain. These include ulceration and obstruction from enteric-coated tablets containing potassium salts[16] and mesenteric vasculitis from oral contraceptives.[43] Corticosteroid therapy has been associated with idiopathic mesenteric vasculitis (arterial and venous), causing acute or chronic GI bleeding or small bowel infarction. The majority of these patients can be identified by other signs of collagen-vascular or autoimmune disease, but occasionally idiopathic thrombophlebitis of the mesenteric vessels is the first serious indication of the presence of such diseases.[64]

During the past decade, small bowel resections and bypass operations have been proposed and tested for treatment of obesity and hypercholesterolemia. At the present time, the ileal bypass operation appears to be a useful procedure in patients with congenital hypercholesterolemia. When performed as described by Buchwald (1968),[7] it is said to produce a 40 per cent decrease in cholesterol at three months, and 61 per cent of patients have a cholesterol which decreases to less than 200 mg per cent. Ileal bypass is not without risk, since intussusception and a variety of metabolic complications have been reported from it, including B-12 deficiency anemia, gastrointestinal bleeding, and electrolyte deficiencies. Jejunal-ileostomy[57] has produced remarkable reduction in weight in patients with intractable obesity, but the bypass or "shunt" has considerable risk, especially from electrolyte depletion, and some of these patients have reportedly died from hypocalcemia, hypomagnesemia and hypokalemia. Patients proposed for operations to control obesity should be evaluated independently by the surgeon, an internist and a psychiatrist, and close, long-term follow-up is mandatory post-operatively.

Mesentery

The mesentery is rarely identified preoperatively as the primary location of disease. However, some mesenteric diseases are known which should be considered as possible causes of obscure abdominal pain, fever, gastrointestinal bleeding, and abdominal masses. The mesenteric diseases most commonly encountered are lesions of the vessels and lymph nodes. In each case, surgery is ordinarily required to confirm the diagnosis or to initiate definitive therapy.

Mesenteric arterial vascular obstruction may be acute (embolus, or thrombosis due to low arterial flow), in which case gangrene and death will ensue unless immediate surgery is performed and repair is possible. Chronic intestinal ischemia due to arteriosclerosis may cause the rare syndrome of intestinal angina (pain and nausea after meals). This diagnosis should be confirmed by selective arteriography and the disease may be alleviated by arterial reconstruction. Mesenteric venous obstruction may be insidious, and usually progresses to infarction before it is recognized. However, in patients with a history of idiopathic thrombophlebitis and hypercoagulability, the illness may be aborted by medical therapy. Treatment should be performed in the hospital, controlled with studies of coagulation parameters. It is the responsibility of the outpatient surgeon to suspect this condition and institute the measures which lead to treatment.

Mesenteric lymph nodes may be involved with a wide variety of infections and neoplasms, and are occasionally the key to the diagnosis of an obscure illness. In fever of unknown origin, for example, laparotomy should be scheduled as a part of the key studies, rather than as an afterthought when all else has failed to provide a diagnosis. Biopsy in such cases may reveal lymphosarcoma, tuberculosis, or occult carcinoma. Arrangements should be made preoperatively to obtain cultures of the nodes for routine and exotic bacteria, fungi, acid fast organisms, and viruses, if a virus laboratory is available. Frozen section should also be arranged, so that additional tissue can be removed if the pathologist suggests it.

Mesenteric adenitis is relatively uncommon in adults, and when laparotomy for appendicitis in adults reveals only this condition, a thorough laparotomy should be planned in addition to diagnostic biopsy of the nodes.

Other conditions of the mesentery which are rarely diagnosed prior to surgery include mesenteric lipoma ("lipodystrophy")[20]—a condition which may simulate aortic aneurysm because of the palpable midabdominal mass which transmits the aortic pulsation—and congenital mesenteric defects which lead to intra-abdominal hernia and bowel obstruction.

Appendix

This useless little structure has been a source of great misery for humans, and its elective removal is frequently performed in the course of uncomplicated laparotomy for a wide variety of conditions. Elective appendectomy should be discussed preoperatively with patients, and may be carried out with relatively little morbidity when the appendix is easily accessible during cholecystectomy, gastrectomy, a variety of gynecological procedures and inguinal herniorraphy. Elective appendectomy is warranted in young people who have undergone one or two episodes of illness similar to classic acute appendicitis. It is also indicated in individuals planning to spend a prolonged period in areas where surgical assistance would be unavailable. It is considered by many surgeons to be safe as an associated procedure during major vascular reconstruction, emergency surgery for abdominal trauma and colon resection. However, appendectomy in these instances is obviously more hazardous and cannot be routinely recommended at this time. The major disease of the appendix which provokes concern is, of course, acute appendicitis, but pinworm infestation, malignant carcinoid tumors, adenocarcinoma, and mucocoele with pseudomyxoma peritonei are also problems which can originate or persist in the appendix. A fecalith in the appendix is a sign of potential trouble (Fig. 18–8) and is an indication for appendectomy.[13] On the other hand, free reflux of barium into the appendix during small bowel x-ray or barium enema does not appear to be a particularly worrisome situation.

Appendicitis should be suspected in every instance of right lower abdominal pain. The usual patient with appendicitis does not require immediate surgery, and critical illness with severe right lower abdominal pain of short duration is more likely to be due to bowel infarction, ruptured ovarian cyst, ectopic pregnancy or some other problem than appendicitis. The typical symptoms of appendicitis usually appear over a period of somewhat less than 24 hours, involving a sequence of midabdominal pain shifting to the right lower abdomen, mild nausea or anorexia, constipation (or occasionally, diarrhea), low grade fever and mild leukocytosis. Such a patient usually can, if necessary, be admitted for a few hours' observation before a decision is made to operate. The delay is sometimes an important means of differentiating nonsurgical diseases from appendicitis, including simple constipation, "mittleschmerz" (pain from rupture of the ovarian follicle), and gastroenteritis. But if appendicitis is strongly suspected, therapy should be directed to prepare for surgery. A critically ill patient with appendiceal abscess and peritonitis will profit by several hours of preoperative preparation by fluid restoration and antibiotics.

Carcinoid tumors of the appendix are usually found incidentally at laparotomy. These are the most common and also the most curable type of carcinoids. Simple appendectomy is ordinarily sufficient, unless obvious metastases are apparent. Pseudomyxoma peritonei is usually caused by relatively slow-growing tumors of the appendix or ovary.

The primary tumor should be removed if it is still in place when the patient presents with pseudomyxoma.[8] An unruptured mucocoele of the appendix is unlikely to be diagnosed preoperatively, and should be removed with caution if encountered unexpectedly. Adenocarcinoma of the base of the appendix should be treated as a carcinoma of the cecum. A difficult preoperative diagnosis is posed by the turned-in appendiceal stump, which may have the smooth, convex surface of a small benign tumor of the cecum. But since it cannot be known with certainty that the lesion is a turned-in stump, exploration is usually advisable.

Colon

The major concern of the surgeon with respect to the colon is cancer. Surgeons are called upon to evaluate and treat many emergencies of the colon, such as bleeding, obstruction, perforation, volvulus and impaction. Regardless of the certainty of diagnosis of a nonmalignant condition, the wise surgeon always keeps in mind the possibility that perhaps a cancer is also present. This thinking is based on the knowledge that carcinoma of the colon and rectum is the most common cancer of humans, and only half of its victims are salvaged even with aggressive surgery, radiation therapy and chemotherapy. With this ominous disease in mind, it is little wonder that frequent examinations and early surgery are recommended for lesions which may appear to be relatively benign. Rectal examinations should be performed as part of all complete physical examinations, and should be a part of all abdominal examinations. A stool specimen should be obtained and examined personally by the surgeon for occult blood during every rectal examination. A sigmoidoscopy, followed by (not preceded by) barium enema should be performed for rather liberal indications, knowing the high incidence of colorectal cancer in our population. Most patients with diverticulosis and diverticulitis,

ulcerative colitis and granulomatous colitis may be managed by internists, but when carcinoma of the colon is suspected, the disease requires hospitalization and surgery.

Carcinoma of the colon occurs most commonly in the rectum and distal sigmoid colon. At least 50 per cent of colorectal cancers are visible through the sigmoidoscope. Constipation is a common symptom of carcinoma of the sigmoid. This tumor may leave blood and mucus streaked on the bowel movements. On the other hand, carcinoma of the cecum may be relatively silent for a long time (Fig. 18–16). It may grow to immense size before perforating or causing obstruction, and it will frequently produce severe anemia from occult bleeding without obvious change in the color or consistency of bowel movements. Carcinoma should be strongly suspected in flat or napkin-ring lesions of the colon. It is relatively uncommon but may also occur in pedunculated polyps (Fig. 18–17). It is present, unsuspected preoperatively, in 3 per cent of resections for diverticulitis.[5] Carcinoma is a significant risk in patients with ulcerative colitis for more than ten years. Early diagnosis is important, for curability decreases as the disease spreads through the layers of the colon. With lesions confined to the mucosa, 85 per cent of patients may be cured. However, only 50 per cent are cured when all of the layers of the colon are invaded, and only 15 per cent when lymph nodes or adjacent organs are involved.[1,44,54,55,59,61] Essentially no patients are cured if residual cancer is left, although aggressive chemotherapy, radiation therapy, and "second look operations" have produced salvage in a few "incurable" cases.[15] The carcinoembryonic antigen described in association with colon cancer may provide a useful serological test for early cancer. It has already been utilized on an experimental basis to identify patients and to follow the progress of disease.

Colonic polyps are a troublesome problem, since sessile polyps may be

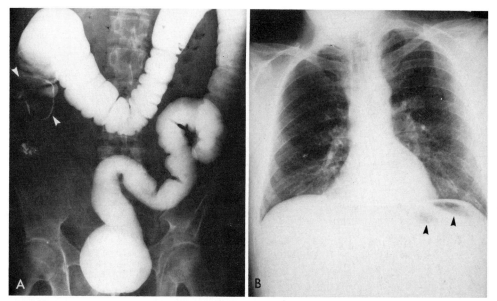

Figure 18-16 Carcinoma of the cecum with perforation and death. Fifty-one year old male psychiatric outpatient with mild bloating and indigestion for several months. GI series normal. Barium enema *(A)* was read as "normal." Patient developed acute collapse 25 days later and was admitted to Emergency Room. Chest x-ray *(B)*, taken during resuscitation, was read as "normal." Patient subsequently complained of abdominal pain and review of x-rays showed cecal lesion (arrows, *A*) and double left subdiaphragmatic air shadow (arrows, *B*) characteristic of gastric bubble and free air. At laparotomy, gangrenous perforated carcinoma of cecum and generalized peritonitis were found. Patient died of septicemia postoperatively.

malignant and even pedunculated adenomatous polyps are not free of the possibility (Fig. 18–17). In general, polypectomy can be recommended for polyps over 1 cm in size, since the operation is relatively safe if the colon is well prepared. A definite demonstration of the polyp on two successive barium enemas is mandatory, however, since a ball of feces may mimic a sessile polyp and produce embarrassment in the operating room.

Villous adenomas are large sessile polypoid tumors which occur most frequently in the distal sigmoid and rectum. Although frequently benign on surface biopsy, they must be excised completely for diagnostic evaluation, since areas of malignancy are frequently found when they are examined completely under the microscope. If malignant, they should be treated as if they were an adenocarcinoma in that particular location. Villous adenomas frequently present with massive loss of fluid, mucus, protein and potassium.

Multiple familial polyposis is a premalignant disease. Patients with a family history of this condition should be scheduled for total colectomy in their twenties or as soon thereafter as possible. Patients with polyposis or ulcerative colitis who have ileorectal anastomoses must have the entire residual rectum visualized through a proctoscope at intervals of three to six months. Resection of the rectum is ideal for protection from cancer, but many patients will not consent to it.

Ulcerative colitis is a disease which requires considerable judgment by the internist and surgeon. Although the dangers of complications are readily apparent (carcinoma, hepatitis, pyoderma, toxic megacolon), the patients are not usually willing to accept total colectomy when the disease is first diagnosed. Proper medical and psycho-

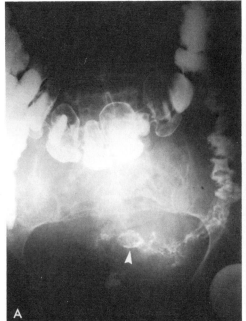

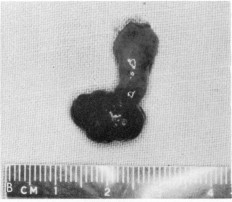

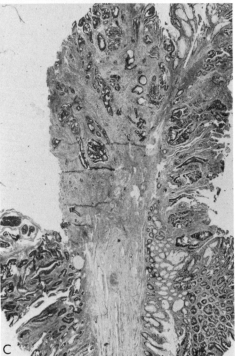

Figure 18–17 Carcinoma in a polyp. Eighty year old woman transferred from nursing home for evaluation of rectal bleeding. Proctoscopy negative. Barium enema *(A)* revealed polyp (arrow) in sigmoid colon, which was removed by transabdominal colotomy. Polyp was 1.5 cm in diameter, and had a stalk 2.0 cm long *(B)*. Although polyp was grossly benign, carcinoma was seen histologically on permanent section *(C*, original magnification 4.5×). Because base of stalk was free of cancer, and because of patient's marginal physical status, no further surgery was performed.

logical management may even lead to complete recovery in some cases. Good management may reduce the risk of life-threatening complications during the period when the patient with chronic ulcerative colitis is adjusting to the necessity for resection. The surgeon may help in providing consultation, sigmoidoscopy (and *cautious* rectal biopsy to establish the diagnosis), and management of the perianal problems which arise. He should recommend surgery when he firmly believes that it is advisable (rather than too early, or after the patient is moribund). He must be prepared to bear the brunt of the patient's displeasure with this recommendation and with the operative result. Elective colectomy is recommended for patients with a history of ulcerative colitis for ten or more years because carcinoma becomes a significant risk after this length of time. Total colectomy (with terminal ileostomy) is indicated if the rectum is diseased. Emergency total colectomy is indicated for toxic mega-colon.[62] This complication occurs in less than 4 per cent of patients with ulcerative colitis, but it can unfortunately be masked by steroid therapy until perforation and peritonitis have developed. The end ileostomy which is fashioned after total colectomy should be matured at the time of surgery. The patient should be taught to manage the appliance before he leaves the hospital. The surgeon should be aware of the value of karaya gum powder, zinc oxide and aluminum paste for skin protection. Each surgeon should become expert in applying the ileostomy appliance for his patients. The patient should be assisted by the local community's "Ostomy Association," which will provide preoperative and postoperative counseling. Ileostomy dysfunction (cramps and diarrhea) commonly results from stricture at the level of fascia or skin. It is an indication for hospitalization if digital examination confirms the existence of a stricture. Herniation of small intestine may occur adjacent to the terminal ileum, and is a cause of "ileostomy dysfunction" or acute bowel obstruction in some patients.

Granulomatous colitis is an inflammatory disease of the muscularis and mesentery of the colon, with secondary erosion of the mucosa. This condition is contrasted to ulcerative colitis in which ulceration begins in the mucosa, forming pseudopolyps and penetration outward into the muscularis. Granulomatous colitis is frequently associated with regional enteritis (Crohn's disease) in which the pathology is similar. It may be difficult to distinguish granulomatous from ulcerative colitis except when colon resection is performed. However, granulomatous colitis does not have the same association with cancer as ulcerative colitis, and may have long periods of spontaneous remission. Conservative management of some patients with ulcerative colitis may therefore be indicated, in the hope that their disease may follow the evolu-tion of granulomatous rather than ulcerative colitis.

Volvulus of the colon is an uncommon but dramatic problem which occurs most commonly in psychotic or elderly patients. The x-ray findings are usually diagnostic of volvulus, although similar findings *may* occur in patients with annular obstructing carcinomas. A dilated loop of colon is usually seen in the mid and right upper abdomen with sigmoid volvulus, and a dilated loop of colon is usually present in the midabdomen and left upper abdomen with cecal volvulus. The x-ray features may be misleading, or as typical as those shown in Figures 18–18 (sigmoid volvulus) and 18–19 (cecal volvulus). A "funnel" or "parrot beak" narrowing of the twisted portion of the colon may be visible on the plain film or may be seen on barium enema. Cecal volvulus is an indication for immediate hospitalization and surgery.[38] Sigmoid volvulus, on the other hand, may be corrected by sigmoidoscopy, rectal tube or barium enema.[71] Many of these patients are senile or otherwise intolerable candidates for surgery, and the nonoperative reduction may be considered sufficient until another episode occurs. Even in properly selected patients, elective resection for sigmoid volvulus has a 30 per cent mortality, and emergency resection has a 58 per cent mortality. Severe coexisting disease has been reported in 90 per cent of patients with sigmoid volvulus. Recurrence may be prevented by dietary counseling and induction of regularity by stool softeners, laxatives and enemas.

Trauma to the colon is a major surgical problem and suspicion of injury to the colon is sufficient indication for immediate hospitalization. Rupture of the sigmoid colon may occur during sigmoidoscopy, especially if the procedure was difficult and air was insufflated. The relative benignancy of the condition in the first few minutes or hours should not lull the surgeon into complacency. The safest procedure is a proximal colostomy and closure of the defect, or exterioriza-

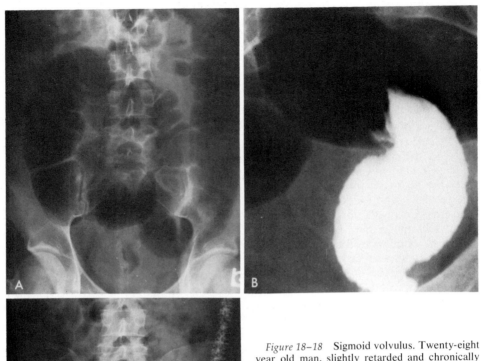

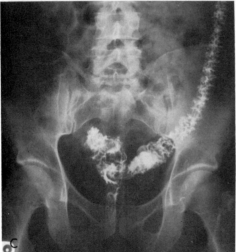

Figure 18–18 Sigmoid volvulus. Twenty-eight year old man, slightly retarded and chronically constipated. No previous history of volvulus. Obstipation and distention when admitted to Emergency Room. Abdominal x-ray shows massive colonic distention and small amount of air in rectum, presumably from a self-administered enema *(A)*. Barium enema showed characteristic inverted funnel as contrast medium was introduced *(B)*. Volvulus was immediately reduced by the barium enema, which then revealed a redundant loop of sigmoid colon *(C)*. Sigmoid resection was performed electively and postoperative course was benign.

tion of the lacerated segment of colon — just as it is for a gunshot or stab wound of the colon.

Free intraperitoneal air may occasionally be discovered in a patient who feels well. The condition may be caused by escape of air from the wall of the intestinal tract in patients with pneumatosis intestinalis, or it may be truly idiopathic. These situations are relatively uncommon in the Outpatient Clinic, so the conservative approach to a patient with free intraperitoneal air usually is to operate rather than to observe him expectantly.

Diverticulosis is a common cause of colonic bleeding. In some cases a small artery at the base of a diverticulum may produce a furious hemorrhage, even though the colon shows no signs of inflammation on barium enema, sigmoidoscopy or even external palpation in the operating room. Diverticulosis or idiopathic ulceration of the right colon may cause sudden severe bleeding without prior symptoms. Most patients with

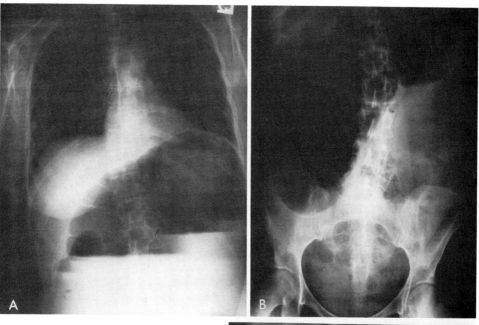

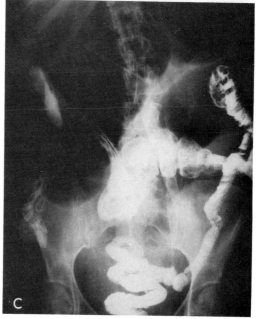

Figure 18–19 Cecal volvulus. Fifty-nine year old woman, a recluse who could not relate a history, was brought to Emergency Room with an acute abdomen. X-rays of chest *(A)* and abdomen *(B)* showed massive dilatation of colon. Diagnosis was immediately clarified by barium enema *(C)* which showed typical tapered narrowing of barium column at hepatic flexure due to cecal volvulus. Laparotomy was immediately performed, and the gangrenous, perforated right colon was resected. She eventually recovered after a stormy postoperative course.

bleeding from diverticulosis of the left colon will give a history consistent with prior episodes of diverticulitis. In most cases, however, diverticulosis is a relatively benign disease, and the patient should simply be cautioned to avoid large particles of roughage (such as whole kernel corn, citrus fruit pulp, celery). He should maintain regularity in bowel movements with appropriate softeners, fluids and exercise, thereby avoiding production of diverticulitis and stercoral ulcers. Diverticulitis can be a devastating disease, especially in elderly patients, because of the complications of hemorrhage, obstruction and abscess. The disease may present for the first time with one of these major complications, or perforation into small bowel, urinary tract or vagina. If the patient has had one episode of definite diverticulitis, and is a reasonably good operative risk, elective resection of the significantly involved area is recommended. A sigmoid colectomy is usually advisable, though a complete resection of areas containing diverticulosis and diverticulitis is the ideal therapy for patients who are in good general health. The overall mortality for resection in 206 patients reported by Botsford and Zollinger (1969)[6] was 7.8 per cent, but most of the fatalities occurred in association with emergency operations.

Preparation for colon surgery is best done in the hospital, where both a mechanical preparation and reduction in fecal bacteria can best be accomplished.[46] For situations in which outpatient preparation is necessary, some or all of the steps shown in Table 18–4 may be utilized. It is recommended that a final plain x-ray of the abdomen be obtained prior to surgery if preparation is done as an outpatient, to look carefully for signs of residual feces. The symptoms of danger in a bowel prep should be pointed out to the patient and his family if outpatient preparation is elected. The signs include depletion of salt and water (dehydration and collapse), deficiency of fat soluble vitamins (especially vitamin K), and pseudomembranous enterocolitis.

Colostomy care is a subject for outpatient consideration, for few patients are perfectly adjusted to a colostomy by the time they leave the hospital after surgery. A left-sided colostomy can usually be managed eventually with only a cloth compress covering the matured stoma, and may rarely require irrigation when it is "trained." But careful guidance and encouragement of the patient is necessary to achieve this goal.

TABLE 18–4   PREOPERATIVE PREPARATION OF COLON (5 days)

1. Low residue diet for 3 days, followed by
2. Clear liquids p.o. for last 2 days before surgery.
3. Sulfathaladine 2.0 gm 4 times per day for 5 days or Sulfasuxadine 2.0 gm 8 times per day for 5 days
4. Neomycin 1.0 gm p.o. q 4 hr for final 36 hours before surgery.
5. Soapsuds enema every 2 days (days 1, 3 and 5) alternating with
6. Magnesium Citrate 8 oz p.o. every 2 days (days 2 and 4)
7. Vitamin B–complex tablets b.i.d. (e.g., B–complex Squibb, with B_1, 2 mg; B_2, 2 mg; B_6, 2 mg and Niacinamide 15 mg)
8. Vitamin C 100 mg t.i.d.
9. Vitamin K 5 mg q.d. (e.g., menadiol, "Synka-vite")
10. KCl elixir, 1 teaspoon 4 to 5 cc t.i.d.

The goal is important for psychological and medical reasons. Avoidance of the irrigation and bag will allow the patient to resume a normal existence and will eliminate the serious hazard of colonic perforation by the irrigating catheter. A colostomy of the transverse or right colon may be a chore to manage. These colostomies commonly have two stomata adjacent to each other, and are relatively "wet." This combination makes it difficult to maintain a satisfactory collection of the feces. These difficult colostomies should be scheduled for conversion to a definitive, manageable colostomy, or resected and closed as soon as possible—usually within four weeks after they are created.

The ideal size of a matured colostomy stoma is determined by the adequacy of its function. The surgeon should not be dismayed if the stoma admits only his little finger, if it has functioned well for a long time. On the other hand, most well-functioning colostomies in adult patients will accept two joints of the index finger if a little patience is used in performing the examination. The postoperative evaluation of a colostomy patient should include digital examination of his colostomy. Even if the stoma was constructed for a benign disease, the patient is usually pleased to have a physician inspect it and comment upon it. Most of these patients are anxious to ask some questions about their colostomy, but will not do so unless the physician is personally interested in examining it. Colostomy stricture may occur at the skin or deep fascia. A skin stricture may be resected under local anesthesia in the clinic; however, bleeding may be unexpectedly brisk, and assistance should be available. A stricture at the fascial level requires hospitalization and general or spinal anesthesia with relaxation for repair.

CONCLUSION

There is probably no other field in which both the art and science of surgery are so important as with diseases of the abdomen and gastrointestinal tract. Many rules and suggestions may be studied as guides to therapy. Nevertheless, the young surgeon must always be ready to ask for advice from his colleagues when the problem is unusual. In lonely clinics or remote regions, the decision may be especially difficult. But inevitably the moment of decision will come.

The trained surgeon must decide whether to operate, or perhaps by hesitation allow his patient to slip into an irreversible condition and an unnecessary death.

References

1. Bacon, H. E., and Gennaro, A. R.: Carcinoma of the transverse colon and splenic flexure. Surg. Gynecol. Obstet., *127*:523–527, 1968.
2. Bell, J. W.: Abdominal exploration in one hundred lung carcinoma suspects prior to thoracotomy. Ann. Surg., *167*:199–203, 1968.
3. Ben-Shoshan, M., Gius, J. A., and Smith, I. M.: Exploratory laparotomy for fever of unknown origin. Surg. Gynecol. Obstet., *132*:994–996, 1971.
4. Bloch, M. A., and Allen, H. M.: Elective repair of esophageal hiatus hernia at the time of cholecystectomy. Surg. Gynecol. Obstet., *132*:46–50, 1971.
5. Botsford, T. W., and Wilson, R. E.: The acute abdomen. Philadelphia, W. B. Saunders Co., 1969.
6. Botsford, T. W., and Zollinger, R. M., Jr.: Diverticulitis of the colon. Surg. Gynecol. Obstet., *128*:1209–1214, 1969.
7. Buchwald, H., Frantz, I. D., Gebhard, R. L., and Moore, R. B.: Effect of ileal bypass versus ileal excision on cholesterol synthesis and whole blood cholesterol concentration in the rabbit. Surgery, *64*:126–133, 1968.
8. Byron, R. L., Jr., et al.: The management of pseudomyxoma peritonei secondary to ruptured mucocele of the appendix. Surg. Gynecol. Obstet., *122*:509–512, 1966.
9. Cleveland, H. C., and Waddell, W. R.: Retroperitoneal rupture of the duodenum due to nonpenetrating trauma. Surg. Clin. N. Amer., *43*:413–431, 1963.
10. Condon, R. E., Granville, G. E., Jordan P. H., Jr., and Helgason, A. H.: Hypercalcemic crisis and intractable gastrointestinal ulceration in a patient with endocrine polyglandular syndrome. Ann. Surg., *167*:185–190, 1968.
11. Cooperman, A. M., Kelly, K. A., Bernatz, P. E., and Huizenga, K. A.: Arteriovenous malformation of the intestine: An uncommon cause of gastrointestinal bleeding. Arch. Surg., *104*:284–287, 1972.
12. Cope, Z.: The early diagnosis of the acute abdomen. 13th Ed. London, Oxford, 1968.
13. Copeland, E. M., and Long, J. M., III: Elective appendectomy for appendiceal calculus. Surg. Gynecol. Obstet., *130*:439–442, 1970.
14. Crile, G., Jr.: Advantages of bypass operations over radical pancreatoduodenectomy in the treatment of pancreatic carcinoma. Surg. Gynecol. Obstet., *130*:1049–1053, 1970.
15. Curreri, A. R., and Mackman, S.: Reoperation in carcinoma of colon following resection and adjuvant chemotherapy. Surg. Gynecol. Obstet., *123*:274–276, 1966.
16. Delaney, T., and Hoxworth, P. I.: Enteric-coated potassium chloride enteropathy. Surg. Gynecol. Obstet., *127*:76–80, 1968.
17. Devlin, H. B., Evans, D. S., and Birkhead, J. S.: Elective splenectomy for primary hematologic and splenic disease. Surg. Gynecol. Obstet., *131*:273–276, 1970.
18. Diaco, J. F., Miller, L. D., and Copeland, E. M.: Role of early diagnostic laparotomy in acute pancreatitis. Surg. Gynecol. Obstet., *129*:263–269, 1969.
19. Ebert, P. A., Gaertner, R. A., and Zuidema, G. D.: Traumatic diaphragmatic hernia. Surg. Gynecol. Obstet., *125*:59–65, 1967.
20. French, W. E., Bale, G. F., and Winborn, W. B.: Lipodystrophy of mesenteric fat.

Surg. Gynecol. Obstet., *122*:1046–1052, 1966.

21. Glenn, F., and McSherry, C. K.: Etiological factors in fatal complication following operations upon the biliary tract. Ann. Surg.: *157*:695–706, 1963.

22. Glenn, F., and McSherry, C. K.: Secondary abdominal operations for symptoms following biliary tract surgery. Surg. Gynecol. Obstet., *121*:979–988, 1965.

23. Glenn, F., McSherry, C. K., and Dineen, P.: Morbidity of surgical treatment for non-malignant biliary tract disease. Surg. Gynecol. Obstet., *126*:15–26, 1968.

24. Goldenberg, I. S., Cohen, J. M., and Skinner, D. G.: Study of survival patterns in patients with gastric carcinoma. Surg. Gynecol. Obstet., *124*:241–250, 1967.

25. Grigsby, W. P.: Surgical treatment of amebiasis. Surg. Gynecol. Obstet., *128*:609–627, 1969.

26. Grossman, M. I., Kirsner, J. B., and Gillespie, I. E.: Basal and histalog-stimulated gastric secretion in control subjects and in patients with peptic ulcer or gastric cancer. Gastroenterology, *45*:14–26, 1963.

27. Hanks, G. E., Terry, L. N., Jr., Bryan, J. A., and Newsome, J. F.: Contribution of diagnostic laparotomy to staging of non-Hodgkin's lymphoma. Cancer, *29*:41–43, 1972.

28. Hendren, W. H., Warshaw, A. L., Fleischli, D. J., and Bartlett, M. K.: Traumatic hemobilia: Non-operative management with healing documented by serial angiography. Ann. Surg., *174*:991–993, 1971.

29. Herrington, J. L., Jr.: Antiperistaltic jejunal interposition for control of dumping. Kaplan, H. J. "Medical Commentary." Hosp. Pract.: January, 1972, 87–97.

30. Hicks, R. E., and Brooks, J. R.: Total pancreatectomy for ductal carcinoma. Surg. Gynecol. Obstet., *133*:16–20, 1971.

31. Hill, G. J., II, Steinberg, H., and Speer, D. S.: Free perforation of the common bile duct. New Eng. J. Med., *259*:1267–1268, 1958.

32. Hollander, F.: The insulin test for the presence of intact nerve fibers after vagal operations for peptic ulcer. Gastroenterology, *7*:607–614, 1946.

33. Howard, J. M., and Ehrlich, E. W.: The etiology of pancreatitis: A review of clinical experience. Ann. Surg., *152*:135–146, 1960.

34. Hughes, C. W., Baugh, J. H., Mologne, L. A., and Heaton, L. D.: A review of the late General Eisenhower's operations: Epilog to a footnote to history. Ann. Surg., *173*:793–799, 1971.

35. Hyatt, D. F., Skarin, A. T., Moloney, W. C., and Wilson, R. E.: Splenectomy for lymphosarcoma. Surg. Gynecol. Obstet., *131*:928–932, 1970.

36. Ibach, J. R., Jr., Hume, H. A., and Erb, W. H.: Cholecystectomy in aged. Surg. Gynecol. Obstet., *126*:523–528, 1968.

37. Jones, C. M.: Digestive tract pain, diagnosis and treatment. New York, MacMillan Co., 1928.

38. Large, A. M.: Partial intermittent volvulus of the cecum. Ann. Surg.: *167*:609–611, 1968.

39. Malt, R. A., Hershberg, R. A., and Miller, W. L.: Experience with benign tumors of the liver. Surg. Gynecol. Obstet., *130*:285–291, 1970.

40. McDermott, W. V., Jr., Bartlett, M. K., and Culver, P. J.: Acute pancreatitis after prolonged fast and subsequent surfeit. N. Eng. J. Med., *254*:379–380, 1956.

41. McVay, C. B.: Hernia: the pathological anatomy of the more common hernias and their anatomic repair. Springfield, Charles C Thomas, 1954.

42. Menghini, G.: Two-operator needle biopsy of the liver. Amer. J. Dig. Dis., *4*:682, 1959.

43. Miller, D. R.: Unusual focal mesenteric venous thrombosis associated with contraceptive medication: a case report. Ann. Surg., *173*:135–138, 1971.

44. Miller, L. D., Boruchow, I. B., and Fitts, W. T., Jr.: Analysis of 284 patients with perforative carcinoma of colon. Surg. Gynecol. Obstet., *123*:1212–1218, 1966.

45. Myren, J.: Gastric secretion following stimulation with histamine, histalog and gastrin in man. In, Semb, L. S., and Myren, J. (Eds.): The Physiology of Gastric Secretion. Baltimore, Williams and Wilkins Co., 1968.

46. Nichols, R. L., and Condon, R. E.: Preoperative preparation of the colon. Surg. Gynecol. Obstet., *132*:323–337, 1971.

47. Nyhus, L. M., and Harkins, H. M.: Hernia. Philadelphia, J. B. Lippincott Co., 1964.

48. Olsen, W. R., and Beaudoin, D. E.: Surgical injury to the spleen. Surg. Gynecol. Obstet., *131*:57–62, 1970.

49. O'Neil, J. A., Scott, H. W., Jr., Billings, F. T., and Foster, J. H.: The role of splenectomy in Felty's syndrome. Ann. Surg., *167*:81–84, 1968.

50. Orcutt, T. W.: Hernia of the superior lumbar triangle. Ann. Surg., *173*:294–297, 1971.

51. Prosnitz, L. R., Nuland, S. B., and Kligerman, M. M.: Role of laparotomy and splenectomy in the management of Hodgkin's disease. Cancer, *29*:44–50, 1972.

52. Rees, J. R., Thorbjanarson, B., and Barnes, W. H.: Achalasia: Results of operation in 84 patients. Ann. Surg., *171*:195–201, 1970.

53. Resnicoff, S. A., Morton, J. H., and Bloch, A. L.: Retroperitoneal rupture of duodenum due to blunt trauma. Surg. Gynecol. Obstet., *125*:77–81, 1967.

54. Reynolds, C. T., LaCoste, C. E., Rogers, W. P., Jr., and Yatsuhashi, M.: Total salvage in adenocarcinoma of the rectum and rectosigmoid. Surg. Gynecol. Obstet., *127*:975–980, 1968.

55. Rosato, F. E., Frazier, T. G., Copeland, E. M.,

and Miller, L. D.: Carcinoma of the colon in young people. Surg. Gynecol. Obstet., *129*:29–32, 1969.

56. Sandusky, W. R., Rudolf, L. E., and Leavell, B. S.: Splenectomy for control of neutropenia in Felty's syndrome. Ann. Surg., *167*:744–751, 1968.

57. Scott, H. W., Jr., Law, D. H., IV, Sandstead, H. H., Lanier, V. C., Jr., and Younger, R. K.: Jejunoileal shunt in surgical treatment of morbid obesity. Ann. Surg., *171*: 770–782, 1970.

58. Seltzer, M. H., and Rosato, F. E.: Mortality following cholecystectomy. Surg. Gynecol. Obstet., *130*:64–66, 1970.

59. Speck R. L., Thomas, W. H., Larson, R. A., Wright, H. K., and Cleveland, J. C.: Analysis of 860 patients with carcinoma of transverse and descending colon. Surg. Gynecol. Obstet., *130*:259–262, 1970.

60. Stone, H. H., Webb, H. W., and Kovalchik, M. T., III: Pneumatosis intestinalis of infancy. Surg. Gynecol. Obstet., *130*: 806–812, 1970.

61. Thomas, W. H., Larson, R. A., Wright, H. K., and Cleveland, J. C.: Analysis of patients with carcinoma of the right colon. Surg. Gynecol. Obstet., *127*:313–318, 1968.

62. Thomford, N. R., Rybank, J. J., and Pace, W. G.: Toxic megacolon. Surg. Gynecol. Obstet., *128*:21–26, 1969.

63. Trimble, C.: Gonococcal perihepatitis simulating acute cholecystitis. Surg. Gynecol. Obstet., *130*:54–56, 1970.

64. Vanway, C. W., Brochman, S. K., and Rosenfeld, L.: Spontaneous thromboses of the mesenteric veins. Ann. Surg., *173*:561–568, 1971.

65. Waddell, W. R.: Exposure of intrahepatic bile ducts through interlobar fissure. Surg. Gynecol. Obstet., *124*:491–500, 1967.

66. Waddell, W. R., and Taubman, J.: Mechanical and chemical methods of opening occluded T tubes. Surgery, *71*:91–96, 1972.

67. Whittaker, L. D., Jr., Judd, E. S., and Stauffer, M. H.: Analysis of use of vagotomy with drainage procedure in surgical management of duodenal ulcer. Surg. Gynecol. Obstet., *125*:1018–1026, 1967.

68. Williams, J. S., and Hule, H. W.: The advisability of inguinal herniorraphy in the elderly. Surg. Gynecol. Obstet., *122*:100–104, 1966.

69. Witte, C. L.: Mesentery and bowel injury from automotive seat belts. Ann. Surg., *167*:486–492, 1968.

70. Wormsley, K. G., and Grossman, M. I.: Maximal histalog test in control subjects and patients with peptic ulcer. Gut, 6:427–435, 1965.

71. Wuepper, K. D., Otterman, M. G., and Stahlgren, L. H.: Appraisal of operative and nonoperative treatment of sigmoid volvulus. Surg. Gynecol. Obstet., *122*:84–88, 1966.

72. Zollinger, R. M., and Ellison, E. H.: Primary peptic ulcerations of the jejunum associated with islet cell tumors of the pancreas. Ann. Surg., *142*:709–723, 1955.

19

Urinary System and Male Genitalia — Urology

By NORMAN E. PETERSON, M.D.
and ALFRED J. DeFALCO, M.D.

INTRODUCTION

Urology is the surgical specialty concerned with the male genitourinary system and the female urinary tract. Ambulatory surgery of the genitourinary organs is mainly performed upon the external genitalia, the prostate and the

696

urinary bladder, access to which is gained through the urethra. The remainder of the genitourinary tract is an internal system and therefore poorly suited to ambulatory surgery. Outpatient urological surgery is also concerned with diagnosis, preoperative evaluation and postoperative care.

Four common urgent symptom complexes which appear in outpatient urological practice are acute urinary tract infection, acute urinary retention, gross hematuria and renal colic. In each case, the symptoms may be severe or mild, and the diagnosis may be immediately apparent or may be thoroughly obscure. The major features of differential diagnosis, outpatient workup and immediate treatment for each of these problems will be considered in this chapter.

A variety of elective operations and chronic diseases which are dealt with in outpatient work will also be presented, and the techniques for local and regional anesthesia of the genitourinary organs will be illustrated.

Urology is unique in its reliance upon endoscopic (cystourethroscopic) and specialized radiographic contrast data. These methods are listed and briefly discussed in Table 19–1.

ANESTHESIA

Penile Block (Fig. 19–1)

Minor surgical procedures can be performed on the penis under local infiltration anesthesia. These operations include circumcision, dorsal preputial slit, urethral meatotomy, cutaneous biopsy, reduction of painful paraphimosis, retraction of painful partial phimosis and so forth. The sensory distribution of the penis occurs subcutaneously, in quadrants at the two, four, eight and ten o'clock positions. Appropriate infiltration of these quadrants at the base of the penis will usually afford total temporary anesthesia distally. The procedure consists of routine surgical cleansing and draping of the penis, after which an appropriate local anesthetic is employed. A skin wheal is raised at one of the four indicated positions. The needle is then advanced through the skin and, after aspiration, infiltration of the subcutaneous tissue is continued. The needle can then be advanced and withdrawn subcutaneously to infiltrate thoroughly the other three positions. After a suitable delay, testing will usually confirm total cutaneous anesthesia, although additional infiltration at the frenulum will occasionally be necessary to complete the block.

Spermatic Cord Block (Fig. 19–2)

Prompt and thorough inspection of every mass lesion of the testis is essential. Inflammatory and traumatic lesions may be extremely painful, and severe discomfort may also be experienced in the uncommon event of hemorrhage into a neoplasm. Such discomfort, in addition to distressing the patient, may interfere with adequate examination by the physician. Relief of the discomfort will therefore assist both the patient and the examiner.

With the patient lying supine a sterile field is prepared, employing every effort to avoid painful scrotal manipulation. Ten cc of appropriate local anesthetic is readied, after which the spermatic cord is gently grasped between the fingers of one hand, and a wheal is raised in the overlying skin. The needle is advanced into the spermatic cord and the cord is thoroughly infiltrated, after sequential aspiration to avoid intravascular injection. Moments later the patient will experience essentially complete relief of pain, and examination may proceed. It is often observed that relief of discomfort may exceed the usual duration of anesthesia obtained by the local anesthetics employed. Local symptoms may ultimately be manageable with non-narcotic analgesics. Resolution of inflammation may also be enhanced by improved circulation and relief of autonomic vasospasm.

TABLE 19–1 GENITOURINARY INVESTIGATIVE PROCEDURES

EXCRETORY UROGRAM (INTRAVENOUS PYELO-GRAM): Renal concentration, excretion of intravenously administered contrast medium. Anatomic, but not a functional study.

Hypertensive: Includes early films (30 sec., 1 min., 2 min.) revealing time and concentration discrepancy between kidneys, which may suggest reduced renal artery flow.

Infusion: Large dose of contrast medium, allowing visualization of kidneys despite elevated BUN and poor preparation. 1 cc per pound contrast medium with 1 cc per pound normal saline, rapidly infused.

CYSTOGRAM

Antegrade: Bladder visualization associated with routine or infusion IVP.

Retrograde: Through urethral catheter or accompanying retrograde urethrogram.

Voiding: May accompany retrograde study; may reveal reflux, diverticulum or valve.

Chain: Outlines posterior urethro-vesicle angle and may assist explanations of stress continence.

Cine: Accompanies fluroscopy; dynamic illustration of voiding act; helpful in demonstrating minimal reflux, pelvic relaxation, diverticula, fistulae, valves.

Double Exposure: Occasionally helpful in demonstration and staging bladder tumors; does not replace cystoscopy/biopsy.

URETHROGRAM

Voiding: Accompanies cystogram; helpful in demonstrating valves, diverticula, fistulae.

Retrograde: Isolated procedure; assists investigation of urethral trauma, stricture, congenital defects.

Cine: Accompanies ciné cystograms; dynamic study of voiding; assists investigation of stricture, valves, fistulae, diverticula.

URETEROPYELOGRAM

Retrograde: Accompanies cystoscopy; delineates ureter and renal pelvis.

Cine: Dynamic study of renal pelvis and ureter; useful for investigation of the presence and effectiveness of peristalsis, obstruction; accompanies fluoroscopy.

RENAL CYSTOGRAM: Accompanies IVP and fluoroscopy; aspiration of cyst fluid and insertion of contrast medium; assists differentiation between renal cyst and tumor; accompanied by cytology of aspirate.

NEPHROTOMOGRAM: Accompanies IVP; elucidates mass lesions (cyst vs. tumor).

ARTERIOGRAM

Translumbar: Percutaneous injection of contrast medium into lumbar aorta.

Seldinger: Percutaneous transfemoral arterial catheterization and advancement.

Midstream Aortic: Outlines the aorta and major branches.

Selective Renal: Selective fluoroscopic catheterization of renal arteries; occasionally used for infusing chemotherapeutic agents.

Selective Adrenal: Selective fluoroscopic catheterization of adrenal arteries.

Selective Hypogastric: Selective fluoroscopic catheterization of hypogastric arteries; occasionally helpful in staging bladder tumor; occasionally used to infuse chemotherapeutic agents.

Epinephrine: Preceding contrast injections; normal vessels constrict and do not fill well; neoplastic vessels do not constrict, remain unchanged.

INFERIOR VENA CAVOGRAM: Percutaneous transfemoral venous catheterization; outlines displacement, effacement, obstruction, compromise of inferior vena cava by lymph nodes, tumor, thrombus.

RENAL VENOGRAM

Selective: Extension of inferior vena cavogram.

Differential Collections: Including renin levels (renal hypertension) epinephrine levels (phenochromocytoma).

VASOGRAM: After surgical exposure of vas deferens, needle or catheter cannulation, contrast injection; to demonstrate displacement, obstruction, inflammation, neoplasia of vas deferens or seminal vesicle.

LYMPHANGIOGRAM

Pedal: Contrast migration from pedal lymphatics to iliac, lumbar, periaortic, renal hilar nodes; useful for evaluation of staging of testis tumor, gynecologic tumor, and so on; may miss lateral sentinal node of metastatic testis tumor.

Testicular: Migration of contrast from testis lymphatics to proximal nodes; may demonstrate lateral sentinel node in metastatic testis tumor.

UROFLOWMETRY WITH/WITHOUT CATHETER: Time/volume evaluation of urine flow; normal flow exceeds 20 cc per minute; may assist evaluation of surgical results.

CYSTOMETROGRAM (BETHANECOL TEST): Dynamic study of bladder pressure plotted against time and volume; significant subjective component; assists evaluation of neurogenic bladder.

ELECTROMYOGRAPHY (RECTAL SPHINCTER, PERIANAL): Helpful in determining muscle activity (innervation) in neurologic lesion affecting lower urinary tract function.

ISOTOPE STUDIES

Renogram: I^{131}-labeled Hippuran; differential concentration/decay curve; helpful in evaluating differential renal function, blood flow, obstruction.

Renal Scan: I^{131} Hippuran or Hg^{203} Chlormerodrin; graphic demonstration of differential renal blood flow, concentration, excretion; helpful in differentiating "hot" and "cold" renal lesions (infarct, tumor, cyst).

OSMOMETRY: Measurement of osmotic activity, commonly employing freezing point technique; helpful in comparing urine and serum values in evaluating oliguria and renal failure.

RADIOXENOGRAPHY: Injection of xenon isotope; decay curve from which can be extrapolated renal blood flow and blood flow per gram of tissue.

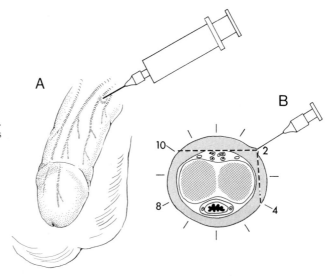

Figure 19–1 Penile block. *A.* Skin wheal raised. *B.* Subcutaneous infiltrations in four quadrants.

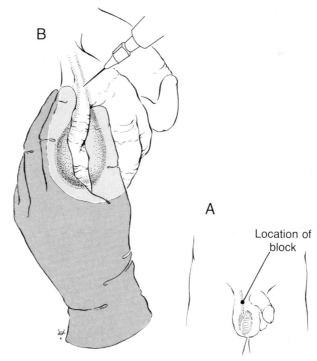

Figure 19–2 Spermatic cord block. *A.* Area of insertion of needle for spermatic cord infiltration. *B.* Spermatic cord is grasped above the testis with thumb and forefinger and infiltrated through a skin wheal with 5–10 cc of appropriate local anesthetic.

Location of block

GENITOURINARY INFECTION

Veneral Diseases

Gonococcal Urethritis

Gonorrhea is the most common reportable communicable disease in the United States. It is important to emphasize the fact that this disease is symptomatic in only 50 per cent of males and 10 to 20 per cent of females; asymptomatic infection is therefore a frequent cause of reinfection. Incidence is rising steadily, with asymptomatic infection estimated to be present in more than one million women at this time. (The National Commission on Venereal Disease has predicted that more than two million Americans contracted venereal disease, principally gonorrhea, in 1971.) The advice of some authorities is to treat prophylactically any female exposed to gonorrhea, regardless of the absence of symptoms and a negative culture.

Gonococcal urethritis typically occurs three to five days after exposure, and is manifested by the classic symptoms of burning dysuria and creamy-yellow urethral discharge. The patient may occasionally experience symptoms of epididymitis and prostatitis, and more rarely systemic symptoms, including arthritis (most commonly involving the wrist, ankle and knee), ophthalmia, endocarditis, perihepatitis and meningitis.

In evaluating patients suspected of harboring *N. gonorrhoeae*, it should be remembered that a negative smear does not exclude gonorrhea, and a culture should be performed before nongonococcal urethritis is considered. Similarly, a negative smear is an inadequate test of cure after antibiotic therapy. In females, an examination of smears of urethral or cervical exudates is inadequate for diagnosis and should not be used except as an adjunct to appropriate culture methods. Also, if a smear is positive while selective culture is negative, a false positive smear should be considered. Cultures should be obtained whenever gonorrhea is suspected, regardless of physical findings. A single cervical culture will detect approximately 82 per cent of infected women, while men with conclusively positive urethral smears will almost invariably have positive cultures. Any patient with a presumptive diagnosis of gonococcal urethritis should receive immediate antibiotic treatment without waiting for diagnostic confirmation.

The Thayer-Martin selective culture medium, incorporating vancomycin, colistimethate and mycostatin, has become the medium of choice for isolation of pathogenic Neisseria (gonorrheae and meningitidis), reducing overgrowth by contaminants and inhibiting saprophytic Neisseria and other organisms (Mima polymorpha) potentially mistaken for gonococci. Thayer-Martin cultures should be taken from the urethra and rectum of males and the cervical canal and rectum of females suspected of gonococcal infection.

All patients treated for gonorrhea should undergo serologic testing for syphilis at the time of treatment and a follow-up test each month for four months to detect syphilis that may have been partially masked by gonorrheal therapy.

Treatment schedules recommended by the U. S. Department of Health, Education and Welfare, Center for Disease Control, are outlined in Table 19–2.

Alternate treatment regimens include:

1. The combination of equal parts of aqueous procaine penicillin G and procaine penicillin G in oil with 2 per cent aluminum monostearate for two separate intramuscular injections of 2.4 million units in each site given at one visit.

2. A single oral dose of 3.5 gm ampicillin with probenecid 1.0 gm, followed by 0.5 gm probenecid at 6, 12 and 18 hours.[1]

3. Adding to the preceding regimen 0.5 gm ampicillin p.o. in 24 hours.[2]

4. 1.0 gm probenecid p.o. followed

TABLE 19–2 GONORRHEA

Although some isolates of *Neisseria gonorrhoeae* have decreased susceptibility to penicillin, this resistance is relative, not absolute, and penicillin in large doses remains the drug of choice. Physicians are cautioned not to use less than recommended doses.

RECOMMENDED TREATMENT SCHEDULES
Uncomplicated gonorrhea in men: aqueous procaine penicillin G, 2,400,000 units in one intramuscular injection.
Uncomplicated gonorrhea in women: aqueous procaine penicillin G, 4,800,000 units intramuscularly divided in two injection sites at one visit.
Prophylactic or epidemiologic treatment for gonorrhea (male and female) is accomplished with the same treatment schedules as for the uncomplicated gonorrhea.

PENICILLIN SENSITIVITY
Gonorrhea patients sensitive to penicillin may be treated effectively with tetracycline, administered as an initial oral dose of 1.5 grams followed by 0.5 grams every 6 hours for 4 days, a total dosage of 9 grams.

RETREATMENT AND COMPLICATIONS
Test of cure procedures are recommended at approximately 5-7 days after therapy. In the male, a gram stained smear is adequate if positive; otherwise, a culture specimen should be obtained from the anterior urethra. In the female, culture specimens should be obtained from both the endocervical and anal canal sites.

Retreatment in the male is indicated if the urethral discharge persists for three or more days following initial therapy and the smear or culture remains positive. Follow-up treatment consists of 4,800,000 units of aqueous procaine penicillin G intramuscularly divided in two injection sites at a single visit.
In uncomplicated gonorrhea in the female, retreatment is indicated if follow-up cervical or rectal cultures remain positive for *N. gonorrhoeae*. Follow-up treatment consists of 4,800,000 units of aqueous procaine penicillin G daily on two successive days.
Treatment of severe complications of gonorrhea should be individualized using large amounts of short-acting penicillin.

SEROLOGIC TESTS FOR SYPHILIS
All patients treated for gonorrhea should have a serologic test for syphilis at the time of treatment and a follow-up test each month for four months to detect syphilis that may have been partially masked by gonorrheal therapy.
Gonorrhea patients who are sexual contacts of infectious syphilis should be given full prophylactic therapy for syphilis (2.4 million units of benzathine penicillin) as well as recommended therapy for gonorrhea.
Gonorrhea patients who concomitantly have syphilis should be given full therapy appropriate to the stage of syphilis in addition to the above recommended treatment for gonorrhea.
While long-acting forms of penicillin (such as benzathine penicillin G) are ideal in syphilotherapy, they are not indicated in routine gonorrhea treatment.

---

in 15 minutes by a single IM injection of 5 million units of benzyl penicillin combined with 8 ml 0.5 per cent lidocaine.[3]

5. 2.0 gm spectinomycin IM as a single dose.[22]

Syphilis

Ranking third among reportable communicable diseases, syphilis is estimated to involve 75,000 new patients in the United States annually. The resurgence of this disease and its potential medical and social complications represent a serious problem which must be challenged by astute medical attention, investigation and therapy.

The primary stage of syphilis becomes manifest after an incubation period of 9 to 90 days, averages 3 weeks and is characterized by a chancre emerging at the site of inoculation, usually on the genitalia. Regional lymphadenopathy is common. A positive darkfield microscopic examination establishes the diagnosis, but a negative conclusion requires repeat examinations on three consecutive days. Since only 25 per cent of patients have positive serologic studies during the first week of appearance of the chancre, such studies may be positive or negative at the time of darkfield evaluation. This figure increases by 25 per cent with each successive week, so that by the fourth week all patients will have positive serologic reactions, at which time most patients will exhibit symptoms of secondary syphilis. The darkfield positive-seronegative patient may become reagin-positive during or shortly after treatment, but will revert to seronegativity by three months, while the seropositive patient may require six to nine months to achieve seronegativity. Those patients who remain seropositive nine months after initial treatment require retreatment, prior to which a spinal fluid examination should be performed. If abnormal, prolonged treatment schedules must be used.

Secondary syphilis generally appears within six months, typically six to eight weeks after exposure, at which time the chancre is usually healing. Symptoms are protean, but may be summarized as a flu-like syndrome, generalized lymphadenopathy, and a generalized eruption which typically involves the palms and soles. Seropositivity is uniform. After treatment, the titre of the serologic test for syphilis rises initially, then declines progressively, becoming negative in 98 per cent of patients within one year following treatment. The remaining 2 per cent should become seronegative during the second year. It is wise to perform spinal fluid examination on patients remaining seropositive one year after treatment. If negative, routine retreatment is initiated; if abnormal, increased retreatment schedules are given. In addition, the Wasserman–fast patient should be examined clinically and serologically each month for the first year, every three months during the second year, and annually thereafter.

Treatment schedules recommended by the U. S. Department of Health, Education and Welfare, Center for Disease Control are outlined in Table 19–3.

Lymphogranuloma Venereum
(Lymphopathia Venereum; Tropical Bubo)

This disease results from venereal contamination by a large virus, following an incubation period ranging from 3 to 30 days. Clinical presentation typically involves the development of a local papule or vesicle which heals spontaneously, with simultaneous development of enlarged inguinal lymph nodes above and below the inguinal ligament. Suppuration and fistula formation from the regional lymph nodes is a frequent occurrence. Diagnosis relies upon the sexual history, the gross appearance and evolution of the lesions, and special studies, including the Frei test (intradermal) and complement fixation tests. Tetracycline in the usual dosage is the antibiotic therapy of choice.

Chancroid

Chancroid is an acute infection caused by *Hemophilus ducreyi*, and is highly contagious if wounds or abrasions are present. Although lesions are usually genital, autoinoculation is common and extragenital lesions occur. Clinically, following an incubation period of one to five days, an inflammatory papule appears, soon thereafter becoming a pustule which then ruptures, leaving a dirty, painful ulcer with undermined, unindurated edges ("soft chancre"). Single or multiple ulcers may appear. Diagnosis relies on the typical history, gross appearance of the lesion, stained smears and special culture techniques for the offending organism. Effective treatment regimens have previously utilized tetracycline and sulfisoxazole, alone or in combination. A significant incidence of treatment failures has shown the need for protracted treatment programs. A regimen consisting only of continuous intravenous cephalothin, 3.0 gm daily, has produced essentially a 100 per cent cure rate after 5 to 15 days of therapy, the average course being 7 days. Local phlebitis may be associated with such therapy in up to 50 per cent of cases and requires routine conservative care.

Herpes Genitalis

Caused by the herpes simplex virus, herpes genitalis is an ulcerative disease

TABLE 19-3 RECOMMENDED TREATMENT SCHEDULES FOR SYPHILIS

Primary, Secondary Syphilis

Rx: Benzathine penicillin G — 2.4 million units total (1.2 million units in each buttock) by intramuscular injection.

or: PAM — 4.8 million units total usually given 2.4 million units at first session, as above, and 1.2 million units at each of two subsequent injections 3 days apart.

or: Aqueous procaine penicillin G — 600,000 units daily for 8 days to total 4.8 million units.

Latent Syphilis

Rx: Benzathine penicillin G — If no spinal fluid examination is done, treatment must encompass the possibility of asymptomatic neurosyphilis. In this case, 6.0 = 9.0 million units total, given 3.0 million units (1.5 in each buttock each session) at 7-day interval.
With nonreactive spinal fluid examination, 2.4 million units (as primary).

or: PAM — Aqueous penicillin G — Same as primary syphilis.

Congenital Syphilis

Rx: Benzathine penicillin G — 50,000 units per kilogram of body weight at one clinic visit.*

or: Aqueous Procaine Penicillin G — 100,000 units per kilogram of body weight divided into daily dosage over 10-day period.*

Late Syphilis

Asymptomatic neurosyphilis
Symptomatic neurosyphilis
Cardiovascular syphilis
Late benign (cutaneous, osseous, and visceral gumma) syphilis

Rx: Benzathine penicillin G — 6.0 to 9.0 million units total, given 3.0 million units at 7-day intervals.

or: PAM — 6.0-9.0 million units total, given 1.2 million units at 3-day intervals.

or: Aqueous procaine penicillin G — 6.0 to 9.0 million units total, given 600,000 units daily. Any benefit from more than 10 million units has not been demonstrated.

Syphilis in Pregnancy

Syphilis in pregnancy should be managed in the same manner as with any non-pregnant patient. Urgency of treatment is the keynote to therapy.

Alternate Antibiotics

When sensitivity precludes use of penicillin, erythromycin and tetracycline are the best alternate drugs. Recommended dosage orally is 30-40 gms. of erythromycin and 30-40 gms. of tetracycline given over a period of 10-15 days.
Treatment with such alternate antibiotics must be accompanied by close followup of the syphilitic patient since none of these drugs has had adequate evaluation in all stages of syphilis. Spinal fluid examinations must be done as part of followup after this type of therapy.

Preventive Treatment

If the patient is known to have been exposed to lesion syphilis, it is a fallacy to wait for the disease to develop to the clinical or reactive serologic stage, meanwhile allowing reinfection of treated patients and the infection of additional persons. However, every effort should be made to arrive at a diagnosis, including a complete physical examination, before administering preventive treatment. Adequate preventive treatment may consist of 2.4 million units of benzathine penicillin G.

*Total dosage not to exceed 5.0-6.0 million units.

---

of the genitalia characterized by 2 to 3 mm vesicular lesions which typically rupture after one to 4 days, following which secondary infection is common. Spontaneous healing usually occurs within one to three weeks. Diagnosis relies upon sexual history, the clinical appearance and evolution of the lesions, and smears of the vesicle fluid. Therapy is limited to improved hygiene and specific treatment of superinfection.

Condyloma Accuminata

Condyloma accuminata is characterized by verrucal warts of viral etiology occurring on the mucous membranes and skin of the genitalia, including the penis, scrotum, perineum and anus. Lesions most commonly occur under the prepuce in the male, and involvement of the frenulum and urethral meatus is not uncommon. Sexual transmission occurs, and an incubation period of several weeks to months may be present. Diagnosis relies exclusively on clinical appearance, while treatment may include surgical excision, electrocautery or, most effectively, local application of 10 to 25 per cent podophyllin suspension in tincture of benzoin. Application of podophyllin should be accompanied by instructions for local soap and water cleansing after four hours in order to prevent chemical burn. In the presence of meatal lesions, panendoscopy is essential to rule out intra-urethral involvement, in which case endoscopic electrofulgeration is indicated.

Molluscum Contagiosum

This is a viral disease which may occur anywhere on the body. Genital occurrence may rely on venereal contact, however. Following an incubation period of three to six weeks, waxy, firm, smooth, umbilicated elevations of various sizes develop. Diagnosis relies on clinical appearance and histopathologic changes, while therapy may include electrodessication, currettement, surgical excision or application of liquid nitrogen.

Other Infections

Nonspecific Urethritis

Clinically similar to gonococcal urethritis although there is a less distinct temporal relationship to venereal exposure, the urethral discharge in this infection is often scant, usually occurring in the morning, and there are no characteristic findings on gram stain and culture. Offending agents are often viral, and occasionally due to more uncommon organisms such as the Bedsonia and Mycoplasma groups.[4,5] When culture and sensitivity studies are positive, appropriate antibiotics can be administered, while in their absence, the most gratifying results have accompanied the use of oral doxycycline (Vibramycin), 50 mg b.i.d. for five days, hot sitz baths, and occasionally the use of nitrofurazone-hydrocortisone (Furacin-HC) urethral inserts.

Prostatitis

A distinction must be made clinically between acute and chronic prostatitis.

Acute prostatitis is a severe, acute bacterial infection, manifested by disabling local symptoms and significant systemic symptoms. Fever, chills and septicemia are not uncommon, while suprapubic and perineal discomfort, urinary frequency, urgency, strangury, dysuria, hematuria, pyuria and positive bacteriologic studies are the rule. Physical examination will reveal a moderately enlarged, tense, exquisitely tender prostate gland. Rectal examination should be performed extremely gently, in deference to the patient's comfort and the potentiality of manually-induced, retrograde epididymitis. Severity of symptoms may dictate hospitalization, when treatment may require parenteral broad-spectrum antibiotics, potent analgesia, intravenous fluid replacement, antifebrile measures and sedation.

Chronic or *congestive prostatitis* is a clinical entity seldom associated with bacteriologic invasion and the pathology typically associated with acute inflammation disorders. It usually involves patients in the fifth and sixth decades, and may also occur following interruption of an active sexual pattern. Acute local or systemic symptoms are seldom severe. Symptoms of vague perineal discomfort, mild symptoms of prostatism or vesical irritability, and reduced sexual potency are frequently experienced. Urinalysis may demonstrate pathognomonic mucus shreds, representing prostatic ductal casts due to stasis. Rectal examination will reveal a moderately enlarged, boggy gland of otherwise benign consistency. Prostatic massage may produce significant volumes of thin, milky secretions which on microscopic analysis contain large numbers of dead spermatozoa and white blood cells exceeding the normal number of 15 per high power field. Occasionally patients may complain of premature ejaculation, which is usually the result of posterior urethritis. Hemospermia, which is less common, usually represents seminal vesiculitis.

Chronic prostatitis may also be due to infection. This should be evaluated by urinalysis and culture of specimens obtained before and after prostatic massage. If the initial urine contains few or no bacteria, and the postmassage specimen has large numbers of bacteria, the diagnosis of chronic bacterial prostatitis is established, and prolonged antibacterial therapy is indicated.

Treatment of chronic congestive prostatitis includes a series of prostatic massages accompanied by hot sitz baths and re-establishment of normal sexual activity. Posterior urethritis may best be treated by adding a brief course of broad-spectrum antibiotic (doxycycline 50 mg p.o. b.i.d. × 5 days), as well as nitrofurazone-hydrocortisone urethral suppositories. Seminal vesiculitis and posterior urethritis may also be improved with a brief course of oral diethylstilbestrol (DES), 5 to 10 mg daily, which acts as a local decongestant. Patients treated with DES should be told that potency will be depressed temporarily. Protracted or recalcitrant seminal vesiculitis may respond dramatically to instillation of antibiotic-antiinflammatory medication through a unilateral or bilateral vasotomy.

Cystitis

The symptoms of cystitis may be summarized as "vesical irritability," and include dysuria, frequency, urgency, pubic discomfort and a sensation of incomplete vesicle emptying. The spectrum of symptoms associated with the clinical entities of cystitis and trigonitis are similar, and initially identical to that described later for the urethral syndrome. While a negative urine sediment is not uncommon with uncomplicated chronic urethritis, infection responsible for cystitis or trigonitis will typically produce micropyuria, bacteriuria, and not uncommonly, microhematuria. In addition, the entity of hemorrhagic cystitis most often involves females in the third and fourth decades and differs from the above-described syndrome only as regards the presence of gross hematuria. Left untreated, the hematuria will usually subside spontaneously within 48 hours, although

the physician is most frequently consulted during its presence.

It is a wise rule to investigate every patient with hematuria, gross or microscopic. This is particularly true in the older age groups. When such an investigation may be difficult or is refused by the patient, and when the clinical impression is overwhelmingly in favor of an infectious or otherwise benign etiology, it may often be reasonable to treat the infection according to sensitivity results by instituting an appropriate preliminary agent while awaiting these results (sulfisoxazole, nitrofurantoin, nalidixic acid, pyridium), and then re-evaluating the urine analysis after completion of treatment. Resistence or recurrence of hematuria is an indication of the first magnitude for thorough evaluation of the entire urinary tract.

Cystitis seldom occurs clinically as a localized entity. An association frequently exists with some form of vesical outlet obstruction or prostatitis in the male, while in the female such factors as urethral stenosis, urethral-hymenal fusion, and local irritants (such as detergents or synthetic fiber under-garments) are often contributory. Treatment, in addition to that indicated by specific culture and sensitivity studies, includes management of the contributing disorder.

Pyelonephritis

From whatever cause, this is a clinically urgent disorder requiring prompt and thorough management. Once the diagnosis is established or even suspected, specific treatment is urgently required, after which thorough investigation should be undertaken to discern all potential contributing factors such as vesicoureteral reflux, urinary tract obstruction and stasis, calculous disease, drug abuse (phenacetin), systemic disorders, septicemia and so on. The clinical syndrome of *acute pyelonephritis* includes fever, chills, diaphoresis, flank pain, lower urinary tract irritability and abnormalities of the urinary sediment. Severe systemic symptoms may dictate hospitalization, while less severe episodes may be adequately treated on an ambulatory basis. Appropriate antibiotics are essential, while the remainder of the treatment program will be dictated by the type and severity of the patient's symptoms. The first attack of acute pyelonephritis is often adequately treated with a single 10 to 14 day course of organism-specific therapy, with recurrent episodes best managed for a longer duration ranging from several months to years. Evidence exists that the failure of many treatment regimens results from reinfection with new and resistant organisms, rather than relapse with the initial pathogen. Relapses indicate that a more prolonged course of therapy is warranted.[6] Reinfection with a new strain requires a short course of a different therapeutic agent. There is little evidence that prolonged antimicrobial therapy is useful in patients with reinfection.

Long-term administration of relatively nonabsorbable sulfonamides (succinylsulfathiazole, phthalylsulfathiazole) has been advocated as an effective means of suppressing *E. coli* in the gut and thereby offering an approach to the control of recurrent coliform infections of the urinary tract. These sulfa drugs have been particularly helpful in female children, pregnant women, and in patients with chronic or recurrent bacteriuria who are at risk from progressive renal damage.[7] This type of treatment is indicated when the organisms responsible for the urinary infections are identical to those recovered in the patient's feces.

Any contributing anatomic or physiologic factors should be corrected promptly, after the acute process has been brought under control.

Chronic pyelonephritis frequently does not produce localizing symptoms and it may therefore result in severe renal parenchymal loss and functional deterioration before clinical clues develop which prompt medical intervention. The only symptoms may be "failure to thrive," chronic lethargy, borderline anemia or urinary frequency caused by limited renal concentrating capacity. Once the diagnosis has been established, a thorough evaluation of renal function is mandatory. An attempt should be made to determine the rate of deterioration and a search for contributing factors must be carried out.

Since chronic pyelonephritis often assumes an indolent, smoldering course, a brief period of chemotherapy is seldom, if ever, helpful. In such cases it may be necessary to continue maintenance chemotherapy for periods extending from six months to two years.[8,9] In such circumstances the best criteria of adequate therapy are stabilization of renal function and consistently negative urine cultures.

Septicemia

Sepsis and shock may result from gram negative bacillary infection arising in any organ of the genitourinary system. These infections demand early recognition and immediate, vigorous, thorough and expectant therapy. Such management can be adequately performed only in the hospital. Gram negative sepsis requires intensive, round-the-clock work by qualified personnel until the crisis has passed. The details of evaluation and management in gram negative septic shock are summarized in Table 19–4.

Acute Intrascrotal Infection (Epididymitis and Orchitis)

Acute inflammatory conditions of intrascrotal organs are discussed below, in conjunction with other acute intrascrotal disorders.

Management of Acute Urinary Tract Infection

Acute discomfort in the bladder or urethra, associated with discomfort on voiding, is readily recognized as symptomatic of urinary tract disease. The first thing which must be done in treating a

TABLE 19–4 GRAM NEGATIVE SEPSIS

EVALUATION	MANAGEMENT

1. Vital signs
   Acute temperature elevation
   Hypotension
   Tachycardia, bradycardia
   Restlessness
   Disorientation
   Air hunger
   Rigors
   Diaphoresis, dry skin
2. Central venous pressure (<6 cm H_2O; often <2 cm H_2O)
3. Urine output (oliguria, reflecting lowered splanchnic perfusion)
4. Pulse pressure lowered (reflecting lowered cardiac output)
5. Chest x-ray (pneumonia, atelectasis, pulmonary edema, embolism)
6. Electrocardiogram (dysrhythmia, ischemia-infaction, pericardial tamponade, pulmonary hypertension)
7. Urinalysis (infection, crystalluria, hematuria, clot, casts, tissue)
8. Blood and urine cultures
9. Laboratory data:
   Hemogram—anemia, hemolysis
   Electrolytes—hyponatremia, hypercalcemia, acidosis, hypocalcemia
   Blood sugar
   BUN, creatinine
   Serial platelet count
 	
   Fibrinogen level ⎫ useful for the recogni-
   Fibrin split products ⎬ tion of diffuse intravas-
   　　　　　　　　　 ⎭ cular coagulation
	1. Early recongition; prompt aggressive intervention
	2. Rapid fluid replenishment
	   Blood, colloid, saline, Ringer's solution
	   Monitor CVP, which reflects volume status and cardiac efficiency
	   Monitor BP, urine output, chest auscultation
	3. Antibiotics
	   Penicillin (20–60 × 10⁶ u/d IV) or cephalothin (1.0 gm IV q 4–6 h)
	   Kanamycin (500 mg IM q 12 h)—Proteus
	   Sodium colistimethate (15 mg IM q 12 h)—Pseudomonas
	   Gentamycin
	   Carbenicillin
	   (Observe indicators of drug intolerances and renal impairment)
	4. Steroids—hydrocortisone (100–500 mg IV stat; 100 mg IV q h)
	   Methylprednisolone (250 mg IV q 4–6 h)
	   (add prophylactic oral antacid therapy)
	5. Oxygen (nasal, mask)
	6. Antifebrile measures (hypothemia blanket)
	7. Sodium bicarbonate IV
	8. Digitalis for cardiac dysrhythmias with rising CVP, pulmonary congestion, hypotension
	9. Isoproterenol (2.5–5 mg/250–500 cc normal saline; titrate infusion for effect)
	   Pulse rate <120
	10. Furosemide (40–80 mg IM or IV; observe response, repeat, increase prn)
	11. Chlorpromazine or phenoxybenzamine to assist micro-circulation
	12. Heparin (in presence of evidence of diffuse intravascular coagulation)

urinary tract infection is to distinguish between an upper and lower urinary tract infection. Lower urinary tract infection is a nuisance, but upper tract infection is a serious threat, particularly in children, who do not handle pyelonephritis well. Next, the possibility of gonococcal urethritis must be considered, particularly if purulent urethral discharge is present.

If the patient is afebrile and if infection is documented on urinalysis, it is usually reasonable to begin treatment immediately with an appropriate antimicrobial agent such as sulfisoxasole (Gantrisin), nitrofurantoin (Macrodantin), or nalidixic acid (Neg-gram). The urine should be cultured and the treat-ment later adjusted to a specific antibiotic if infection does not subside promptly. In females these infections are usually caused by cystitis or urethritis, both of which are discussed above. In males, acute urinary tract infections are usually due to prostatitis, which tends to be a more serious infection and is associated with fever and constitutional symptoms.

Urinary tract infection in males is also caused by chronic vesical outlet obstruction, which is usually caused by median bar hypertrophy. Most of these men have a long history of symptoms, with enuresis, slow stream and urinary frequency. Antibacterial treatment is preferable to resection in most of these patients since the consequence of resection in young men is often a distressing degree of retrograde ejaculation.

The symptoms of acute urinary tract infection usually subside promptly with fluid-loading and antibacterial treatment, and pyridium is not necessary in most cases.

If acute upper urinary tract infection is also present, fever will usually accompany it, and these patients should be hospitalized until the infection is under control. The antibiotics most commonly effective in outpatient urinary tract infections with coliform organisms are tetracycline and ampicillin, but these drugs are usually reserved for resistant infection or for patients who are allergic or otherwise intolerant to the antimicrobial agents mentioned above. Recurrent or persistent urinary tract infection is an indication for complete urological work-up, since these patients often have congenital or acquired lesions, such as posterior urethral valves, median bar, diverticulum, ureteral reflux and so forth.

URINARY RETENTION

The patient presenting with urinary retention poses two basic problems: (1) whether the retention represents an acute or a chronic phenomenon, and (2) how best to relieve it.

Acute Retention

This condition may present abruptly as inability to void preceded by a history of outflow obstruction, including diminished size and force of urinary stream, hesitancy, postvoid dribbling and nocturia. In these patients a physiologic balance between outflow obstruction and increased vesical effort has been established to maintain satisfactory voiding performance. Any situation which then interferes with optimum bladder contractility will upset this balance, causing diminished efficiency of voiding power. Typical precipitating events include alcoholic overindulgence, a lengthy motor trip or other similar circumstances. Even mild vesical overdistention in some patients may produce diminished efficiency of the bladder musculature, resulting in the acute retention syndrome. Such patients are usually totally anuric, experience severe discomfort and exhibit few physical findings other than the palpably distended bladder. Relief is immediate with the passage of a urethral catheter, and prompt and complete decompression can be performed with impunity. Following decompression the catheter may be removed immediately. Prompt restoration of the predistention voiding pattern will frequently occur. Complete urologic evaluation should be carried out.

Occasionally, vesical outlet obstruction will resist easy passage of a urethral catheter, in which case a Coudé-tipped catheter may be successful (Fig. 19–3 A, B). Another alternative is a sterile flexible wire catheter guide (mandrin) inserted inside the urethral catheter (Fig. 19–3 C). The mandrin gives the catheter the semirigid curvature of a urethral sound, which with perineal or rectal pressure as an added guide, facilitates successful passage into the bladder.

Chronic Urinary Retention

Chronic urinary retention is generally seen in older, more debilitated and mentally obtunded patients. A history of prostatism may be obtained, and there is characteristically a varying history of frequent dribbling urinations and incontinence. Despite a palpably distended bladder, discomfort may be absent. Edema of the lower extremities is often present, due to lymphatic and venous obstruction produced by prolonged vesical distention. The chronic increase in intravesical pressure may also result in vesicoureteral reflux and transmission of hydrostatic pressure proximally to the kidneys. Serious sequelae are not infrequent in such cases. Infection, uremia and advanced renal deterioration may result.

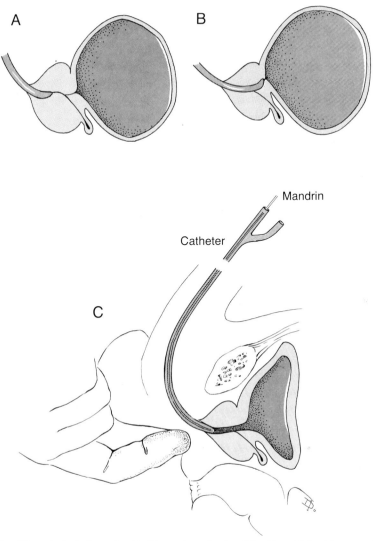

Figure 19–3 Alternate techniques for bladder catheterization (Coudé and Mandrin). *A* and *B*. Coudé-tipped catheter more easily maneuvered through posterior urethra in the presence of enlarged middle lobe of prostate *(A)* or median bar at vesical neck *(B)*. *C*. Mandrin guide technique. Lubricated mandrin is inserted inside catheter and bent into desired shape. Catheter is then inserted, as is a urethral sound (see Fig. 19–9), with perineal digital pressure aiding advancement through posterior urethra.

Although drainage is obviously necessary, prompt and complete decompression must be avoided, since abrupt relief of the hydrostatic pressure can result in vesical hemorrhage and severe fluid and electrolyte imbalances. Vesical hemorrhage is probably caused by acute engorgement and rupture of venous channels as the intravesical pressure suddenly falls. Electrolyte imbalances are thought to be owing to a lag in return of physiologically active renal tubular activity. Passive glomerular filtration results in a large volume of fluid passing into the renal collecting tubules. Reabsorption is impaired in these patients and electrolytes are lost in the urine. In such circumstances, gradual decompression is necessary and can be achieved in several ways. Release of a small volume of urine from the clamped catheter can be performed at periodic intervals (100 cc per hour) until decompression is complete. This is an effective although tedious method. The retained volume and the postretention diuresis may total several liters of urine, representing several days of hourly aliquots. Another technique involves the use of a smaller catheter, to which is applied a screw clamp, adjusted to limit the efflux to a rapid drip. A No. 10 F. ureteral catheter or the traditional indwelling Foley catheter can be used for this purpose. Although this technique will require just as long for complete vesical decompression, the demands on nursing personnel and the opportunities for error are lessened. Another effective technique involves the attachment of the urethral catheter to the drainage tubing through a three-way glass or plastic adaptor with one limb of the adaptor open to the air, thus preventing the establishment of a siphon (Fig. 19–4). The tubing is then attached to an intravenous pole at the bedside at an initial height of 20 cm above the pubic symphysis and remains there for 24 hours. It is

then lowered to 10 cm above the symphysis for another 24 hours, after which it is placed for routine gravity drainage. Regardless of the technique employed, close attention must be maintained for potential electrolyte imbalances.

Occasionally the patient with urinary retention will present with urethral pathology preventing catheterization by any of the maneuvers described above. In such circumstances prompt relief can be gained by the passage of a *suprapubic drainage tube* through a large bore needle. This maneuver provides gradual decompression. It is an efficient means of obtaining urine for bacteriologic examination while avoiding possible urethral contamination. The procedure should be employed only when the bladder is easily palpable above the pubic symphysis. The procedure is contraindicated in patients with prior lower abdominal surgery, because of the possibility of adhesions of peritoneum and bowel to the anterior vesical surface.

After preparation of the lower anterior abdominal wall, a site is selected in the midline two finger-breadths above the pubic symphysis. Local anesthetic is

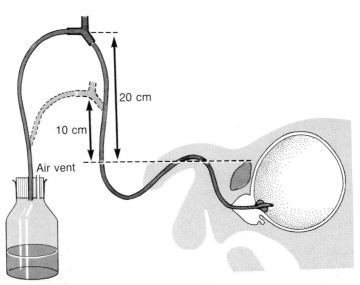

Figure 19–4 Gradual vesical decompression. Drainage tubing attached to catheter through **Y**-adapter open to the air. Adapter initially placed 20 cm for 24 hours, lowered 10 cm for 24 hours, then placed to gravity drainage.

infiltrated into the skin and deeper tissues along the intended tract of the catheterizing trocar. The procedure involves the use of a long polyethylene catheter which can pass through the bore of a large caliber needle. A pre-assembled apparatus (Cystocath) is now commercially available. The trocar needle is passed through the anesthetic wheal and directed caudally at a 45° angle behind the pubic symphysis until urine is returned. The polyethylene catheter is then threaded through the needle until urine is seen in its lumen, after which the needle is removed over the catheter. The catheter is secured to the skin with an appropriate silk or poly-ethylene suture, and drainage tubing is attached. A local antibiotic (neomycin-bacitracin) ointment is applied, and the skin is covered with a sterile dressing.

Suprapubic Cystostomy (Fig. 19–5)

One may occasionally encounter a situation requiring prolonged drainage of the bladder in which urethral catheterization is best avoided. Indications include intolerance to a urethral catheter, severe urethritis, and sensitivity to chemicals and materials of which the catheter is composed. In such circumstances a suprapubic catheter is preferable and often mandatory. Nonoperative supra-pubic catheterization technqiue utilizes the Lowsley retractor, an instrument commonly employed in perineal pros-tatic surgery. This instrument is shaped like a urethral sound, and has retractable blades at the leading edge which can be opened and retracted by the operator. This method is contraindicated in pa-tients who have had prior lower ab-dominal surgery. Vesical distention may be produced by fluid instilled through a urethral catheter.

After appropriate sedation and instil-lation of local urethral anesthetic, the Lowsley instrument is passed into the distended bladder and manipulated until it can be palpated through the skin in the midline suprapubically, after which the skin and deeper subcutaneous tis-sues are thoroughly infiltrated with local anesthetic. A short incision is made over the retractor's leading edge until it can be delivered through the abdominal wound. The retractable blades are then opened, and a No. 24 F. Foley catheter is grasped by the retractor blades as they are closed. The instrument is with-drawn until the catheter tip is located inside the bladder, as indicated by the efflux of urine or irrigating solution from the catheter. The retractor blades are then opened slightly to release the cathe-ter. The balloon of the catheter is in-flated and placed on slight tension. The retractor blades are then closed, and the instrument is removed. The catheter is secured to the skin, covered with anti-biotic ointment, and a dry sterile dress-ing is applied. Gravity drainage is then instituted.

Although suprapubic catheters are frequently better tolerated than urethral catheters, they should nevertheless be changed at periodic intervals. Latex catheters will usually require changes as frequently as every two to three weeks, whereas siliconized and Teflon-coated catheters are often tolerated well for periods of up to eight weeks. Irrigation should be performed daily with sterile saline, 0.25 per cent acetic acid, or solu-tion G to assure patency. In the ab-sence of irrigations, vesical detritus accumulates which may encourage in-fection and serve as a nidus for cal-careous encrustation and calculus forma-tion. Suprapubic catheters are easily changed if a catheter of similar size is immediately inserted after removal of the prior catheter. However, despite prolonged catheterization, the suprapubic vesicocutaneous fistula will usually close spontaneously within a day or two, unless there is concomitant vesical outlet obstruction.

Perineal Urethrostomy (Fig. 19–6)

Proximal urinary diversion may be required in patients undergoing urethro-plastic surgical procedures or in patients with pendulous urethral strictures. Other

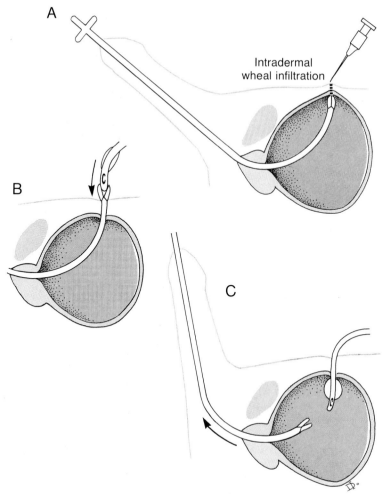

Figure 19–5 Suprapubic cystostomy (Lowsley). *A*. Lowsley retractor passed into distended bladder as with a urethral sound and maneuvered until it is palpable in the midline suprapubically. Cutaneous and subcutaneous anesthetic infiltration. *B*. Incision through anesthetized tissues and delivery of the retractor through the suprapubic wound. Retractor blades opened to grasp Foley catheter. *C*. Catheter withdrawn into bladder. Foley balloon inflated. Retractor withdrawn with blades closed. Suprapubic wound closure as necessary.

indications include trauma and poor tolerance to urethral catheterization. Methods of diversion include either suprapubic or proximal urethral (perineal) drainage. Perineal urethrostomy is performed in the frog-legged supine or lithotomy position. Following appropriate preparation a metal sound is introduced into the urethra. The scrotum and its contents are retracted appropriately, according to the site selected. The sound is stabilized in the perineum between the

thumb and forefinger of the left hand. Local anesthesia is thoroughly infiltrated, after which a 2 cm incision is made in the midline over the sound and is carried down onto the sound. Sufficient exposure is obtained to allow each lateral edge of the wound to be grasped with Allis clamps, including skin, fascia and the incised edges of urethra. Absorbable sutures are used to secure the minor bleeding which occurs and to assist retraction. The sound is then re-

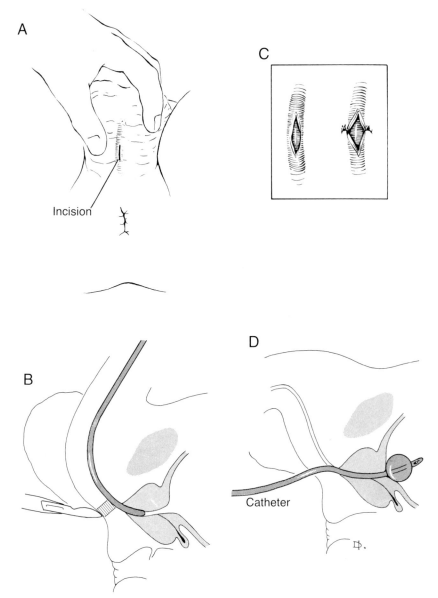

Figure 19–6 Perineal urethrostomy. *A.* Urethral sound is grasped in the perineal midline between thumb and forefinger. *B*, and *C*. Longitudinal incision is made over the sound until sound is visible. *D*. Urethral mucosa sutured to cutaneous margin with single absorbable suture on either side. *E*. Sound withdrawn and retention catheter inserted into the bladder.

moved and the catheter is introduced retrograde into the bladder. In the absence of distal urethral obstruction, this type of perineal fistula will usually close promptly following removal of the catheter.

In the presence of pendulous urethral strictures preventing introduction of metal sounds, the midline structures of the perineum should be grasped manually, including the proximal penile urethra, which is situated close to the surface in this region. Successful incision into the urethra can be made while maintaining a secure grasp of these tissues. The urethra can be identified by its pearly glistening surface. The procedure is continued as described above. In such cases, a retrograde urethrogram will assist in proper positioning of the fistula, avoiding opening into a strictured area unsuitable for catheter placement.

Percutaneous Nephrostomy

A critical situation is presented by either simultaneous bilateral urinary obstructive disease, or by obstruction to a solitary functioning kidney. Several surgical alternatives are available for such patients. Occasionally patients are encountered in whom advanced renal decompensation, sepsis or the critical sequelae of uremia have produced a prohibitive hazard to general anesthesia and major surgery. Percutaneous renal decompression and drainage under local anesthesia is a valuable maneuver in such patients.

The safest and least traumatic technique for percutaneous nephrostomy utilizes identification of the renal pelvis with a No. 21 gauge spinal needle. A Vim-Silverman needle is then introduced alongside the spinal needle and advanced into the renal pelvis.[20] Next, a No. 5 F. ureteral catheter is inserted through the lumen of the Vim-Silverman needle. Fluoroscopic control may be used for positioning of the needles and catheter. Following removal of the needles, the catheter should be taped to the skin to maintain its position.

A slightly more complicated procedure employs the introduction of a drainage tubing over a guidewire, thus giving the advantage of a catheter of greater diameter than its trocar tract. This technique minimizes hemorrhage and urinary leakage and provides drainage equal to that of a No. 18 F. nephrostomy tube.[21] A commercially available pack provides all the necessary equipment and materials.

The patient is positioned prone on the fluoroscopy table. After suitable preparation and draping, a point is located 5 to 7 cm lateral to the midline below the twelfth rib. The skin and fascia are infiltered with local anesthesia. A No. 22 gauge spinal needle attached to a syringe is then advanced at right angles to the skin in a direction 15° cephalad, with further infiltration as required. Gentle aspiration is performed as the anticipated position of the kidney is approached. A sudden diminution in pressure will signal entry into the renal pelvis or a vein. Aspiration of blood will usually indicate positioning in the paracalyceal venous plexus, in which case minimal advancement will result in entry into the renal pelvis, indicated by aspiration of urine. Rocking of the needle with respiration will verify its position within the renal substance. At this point the needle may be attached to an intravenous tubing and contrast medium may be introduced to confirm its position fluoroscopically. Prior addition of methylene blue to the contrast medium will assist later maneuvers. A 1 cm incision is then made through the skin and fascia adjacent to the spinal needle with a special fascia-cutting needle. A 4½″ 18 gauge thin-walled needle is then introduced adjacent to the spinal needle. Its entry into the renal pelvis is indicated by return of methylene blue-colored fluid. A flexible plastic-tipped guidewire is then introduced through the second needle to a depth sufficient to allow it to pass easily, after which the No. 18 gauge needle is removed. Care is taken to avoid withdrawing the guidewire with the needle, which could shear off its tip. The fascia-cutting needle is then passed along the guidewire to its full depth and removed. A No. 12 F. polyethylene catheter is then inserted over the guidewire and advanced into the renal pelvis to the depth of easy passage, and at least 2 cm beyond the guidewire tip. All its holes are then within the renal pelvis. If it can be introduced into the proximal ureter, stability is improved. Return of blue fluid will again verify position of the catheter, after which the guidewire and spinal needle can be removed. Fluoroscopic studies may then be obtained. Urinary drainage is accomplished with an intravenous tubing attached through an appropriate adapter, the tubing being secured to the skin.

The insertion of a small catheter or tubing through a percutaneous trocar introduced into the renal collecting system may be considered, but it requires a dilated or an extrarenal pelvis. A large bore trocar is necessary, and this is prone to produce hemorrhage. The drainage conduit is smaller in caliber than the trocar tract and may be associated with urinary leakage along the tract. Inefficient drainage and obstruction by clots are frequent occurrences. Obviously, this means of decompression and drainage is limited in its application.

Ileal Conduit — Indications and Long-Term Management

The major indications for this form of urinary diversion are cancer of the bladder, myelomeningocoele and severe renal damage due to chronic lower urinary tract obstruction. In the latter condition, emergency skin ureterostomies are frequently done, and the diversion is converted to an ileal "loop" when the situation has been stabilized.

One of the complications of ileal loop diversion is obstruction, which is usually due to poor surgical technique and in which stricture occurs at the ureteral orifices, the fascia or the skin. Occasionally, when the loop is too long, it may serve as a reservoir instead of as a conduit. The symptoms of dysfunction are those of infection, uremia or — rarely — stone formation. The patients may have poor appetite, fever, pyuria, poor urinary output or pain. The evaluation of such patients should include urinalysis and culture, and x-ray studies (retrograde "loop"-o-gram) or intravenous pyelogram. When complications arise, the loop should usually be catheterized

and the patient hospitalized for further studies and revision if necessary.

The patient who has an ileal conduit should maintain longterm contact with an ostomy association or the manufacturer's representative for ileostomy appliances. This association should begin before the patient leaves the hospital for the first time. Each appliance has its own instructions, cement and special techniques required for its use. All appliances require that the skin be meticulously cleaned and dried before the cement is applied. The ileostomy should be dilated whenever the appliance is replaced, usually at weekly intervals. In an adult, the ileostomy should be dilated through the fascia, and usually it will accept the index finger through the proximal interphalangeal joint.

Bladder Irrigation

Catheters should be irrigated and changed as indicated for each specific patient. The intervals vary with the size and type of catheter used, and with the degree of infection present. Large catheters, and those made of Teflon, may not require changing for periods of 4 to 12 weeks. Nephrostomy catheters should be irrigated daily, but should be changed as infrequently as possible, since it is often difficult to reinsert the catheter within the renal pelvis. All patients with urinary draining catheters should have on hand an extra sterile catheter, so that it can be replaced promptly if it becomes dislodged.

The best irrigating solution is Neosporin solution, but its use encourages resistant bacterial overgrowth. Other useful solutions are $1/4$ per cent acetic acid, normal saline, Solution G or Solution M. Bladder irrigation should be performed as needed to guarantee patency of the catheter and to reduce sludge. Spastic bladder does not respond to irrigation. It is a neurogenic problem and requires pudental block or rhizotomy for control.

HEMATURIA

Evaluation of the patient with hematuria must take into consideration the age and sex of the patient and the associated symptoms. In pediatric urology, the commonest causes are urethral meatitis (in infants), and acute glomerulonephritis (in childhood). Meatitis occurs predominantly in infants under two years of age and is caused by irritation from the diapers. Acute glomerulonephritis is usually seen in older children and adolescents, who usually are ill with fever and malaise. Wilms' tumor must always be considered in any infant or child with sudden, gross hematuria. These children may be completely free of other symptoms but may have a palpable abdominal or flank mass, and the intravenous pyelogram will confirm the presence of a tumor.

In young female adults, gross hematuria is usually due to hemorrhagic cystitis. The patient may initially have no other complaint than hematuria, but discomfort and urinary frequency usually appear within a short time. The treatment of cystitis is discussed above. In males the commonest cause is acute prostatitis, which is also discussed above. These patients are usually acutely ill. Chronic prostatitis may also cause hematuria, which is associated with perineal discomfort. In both males and females, carcinoma of the kidney is always a possibility, though it is not common. In older patients, carcinoma of the bladder is always considered a possibility until it is ruled out by cystoscopy. For these reasons, it is wise to consider and recommend immediate cystoscopy unless the symptoms and signs clearly point to cystitis or prostatitis. In this case, the patient may be treated initially with antibiotics and a high fluid intake, but if hematuria persists or recurs, cystoscopy or intravenous pyelography must be performed.

Patients are frequently referred for evaluation of microscopic hematuria which is discovered in the course of a routine physical and laboratory examination, or in the laboratory evaluation of some other illness. In young adults it is usually reasonable to have the patient simply return in a week for repeat urinalysis. If the microscopic hematuria persists, a full work-up should be done, including culture, cystoscopy and intravenous pyelography. In an older person, the likelihood of malignancy of the kidney, ureter, bladder or prostate is increased.

It is frequently impractical to perform the complete work-up immediately, or the patient may refuse it if he or she is completely asymptomatic. Therefore, the most important thing to remember is that a good relationship with the patient must be established, so that follow-up studies can be obtained even if the full work-up is deferred temporarily for some reason. If there are associated symptoms such as vesical irritability or flank pain, a complete work-up should be done promptly, since these symptoms increase the likelihood of the presence of a serious underlying disease. Painless hematuria of sudden onset in a middle-aged man or woman means a bladder tumor until it is proved otherwise.

RENAL COLIC

Acute, intermittent, extremely severe pain along the course of the urinary tract suggests the presence of renal colic. Prompt medical intervention is needed to alleviate the patient's suffering and to prevent more serious sequelae, including sepsis and permanent renal dysfunction. Renal (ureteral) calculus is the commonest cause of renal colic. Other causes include blood clot, sloughed renal papillae and mycelioma. Examination of the urinary sediment will assist in verifying the clinical impression. Intravenous pyelography will confirm the presence of obstruction and may identify the underlying cause as well.

The intensity of the pain of renal colic makes it a urologic emergency, and efforts should be directed toward prompt clinical relief. Nausea and vomiting are commonly experienced. The patient engages in restless activity in an effort to find a position of relief, and this frequently differentiates renal colic from intra-abdominal calamities—in which relief is usually afforded by avoidance of movement. Chronic, progressive urinary tract obstruction may be silent or may produce only dull discomfort, localized to a specific anatomic area. In contrast, renal colic is acute, intense, waxing and waning, and will frequently shift as the obstruction advances down the ureter. Pain commonly originates in the area of the costovertebral angle, and involves sequentially the flank, loin and groin, radiating into the ipsilateral testis or labium majus and medial thigh. Urinary tenesmus may be experienced as the obstruction nears the ureterovesical junction. Sudden relief typically occurs with passage of the obstruction into the bladder, after which expulsion in the urinary stream may occur within the first several voidings.

Examination of the urinary sediment may reveal microhematuria and, less commonly, crystalluria with ureteral calculi, and occasionally other components compatible with the obstructing process. Total ureteral obstruction may render the urine essentially normal, however. Therefore the diagnosis of renal colic should never be dismissed without excretory urography to confirm the site and degree of obstruction. Delayed films may be necessary to evaluate the renal systems adequately. Contrast studies are incomplete without films which evaluate delayed function due to acute obstruction. Opaque calculi within the ureter can be measured on the x-ray film. A calculus measuring less than 6 mm in diameter will pass spontaneously in 90 per cent of patients, while calculi greater than 6 mm will pass spontaneously in less than 10 per cent of cases. Radiolucent calculi may be followed clinically by excretory urography in order to chart progress. Retrograde contrast studies are occasionally required. Large calculi obstructing the ureteropelvic junction offer little hope for spontaneous ureteral passage. In these cases, Trendelenburg positioning on the side of the calculus may relieve the obstruction and the symptoms until appropriate surgery can be arranged.

Acute management of renal (ureteral) colic requires prompt administration of analgesia. Narcotics are nearly always necessary (hydromorphone, 1.0 to 2.0 mg IM). Antispasmodics and anticholinergics are not of benefit. The potential ureterospasm produced by narcotic medication is outweighed by its analgesic properties. Antiemetics are occasionally necessary, although relief of pain will also commonly relieve nausea. Dehydration may require intravenous rehydration, and in these cases hospitalization will be necessary.

A patient may be discharged with oral analgesic medications if he demonstrates no evidence of infection, a satisfactory response to analgesic medication, and a calculus measuring less than 6 mm in diameter which progresses down the ureter. Instructions for follow-up care include straining all voided urine. Follow-up evaluations should also include urinalysis, plain abdominal x-ray for opaque calculi, isotope renography if indicated, evaluation of symptoms, and the need for relief of pain. If the calculus can be captured it should be studied by chemical analysis in order to assist formulation of a diet which will discourage further development of calculi, and to investigate metabolic contributions to calculogenesis. At initial presentation, screening laboratory data should include serum calcium, phosphorus, uric acid, alkaline phosphatase and serum proteins. Urinary pH determination is essential, and a 24 hour urinary study of calcium excretion may be indicated.

Uric acid calculi may dissolve during treatment, which includes urinary alkalinization with sodium bicarbonate, potassium citrate, and sodium citrate and administration of uric acid antagonists (allopurinol). Cystine calculi are often managed successfully by a maintenance regimen of diuresis, urinary alkylinization and penicillamine. All patients with urinary tract calculi should be encouraged to increase fluid intake to a level resulting in a urine output of 2500 to 3000 cc daily.

Ureteral obstruction by mycelioma (fungal ball), blood clot or sloughed papilla obviously suggests more significant disease. In these cases hospitalization will be warranted at the outset. Retrograde ureteral catheter drainage and irrigations may be of great importance in such obstructions.

Indications for operative intervention include infection or sepsis, intractable pain, failure of the calculus to progress further distally, and diminishing renal function, which is best evaluated with serial isotope renograms.

ACUTE INTRASCROTAL DISORDERS

The differential diagnosis of acute, unilateral inflammatory intrascrotal disorders includes acute epididymitis, orchitis, torsion of the spermatic cord or testicular appendages, hematocele, scrotal abscess, leukemic infiltration, spermatic cord hematoma, hemorrhage into neoplasm, and strangulated indirect inguinal hernia. Such lesions are nearly always unilateral. The most common exception is mumps orchitis, which can occur bilaterally in 6 per cent of involved cases. The diagnosis of mumps orchitis is assisted by the fact that this disease rarely occurs prior to puberty, is typically preceded by parotitis and is associated with a rising mumps antibody titer.

Acute Epididymitis

Acute epididymitis is the most common acute intrascrotal inflammation in the adult. This disorder seldom occurs prior to the third decade. Its documented presence in a child or adolescent should raise the suspicion of underlying disease elsewhere in the urinary tract. Similarly, acute epididymitis in a young adult is often related to vesical outlet obstruction, most often a congenital median bar at the posterior vesical neck. Appropriate questioning and further evaluation will often confirm this correlation. Chronic infections of the vas and epididymis by lues (gumma) and tuberculosis are rare at this time.

Symptoms of acute epididymitis include acute—though not precipitous—onset of unilateral pain, tenderness, swelling and induration, initially localized to the epididymis at the posterior aspect of the testis. Symptoms may occasionally be limited to a single epididymal pole. Further enlargement and induration will result in obliteration of the epididymal sinus, giving the clinical impression of a solitary mass. Dimensions of the lesion may vary from minimal polar induration to enlargement to grapefruit size. Scrotal edema and erythema is common. These features are usually localized to the side of the lesion, but may involve the entire scrotum. Pain and tenderness may be intense, frequently extending along the spermatic cord. In this case, adequate clinical evaluation may be difficult or impossible without spermatic cord block. Development of a secondary hydrocele may further interfere with effective clinical evaluation. Manual elevation of the testis will frequently produce symptomatic relief (Prehn's sign), assisting differentiation from other scrotal disorders. Urinalysis, urine culture and examination of prostatic secretions may be positive or negative. If fever and leucocytosis develop, an associated prostatitis may be present.

Since it is difficult to prove the diagnosis of acute epididymitis in children or adolescents, prompt exploration is often required in young people in order to rule out spermatic cord torsion. Exploration may occasionally be necessary in older age groups in order to rule out testicular tumor, which may mimic an acute inflammatory process if a hemorrhage into it occurs.

The treatment of acute epididymitis includes institution of oral or parenteral broad-spectrum antibiotics, according to the severity of the condition. If urine cultures are ultimately positive, therapy can be altered according to specific sensitivities. Bed rest is recommended during the acute stage. Scrotal elevation usually provides significant relief, and may be further improved by local application of heat or ice, whichever is subjectively more effective. Effective support is provided by the Bellevue bridge, a broad strip of adhesive tape passed between the upper anterior thighs. A pillow may be equally beneficial. Analgesic and antifebrile measures may be required. After the acute stage has subsided and the patient is allowed to ambulate once again, continued scrotal and systemic symptoms will usually subside after three to five days, with resolution of the enlargement and induration over several weeks thereafter. Continued sepsis after several days of adequate treatment raises the possibility of testicular or epididymal abscess, management of which is surgical.

Orchitis per se is exceedingly rare, and occurs as a primary infection only in disseminated infectious diseases such as mumps and syphilis. It may develop secondary to epididymitis, in which case the treatment is as described for epididymitis.

Spermatic Cord Torsion

This disorder may occur in all age groups, but affects primarily children and adolescents. Two types of spermatic cord torsion may occur: intravaginal ("bell clapper"), and extravaginal. Intravaginal torsion occurs in testes lacking the normal epididymal attachment of the tunica vaginalis, which attaches proximally on the spermatic cord. Such testes are thus allowed to swing freely within the tunica. Extravaginal torsion occurs when the entire parietal tunica vaginalis twists within the scrotum. This occurs primarily in newborns, presumably due to the greater mobility of the testis and spermatic cord at this early age.

Trauma and exertion frequently contribute to the development of spermatic cord torsion, although onset during sleep is not uncommon. Other factors reported as contributory include cryptorchidism,[15] Marfan's syndrome,[16] and Henoch-Schönlein purpura.[17]

The clinical syndrome typifying spermatic cord torsion includes the acute onset of unilateral testicular pain and tenderness, often with abdominal pain, nausea and vomiting. On the other hand, some patients exhibit a gradual onset of symptoms. Repeated episodes of torsion and spontaneous detorsion apparently occur in a significant number of patients. Acute painless scrotal swelling in an infant is sufficient cause for prompt surgical intervention because of the possibility of torsion of the testis.

Fever and abnormal urinary sediment are rare, while hemiscrotal edema and erythema, and woody induration of the testis are common. Testicular retraction (testis redux), if present, will assist diagnosis. Prehn's sign is absent.

Spermatic cord torsion will initially obstruct only venous circulation, resulting in obstructive edema of the testis and spermatic cord. Persistence of occlusion will ultimately result in hemorrhagic infarction of the testicle. The need for prompt detorsion is obvious. Manual external derotation is often unsuccessful due to early local fibrin deposition. Diagnosis of spermatic cord torsion requires prompt surgical exploration, with detorsion or orchiectomy depending on the status of the involved testis. Intrascrotal fixation of both testes should be performed, since the developmental defect predisposing to torsion exists bilaterally. The importance of prompt intervention is demonstrated by statistics indicating an 83 per cent salvage rate in patients explored within five hours of onset of symptoms, falling to 70 per cent if exploration is performed between five and ten hours after onset, and falling further to 20 per cent if further delayed beyond ten hours.[18]

Torsion of the Testicular Appendages

This presents a clinical syndrome similar to that associated with acute epididymitis and torsion of the spermatic cord. Surgical intervention will frequently be indicated. Differential diagnosis is similar to that described for acute epididymitis.

The incidence of at least one unilateral pedunculated testicular appendage has been reported as 74 per cent, with the bilateral presence of such appendages reported as exceeding 50 per cent. Such appendages include the appendix testis, responsible for 95 per cent of torsion of testicular appendages, and the appendix epididymis, responsible for the majority of the remainder.[19] Both of these appendages reside near the junction of the globus major of the epididymis and the superior pole of the testis anteriorly. Other appendages include the paradidymis, residing at the inferior (proximal) aspect of the spermatic cord, and the vas aberrans, typically occupying the junction of the body and tail of the epididymis.

The clinical presentation includes the onset of unilateral pain, usually severe and often localized to the upper pole of the involved testis. Lower abdominal pain is not uncommon and confusion with appendicitis has been reported. Hemiscrotal erythema and edema may be extensive, although usually less than that associated with spermatic cord torsion. Transillumination may demonstrate a blackish body in the region of the upper pole of the testis, despite the presence of an inflammatory hydrocele. Clinical abnormalities will usually subside spontaneously without sequelae within 5 to 12 days, although occasionally infarction and calcification may later present the diagnostic problem of a free or attached, firm, nontender intrascrotal mass. The acute process will commonly justify prompt emergency exploration.

Cremaster Muscle Spasm

Another lesion occasionally masquerading as spermatic cord torsion is cremaster muscle spasm. This condition is a recurrent unilateral disorder of slow onset, producing retraction or elevation of the involved testis. Aching pain occurs in the testis and groin. Clinical findings are otherwise absent. Treatment is primarily limited to symptomatic care, plus spermatic cord block in some cases. Recurrent or recalcitrant episodes may warrant exploration and division of the cremaster muscle fibers investing the spermatic cord.

CUTANEOUS LESIONS

The skin of the external genitalia is subject to inflammatory, infectious, traumatic and neoplastic disorders affecting the skin elsewhere. The scrotum is seldom involved by neoplasia but is frequently affected by inflammatory lesions, and typically responds with extensive edema and erythema. Intrascrotal disorders, specifically epididymitis and torsion of the testicular appendages, may in turn be accompanied by scrotal edema and erythema which can often either confuse the clinical impression or assist correct diagnosis. Although the circumcised penis is less likely to develop cutaneous abnormalities than the uncircumcised, it nonetheless may respond with edema and erythema to inflammatory and allergic insults. Any suspicious lesion of the prepuce, glans or scrotum should undergo biopsy immediately. Biopsy is frequently best done under appropriate general or regional anesthesia. It is also permissible under local anesthesia if the basic principles for such surgery are remembered; namely, gentle manipulation and adequate tissue for pathologic study.

Preputial Dorsal Slit (Fig. 19–7)

Phimosis occurs in association with infection or inflammation due to accumulation of smegma, trauma of intercourse, or systemic disorders (e.g., diabetes). Phimosis will persist until local cleaning

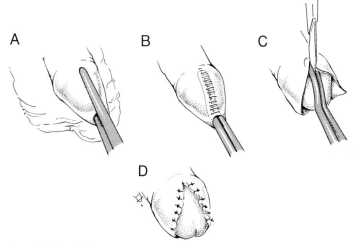

Figure 19–7 Preputial dorsal slit. *A*. Application of hemostat in vertical midline to depth of ½ to 1 cm distal to corona. *B*. Insertion of grooved director. *C*. Incision of clamped tissue. *D*. Application of absorbable suture. A running hemostatic suture is usually preferable to the interrupted stitches shown here.

and treatment can be instituted. Immediate circumcision is often contraindicated because of the local inflammation. In such situations preputial retraction will be easily accomplished after a simple dorsal incision, performed under total penile block (Fig. 19–1), or after infiltration of local anesthesia along the proposed line of incision. Following routine preparation and draping, local anesthesia is instilled. A straight hemostat is inserted into the phimotic preputial meatus and extended vertically in the midline to a distance sufficient to allow retraction. The hemostat is not inserted beyond one cm distal to the corona, which is the appropriate margin for later elective circumcision. After a few minutes the clamp is removed and the crushed tissue is divided. Care must be taken to avoid inserting the probing blade of the clamp or scissors into the urethral meatus. Bleeding is controlled with a running suture of 3-0 chromic gut along the cut edges of the incision. Inflammatory reaction and edema will usually subside promptly, after which consideration can be given to completion of circumcision.

Paraphimosis

This disorder exists when the prepuce is retracted sufficiently proximal to the glans to allow the development of circumferential edema. Reduction becomes progressively difficult and painful. Paraphimosis frequently develops in unconscious or debilitated patients, in whom the prepuce has been retracted to allow cleansing, inspection or catheterization, after which immediate reduction was neglected. Despite severe edema, the disorder is not initially uncomfortable. If untreated, the edema may evolve into a constrictive band.

Treatment consists of several maneuvers which are performed sequentially until reduction is obtained. The first technique (Fig. 19–8) involves placing the thumbs on the glans, producing counter traction against the second and third fingers of both hands placed on either side and behind the preputial contraction ring. Counter pressure is then exerted until reduction occurs. The application of liquid soap or mineral oil about the corona may facilitate this maneuver. Circumferential or quadrantic injection of hyaluronidase (Wydase: 150 turbidity-

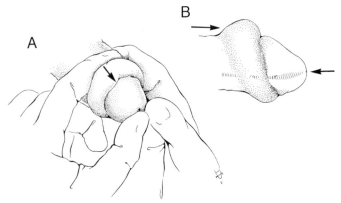

Figure 19–8 Reduction of paraphimosis. *A*. Manual reduction, demonstrating counter-pressure between thumbs and fingers *(B)*.

reducing units in 2 cc normal saline) around the constricting band may facilitate reduction, which may occur spontaneously.[12,13] Fifteen minutes are usually required for optimum enzymatic activity. Success has also been described with the quadrantic application of Babcock clamps to the retraction ring, with continuous gentle and equal traction on the clamps resulting in rapid and relatively painless reduction.[19] Should these maneuvers fail a dorsal preputial slit will usually be successful. A two or three cm midline vertical incision is carried from a point proximal to the constricting band, across the band and onto the distal aspect of the edematous retracted prepuce. Reduction can then be effected, after which the incision is closed transversely to maintain the added circumference.

Circumcision

In the older child and adult this procedure is usually performed without the Gomco clamp typically used for infant circumcisions. Unless phimosis with inflammation or urinary obstruction dictates earlier intervention, it is wise to defer childhood circumcision until after 12 months of age in order to avoid potential anesthetic problems. The technique of circumcision in children is shown in Fig. 23–11. The technique in

adults is similar, except that local anesthesia may be used.

After appropriate preparation and draping, the penis is anesthetized as shown in Figure 19–1. After testing for anesthesia a vertical midline dorsal incision is made, maintaining a 1.0 cm margin from the coronal sulcus. Care should be taken to avoid unnecessary traction on the prepuce, which may result in an exaggerated proximal extension of the dorsal slit. The prepuce is then everted to assure a similar margin on the internal aspect, which should be adjusted as necessary. A suture of 3-0 plain gut approximates the outer and inner apices of the dorsal incision. The procedure is then repeated in the midline ventrally, extending to the frenular attachment only. More proximal extension results in excessive bleeding and may damage the sensory innervation of the glans. A ventral horizontal mattress traction suture may be helpful in securing frenular bleeding which may occasionally be troublesome. By everting the prepuce from side to side away from the glans the corona can be exposed completely. Excision of the redundant prepuce can then be easily and accurately performed. Undue tension on the prepuce should be avoided during excision in order to prevent excessive excision of prepuce. An even incision is easily obtained if it is begun as far proximal on the blades of the scissors as possible. Hemicircumcision is thereby performed with a single maneuver rather than a series of smaller maneuvers, which tend to result in scalloping. Following hemicircumcision, bleeding vessels are identified and secured with electrocautery or interrupted 3-0 plain gut ligatures. The procedure is then repeated on the opposite side. An excessive number of sutures should be avoided by bisecting each remaining distance. More than a dozen stitches are seldom required. The suture line is then protected with a dressing of Vaseline gauze or plain sterile gauze which is cut and folded appropriately. Dressings can be removed later the same day. Circumcisions are not particularly painful in adults. The patient will adapt quickly to the discomfort, which diminishes rapidly.

Urethral Stricture and Stenosis

Urethral obstruction in the female may result from such causes as meatal stenosis, a distal fibrous ring and inflammatory urethritis, whereas in the male causes may include fibromuscular vesical neck contraction, posterior bar formation at the vesical neck, prostatic hypertrophy and neoplasia, prostatitis, urethral valve, urethral diverticulum and postinflammatory and post-traumatic strictures.

Urethral Stricture

Straddle injuries usually produce strictures of the bulbous urethra, while those accompanying deceleration injuries and pelvic fracture most commonly involve the area of the membranous urethra. Strictures associated with gonococcal urethritis will usually involve the bulbous and proximal pendulous urethra. Strictures due to urethritis from indwelling catheters typically involve the distal pendulous urethra at the level of the fossa navicularis and the urethral meatus. Strictures associated with periurethral abscess due to pressure

necrosis from chronic indwelling catheters usually involve the distal bulbous and proximal pendulous urethra at the penoscrotal junction.

Evaluation and treatment of urethral stricture will depend upon the site and severity of the lesion. This may bear little relationship to the symptoms experienced or the sequelae produced. Symptoms may range from urinary tract infection and outflow obstruction to vesicoureteral reflux and deterioration of the upper urinary tract. Urethral meatal strictures can be managed by simple urethral meatotomy. Fossa navicularis strictures may be managed by dilatation and internal urethrotomy. An alternate technique is careful insertion of a No. 11 scalpel blade through the meatus and stricture. Meatotomy is frequently necessary before the scalpel blade can be introduced. Ultimately, dilatation is carried out to a No. 24 French with bougie or metal sound. This technique should be performed only by experienced personnel, under adequate local anesthesia. More proximal urethral strictures require thorough investigation prior to intervention, including bougie-a-boule calibration in the less severe strictures. Calibration yields information regarding the site, density, pliability, and extent of the fibrous obstructions. More severe strictures and those not amenable to such calibration are best delineated preoperatively by urethrography. Vesical outlet obstruction due to prostatic disease and stricture at the vesical neck are best investigated cystographically and endoscopically.

Nonoperative management of urethral strictures includes the use of urethral sounding, filiforms and followers, and internal urethrotomy.

Urethral Sounding (Fig. 19–9). This procedure should be preceded by filling the urethra with a water-soluble lubricant such as K-Y Jelly, Lubasporin, or a topical anesthetic such as Xylocaine jelly. In apprehensive male patients, topical anesthetic is usually not as useful as intravenous sedation with Valium. In such patients, we fill a syringe with 10

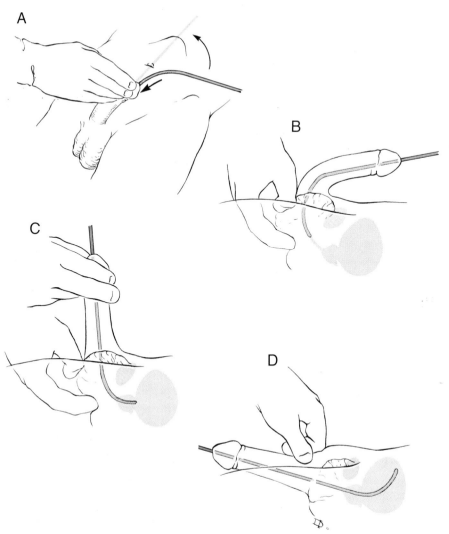

Figure 19–9   Urethral sounding technique. *A.* Sound introduced through meatus with handle over left iliac crest to facilitate passage. *B.* Sound maneuvered to midline vertical position, and advanced to the level of the urethral bulb. *C.* Sound maneuvered gently to horizontal position to facilitate advancement through external splinter and vesical neck. Digital perineal pressure may assist. *D.* Sound advanced through vesical neck.

mg of Valium and administer 5 mg slowly over a period of 30–60 seconds. Drowsiness will usually be achieved with this dose, although in large or unusually apprehensive patients, an additional 2–3 mg may be needed. In females, urethral sounding is relatively quick and painless, especially if preceded by application of Xylocaine jelly for a few seconds on a sterile cotton swab.

Filiforms and Followers. With dense and tortuous strictures it may be necessary to employ the use of filiforms and followers in order to carry out therapeutic dilatation or incision. Urethral filiforms are merely flexible guides of small caliber and varying tips (olive or pig tail, for instance) which may be introduced into the urethra until an obstruction is met or until the urethral lumen at the level of obstruction is encountered and traversed. If obstruction

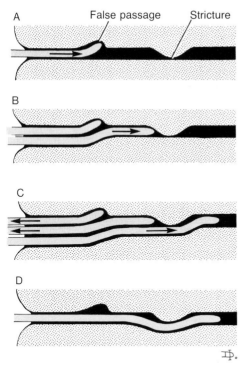

A False passage Stricture

B

C

D

Figure 19–10   Insertion of urethral filiform guide. Insertion of multiple filiform guides will obliterate false passages *(A, B)* while further diameters allow passage through strictured urethral segments *(C)*. The vesical filiform is then stabilized while the remaining filiforms are removed.

is met, the filiform is left in place and another inserted. This process is repeated until the obstruction is traversed, at which point the final filiform is maintained in position while the others are removed (Fig. 19–10). Each filiform has a proximal fitting to which can be attached appropriate followers of varying dimensions for dilatation, including the Phillips woven silk catheters and the LeFort metal sounds (Fig. 19–11). Beginning with an appropriately small-caliber follower, the area of the stricture is sequentially dilated with the replaceable followers until an appropriate caliber has been attained or until the operator's experience indicates that further dilatation would be hazardous. A similar technique is employed for relief of urinary retention associated with urethral strictures which preclude

easy catheterization. It is to be emphasized that such a maneuver should be performed under the strictest aseptic technique with attention to the patient's comfort and anxiety, and with maximum observation for potential infection and sepsis. Antibiotics are essential following the procedure, and the patient should be instructed to notify the physician immediately upon experiencing any prodromal symptoms of septicemia. In employing the LeFort follower, gentle digital perineal pressure will assist in diverting the instrument anteriorly away from the rectum and through the vesical neck. At no time should exertion be used with any dilating instrument. Dilatation above a No. 24 French caliber is unnecessary in males.

Internal Urethrotomy. Longer or more proximal areas of fibrous strictures and those which respond poorly to repeated dilatations are often more responsive to internal urethrotomy. This technique utilizes the Otis urethrotome (Fig. 19–12). This instrument combines a variable caliber and a nontraumatic, movable cutting blade restricted to a single plane. After routine preparation of the patient in the lithotomy position, the instrument is introduced in its smallest caliber in the manner shown in Fig. 19–12A. The gauge is then set at the desired caliber, and the knife is withdrawn from its shielded position along its track. Depending on the severity of the stricture, incisions may be repeated at the three, nine and twelve o-clock positions. Caliber in the male need not exceed a 24 French, while in the female calibers up to 40 French are employed. A 24 French retention catheter of inert material should be left in place for three to six weeks to prevent coaption of the incisions, and routine attention to catheter hygiene should be observed.

Urethral Stenosis

Meatal Stenosis and Meatotomy. Urethral meatal stenosis in the male is usually seen as a congenital defect in infants and children in which the orifice

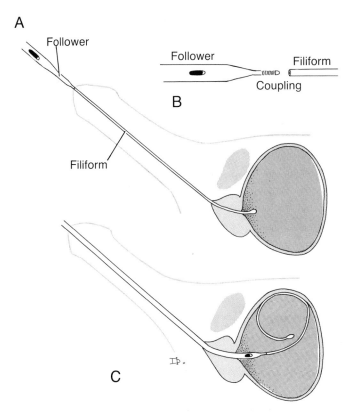

A

Follower

Follower

Filiform

Coupling

B

Filiform

C

Figure 19–11 Insertion of filiforms and follower. *A.* Filiform
guide advanced into bladder. *B.*
Follower (draining catheter or
dilating sound) attached to filiform. *C.* Follower advanced into
bladder.

is restricted to pinpoint dimensions. It may also occur as a result of progressive fibrous contraction resulting from meatitis accompanying ammoniacal diaper dermatitis, in which case gross hematuria may occur. In such cases therapy is directed toward the dermatitis, including urinary acidification. Symptoms include recurrent urinary infections, dribbling urination, a fine forceful urinary stream, or discomfort and straining at voiding. Thorough evaluation of such children should include intravenous pyleography and voiding cystourethrography. Other congenital lesions and related sequelae such as vesicoureteral reflux and upper urinary tract disorders should be ruled out. Cystoscopy is also advisable. The procedure is difficult to perform in children under local anesthesia, so general anesthesia is advisable.

Urethral meatal stenosis in the adult male is generally the result of fibrous narrowing due to inflammatory disorders or chronic irritation. Stenosis is not uncommon following even brief episodes of indwelling catheterization.

Meatotomy can be performed under local anesthesia in the adult male and the cooperative child. After appropriate preparation and draping, anesthetic is introduced through a 25 gauge needle into the lateral and ventral aspect of the urethral meatus, extending ventrally in the midline to the frenulum. A straight hemostat or appropriately larger clamp is then applied for several minutes to the anesthetized tissue (Fig. 19–13), after which the crushed tissue is incised over a metal sound, a grooved director or an appropriate clamp passed into the proximal urethra. Bleeding is usually minimal and may be controlled with application of a silver nitrate stick. A helpful maneuver is to suture the cut edges of the new meatus laterally to the

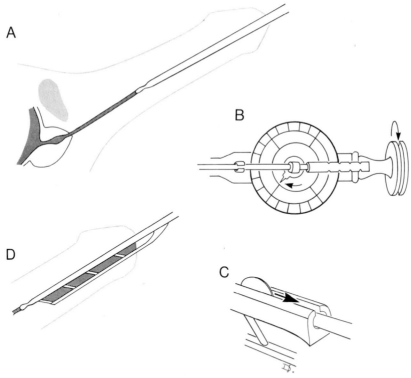

Figure 19–12 Internal urethrotomy technique. *A.* Urethrotome in closed, shielded position advanced through area of stricture. *B.* Dilator gauge advanced to desired setting, resulting in urethral dilatation (*C*). *D.* Withdrawal of the unshielded urethrotome, resulting in incision of the strictured area.

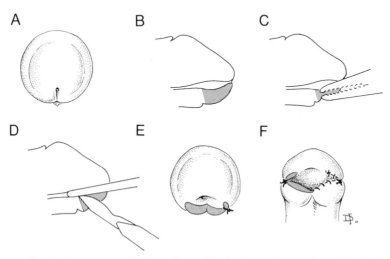

Figure 19–13 Urethral meatotomy in the male. *A.* Urethral meatal stenosis. *B.* Depth of meatotomy (shaded area). *C.* Application of hemostat. *D.* Incision of clamped tissue over grooved director or metal sound. *E, F.* Suture of neomeatus laterally to each corona to impede coaptation.

corona on either side with 3-0 or 4-0 absorbable suture in order to prevent coaptation and restenosis.

Urethral meatotomy in the female is performed only after demonstration of urethral stenosis at the meatus, by calibration with bougie and metal sounds. Once demonstrated, a straight hemostat is applied for several minutes to the meatus at the twelve o'clock position and the crushed tissue is incised over a metal sound. Repeat sounding will then demonstrate significant increase in caliber if the meatotomy has been adequate. Application of a silver nitrate stick again may be helpful, although further maneuvers are usually unnecessary.

Proximal Stenosis and Urethrolysis; the Urethral Syndrome. Perhaps the most common pathologic entity in female urology is urethral stenosis, in turn producing the urethral syndrome. The latter is characterized by intermittent episodes of lower urinary tract irritability with occasional infection, burning dysuria, frequency, tenesmus and nocturia. Although recurrent lower urinary tract infections may be documented in some patients, negative urinalyses may be the rule in others. Some patients can describe no precipitating factors while others attribute symptomatic exacerbations to sexual intercourse, the use of certain bathing soaps and bubble baths, contraceptive medication, constipation, various types of underclothing, toilet tissue and so on. These potential factors should be sought out. A trial of specific avoidance should be resorted to if a specific cause is suspected.

Endoscopy may reveal an inflammatory pseudomembrane or vascular injection involving the urinary trigone, compatible with chronic trigonitis. The vesical neck and urethra may exhibit pseudopolypoid changes, edema and erythema indicative of chronic urethritis. Palpation of the urethrovaginal septum over the endoscope or metal sound may reveal tenderness or thickening. These findings indicate the presence of edema and scarification due to the prolonged or recurrent inflammatory process. Calibration will usually reveal tenderness and snugness to smaller calibers, while dilatation to 36–40 French may produce prompt improvement, lasting for varying periods of time. Acute urethritis will often respond to a course of hot sitz baths and the temporary use of urethral suppositories (nitrofurazone-hydrocortisone). The subacute and chronic problem is best managed by a short course of specific antibiotics postdilatation, and a more prolonged course of oral conjugated estrogen preparation (Premarin, 2.5 mg daily). Such patients are seldom improved permanently after a single dilatation. In many patients, periodic dilatations are required at varying intervals when symptoms recur. If sexual intercourse continues to result in acute exacerbations, a single antibiotic tablet (pencillin, ampicillin or tetracycline) should be taken at the time of sexual relations, and postcoital micturition should be carried out, to assist in aborting these episodes. Local application of antibiotic ointment to the urethral meatus following voiding or intercourse may also be beneficial. Ointments which we have found to be helpful are neomycin-polymyxin (Neosporin) and povidone-iodine (Betadine).[10]

Severe chronic urethritis requiring frequent urethral dilatations without prolonged benefit may respond favorably to internal urethrotomy (Fig. 19–12).

When all these maneuvers have failed to produce significant or lasting relief, it may be noted that the chronic urethritis has resulted in the development of periurethral fibrosis, manifested clinically as a thickened urethrovaginal septum. The recently described operative technique of *urethrolysis* (Fig. 19–14) has been effective in relieving the urethral syndrome in up to 80 per cent of properly selected patients.[11] After appropriate sedation, the patient is placed in the lithotomy position and routinely prepared. With an assistant exposing the urethra by manual separation of the labia, local anesthetic is infiltrated about the urethral meatus ventrally. Anesthetic is

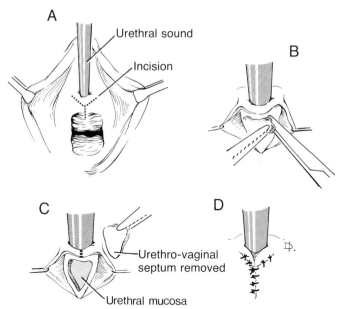

A
Urethral sound
Incision

B

C
Urethro-vaginal
septum removed
Urethral mucosa

D

Figure 19–14 Urethrolysis in the female. *A*. Urethral sound in position; labia minora retracted. Para-urethral and vaginal incisions as indicated (dotted lines). *B*. Fibrous investment of urethrovaginal septum excised. *C*. Urethral mucosa visible through septal defect. *D*. Re-approximation of vaginal mucosa.

then injected proximally along the length of the urethra and bilaterally into the adjacent urethrovaginal septum. A urethral sound is introduced, and the urethral meatus is sharply semicircumcised ventrally. The incision is then continued in the midline proximally through the vaginal mucosa along the length of the urethra. The vaginal mucosa is reflected bilaterally, thus exposing the thickened plaque of fibrous tissue. Beginning approximately one cm lateral to the urethra, the plaque is resected proximally to the junction of the proximal and the middle thirds of its length. The urethra is gradually divested of all such tissue. After excision of the fibrous plaque, the urethral sound will be visible through the normally translucent urethra. The vaginal mucosa is re-approximated with 4-0 chromic gut sutures after performance of a short ventral urethral meatotomy. A vaginal pack and a 24 French urethral catheter are left in place for one day. These patients are typically improved almost immediately. Dilatation of the urethra is possible

postoperatively to calibers well in excess of preoperative tolerances. While relief may be temporary, employment of this procedure in properly selected patients often produces dramatic benefit.

Failure of all medical and surgical attempts to relieve the female urethral syndrome may indicate a psychogenic source of symptoms, in which event psychotherapy may succeed where other modalities have not.

Urethral Caruncle

This lesion is a pyogenic granuloma. It is characteristically the result of chronic urethritis. It is typically seen in elderly females as a reddened tumor mass at the urethral meatus and accompanies a history of burning dysuria of varying, occasionally extreme, severity. Urethral stenosis is also often present, probably due to the chronic urethritis. Atrophic vaginitis is another frequent component, suggesting estrogen depletion. This is thought to explain the high incidence of caruncles in elderly females and their association with chronic urethritis and urethral stenosis.

Urethral caruncles frequently respond promptly to the institution of a conjugated estrogen vaginal cream (dienestrol), after which a daily dosage of similar oral medication (Premarin, 2.5 mg) will often prevent recurrence. Should surgery be necessary, the lesion can be cauterized with the coagulating electrode after appropriate preparation and local infiltration anesthesia, or it can be surgically excised. The latter maneuver requires an assistant for appropriate retraction and exposure. A urethral meatal circumcising incision is made through the mucosa, after which the urethral mucous membrane is separated from the muscularis for a reasonable margin around the tumor. The vaginal mucosa is then undermined around the meatus. The lesion is then amputated and the urethral and vaginal mucosa are approximated with interrupted 4-0 chromic gut sutures.

Urethral caruncle is differentiated from *urethral mucosal prolapse* by the quadrantic distribution of the former, compared with the circumferential nature of the latter. Differentiation from urethral neoplasm is mandatory, and pathologic confirmation is therefore essential.

CYSTOSCOPY

Outpatient urological practice utilizes cystoscopy extensively for diagnosis, and to a lesser extent in therapy. Cystoscopy should be performed only under supervision by an experienced urologist, with full understanding of the hazards of the procedure. When performed properly, outpatient cystoscopy can be helpful in providing immediate answers to diagnostic questions. It may eliminate the cost and time of hospitalization in selected patients with certain types of recurrent bladder diseases, which are amenable to transurethral biopsy or fulguration.

The indications for cystoscopy include any type of voiding dysfunction, such as vesical irritability, reduced size of stream, infection, nocturia, incomplete emptying, hematuria, pain and so forth. There is essentially no contraindication to cystoscopy in patients who require a urological evaluation.

Cystoscopy requires right angle and foroblique cystoscope optical adaptors and at least four sizes of cystoscopes for children and adults (8, 12, 16 and 22 French). Cystoscopes are stored in liquid germicide such as Cytal, and are rinsed in water immediately before use. The safest and most common irrigating solution is normal saline, which eliminates the risk of hemolysis which is present when water is used. However, for resection and fulguration a nonelectrolyte solution is required; such solutions usually contain mannitol or sorbitol for isotonicity.

The patient for cystoscopy should be positioned and sedated as for urethral sounding. The cystoscope is passed in a fashion similar to the urethral sound (Fig. 19–9). The entire bladder should always be inspected, including the dome, trigone, bladder neck and ureteral orifices. Biopsy may be performed cautiously with a transurethral cup or alligator forceps. However, since the entire lesion must be removed if there is any suspicion of malignancy, it is usually wisest to admit the patient to the hospital and perform the biopsy as deeply as is necessary. Deep biopsy will often be followed by a moderate amount of bleeding, and a urethral catheter is indicated in such patients until all bleeding has ceased.

HYDROCELE

Small or moderately large hydroceles are seldom symptomatic and rarely require excision or decompression. When symptoms dictate, surgical resection is indicated. The procedure is usually brief and benign, with minimal morbidity and rapid convalescence. Occasionally the situation will exist where symptoms are troublesome, and yet the patient is a poor risk for general or regional anesthesia. Although such lesions are amenable to excision under local anesthesia, periodic percutaneous needle aspiration may be considered a more acceptable means of management. Correct diagnosis is essential. The major differential diagnosis of hydrocele is spermatocele, since both lesions are translucent, smooth, cystic structures. Hydrocele is formed by the collection of clear straw-colored fluid within the tunica vaginalis, thereby surrounding and often obscuring the testis. On the other hand, a spermatocele develops as a result of obstruction of an epididymal duct, therefore occurring distinctly above the testis. It is filled with milky fluid containing spermatozoa.

After routine sterile preparation of the scrotum, the skin is stretched over the intrascrotal mass and a skin wheal raised anteriorly. A large caliber plastic intracath needle is then introduced into the sac. Anterior insertion of the trocar is mandatory. The beveled obturator is removed and the hydrocele contents aspirated. Sclerosing agents should not be injected.

VASECTOMY

Vasectomy is performed for prevention of retrograde epididymo-orchitis, and as an elective sterilization procedure (Fig. 19–15). Vasectomy is commonly employed at the time of open prostatectomy, and has produced a significant decline in the incidence of postprostatectomy epididymitis. The advent of more inert catheter materials and more efficient antibiotic therapy may render this procedure less necessary in the future. Patients who require long-standing indwelling catheterization who have no desire or need for family expansion may also benefit from vasectomy.

Vasectomy is increasingly utilized as an elective sterilization procedure. It is desired by many young adults who wish to limit the size of their families and to avoid the expense, inconvenience, discomfort and possible hazards of other methods of contraception. The philosophy of the procedure is a private matter between the physician, the patient and the patient's wife. The legal aspects vary from area to area and should be understood by all parties concerned. The operation should always be preceded by a consultation with both husband and wife, during which time an opportunity for free and thorough discussion is encouraged. It is important to emphasize that the procedure should be undertaken with irrevocable and permanent intent. (Reanastomosis and recanalization is occasionally possible later by a more difficult procedure, but reliance on this possibility is imprudent and unwise.) The patient should be informed that sterility is not immediate. Contraception should be continued until 10 to 12 ejaculations have occurred, in order to allow emission of viable sperm distal to the point of vasal interruption. A semen inspection by the physician should then be performed to assure aspermia. Finally, it should be emphasized that spontaneous recanalization occasionally occurs, despite the use of proper surgical technique. The patient must be willing to accept this risk. Recanalization will usually occur within six months. A semen analysis should be performed at that time to verify continued sterility. Permission for elective vasectomy for sterilization should ideally include witnessed consent of both husband and wife.

The surgical procedure should be preceded by shaving the scrotum and the base of the penis, best accomplished by the patient at home. After routine sterile preparation the vas deferens is isolated on either side through the scrotal skin at a convenient site above the globus major of the epididymis. A skin wheal is raised and the needle is advanced to the region of the vas deferens. Infiltration is continued after aspiration to avoid intravascular injection. The needle is then

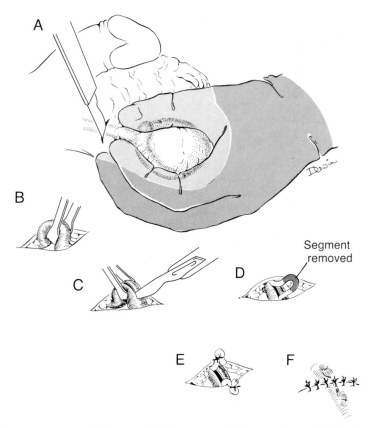

Figure 19–15 Vasectomy technique. *A.* Incision over vas deferens after anesthetic infiltration of skin and spermatic cord. *B.* Vas deferens, in its fibrous sheath, grasped with Allis clamp and delivered through incision. *C.* Longitudinal incision in fibrous sheath, exposing vas deferens. *D.* Vas deferens delivered with fine-toothed forceps. Segment excised (shaded area). *E.* Vasal remnants suture ligated. *F.* Scrotal skin closed with interrupted absorbable sutures.

withdrawn and a scratch is made in the skin over the wheal to allow later identification of the site of anesthesia. The procedure is repeated on the opposite side, after which a one cm transverse incision is made through either wheal. The tissue investing the vas deferens is separated with a hemostat. An Allis clamp is then introduced through the incision, grasping the vas and delivering it into the wound. The fibrous investment of the vas is incised longitudinally, exposing its glistening fibrous sheath. The vas is then grasped with a fine-toothed forceps and withdrawn sufficiently to allow resection of two to three cm of its length. The cut edges of the vas are then turned upon themselves and suture ligated with 000 chromic gut. Local hemo-

stasis must be assured to prevent development of a hematocele which may occur from apparently insignificant capillary bleeding. Electrocoagulation of the lumen of the vas is sometimes practiced and appears to be equally effective. Electrocoagulation is cumbersome, since special equipment is required. It is also more likely to produce an uncomfortable temporary local inflammation in the vas. The vasal remnants are returned to their normal intrascrotal position, and the scrotal incision is closed with absorbable sutures. The procedure is then repeated on the opposite side. The patient is re-instructed and discharged. Aspirin is usually sufficient to manage the discomfort which is commonly experienced. Antibiotics and scrotal support are seldom necessary, although an occasional patient will experience symptomatic benefit with the temporary use of a support. Vigorous activity should be avoided for a day or two to discourage capillary bleeding.

PROSTATE BIOPSY

The importance of digital rectal examination (Fig. 19–16) cannot be overemphasized, particularly in men over the age of forty. Prostatic carcinoma ranks as the third most common cause of death from cancer in men, and it was estimated that over 17,000 deaths were caused by this disease in 1971.

Any patient demonstrating nodularity or induration of the prostate gland, whether symptomatic or asymptomatic, requires investigation by prostatic biopsy. Four methods are available for prostate biopsy. Open perineal biopsy is reserved for clinical confirmation of malignant disease prior to total perineal prostatectomy in patients potentially amenable to surgical cure. Transurethral resection is restricted to selected patients in whom urethral obstruction requires relief. The other two biopsy techniques

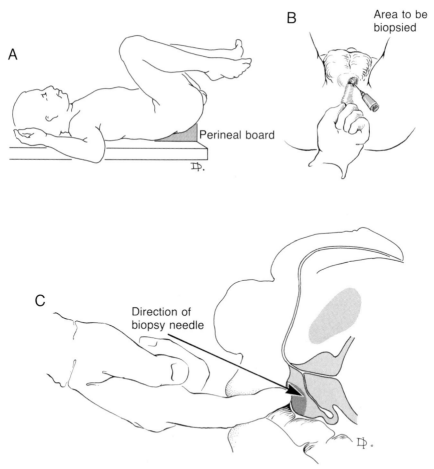

Figure 19–16 Prostate biopsy. *A.* Extreme lithotomy with perineal board (shaded area). *B.* After perineal skin wheal is raised, rectal finger guides infiltrating needle to the suspicious prostatic area. Prostatic capsule is infiltrated at this area. *C.* Lateral view, demonstrating direction of biopsy needle.

are transrectal and transperineal needle biopsy, utilizing the Franklin modification of the Vim-Silverman biopsy needle or the Travenol disposable biopsy needle. Needle biopsy of the prostate can be performed in the Outpatient Department under local infiltration anesthesia by a physician who is acquainted with the technique and familiar with the local anatomy. The accuracy of needle biopsy is reported to range from 70 to 95 per cent, compared with open perineal biopsy.

The technique involves the extreme lithotomy position, in which the perineum is essentially parallel with the floor (Fig. 19–16 *A*). This position is best accomplished with a wedgeshaped, padded support placed under the patient's lumbosacral spine. In the transperineal technique, after suitable preparation, a skin wheal is raised in the midline, two fingerbreadths anterior to the rectum at the approximate site of the perineal body, and infiltration is continued as the needle is advanced to the prostate gland (Fig. 19–16 *B*). Periodic aspirations will prevent intravascular injection. A rectal finger guides the needle to the intended area, which is thoroughly infiltrated. The needle is then withdrawn and the area of the original wheal nicked with a scalpel blade to facilitate introduction of the biopsy needle, which is then advanced into the lesion (Fig. 19–16 *C*). Several cores of tissue are removed for pathologic inspection. It is also wise to remove tissue from the opposite prostatic lobe. Hematuria occurs in 7 per cent of cases and is typically mild and self-limited. Bleeding from the perineum is seldom troublesome, and pain is generally minimal. Efflux of urine from the needle indicates that the bladder was inadvertently punctured. In such cases, indwelling catheterization and antibiotic coverage is advisable for a day or two. We are aware of only five cases in which seeding of the needle tract with tumor cells has been reported.

The transrectal biopsy technique requires rectal evacuation. The biopsy needle is then introduced into the rectal ampulla, guarded by the index finger, until it can be introduced into the lesion. Sedation is advisable, but local anesthesia is not required. The remainder of the procedure is as described in the perineal biopsy technique.

Percutaneous Renal Biopsy

This procedure (Fig. 19–17) is a reasonably safe and efficient means to obtain renal tissue for pathologic evaluation in patients of all ages. Since anesthesia is seldom necessary when sedation is adequate, percutaneous renal biopsy may be performed in the Outpatient Department. The most common indications for renal biopsy are hematuria, proteinuria and hypertension of obscure or uncertain diagnosis. The histologic diagnosis provides a guide to a prudent and rational therapeutic regimen.

An oral or intravenous water load of approximately 3 per cent of body weight should be given during the two hours prior to biopsy. A similar oral or intravenous volume should be given postoperatively. This will produce sufficient diuresis to allow monitoring of urine color changes and will reduce clot formation, which may cause colic or urinary retention. Excretory urography, hemoglobin, hematocrit and coagulation studies are routinely obtained preoperatively.

Biopsy is performed on a fluroscopy table with the patient in the prone position. The right kidney is selected whenever possible because of its caudal position. A sand bag is fitted snugly under the abdomen against the lower border of the rib cage (Fig. 19–17 *A*). This tends to fix the kidney and is an important adjunct to successful biopsy. Many techniques have been used to localize the kidney, including application of lead markers and sterile needles on the skin. The procedure should include intravenous administration of contrast medium for visualization of the renal collecting system. Renal

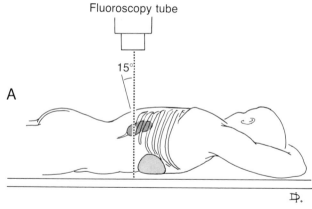

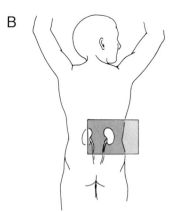

Figure 19–17 Percutaneous renal biopsy. *A*. Patient in prone position with sandbag under lower rib cage on side of biopsy (preferably right) to stabilize kidney. Fluoroscopy tube indicated. Arrow indicates 15° cranial angulation of biopsy needle. *B*. X-ray grid in place to localize kidney for biopsy.

biopsy in the presence of severe functional depression may require retrograde pyelography for appropriate preoperative radiographic localization. This technique will also be useful in the presence of allergy to organic iodides. When image intensification is used, IVP alone will often provide sufficient visibility for accurate biopsy from the inferior renal cortex. The development of a disposable radiopaque grid (Bio-Medical Systems, Inc., Danbury, Conn.) applied over the desired area, however, has further simplified the procedure, while encouraging accuracy and safety (Fig. 19–17 *B*).

The procedure includes adequate prebiopsy sedation, routine preparation and draping of the skin, and the Franklin modification of the Vim-Silverman needle or Travenol disposable biopsy needle. The biopsy specimen should be immediately studied under a dissecting microscope to assure presence of glomeruli, as this will reduce the need for rebiopsy later due to inadequacy of the specimen. Postoperative diuresis can be further enhanced by administration of potent diuretics (furosemide 40–80 mg for adults). Routine postbiopsy care should also include temporary bed rest, observation of serial urine specimens, and hematocrit and hemoglobin determinations four to six hours postoperatively.

Contraindications to percutaneous renal biopsy include the presence of a solitary kidney, a hemorrhagic diathesis or a cutaneous lesion at or near the biopsy site.

Complications from needle biopsy include perirenal hematoma, renal colic, vesical clot retention, leakage of urine outside the collecting system, entrance into the pleural space, splenic, hepatic and bowel injuries, and arteriovenous fistulae. Microhematuria is common and generally self-limited. Gross hematuria, which may be immediate or delayed in onset, will usually subside with bed rest, although blood transfusion may occasionally be necessary. An arteriovenous fistula may produce significant hypertension, particularly in children, but will usually subside spontaneously with the passage of time. Preoperative and postoperative auscultation over the renal arteries should be routine. Any patient with postbiopsy pain after 24 hours should undergo intravenous pyelography. Inadequate biopsy specimens after three repeated attempts, atrophic or hypoplastic kidneys, or excessive subcutaneous or muscular thickness may result in the need for open surgical biopsy.

PERCUTANEOUS RENAL CYST ASPIRATION

Although diagnosis of a renal cyst can be made correctly radiographically in over 95 per cent of cases, and although continued diagnostic uncertainty after routine studies is usually ample justification for exploration, occasionally a patient will be encountered in whom added measures must be taken in order to avoid surgery if at all possible, particularly when the clinical suspicion of cystic disease exists. In such patients, percutaneous aspiration affords an excellent means of confirming the diagnosis, obtaining cystic fluid for special studies, and providing more definitive radiographic information.

The technique follows that described for percutaneous renal biopsy, utilizing intravenous contrast medium, the sterile disposable cutaneous x-ray grid, and image intensification. A 4½ inch 22 gauge needle on a syringe is employed rather than a biopsy needle. The needle can be advanced into the desired area under fluoroscopic control. The cyst contents can be partially aspirated and replaced with contrast medium, and permanent radiographs can be obtained. Aspirated fluid can then be submitted for special studies, including cholesterol and triglyceride determinations, and cytologic examination.

RENAL HYPERTENSION

The urological aspects of the work-up of a patient with hypertension can be performed in part in the Outpatient Department.

Patients with renal hypertension usually have a family history of similar disease. In most of these patients the hyper-

---

TABLE 19–5 INDIVIDUAL KIDNEY FUNCTION TESTS FOR
EVALUATION OF HYPERTENSION*

Preparation
  For one week prior to the test, a normal sodium diet is taken, and all diuretic medications are discontinued if possible. On the morning of the test, breakfast is omitted. Beginning two hours before cystoscopy, the patient is hydrated with 240 ml of water by mouth or 120 ml of 5 per cent dextrose and water intravenously at half-hour intervals, continuing throughout the test. General anesthesia is usually necessary in children. Saddle block or adequate urethral anesthesia will usually suffice in adults.
 	
Catheterization
  The ureters are catheterized through a No. 24
	Brown-Buerger cystoscope. The possibility of postcatheterization edema should be considered, and for this reason only the kidney suspected of being abnormal should be catheterized in some patients. This complication is more common in males than females. The other kidney in these patients can be drained through a bladder catheter.
	
	Collection of Specimens
	  Urine collection is started 15 minutes after insertion of the catheters. The normal kidney should excrete 1 ml per minute or more. Collection periods are timed to the nearest 15 seconds, and should allow for collection of at least 20–30 ml of urine from the better kidney in each period.

*Adapted from Protocol of the Cooperative Renal Hypertension Study Group.

Urine is collected directly into 50 ml graduated cylinders, for at least three collection periods. The bladder is emptied and measured at the end of each collection period. Blood specimens include appropriate pre-infusion and mid-collection period specimens as well as a final specimen at the end of the test. A record is made of blood pressure every 15 minutes, and each urine specimen should have its color and volume recorded before it is centrifuged for chemical analysis.

RAPOPORT TEST (Tubular Rejection Fraction Ratio)

This is the shortest and simplest of the split function tests. Urine is measured for sodium and creatinine. Glomerular filtration rate (GFR) is calculated for each kidney, utilizing a blood specimen obtained at the midpoint of each urine collection, and the formula:

$$GFR = C_{cr} = \frac{U_{cr} \times \dot{V}}{P_{cr}}$$

C_{cr}　Creatinine clearance (ml/min)

U_{cr}　Urinary creatinine concentration (mg/ml)

$\dot{V}$　Urinary flow (ml/min)

P_{cr}　Plasma creatinine concentration (mg/ml)

The tubular-rejection-fraction of sodium (TRFNa) of the left kidney is divided by that of the right. The result is Tubular Rejection Fraction Ratio (TRFR):

$$TRFR = \frac{L\ U_{Na}}{L\ U_{Cr}} \times \frac{R\ U_{Cr}}{L\ U_{Na}}$$

A positive test consists of a TRFR of less than 0.7 or greater than 1.5. A low TRFR (0.6 or less) indicates involvement of the right renal artery.

HOWARD TEST

Urine from each kidney is measured for volume, sodium and creatinine. For volume and sodium the formula used is:

$$\frac{normal - diseased}{normal} \times 100$$

For creatinine calculations, the formula used is:

$$\frac{diseased - normal}{diseased} \times 100$$

A positive test consists of (1) reduction of 40 per cent or more in urine volume, coupled with 15 per cent or more reduction in sodium concentration; or (2) reduction of 40 per cent or more in urine volume, with creatinine concentration at least 50 per cent higher from the affected kidney than from the nonaffected kidney.

STAMEY TEST (Urea-PAH)

Salicylates, penicillin, chlorothiazide and sulfonamides must not be administered for 48 hours prior to this test, and procaine must not be used during the procedure. These substances interfere with determination of para-amino hippurate (PAH). Ten ml of blood is needed for determination of PAH in the blood specimens.

A single priming dose of PAH is given intravenously. The desired plasma concentration of PAH is 2.5 mg/100 ml. The volume of 20 per cent PAH injected is determined by multiplying the patient's weight by 0.04. For example, a 70 kg man would receive 2.8 ml of 20 per cent PAH solution.

Urea is given in an 8 per cent solution at the rate of 10 ml per minute. The solution used is a "urea-PAH-ADH solution." It is prepared by withdrawing 160 ml of saline from a 1000 ml bottle of normal saline; 60 ml are discarded and 50 ml are injected into each of two 40 gm bottles of crystalline urea U.S.P. The saline-urea mixture from the small bottles is reinjected into the liter bottle of saline. PAH must then be added to this bottle to maintain a plasma level of approximately 2.5 mg per cent during the test. The amount of 20 per cent PAH added depends on the patient's renal function. If the serum creatinine is 2.0 mg per cent or less, 5.3 ml of PAH solution is added; if the serum creatinine is greater than 2.0 mg per cent, 2.6 ml of PAH is added. Pitressin is then added, in a total dose of 9 milliunits per ml. The dose desired is measured with a tuberculin syringe; for example, for a 70 kg man, 0.63 ml (630 milliunits) would be added to the liter bottle.

Collection periods are begun 45 minutes after the urea-PAH-ADH infusion has been started. Each collection lasts at least 10 minutes, and a urine flow of at least 2 ml per minute is necessary. At least 30 ml of urine must be obtained from each ureter during each collection period. A blood specimen for PAH should be obtained in the midpoint of each urine collection period, or at least at the midpoint of the second collection period.

Because the patient has received an osmotic diuresis in this test, the bladder should be catheterized for at least six hours after the test, and he should receive 2000 ml of 5 per cent dextrose in water at a rate of 300 ml per hour.

A positive test consists of at least a 3:1 difference in urine flow rates and a 100 per cent or greater difference in PAH concentrations. Flow rate is *decreased* on the affected side and PAH concentration is *increased* on the affected side. A 2:1 difference (decrease) in urine flow rate on the affected side and an increase of less than 100 per cent in PAH concentration on the affected side are compatible with any of the following:

1. Essential hypertension with disparity in nephrosclerosis
2. Segmental renal hypertension (branch lesion) in one kidney
3. Bilateral renal arterial stenosis with disparity in ischemia.

tension will have appeared or increased abruptly. Renal artery stenosis due to fibromuscular hyperplasia is most common in women in their late twenties, thirties and early forties.

The steps in evaluation for renal hypertension include intravenous pyelogram, radioactive renogram, "split function" tests, arteriography and renal vein renin collections.

Intravenous pyelography should be performed with early (one minute) and delayed films, looking for a differential delay in initiation of excretion, and a differential delay in clearance of dye from the renal pelvis, both of which are characteristic of the diseased kidney. A difference in renal size may, however, be the only abnormality observed. If differential alteration of more than 1.5 cm in length from the normal is present, it is considered an abnormality. It should be remembered that the left kidney is usually 1.0 cm longer than the right.

Renogram is performed by injection of I^{131}-labeled Hippuran, followed by scanning over both kidneys. The excretion from both kidneys is monitored simultaneously. An abnormal curve suggestive of unilateral renal disease is seen when the initial slope is not steep, the peak is low and the disappearance of radioactivity from the area of the kidney is delayed.

"Split function" studies are performed by transurethral insertion of bilateral ureteral catheters. Simultaneous urine collections are studied for volume, sodium content and concentration, creatinine (for clearance), osmolarity and para-amino hippuric acid (for clearance). The techniques have been described in detail by Rapoport (1960),[23] Howard (1962)[24] and Stamey (1961).[25] They have been reviewed by Stewart (1965),[26] and Maxwell (1968),[27] and are summarized in Table 19–5. Spinal anesthesia is usually required for this test in the male, since he is required to lie quietly for several hours with the bladder and ureters catheterized.

Renal arteriography and renal vein catheterization can be performed by the percutaneous transfemoral approach in outpatients. Most of these patients are admitted to the hospital for the studies since they are tedious and uncomfortable, and additional aspects of the work-up can be performed during the same hospitalization. Renal vein samples are analyzed for renin. If there is any suggestion of an adrenal adenoma on physical examination or by other laboratory studies, adrenal arteriography and adrenal vein sampling should also be performed.

References

1. Kvale, P. A., Keys, T. F., Johnson, D. W., and Holmes, K. K.: Single oral dose ampicillin – probenecid treatment of gonorrhea in the male. J.A.M.A., *215*:1449–1453, 1971.
2. Shapiro, L. H., Lynn, D. R., DiGiacomo, A. M., and Adrian, D. C.: One-day oral ampicillin – treatment of gonorrhea in young adults. Obstet. Gynecol., *37*:414–418, 1971.
3. Gray, R. C. F., Phillips, I., and Nicol, C. S.: Treatment of gonorrhea with three different antibiotic regimens. Br. J. Vener. Dis., *46*:401–403, 1970.
4. Phillips, W. R., and Biggs, A. W.: The incidence of cytoplasmic and nuclear inclusions in non-specific genital infections in men. J. Urol., *104*:470–473, 1970.
5. Shepard, M. C.: Nongonococcal urethritis associated with human strains of "T" mycoplasmas. J.A.M.A., *211*:1335–1340, 1970.
6. Turck, M., Anderson, K. N., and Petersdorf, R. G.: Relapse and reinfection in chronic bacteriuria. N. Eng. J. Med., *275*:70–73, 1966.
7. Schwarz, H.: Rationale for the use of non-absorbable antibiotics to treat urinary infections: Preliminary report. South. Med. J., *63*:930–934, 1970.
8. Freeman, R. B.: Medical management of chronic pyelonephritis: acute and chronic. Mod. Treat., *7*:271–282, 1970.
9. Fischer, R., Richter, H. P., and Berning, H.: Long-term treatment of chronic pyelonephritis. Ger. Med. Mon., *13*:165–169, 1968.
10. Landes, R. R., Melnick, I., and Hoffman, A. A.: Recurrent urinary tract infections in women: Prevention by topical application of antimicrobial ointment to urethral meatus. J. Urol., *104*:749–750, 1970.
11. Richardson, F. H., and Stonington, O. G.:

Urethrolysis and external urethroplasty in the female. Surg. Clin. N. Amer., *49*:1201–1208, 1969.

12. Ratliff, R. K.: Hyaluronidase in treatment of paraphimosis. J.A.M.A., *155*:746, 1954.

13. Williams, T. H., and Nichols, R. K.: A method of treating paraphimosis. J. Med. Assoc. State Ala., *21*:233–234, 1952.

14. Skoglund, R. W., Jr., and Chapman, W. H.: Reduction of paraphimosis. J. Urol., *104*:137, 1970.

15. Adams, A. W., and Slade, N.: Torsion testis and its treatment. Report of a bilateral case. Br. Med. J., *1*:36–38, 1958.

16. Wightman, J. A. K.: Genito-urinary aspects of Marfan's Syndrome with case report. Br. J. Urol., *35*:143–146, 1963.

17. Eadie, D. G. A., and Higgins, P. M.: Apparent torsion of the testicle in a case of Henoch-Schönlein purpura. Br. Surg., *51*:634–635, 1964.

18. Alan, W. R., and Brown, R. B.: Torsion of the testis: A review of 58 cases. Br. Med. J., *1*:1396–1397, 1966.

19. Skoglund, R. W., McRoberts, J. W., and Ragde, H.: Torsion of testicular appendages: Presentation of 43 new cases and a collective review. J. Urol., *104*:598–600, 1970.

20. Cobb, B.: Silverman needle nephrostomy. J. Urol., *98*:309–313, 1967.

21. Petersen, R. A.: Percutaneous nephrostomy. Eaton Laboratories Film Series, 1972.

22. Pedersen, A. H. B., Wiesner, P. J., Holmes, K. K., Johnson, C. J., and Turck, M.: Spectinomycin and penicillin G in the treatment of gonorrhea. A comparative study. J.A.M.A., *220*:205–208, 1972.

23. Rapoport, A.: Modification of the "Howard test" for the detection of renal-artery obstruction. N. Eng. J. Med., *263*:1159–1165, 1960.

24. Howard, J. E., and Connor, T. B.: Hypertension produced by unilateral renal disease. Arch. Intern. Med., *109*:8–17, 1962.

25. Stamey, T. A., Nudelman, I. J., Good, P. H., Schwentker, F. N., and Hendricks, F.: Functional characteristics of renovascular hypertension. Medicine, *40*:347–394, 1961.

26. Stewart, B. H., Schacht, R. A., Bishop, R. C., and Conway, J.: Differential function studies in renal hypertension: Indications and techniques. J. Urol., *94*:7–14, 1965.

27. Maxwell, M. H., Lupu, A. N., and Kaufman, J. J.: Individual kidney function tests in renal arterial hypertension. J. Urol., *100*:384–394, 1968.

20

Female Genitourinary Tract and Obstetrics — Outpatient Gynecological Surgery

By WATSON A. BOWES, Jr., M.D.
and WILLIAM DROEGEMUELLER, M.D.

INTRODUCTION

The gynecologist's endeavor is largely one of outpatient evaluation and minor surgical procedures.[16] Evaluation of pelvic pain, both acute and chronic, investigation of pelvic masses, determining the source of abnormal uterine or vaginal bleeding, the differential diagnosis of chronic and acute vaginal discharge, the appraisal of infertility problems, counseling about contraceptive and sexual problems and conducting tests to establish intrauterine diagnosis comprise the greatest part of an obstetrician-gynecologist's daily work. Most of these tasks can be accomplished on an outpatient basis. Because the text will be used in countries where hospital delivery is not feasible, a section on home delivery will be included. For a more complete discussion of many of the problems touched on in this chapter, the reader is referred to texts such as those of Ball and TeLinde.[1,18]

VULVA AND PERINEUM

Patients with lesions of the vulva or perineum often present because of chronic irritation, itching or unusual discharge. Many times, however, lesions of the external genitalia are discovered in an asymptomatic patient at the time of routine gynecological examination.[7]

The thorough examination of the vulvar region includes careful examination of the external genitalia, description of the hair distribution, awareness of unusual erythema, atrophy, pigmented lesions or vesicles. Careful palpation along the labia major will often disclose subcutaneous nodules which should undergo biopsy. These are usually hydradenomas or sebaceous cysts. Women who complain of chronic pruritis, particularly women in the postmenopausal years, should have toluidine blue staining of the perineum included in the examination. This is a simple procedure which will often demonstrate lesions that would be overlooked by the usual inspection of the genitalia.[3]

Toluidine Blue Staining

The vulva and perineum are cleansed with 1 per cent acetic acid solution. An aqueous solution of 1 per cent toluidine blue is then sponged over the vulva and perineum. Care should be taken to introduce the stain into any folds of skin or mucous membrane. One per cent acetic acid is then used again to sponge the vulvar region and remove the toluidine blue. Areas in which the stain remains should be considered potentially malignant and a biopsy of them should be performed by the technique described below. Toluidine blue is a nuclear stain and marks tissues in which there is abnormal cellular activity.

Biopsy of Vulvar Lesions

Vulvar nevi irritated by clothing, areas of leukoplakia or atrophy, nonhealing ulcerations, or any other suspicious vulvar lesion should undergo biopsy examination. This usually can be accomplished with dermatological punch biopsy instruments (Fig. 20–1). The area surrounding the lesion is cleansed with a suitable skin antiseptic. The skin adjacent to the lesion is infiltrated with 1 per cent lidocaine using a 25 gauge needle. The diameter of the punch biopsy instrument should include tissue from the lesion itself as well as adjacent

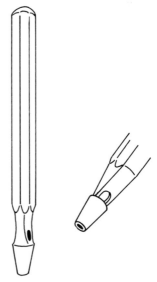

Figure 20–1 Punch biopsy instruments for vulvar biopsy.

normal tissue. Pressure is applied with a rotary, clockwise motion of the instrument. The biopsy can then be lifted from the underlying tissue and removed with a small pair of scissors or a scalpel blade. Bleeding can be controlled by touching the biopsy site with an astringent solution. Rarely is a suture necessary except in very large punch biopsies, and epithelialization occurs rapidly following the biopsy. This technique is used predominantly for diagnostic purposes.

Excisional biopsies for larger lesions should be accomplished with wide elliptical incisions in a manner similar to that used for biopsies of superficial or other subcutaneous lesions. The two subcutaneous lesions most commonly encountered by the gynecologist for excisional biopsy on the vulva are sebaceous cysts and hydradenomas. Also found in this area are fibromas, lipomas and hemangiomas. It is frequently difficult to distinguish one lesion from another without biopsy, since they will appear as asymptomatic subcutaneous masses. The hydradenoma, which is a benign neoplasm of sebaceous gland origin, is more firm than the usual sebaceous cyst and occasionally is characterized by erosion of the superficial epithelium. The indications for removal of masses within the external genitalia are dyspareunia pressure symptoms, and the necessity to rule out the diagnosis of the rare primary or metastatic malignant neoplasm which may occur in this area, for example, malignant melanoma, hemangiopericytoma, and granular cell myoblastoma.

Excisional biopsy of vulvar lesions can usually be performed adequately under local infiltration anesthesia. The patient is placed in a comfortable dorsal lithotomy position, preferably with her knees resting on padded supports rather than placing her feet in stirrups. The pubic hair surrounding the lesion should be shaved, and the vulva cleansed with an appropriate skin antiseptic. The skin surrounding the lesion should be infiltrated with 1 per cent lidocaine. An elliptical incision with a scalpel blade is made surrounding the mass. The mass is grasped with an Allis clamp, and a plane can usually be developed that allows blunt dissection around the mass. The major blood supply is usually at the base of the lesion, and a clamp should be placed at this point before completely removing the mass. All bleeders should be tied with 000 plain catgut sutures and the subcutaneous tissue approximated with similar suture. The skin edge is approximated with a subcuticular suture of 000 plain catgut or interrupted skin sutures. A small pressure dressing is often advisable for three to six hours and can be placed beneath the patient's perineal pad. For larger biopsies application of an ice pack will alleviate symptoms of swelling.

Venereal Warts

Venereal warts or condylomata acuminata are benign vulvar growths thought to be due to a viral infection that usually occurs as a result of poor perineal hygiene. When these growths are localized to a small area, they may be satisfactorily treated by applications of 10 to 25 per cent podophyllin. This solution must be painted on the lesion sparingly with a cotton applicator. The patient is advised to wash the affected area with warm water within four hours to minimize the chemical irritation of the podophyllin. Occasionally the entire perineum may be covered by the pedunculated masses, and in these situations surgical removal is necessary. The patient must have adequate regional or general anesthesia. The lesions are then removed at their base with a scalpel and the base superficially cauterized with electrocautery. It is also important to treat simultaneously any local vaginitis or vaginal discharge, which is most often due to trichomonas vaginalis.

The benign disorders of the vulva and vagina are comprehensively reviewed in the book by Gardner and Kaufman (1969).[7]

Enlargement of Bartholin's Gland

One of the most common vulvar lesions encountered by the gynecologist is enlargement of one of the Bartholin's glands. These are two superficial compound racemose glands that appear at the vulvovaginal ring and have a single excretory duct. Infection of these glands occurs frequently and painful enlargements in this area are usually secondary to Bartholinitis. A Bartholin cyst is usually the result of infection which has obstructed the excretory duct. The enlarged gland is identified as a swelling involving both the labium majus and the labium minus. It may extend into the perineum near the rectum and must be differentiated from an ischiorectal abscess or an inguinal hernia. Bartholin's gland cysts or abscesses will not impinge on the rectum, and rectal exam is the most helpful means of differentiating these from an abscess in the ischiorectal space.

Simple incision and drainage is not a satisfactory method for handling these lesions, for they frequently recur. Complete excision of a Bartholin cyst in the noninfected state has been advocated but is a more extensive procedure than

is necessary to manage the majority of these lesions. The most simple and effective measure with a Bartholin's gland abscess or cyst is marsupialization.

Marsupialization. The perineum and vulva are cleansed with an aseptic solution. Shaving is not necessary. The skin and subcutaneous tissue over the lesion are infiltrated with 1 per cent lidocaine so that a generous linear incision may be made over the abscess or cyst along the mucocutaneous junction of the vagina and the vulva. The incision is carried down into the cyst as shown in Figure 20–2. After opening the cyst wall, draining its contents and irrigating the cavity, the lining of the cyst is everted and sutured to the skin with interrupted 000 chromic catgut.[1] Drains and packs are not necessary, but frequent sitz baths are advised for three to four days following the procedure. The patient should be seen in 48 to 72 hours to insure that the edges of the incision are not agglutinated, thus closing the marsupialized cyst. After several weeks a small dimple will remain in the area of the marsupialization.

A more recent innovation in the management of a Bartholin's gland cyst is a bulb-tipped catheter supplied by The

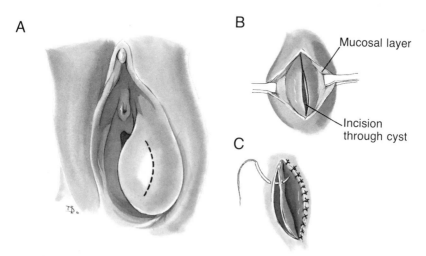

Figure 20–2 Marsupialization of Bartholin's cyst. *A*. Longitudinal incision is made along mucocutaneous junction of vulva and vagina, overlying the cyst. *B*. Incision is carried down through cyst wall and contents are drained. *C*. Cyst lining is everted and sutured to skin, with interrupted 3-0 chromic catgut sutures.

American Cystoscope Makers, Inc. (Pelham Manor, New York). This catheter, resembling the distal end of a Foley catheter, is inserted into a small incision in the cyst and the catheter inflated. The distal end of the stem is tucked in the vagina. The device is then left in place for four to six weeks and marsupialization of the cyst results when epithelialization occurs around the catheter.[20]

Bartholin's Gland Excision. In the excision of a Bartholin's gland, preparation of the skin and anesthesia for the patient are similar to those used for marsupialization, except that it is difficult to carry out excision under local anesthesia. Adequate general or regional anesthesia should be used. A vertical incision is made over the cyst just inside the labium minus (Fig. 20–3). The incision is carried down to, but does not include, the cyst wall. When the cyst wall is identified, it can be grasped with an Allis clamp and the remainder of the cyst freed by blunt dissection. Any bleeders should be clamped and ligated with 000 chromic catgut. A wedge of mucosa should be excised around Bartholin's duct. The cyst bed is then oblit-erated with interrupted 000 chromic catgut sutures. Excessive mucosa is trimmed off, and the mucosa is approximated with 000 chromic sutures. Frequent hot sitz baths are recommended until tenderness subsides. Antibiotics are necessary only if there is cellulitis present.

Laceration of the Vulva

One of the most common emergencies encountered in adult and pediatric gynecology is laceration of the vulva or vagina. In children these are frequently bicycle injuries or injuries sustained when the child falls on a fence or a stick. General anesthesia is usually necessary in children for adequate visualization of the traumatized tissues. Unless the laceration is superficial, the child will have enough reflex pain that thorough examination is precluded. Postoperatively, conjugated estrogens (2.5 mgm daily for seven days) are given to premenarchal girls to facilitate healing.

In adults superficial lacerations may be debrided and irrigated under local anesthesia, and admission to the hospital

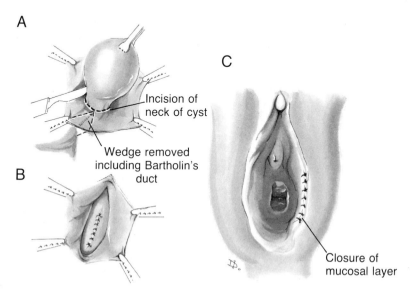

Incision of neck of cyst

Wedge removed including Bartholin's duct

Closure of mucosal layer

Figure 20–3   Excision of Bartholin's cyst. *A.* The cyst is elevated by blunt dissection and its neck identified. A wedge of the neck is removed, which prevents recurrence. *B.* Submucosa is approximated with 3-0 chromic catgut sutures. *C.* Mucosa is closed with interrupted chromic.

is seldom required. However, if the trauma appears to involve either the urethra, bladder, rectum, or upper third of the vagina, the patient should be admitted to the hospital, and examination under general anesthesia carried out with a Foley catheter in the urinary bladder. Débridement and repair of the laceration can be accomplished under the same anesthesia. Deep vaginal lacerations occur as the result of intercourse or the introduction of foreign bodies as used in self-abortion.

VAGINA

Examination of the Vagina in Children

Adequate visualization of the vagina in children is extremely important in making a differential diagnosis of vaginal discharge. The most common source of vulvovaginitis in children is a foreign body.[10] Often these can be palpated on rectal examination, but small particles, such as sand or paper clips, may escape detection. An instrument for visualizing the vagina in small children is the Kelly air cystoscope with a light source at the tip. Mild sedation is occasionally necessary and should be given in recommended pediatric dosage.

Before inserting the instrument, it should be recognized that a child's vagina does not have the distensibility or the pliability of the adult vagina. The instrument should be adequately lubricated with surgical jelly and introduced one to two inches until gentle resistance is met. The obturator is removed and the examiner then visualizes the cervix. At this point, sterile swabs should be introduced through the scope, and specimens obtained for cytology, culture and wet smear. The scope is gently withdrawn as the examiner visualizes the walls of the vaginal mucosa. Small foreign bodies can be picked up with a pair of forceps, or can be removed by irrigating with warm water.

The Evaluation of Vaginal Supports and Stress Incontinence

A common complaint of gynecological patients is loss of urine with increase in intra-abdominal pressure. While the surgical correction of urinary stress incontinence should be performed within the hospital, much of the preoperative evaluation of this condition is appropriate in the outpatient department.[8] Patients should not be admitted to the hospital until a clear-cut diagnosis has been made, and other causes of urinary incontinence are excluded. The most common anatomical cause of urinary stress incontinence in females is a loss of the posterior urethrovesical angle. This is usually due to injury or relaxation of the supports following childbirth or aging. However, women with trigonitis, urinary tract infections, various forms of neurogenic bladder dysfunction, or even some women with poor voiding habits will complain of symptoms interpreted as stress incontinence. Consequently, it is important that every patient with a chief complaint of urinary stress incontinence be systematically evaluated to eliminate causes other than inadequate pelvic supports.

Some descensus of the uterus and the appearance of a cystourethrocele will be evident by simply inserting a speculum into the vagina, having the patient bear down, and slowly withdrawing the speculum. An enterocele or a rectocele will also become apparent during this examination. However, these facts themselves do not mean that the incontinence is due to loss of the posterior urethrovesical angle. Frequently, patients with an extensive cystocele will have no stress incontinence because of the acute angle between the bladder floor and the urethra. An impression of the adequacy of the levator muscles (pubococcygeus) can be ascertained by inserting two fingers in the vagina, and asking the patient to draw up the muscles that would prevent her from urinating. If the muscles can be palpated when the patient performs this exercise and the tone is poor, exercises will in many cases correct the patient's stress incontinence and improve her symptoms of pelvic relaxation.[11] These isometric exercises are performed by having the patient tighten this muscle intermittently 100 to 200 times a day.

Further evaluation of the patient's urinary stress incontinence can be accomplished by having the patient void and immediately inserting a Foley catheter. The volume of residual urine is measured and a specimen obtained for culture and urinalysis. If over 50 ml of residual urine are found, the diagnosis of a neurogenic bladder must be ruled out before performing surgery. A bottle of 1000 ml of normal saline is attached to the catheter. As the solution slowly fills the patient's bladder, she acknowledges the first sensation of bladder fullness (150–200 ml) and the point at which she feels her bladder can hold no more (500–700 ml). If the patient's first urge to void is at 50 ml or less, she should be suspected of having trigonitis or a small, spastic bladder. If the bladder capacity is over 700 ml, a flaccid, neurologic bladder may be the problem and more sophisticated urological investigation should be undertaken before any pelvic surgery is performed.[9]

After the bladder capacity has been reached, saline is drained from the catheter until 250 ml remain within the bladder, and the catheter is removed. In the lithotomy position, if the patient loses urine when she coughs, two fingers are inserted into the vagina, elevating the urethrovesical angle beneath the symphysis pubis. Care should be taken not to occlude the urethra. The patient again coughs and if urine is not expelled, it suggests that one of the surgical procedures to elevate the posterior urethrovesical angle will be successful in correcting the incontinence. The test should be repeated in an upright position if incontinence cannot be demonstrated when the patient is lying down. If loss of urine with coughing cannot be demonstrated with 250 ml of saline in the bladder, the diagnosis of stress incontinence due to poor anatomical support should be questioned. Under these circumstances, attempts at surgical correction will not improve the patient's symptoms and, in fact, may aggravate her problem.

A further refinement in identifying the type of stress incontinence and measuring the posterior urethrovesical angle is the bead-chain cystogram.[8]

Use of Pessaries for Vaginal Support

There are several occasions on which a physician can use vaginal pessaries to great advantage: to temporarily relieve symptoms of the retroverted or retroflexed uterus, or to correct uterine descensus in the pregnant patient, in the immediate postpartum period, and in the elderly patient who is a poor operative candidate. Some authors have advised the use of a pessary to manage the syndrome of incompetent internal cervical os, one of the causes of second trimester pregnancy loss.

There are several shapes and sizes of pessaries, the most common being the Smith-Hodge type (Fig. 20–4). The Smith-Hodge pessary will serve most patients well; occasionally doughnut or cube pessaries with strings attached to facilitate removal are best for the elderly patient.

The pessary should be selected so that it is large enough to fit beneath the symphysis and behind the cervix without shifting in the vagina or being expelled when the patient exerts intra-abdominal pressure. It should not be so large as to cause pressure symptoms or difficulty in voiding. The pessary should be well lubricated and should not be inserted if there is acute vaginitis. It should remain in place without symptoms to the patient. The patient should remove, clean, and reinsert the pessary at weekly intervals. If the patient suddenly begins to complain of vaginal discharge, it should be removed until the vaginitis can be treated. In menopausal women using pessaries, bi-

A

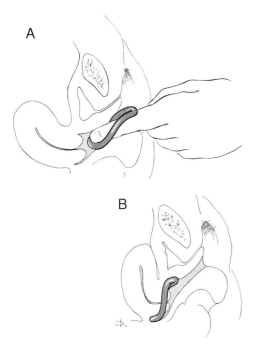

B

Figure 20–4 Pessaries: Smith-Hodge type. *A.* Pessary is inserted behind cervix. *B.* Pessary in place.

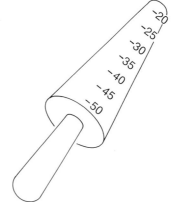

Figure 20–5 Kelly dilator for self-dilatation of hymen.

weekly vaginal application of estrogen cream reduces the incidence of vaginitis.

DISORDERS OF THE HYMEN

The physician involved in premarital counseling has an opportunity to anticipate and prevent the dyspareunia associated with the undilated hymenal ring. One of the most successful forms of treatment is self-dilatation with the Kelly dilator (Fig. 20–5).[2] The patient is advised to use the dilator once a day. The instrument should be gently inserted into the hymenal ring and advanced to the point of slight pain. By gradually increasing the pressure on the dilator each evening over a period of two to three weeks, nontraumatic but very adequate dilatation of the hymenal ring will occur.

Occasionally, the patient will present with almost complete obliteration of the hymenal opening. She may have dis-covered the problem with attempts to insert tampons at the time of menstruation or by self-examination.

The technique for hymenotomy or hymenectomy should begin with adequate regional or general anesthesia. The perineum and external genitalia are cleansed with an appropriate skin disinfectant. Through the largest opening in the hymenal structure, a probe is passed to delineate the vaginal canal from surrounding structures. It is important to identify the urethra so that there will be no trauma to the urethra or bladder. It is not necessary to catheterize the bladder. In the case of total absence of an opening in the hymen, an incision is made directly into the area, usually well defined by menstrual blood, which causes a bluish protrusion of the hymen. A wedge-shaped area is excised (Fig. 20–6), and bleeding is controlled by interrupted 000 chromic sutures.

Labial agglutination in a child rarely requires surgical correction. It is best treated by the mother applying estrogen cream once daily to the labial area for two to three weeks.

CONTRACEPTION

Diaphragm

The use of the vaginal diaphragm for contraception is less common than either

A   B

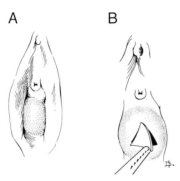

Figure 20–6   Hymenotomy technique. *A.* Hematocolpos due to imperforate hymen. *B.* A triangular wedge of mucosa is excised, approximately 1.5 cm on each side.

the contraceptive hormones or the intrauterine device. The pregnancy rate for the diaphragm is 10 to 12 per hundred women years. However, there are times when both of the latter methods are contraindicated or the patient by personal choice requests a diaphragm for birth control. It is important that the diaphragm be fitted properly. Sets of fitting rings are available from the manufacturers of diaphragms, or a very satisfactory set can be made from diaphragms themselves. The latter has the advantage of allowing the patient to insert the diaphragm so that the physician can be absolutely certain she understands the method of introduction and that the diaphragm is in the proper place. The largest diaphragm that will be accommodated by the vagina and will not cause discomfort is the most satisfactory. There is evidence that during orgasm enlargement of the upper third of the vagina occurs which may dislodge a diaphragm that is too small. The fitting ring or the test diaphragm should be well lubricated and inserted in the same manner as the vaginal pessary. The physician should be certain that the diaphragm extends from behind the symphysis pubis to the posterior vaginal fornix, thus covering the cervix. A retroverted or retroflexed uterus is not a contraindication for the use of a dia-

phragm, unless the diaphragm cannot be fitted properly. The diaphragm should be inserted prior to intercourse and removed not sooner than six hours after coitus. The diaphragm should always be used with a spermicidal jelly or cream applied to the surface of the diaphragm in contact with the cervix. It can be washed with soap and water, and during the day it should be protected from direct sunlight. Periodic inspection of the latex surface will detect tears or small holes in the diaphragm.

Intrauterine Device

There are many shapes and sizes of intrauterine devices, and most of them are packaged in sterile, disposable units with the introducer included.[19] The pregnancy rate for the intrauterine device is two to three per hundred women years. The major side effects are irregular bleeding and cramping, and the major complication is perforation of the uterus at the time the device is inserted. If recognized, this requires laparotomy.

Relative contraindications for insertion of an intrauterine device are active pelvic infection, large or submucous leiomyomas and uterine anomalies. There has been a high expulsion rate in nulligravidas, but with newer designs in intrauterine devices even the nulligravid patient will find this an excellent means of contraception.

Careful pelvic examination will detect pelvic disease and ascertain the direction of the uterine fundus. A speculum is inserted into the vagina, and after cleansing the cervix, the anterior lip of the cervix is grasped with a tenaculum. The uterine cavity is explored with a uterine sound. After the intrauterine device is drawn into the appropriate introducer, traction is placed on the tenaculum to help straighten the uterine cavity. The introducer with the device within is then directed through the cervix into the uterine cavity up to the flange on the introducer. The device is then gently pushed out as the introducer is advanced. Most intrauterine devices have a string attached to the device and this should be cut as long as possible. There is a tendency for intrauterine devices to retract and draw the string into the uterine cavity. A pelvic examination should be done immediately after removal of the speculum and the tenaculum and the patient warned that there will be bleeding for several days.

Because most of the perforations occur in the soft postpartum uterus, it is ideal to wait at least ten weeks following delivery before introducing an intrauterine device and to insert it at the end of a menstrual period. This takes advantage of the physiological dilatation of the cervix which occurs at this time and assures the physician that the patient is not pregnant.

Removal of an intrauterine device is a simple task if the synthetic thread is visible, in which case it may be grasped and withdrawn gently. If much force is required, a tenaculum should be put on the anterior lip of the cervix and traction on the uterus used to straighten the uterine cavity. If the string of the device cannot be visualized or if it is the type of device that does not have a thread, a special hook or forceps is necessary to grasp the device.

There are instances when a patient feels she has expelled her intrauterine device and the physician cannot visualize the string. Frequently a uterine sound will be successful in touching the device, thus assuring the physician and the patient that the device is *in situ*. However, if there is still some doubt after this maneuver, the best procedure is to perform an AP x-ray of the pelvis with a sound in the uterus. This not only confirms the presence of the device, but assures the physician that the device is within the uterus. If the intrauterine device results in abnormal bleeding, ascorbic acid (500 mgm, four times daily), is prescribed for ten days. If this does not resolve the bleeding, treatment with conjugated estrogens (1.25 mgm

daily, day 5 through day 24) is often successful.

CERVIX

Vagnal and Cervical Cytology Tests

The cervical and vaginal cytological smears for the detection of abnormal desquamated cells have become a routine part of any gynecological examination. Necessary equipment for making adequate smears includes clean glass slides, cotton-tipped applicators or cervical spatulas, and a container of equal parts 95 per cent alcohol and ether. We prefer the cotton-tipped applicator to obtain the smears because it avoids unnecessary trauma to the cervix.

After inserting a nonlubricated speculum, the applicator is turned within the cervical canal to insure adequate sampling from the endocervix and the squamocolumnar junction. If the squamocolumnar junction has been everted, as in pregnancy, one should swab this area with the applicator. The cells are then transferred to the clean glass slide by carefully rolling out a thin smear. Thick smears and blood make cytological screening much more difficult and should be avoided. The slide is immediately placed in the alcohol-ether solution for fixing. A second slide is taken from the posterior vaginal pool in a similar manner. After the smears have been fixed for one or two hours in the alcohol, they may be removed, dried, and sent to the pathology laboratory.

While the Papanicolaou technique for cytological diagnosis is an excellent screening technique, it should not replace other clinical measures for the detection of malignancies. A biopsy should be made of any gross lesion of the cervix or vagina. The cytological methods have their greatest value when there are no visible lesions. It is not uncommon to find invasive carcinoma of the cervix with an inflammatory exudate so that the abnormal epithelial cells are not found in the cytological specimens.

Biopsy of Cervix

Biopsy of the cervix is mandatory for any suspicious lesion. There is no evidence that it causes any dissemination of malignant disease. Prior to biopsy the cervical and vaginal epithelium should be stained with Lugol's solution or Gram's iodine (Shiller test). These stains are rapidly absorbed by glycogen-containing stratified epithelium. Nonstaining areas should be examined by biopsy. Neoplastic cells will not incorporate the stain nor will areas of rapid regeneration following infection or trauma. Everted endocervical columnar epithelium also will not stain.

The Schubert cervical biopsy forceps has been the most satisfactory instrument in our experience (Fig. 20–7). Biopsies are made of areas of suspicious erosion or nonstaining areas, and any bleeding points should be controlled with chemical or electrocautery. Biopsy specimens are placed in 10 per cent formalin and sent to the pathologist.

Cone Biopsy of the Cervix. Cone biopsy of the cervix is used most often with patients whose cells are abnormal and who have no gross lesion of the cervix. The cone biopsy removes the entire squamocolumnar junction, allowing the pathologist to examine a wide selection of tissue. Cold knife cone biopsy should be performed rather than the older meth-

ods of cone biopsy with a cautery instrument. At all times except during pregnancy, this procedure is combined with dilatation and curettage of the uterus to establish the source of the abnormal cells and the extent of the disease.

While it is possible to accomplish this procedure under local anesthesia or uterosacral block, it is preferable to use regional or general anesthesia. Shaving the perineum is definitely unnecessary and only causes the patient undue discomfort after the procedure. The patient is placed in the dorsal lithotomy position and the perineum and vagina are prepared with an appropriate skin antiseptic. Care should be taken during the preparation to avoid the cervix and upper vagina so that superficial cells will not be dislodged. Pelvic examination should be done to confirm the preoperative findings. A weighted speculum is placed in the vagina to depress the posterior vaginal wall, and narrow retractors are utilized to visualize the remainder of the vagina and cervix. With a tenaculum on the anterior lip of the cervix, the cervix and vagina are stained with Lugol's solution or Gram's iodine. The cervical canal and the uterine cavity should be gently probed with a uterine sound to determine the direction of the cervical canal before biopsy. One of two methods of hemostasis should be accomplished before making an incision in the cervix. Many surgeons prefer to place a single 0 chromic suture in each lateral portion of the cervix to occlude the major blood supply to the cervix. These sutures are left quite long so that they can be used for traction during the procedure. An alternate method is the injection of the cervix with a dilute solution of vasopressin. A solution containing 1 unit vasopressin in 10 ml saline can be injected at several points in the cervix prior to making the incision. This provides excellent hemostasis throughout the procedure, does not cause untoward cardiovascular changes in the patient, and it has not been associated with an increase in postoperative complications (Fig. 20–8).

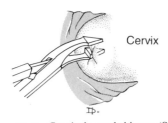

Cervix

Figure 20–7　Cervical punch biopsy (Schubert forceps). Biopsy must include squamocolumnar junction. With this instrument, it is possible to include tissue within the endocervical canal in the biopsy.

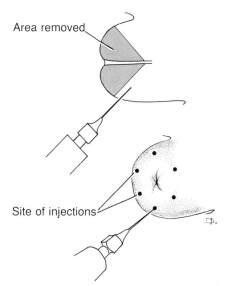

Figure 20–8 Cervical cone biopsy #1: Vasopressin injection for hemostasis, 10 ml of saline containing 1 unit of vasopressin are injected in multiple sites outside the biopsy site. The needle is angled as shown.

After one of the hemostatic measures is performed, a conelike incision is made in the cervix with a scalpel blade, the margins of the cone including all non-staining areas. A shallow incision is carried far enough to include the squamocolumnar junction but not the internal os, which has previously been identified with the uterine sound. After the initial incision is made, the upper limits of the cone biopsy can be removed from the cervix with curved scissors (Fig. 20–9). To help orient the pathologist, the cone biopsy should be marked with a suture at 12 o'clock, pinned to a small cork board, and floated in 10 per cent formalin. If vasopressin has been injected, further sutures are usually unnecessary. However, any bleeding points on the cervix should be controlled with "figure of 8" sutures of 0 chromic. If a large portion of the cervix is removed with the cone, the Sturmdorf mattress type of suture will help reconstitute the epithelium and at the same time control bleeding (Fig. 20–10).

Antibiotics, packing and douches are unnecessary following a cone biopsy. The patient should be advised to abstain from intercourse for one month, and she should be seen by the physician at two weeks and six weeks after the procedure so that the cervical canal can be sounded to prevent stenosis or adhesions.

A small percentage of patients with a cone biopsy will have excessive postoperative bleeding. Usually this occurs about ten days after the procedure when the escar is expelled. In these cases the bleeding areas must be resutured or cauterized.

Cauterization of the Cervix

One of the most successful treatments for chronic inflammation of the cervix is electrocauterization.[18] Prior to cauterization, cytological examination and biopsy of the cervix should be performed to rule out a malignant lesion. A nasal cautery tip is introduced into the

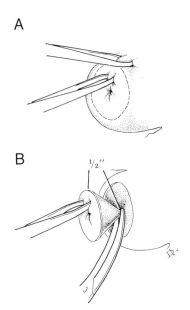

Figure 20–9 Cervical cone biopsy #2: Removal of specimen. *A.* The cervix is grasped with a tenaculum. Circular scalpel incision should include squamocolumnar junction, but not the internal os. *B.* Removal of specimen is completed with curved Mayo scissors.

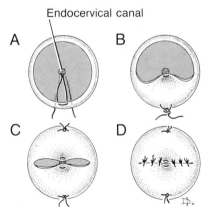

Endocervical canal

Figure 20-10   Cervical cone biopsy #3: Closure with Sturmdorf mattress suture. *A.* An 0-chromic suture on a heavy, curved, noncutting needle is passed from the posterior aspect of the *portio vaginalis* to the apex of the cone in the endocervical canal. The suture is then brought back to the superficial margin of the biopsy. It is returned to the apex of the cone and again brought out to the *portio vaginalis*. *B.* The suture is tied, inverting the mucosa over the biopsy site. *C.* Similar suture is placed anteriorly. *D.* Additional sutures may be used as necessary for hemostasis and to close the mucosal defect.

endocervical canal and six or eight radial strips are cauterized over the eroded surface of the cervix (Fig. 20–11). After cauterization, the patient will note an increase in vaginal discharge during the healing process. Nightly applications of

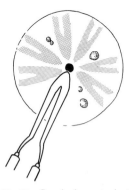

Figure 20-11   Cervical cauterization. Nasal cautery tip is introduced into the endocervical canal. Six or eight radial strips are cauterized over the eroded surface. "Actual" cautery is used, with a glowing red cautery tip.

a vaginal antibiotic cream will improve the symptoms.

Some of the long-term complications of extensive cautery of the cervix or of cone biopsy are cervical stenosis, infertility due to the destruction of the mucus-producing portion of the cervix, and incompetent cervical os in a subsequent pregnancy. In any operation performed on the cervix, every effort must be made to avoid trauma to the internal os, particularly in women of child-bearing age. Correction of chronic cervicitis may play a significant role in reducing the incidence of invasive cancer of the cervix.

Cryotherapy of the Cervix

Since 1964 cryotherapy has been used to treat chronic cervicitis and cervical erosion. The indications for its use are similar to those for electrocautery of the cervix. The procedure can be performed without anesthesia, although occasionally a mild analgesic is necessary immediately after the procedure. The probe of the cryosurgery unit is inserted into the cervical os, including most of the exocervix. Freezing temperatures and time necessary to produce coagulation necrosis depend upon the agent used (liquid nitrogen, nitrous oxide, Freon, or carbon dioxide). The probe tip should be placed directly on any abnormal area for coagulation. Once the probe is in contact with the affected area, the cooling agent flows through the probe, which assumes its operating temperature over the next 30 to 45 seconds.

Following the procedure, the patients develop a profuse, clear vaginal discharge beginning on the first postoperative day, reaching a maximum by the sixth day, and lasting from 1 to 13 weeks. Because the discharge has a high potassium content, patients are encouraged to increase dietary potassium. One can expect complete healing of the cervix in 80 per cent of patients within eight weeks of treatment. Cervical canal stenosis following this procedure is extremely rare.[14,15]

*Postcoital Test for Infertility
Investigation*

The investigation of the infertile couple includes a systematic evaluation of the reproductive tracts of both individuals. One of the most important tests performed is the postcoital test which determines if spermatozoa are penetrating the cervical mucus.[12] The patient should be seen at midcycle as determined either by her menstrual calendar or by a basal body temperature rise. She is instructed to have intercourse within eight hours prior to the time of examination and to use no lubricants or douches. A speculum is introduced into the vagina and the cervix visualized. At midcycle there should be copious amounts of cervical mucus. A small portion of cervical mucus is applied to a clean glass slide with either a glass pipette or a saline-saturated, cotton-tipped applicator. A cover slip is placed over the cervical mucus and the specimen examined under the microscope. Between 5 and 20 motile spermatozoa will be seen per high power field in a normal examination. If all spermatozoa are nonmotile the differential diagnosis is between a defect in cervical mucus, poor sperm motility and an antibody-antigen response. When one has to scan several fields to discover spermatozoa, oligospermia or poor coital techniques should be suspected. The cervical mucus pH at midcycle should be between 6.5 and 7.5 and bacteria and leukocytes rarely visualized.

hormonal therapy rather than the prescription of hormones without any consideration of the endometrial histology. In the infertile patient the endometrial biopsy is used to establish indirectly that ovulation is occurring and to evaluate the adequacy of the corpus luteum. Many physicians prefer doing the endometrial biopsy on the first day of a menstrual period. This has the advantage of excluding an early pregnancy. It has the disadvantage of being inconvenient, occasionally giving poor tissue for examination, and providing little information about the progesterone effect on the endometrium. A timed endometrial biopsy performed during the 21st through the 24th day of the cycle provides more information and rarely interferes with pregnancy.

Except in unusual situations, the procedure requires no anesthesia. The instrument used is a Novak curette (Fig. 20–12). The patient's anxiety can be relieved by carefully explaining the procedure and warning her that she will briefly experience pain similar to menstrual cramps. The pain will disappear as soon as the curette is withdrawn from the uterus.

Prior to performing the biopsy, a bimanual examination is performed to ascertain the direction of the uterine fundus. A speculum is placed in the vagina and a tenaculum is placed on the

UTERUS

Endometrial Biopsy

The endometrial biopsy has its greatest use in the evaluation of the infertile patient. Patients with abnormal bleeding, particularly those under the age of 40 in whom endometrial carcinoma is not a major consideration, can be evaluated satisfactorily with endometrial biopsy. The biopsy will allow knowledgeable

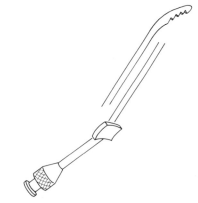

Figure 20–12   Novak curette for endometrial biopsy.

cervix. After the cervix is cleansed, a 10 ml syringe is attached to the Novak curette, which is then gently inserted through the endocervix so that the curve of the curette will conform to the position of the uterine fundus. Gentle pressure should be applied until the curette has reached the furthermost point of the uterine cavity. With suction on the syringe, the curette is withdrawn. A single strip of tissue from the anterior wall is sufficient for infertility investigations. However, if one is performing the endometrial biopsy to evaluate abnormal bleeding, the curette should be turned in all four quadrants of the uterus and the withdrawal motion repeated while suction is maintained on the syringe. The biopsy specimen is expelled into 10 per cent formalin and the syringe flushed with formalin to remove any remaining particles of tissue. The patient may have spotting for 24 hours but should experience no other difficulty.

The major complication of endometrial biopsy is perforation of the uterus. This can be avoided if one does not exert undue pressure when inserting the curette and abandons the procedure if the curette does not advance with ease into the endometrial cavity. The average uterine cavity measures 2½ to 3½ inches, and if the curette passes beyond this in the normal uterus, perforation of the uterus should be suspected and the procedure discontinued. There is one very promising modification of the endometrial biopsy which may broaden its use. By attaching a suction apparatus and introducing a sputum collection trap, one can sample the entire uterine cavity efficiently. It has been shown that this procedure performed on an outpatient basis without anesthesia will remove as much tissue as the standard curettage.

Uterosacral Block

Uterosacral block is satisfactory anesthesia for most procedures requiring dilatation of the cervix. Minor dilatation of the cervix such as that required for

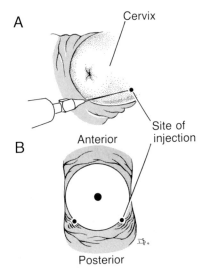

Figure 20–13 Uterosacral block. *A*. Sites of injection in the uterosacral ligaments are 4:00 and 8:00 with the patient in the lithotomy position. *B*. Gentle traction on the cervix permits identification of the uterosacral ligaments. 5 to 10 ml of 1% lidocaine are injected with a 22 gauge, 3½ inch spinal needle. Each uterosacral ligament is injected to a depth of 0.5 cm.

endometrial biopsy is tolerated well by most patients without anesthesia.

A speculum is placed into the vagina and the cervix is grasped with a tenaculum. Gentle traction on the cervix will usually identify the uterosacral ligaments which are at 4 o'clock and 8 o'clock. A 10 ml syringe with a 22 gauge, 3½ inch spinal needle is used. Five to ten ml of 1 per cent lidocaine is injected into each uterosacral ligament after the needle has been inserted ½ cm into the ligament. A submucosal swelling should be visible at the injection site. The needle is introduced about 2 cm. from the external os (Fig. 20–13). Aspiration on the syringe is important before injecting the solution to avoid a sudden intravenous injection in this highly vascular area.

Dilatation and Curettage of the Uterus

Dilatation and curettage of the uterus, fondly referred to as D and C, is perhaps the most common procedure performed by gynecologists. It is used to evaluate abnormal bleeding and cytology, and to terminate incomplete abortion and postpartum hemorrhage. Dysfunctional uterine bleeding is related to a hormonal imbalance and is not associated with pregnancy, cancer, benign growths, or pelvic inflammation. This diagnosis is made by excluding the other conditions at the time of curettage, which in 75 per cent of patients will be not only diagnostic but therapeutic.

For incomplete and therapeutic abortion prior to 12 weeks gestation, the classical curettage of the uterus is being replaced by suction curettage. Curettage of the uterus is also performed for abnormal postpartum bleeding. The most common causes are subinvolution of the placental site or retained placental fragments.

Dilatation and curettage of the nonpregnant uterus can be performed as an outpatient procedure but it does require anesthesia. The pain of the procedure is associated with dilatation of the cervix. The afferent pathways for cervical pain are through Frankenhauser's plexus and traverse the uterosacral ligaments; consequently, the procedure can be accomplished using the uterosacral block. Many clinics are performing this procedure with light general anesthesia. In these situations one can facilitate the patient's recovery by avoiding narcotics and sedatives as premedication.[16]

The patient is placed in the lithotomy position and the perineum and vagina are washed. Shaving the perineum is entirely unnecessary. A weighted speculum is inserted in the vagina and the cervix visualized. A single-tooth tenaculum is used to grasp the anterior lip of the cervix. The uterine cavity is explored with a sound and the depth of the cavity measured. If the curettage is being performed to evaluate abnormal cytology, the cone biopsy should be done prior to dilatation of the cervix to avoid trauma to the endocervical tissues.

A

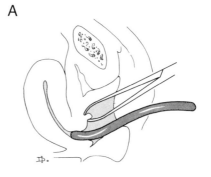

B

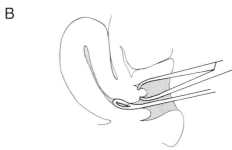

Figure 20–14 Dilatation and curettage of the uterus. *A.* Progressively larger Hegar dilators are used to overcome resistance at internal os. Forcep type dilators should not be used. *B.* The largest sharp curette which can be passed through the endocervix is passed to the fundus. Strips of endometrium are removed from the uterine cavity in a clockwise fashion. The illustration shows the curette in the endocervix, which should be curetted as a separate specimen prior to introduction of the curette to the fundus.

Hegar dilators are used to dilate the cervix (Fig. 20–14). One begins with the smallest dilator that meets resistance at the endocervix. When resistance is felt, constant pressure is applied with the hand of the operator resting on the patient's perineum. This will avoid a sudden thrust resulting in perforation when resistance at the endocervix is overcome. The graduated dilators are inserted up to size 8, with further dilatation usually unnecessary. Dilatation beyond this point may damage the endocervix, especially in women who are of child-bearing age. The endocervix is then curetted with a small serrated curette, and this tissue is saved as a separate specimen. Endometrial cancer which has extended to the endocervix will spread like a cervical cancer into the perimetrial and pericervical lymphatics; consequently, it is important to curette this area separately for diagnostic, therapeutic and prognostic purposes. The uterine cavity is explored with an ovum forceps to detect any large uterine polyps prior to the curettage. Thereafter, as large a sharp curette as can be introduced through the endocervix is inserted until the fundus of the uterus is contacted. Strips of endometrium are withdrawn in a clockwise fashion so that the full extent of the uterine cavity is sampled. Soft areas in the uterine wall and areas abundant in tissue should be noted. These may suggest an area of endometrial cancer, the presence of a submucous myoma, or the base of an endometrial polyp. The tissue is collected on a gauze sponge which has previously been inserted into the vagina. After removing the curette and the tenaculum from the cervix, a pelvic examination is repeated, and the procedure is terminated.

Suction Curettage of the Uterus

Suction curettage of the uterus is useful in the treatment of incomplete abortion, and termination of pregnancy within the first twelve weeks of gestation.[5] Suction curettage does not allow the surgeon to discriminate the area from which tissue is being obtained, and for this reason it should not be used in place of fractional curettage in the evaluation of abnormal cytology or suspected endometrial carcinoma.

In the case of spontaneous incomplete abortion suction curettage can frequently be performed without anesthesia. The cervix, having been dilated by the products of conception, usually admits a medium-sized suction cannula which suffices in evacuating the remaining tissue from the uterus. The patient is placed in a comfortable lithotomy position and pelvic examination is performed to determine the position of the uterus. The

perineum, vagina and cervix are cleansed with an antiseptic solution and the legs and perineum are covered with sterile drapes. A weighted speculum is gently placed in the vagina and the anterior lip of the cervix is grasped with ring forceps. It is best to avoid a single tooth tenaculum in grasping the soft pregnant cervix. This will often lacerate the cervix when minimal traction is applied or will result in undue bleeding when it is removed. The depth of the uterus is determined with a uterine sound. The largest suction cannula that can be admitted without meeting resistance at the internal cervical os is selected. Before introducing the cannula into the cervix, the suction should be checked by immersing the tip of the cannula into a pan of sterile water. The maximum pressure of the apparatus should also be checked by occluding the suction tubing and determining that no more than 50 mm of mercury pressure is maintained.

With traction on the cervix the uterine cavity is explored with an ovum forceps and any large fragments of tissue are removed. The suction cannula is then gently introduced to the full extent of the uterine cavity and the escape valve is closed so that suction is applied to the cannula. By gently withdrawing the cannula in each of the four quadrants of the uterus, the products of conception will be evacuated. The suction curette is efficient in removing all tissue from the uterus and a sharp curettage following this procedure is unnecessary. The patient should be warned that minimal vaginal bleeding will be noted for one to two days following the procedure. The only serious complication of this procedure is uterine perforation which usually occurs when the uterine sound is passed. If this occurs, the patient should be observed for a 24-hour period, and if there are no signs of peritoneal irritation, no further treatment is necessary. If there is any evidence that omentum or bowel has been damaged, exploratory laparotomy must be carried out.

If the surgeon feels that the suction curettage cannot be accomplished under analgesia or with the aid of a para-cervical block, general or regional anesthesia can be used.

In the case of missed abortion or termination of pregnancy within the first twelve weeks of gestation, the suction curettage can be facilitated by introducing a No. 18 Foley catheter with a 30 ml balloon on the evening prior to the procedure. This is done by placing the patient in the lithotomy position and cleansing the cervix and vagina. The Foley catheter is then introduced into the cervix beyond the internal cervical os. The Foley catheter balloon is inflated and the patient is returned to her room. No further precautions are necessary and traction on the catheter is not required. This allows dilatation of the cervix through the night, and further dilatation on the following day is usually unnecessary. The curettage is then carried out in a manner similar to that for incomplete abortion.

Recently, laminaria coated with antibiotic cream have replaced other mechanical methods of "softening" the cervix prior to curettage.

AMNIOCENTESIS

Amniocentesis is the removal of a sample of amniotic fluid, usually performed transabdominally, for diagnostic or therapeutic purposes.[6] There are several indications for the use of diagnostic amniocentesis, the most common being the evaluation of patients with isoimmunization. Amniotic fluid analysis of the concentration of unconjugated bilirubin will determine the need for premature delivery or fetal transfusion. Questions of gestational age can be clarified by determining the creatinine content of amniotic fluid as well as evaluating the percentage of fat-containing cells in the amniotic fluid. Other tests for fetal maturity are presently being evaluated, including the ratio of lecithin to sphingomyelin. In pregnancies of 42 weeks or more, the presence of me-conium in amniotic fluid will often forewarn the obstetrician of chronic intra-uterine distress. During the second trimester amniocentesis is performed to establish the diagnosis of a variety of chromosomal and metabolic disorders of the fetus.

Technique of Amniocentesis During First Twenty Weeks of Pregnancy

After the patient voids, a pelvic examination is done to determine the size of the uterus. The uterus must be at least 14 weeks in size before amniocentesis is attempted. If the uterus is still within the pelvis, a small area above the symphysis pubis is shaved because the amniocentesis will have to be performed just above the symphysis. The skin is prepared with an antiseptic solution and the skin and subcutaneous tissue are infiltrated with a local anesthetic agent about one inch above the symphysis pubis in the midline. With one hand in the vagina elevating the uterus, the other hand is used to direct a 22 gauge, $3\frac{1}{2}$ inch spinal needle through the skin into the uterus. There is a characteristic change in resistance when the needle enters the amniotic cavity. The assistant attaches a syringe to the needle, and the amniotic fluid is withdrawn. There are no unusual precautions that the patient must observe following this procedure. In about 10 per cent of the cases, fluid is not obtained in the first attempt. In these situations, the patient returns in one week and the procedure is repeated.

If the amniocentesis is being performed at a time when the uterus is easily palpable in the abdomen, it is unnecessary to elevate the uterus. The amniocentesis, in these situations, can be carried out in a manner similar to the procedure used after 20 weeks gestation.

Amniocentesis After Twenty Weeks Gestation

After the patient voids, the position of the fetus is determined by palpation.

A site near the fetal small parts is selected for the amniocentesis. This usually is one or two inches below the umbilicus and one or two inches to the left or right of the midline. The abdomen is prepared with an antiseptic solution, and the skin and subcutaneous tissue are infiltrated with a local anesthetic agent. A 22 gauge, 3½ inch spinal needle is introduced past the skin resistance and then up to the hub of the needle with a single deliberate motion, or until the needle meets definite resistance. A syringe is attached and the amniotic fluid is aspirated. If initially the fluid cannot be withdrawn into the syringe, the needle is gently withdrawn and rotated with negative pressure on the syringe. After aspirating the fluid, the needle is withdrawn. If blood is obtained or if no fluid can be obtained at the site first chosen for the amniocentesis, an alternative method is the suprapubic approach. The subrapubic hair is shaved, and the area prepared with an antiseptic solution. A site 1 to 2 inches above the symphysis pubis in the midline is infiltrated with local anesthetic agent. The fetal presenting part is elevated with one hand, and the needle is introduced with the other. An assistant must aspirate the fluid while the needle is held firmly in place.

The most common complication of amniocentesis is fetal-maternal transfusion, which occurs in about one out of every ten procedures. We feel placental localization is unnecessary unless the fluid cannot be obtained by either of the methods described above. Other reported complications are amnionitis, fetal bleeding, separation of the placenta, rupture of membranes and premature onset of labor. These are rare complications, and there are several series with well over 1000 amnioceneses in which none of these complications have been encountered.

Amniocentesis for Therapeutic Abortion

Therapeutic termination of pregnancy after 12 to 14 weeks gestation must be carried out by methods other than curettage of the uterus. The introduction of hypertonic solutions into the amniotic cavity is an effective method of terminating a pregnancy. The amniocentesis is performed in a manner described above, but in these situations it is best to use an 18 gauge needle. Amniotic fluid is drained by gravity until 100 to 150 ml have been removed and then replaced with 200 ml of 20 per cent sodium chloride (NaCl). Two or three times during the infusion, aspiration should be performed to insure that the needle remains within the amniotic cavity. After installation of the hypertonic solution, a latent period of approximately thirty hours follows before the labor ensues.[4] The most serious complication of termination of pregnancy with hypertonic saline is hypernatremia due to inadvertent intravascular infusion of the solution or too rapid uptake of the sodium from the uterus. This complication should be suspected in patients who develop a headache, thirst or sudden hypertension during the infusion. The immediate intravenous infusion of large amounts of dextrose and water should be instituted as well as the administration of furosemide to promote diuresis. Post-abortal infection, retained placenta, and hemorrhage during or following the abortion are occasional complications of second trimester abortion. Curettage of the uterus is necessary for retained placental fragments or delayed hemorrhage.

Amniocentesis is occasionally employed to relieve the pressure and respiratory symptoms of acute polyhydramnios. Because this procedure usually results in the onset of labor, it should be performed only in situations that cannot be managed with bed rest or diuresis. The fluid should be allowed to drain slowly to avoid sudden decompression of the uterus. In these cases the amniocentesis is done with an 18 gauge Touhy needle and an epidural catheter. The catheter is threaded through the needle and the needle withdrawn. This allows a slow, controlled removal of a large volume of fluid. Because of the danger of infection, the catheter should be removed within eight hours. When the complication occurs with twins it is usually the lower twin in which the polyhydramnios has occurred; thus amniocentesis should be done near this twin. When acute polyhydramnios occurs there is a 30 to 50 per cent chance of a fetal anomaly.

Amniography

Amniography is a technique which can be used to detect fetal hydrops, establish the placental site, confirm fetal death, or determine abnormalities of the gastrointestinal tract of the fetus.[13] Amniocentesis is performed in the routine fashion. After withdrawing 10 to 20 ml of amniotic fluid, 10 to 20 ml of a suitable contrast material are infused. These hypertonic iodinated compounds are the same as those used for intravenous pyelography. The first x-ray should be taken within 1 hour after injecting the material and a second x-ray is taken after 12 hours. The first x-ray will show the fetus and placenta well outlined by contrast material and will detect soft tissue fetal abnormalities such as the edema of hydrops fetalis. If the scalp thickness is greater than 0.5 cm this condition should be suspected. Contrast material should be seen in the gastrointestinal tract in the film taken after 12 hours. If contrast material cannot be detected in the fetal gastrointestinal tract, fetal death, anencephaly, or gastrointestinal malformations must be suspected.

The complications of amniography are the same as those for amniocentesis except that premature labor or rupture of the membranes may be induced if large amounts of the hypertonic contrast material are used.

FALLOPIAN TUBES AND OVARIES

Evaluation of the patency of the fallopian tubes is an important part of an infertility investigation.[17] All of the tests used for this purpose employ the basic principle of a solution or a gas injected through the fallopian tube, with visualization of this material entering the peritoneal cavity, or causing symptoms of its presence within the abdomen. One of the most popular tests is tubal insufflation with carbon dioxide, known as the Rubin test.

Rubin Test

The patient will experience cramping during this procedure, and the steps involved must be carefully explained to alleviate anxiety. An olive-tipped cannula is attached to the pressure monitoring device and to a source of carbon dioxide. It is important that the entire system be filled with carbon dioxide before the test is begun. A pelvic examination must be performed to establish the position of the uterine fundus and to eliminate the presence of acute pelvic inflammatory disease. After a speculum is placed in the vagina and the anterior lip of the cervix is grasped with a tenaculum, the cervix is cleansed with an antiseptic solution. The sterile, olive-tipped cannula is then inserted into the cervix until the olive portion is firmly in contact with the cervix (Fig. 20–15). This ensures that gas will not exit

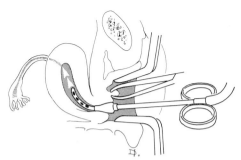

Figure 20–15 Technique for instillation of CO_2 or contrast material into uterus and fallopian tubes. Traction is placed on cervix with tenaculum. Olive-tipped cannula is inserted into cervix to achieve air-tight apposition of cervix to the olive portion. CO_2 or contrast material is introduced, depending on the test desired, as described in the text.

through the cervix. The insufflation is begun slowly and the pressure device is observed. Initially there is a gradual rise in pressure as the gas fills the intrauterine cavity. A flow rate of 30 ml per minute is recommended. During the insufflation an assistant listens to the abdomen with a stethoscope. A definite souffle can be heard as the gas enters the peritoneal cavity through the fallopian tube; there will be a distinct plateau of pressure and eventually a decrease in pressure as the gas passes through the tube. The configuration of the pressure patterns, if these are recorded, cannot be relied upon to determine the degree of tubal spasm, the extent of tubal adhesions or other tubal pathology. A symptom of tubal patency is shoulder pain which the patient will experience upon sitting up. Pressures above 200 ml of mercury must be avoided. If there is no evidence of gas escaping into the peritoneal cavity either by auscultation, change in the pressure pattern, or symptoms of peritoneal irritation, one cannot assume that anatomical obstruction is present. Tubal spasm may produce the same result. On the other hand, if symptoms and signs of tubal patency are present, it does not eliminate the possibility of other tubal disease such as peritubal adhesions.

Contraindications for this test are acute pelvic inflammation or pregnancy. It is best to perform the test in the preovulatory phase of the menstrual cycle to avoid interfering with an early conceptus.

Complications of this procedure include uterine perforation and inadvertent vascular injection of the gas. For this reason carbon dioxide must be used rather than air.

Hysterosalpingography

A more complete evaluation of the fallopian tubes as well as the uterine cavity can be performed by hysterosalpingography. The indications are infertility, abnormal uterine bleeding following curettage to rule out endometrial polyps, and the need to rule out uterine abnormalities following midtrimester pregnancy loss or habitual abortion. The contraindications for the procedure are identical to those for tubal insufflation.

Mild analgesia is often of value when performing this procedure. A laxative or enema on the evening prior to the procedure is advisable. A scout film of the abdomen and pelvis is taken prior to beginning the procedure. The patient is placed in a comfortable lithotomy position on the x-ray table, and a speculum is introduced into the vagina. The anterior lip of the cervix is grasped with a tenaculum and the cervix is cleansed. A cannula similar to that used for tubal insufflation is filled with contrast media eliminating air bubbles from the cannula and syringe. The cannula is inserted in the cervix and secured either by hand or by attaching the cannula to a special clamp on the tenaculum.

The contrast media used may be either water-soluble or oil-soluble. The water-soluble material is rapidly absorbed and is not associated with the rare but perplexing complication of oil granuloma. The oil-soluble material has the advantage of causing less uterine and tubal spasm and allows a delayed film to ascertain peritoneal spill.

After proper placement of the cannula 1 to 2 ml of media are slowly injected into the uterus, and the first film is exposed. A second injection of 1 to 3 ml of media is slowly carried out, and another film is taken ten seconds after the second injection. Usually the two films are sufficient to show satisfactory tubal patency; however, if these films fail to visualize both fallopian tubes well, the patient is turned to either oblique position and a third injection of 1 to 3 ml is made to adequately visualize the fallopian tube which may have been obscured by the position of the uterus. Defects in the uterine cavity must be differentiated from air bubbles by persistence of the defect on all films. Spill of the material into the peritoneal cavity is evidence of tubal patency. One must still be suspicious of peritubal pathology if the passage of the contrast material into the peritoneal cavity is delayed or if the material becomes restricted to one area. A 10 minute delayed film will be satisfactory with water-soluble media, and if oil-soluble media are used, a 24 hour delayed film will be helpful in determining peritoneal spill of the contrast material.

Complications of this procedure are uterine perforation, occasional pelvic granuloma, and intravascular injection of contrast material if excessive force is used during the injection. The ideal time for performing hysterosalpingography is seven to ten days following the onset of the last menstrual period.

CULDOCENTESIS

Direct sampling or direct visualization of the peritoneal cavity is an important diagnostic aid in many clinical situations. Culdocentesis is the needle aspiration of peritoneal fluid from the posterior culdesac. This is a procedure which can be performed by any physician. Culdoscopy and laparoscopy, both of which allow direct visualization of pelvic structures through endoscopes, are procedures which require technical proficiency and special equipment not available in many outpatient departments.

The indications for culdocentesis are suspected ectopic pregnancy, or the need to confirm the presence of blood, pus or malignant cells in the peritoneal cavity.

Anesthesia and analgesia are unnecessary for this procedure. A bimanual pelvic examination is performed prior to the procedure. One contraindication to the procedure is a mass which is fixed in the culdesac. Pelvic infection is not a contraindication, and this procedure will often be helpful in establishing a differential diagnosis when pelvic inflammatory disease is being considered.

A speculum is inserted into the vagina, and the posterior lip of the cervix is grasped with a tenaculum. The cervix is elevated, allowing adequate visualization of the culdesac. A 3½ inch 18 gauge needle is attached to a syringe containing 1 ml of saline or local anesthetic solution. The needle is then advanced through the vaginal mucosa into the culdesac with a single deliberate motion (Fig. 20–16). At this point, the patient will experience a sudden but brief pain when the needle traverses the peritoneum. The patient

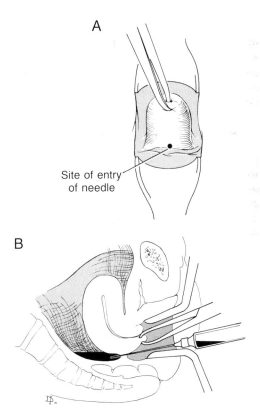

Figure 20–16 Culdocentesis *A.* Traction on posterior lip of cervix exposes posterior culdesac. *B.* Syringe containing 1 ml of saline or local anesthetic is attached to 18 gauge, 3½ inch needle. Needle is introduced into posterior culdesac. Fluid is injected to clear tissue from the needle, followed by aspiration of culdesac contents. Needle is introduced parallel to the sacrum, to avoid entry into uterus or rectum.

should then be positioned so that any abdominal fluid will pool in the culdesac of Douglas. The solution within the syringe is injected to clear the needle, and the needle is then slowly withdrawn while aspirating the syringe. In normal patients, a small amount of yellowish peritoneal fluid can be obtained. A hematocrit of any bloody fluid should be performed. If it is less than 10 per cent, needle trauma of the uterus or adjacent structures or a ruptured ovarian cyst must be suspected. If the hematocrit is greater than 10 per cent, the source of intra-abdominal bleeding must be determined by surgical exploration. No special precautions are necessary following culdocentesis.

OUTPATIENT OBSTETRICAL DELIVERY

There can be little argument that if cost, availability of personnel and facilities permitted, all obstetrical patients should be delivered in a hospital setting where operating room facilities, a blood bank and an adequate laboratory are available. Although careful prenatal evaluation can identify the patients who are unlikely to have complications in labor and delivery, there are those occasional situations in which the most carefully followed, low-risk patients suddenly develop complications in labor which require intensive in-hospital care. Nevertheless, the necessity for home or outpatient delivery of a baby often occurs because of geographic isolation, an unexpectedly rapid labor, or perhaps cultural suspicion of modern medical facilities. The physician attending such a patient should have available the following items:

Clean towels and receiving blanket
Sterile gloves (several pairs)
Rubber half sheet
Equipment for administering an enema
Stethoscope
Sphygmomanometer
Urethral catheter

Instruments
  Syringes—Several 2 ml syringes; 22 gauge needles
    Several 10 ml syringes; 22 gauge needles
  Mayo-type scissors
  Needle holder
  4 Kelly clamps
  Cord clamps or umbilical tape
  (If the preceding four items are not sterile they can be cleansed in boiling water before use)
  Several packs of 000 chromic suture with swedged-on noncutting needle
  Soft rubber bulb-suction
  Infant laryngoscope
  Cole infant endotracheal tube with stylet

Medications
  Morphine or meperidine
  Oxytocin (10 units per 1 ml vial)
  Methylergonovine (0.2 mg per 1 ml vial)
  Magnesium sulfate (50 per cent solution in 10 ml vials)
  Lidocaine 1 per cent
  Antibiotic ophthalmic ointment (1 gm tube)
  Alcohol sponges

Labor

When the patient is in labor a vaginal examination is performed with a sterile glove. The dilatation and effacement of the cervix and the position of the presenting part are determined. If delivery is not imminent, a soapsuds enema is administered to avoid fecal contamination of the perineum and the infant at the time of delivery. Thereafter, as few vaginal or rectal examinations as possible are done. This is particularly important after rupture of the membranes has occurred to minimize the risk of intra-amniotic infection. Meperidine (100 mg) or morphine sulfate (10 mg) may be administered intramuscularly to relieve pain. If the cervix has not become fully dilated in 12 hours after the onset of labor in a primiparous patient (8 hours in a multiparous patient) cephalopelvic disproportion or an abnormality of uterine contractions should be suspected. The same is true if there is no progress in cervical dilatation or descent of the presenting part in a two hour period. In either case, one should prepare to transfer the patient to a hospital.

Throughout the first stage of labor the fetal heart rate is determined at least hourly. Any persistent change of fetal heart rate to over 160 per minute or under 100 per minute indicates fetal distress. The patient should be turned on her side to allow adequate venous return through the inferior vena cava. If this does not result in an improvement in fetal heart tones, preparation should be made for delivery of the infant or transfer of the patient to an obstetrical unit.

If at any time during labor the blood pressure reaches levels of 140/100 and the deep tendon reflexes are hyperactive one should suspect pre-eclampsia and administer magnesium sulfate (10 ml of 50 per cent solution given as a deep intramuscular injection into each buttock — total dose of 10 gms). Thereafter 5 gm of magnesium sulfate are given every four hours throughout labor and delivery for 24 hours after delivery, as long as reflexes are active.

The second stage of labor (the time from full dilatation to delivery) should last no longer than two hours in the primiparous patient and one hour in a multiparous patient. A second stage of labor lasting longer than these limits suggests cephalopelvic disproportion or abnormal presentation of the fetus (brow, face, shoulder or compound presentation).

Delivery

When delivery is imminent as evidenced by perineal crowning of the presenting part, the delivery area should be prepared. A rubber half sheet or a generous covering of newspapers is applied to the bed or table, and the perineum is washed with soap and water. The patient is delivered in the most comfortable position whether this be on her left side with the physician standing behind the patient or with the patient on her back with knees flexed and the physician standing at the foot of the bed or table.

The left lateral position avoids vena cava compression by the pregnant uterus, while the supine position allows more effective pushing efforts by the patient as she grasps her flexed knees and brings her head forward during contractions.

As the head distends the perineum, counter pressure should be applied to prevent the explosive exit that results in extensive lacerations. If the head is carefully controlled at this point, there will usually result only a small perineal laceration near the midline. This can be easily approximated with interrupted 000 chromic sutures after local infiltration with 1 per cent lidocaine. When the head is delivered, the mouth and nares of the infant are gently aspirated with a soft rubber bulb-suction. With the next contraction gentle downward traction will bring the anterior shoulder under the symphysis pubis. By then directing the head toward the symphysis the posterior shoulder will deliver over the perineum, and the remainder of the birth is inevitable.

The umbilical cord is clamped or tied and cut about 1 inch from the abdomen. A rapid evaluation of the baby will indicate if there is need for resuscitation. A baby who is breathing spontaneously, has a vigorous cry, good tone, a plethoric-pink appearance, and a pulse rate over 100 per minute requires no further resuscitation. If the baby does not breathe spontaneously, has poor tone, a mottled blue and pale color, and the pulse is less than 100, resuscitative efforts should be instituted at once. When available, an infant laryngoscope is used to visualize the vocal cords to rule out an obstruction, and an endotracheal tube is passed for mouth-to-tube ventilation. Mouth-to-mouth resuscitation will suffice if intubation equipment is not at hand. In most depressed infants who have no congenital abnormalities, maintenance of ventilation and body warmth will result in rapid improvement in a few moments. After the infant's condition is stable, body temperature should be maintained by wrapping him in warm blankets, and an antibiotic ointment applied to the eyes to prevent gonococcal ophthalmia.

Third Stage of Labor—Delivery of the Placenta

Gentle traction on the umbilical cord will suffice to deliver the placenta after it has descended into the lower uterine segment. If the placenta has not been delivered within 30 minutes, a hand wearing a sterile glove should be inserted into the uterus. If the cervix is tightly closed or if the placenta within the uterus seems adherent, further, more vigorous efforts to remove the placenta should await the patient's transfer to an obstetrical unit. Hemorrhage at this stage can be catastrophic. Immediately after the placenta is removed oxytocin (10 units) or methylergonovine (0.2 mg) is given intramuscularly to maintain uterine tone. Gentle massage of the uterine fundus will also improve uterine tone.

The perineum is inspected for lacerations which can be repaired with interrupted 000 chromic sutures after local infiltration with 1 per cent lidocaine. Two-layer closures are quite satisfactory with the first sutures approximating the submucosal and subcutaneous tissues. If it appears that the external anal sphincter or the rectal mucosa has been lacerated (third and fourth degree lacerations respectively) it must be meticulously repaired in a three-layer closure with interrupted 000 chromic sutures. The closure begins with approximation of the rectal submucosa in two layers. One should avoid placing sutures through the rectal mucosa. The ends of the external anal sphincter are identified and several sutures are placed in the surrounding capsule to approximate the torn ends of the muscle. Sutures within the muscle itself are unnecessary. The remainder of the perineum and vagina are closed in two layers. Antibiotics and laxatives are unnecessary following an episiotomy repair or the repair of a third or fourth degree laceration.

Immediate Postpartum Period

Care during the immediate puerperium includes frequent observations to detect hemorrhage from uterine atony, prolonged urinary retention, or hypertension or postpartum eclampsia. Uterine atony can be avoided by administering methylergonovine tablets (0.2 mg) every 4 hours for 24 hours. Urinary retention manifested by a distended bladder and inability to void, and usually due to urethral edema or reflex perineal pain, should be relieved by catheterization. Hypertension is a sign of potential postpartum eclampsia which can be avoided by administering magnesium sulfate in a manner similar to its use in labor.

Early ambulation of postpartum patients should be encouraged to avoid venous stasis which may lead to thrombophlebitis or pulmonary embolism.

References

1. Ball, T. L.: Gynecologic Surgery and Urology. St. Louis, C. V. Mosby Co., 1963.
2. Barter, R. H., and Yochelson, L.: Psychophysical indications for hymenal dilatation. Am. J. Obstet. Gynecol., *82*:1134–1140, 1961.
3. Collins, C. G., Hansen, L. H., and Theriot, E.: A clinical stain for use in selecting biopsy sites in patients with vulvar disease. Obstet. Gynecol., *28*:158–163, 1966.
4. Droegemueller, W., and Greer, B. E.: Saline versus glucose as a hypertonic solution for abortion. Am. J. Obstet. Gynecol., *108*: 606–609, 1970.
5. Eaton, C. J.: Uterine aspiration for evacuation of the pregnant uterus. J.A.M.A., *207*: 1887–1889, 1969.
6. Fuchs, F., and Cederqvist, L. L.: Recent advances in antenatal diagnosis by amniotic fluid analysis. Clin. Obstet. Gynecol., *13*: 178–201, 1970.
7. Gardner, H. L., and Kaufman, R. H.: Benign Diseases of the Vulva and Vagina. St. Louis, C. V. Mosby Co., 1969.
8. Green, T. H., Jr.: The problem of urinary stress incontinence in the female: An appraisal of its current status. Obstet. Gynecol. Surg., *23*:603–634, 1968.
9. Hodgkinson, C. P.: Urinary stress incontinence in the female: A program of preoperative investigation. Clin. Obstet. Gynecol., *6*:154–177, 1963.

10. Huffman, J. W.: The Gynecology of Childhood and Adolescence. Philadelphia, W. B. Saunders Co., 1968.
11. Kegal, A. H.: Progressive resistance exercise in the functional restoration of the perineal muscles. Am. J. Obstet. Gynecol., *56*: 238–248, 1948.
12. Kleegman, S. J., and Kaufman, S. A.: Infertility in Women: Diagnosis and Treatment. Philadelphia, F. A. Davis Co., 1966.
13. McLain, C. R., Jr.: Amniography, a versatile diagnostic procedure in obstetrics. Obstet. Gynecol., *23*:45–50, 1964.
14. Ostergard, D. R., Townsend, D. E., and Hirose, F. M.: The long-term effects of cryosurgery of the uterine cervix. J. Cryosurg., *2*:17–22, 1969.
15. Ostergard, D. R., Townsend, D. E., and Hirose, F. M.: The treatment of chronic cervicitis by cryotherapy: A preliminary report. Cryobiology *4*:97–102, 1967.
16. Shields, L. V.: Outpatient or hospital day-care for minor gynecologic procedures. Am. J. Obstet. Gynecol., *104*:809–811, 1969.
17. Sweeney, W. J., III, and Gepfert, R.: The fallopian tube. Clin. Obstet. Gynecol., *8*: 32–47, 1965.
18. Te Linde, R. W., and Mattingly, R. F.: Operative Gynecology. Philadelphia, J. B. Lippincott Co., 1970.
19. Tietze, C.: Contraception with intrauterine devices: 1959–1966. Am. J. Obstet. Gynecol., *96*:1043–1054.
20. Word, B.: New instrument for office treatment of cyst and abscess of Bartholin's gland. J.A.M.A., *190*:777–778, 1964.

21

Anus and Rectum—
Proctology

By J. E. L. SALES, M.A., M.B., M.Chir., F.R.C.S.

INTRODUCTION

Anorectal conditions requiring treatment are a common outpatient problem. This chapter describes the diagnostic evaluations and surgical procedures which may be carried out in outpatients. The chief complication of most of these surgical procedures is reactionary hemorrhage. It is, therefore, important to warn the patient that bleeding may occur and to provide facilities, especially at night, for its emergency treatment.

ANATOMY

This section describes the anatomy of the anorectal region. It is not intended to be a comprehensive account, but those aspects of the anatomy which are of practical importance in examination and surgery of the region are described in detail.

The Rectum

The rectum starts in front of the third piece of the sacrum at the rectosigmoid junction. It follows the curvature of the sacrum and coccyx inferiorly and anteriorly until at 1½ inches anterior to the coccyx it makes a right-angled bend posteriorly to become the anal canal (Fig. 21–1). It is approximately 5 inches (12.5 cm) long. In addition to its anteroposterior curvature, it has three lateral curves, one right and two left, which produce shelves within the rectum—the valves of Houston (Fig. 21–2).

The upper third of the rectum is covered with peritoneum anteriorly and laterally, the middle third anteriorly only. The lower third, which is dilated to form the ampulla of the rectum, lies below the level of the rectovesical pouch and is therefore devoid of peritoneum (Fig. 21–2). The distance from the anal verge to the rectovesical pouch is 3 inches (7½ cm).

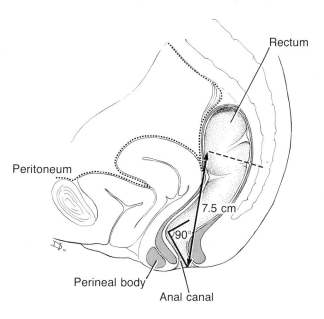

Figure 21–1 Sagittal section of the female pelvis showing the relationship of the peritoneum and pelvic structures to the rectum.

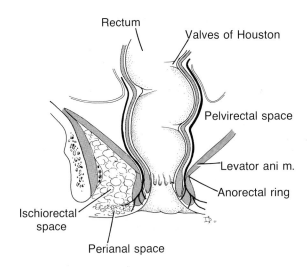

Figure 21–2 Coronal section of the pelvis showing the rectal curves and the tissue spaces surrounding the rectum and anal canal.

The rectum is lined with columnar epithelium, which is pink in color. In the normal bowel, the submucosal vessels can be seen clearly through the mucosa.

The Anal Canal

The anal canal in the adult is approximately 1½ inches long, and it extends from the anal verge to its junction with the rectum at the level of the anorectal ring (Fig. 21–3). The lining of the canal may be divided into two parts: an upper or proximal mucosal, and lower or distal cutaneous, and these are separated by the dentate line some ¾ inch from the anal verge.

The mucosa of the upper anal canal is folded into approximately ten longitudinal folds—the anal columns. These become less distinct with increasing age of the patient. The distal end of these columns fuse to form the anal valves, and behind each is a small pocket, the anal sinus or crypt (Fig. 21–3). The mucosa is principally simple columnar epithelium in type, and appears plum-colored due to the underlying internal hemorrhoidal venous plexus.

Below the dentate line, the canal is lined by stratified squamous epithelium, which contains no hair follicles or sebaceous glands. It merges with normal skin at the anal verge.

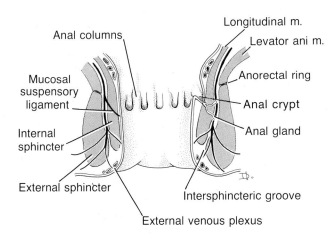

Figure 21–3 The anatomy of the anal canal and anorectal ring. The dentate line is the row of anal crypts which separates the stratified squamous epithelium of the anal canal from the columnar epithelium of the rectum.

Anal Glands

These small branching glands, usually four to eight in number, open into the anal crypts and extend for a variable distance into the anal musculature (Fig. 21-3). They are lined with stratified columnar epithelium and do not secrete. However, it has been suggested that infection occurring in these glands is the underlying cause in the majority of cases of anal fistula.[30] Nesselrod (1964)[27] believes that anal crypt gland infection is also a principal cause of hemorrhoids and fissure. This view, however, is not generally accepted.

The Anal Sphincters

The Internal Sphincter

This is a thick cylinder of smooth muscle surrounding the anal canal. It is a localized thickened portion of the circular muscle of the rectum, extending just distal to the dentate line. It has a well-marked and palpable rounded lower edge.

The External Sphincter

This is composed of striated muscle, surrounding the internal sphincter and extending distally to it. It blends with the puborectalis superiorly, inferiorly it is inserted into the perianal body, and posteriorly with the anococcygeal raphe. There is no suggestion histologically that it is divided into three separate parts as traditionally described.[13] Its lower border can be felt on digital examination just inferior and lateral to that of the internal sphincter. There is a palpable interval between the two sphincters in the wall of the anal canal, the so-called intersphincteric or intermuscular groove.

The Longitudinal Muscle

This is a continuation of the longitudinal muscle of the rectum. It passes downward between the internal and external sphincters. At its lower end it splits up into many fibers which pass through the lower borders of the internal and external sphincters. Some fibers passing through the internal sphincter bind the anal mucosa firmly to the sphincter just below the dentate line, the mucosal suspensory ligament[29] (Fig. 21-3). Although the presence of a definite ligament is disputed, the mucosa is firmly bound at this point and this forms the boundary between the internal and external hemorrhoids — the inter-hemorrhoidal groove (Fig. 21-8). The fibers passing through the external sphincter are inserted into the skin of the anus and perianal region, and this constitutes the corrugator cutis ani.

The Levator Ani Muscles

This group of muscles which form the pelvic diaphragm also constitute part of the anal sphincter mechanism (Figs. 21-2 and 21-4). The two major parts of the muscle are:

1. Iliococcygeus
2. Pubococcygeus

These arise from the pelvic wall fascia and pubis and are inserted into the lower pieces of the sacrum, fusing with the muscle of the opposite side to form the anococcygeal raphe. The innermost fibers of the pubococcygeus are usually separately described as the puborectalis. They arise from the posterior aspect of the pubis and form a sling around the anorectal junction, producing the anorectal angle. At the anorectal junction, these fibers combine with those of the internal and external sphincters to form the anorectal ring (Fig. 21-3). This ring of muscle, which is stronger laterally and posteriorly than it is anteriorly, constitutes the principal part of the anal sphincter mechanism.

Although the internal and external sphincters are important in the preservation of continence, they can, if necessary, be divided with no loss of normal control. If, however, the anorectal ring

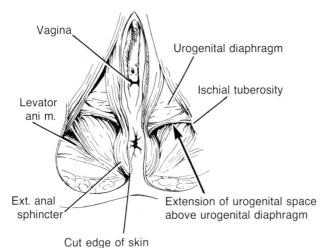

Figure 21–4   The female perineum.

Vagina

Urogenital diaphragm

Ischial tuberosity

Levator
ani m.

Ext. anal
sphincter

Extension of urogenital space
above urogenital diaphragm

Cut edge of skin

is completely divided, incontinence results. It is therefore vitally important to identify this ring of muscle before performing any surgery.

Tissue Spaces

There are several tissue spaces related to the anal canal which are important as they are frequent sites of infection.

The Ischiorectal Fossa

This is a wedge-shaped space filling the lateral part of the anal triangle and extending forward above the urogenital triangle (Fig. 21–4). Its lateral wall is formed by the fascia over the lower part of obturator externus, the falciform margin of the sacrotuberous ligament and the ischial tuberosities. Medially, the two fossae are separated by the perineal body, the anal canal and the anococcygeal body. The roof is formed by the levator ani muscles. The fossa is filled with coarsely lobulated fat into which the anal canal can expand during defecation. It is important to remember that infections of this space may also involve the extension of the fossa above the urogenital diaphragm. The inferior rectal artery and vein and inferior rectal

nerve (S3,4) arise from the neurovascular bundle in the pudendal canal, cross the floor of the fossa to supply the external sphincter, the posterior part of levator ani and the perianal skin.

The Perianal Space

This is the subcutaneous space which extends from the lower part of the anal canal to the buttocks (Fig. 21–2). The fat in the space is finely lobulated in contrast to that of the ischiorectal space, since the lobules are separated by fibrous septa. Whether there is a definite layer of fascia separating these two spaces is disputed. Infection or hematomas in this space give rise to considerable tension and hence are exquisitely painful.

The Submucous Space

This lies under the mucosa of the upper two-thirds of the anal canal. It contains the internal hemorrhoidal plexus and is the site of sclerosant injections in the treatment of hemorrhoids (Fig. 21–8).

The Pelvirectal Space

This is a potential space containing connective tissue lying between the peritoneal floor of the pelvis and the upper surface of the levator ani muscles (Fig. 21–2). On rare occasions, it is the site of infection.

Blood Supply to Rectum and Anal Canal

Arterial Supply

The principal arterial blood supply to the rectum and anal canal is the superior rectal artery, which is the terminal branch of the inferior mesenteric artery. At the rectosigmoid junction, it divides into right and left branches, which run forward around the rectum and branch into it. The branches of the superior rectal artery then pierce the muscle layer and run into the submucosa. The right branch divides into two parts while the left remains single, and these branches continue as far as the anal columns. This arrangement accounts for the position in which the primary hemorrhoids occur in the anal canal (Fig. 21–8 *B*). The middle rectal arteries are variable in size. They arise from the internal iliac and pass to the rectum in the lateral ligaments. The inferior rectal artery arises from the internal pudendal artery in the pudendal canal, crosses the ischiorectal fossa and supplies the anal canal below the dentate line and the perianal skin. It anastomoses with the superior rectal artery.

Venous Drainage

This follows the arterial supply. The submucosal hemorrhoidal plexus of the anal canal above the dentate line and the plexus in the rectal wall drain into the superior rectal veins. These veins unite at the level of the rectosigmoid junction to form a single superior rectal vein which drains into the inferior mesenteric vein. The middle rectal veins chiefly drain the muscular wall of the rectal ampulla and end in the internal iliac veins. The inferior rectal vein drains the anal canal below the dentate line to the pudendal vein. The venous plexus which lies between the lower border of the external sphincter and the perianal skin is called the external hemorrhoidal plexus (Fig. 21–8 *A*). The rectal veins do not contain valves.

Lymphatic Drainage

Lymphatic drainage also follows the arterial supply and therefore flows principally upward. The lymphatic plexuses of the rectal wall and upper anal canal drain into the pararectal nodes which lie behind the rectum, and then to the superior rectal and inferior mesenteric nodes. The lymphatics following the middle rectal vessels drain into the internal iliac nodes. The upper part of the anal canal also drains into the internal iliac nodes by lymphatics which pierce the levator ani. The anal canal below the dentate line drains via the cutaneous lymphatics to the inguinal nodes.

Nerve Supply

The rectum and upper anal canal is supplied by the rectal plexus, which is derived from the pelvic plexus. It contains sympathetic and parasympathetic fibers. The parasympathetic nerves, derived from the pelvic splanchnic nerves (S2–4) contain both afferent and efferent fibers. The afferent nerves are sensory from the rectum, while the efferent are motor. The anal canal below the dentate line is innervated by the inferior rectal nerve (S2, 3 and 4).

Anal Sphincters

The levator ani muscles are innervated on their pelvic aspect by branches from S4 and on the perianal aspect by the inferior rectal nerve.

The internal sphincter has sympathetic and parasympathetic innervation. The sympathetic system is motor and the parasympathetic system is inhibitory.

The voluntary external sphincter is supplied by the perineal branch of the inferior rectal nerve (S4).

HISTORY

The patient frequently finds difficulty in describing his symptoms accurately. Therefore, although a well-taken history is essential, it usually is of less significance than a careful clinical examination. It is advisable and quicker then, to take the history in the form of a series of leading questions put to the patient. Most clinics have a form pre-printed for this purpose. The main symptoms about which the patient must be asked are:

1. *Nature of complaint* and its duration.
2. *Bleeding.* When it occurs, amount, whether bright or dark red and whether or not it is mixed with the stool.
3. *Pain.* Its nature, location (i.e., whether it occurs in anus, rectum or abdomen), and its relationship to defecation.
4. *Prolapse.* Whether it occurs with defecation or at other times. Whether it will reduce spontaneously or must be replaced.
5. *Swelling.* Mode of onset, duration and degree of pain, if any. Any discharge of blood or pus.
6. *Pruritus.* Is it constant or does it occur only after defecation? Is it worse at night? Does it involve the vulva, groins or toes?
7. *Incontinence.* Its degree and nature.
8. *Bowel habit.* Any recent change in habit. Constipation or diarrhea. If diarrhea, its frequency and presence of any associated blood or mucus.
9. *Micturition.* Any recent evidence of cystitis or pneumaturia.
10. *General health.* Any recent deterioration, loss of appetite or weight.
11. *Past history.* Illnesses or previous operations.
12. *Family history.* Any history of bowel diseases.
13. *Therapy.* Any drugs being taken. Any anal suppositories or creams being used.

EXAMINATION

A general physical examination must be carried out. It is important to remember that anorectal symptoms can be a manifestation of systemic disease. The principal points that should be noted in the examination are:

1. General condition, any weight loss or evidence of anemia.
2. Cardiopulmonary status, with a view of anesthesia.
3. Abdomen—presence of any distension, fluid, tenderness or masses.
4. Lymphadenopathy, cervical and inguinal.

When the general examination has been completed, the rectal examination should be carried out.

Position for Rectal Examination

The three positions for rectal examination are shown in Figure 21–5 *A*, *B* and *C*: (1) Left lateral or Sims' position; (2) Knee-shoulder; and (3) Prone on proctoscopic table.

The position one uses for the examination depends, of course, on personal preference. I feel that the left lateral is the best, both for the comfort of the patient and for the performance of the examination.

Inspection

It is most important to examine the perianal region carefully, as many of the common anal conditions can be diagnosed on inspection alone. Rubber gloves should be worn on both hands

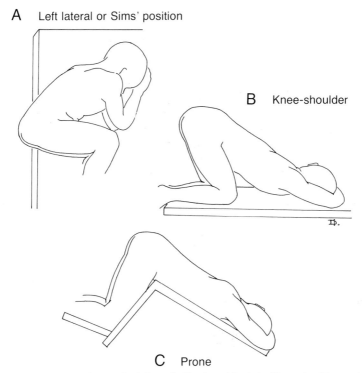

A Left lateral or Sims' position

B Knee-shoulder

C Prone

Figure 21–5 Rectal examination. *A*. Left lateral (Sims' position). *B*. Knee-shoulder position. *C*. Prone position.

at all times. The chief points to notice are:

1. The condition of the perianal skin. Notice whether there are any skin changes, their extent and characteristics, and whether there are any other skin lesions on the body. Are there scars from previous operations?

2. Note whether there is any discharge. If so, what is its nature and origin? A careful look for a fistulous opening must be made if the discharge is purulent. If there is a fecal leak and soiling of clothes, note whether this is due to poor hygiene or incontinence.

3. The presence of swellings, e.g., perianal hematoma, external hemorrhoids, skin and sentinel tags, condylomata acuminata, and so on.

4. The tone of the sphincters, which may be gauged by lateral separation of the buttocks. If lax, the patient should be asked to strain down to see whether there is any prolapse. If there is spasm, note whether there is a fissure present.

Rectal Examination

A well-lubricated finger cot must be used over the glove. The perianal region should first be gently and carefully palpated for evidence of tenderness and induration.

The finger should then be gently inserted into the anal canal. It is very important to tell the patient exactly what you are going to do in order to retain his confidence and keep him relaxed. Relaxation is facilitated by asking him to breathe slowly and deeply through the mouth. He should be warned that it may be uncomfortable. If an acute anal fissure is present with spasm of the sphincter, the examination should be postponed. When the finger is in the anal canal, the tone of the sphincters and any narrowing of the canal must be noted. The perianal structures should then be palpated between finger and thumb for any evidence of inflammation, and also to determine the direction of a fistulous tract if present. The finger should then be advanced into the rectum. The depth to which the finger can be inserted depends on its length and the size of the patient, but usually it is some 8 to 10 cms.

The lumen of the rectum should first be examined for fecal contents and for any evidence of stricture. Hard feces may sometimes feel like a tumor but usually can be indented. The rectal wall is next carefully palpated. It is good practice to start with an assessment of the prostate in the male and cervix in the female in order to get one's bearings in the rectum. The finger is then swept round the bowel wall to detect any irregularity, e.g., the cobblestone mucosa of Crohn's disease, polyps, soft villous adenoma. The indurated edge of a carcinoma has a characteristic feel. Its site, extent and mobility should be assessed. Pedunculated polyps may be difficult to feel if they have a long stalk. It is very important to feel posteriorly just above the anorectal ring, as lesions in this site may easily be missed on endoscopy.

The extrarectal structures should be palpated, starting with the rectouterine or rectovesical pouch. This should be a bimanual examination. In the female, the size and position of the uterus and the presence of any adnexal swellings should be determined. Are there any swellings in the sigmoid colon or secondary carcinoma deposits in the pouch? Laterally and posteriorly the walls of the pelvis, sacrum and coccyx should then be palpated.

Finally, on withdrawal of the finger, the color and consistency of the feces, and the presence of any blood, mucus or pus, should be noted. The feces should also be tested chemically for the presence of occult blood with guaiac, benzidine or Hematest.

PROCTOSCOPY

The patient is put in the left lateral or Sims' position. The upper or right but-

tock is retracted with the left hand. The proctoscope is held in the right hand with the handle in a horizontal position pointing toward the patient's back in the line of the natal cleft. The obturator is held in position by the right thumb. The proctoscope, which must be well lubricated, is gently inserted in the direction of the umbilicus. Once fully inserted, the handle is grasped by the left hand and the obturator is removed with the right. Cotton wool pledgets held in long nontoothed forceps can be used to clean the anal canal of excess mucus or feces.

When the proctoscope is fully inserted, it lies above the anorectal ring (Fig. 21–6 *A*). On removing the obturator, the lumen of the rectum is examined. A note is made of the color and consistency of the feces, and whether or not any blood or mucus is present in or around the stool. The mucosa is next examined for any inflammatory changes, as shown by changes in color, ease of bleeding, ulceration or edema. Occasionally, lowlying tumors can be seen and a biopsy can be undertaken. The proctoscope is then slowly withdrawn. As it passes

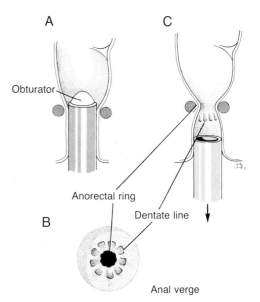

Figure 21–6 Technique of proctoscopy. *A–C.* Views of anal canal seen on withdrawal of the proctoscope.

from the rectum into the anal canal, the anorectal ring closes above it (Fig. 21–6 *B* and *C*). The upper canal is surrounded by the submucous hemorrhoidal plexus, which gives it a plum color. If hemorrhoids are present, they will be visible in the lumen as bulges of varying sizes. It is advisable to ask the patient to strain down gently at this point to ascertain the degree of prolapse of any hemorrhoids, or to detect any potential prolapse. The anal valves are usually clearly visible and a note should be made of any hypertrophied papillae or fibrous polyps arising in this area. Below the valves, a fissure, if present, may be seen in the midline posteriorly. The internal opening of a fistulous tract usually occurs at the level of the anal valves, and this may be confirmed by pressing on the tract either by finger or proctoscope, at which time a bead of pus will appear at the opening.

SIGMOIDOSCOPY

A sigmoidoscopy must be carried out in all cases.

Bowel Preparation

Sigmoidoscopy is best carried out, if possible, without any previous bowel preparation by laxatives and enemas. These produce fluid stools which irritate the rectal mucosa with resulting congestion and excess mucus production. This leads to obvious problems with the procedure and often to difficulties in diagnosis. Ideally, the patient should be asked to have a bowel movement a few hours prior to the examination. If the bowel is so loaded that examination is impossible, the patient should be sent away to defecate or return at a suitable time after a bowel action with or without the aid of laxatives.

If a more intensive preparation is desired or required, the following instructions may be given:

INSTRUCTIONS FOR PATIENTS TO PREPARE FOR PROCTOSIGMOIDOSCOPY

Report to the clinic at_____on_____
Eat as follows:
  For *supper* the evening before:
      You may have meat, fish, eggs or cottage cheese. Crackers, bread and butter. Rice. Tea, coffee or milk. Cream and sugar. Strained fruit juice, plain cupcakes, ice cream for dessert.
  Do not eat at bedtime.
  For *breakfast* the morning of coming:
      Eat only crackers, butter or margarine, tea or coffee with cream and sugar if desired.
  Drink all the water you wish.
      You may have "cokes," "pop" or gingerale, if desired.

Prepare as follows:
  At 8:00 P.M. the evening before:
      Take a two quart, warm water enema to which you have added two teaspoons of baking soda.
  At 10:00 A.M. the morning of coming:
      Take another two quart enema, prepared in the same way.

Technique

The patient may be placed for this examination in one of the following positions (Fig. 21–5): (1) Left lateral or Sims' position; (2) Knee-shoulder; (3) Prone on the sigmoidoscopy couch.

The left lateral is probably the most convenient and comfortable position for the patient. In order to prevent complications caused by blind passage of the instrument, a digital examination must always be carried out prior to instrumentation. The digital examination must be done to exclude a stricture or any gross pathology in the anal canal and lower rectum. A well-lubricated sigmoidoscope should then be gently introduced in the direction of the umbilicus (Fig. 21–7, position 1). The progress of the sigmoidoscope will be stopped by the anterior wall of the rectum just above the anorectal ring. The obturator should

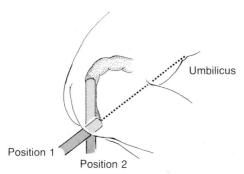

Figure 21–7 Sigmoidoscopy, showing the change of axis of the instrument required following insertion into the rectum.

then be withdrawn, and the light and bellows attached. Further progress of the sigmoidoscope must be performed under direct vision. Using the minimum of inflation with the bellows, the sigmoidoscope should be gently advanced up the rectum following the sacral curve past the valves of Houston (Fig. 21–7, position 2). Any small amounts of feces obstructing the passage or impeding a view of the mucosa should be cleared with pledgets of cotton wool held in long alligator forceps. Liquid stool may be removed by a suction tube. It is important not to overinflate the rectum, as this produces an intense desire to defecate, which may unsettle the patient and make him uncooperative. The rectosigmoid junction is reached when the sigmoidoscope has been inserted to about 15 cm. Here the bowel bends at an acute angle into the left iliac fossa. It is usually possible to pass it into the sigmoid colon by gentle inflation and manipulation of the sigmoidoscope. In some cases, however, there may be acute angulation of the bowel at this point due to a short mesosigmoid. The rectum may also be narrow due to spasm or rigid due to inflammatory changes produced by, for example, diverticulitis, or extracolonic pelvic pathologic process. It is then difficult, and often very distressing to the patient, to try and negotiate the bend. Force should not be used, and in these cases the procedure should be abandoned at this level. A barium enema may be used to display the sigmoid colon.

During the procedure, usually when withdrawing, great care should be taken to examine all parts of the rectum and the visible sigmoid colon, and the following points must be noted:

1. Distance to which the instrument was inserted.

2. The nature of the feces in the rectum and whether or not there is any blood, pus or excess mucus present in or on the stool.

3. The state of the mucosa and the nature and extent of any inflammatory changes., i.e. color, friability, edema, ulceration and extent of bleeding when rubbed with a cotton pledget.

4. The presence of any intraluminal polyps, villous adenomas or carcinomas, their size and their level measured from the anal verge.

5. Mobility of gut wall when inflated and whether there is any evidence of rigidity in the wall.

If, for reasons such as nervousness of the patient or excessive pain and discomfort, sigmoidoscopy is unsatisfactory, the procedure should be carried out under general anesthetic.

RECTAL BIOPSY

A biopsy must be performed for all suspicious lesions of the rectum before making a tissue diagnosis. Biopsy may also be used as a follow-up procedure in chronic ulcerative colitis when the development of histological precancerous changes in the rectum reflect the general condition of the colonic mucosa.[26]

Punch Biopsy

This may be used for mucosal lesions, small sessile polyps and carcinomas.

Technique. The forceps are introduced through the sigmoidoscope under direct vision. The lesion is grasped and the handles closed to cut the biopsy. This usually is easy in friable lesions, but is sometimes difficult when normal mucosa is included in the biopsy. In these cases, the forceps should be rotated so that the biopsy is twisted off the surrounding mucosa. Great care should be taken when making biopsies above the peritoneal reflection, as perforation is a risk.

A disadvantage of this technique is that it often provides the pathologist with a damaged piece of tissue which is difficult to assess.

Suction Biopsy

This method is preferable for inflammatory lesions when the mucosa is friable. It provides a relatively undamaged piece of mucosa for histological examination.

Technique. The Truelove-Salt or Dick instrument should be used. A sigmoidoscope is passed and the site of biopsy is selected. The biopsy instrument is then passed, suction applied and the tissue taken. The piece of tissue obtained should always be orientated by the examiner before fixation so that the pathologist can take a truly transverse section. This can best be done by pressing it on to a ground glass slide or piece of blotting paper with the epithelium uppermost to prevent curling.

Complications. The site of the biopsy must be carefully inspected after removal of the tissue. It there is excessive bleeding, then a pledget of cotton wool soaked in 1:1000 solution of epinephrine should be applied to the site and held in position for a few minutes until the bleeding stops. The patient should not be sent home for at least an hour or until further examination after this time shows that the bleeding has completely stopped. Rarely, blood transfusion may be required for persistent bleeding.

Incisional Biopsy

This method is used to confirm the diagnosis of Hirschsprung's disease. A strip of mucosa, submucosa and muscle is excised from the rectal wall and anal canal below the peritoneal reflection.

Technique. The bowel should be prepared with enemas before the operation, a procedure which should be carried out under a general anesthetic with the patient in the lithotomy position. A bivalve speculum is placed in the anal canal and a chromic catgut stitch is then inserted into the left posterior wall 1 inch above the anorectal ring. Another catgut stitch is inserted vertically below in the anal canal just above the dentate line. Traction is then applied to both sutures to raise a ridge of rectal wall. A strip of mucosa, submucosa and muscle approximately 5 mm wide is excised. The defect is closed with a running chromic catgut stitch. The patient may go home after recovering from the anesthetic.

Complications. Bleeding may occur. This should be stopped either by direct pressure through a proctoscope or underrunning the bleeding point with a catgut stitch.

Anal and Perianal Biopsy

Any lesion in this area should be subjected to biopsy by taking a small wedge of tissue with a scalpel after previously infiltrating the area with a local anesthetic. A hemostatic catgut stitch may be inserted afterwards if necessary.

INVESTIGATIONS

Further tests may be required to establish the diagnosis. The principal ones are:

1. *Radiology.* A barium enema should be carried out if a lesion is suspected higher in the colon, or to find the extent of a mucosal lesion or polyposis present in the rectum. The barium enema with air contrast is the most accurate technique for assessing the colon. If facilities are available, an "instant" barium enema[37] may be performed without preparation for immediate information regarding the extent of the mucosal le-

sions seen on sigmoidoscopy. A barium meal and follow-through should be carried out for small bowel lesions. Sigmoidoscopy should *always* be performed before barium enema to rule out the presence of a lesion in the rectosigmoid colon. If a constricting rectal or sigmoid lesion is present, barium must be instilled with great caution to prevent impaction which may require an emergency colostomy for decompression. Likewise, proctosigmoidoscopy and barium enema should ordinarily precede barium meal and small bowel examination to prevent inadvertent impaction of barium above a lesion of colon or rectum.

Barium enema should not usually be performed on the same day as a biopsy of the rectum, in order to prevent the occurrence of perforations.

2. *Examination* of stools for cysts, ova, protozoa and occult blood.

HEMORRHOIDS ("PILES")

Hemorrhoids are varicosities of the venous plexus lying in the wall of the anal canal. They may be classified according to their site of origin (Fig. 21–8):

1. *Internal.* These are varicosities of the internal hemorrhoidal plexus in the submucous space of the upper anal canal above the mucosal suspensory ligament. They are covered with columnar epithelium.

2. *External.* These arise in the external hemorrhoidal plexus of the lower third of the anal canal and anal verge. They are therefore covered by skin.

Internal Hemorrhoids

Internal hemorrhoids are one of the commonest conditions requiring surgical treatment. It is difficult to estimate their true incidence, as they are often asymptomatic and patients are frequently reluctant to consult the doctor about them. They may occur at any age, but the incidence increases over the age of 50 years. Men are more commonly affected than women, although temporary prominence of hemorrhoids is a common complaint of pregnant women. Primary hemorrhoids arise in the left lateral, right

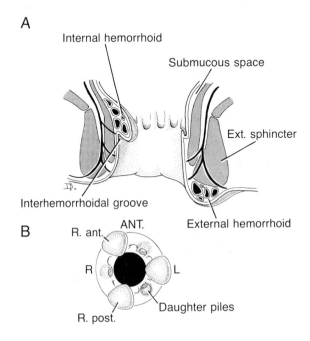

Figure 21–8 Hemorrhoids — anatomical location. *A.* Anatomical relationship of internal and external hemorrhoids. *B.* Arrangement of primary internal and accessory hemorrhoids as seen from below.

anterior and right posterior positions (Fig. 21-8 *B*) which corresponds to the anatomical position of the terminal branches of the superior hemorrhoidal artery. Secondary and daughter piles, however, occur between them.

Classification

They are classified according to their size:

First degree: bleed but do not prolapse.

Second degree: prolapse on defecation, but return spontaneously.

Third degree: prolapse on defecation or spontaneously, and have to be replaced manually.

Clinical Features

Hemorrhoids commonly present with bleeding and prolapse.

Bleeding. This occurs during and after defecation. It is bright red and is not mixed with the stool. It usually is only a small amount, but occasionally can be profuse, particularly from a prolapsed bleeding hemorrhoid. Bleeding may occur without defecation and stain the underclothes. It is important to remember that chronic blood loss from hemorrhoids is a common cause of hypochromic anemia.

Prolapse. This usually occurs when straining at stool. Third degree hemorrhoids may prolapse on walking or coughing. Prolapse is painless unless thrombosis occurs.

Discharge. A mucous discharge is common in patients with prolapsed piles. There may also be a fecal leak.

Examination

A general examination should be carried out to exclude anemia and primary cause for the hemorrhoids, e.g., abdominal tumors, pregnancy or portal hyper-tension. Inspection of the perianal tissue will reveal the extent of any external hemorrhoids, skin tags, third degree hemorrhoids and pruritic skin changes.

A rectal examination will exclude a rectal carcinoma, as hemorrhoids are not palpable unless thrombosed.

Proctoscopy determines the size and degree of prolapse. The proctoscope should be inserted above the anorectal ring, then slowly withdrawn. The patient should be asked to strain down and the degree of prolapse noted.

Sigmoidoscopy must be carried out in all cases to exclude any lesion in the rectum and lower sigmoid.

If there has been any recent alteration in bowel habit, a barium enema must be carried out to exclude a colonic lesion before the hemorrhoids are treated.

Complications

Thrombosis (Strangulated Hemorrhoids). This may occur in second degree or third degree hemorrhoids. They prolapse and are gripped by the anal sphincters, producing thrombosis in the hemorrhoids and edema of the perianal tissues. It is a very painful condition which may be aggravated by simultaneous thrombosis of external hemorrhoids.

Rectal examination reveals the prolapsed internal hemorrhoids with marked edema of the perianal tissues. Proctoscopy and sigmoidoscopy should not be attempted until the condition has resolved.

The majority will resolve spontaneously. If untreated, a few will sclerose and slough ("auto hemorrhoidectomy"). Occasionally, abscess formation may occur as a result of secondary infection.

Treatment. There are two effective safe methods for the outpatient treatment of uncomplicated hemorrhoids:

1. Injection of sclerosant.
2. Ligation (Blaisdell-Barron technique).

Before treatment is started, any constipation should be corrected by diet and laxatives, so as to establish a regular bowel habit.

Injection Therapy

The aim of injections is to produce a submucosal fibrosis around the vessels of the internal hemorrhoidal plexus, which obliterates them and thereby causes the hemorrhoid to shrink. The most effective solutions commonly used are 5 per cent phenol in almond or arachis oil, 5 per cent aqueous solution of quinine urea hydrochloride, or 50 per cent glucose in water. Quinine urea perhaps should be avoided in pregnant women because of reputed danger of inducing miscarriage.

Indications

This technique is suitable for all first degree and the smaller second degree hemorrhoids. In these cases it will give either a complete cure or a prolonged relief from symptoms. It may be used also as a temporary palliative measure in third degree hemorrhoids.

Contraindications

1. When there are associated pathological conditions in the anal canal or rectum, e.g., anal fissure or fistula.
2. If there are strangulated hemorrhoids present.
3. When the submucosal tissue plane is completely fibrosed following several injections. Further injections are liable to produce mucosal ulceration.

Preoperative Preparation

The rectum should be empty before injections are given.

Technique

The procedure is described with the patient supine, in the lithotomy position,

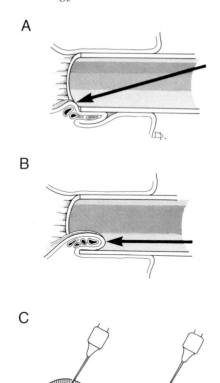

Figure 21–9 Techniques of injecting hemorrhoids. *A*. Injection into the submucosa at the back of the anorectal ring. *B*. Injection directly into hemorrhoid. *C*. Care must be taken in both techniques to inject the sclerosant into the submucosa. Injection into the mucosa produces blanching and subsequent necrosis and ulceration. Record the site and amount of sclerosant injected.

although the prone or Buie position may also be used.

The sclerosant must be injected into the submucous space over the pedicle of the hemorrhoid, which lies immediately above the level of the anorectal ring. The technique is illustrated in Fig. 21–9 *A*. The proctoscope is inserted into the rectum, and then withdrawn until its tip lies just below the anorectal ring. Then at 3, 7 and 11 o'clock, the sclerosant is injected slowly into the submucosal space, approximately 5 ml of phenol in almond oil. The injection should continue until the distended mucosa blanches and the small capillary vessels become visible over it. If a 5 per cent aqueous solution of quinine urea hydrochloride is used, 1 ml is given directly into or in the submucous tissue adjacent to the hemorrhoid, Fig. 21–9 *B* and *C*. A record should be made of the sites and amount of sclerosant injected. Great care must be taken not to inject the sclerosant into the mucosa or too deeply, i.e., outside the bowel wall. Injection into the mucosa produces an intense white area, and this should be a warning to stop. If injection is too deep, no distension occurs and there is also resistance to the injection.

Postoperative Management

The patient should be advised not to move his bowels until the day after injection, as this may precipitate bleeding. Otherwise, there are no special precautions, and the patient may return to work immediately.

The patient should be re-examined again in six weeks, by which time all swelling and induration in the anal canal caused by the injections usually has resolved. Further injections may then be given if the symptoms still persist. Two series of injections are usually enough to control bleeding, but may not be sufficient if prolapse is the prominent symptom. The limiting factor in this therapy is the submucosal fibrosis which is produced and prevents further injections. Injections can be given between the primary pile sites until these sites are also fibrosed.

When submucosal fibrosis prevents further injection in the pedicle of the hemorrhoid, injections may be given directly into the hemorrhoid. The 5 per cent aqueous solution of quinine urea hydrochloride is probably the best for this treatment, given 1 cc at a time. This technique may produce brisk bleeding, or, if too much solution is injected, prolapse and occasionally thrombosis of the hemorrhoid. It does, however, allow injection therapy to be prolonged. Care must be taken to keep injections above the dentate line in order to avoid pain and discomfort. If carefully used in prop-

erly selected patients, injection therapy can control the patient's symptoms for many years.

Complications

The following complications may occur. Serious complications are, however, rare.

Faintness. Occasionally the patient may feel faint after the injections.

Bleeding. An injection made straight into the hemorrhoid may puncture a hemorrhoidal artery radicle and produce brisk bleeding.

Treatment: This usually can be easily controlled by either injecting more sclerosant submucosally around the bleeding site, or by applying pressure with a pledget of cotton wool soaked in 1:1000 epinephrine.

Prolapse. If a large second degree or third degree hemorrhoid has been injected, the swelling in the anal canal may give the patient the desire to defecate. In trying to do so, the hemorrhoid may prolapse, bleed and subsequently thrombose if not replaced.

Treatment: The hemorrhoid should be replaced if possible and the patient confined to bed for 24 to 48 hours until swelling has resolved.

Injection Ulcer. This occurs at the site of injection by either injecting the sclerosant directly into the mucosa or occasionally putting too much sclerosant in one spot. Ulceration occurs after about a week. It is well-circumscribed, usually with surrounding induration, and may feel and look like a small carcinoma. It may be asymptomatic and found on follow-up, or it may present with bleeding. Usually this is small in amount, but occasionally it may be massive enough to require transfusion. The hemorrhoids take a further three to six weeks to heal, and obviously no further injections should be given during this period.

Treatment: Pressure with a pledget of cotton wool soaked in 1:10,000 epinephrine is usually sufficient.

Rare Complications. (a) Submucosal abscess produced by injection at site of injection. This usually discharges spontaneously; and (b) hematuria and prostatic abscesses have been reported when injection has been made too deeply.

Ligation of Hemorrhoids

The technique of outpatient ligation of hemorrhoids was first described by Blaisdell[3] in 1958 and subsequently modified and developed by Barron (1964).[2] The objective is to place a latex band around the mucosal part of the internal hemorrhoid so that it becomes ischemic, necroses and sloughs away, leaving a clean granulating wound. The ring must not include the lining of the anal canal below the dentate line, as this is somatically innervated and inclusion produces severe pain.

The advantage of this technique is that it is simple and almost painless. There are no medical contraindications, and no local or general anesthetic is required. There is also no need for hospitalization or time off work.

Indications

1. Any patient with internal hemorrhoids may be treated by this method. The most suitable are those with secondary or small third degree hemorrhoids. Those patients with large third degree hemorrhoids and associated external hemorrhoids are less likely to have a successful result. However, Barron (1964)[2] and Rudd (1970)[32] have found that in the large majority of patients with combined internal and external hemorrhoids, the external hemorrhoid will shrink or disappear when the internal hemorrhoid is removed. Any residual skin tags can be removed under local anesthetic.

2. Acute prolapsing hemorrhoids may be safely treated by this method.[33] Salvati had no complications in 32 cases treated by this method.

3. Small degrees of rectal mucosal prolapse may be effectively treated.

Contraindications

1. Associated pathological conditions in the anal canal or rectum, e.g., anal fissure or fistula.

2. Obese patients with large associated external hemorrhoids, as they frequently have a short anal canal and require repeated ligations.[33]

Preoperative Preparation

The rectum should be empty, as it is important to have a clear view of the rectum and anal canal to permit accurate placement of the latex band. The patient should be placed in the left lateral position.

Technique (Fig. 21–10 A-F)

The latex rings are first loaded onto the ligator. Two rings should be used for each hemorrhoid. The proctoscope is then inserted into the anal canal to the level of the dentate line and positioned so that the hemorrhoid protrudes into it. The ligator is then inserted so that the drum surrounds the hemorrhoid, which is then grasped and drawn into it by a pair of grasping forceps. The inferior edge of the drum should be at least 1/4 inch above the dentate line to avoid including the skin of the lower end of the anal canal in the ligature. The two rubber bands are then pushed off by closing the handles of the ligator. This produces a cherrylike internal hemorrhoid which rapidly becomes cyanotic. A little local anesthetic solution can be injected into the cherry. This causes quicker separation, and diffusion may reduce late pain. The ligated hemorrhoid sloughs in three to six days.

Postoperative Management

It is advisable to ligate one hemorrhoid at a time. The procedure may be repeated after two weeks. There is no limitation to the number of ligations. Salvati (1967)[33] reporting his results of 625 ligatures in 190 patients, found that the

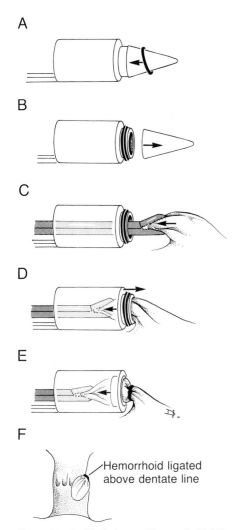

A

B

C

D

E

F

Hemorrhoid ligated
above dentate line

Figure 21–10 Technique of hemorrhoidal ligation. *A* and *B*. Method of rolling the rubber rings onto the drum of the ligator. *C*. The ligator is inserted through a proctoscope and the mucosal part of the hemorrhoid is drawn into it with the forceps. The inferior margin of the ligator drum must be at least ½″ above the dentate line. *D* and *E*. The rings are pushed off the drum onto the hemorrhoid by closing the handles of the ligator. *F*. Rings in place around base of the hemorrhoid.

number of ligations varied from one to nine, with an average of 3.3 per patient.

Complications

These are unusual if the correct technique has been used.

Pain. At the time of application of the band, the patient may feel some discomfort, but this should last only a few minutes. A few patients have more persistent, dull, aching pain in the rectum which lasts for about 48 hours, and can be controlled with analgesics. If the anal canal below the dentate line is caught in the band the pain will be immediate, severe and persistent. The latex band must then be removed. Occasionally, when the band fails to separate, pain may occur about seven days postoperatively. The band may be removed if symptoms are severe.

Bleeding. Bleeding may occur from tearing the hemorrhoid with the grasping forceps. This is controlled when the latex band is in place. Secondary hemorrhage occurs in about 2 per cent of cases 10 to 16 days postoperatively. If the hemorrhage does not stop spontaneously or is severe, the patient should be admitted to the hospital. A simple quick way to stop the bleeding is to insert a well-lubricated 30 F Foley catheter into the rectum and inflate the bag with 20 to 30 cc of water (Fig. 21–11 *A*). Traction is then applied to the catheter, which compresses the internal hemorrhoidal vessels at the level of the anorectal ring. It should be kept in position by strapping to the thigh for 48 hours, then slowly re-

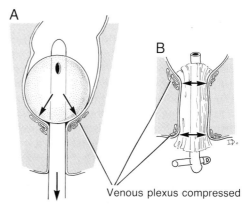

A

B

Venous plexus compressed

Figure 21–11 Methods of controlling secondary hemorrhage after hemorrhoidectomy. *A*. Traction on a large Foley catheter. *B*. Direct pressure on bleeding point by paraffin gauze surrounding a rubber tube.

moved. Alternatively, a thick rubber tube with paraffin gauze wrapped round it may be placed in the anal canal through a proctoscope, which is firmly gripped by the anal sphincter when the proctoscope is removed (Fig. 21–11 *B*). This also should be removed after 48 hours. The rubber tube is very uncomfortable and has no great advantage over the Foley catheter. Otherwise, the bleeding vessel must be ligated under a general anesthetic.

It is important to keep the bowel movements soft temporarily, as a constipated stool may cause a recurrence of the bleeding.

These techniques are also applicable to secondary hemorrhage following hemorrhoidectomy.

Thrombosed External Hemorrhoids. This occurs in about 3 per cent of cases. Interestingly, it does not necessarily occur adjacent to the previously treated internal hemorrhoid and is probably related to altered hemodynamics in the area.[32] It may be precipitated by straining at stool.

Treatment of Thrombosed Hemorrhoids

They may be managed conservatively or by immediate hemorrhoidectomy.

Conservative Treatment. The patient should be put to bed with the foot elevated on 9 inch blocks. Dressings soaked in ice cold saline should be applied to the prolapsed hemorrhoids every one to two hours. Analgesics, e.g., Demerol, should be given initially to control pain and also prior to the first defecation. Stool softeners should also be given. Systemic antibiotics should be administered if sloughing or sepsis occurs. On this regime, the acute symptoms and perianal edema will usually settle in three to seven days. The patient will then be well enough to return to work in 14 to 21 days. If sloughing or sepsis occurs, the convalescence will be longer.

The patient should be reviewed four to six weeks after the acute episode has subsided, and the residual hemorrhoids treated either by injection, ligation or hemorrhoidectomy.

Hemorrhoidectomy. Immediate hemorrhoidectomy is widely practiced on the grounds that it rapidly relieves the symptoms. The convalescence is no longer than with the conservative method, and a second hospital admission is not required.

The operation is usually very straightforward, but great care must be taken in the presence of perianal edema not to excise too much skin and risk the subsequent development of a stricture. If there is extensive perianal edema, it is probably safer to treat the initial episode conservatively.

External Hemorrhoids

External hemorrhoids occur at the anal verge and in the perianal region. According to the symptoms and signs they produce, they are usually divided into two groups — chronic skin tags and thrombosed external hemorrhoids (anal hematomas).

Chronic Skin Tags

These may be classified into two groups according to their etiology:

1. Primary or idiopathic. The majority of people examined have skin tags. In this group, there are no obvious etiological factors.

2. Secondary. These occur in association with internal hemorrhoids, anal fissure, chronic pruritus ani, or following the resolution of an anal hematoma.

Examination. A full local rectal examination must be carried out to exclude any associated pathology.

Treatment. Idiopathic skin tags which do not give trouble require no treatment. Frequently, however, they may cause discomfort and difficulty in cleansing the anal region after defecation. They may be removed under local anesthetic. Care must be taken not to excise too much skin and to make sure that the wound is pear-shaped, the narrow end toward the anus so that it will heal flat, from the anus out. If the tag is simply cut off without attention to the shape of the wound, it will result in the formation of more skin tags.

The treatment of secondary skin tags is primarily directed at the causal lesion. If they are still troublesome when this has been treated, then they may be removed as above.

Thrombosed External Hemorrhoids (Anal Hematoma)

In this condition, rupture occurs of one of the veins of the external hemorrhoidal plexus lying subcutaneously at the anal verge (Fig. 21–12 A). The blood clots and a tense, painful swelling is produced. It may be caused by straining at stool or prolonged sitting, squatting or other effort with legs apart. Frequently there is no obvious precipitating cause.

Clinical Features. The condition usually presents with the sudden onset of an exquisitely painful swelling at the anal verge. Sometimes, however, there is no associated pain and it is not diagnosed until the patient notices the swelling. The hematoma may rupture spontaneously, producing bleeding and relief of pain. If untreated, the pain generally subsides after 48 hours. The untreated hematoma gradually resolves leaving a residual skin tag.

Examination. On examination there is a small, tense, bluish-tinged swelling at the anal verge. Occasionally there may be more than one hematoma (conglomerate hematomata).

Treatment. Treatment depends upon the degree of pain experienced by the patient.

1. *Expectant.* If the patient presents after 48 hours with subsiding symptoms or a painless hematoma, it is best to use conservative treatment. The patient should be reassured that the swelling will resolve spontaneously and that no treatment is required. The treatment should also be conservative if the hematoma is in the midline either anteriorly or posteriorly, as these wounds take a long time to heal, and also if multiple hematomas are present.

2. *Operative.* If the patient presents within 48 hours of the onset of the pain and swelling, then evacuation of the clot will produce instant relief of symptoms.

Technique (Figs. 21–12 A and B). The skin and subcutaneous tissues around and beneath the hematoma are infiltrated with 1 per cent lidocaine containing epinephrine 1:100,000. A small radial elliptical incision is made over the swelling and the skin and clot are excised. The incision should not extend into the anal canal.

The patient should take daily sitz baths and stool softeners until the wound is healed. If internal hemorrhoids are

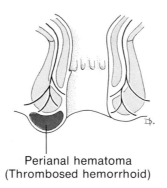

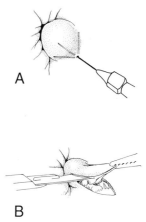

Figure 21–12 Excision of perianal hematoma. *A.* Technique of injecting local anesthetic. *B.* Excision of clot through an elliptical skin incision.

Perianal hematoma
(Thrombosed hemorrhoid)

A

B

present, they should be treated by sclerosant therapy if suitable. If they are of third degree, elective hemorrhoidectomy should be carried out when the wound has healed.

ANAL FISSURE (FISSURE-IN-ANO)

An anal fissure is a crack in the skin lining of the lower part of the anal canal (Fig. 21–13 *A* and *B*). It is a common and exquisitely painful condition. The majority occur in the midline posteriorly. Some 20 per cent occur anteriorly in females, but only 1 per cent in males.

Etiology

Fissures-in-ano are most probably produced by a combination of straining at stool and constipation. The passage of hard stool tears the squamous epithelium of the anal canal because it is firmly attached to the underlying internal sphincter by the mucosal suspensory lig-ament and therefore is relatively unelastic. It is believed that the tear occurs in the midline posteriorly because there is a deficiency of the subcutaneous external sphincter at this site.

Pathology

In the acute state the condition consists of a crack in the skin, the base being formed by the fibers of the longitudinal muscles. If it persists and fails to heal, the fissure deepens, exposing the white circular fibers of the lower quarter of the internal sphincter. This chronic fissure is usually associated with a tag of skin at its inferior end, the sentinel pile. The anal valve above this fissure may also become edematous and subsequently fibrose, producing a hypertrophied anal papilla. Persistent untreated fissure may produce fibrosis and stricture formation in the inferior part of the internal sphincter.

Clinical Presentation

The classical symptom is severe pain during and after defecation. The pain,

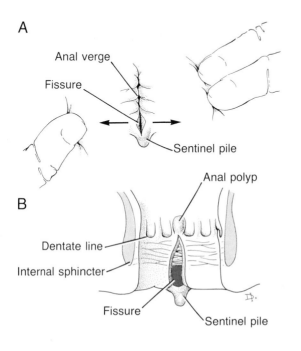

A

Anal verge

Fissure

Sentinel pile

Anal polyp

B

Dentate line

Internal sphincter

Fissure

Sentinel pile

Figure 21–13 Anal fissure. *A*. Demonstration of a chronic anal fissure on lateral separation of the anal verge. *B*. Anatomy of a chronic anal fissure.

which produces sphincter spasm, may be such that the patient becomes afraid to defecate. Constipation develops and aggravates the condition. Often associated is bright red bleeding on defecation which streaks the outside of the stool and appears on the toilet tissue, and there may also be a mucus discharge.

Examination

This should be carried out with great gentleness. The fissure can usually be seen by lateral separation of the anal verge (Fig. 21–13 *A*). However, this may be difficult owing to the associated spasm of the anal sphincter. The use of topical anesthetic jelly, e.g., 4 per cent Xylocaine, may make the examination easier. If there is much spasm, digital and proctoscopic examination should be avoided at the first visit. In these cases, it is often possible to pass, without causing too much discomfort, a well-lubricated, small-bore sigmoidoscope in order to examine the rectum. A complete examination should be carried out on the second or third visit when the fissure is healing, or under general anesthetic during operative treatment.

Differential Diagnosis

The diagnosis is usually self-evident. It must be remembered, however, that fissures are commonly associated with ulcerative colitis and Crohn's disease. These are usually atypical, chronic and fail to heal. There may or may not be evidence of colonic disease. Fissures in these conditions should not be treated until the colonic lesions have been fully evaluated. Rarely, carcinoma of the anus may present as a fissure, but it is usually atypical and its edges are hard and raised.

The anus is not an uncommon site for the primary chancre of syphilis and acute inflammation due to gonorrhea. If there is any doubt about the nature of the anal fissure, a biopsy should always be made.

If syphilis is suspected, a smear should be prepared for dark-field examination.

Treatment

Conservative

Conservative treatment should be tried first in cases of acute fissure. The most important factor is the avoidance of constipation, as the repeated trauma of hard feces on the anal canal will prevent the fissure from healing. The bowels should be regulated with a mild laxative, e.g., Milpar or Metamucil, to produce a soft, formed stool. Care must then be taken to make sure that a regular bowel habit is maintained.

The use of an anal dilator will also facilitate healing. It is used to overcome the anal spasm so that the fissure can heal with the sphincters relaxed. A fissure will not heal with the sphincters in spasm, as each bowel action will reopen it.

The dilator, lubricated with 4 per cent Xylocaine ointment, should be inserted up to the flange and left in position for two minutes. It should be passed by the patient twice a day and also after defecation, and he should be thoroughly familiar with the technique before leaving the clinic. This method of treatment may be tried for two to three weeks, or longer if the fissure shows signs of healing. If, after this time, the patient is still experiencing pain and the fissure remains unhealed, operative treatment should be carried out.

Operative Treatment

Anal Sphincter Stretch. This is the simplest method, with only a 16 per cent recurrence rate.[36] The procedure must be carried out under general anesthesia with a short-acting muscle relaxant. The patient is placed in the left lateral or lithotomy position. The index fingers of both hands are first inserted into the anus and traction is applied gently in a lateral direction (Fig.

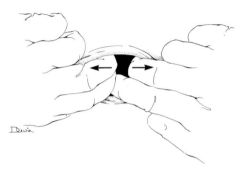

Dewin

Figure 21–14 Anal sphincter stretch. Four fingers are inserted into the anus, which is then stretched for three minutes.

21–14). As the sphincters stretch, the middle fingers of both hands are then inserted, making four fingers in the anus. The stretching should be maintained for three to four minutes. This is a tiring process for the fingers and arms and can be done equally well by inserting a bivalved anal speculum and slowly winding it open until the sphincters are maximally stretched. It should be left in position for three to four minutes.

The stretching tears the anal skin and undoubtedly some of the fibers of the internal sphincter. The patient may go home after recovering from the anesthesia and should be reexamined in one month.

Internal Sphincterotomy. The use of internal sphincterotomy for chronic fissure was first described by Eisenhammer. Under local anesthetic, he divided the lower part of the internal sphincter in the midline posteriorly, usually through the fissure. Although the recurrence rate was only 7 per cent, the wounds took a long time to heal and there was a high incidence of minor imperfections of anal continence. Eisenhammer (1959)[10] suggested that lateral sphincterotomy might have fewer complications. Hawley (1969)[18] reported no recurrence, fecal leak or soiling in 24 patients on whom this technique was used.

Operative Procedure. The simplest and most satisfactory outpatient technique is that of lateral subcutaneous internal sphincterotomy.[20] The operation is performed under general or local anes-

thetic. The patient is put in the lithotomy position and a bivalve speculum is inserted into the anal canal. Its handle is then rotated to the patient's right, so that the blades lie anteriorly and posteriorly (see Fig. 21–15 *A*). The blades are then gently opened to approximately two finger breadths. This exposes the left lateral wall of the anal canal and makes the lower edge of the internal sphincter in that region taut and therefore easily palpable. The sphincterotomy is performed with a Von Graefe knife or a No. 10 blade on a long Bard-Parker handle. It is inserted through the perianal skin immediately lateral to the lower edge of the internal sphincter and passed vertically upwards in the intersphincteric plane until its point lies at, or just above, the

A

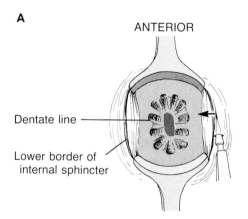

ANTERIOR

Dentate line

Lower border of internal sphincter

B

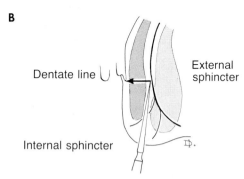

Dentate line

External sphincter

Internal sphincter

Figure 21–15 Lateral subcutaneous internal sphincterotomy. *A.* Bivalve speculum in position, displaying the left lateral wall of the anal canal. *B.* Knife inserted lateral to lower edge of internal sphincter which is divided up to the level of the dentate line.

dentate line (Fig. 21-15 *B*). The lower half only of the internal sphincter is then divided by gentle cutting strokes made toward the anal canal.

Care must be taken not to penetrate the lining of the anal canal. Hoffmann and Goligher suggest that this may be avoided by leaving a few of the innermost fibers undivided; these may then be ruptured by lateral pressure of the finger in the anal canal after the knife has been removed. Firm pressure is then maintained over the myotomy site to achieve hemostasis. Sentinel tags and hypertrophied anal papillae should then be removed if large and troublesome. A cotton wool pad and T-binder are then employed.

Postoperative Management. The patients may go home after they have fully recovered from the anesthetic. They are given Demerol to control pain for 48 hours, and they should be advised to take a mild aperient such as mineral oil to soften the stool. They should have frequent sitz baths, preferably after defecation, and should apply a dry gauze or cotton dressing if there is any discharge. The use of toilet paper should be avoided until the wound has healed. Patients should be encouraged to return to work in about four to seven days.

Complications. These are minimal. Reactionary hemorrhage may occur rarely and this can easily be controlled by pressure. Alterations in anal sphincter function, such as flatus control, occur temporarily in 5 per cent of cases.

This technique gives complete and permanent relief of pain in the majority of cases, and the fissure usually heals within a month. Hoffmann and Goligher (1970)[20] had a 3 per cent failure rate in 99 cases which were followed for an average of 11 months.

ANORECTAL ABSCESS

This is a common painful condition in which suppuration occurs in the tissue around the anus and rectum. Anorectal

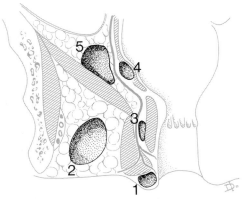

Figure 21-16 Classification of anorectal abscesses. (1) Perianal. (2) Ischiorectal. (3) Intersphincteric. (4) Higher intermuscular. (5) Pelvirectal.

abscesses are classified according to their site (Fig. 21-16): (1) perianal; (2) ischiorectal; (3) intersphincteric; (4) high intermuscular; and (5) pelvirectal.

Perianal and ischiorectal abscesses are the commonest and occur more frequently in men than in women. The common infecting organisms are *E. coli* and *Staph. aureus.*[15]

Etiology

In the majority of cases, no obvious cause can be found. However, perianal infections are a common complication of ulcerative colitis and Crohn's disease. Other systemic disease, such as diabetes or leukemia, may also predispose to these infections. Therefore, before treatment, conditions such as these should be excluded. The most accepted theory is that the infection starts in the anal glands.[11, 30] Suppuration in these glands produces an intersphincteric abscess lying between the internal and external sphincter muscles. From this site, it may then extend through the external sphincter to the ischiorectal space, inferiorly to the perianal space and superiorly, giving a high intermuscular abscess. However, this theory of etiology is disputed by Goligher, Ellis and Pissidis (1967),[14] who carefully examined 29 cases of anorectal abscess for evidence of an internal opening at the level of the anal valves. They could find only five cases with an internal opening, and these were associated with perianal abscess; none were demonstrated with ischiorectal abscess.

Clinical Features

Perianal. This abscess presents as an exquisitely tender swelling immediately adjacent to the anus. It is red, well localized, and may or may not be fluctuant. There is usually no constitutional upset. Rectal examination reveals no induration or tenderness deep in the ischiorectal fossa.

Ischiorectal. These abscesses also present with perianal pain. In the early stages, there may be few clinical signs apart from tenderness in the perianal region, localized to the ischiorectal fossa on rectal examination. If untreated, a diffuse tender indurated area develops in the perianal skin with similar findings on rectal examination. Fluctuation occurs late. There is frequently an associated pyrexia. In patients who have received antibiotics, the abscess may become cold and nontender, and may not be diagnosed until fluctuation occurs.

Intersphincteric. An intersphincteric abscess presents with acute pain in the anal region. There is no obvious swelling in the perianal or ischiorectal spaces. However, it can be diagnosed by finding an exquisitely tender spot on palpating the lower border of the internal sphincter, usually within the anal canal at the level of the dentate line.

Intermuscular. This kind of abscess is usually called a submucous abscess but is in fact a rectal wall abscess. It usually presents with rectal pain and may be difficult to diagnose. There are no signs in the perianal region, but rectal examination may reveal a smooth, tender indurated swelling in the rectal wall. Occasionally these abscesses have ruptured by the time of presentation. They are rare.

Pelvirectal. Pelvirectal abscesses are very rare. Their presentation is usually insidious with a pyrexia but no anal or rectal symptoms. There may be a recent history of pelvic infection. Rectal examination reveals a tender mass high in the pelvis.

Treatment

The treatment is surgical. Antibiotics may theoretically abort the early infection process, but usually by the time patients present at the clinic, pus is present and must be drained. A full rectal and sigmoidoscopic examination must be carried out. This preferably should be done while the abscess is being drained, or shortly after, since anesthesia is usually required for the examination.

Perianal. This may be drained under local anesthetic. If, however, there is any doubt as to the site of the abscess, then the procedure should be carried out under general anesthetic.

A very small radial or cruciate incision over the abscess (Fig. 21–17 *A* and *B*) is all that is necessary. A Eusol dressing is then applied. Daily sitz baths should be taken until the wound is healed.

Ischiorectal. This should be drained through a small pear-shaped or cruciate incision (Fig. 21–17 *C*), and the minimum of skin should be removed. A finger may be inserted into the ischiorectal fossa to break down adhesions. Under no circumstance should the cavity be probed with a clamp or a pair of sinus forceps, for if undue force is used, a fistulous opening may be made into the rectum or into the supralevator space. It is important to remember that the abscess may extend above the urogenital diaphragm. Rarely, the abscess may extend posteriorly to the other ischiorectal fossa. In this case, a more extensive incision should be made passing posterior to the anus in order to drain both sides, or a separate drainage incision may be made on the opposite side.

The wound should be covered with a gauze dressing soaked in Eusol backed with a cotton wool pad and held in position with a T-binder. It is not necessary

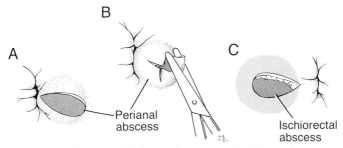

Figure 21–17 Methods of drainage of perianal and ischiorectal abscesses.

to pack the ischiorectal cavity with gauze, as there is natural dependent drainage and it is also very uncomfortable for the patient. Antibiotics may be given if there is an associated constitutional upset, but usually such symptoms are relieved by drainage. The patient should take daily baths, after which the wound should be redressed. Stool softeners are helpful in the first postoperative week. The wound should be inspected twice a week to make sure that the wound edges do not heal prematurely. They usually take four to six weeks to heal completely. Ideally, the patient should be hospitalized for the first three to six postoperative days.

Intersphincteric. The site of maximum tenderness should be marked before the anesthetic is given. With the patient in the lithotomy position, a small incision is made over this site and a pair of sinus forceps is pushed up in the intersphincteric plane until the abscess is entered (Fig. 21–18). A small rubber drain may be left in the cavity for 48 hours and then removed. Daily sitz baths should be taken until the wound is healed. The patient should be hospitalized for 24 to 48 hours.

High Intermuscular and Pelvirectal. The patient must be admitted to hospital for the treatment of these abscesses and their underlying causes.

Associated Fistula-in-Ano

In the majority of cases of perianal and ischiorectal abscess, no fistula can be demonstrated at the time of abscess drainage. It is commonly taught that these patients should be reexamined after a week to see if a fistula is present, and if so, laid open. I do not think that this is necessary, as the majority of these abscess cavities heal uneventfully. In a small percentage, the abscess may recur, and in these patients a fistula should be sought.

Immediate Fistulotomy

If there is an obvious low level fistula present, i.e., with an opening at or below the anal valves, the fistula can be laid open when the abscess is drained.[35] The procedure, however, is only for the experienced surgeon, as careless division of the internal sphincter may lead to incontinence.

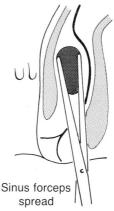

Sinus forceps spread

Figure 21–18 Method of drainage of an intersphincteric abscess.

Immediate fistulotomy is contraindicated:

1. In the presence of a high level fistula with opening above anal valves.

2. When the fistula is associated with ulcerative colitis, Crohn's disease or anorectal tuberculosis, the latter condition now being rare.

3. When there is doubt as to the level of the fistula.

4. If the abscess is large and there is gross perianal induration and edema.

Technique. A general anesthetic should be given and the patient placed in the lithotomy position. A bivalve speculum is then placed in the anal canal and an attempt is made to identify the internal opening before the abscess is drained. In a posterior abscess, the internal opening of a fistula is almost always in the midline. An anterior abscess usually has the opening within a crypt directly adjacent to the point of maximum swelling (Goodsall's rule). If an internal opening is present, pus may frequently be seen oozing from it, especially if pressure is applied to the abscess. A probe may then be gently inserted into the tract — no force should be used. The abscess is then drained as above. If the probe is visible in the abscess cavity, the fistulotomy is carried out by first dividing the skin, subcutaneous tissue and the sphincter muscle down to the probe. The probe should be positioned so that the sphincter muscle is cut in a radial rather than an oblique plane. This causes minimal damage to the sphincter and facilitates healing.

If no internal opening can be found, the abscess cavity is first drained. A probe is then passed gently from the abscess cavity toward the suspected crypt in an attempt to identify the fistulous tract. If a tract is found, fistulotomy is carried out as above (Fig. 21-19 *A*, *B*, and *C*). Great care, however, must be taken not to create a false tract with forceful use of the probe.

Postoperative Management

The wound is covered but not packed with a gauze dressing soaked in Eusol.

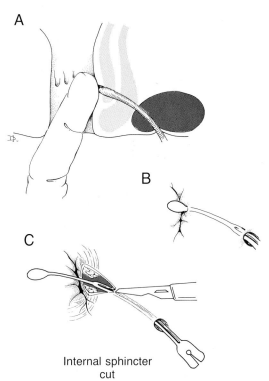

A

B

C

Internal sphincter
cut

Figure 21–19 Method of immediate fistulotomy for low level anal fistula associated with ischiorectal abscess. *A.* Grooved probe is passed through fistula into the anal canal. Great care must be taken not to create a false tract. *B.* Probe in position. *C.* Fistula layed open by cutting onto probe.

This should be removed after 24 hours and daily sitz baths taken. Stool softeners should be given. The patient is kept in the hospital for at least 48 hours. The wound should be examined initially twice a week to make sure that it is healing from its base and to prevent premature closure of the wound edges.

FISTULA-IN-ANO

A fistula-in-ano is an abnormal tract between the anal, rarely rectal, mucosa and the perianal skin. It has a fibrous wall and is lined with granulation tissue.

Etiology

It probably arises in the majority of cases as a sequel to anal gland infection, as was discussed in the etiology of anorectal abscess.[30] Some 10 to 20 per cent occur secondary to lesions of the bowel such as ulcerative colitis, Crohn's disease or tuberculosis.

Classification

They may be classified as follows:

    Anal   Subcutaneous
                Submucosal
                High and low anal
    Anorectal

The fistulous tracts may be single or multiple, and the posterior ones commonly have a horseshoe configuration.

The important distinction between the two groups is the relationship of the internal opening to the anorectal ring. In the anal group, the internal opening is below the ring, usually at the level of the dentate line. The anorectal group, in which the opening is above the anorectal ring, is fortunately rare. These are much more difficult to treat because if the anorectal ring is divided, incontinence will result (Fig. 21–20 *A*).

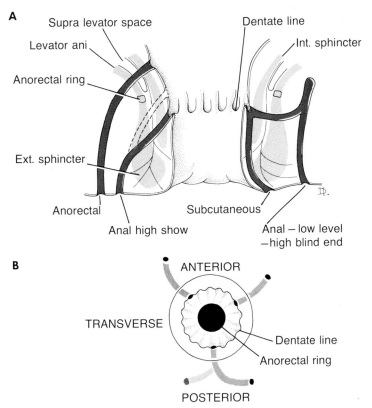

Figure 21–20   *A.* Classification of fistula-in-ano. *B.* Diagram illustrating Goodsall's rule.

The horizontal disposition of the fistulae follow, in the majority of cases, Goodsall's rule.[16] He said that if a transverse line is drawn across the midpoint of the anus, fistulae with their external openings anterior to this line usually run directly to the anal canal, while those with openings behind the line tend to take a curved course to an opening in the midline of the posterior wall of the anal canal (Fig. 21–20 *B*). The tracts of posterior and horseshoe fistulae lie at the level of the anorectal ring, to which they are closely applied. However, their internal openings are usually at the level of the dentate line.

Clinical Features

The patient presents with a chronic purulent anal discharge. In patients with anal fistulae the onset of symptoms may or may not be related to a perianal abscess. Patients with anorectal fistulae, however, usually give a history of abscess drainage, followed by recurrent abscess or intermittent discharge. The discharge is irritating and is therefore often associated with pruritus ani. If the fistulae are secondary to ulcerative colitis or Crohn's disease, for example, there may be associated symptoms of these diseases.

Examination

A full examination should be made to exclude any cause for the fistula. Inspection of the perianal skin will show one or more fistulous openings. These are usually marked by a little spout of granulation tissue and pressure will produce a discharge from the opening. A note should be made of any scars from previous operations.

The perianal tissues and anal glands should then be palpated to determine the direction of the tract. In the low anal fistula, it can be felt as a hard subcutaneous cord.

Proctoscopy is important to determine the level of the internal opening, whether it is above or below the anorectal ring.

The internal opening may be revealed by pressure on the tract expressing from it a bead of pus. A fine rectal probe may be used to define the tract. Great care and gentleness must be used to avoid creating a false passage. The probe may be passed from either the internal or external opening. If there is any difficulty, the probing must be stopped until the patient can be fully examined under anesthetic.

Sigmoidoscopy and barium enema are used to exclude a lesion of the bowel.

Differential Diagnosis

Chronic suppurative hidradenitis may produce a picture resembling anal fistula. However, there is no internal opening to the sinuses and no associated induration in the anal canal.

Treatment

Associated bowel lesions must first be treated, or there may be difficulty in healing of the anal wound, especially in ulcerative colitis and Crohn's disease.

The ancient treatment of laying open a fistula (Fig. 20–19 *A, B* and *C*) and allowing the wound to granulate is still the treatment of choice. This should not be undertaken in outpatients, except perhaps in the anal fistulae of the subcutaneous type.

POLYPS OF COLON AND RECTUM

A polyp is a tumor which projects from the surface of the intestinal mucosa. It may be either sessile or pedunculated, multiple or single.

Pathology

Polyps may be classified into four main groups:[24] neoplastic, hamartomatous, inflammatory and unclassified (metaplastic).

TYPE	SOLITARY	MULTIPLE
Neoplastic	Adenoma Papillary adenoma Villous adenoma	Familial, adenomatous, polyposis
Hamartomatous	Juvenile Peutz-Jeghers syndrome	Juvenile polyposis Peutz-Jeghers syndrome
Inflammatory	Benign lymphoid polyp	Benign lymphoid polyposis Inflammatory polyposis
Unclassified	Metaplastic polyp	Multiple metaplastic polyps

Neoplastic Polyps

Solitary. Although these tumors have a varying gross appearance, microscopically they all present the same features in that they are all part of the spectrum of intestinal mucosal neoplasia. There is considerable evidence that these lesions are premalignant,[12] but the incidence of malignant change is difficult to estimate. However, the size of the polyp is a useful guide to its malignant potential. Grinnell and Lane (1958)[17] found that the benign adenomatous polyps were usually 1 to 2 cm in size and the average diameter of polyps with carcinoma was 2.1 cm. Although invasive carcinoma can develop in small polyps, a useful rule to follow is that polyps less than 1 cm in size rarely become malignant, polyps 1 to 2 cm in diameter should be carefully watched, and polyps over 2 cm should be excised. All polyps within reach of the sigmoidoscope should be excised regardless of their size.

A high percentage of villous adenomas will develop an area of invasive carcinoma, particularly if the lesion is over 6 cm in diameter.

Clinical Features. Adenomatous polyps may present with bleeding. In the majority of cases they are, however, asymptomatic. Villous adenomas usually present with a mucous discharge. If the lesion is large, this discharge may be so profuse as to produce a spurious diarrhea and occasionally weakness and lassitude due to electrolyte depletion, especially of potassium.

Examination. On rectal examination, adenomatous polyps are smooth, lobulated and firm to palpation. However, they may be difficult to feel, particularly if they are small or have a long stalk. A villous adenoma feels soft, and because of this it may be difficult to detect, or to define its extent. It is important to remember that the presence of palpable induration in the polyp or its base may be the first sign of malignancy. The presence of a nodule or induration at the site of a previously excised polyp should also be regarded with suspicion.

Sigmoidoscopy is mandatory, as the majority of these lesions occur in the rectum and lower sigmoid, and excisional biopsy will give a tissue diagnosis. It is usually possible to distinguish grossly between adenomatous and villous polyps, although this may be difficult if bleeding occurs. A villous adenoma is generally larger and is characterized by a purple, pink color and a shaggy surface.

Investigations. 1. A biopsy should first be made of all sessile polyps, but pedunculated polyps must be removed together with their stalks (Fig. 21–21). A villous adenoma biopsy may initially be undertaken to confirm the diagnosis, but it must subsequently be removed completely to exclude malignant change.

2. An air contrast barium enema should be carried out to determine whether other polyps are present in the colon.

Treatment. Diathermy excision or coagulation is the treatment of choice for those adenomatous polyps within reach of the sigmoidoscope (Fig. 21–21). This technique may be used on small villous

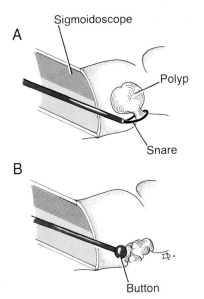

A — Sigmoidoscope, Polyp, Snare

B — Button

Figure 21–21 Methods of removing rectal polyps. *A.* Diathermy snare. *B.* Diathermy button.

lesions, but preferably these should be excised completely through the anus, if small, or by either the Kraske approach, the transphincteric approach, or abdominoperineal excision if large.

Familial Adenomatous Polyposis (Polyposis Coli). This condition is transmitted by a dominant gene and therefore affects both sexes.[9] The polypoid changes first appear in the colon and rectum around the age of puberty and, if left untreated, will usually undergo malignant change by the age of 35 years.

A full family history must be obtained and all potentially involved members examined.

Clinical Features. Symptoms such as mild diarrhea first occur between the ages of 15 and 20. Later, mucous discharge and bleeding occur, and are frequently a sign of malignant change.

Diagnosis. On sigmoidoscopy, multiple small sessile and pedunculated polyps are present in the rectum and lower sigmoid. A barium enema should be carried out to ascertain their extent in the colon and a biopsy should be done to confirm the diagnosis.

Treatment. If no carcinoma is present in the rectum, then a colectomy and ileorectal anastomosis should be performed, ideally between the ages of 15 and 20 years. The polyps in the rectum are treated by fulguration. The patient must then be reexamined indefinitely at six-month to yearly intervals so that any new polyps can be fulgurated as they appear, or if malignant change occurs, the rectum can be removed at an early stage.

Hamartomatous Polyps

A hamartoma is a tumor composed of an abnormal mixture of normal tissues. There is no evidence that they are premalignant.

Juvenile Polyp. The juvenile adenoma is commonly found in children, but occasionally in adults. It is a smooth round bright scarlet polyp with characteristic histological features.[22]

Treatment. A biopsy should be performed to confirm the diagnosis and the polyp should be removed if causing symptoms.

Juvenile Polyposis. This condition presents before the age of 10 years in contradistinction to familial adenomatosis. It is a pathologically distinct entity often associated with congenital abnormalities.[34]

Treatment. Polyps should be removed if they cause symptoms.

Peutz-Jeghers Syndrome. This syndrome is inherited as an autosomal dominant trait. It is characterized by melanin spots on the buccal mucosa and lips, and multiple polypoid lesions in the small intestine. In 50 per cent of cases, the large bowel is also involved. The polyps occasionally become malignant.

The syndrome usually presents with intermittent abdominal pain, episodes of bleeding and small bowel intussusception.

Treatment. The polyps are usually left alone until symptoms occur, at which time the polyps should be excised through multiple enterotomies.

Inflammatory Polyps

Benign Lymphoid Polyp. This polyp is commonly found in the rectum and terminal ileum and is pale or yellowish in color. Occasionally it can be multiple. It is composed of normal lymphoid tissue.[8]

Treatment. Perform biopsy to make the diagnosis.

Inflammatory or Pseudopolyps. Occurring principally in chronic ulcerative colitis, these polyps are islands of inflamed mucosa produced by extensive mucosal ulceration. They occur in the lower sigmoid, but may extend into the rectal ampulla.

Treatment. Directed at primary pathology.

Metaplastic Polyps

These are the very small, often multiple, mucosal-colored polyps which are frequently seen in the rectum or during an otherwise normal sigmoidoscopy. Histologically, they have a distinct structure and are benign.[1]

Treatment. None is necessary except a biopsy if the diagnosis is in doubt.

Rectal Polypectomy

Pedunculated Polyp

Adenomatous pedunculated polyps should be treated in the first instance by local excision, subsequent treatment being based on the histological report. The whole polyp and stalk must be removed together. Biopsy should be avoided unless the size precludes primary local excision. The reason is that a biopsy will remove only a superficial part of the polyp, and this may not be representative of the whole lesion. In addition, by removal of the whole polyp, the pathologist can ascertain the completeness of excision if an invasive carcinoma is found.

In all cases where a polyp is found, the whole colon must be examined by double contrast enema for other polyps and any associated neoplasms.

Instruments. A wide-bore operating sigmoidoscope, approximately 1 inch in diameter, should be used so that a good view can be obtained. A wire diathermy loop, as illustrated, should be used for removing the polyp. Ideally, a nonconductive sigmoidoscope of bakelite or plastic should be used. The same effect may be achieved when using a metal sigmoidoscope if the sheath of the diathermy loop is insulated with plastic or rubber tubing, and care is taken to avoid grounding the metal tip on the sigmoidoscope.

Preoperative Preparation. The rectum should be cleared, if necessary, by a disposable enema, e.g., Fleet's enema given one to two hours prior to operation. A general anesthetic is preferable for the procedure. The patient may be placed in either the Sims' or the lithotomy position.

Technique. The sigmoidoscope is introduced. The wire snare is then passed over the polyp and tightened round the stalk (Fig. 21–21 *A*). The polyp is then gently pulled away from the wall, at the same time a low cutting diathermy current is applied intermittently until the stalk is divided. After the removal of the polyp, the site should be checked for bleeding. If there is a brisk oozing, this may be controlled by pressure with a pledget of cotton wool soaked in epinephrine 1 : 1000.

Postoperative Management. It is advisable to admit the patient overnight. If the lesion, however, is below 7 cm, i.e., below the peritoneal reflection, he may be allowed to go home.

Sessile Polyp

It is not safe to use a diathermy snare on these polyps, as perforation is a very real risk, especially above the peritoneal reflection.

Technique. The procedure is the same as for the pedunculated polyp, only a diathermy button electrode is used and the polyp is fulgurated (Fig. 21–21 *B*). The polyp should be touched at several points on its surface and short bursts of a low coagulating current applied. It is important not to overfulgurate the lesion, as subsequent tissue destruction is always greater than appears at time of treatment.

Postoperative Management. Patients with lesions treated above the peritoneal reflection should be admitted overnight. Another sigmoidoscopy should be done in three weeks and any residual tumor cauterized again with diathermy.

Villous Adenoma

These lesions are rarely suitable for primary outpatient treatment. If, however, they are small or have occurred after previous treatment, then they may be fulgurated, provided biopsy shows no evidence of malignant change.

Complications

Secondary Hemorrhage. This may occur from the sixth to the tenth day and may be minor or profuse. If profuse, it is advisable to give a short general anesthetic, so that the rectum can easily be cleared of blood clots and the bleeding point identified. The bleeding may then be stopped by pressure with an epinephrine-soaked swab, or by diathermy or suture-ligation to the bleeding point. The patient should be admitted until the bleeding has completely stopped for 48 hours.

Perforation of the Bowel. Great care should be taken with all polyps above 7 cm, i.e., above the peritoneal reflection, as excessive traction on the polyp and too high a current when dividing the stalk of a pedunculated polyp or fulgurating a sessile polyp may easily perforate the bowel. If perforation is recognized immediately, laparotomy should be carried out and the perforation sutured. It is not always necessary to carry out a proximal colostomy in these cases. However, if the perforation is missed and peritonitis develops subsequently, a laparotomy, drainage and proximal colostomy must be carried out.

RECTAL PROLAPSE

Prolapse of the rectum is defined as a protrusion of the rectum through the anus. If only mucosa prolapses, it is called mucosal or incomplete prolapse (Fig. 21–22 *A*). If all layers of the rectum prolapse, then it is a complete prolapse (Fig. 21–22 *B*).

Incidence

Prolapse commonly occurs at the extremes of life. In children, the highest incidence occurs in the first two years of life and is rare after the sixth year.[7] The majority of these prolapses are of the mucosal type.

In adults, however, the majority of prolapses are complete. Eighty percent occur in women, with increasing incidence after the fifth decade. In men the maximum incidence is before the age of 40.[21]

Etiology

The etiology is not fully understood. In children, it is probably produced by constipation or persistent coughing. Obsessive toilet-training may be a factor. In adults there is no obvious cause in the majority of cases. In a small percentage, there may be a neurological cause, e.g., a cauda equina lesion. The principal etiological factors in adults are thought to be a weakness of the muscles of the pelvic diaphragm and straining due to constipation. Constant straining at stool causes the weak pelvic muscles to stretch and the rectum to descend. In support of this concept, Parks, Porter and Hardcastle (1966)[31] have shown that there is a tendency of the muscles of the pelvic floor to respond to straining by a sustained decrease in tone.

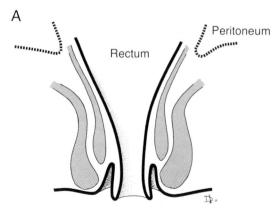

A

Peritoneum

Rectum

Mucosal (incomplete) prolapse

Figure 21–22 Coronal section of rectum and anal canal showing *A*, mucosal (incomplete) prolapse, and *B*, complete prolapse.

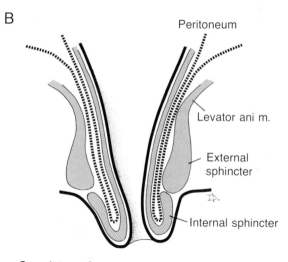

B

Peritoneum

Levator ani m.

External sphincter

Internal sphincter

Complete prolapse

Clinical Features

On physical examination, it is important to establish three facts: (1) the degree of prolapse; (2) the state of continence; and (3) the exclusion of any pathology in the rectum and colon.

The degree of prolapse may be determined by asking the patient to strain down. (A receptacle should be placed at the anus!) In complete prolapse, the rectum protrudes to a length of 4 inches. The mucosa is usually inflamed and edematous and is thrown into concentric circular folds. If a finger is inserted into the lumen of the prolapsed bowel, the double layer of rectal wall can be palpated. This characteristic feature is missing in the cases of mucosal prolapse. However, a large mucosal prolapse may sometimes be difficult to distinguish from an early complete prolapse. A patulous anus, which may easily admit three or four fingers, is commonly found in complete prolapse.

It is important to establish whether the patient has had any history of incontinence. A history of previous anorectal surgery may be important in this context. If the patient has true fecal incontinence, he is very unlikely to benefit from any surgical treatment. Patients frequently have a profuse mucus discharge, which may be stained by feces or blood produced by the prolapse. The prolapse may also make control of defecation difficult, especially if the patient is constipated. However, these patients are usually aware of any fecal soiling, whereas those with true incontinence are not. All patients must have a full proctoscopic and sigmoidoscopic examination to exclude any pathology in the rectum and lower colon. If surgical treatment is contemplated, a barium examination of the colon must also be carried out.

Differential Diagnosis

In children, the apex of an intussusception may rarely present at the anus. This is usually easily distinguished from a prolapse by the history and the fact that the examining finger will pass into the rectum lateral to the intussusception but will not in a prolapse. In adults, large third degree piles or a prolapsing rectal polyp may simulate a prolapse.

Treatment

Outpatient treatment is limited to small mucosal prolapses and to the occasional early complete prolapse in the elderly. Before any treatment is undertaken, it is important to correct constipation to prevent the patient from straining at stool.

Mucosal Prolapse

Children. Correction of constipation and bowel training is of paramount importance along with psychiatric consultation in selected cases. On this regime, the condition will resolve spontaneously in the majority.

Operative Treatment. Submucosal injection of 5 per cent phenol in almond oil given at the level of the anorectal ring as for hemorrhoids, is the simplest and most effective treatment. The submucosal fibrosis produces retraction of the mucosa.

The injection should be given under a short general anesthetic with the patient either in the lithotomy or left lateral position. About 3 ml of sclerosant should be given submucosally in four quadrants at the level of the anorectal ring. The patient should be reassessed in six weeks and further injections given as necessary.

Adults. Submucosal sclerosant therapy is also the most simple and effective treatment for small degrees of mucosal prolapse. The technique employed is the same as for children, but it may be carried out without anesthetic. Patients with greater degrees of mucosal prolapse or those who have failed to respond to sclerosant therapy should be treated by hemorrhoidectomy.

Complete Prolapse

For those patients with a complete prolapse, abdominal repair should be carried out. However, in a small percentage of patients, who are usually aged and unfit for operation, the Thiersch operation may be tried. It may also be used to correct a patulous anus after an abdominal repair.

Thiersch Operation (Fig. 21–23 *A* to *C*). This may be carried out under local anesthetic by infiltration of the perianal tissues with 1 per cent lidocaine containing epinephrine 1 : 100,000.

The patient should be placed in the lithotomy position and the perianal tissues cleansed. Two small incisions are made in the midline 1 inch in front and behind the anal verge. A half circle needle is passed from the posterior to the anterior wound in the subcutaneous plane. One end of either a 20 S.W.G. silver wire or a monofilament No. 1 nylon is passed through the eye of the needle which is then withdrawn through the posterior wound. The needle is then reinserted on the opposite side of the anus and the other end of the wire or

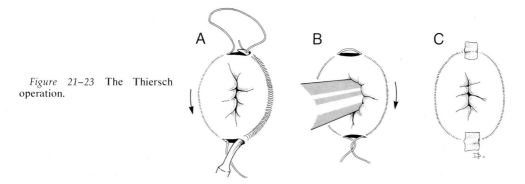

Figure 21–23 The Thiersch operation.

nylon is also withdrawn through the posterior wound. It is advisable to use three strands of the monofilament nylon. An 18 Hegar dilator or an assistant's index finger is inserted into the anus. The wire or nylon is then pulled up around the dilator or finger, making sure it is not kinked, and tied. The proximal interphalangeal joint of the index finger should be able to pass comfortably through the anus.

The knot should be buried and the skin incision closed with a silk stitch or Michel's clips.

Postoperative Management. Fecal impaction is the major problem. Therefore, mild aperients, e.g., Senna, milk of magnesia and suppositories if necessary should be given from the first postoperative day. A rectal examination should be carried out at least at weekly intervals initially to ensure that the rectum is being emptied and the patient's bowel movements are regular. The skin sutures may be removed after seven days. The patient should have regular follow-up to ensure that the wire remains intact, that the prolapse is controlled and that fecal impaction does not occur. The wire may be replaced on several occasions if necessary.

POSTANAL (PILONIDAL) SINUS DISEASE

A pilonidal or postanal sinus is a tract lined by squamous epithelium which occurs in the natal cleft overlying the sacrococcygeal region (Fig. 21–24 *A*). There may be one or several openings to the tract. Frequently in this condition there are several shallow midline pits in the natal cleft, which may or may not communicate with the sinus. The sinus characteristically contains loose hairs and debris (Fig. 21–24 *B*). Occasionally there may be only a cyst at this site containing fluid and epithelial debris.

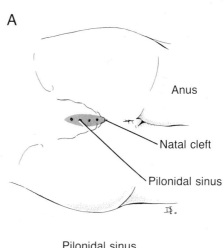

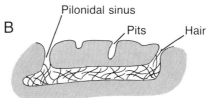

Figure 21–24 Pilonidal sinus. *A.* Sinuses occur in midline some two inches above the anus in the natal cleft. *B.* Longitudinal section showing sinuses and pits.

Etiology and Incidence

Hodges (1880)[19] suggested that the primary postanal sinus may be the result of a congenital predisposition due to hirsutism, or a deep sacrococcygeal pit or a combination of these factors. Although some sinuses may be congenital in origin, it is now believed that the majority are acquired.[5] Buttock movements drill loose local hair into the skin of the natal cleft. Squamous epithelium proliferates into this puncture wound to form the primary pit in which hairs and debris accumulate. Pilonidal sinuses occur most frequently in males between the ages of 18 and 30. The majority are dark and hirsute, although the lesion is rare in Negroes.

Pathology

Once the sinus is formed, the majority sooner or later become secondarily infected, and the subcutaneous cavity then becomes lined by granulation tissue. The natural history is then one of intermittent suppuration and discharge, with incomplete healing. This in turn causes a gradual extension of the sinus in a cephalad direction, and — if left untreated long enough — laterally out into the buttocks.

Clinical Presentation

The patients usually present with either an intermittent or chronic purulent discharge or an acute abscess in the natal cleft. The diagnosis is made on the site, the presence of hair and the direction of the sinus away from the anus. Rectal examination is generally normal.

Treatment

A pilonidal sinus is a foreign body sinus and the principle of treatment, therefore, is to remove all the hair and facilitate free drainage by laying it open. The techniques described below are, in my experience, the simplest and most effective, and are suitable for use in outpatients.

Uncomplicated Pilonidal Sinus

Ideally, the sinus should be treated in the early stage of its development before extensive tracts have formed.

Operative Procedure (Fig. 21–25 *A–D*). The patient may be given a short general anesthetic, although local infiltration with 1 per cent lidocaine containing 1 : 10,000 epinephrine is very effective. The patient is placed on the table in either the left lateral position with an assistant retracting the right buttocks, or prone. The area should be thoroughly shaved and cleansed.

The sinus opening and midline pits are excised with an elliptical incision down the underlying cavity approximately 0.5 cm to each side of the midline removing a minimum of skin. All hair and debris

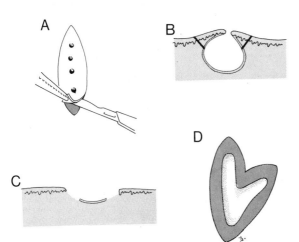

Figure 21–25 Excision of pilonidal sinus. *A–D*. The sinus openings and pits should be excised down to the underlying cavity. Any lateral extensions of the cavity should also be laid open.

are removed by curettage. Any lateral tracts should be laid open in a similar way. The wound should then be packed with a Eusol dressing and the patient sent home when he has recovered from the anesthetic. The pack should remain in position for 24 to 36 hours, after which time it may be removed and frequent sitz baths taken. The patient should be seen once a week until the wound has healed, usually in four to six weeks. Care must be taken to see that the wound heals from the bottom. Any regrowth of surrounding hair should be shaved until the wound is healed. The patient may, however, return to work in two or three days.

Complications. The only major complication likely to be encountered after this procedure is hemorrhage, and this can easily be controlled by pressure dressings. The patient should therefore be instructed that if this occurs at home, he should apply more gauze to the wound and sit on it! In a series of 33 patients treated by this technique and followed-up for six months to two years, there was apparent cure in 32.[23]

Acute Pilonidal Abscess

Simple incision results in a high recurrence rate. Simple incision plus excision of the midline pit and sinus openings does not predispose to recurrence.[25]

Operative Procedure. A general anesthetic is preferable, but local anesthetic can be used if there is no extensive surrounding inflammation. The position of the patient and the technique of excision of the sinus openings and pits are the same as those described for uncomplicated pilonidal sinus. All pus and debris are removed from the cavity, and the region is thoroughly shaved. It is not necessary to remove the granulation tissue from the wall of the sinus. The wound is packed with Eusol dressing for 24 to 36 hours, then removed and daily sitz baths taken.

There is no need subsequently to pack the wound provided the skin edges remain apart, but it should be covered with a dry gauze dressing. It should be inspected at weekly intervals to make sure that it is healing from the bottom of the cavity and to break down any fibrinous bridges which may prematurely close the wound. If these precautions are not taken, there is a high incidence of recurrence. The patient can usually return to work in two to three days.

If extensive infection of the tracts and local cellulitis occur, it is advisable to admit the patient to the hospital.

Recurrent Pilonidal Sinus

The late recurrence rate appears to be equal despite the method of treatment used. Recurrences are principally caused by failures of technique and adequate follow-up, although some late recurrences may be new sinuses.[28] If the recurrent sinus is small, it may be treated on an outpatient basis, as described earlier. If, however, the sinus is multiloculated and infected, or if there have been multiple unsuccessful operations, the patient should be admitted for treatment.

Alternative Techniques

Marsupialization. This is a popular modification of the basic operation described above for the uncomplicated case. The skin edges are sewn to the floor of the sinus with silk or nylon for eight days.[6] This technique usually necessitates the removal of more skin than is necessary and may be difficult to achieve in the obese person. I do not think that it makes the basic operation any more effective.

Excision and Primary Suture. In this technique the sinus cavity and tracts are widely excised and the defect closed with deep tension sutures. This method is not suitable for outpatient treatment.

PROCTITIS

Proctitis is a nonspecific term used to describe inflammation of the rectal mucosa. It may be limited to the rectum or it may be part of a more extensive colitis (proctocolitis).

Etiology

The condition may be primary or idiopathic, or secondary.
1. Primary
   a. Idiopathic proctitis
   b. Ulcerative colitis
   c. Crohn's disease
2. Secondary
   a. Infection:
      (1) Bacillary — Shigella, dysentery, gonorrhea
      (2) Viral — lymphogranuloma venereum
      (3) Protozoal — amebiasis, balantidiasis
      (4) Helminthic — schistosomiasis
   b. Radiation
   c. Carcinoma

Clinical Features

Symptomatology depends on the causative condition. A mild proctitis is essentially asymptomatic except for a slightly increased frequency of bowel movements, whereas in severe cases frequent small loose motions with tenesmus, hemorrhage and mucus are the main symptoms.

Investigations

1. Full medical history
2. General examination
3. Rectal examination

Inspection. The presence of perianal infection, fistula or fissures in association with proctitis is suggestive of Crohn's disease or ulcerative colitis.

Rectal Examination. This is usually normal in mild cases, but if acute, the mucosa may be tender and feel swollen. In Crohn's disease, the lower rectal mucosa may feel thick and nodular. The mucosa may also feel nodular in lymphogranuloma venereum and there may be evidence of a tubular stenosis in the late stage of the disease.

Sigmoidoscopy. Proctoscopy is of little diagnostic help, but sigmoidoscopy is most important to determine the nature and extent of the mucosal inflammation.

In idiopathic proctitis and ulcerative colitis, mucosal changes may range from mild inflammation with mucosal vessels visible, to red and granular with loss of mucosal vessels, and finally to friable edematous mucosa with contact bleeding and purulent discharge. In idiopathic proctitis these changes are confined to the rectum and do not generally extend more than 8 to 10 cm from the anus.

In Crohn's disease, the main feature is edema with scattered areas of ulceration in normal-looking mucosa. In severe cases, however, it may be difficult to distinguish Crohn's disease from ulcerative colitis. Bacillary dysentery produces mucosal edema, and, if severe, superficial ulceration which may become confluent with an associated fibropurulent exudate.

Acute gonococcal proctitis is rarely seen. It produces a very irritating yellow frothy discharge. The chronic form is difficult to diagnose, as the mucosa is only mildly red with streaks of pus. It should be suspected in all male homosexuals.

The acute stages of lymphogranuloma venereum produce a hyperemic, swollen mucosa covered with nodules and variably sized shallow ulcers.

Ulcers of *Entamoeba histolytica* or *Balantidium coli* occur early in the disease and are found predominantly in the sigmoid and upper rectum. They are multiple and small, with undermined hyperemic edges and a yellow necrotic floor which discharges pus. However, the changes may be nonspecific and diagnosed on biopsy. An ameboma of the rectum appears as a soft dark red mass with a friable ulcerated surface. Balantidiasis should be diagnosed and treated as early as possible, for perforation is the ultimate result of an untreated infection.

Rectal Biopsy

Mucosal biopsy should be carried out in all cases especially of ulcerated regions, if present. Multiple small snips of mucosa should be taken if schistosomiasis is suspected.

Examination of Stools

For cysts and ova of *Entamoeba histolytica, Balantidium coli* or schistosoma.

Stool Culture

For bacillary dysentery and gonorrhea. If gonorrhea is suspected, a smear of pus should be examined directly for gram negative intracellular diplococci, in addition to the cultures.

Barium Enema

This should be carried out in all cases to ascertain the extent of the mucosal changes and to exclude any other pathology in the colon.

Blood Tests

Hemoglobin, white count and sedimentation rate.

Specific serological tests may include complement fixation tests for lymphogranuloma venereum, schistosomiasis, gonorrhea and serological tests for syphilis.

Skin Test

The Frei test is an intradermal antigen–antibody reaction specific for lymphogranuloma venereum. A specific skin test can also be used in schistosomiasis.

Treatment. The treatment of proctitis is directed at the primary cause. Idiopathic proctitis may be controlled by prednisolone or acetarsal (triple arsenical) suppositories. Salazopyrine, 2 to 4 grams per day in divided doses, and prednisolone retention enemas may be given if suppositories are not effective. Systemic steroids may be needed if symptoms are not controlled. The benign but recurrent nature of the condition should be explained to the patient.

Crohn's disease and ulcerative colitis, once diagnosed, should be referred to the Gastroenterology Department.

Bacillary dysentery may be treated with either streptomycin 1 gram intramuscularly every six hours or chloramphenicol 250 mg four times a day — both for five days.

Gonorrhea usually responds to penicillin, but antibiotic treatment and its duration should be determined by the sensitivity of the organism.

Lymphogranuloma venereum may be effectively treated by chloramphenicol or erythromycin given in the acute stage.

Amebiasis should be treated with emetine hydrochloride injections 60 mg per day for an adult for three days, then oral emetine bismuth iodide 180 mg daily for ten days. It should be remembered that emetine, besides having a tendency to make the patient vomit, has a toxic effect on the myocardium. Metronidazole has recently been used with satisfactory results and less toxicity (page 104).

Balantidiasis requires immediate hospitalization and treatment as outlined by a specialist in tropical diseases. Schistosomiasis is treated with either trivalent organic antimony compounds or new oral agents such as Neridazole.

Radiation proctitis has no specific treatment. Symptomatic treatment with stool softeners and prednisolone enemas may be helpful.

Carcinomas should be treated by radical surgical excision on an inpatient basis.

PRURITUS ANI

Pruritus ani is the condition of itching of the anal and perianal skin. It is a troublesome condition which may occur at any age in either sex, and is frequently difficult to treat.

Etiology

It occurs in association with many conditions, which may be classified as follows:

1. *Anorectal conditions,* for example: skin tags, anal fissures and fistulae, hemorrhoids and prolapse.

2. *Dermatological lesions,* which may be either localized to region or manifestations of a generalized condition.

Examples are intertrigo, seborrheic dermatitis, psoriasis, contact dermatitis, leukoplakia and the rare lesions, Bowen's disease and extramammary Paget's disease, both of which are "premalignant."

3. *Infections,* which may be of several types.

Bacterial: usually mixed. Erythrasma[4]
Specific: primary chancre of syphilis
Yeast: *Candida albicans*
Fungi: not common, often associated with tinea pedis
Parasites: pediculosis, scabies, pinworm *(Oxyuris vermicularis)*
Viral: condylomata acuminata

It is important to exclude a vaginal discharge as the source of the perianal infection.

4. *General diseases,* for example, uncontrolled diabetes, Hodgkin's disease, jaundice, uremia, and gout.

5. *Idiopathic.* A significant group exists in which no associated organic lesion can be found. Some of these cases are undoubtedly psychological in origin, but great care must be taken not to assign a patient to this group without an exhaustive search for a primary cause.

Clinical Features

Itching is the main complaint. It may be transient or persistent. In severe cases there may be associated soreness, bleeding and a weeping discharge.

Investigations

All patients with persistent symptoms must have:
1. Full medical history
2. General, vaginal and rectal examination
3. Skin scrapings for candida and fungi
4. Bacteriological swab
5. Ultraviolet light examination for erythrasma
6. Scotch tape test for pinworms
7. Urinalysis for glucose
8. Further tests dependent on above findings

Treatment

Specific Treatment. If there is a demonstrable cause for the pruritus, it should be treated. A biopsy should be made if there is any doubt about the nature of the lesion. Anorectal conditions should be treated surgically. Contact dermatitis is commonly caused by prolonged use of local anesthetic, antiseptic and antibiotic creams. If their use is stopped, the condition usually resolves rapidly, but improvement may be accelerated by a short course of 1 per cent hydrocortisone or 0.1 per cent betamethasone cream.

Erythrasma, caused by Corynebacterium minutissimum, responds to oral erythromycin 250 mg four times per day for 14 days. Candidiasis may be treated by local nystatin, and other fungi by systemic griseofulvin or topical Whitfield's ointment. Scabies may be treated with benzyl benzoate. Pediculosis should be treated with baths and DDT powder. Pinworms respond to piperazine, but may require several doses at two week intervals. If pinworm infestation is present, all members of the family should be treated and careful hygiene observed.

Condylomata should be treated by podophyllin or excision.

The idiopathic group is the most difficult to treat. If there are obvious psychological problems, psychotherapy should be given. Symptoms can usually be controlled by hygiene, sitz baths, judicious use of cortisone creams and topical anesthetic (e.g., Nupercaine) and sympathetic handling. The operations of tattooing, undercutting and subcutaneous injection of ethyl alcohol have all been recommended for intractable pruritus ani. Their value, however, is doubtful and most cases can be controlled as described above. The diagnosis must be kept constantly under review in these cases, and it is advisable to seek a dermatological opinion.

General Treatment. The patient should first be instructed on the importance of anal hygiene and given a simple regime to follow. He should be advised to avoid those factors which aggravate the condition, e.g., scratching, heat, tight underclothes, prolonged sitting, excessive use of topical preparations and scented or harsh soaps to wash the anal region. If the symptoms disturb his sleep or work. a hypnotic and a tranquilizer may be prescribed.

Diet plays an important but variable role in pruritus ani. In general, patients should reduce or eliminate spicy foods, coffee and tea from their diets. Some patients have allergies to specific foods, which should be removed from the diet, especially if they cause diarrhea. Tomatoes, garlic, gin, fresh fruits and shellfish are common offenders. Sweets, particularly chocolate, and tobacco may provoke pruritus ani in some patients.

solution should dry before the patient is allowed to dress. A pledget of cotton wool should then be placed at the anus to prevent the podophyllin on the warts coming into contact with the skin. The patient should be told to have a bath four hours after the application. He should be examined at weekly intervals, and further applications made if necessary. The warts have a strong tendency to recur, but they can be effectively treated by the meticulous use of this method.

Operative. Under local anesthetic, the warts may be cut off with a pair of scissors and the base excised by diathermy. Care should be taken to remove any warts in the anal canal, for if these are not removed, a general recurrence will take place. *Postoperative Care:* Daily baths should be taken and a dry dressing applied. The patient should be reexamined after two weeks and any remaining warts removed.

CONDYLOMATA ACUMINATA (ANAL WARTS)

These arise in the skin of the anal canal and perianal region, are multiple and occur more commonly in men. Anal warts are very common in homosexuals. They are viral in origin.

The diagnosis is usually obvious. Rarely, however, they may be confused with the condylomata lata of secondary syphilis. If these are suspected, serology and dark ground illumination of a smear should confirm the diagnosis.

Treatment

Conservative. The application of a 25 to 40 per cent solution of podophyllin in tinct. Benzoin compound on the surface of the wart is the simplest and most effective treatment. The solution should be carefully painted on each wart with a cotton-tipped swab. Care should be taken not to get it on the perianal skin, as it is highly irritating. The podophyllin

References

1. Arthur, J. F.: Structure and significance of metaplastic nodules in the rectal mucosa. J. Clin. Pathol., *21*:735–743, 1968.
2. Barron, J.: Office ligation of internal hemorrhoids. Amer. J. Surg., *105*:563–570, 1963.
3. Blaisdell, P. C.: Prevention of massive hemorrhage secondary to hemorrhoidectomy. Surg. Gynecol. Obstet., *106*:485–488, 1958.
4. Bowyer, A., and McColl, I.: The role of erythrasma in pruritus ani. Lancet, *2*:572–573, 1966.
5. Brearley, R.: Pilonidal sinus. A new theory of origin. Br. J. Surg., *43*:62–68, 1955.
6. Buie, L. A.: Practical Proctology. Springfield, Ill., Charles C Thomas, 1960.
7. Carrasco, A. B.: Contribution à l'Étude du Prolapsus du Rectum. Paris, Masson, 1935.
8. Cornes, J. S., Wallace, M. H., and Morson, B. C.: Benign lymphomas of the rectum and anal canal. A study of 100 cases. J. Pathol. Bacteriol., *82*:371–382, 1961.
9. Dukes, C. E.: Familial intestinal polyposis. Ann. Roy. Coll. Surg. Engl., *10*:293–304, 1952.
10. Eisenhammer, S.: The evaluation of internal anal sphincterotomy operation with special reference to anal fissure. Surg. Gynecol. Obstet., *109*:583–590, 1959.
11. Eisenhammer, S.: The anorectal and anovulval

fistulous abscess. Surg. Gynecol. Obstet., *113*:519–520, 1961.

12. Enterline, H. T., Evans, G. W., Mercado-Lugo, R., Miller, L., and Fitts, W. T.: Malignant potential of adenomas of colon and rectum. J.A.M.A., *179*:322–330, 1962.

13. Goligher, J. C., Leacock, A. G., and Brossy, J. J.: The surgical anatomy of the anal canal. Br. J. Surg., *43*:51–61, 1955.

14. Goligher, J. C., Ellis, M., and Pissidis, A. G. A critique of anal glandular infection in the aetiology and treatment of idiopathic anorectal abscesses and fistulas. Br. J. Surg., *54*: 977–983, 1967.

15. Goligher, J. C.: Surgery of the Anus, Rectum and Colon. London, Bailliere, Tindall and Cassell, 1967.

16. Goodsall, D. H., and Miles, W. E.: Diseases of Anus and Rectum. Part 1. London, Longmans, 1900.

17. Grinnel, R. S., and Lane, N.: Benign and malignant adenomatous polyps and papillary adenomas of the colon and rectum: An analysis of 1,856 tumors in 1,335 patients. Int. Abstr. Surg., *106*:519–538, 1958.

18. Hawley, P. R.: The treatment of chronic fissure-in-ano. A trial of methods. Br. J. Surg., *56*:915–918, 1969.

19. Hodges, R. M.: Pilo-nidal sinus. Boston Med. Surg. J., *103*:485–486, 1880.

20. Hoffmann, D. C., and Goligher, J. C.: Lateral subcutaneous internal sphincterotomy in the treatment of anal fissure. Br. Med. J., *3*: 673–675, 1970.

21. Hughes, E. S. R.: Discussion on prolapse of the rectum. Proc. R. Soc. Med., *42*:1007–1011, 1949.

22. Knox, W. G., Miller, R. E., Begg, C. F., and Zintel, H. A.: Juvenile polyps of the colon: A clinicopathological analysis of 75 polyps in 43 patients. Surgery, *48*:201–210, 1960.

23. Lord, P. H., and Millar, D. M.: Pilonidal sinus: A simple treatment. Br. J. Surg., *52*:298–300, 1965.

24. McColl, L., Bussey, H. R. J., Morson, B. C. Polyps and polyposis. In Morson, B. C. (ed.): Diseases of Colon, Rectum and Anus. New York, Appleton-Century-Crofts, 1969.

25. Millar, D. M., and Lord, P. H.: The treatment of acute postanal pilonidal abscess. Br. J. Surg., *54*:598–599, 1967.

26. Morson, B. C., and Pang, L. S.: Rectal biopsy as an aid to cancer control in ulcerative colitis. Gut, *8*:423–434, 1967.

27. Nesselrod, J. P.: Clinical Proctology. Philadelphia, W. B. Saunders Co., 1964.

28. Notaras, M. J.: A review of three popular methods of treatment of postanal (pilonidal) sinus disease. Br. J. Surg., *57*:886–890, 1970.

29. Parks, A. G.: The surgical treatment of haemorrhoids. Br. J. Surg., *43*:337–351, 1956. (Anatomy)

30. Parks, A. G.: Pathogenesis and treatment of fistula-in-ano. Br. Med. J., *1*:463–469, 1961.

31. Parks, A. G., Porter, N. H., and Hardcastle, J. D.: The syndrome of the descending perineum. Proc. R. Soc. Med., *59*:477–482, 1966.

32. Rudd, W. W. H.: Hemorrhoidectomy in the office: Method and precautions. Dis. Colon Rectum, *13*:438–440, 1970.

33. Salvati, E. P.: Evaluation of ligation of hemorrhoids as an office procedure. Dis. Colon Rectum, *10*:53–56, 1967.

34. Veale, A. M. O., McColl, I., Bussey, H. R. J., and Morson, B. C.: Juvenile polyposis coli. J. Med. Genet., *3*:5–16, 1966.

35. Waggener, H. U.: Immediate fistulotomy in the treatment of perianal abscess. Surg. Clin. N. Amer. *49(6)*:1227–1233, 1969.

36. Watts, J. M., Bennett, R. C., and Goligher, J. C.: Stretching of the anal sphincters in the treatment of fissure-in-ano. Br. Med. J., *2*:342–343, 1964.

37. Young, A. C.: The "instant" barium enema in proctocolitis. Proc. R. Soc. Med., *56*:491–494, 1963.

22

The Foot—Podiatry

By WILLIAM R. ROSS, D.P.M.
and DAVID S. WOLF, D.P.M.

INTRODUCTION

Podiatric medicine is the allied medical branch of the healing arts concerned with the examination, diagnosis and treatment, both medical and surgical, of ailments manifesting themselves in the human foot.[18]

This chapter is designed to be used by physicians in their offices, in Outpatient Clinics and Emergency Rooms in which ambulatory procedures may be performed with ease by the busy practitioner. These outpatient procedures may be performed with minimal postoperative discomfort and disability of the patient. Early ambulation lessens the chance of phlebitis and other circulatory complications.

We will illustrate techniques of diagnosis and treatment which have evolved through years of practice with outpatients at the Podiatry Clinics of the University of Colorado Medical Center. It is not our purpose to give a thorough review of the historical backgrounds of foot disorders, but to demonstrate practical applications on an outpatient basis.

DEVELOPMENTAL DISEASES

Corns (Dorsal Helomas)

A corn is a localized overgrowth of skin with or without a central core. It is a circumscribed, cone-shaped impaction of the horny layer of the epidermis. When external pressure impinges on the sensitive papillae, pain is produced.

The authors wish to thank their colleagues at Denver General Hospital: Edward G. Dreyfus, M.D., Manager, Denver Dept. of Health and Hospitals; Ben Eiseman, M.D., Chief of Surgery; and Robert Beck, M.D., Director of Medical Education. Suggestions and constructive comments have also been given by Frank Weinstein, D.P.M., E. Dalton McGlamry, D.P.M., and the American Podiatry Association.

Corns occur due to the continuous or intermittent pressure produced by shoes. In many instances the style, design or dimension of the shoe causes pressure on the foot, contributing to corn formation. However, all corns are not due solely to poorly-fitting shoes. Very often, elongation, pronation or supination of the foot inside the shoe will also produce pressure, hence a corn. The most common locations of corns are on the sites of the foot where the greatest localized pressures are exerted, such as the lateral side of the fifth toe, the dorsum of the middle toes, or the medial sides of the hallux. In a contracted or hammertoe, the location of the painful helomata is frequently at the distal end of the toe just inferior to the distal margin of the toenail or at the highest part of the toe.

Conservative Treatment

The corn is softened with a wet pledget immersed in warm tincture of green soap solution. The wet pledget will soften or macerate the hardened underlying callus, thus facilitating débridement. Then, using a Bard-Parker No. 10 blade, the surface of the corn is debrided

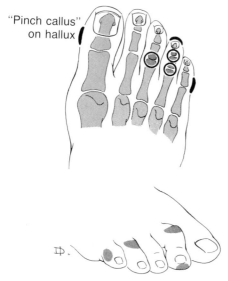

"Pinch callus" on hallux

Figure 22–1 Corn (heloma)—locations. Common locations are on great toe (medial), fifth toe (lateral) and middle toes (dorsal or at distal aspect).

carefully without penetrating vital underlying tissue and creating capillary hemorrhage or pain for the patient. When the superficial layers of the impacted epithelial tissue or corn have been removed, the deeper segment of the corn may be enucleated using a smaller No. 15 blade. The work should be done carefully and deftly to avoid pressing on the inflamed subcutaneous tissue. When most of the corn has been debrided, the toe is then dried and prepared to accept an aperture pad. The skin around the corn is painted with either tincture of benzoin or rubber cement which acts as an adherent. The skin is permitted to dry and a corn pad is then applied. These pads may be purchased ready-cut or fashioned from adhesive felt of varying thicknesses. Adhesive felt or moleskin $1/16$ inch thick is preferred. Soothing medication can be placed on the irritated lesion within the aperture. An anesthetic ointment such as americaine, benzocaine, nupercaine, or diothane may be applied. A thin piece of adhesive tape is then placed over the aperture to retain the ointment and the padding in place. Next, the corn pad itself is wrapped to the toe using lamb's wool or self-adhering gauze, i.e., gauze tape or Gauztex. If a lamb's wool wrapping is used, it can be made to adhere more firmly by brushing the surface lightly with flexible collodion. This creates a water-resistant dressing. It is bulky but very soft and conforms to the interior of the shoe.

Operative Treatment—Dorsal Helomas

Before attempting any surgical procedures for corns, x-ray studies should be made during weight-bearing. In order to delineate the position of the corn in relation to the underlying osseous tissues, each corn is encircled with a piece of soft copper wire held in place with scotch tape. On the film, a white identifying ring may be seen which encircles each lesion, specifically locating the corn and the underlying osseous tissue or condyle which is the etiological factor.

There are various surgical techniques

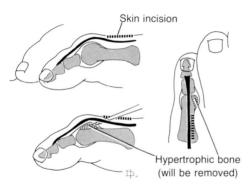

Skin incision

Hypertrophic bone
(will be removed)

Figure 22–2 Subdermal rasping technique. Dorsal skin incision parallel to extensor tendon, preserving tendon from injury. Hypertrophic bone (shown cross hatched) removed with No. 8 Bell dental file.

to permanently eradicate chronic corns (helomata). Those which we perform on an outpatient basis are:

Subdermal Rasping. This procedure is indicated when a dorsal corn is evident and secondary joint changes, such as subluxation, contracture and loss of joint mobility are not present.

The toe is anesthetized with .75 cc of 1 per cent Xylocaine plain plus .25 cc of Celestone or any other short-acting steroid. A rubber band is placed as a tourniquet at the base of the toe for about two minutes.

A 3 mm opening is made through the skin with a No. 15 blade. The incision is placed so that it is parallel to the extensor tendons, approximately 1.5 cm proximal to the excrescence (Fig. 22–2). With another No. 15 blade serving as a deep knife, the incision is carried down below the extensor tendons, care being taken not to damage these tendons. The incision is then carried through the joint capsule to expose the involved condyle, which usually rests below or inferior to the painful corn. A small dental bone rasp (No. 8 Bell file) is inserted into the incision. This rasp has teeth arranged to scrape and remove bone on the withdrawal stroke. Sufficient strokes are made to remove the bony enlargement on the condyle. When this procedure is done correctly, there is a definite inden-

tation or depression directly inferior to the corn. The margins of the wound are opened slightly, using a mosquito hemostat, and are then lavaged. Closure of the wound is usually accomplished with a small compression dressing, a single interrupted suture or a plastic Steri-Strip. A 2 inch square sponge held by a 1 inch Kling bandage makes a very simple, quickly applied dressing. The patient is then advised to go home, elevate the foot, and apply ice packs for the first three to four hours. Little or no pain is experienced by the majority of patients with this type of lesion. The patient wears a shoe with a cut-out aperture or an open-toe sandal for the first two weeks.

Digital Arthroplasty (Fig. 22–3). The toe is anesthetized at its base with 1 cc or less of .75 cc of 1 per cent Xylocaine plain with .25 cc of Celestone added. After the digital block is accomplished, a rubber band tourniquet is placed proximal to the point of injection for about two minutes to retain the anesthesia in the desired area. After anesthesia has

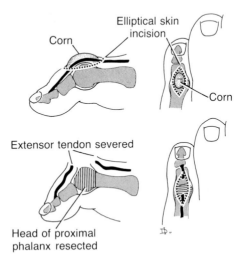

Corn

Elliptical skin incision

Corn

Extensor tendon severed

Head of proximal phalanx resected

Figure 22–3 Digital arthroplasty. Elliptical incision around dorsal corn. Exterior tendon severed. Proximal phalangeal head grasped with towel clamp, resected at surgical neck with large double action rongeur. Bone edges are smoothed with rasp. Capsule, tendon and skin are coapted with three deep mattress sutures.

been accomplished and the foot and toes are carefully shaved, scrubbed, prepped and draped, the tourniquet is then removed. Hemostasis is achieved by a Martin (Esmarch) bandage or a pneumatic cuff applied just proximal to the malleoli and inflated to 50 mm Hg above the patient's systolic blood pressure.

The corn is encircled with two semi-elliptical incisions transversely through the skin using a No. 10 blade. The outlined corn is then grasped with a small Allis clamp and resected, using a deep No. 15 blade. The skin margins are next underscored and the toe is then plantar-flexed, exposing the involved interphalangeal joint directly below the resected corn. The joint space is located and opened, simultaneously severing the extensor tendons. A small-sized dental collar and crown scissors is then inserted into the joint to free the collateral ligaments. Next, a closed Backhaus towel clamp is looped around and under the head of the proximal phalanx. The head of the phalanx is then elevated out of the wound to enable a bone rongeur to sever it at its surgical neck. The phalangeal head is removed and the shaft is smoothed with a rasp. Three deep vertical mattress sutures are used to close the wound. The sutures are inserted so that the base of each stitch includes capsule and tendon while the superficial part of the suture includes only the skin. A helpful hint in placing mattress sutures is to leave 1 cm of suture material exposed at its distal loop where it appears outside the skin. This serves to prevent strangulation of the tissue and allows ready access to the sutures when the time comes to remove them. The wound is dressed with sterile 2 inch square sponges and 1 inch Kling bandage. Sutures are removed in 10 to 14 days.

Soft Corns (Heloma Molles)

Soft corns may occur between any of the toes. The causes of soft corns are: (1) the apposition of adjacent skin surfaces; (2) the excess production of heat or fric-

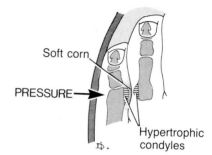

Figure 22–4   Soft corn (heloma molles). Lateral pressure on fourth interdigital space causes soft corn to form as shown. Adjacent bone surfaces (cross hatched) become hypertrophic.

tion; (3) excess production of moisture, either by perspiration or retention of bath water which cannot evaporate; and (4) bony prominences or exostoses on the phalangeal bones producing pressures upon the impinged skin.

This lesion can be one of the most painful and insidious conditions of the foot. The most common site is the fourth interdigital space where moisture accumulates (Fig. 22–4).

Chronic irritation and pressure from narrow footgear causes the condyles on adjacent bone surfaces to enlarge and lie in close apposition, thereby precipitating this interdigital lesion. Frequently, sinus formation in the interdigital web may lead to an acute infection. Subsequently, cellulitis develops which forces the patient to seek treatment.

Lesions which are left untreated often develop an underlaying bursa or cyst. Roentgenograms of the area are necessary and will reveal the underlying osseous hypertrophy.

Fungal infection is the main problem in differential diagnosis.

Conservative Treatment

Separating the toes with properly applied pads and prescribing wider shoes will encourage resolution of these lesions. Symptomatic, temporary relief is also obtained by injecting a solution of $\frac{1}{8}$ cc Xylocaine plus $\frac{1}{8}$ cc Dexamethasone into the base of the digit at periodic intervals. Prior to employing this treatment, the patient's pedal circulation as well as his peripheral and neurological status must be thoroughly evaluated. The justification for steroid therapy in conjunction with the anesthetic agent is the premise that the soft corn is diminutive bursitis without infection.

Surgical Treatment

It is our experience that when the soft corn is of a chronic nature, i.e., the condyles are enlarged and the digits in close apposition, the following surgical procedure is recommended for best results.

Under local anesthesia obtained by means of a digital block, a linear incision is made over the dorsomedial aspect of the digit. The incision commences at the base of the distal phalanx and terminates at the base of the proximal phalanx. The collateral ligament and capsular tissue of the involved articulation are dissected free. The underlying osteophytic hypertrophy is then completely excised. It is usually necessary to excise the contiguous condyles of each phalanx of the involved articulation so that the entire surface remaining presents a smooth flat plane. This can be accomplished either with bone rongeurs or with an air motor drill with bone bit to reduce the condylar enlargement. Pre-op radiographic studies and digital palpation during surgery reveal the necessity of the latter phase of the procedure.

Plantar Callus (Keratosis, Keratoma)

Diagnosis

Calluses are differentiated from corns by their anatomic location on the foot. Routinely, the corn (heloma) is found on the dorsum of the digits. The callus or plantar keratosis is found on the plantar aspect of the foot, usually under weight-bearing areas.

On microscopic examination, the plantar callus presents the following findings: the epithelium on the central portion of the lesion is indented and there is striking hyperkeratosis of the center in comparison to the marginal portions. There is localized elongation of the rete pegs which extend into the corium. Throughout the thickened stratum corium many small shrunken nuclei can be seen. The corium does not show any abnormality.[10]

On an outpatient basis, this lesion is often misdiagnosed as a plantar wart (verrucae). (See discussion of verrucae plantaris under *Neoplasm.*) The verrucae plantaris is caused by a filterable virus, whereas the plantar callus is produced by pressure. Microscopically, these lesions appear similar and for this reason they are often misdiagnosed and subsequently mistreated.

On clinical examination, the plantar callus is found on weight-bearing areas, whereas the plantar verrucae usually are not. The plantar callus is found primarily in female adults since high heeled shoes transfer weight bearing to the metatarsal heads. The plantar keratosis is heavily cornified. When debrided, it presents a small pearl-gray avascular center. The verrucae plantaris has multiple papillae which are discernible upon superificial débridement. Verrucae are also distinguished by the multi-dotted appearance caused by numerous coagulated capillary endings, plus an encircling connective tissue capsule. These lesions are acutely sensitive to pressure.

Treatment

Conservative. Conservative therapy should invariably be tried for relief of symptoms. Conservative measures are identical to those used for corns. A plaster impression can be taken of the foot and a molded inlay fabricated from it to redistribute pressure away from the metatarsal heads. The pad may also be placed proximal to the metatarsal head to alleviate forefoot imbalance.

Surgical. (1) *Plantar Condylectomy* (Fig. 22–5). This procedure is indicated

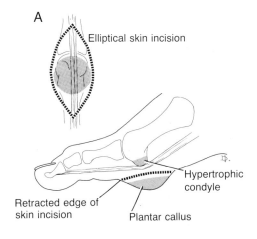

A

Elliptical skin incision

Hypertrophic condyle

Retracted edge of skin incision

Plantar callus

B

Hypertrophic condyle removed with osteotome

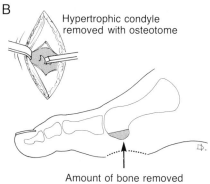

Amount of bone removed

Figure 22–5 A. Plantar condylectomy for plantar callus. Procedure is indicated for intractable callus on metatarsal heads 2, 3, 4 or 5. Elliptical incision is made around the keratoma (callus), which is then removed. Flexor tendons are retracted laterally. Hypertrophic condyle on metatarsal head is removed with osteotome. Bone is smoothed and skin closed. Another technique (osteoclasis) is described in text.

when the metatarsal head is enlarged and/or rotated in its axis and causes an intractable plantar keratoma.

The operative technique is adapted from Duvries (1959).[5] An elliptical incision large enough to include the entire keratoma is made on the plantar aspect of the foot. Sharp dissection is carried down into the fatty tissue, freeing the lesion so that it pops up and out into the wound space. The keratoma is then grasped with a tenaculum and dissected in one piece. Through this opening, the dissection is extended to the flexor tendons which are retracted laterally to expose the joint capsule. The capsule is then incised, and with the aid of a bone elevator, the metatarsal head is brought into view. Then using an osteotome, bone cutting instrument, rasp and chisel, the plantar condyle is removed and the bone surface rasped smooth. The metatarsal is repositioned and the joint capsule closed. The wound is closed in layers. The superficial gap caused by removal of the keratoma is filled with chromic sutures prior to coaptating the skin edges. The area is then covered with a sterile, nonpressure dressing. Ambulation may be permitted 48 hours postoperatively in a cut-out shoe.[1]

(2) *Floating head osteotomy (osteoclasis)*. This is a relatively new procedure for plantar keratosis in which the metatarsal head, just proximal to the surgical neck, is fractured without stabilization. The rationale of metatarsal osteotomy without stabilization is based on our experience that patients with plantar keratomas experienced resolution of their lesions when fractures of the metatarsals occurred after physical injury, i.e., march fractures.

The metatarsal head should be pushed back or up into its proper position by natural pressure forces. The exact amount and degree will be determined by postoperative ambulation (upward pressure from the ground). After osteotomy a hard bony callus is formed around the fracture site.[4] This has the advantage of maintaining the integrity of the metatarsophalangeal joint which has caused the subluxated toes, the shortened toes, and toes that do not function fully. The patient may walk from the office in a postoperative shoe.[4]

(3) *Complication*. Keratotic lesions may be transferred to other metatarsal heads and subluxated or shortened toes. This condition can be obviated with careful preoperative evaluation as well as standard weight-bearing x-ray evaluation of the metatarsal length pattern. We have found excellent results with proper postoperative follow-up, balancing the

patient's foot with orthotics or molded inlays.

Disorders of the Nail Plates

The function of the nail plate is to protect the distal end of the toe and its ungual phalanx. Poor hygiene and improper trimming are not the only underlying causes of nail pathology.

Incurvation is the most frequent affliction of the nail plates and occurs at any age. The medial side of the hallux is generally first involved. Anterior elongation of the first metatarsal and the valgus rotation of the hallux increase the trauma on the nail plate. At first the patient complains of tenderness in the nail groove. As time advances, the nail plate commences to incurvate, and the removal of a small edge of nail plate is necessary. If temporary removal of the nail spicule is the sole method employed to relieve the symptoms, incurvation is destined to become increasingly chronic and severe. Incurvation is also associated with hormonal imbalance, particularly in females at or past the menopause.

Ingrown Toenail (Onychocryptosis)

A confusing variety of procedures has been advocated for this condition in the podiatric, surgical and orthopedic literature.[7, 8, 9, 16, 25]

Pathology (Fig. 22–6). The nail is formed on the dorsal aspect of the distal phalanx in a manner which corresponds to the hair root. The margins of the nail do not ordinarily connect with the adjacent soft tissue.

Ingrown toenails are largely caused and made symptomatic by shoes, which wedge the forefoot into the compressing toe of a shoe. High heels compound the problem by directing the weight onto the forepart of the foot. Pronation of the foot produces increased pressure on the forepart of the foot.

An ingrown toenail is often made worse by improper treatment. Improper trimming destroys the nail groove, which then becomes hypertrophied and may overgrow the nail margin. Infection of the soft tissue complicates the clinical picture.

There are three major types of ingrown toenail:

Subcutaneous nail. As a result of improper trimming of the nail, a prominence may grow distally beneath the soft tissue surrounding the nail. The nail is normal, but it produces irritation by growing into the soft tissue.

Inward distortion of nail plates. The lateral margins of the nail plate may be pressed inward by the surrounding soft

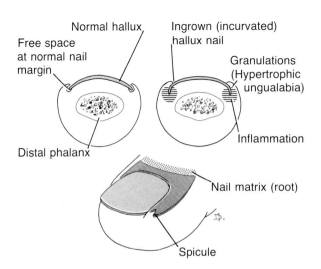

Figure 22–6 Pathology of ingrown toenail. The normal free space at nail margin is obliterated by inflammation and granulation tissue, which is caused by improper nail trimming, trauma to matrix and faulty foot gear.

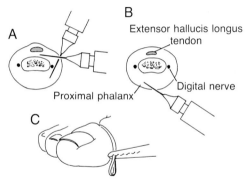

Figure 22–7 Anesthesia for surgery on ingrown toenail. Disposable 25 gauge ⁷/₈ inch needle used to inject lidocaine 1 per cent, and to block lateral, dorsal and plantar aspects, as shown. Maximum volume of lidocaine is 1.5–3.0 ml. Tourniquet is then applied and removed when operative procedure is completed.

tissues. The interfaces between the soft tissue and the nail plate become inflamed. A dorsal extension of the nail plate usually forms a subungual exostosis. The displaced nail hypertrophies.

Hypertrophy of lateral lips of nail. The nail may be normal, but the lips of the nail wall overgrow the nail. Inflammation occurs beneath the hypertrophied soft tissue.

Surgical Treatment. After preparation the toe is anesthetized approximately 1.5 to 3 ml of lidocaine or Carbocaine (Fig. 22–7). A dry field should be obtained with a tourniquet. Anesthesia is produced by injecting the great toe at its fibular side, toward its plantar aspect. The needle is then retracted slightly and redirected horizontally, dorsiflexing the toe so that the needle will pass under the extensor hallucis longus tendon. The dorsum of the toe is infiltrated toward its tibial side. The needle is next inserted on the plantar side of the great toe at its fibular side, directed diagonally upward, until an anesthetic wheal has been created around the base of the toe.

A constricting rubber band or small rubber tubing held with a hemostat acts as a tourniquet at the base of the toe, and is left in place for two minutes. The hemostat acts as a reminder for removal of the tourniquet when the toe is draped.

The offending nail margin is then split from its distal end back almost to its base with an English nail splitting forceps, taking care not to incise the epidermal tissue (Fig. 22–8). The remainder of the nail is split with a T-shaped nail chisel. A small elevator similar to a dental spatula is inserted under the offending section of nail, which is lifted from its bed. The exposed nail bed is then rubbed with 88 per cent carbolic acid applied with a cotton-tipped applicator for two minutes. The applicator must be vigorously applied to the nail bed, without spilling excess phenol on the adjacent normal tissues. If this happens, wipe off spillage with an alcohol-soaked sponge. Chemical cautery produces a mild sloughing of the nail

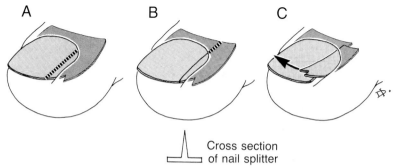

Cross section of nail splitter

Figure 22–8 Surgery for ingrown toenail. Nail is split with nail forceps or sharp, heavy scissors. T-shaped chisel or nail splitter completes division of nail deep to eponychium following nail striations, and loose nail segment is then removed. Exposed nailbed cauterized with 88 per cent phenol (carbolic acid).

bed and matrix, inhibiting recurrence of the nail margin. The patient will rarely complain of postoperative pain after adequate phenol cautery.

After two minutes the area is sponged dry with another cotton-tipped applicator and the wound is dressed with Cortisporin ointment and a compression bandage for 24 hours. The patient then returns to the office for redressing, which usually consists of a bandaid and more of the Cortisporin ointment. In several days a straw-colored exudate will appear. Slight drainage may be experienced for several weeks. Showers and baths are permitted.

The same technique can be used for complete matrix destruction of the entire toenail.

This technique can also be used for diabetics when glucosuria is well controlled. It can also be used in the presence of fungus infections, in which case Fulvicin U/F, 500 mg per day is given for 30 days starting in one week.

Fungal Infection (Onychomycosis)

This is the most common disease entity of the nail plate. Nail growth is affected by the invasion of a fungus. The most common types of fungi that affect the nail plate are tinea rubrum, tinea mentagrophytes and *Candida albicans.*

Diagnosis. Onychomycosis simulates a number of nail conditions and must be differentiated from the following: psoriasis, atopic dermatitis, eczema and lichen planus. Many patients will present a history of trauma followed by distortion and incurvation of the nail plate, which may become infected with fungus.

Fungus involvement of the nail causes elevation of the nail plate from the nail bed, makes the nail plate thickened, yellow and brittle, and may predispose to nail incurvation (onychocryptosis) and secondary cellulitis.

Fungus first appears at the distal tip of the nail plate as a scaley striation with radiating strains along the nail plate. This progresses until the nail plate is brittle and hypertrophic, and has a powdery consistency involving all of the nail components, including the nail matrix.

Before commencing therapy, fungal infection must be differentiated from a pathological condition or trauma, through culture and microscopic examination of the nail tissues. Some offices employ Saboraud's agar or Myco-kit culture tubes to obtain a faster growth.

Treatment. In 1956, Pillsbury stated that onychomycosis of the toenails was incurable.[17] Riehl[19] was the first to describe the value of griseofulvin two years later. It was first administered in tablets of 250 mg four times daily for 16 to 18 months. We have found that Fulvicin U.F. (Ultra Fine) administered in 500 mg tablets twice a day results in resolution of the nail mycosis in approximately 9 to 12 months. If Fulvicin causes undue gastric upset, headaches or nausea, it should be discontinued or the dose reduced. Onycho-Phytex has been used widely for the topical treatment of nail fungus. This preparation is composed of a borotannic complex derived from boric and tannic acid with salicylic acid, dissolved in ethyl alcohol. Frost (1960)[6] recommends treating mycotic nails by atraumatically avulsing the nails and then applying Onycho-Phytex (Wynlett) twice a day for at least four weeks. Treatment with Onycho-Phytex was not effective without avulsion of the nail. If the fungus radiates to the eponychian and nail matrix, topical application will be ineffective.

Other modes of therapy include disinfection of the shoes with formalin, routine débridement of the nail plate with Betadine scrubs and complete avulsion of the nail plate.

For hypertrophic onychomycotic nails associated with brittle, yellow discoloration involving all the nail components, the most effective treatment is atraumatic avulsion of the nail plate and phenolization of the matrix[20] (Fig. 22–7, 22–8).

Neoplasms

Neoplasms in or around the nail plate may affect its blood or nerve supply.

Neoplasms thus produce disturbances of the nail matrix (root cells) causing abnormal color or growth patterns. Many benign neoplasms and even some malignant entities have been misdiagnosed as calloused nail grooves. The following neoplasms should be considered before any treatment is instituted:

Chondroma. Chondroma is a new growth consisting of cartilage. It usually develops directly under the nail plate and causes elevation or deformation of the nail. It is not as dense as subungual exostosis, which is a true bony proliferation. Pain may be severe when pressure is applied to the nail. Treatment consists of surgical excision of this tumor. It is often seen in patients with chronic recurrent ingrown toenails when there is an irritation of the underlying dermal structures.

Glomus Tumor. Glomera are small benign tumors, always excruciatingly painful. They consist of convoluted blood vessels surrounded by muscle and epithelial cells, and they may contain nail tissue. They are reddish purple in color. When one occurs under the nail bed, a bluish red spot under the nail plate is visible. Because of the extreme pain and tenderness caused by this lesion, the diagnosis is easy to render. The slightest touch of the finger or a breath of air directed to the toe may cause the patient to cry out. Steinberg (1956)[22] reported 24 cases of glomus tumor. He points out that very frequently the diagnosis is missed because the lesion is so small that it is not seen by the doctor.

Burleson (1964)[3] believes that xanthoma, felon, fibroma, fracture of the distal phalanx or subungual exostosis can be misdiagnosed as a glomus tumor.

Glomus tumors should be surgically excised.

Granuloma Pyogenicum. This is a pendunculated, red, fungating, benign tumor in which the granulation consists of masses of staphylococci. It is most frequently seen in the nail groove and may range in size from that of a pinhead to that of a coffee bean. Occasionally covering the entire nail surface, it bleeds easily and is ordinarily not too painful. It is one of the complications of the common ingrown toenail but must be differentiated from the granulations found in ingrown toenail infections because wet dressings and antibiotics will not cure granuloma pyogenicum.

Resection of the offending portion of the nail plate is the treatment of choice, followed by electrodesiccation of the granuloma.

Melanoma. Melanomas are highly malignant tumors of pigmented melanocytes. They usually develop in the matrix or in the nail fold. When found under the nail, the bluish color of the lesion will show through the nail plate; also, the lesion will cause elevation of the nail from the bed and distortion of the nail. While most melanomas are black, bluish black or dark brown, rarely one will be found with no particularly distinguishing color. Melanomas metastasize early. Amputation of the involved digit is the recommended treatment. A general surgical consultation should be obtained so that further evaluation and therapy may be performed as indicated.

Verrucae. Verrucae are benign tumors caused by a filterable virus. When seen around the nail, they usually elevate the structure. They are fairly common and resemble any other type of verrucae, bleeding profusely upon superficial débridement. Because of the potential danger to the nail bed, we suggest chemotherapy utilizing mono or trichloroacetic acid as the destructive agent.[2] We have recently been pleased with the results obtained using Canthrone, which is well tolerated, even by children.

Subungual Exostosis

Diagnosis

A subungual exostosis is an osteogenic growth usually found on the dorsum of the distal phalanx of the great toe. Lateral radiographic projections readily identify it as a dome-shaped elevation, creating pressure under the nail plate. Frequently, the exostoses are distal to the nail plate. Upon pressure, pain is felt equally at the site of the exostosis and on the nail plate. Both areas are subject to weight bearing and shoe pressures which accentuate the discomfort. Subungual exostoses are benign and are often associated with a prior history of trauma.

The overlying nail plate is frequently involved and is often elevated and tender upon pressure. This condition is often misdiagnosed as an ingrowing nail but attempts to gain relief by resecting the nail margins will be unsuccessful.

Surgical Procedure: Bone planing (Fig. 22–9)

A 1 cm incision is made at the distal end of the hallux, just below the level of the ventral plane of the distal phalanx. With a No. 15 blade the opening is extended to the distal tip of the phalanx and soft tissue is separated at periosteal level. Care must be exercised to minimize soft tissue damage.

A small curved tenotomy forceps is then inserted into the wound to further detach soft tissue proximal to the exostosis. The reason for starting below the distal phalangeal level is to prevent embarrassment of the nail blood supply. A dental "bell-file" is inserted into the wound and the exostosis is rasped

smooth to slightly below the level of the phalangeal surface.

The wound is then irrigated and closed, using one interrupted dermal suture or $1/8$ inch Steri-Strip. The patient is advised to rest and elevate the foot until the following day, when normal work may be resumed.

This procedure is far less traumatic than the accepted "fish-mouth incision." It avoids laceration of small blood vessels and healing occurs more rapidly. The nail plate, bed, and matrix are not injured so there is no distortion of nail growth and little postoperative pain.

Hallux Valgus

Definition: Hallux Valgus and Bunion (Fig. 22–10)

Hallux valgus is one of the most common chronic disorders seen in our podiatric practices. Hallux valgus is an angulation of the great toe away from the midline of the body or toward the other toes, with a valgus or tibial rotation of the great toe.

A *bunion* is an inflammation of the great toe joint. It is not an exostosis of the medial condylar process of the metatarsal head. Therefore, "exostectomy" is incorrect and "condylectomy" is cor-

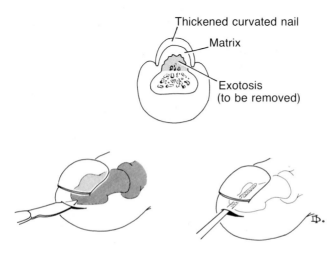

Thickened curvated nail

Matrix

Exotosis (to be removed)

Figure 22–9 Subungual exostosis. Nail is thickened, encurvated, overlaping the rough exostosis (shaded area). This is removed by rasping with a No. 8 Bell dental file, which is inserted through a small transverse incision at distal aspect of the toe. The incision should be just ventral to the plane of the terminal phalanx.

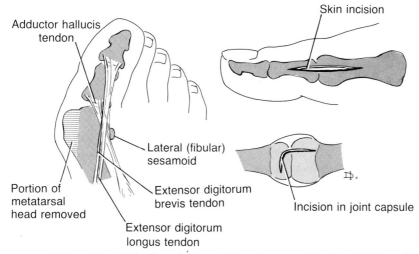

Figure 22–10 Hallux valgus. Hallux is angled toward the other toes, with valgus (tibial) rotation of great toe and partial dislocation of M-P joint. When joint is inflamed, the lesion is termed a "bunion." Surgery is usually necessary for correction.

McBride procedure (illustrated here) uses longitudinal skin incision, inverted "L" capsulotomy, and resection of shaded area of metatarsal head with rongeur. The lateral (fibular) sesamoid is then removed completely and the dorsal tendons inserting at the base of the proximal phalanx are severed. The tendons to be severed are adductor hallucis and extensor digitorum brevis, which lies deep to extensor digitorum longus. Tendons and sesamoid are exposed by retracting skin incision dorsally and laterally.

rect. "Bunionectomy" is also a misnomer. There is, at best, no more than ⅛ inch cortical hypertrophy over the medial condyle. The condition is therefore one primarily of partial dislocation.

Etiology

Predisposing Factors. There is a hereditary tendency to flaccid ligamentous structures as well as long narrow feet. Also inherited may be variations in the morphology of the articular surface of the first metatarsophalangeal joint (an increased obliquity). An increase in the angle of the first metatarsocuneiform articulation is also a contributing factor. The more oblique the angle, the more the individual is predisposed to the hallux valgus formation.

Direct Factors. (1) *Short shoes* are the most important direct factor. (2) The abducted gait, pronation, flatfoot, and the patient's occupation may predispose to the development of hallux valgus. (3) Fatigue factors may cause elongation and pronation of the foot, with resultant progression of the forefoot in the narrow confines of the toe box of the shoe.

Pathological Anatomy

The proximal and distal phalanges of the great toe are directed toward the fibula and occasionally rotated toward the tibia, i.e., overlapping the second toes or underlying first toes. The first metatarsal is directed medially (tibially) and exhibits slight tibial rotation. The tibial capsule of the first metatarsophalangeal joint is stretched and the fibular aspect of the base of the proximal phalanx of the hallux is shortened. The abductor hallucis tendon which inserts into the medial aspect of the base of the proximal phalanx of the hallux is stretched and the extensors hallucis longus and brevis are sometimes shortened.

Treatment

Palliative. One or more of the following may be rendered to accommodate the condition, but will not correct the hallux valgus deformity.

1. *Physical therapy* modalities: (a) hydrotherapy, i.e., whirlpool baths, hydrocollation to increase hyperemia, reducing congestion, stress and inflammation; (b) paraffin baths; and (c) diathermy and ultrasound.

2. *Injection* of steroid hormones in combination with local anesthetic agents to break up the pain cycle and institute an anti-inflammatory effect.

3. Applying an *accommodative shield* utilizing soft felt or sponge to prevent further irritation.

4. *Shoe therapy* is necessary. Consult a reliable shoe fitter for proper foot gear. In fitting of shoes, it must be noted that the size of the shoe is measured from the ball (the metatarsal phalangeal joint) to the posterior aspect of the heel. Therefore, the ball of the foot must be contiguous with the break of the shoe (a diagonal transverse line drawn across the sole from the first metatarsal phalangeal joint to the fifth metatarsal phalangeal joint). Flexion of the forepart of the foot (metatarsal phalangeal joints one through five) with the break of the shoe will cause binding and secondary restrictions of movement, with blistering and subsequent calluses along the dorsum of the foot. If the metatarsals flex at the break of the shoe, there must be a finger's breadth of room distal to the toes upon weight bearing. This defines the long vamp shoe. The higher the heel, the greater the propulsive driving force influences the force of the foot in the toe box. When all these conditions are met, the patient's foot is comfortable and symptoms are alleviated. If none of these procedures are effective, the practitioner should resort to surgical treatment.

Philosophy of Bunion Surgery. Before listing the different surgical approaches that we have found effective in permanent treatment of this disorder, we would like to outline our philosophy of bunion surgery. In our hands, unilateral uncomplicated hallux surgery on an outpatient basis has been more successful than prolonged hospitalization with subsequent circulatory complications, i.e., phlebitis, osteoporotic demineralization and other changes associated with disuse atrophy. The patient may ambulate immediately with a postsurgical shoe (Reese or Ortho mold) which promotes blood flow and ventilation, but without loss of muscle tone due to immobilization of the affected part. With the following unilateral surgical approaches, the patient may use the other foot without suffering excessive emotional or physical disability.

The surgical correction of any foot deformity should be performed with caution since the foot is the most distant organ in the vascular tree. Diminution of circulation and weight bearing are factors which interfere with wound healing.

Surgical Reduction

Silver Procedure (Jones Operation). This procedure is indicated only when there is a mere prominence of bone at the metatarsophalangeal joint without any partial dislocation of the joint. If the patient is elderly or debilitated, surgical relief is indicated, but functional realignment is not necessary. This procedure is the least traumatic and will remove the original symptoms.

The technique commences with a curvilinear incision medial to the extensor digitorum longus tendon. The medial capsule is incised and shortened by making a reverse L-shaped incison which is followed by a medial osteotomy. This is varied by severing the adductor hallucis through a stab wound to help take the hallux out of valgus.

After-care consists of splinting the toe for approximately six weeks to maintain proper alignment. Osteotomy and capsule shortening alone will not straighten the toe. In a very short time, the position of the bones will revert to their preoperative state.

Modified McBride Procedure (Fig. 22–10). The rationale behind a McBride bunionectomy is the removal of the lateral sesamoid. Its resection actually removes part of the internal cubic content of the fibular aspect of the first metatarsophalangeal joint. Upon resection of the lateral sesamoid, the joint capsule is released on its fibular aspect permitting the first metatarsal to move back into proper approximation to the second metatarsal. The primus varus angle is thereby reduced.

A dorsal longitudinal midline incison is made in the skin over the first metatarsophalangeal joint, extending from midshaft of the first metatarsal distally to midshaft of the proximal phalanx. The incision is deepened through the fascial plane and is undermined to the medial and lateral aspects of the joint. The extensor hallucis brevis tendon is next located deep to the longus tendon. The brevis tendon is elevated and a section of it is excised. An inverted L capsulotomy is performed along the dorsal and tibial aspects of the joint. The flap thus created is freed and retracted. The metatarsal head is also freed from capsule along the dorsum. The head is then elevated out of its capsule with a periosteal elevator. The redundant bone is resected with a bone rongeur from the dorsal and tibial aspects of the head. The remaining surface is smoothed. Care is taken to smooth the tibioplantar aspect of the head without sacrificing the condyle at that point. The presence of the condyle is helpful in protecting against overcorrection of the position of the tibial sesamoid, which could result in a hallux varus.

The incison is then retracted to the fibular side of the joint and a self-retaining retractor is inserted in the first metatarsal interspace. Dissection is carried down to the floor of the interspace. An incision is then made parallel to and just dorsal to the fibular sesamoid. This incision in the capsule is approximately parallel to the long axis of the first ray. It extends distally to a point just dorsal to the insertion of the adductor hallucis tendon. The scalpel is re-introduced in the same incision and is backed up in the incision until the cutting edge of the blade is just proximal to the sesamoid. The flat edge of the blade is pressed against the plantar surface of the tendon. A short stroke sawing action is begun distally with the instrument. The edge of the sesamoid is encountered as the blade begins to cut between the sesamoid and the tendon fibers. As cutting progresses distally, the blunt edge of the blade is gradually raised so that the cutting edge of the instrument contacts the sesamoid at approximately a 35 to 45 degree angle. In this way, the flat edge of the blade retracts the tendon while the cutting edge separates the tendon from the sesamoid. This permits freeing of all the attachments of the sesamoid with the exception of the intrasesamoidal ligament.

The hallux should be flexed sharply and the metatarsal head elevated. The blade can then be placed plantarly and parallel to the sesamoid bone with the blade's cutting edge directed against the ligament from beneath. The sesamoid can then be grasped and removed. The adductor hallucis tendon is then grasped with a clamp and is sharply cut from its attachment to the phalanx. The tendon is freed adequately to permit its attachment under physiologic tension into the bone at the neck of the first metatarsal. The hallux is manipulated into overcorrection to ensure that no deforming influence remains and to be certain that the first metatarsal moves into position beside the second metatarsal.

Returning to the tibial side of the joint, the hallux is placed in correct alignment and held while the capsule is closed. The longitudinal portion of the L-shaped capsular incision is closed first along the dorsum of the metatarsal head. With the hallux in correct alignment, the excess joint capsule is then removed with a vertical capsulectomy. The vertical portion of the joint incision can now be closed. In instances where rotation of the hallux may have been present along with valgus, the sutures are placed obliquely in closing the vertical portion of the capsular incision. Oblique placement of sutures will retain correction of the derotation which has been accomplished by this surgery.

When the extensor hallucis longus is excessively short, it is lengthened by Z-plasty. More often, it is simply positioned in its best alignment and sutured to the joint capsule at the metatarsal neck with a double turn 000 plain or chromic catgut. This retains the position of the tendon in relation to the joint during the initial weeks of healing and prevents malposition of the hallux postoperatively as a result of extensor muscle spasm. The fascial plane is next replaced and sutured carefully and completely with multiple 000 plain catgut sutures. The skin is closed with nonabsorbable sutures.

Sterile gauze bandaging is applied over suitable sterile padding. The bandaging is applied is such a way that it assures retention of the correct alignment. A fresh dressing is usually applied after three or four days and a similar bandage is reapplied. One-half of the sutures are removed at five to seven days and the remainder of the sutures at the next redressing, usually at 10 to 14 days after surgery. Once sterile bandaging is unnecessary, the foot is painted with skin adherent and a cohesive gauze supportive bandage is applied so that it will retain the correction. In instances where drifting of the toe may seem evident, the cohesive gauze is reinforced with multiple corrective layers of adhesive tape. Such a bandage can remain in place for up to two full weeks. It may be replaced in problem cases. More often, we apply molded polyurethane retainers three weeks postoperatively and return the patient to a closed, newly fitted, round toe oxford. We require the wearing of such a shoe for approximately two full months from fitting. Orthotic needs are met as required by the patient.[15]

Hiss Bunionectomy. The Hiss bunionectomy is a tendon balance procedure designed to transplant the abductor hallucis tendon into the dorsal aspect of the proximal phalanx. The hallux is thereby brought into normal alignment, while at the same time the sesamoids are brought back to their original articulating facets.

Procedure. A linear incision is made 0.5 cm on the fibular side of the tuberosity of the base of the first proximal phalanx. A short Sistrunk dissecting scissors is inserted into the incision and

the adductor hallucis tendon is severed at its attachments by following the contour of the bone. The scissor points are now utilized to sever the fibular portion of the joint capsule. A medial longitudinal incision approximately 5 cm long is made just above the heavy skin of the sole of the foot and below the calloused area of the metatarsal head. Retraction is accomplished to expose the abductor hallucis tendon while it is dissected free. Note the location of the medial branch of the medial plantar nerve which runs along the lower border of the adductor tendon. The abductor hallucis is reflected back at its insertion into the inferior aspect of the proximal phalanx. The joint capsule is opened with a longitudinal incision. The edges of the joint capsule are then detached and an exostectomy is performed at the enlarged head of the first metatarsal. The sesamoid bones are brought back to their normal alignment by replacing the abductor tendon into the base of the proximal phalangeal base, thereby taking the hallux out of the valgus.

Keller Bunionectomy. Three procedures have been recommended for correction of hallux limitus or rigidus with or without hallux valgus: the Mayo, Keller and Stone procedures. The Mayo procedure has generally been discredited because of the infliction of trauma to the first metatarsal-phalangeal joint. The Keller procedure is most widely used. It is indicated in patients over 50 years of age in whom the metatarsal joint is destroyed or the normal joint space is lost. The Stone procedure is little known, but we have found it generally preferable to the Keller procedure because of the loss of function which follows the latter.

Technique. A medial osteotomy of the first metatarsal is performed in the Keller procedure, along with amputation of the proximal one third to one half of the base of the proximal phalanx. A curvilinear incision is made over the first metatarsophalangeal joint, followed by a U-shaped incision through the capsule with the apex distally. A medial osteotomy is accomplished, followed by resection of the base of the proximal phalanx. The toe is then sutured into proper alignment.

Complications. (1) All four insertions (flexor hallucis brevis, extensor hallucis brevis, adductor hallucis, abductor hallucis tendons) to the base of the proximal phalanx are destroyed. (2) The great toe has little residual function and is frequently dorsiflexed. (3) Calluses develop presently under second, third, and fourth metatarsal heads with possible marked proximal shifting of second, third, and fourth digits. (4) Marked proximal shifting of the sesamoids occurs along the metatarsal shaft.

Stone Procedure. The Stone procedure is a modification of a procedure first described by Fessler in 1926. Fessler removed the prominence of the medial aspect and lateral corner of the first metatarsal head, but left the plantar weight-bearing area intact.

The main advantage of the Stone procedure over the Keller is functional. Shortening of the hallux is minimal and metatarsus primus varus is overcome when a hallux valgus is present. Full function of the first metatarsophalangeal joint is maintained because the intrinsic structures are left intact.[14]

Technique. Make a longitudinal incision approximately 6 cm long medial to the extensor hallucis longus. The incision extends from midshaft of the hallux's proximal phalanx to just behind the head of the first metatarsal. This incision is carried deep through the fascial layers to the capsule both medial and lateral to these fascial structures.

The capsule is opened with a longitudinal incision extending from the metatarsophalangeal joint to just behind the head of the metatarsal. The head of the metatarsal is freed with care from the surrounding capsular structures completely enough so that the head can be retracted free from the wound.

The medial prominence of the head is excised with a mallet and osteotome if a hallux valgus is present. A dorsal cut is made on the bone with a mallet and osteotome extending dorsally downward at approximately a 45° angle. The dorsal cut extends to the articular margin of cartilage on the plantar surface of the metatarsal head. Nearly 1 cm of space should be left between the cut metatarsal head and the articular surface of the base of the proximal phalanx.

The exposed area of bone left after excision is denuded of any sharp edges and rasped smooth. Care should be made to leave the articular surface of the base of the phalanx alone. Any lipping on the dorsum or sides of the base of the phalanx may be removed.

At this time, the hallux should be dorsiflexed 90 degrees. Any limitations of movement should be evaluated and corrected at this time. If a hallux valgus is present, it may be necessary to do a Z-plasty to the extensor hallucis longus to prevent the proximal phalanx from drifting into a valgus position again.

The joint capsule is then closed with 3–0 chromic catgut sutures. Subcutaneous tissue is closed with 4–0 plain catgut. The skin is closed with nonabsorbable sutures and a sterile compression dressing is applied, with the toe maintained in a corrected position.

Postoperative care. Postoperative care consists of letting the patient ambulate with a Reese shoe within 36 hours. Sutures should be left in approximately ten days to two weeks. Physical therapy must be given soon after suture removal to retain motion of the first metatarsophalangeal joint. Patients may return to foot gear two days following suture removal with appropriate splinting. The patient may return to work in four to six weeks.

Tarsal Conditions

Heel Spur (Inferior Calcaneal Spur; Calcaneal Exostosis)

Description. A heel spur is an osteophytic outgrowth just anterior to the tubercle of the calcaneus. The mass extends over the entire width of the tuberosity. It is approximately 2 cm wide with its apex in the plantar fascia.

Etiology. The exact cause is unknown, but heel spur is probably due to mechanical trauma and stress. The condition often is associated with weakfoot or strainfoot. Patients standing or working on concrete floors often develop this condition.

Occurrence. Heel spur is found most commonly in middle age (40 to 60 years). It is more prevalent in females (often concomitant with menopause), but it is also seen in males. It is seen most frequently in obese persons, and it is often unilateral.

Anatomy. The plantar fascia arises from the plantar surface of the calcaneus and the area immediately above it. The area of attachment, over the medial and lateral tubercles, is about 2 cm wide and $1/2$ cm thick. From its origin, the plantar fascia fans out over the entire plantar surface of the foot and inserts into or blends with the soft tissues of the five metatarsal heads. The plantar fascia acts as a bowstring to the longitudinal arch. Therefore, excessive strain will be absorbed by the origin of the fascia. This strain will gradually tend to induce osteophytic proliferation, ultimately producing a characteristic spur. The plantar fascia resembles a trapezoid; the spur resembles a wedge.

Pathology. The earliest change is mild chronic inflammation, with or without pain. As the condition advances, osteophytic changes take place in the sulcus anterior to the tuberosity. The accumulation of bone is self-limiting and the final spur may vary greatly in size and shape, the most common shape being a triangular block.

Types: (1) those which are *massive* in size but *asymptomatic* because the angle of growth is on a plane with the plantar fascia: these often are discovered inadvertently; (2) those which are *massive* in size and *symptomatic:* they are painful because angle of gravity crosses the plane of the plantar fascia; (3) *acute pain,* but *no visible spur* ascertainable in a radiograph.

Symptoms and Signs. The patients state that they have excruciating pain when they get up in the morning, and again late in the afternoon. The onset is usually insidious and if untreated the heel may be painful for years. The patients usually exhibit: (1) pinpoint *pain* and tenderness under the heel at the area of the *medial tubercle;* (2) mild *discomfort* and tenderness in the *arch;* (3) mild *discomfort* and tenderness in the medial side of the heel *up to the ankle.* When the condition is treated, the heel gets better first, but there still will be mild pain in the arch and ankle for some time. Infrequently, bursitis develops deep to the plantar fascia, simulating heel spur symtoms.

Palliative Treatment. 1. *Removal of stress* or weight on the heel. Fitting proper shoes, e.g., laced oxfords with wide Thomas heels.

2. *Elevation of heels* adds to relief pattern: (a) insertion of felt or sponge *heel lifts* in shoes; (b) wearing of shoe types which have *raised* heels, e.g., cowboy boots or lumberjack boots.

3. Injection techniques. (a) *Posterior tibial block* (Fig. 22–11) breaks the pain cycle, and permits painless injection of steroids. (b) Inject *steroids* directly into central pain area.

4. Physical therapy: (a) whirlpool baths; (b) diathermy; (c) ultra-sound radiation; (d) paraffin baths.

Surgery. Many authorities believe that there is no need for corrective surgery as results may be obtained palliatively. If symptoms persist following conservative management, excision of the spur and plantar fasciotomy is indicated.

Haglund's Disease (Albert's Disease, "Pump Bump")

Description and Discussion. Haglund's Disease is a protuberance of the posterior-superior surface (usually the fibular aspect) of the calcaneus. It usually occurs in young girls (ages 14–21) when they start to wear high heels (Fig. 22–12).

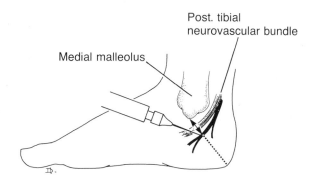

Post. tibial
neurovascular bundle

Medial malleolus

Figure 22–11 Posterior tibial nerve block. Injection site is identified 4 cm postero-inferior to medial malleolus, on the line between medial malleolus and posterior projection of heel. Usual volume required is 5–10 ml 1 per cent lidocaine. Hyperemia of the sole is present when anesthesia is obtained.

Symptoms and Signs. 1. *Callus* at the posterior-lateral aspect of calcaneous. 2. *Pain* over heel cord. 3. Occasional *sinus tract.* 4. Retrocalcaneal *bursitis.*

Treatment, Conservative. (a) *Pad* the foot and later pad the counter of the shoe. (b) Employ a heel lift. (c) *Use physiotherapy.* (d) *Steroid injections.*

Surgical Treatment. With the patient prone, the bursa and the protruding bone

are removed carefully, so as not to sever the sural nerve. A posterior splint is applied with the foot in plantar flexion.

CONGENITAL CONDITIONS

Hammertoe

Definition

Hammertoe is a contraction type of toe deformity in which one or more bones of a toe are subluxated or ankylosed, resulting in limited motion.

Etiology

Static Deformities. Hammertoes often were originally long flaccid toes confined in short fitting shoes. This condition may also be caused by an imbalance in the intrinsic musculature of the foot.

Systemic Diseases. Other forms of muscular imbalance may result from high fever, such as scarlet fever or measles.

Congenital Types. These are usually multiple and are associated with different types of talipes equinus or pes cavus.

Post Poliomyelitis. This type usually involves paralysis following poliomyelitis. The digital deformities usually are multiple and there is a pathological contracture.

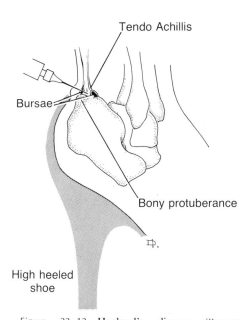

Tendo Achillis

Bursae

Bony protuberance

High heeled shoe

Figure 22–12 Haglund's disease ("pump bump"). Bony protuberance develops on postero-superior aspect of calcaneus in young women wearing high heeled shoes. Treatment is by injection therapy (as shown), or resection of bursae and the protuberance (see text).

Great Toe. When the great toe is involved, it is usually the result of muscular imbalance or high fever.

Anatomy

Great Toe. The head of the proximal phalanx is displaced dorsally and the inferior surface lies immediately above the head of the metatarsal. The dorsal capsule of the interphalangeal is stretched and the plantar capsule is contracted. The extensor hallucis longus is also contracted (Fig. 22–13).

Three Lesser Toes (Middle). There are three types affecting the lesser toes:

1. The *proximal phalanx is dorsiflexed* with the head dislocated dorsally in 90 per cent of the lesser toe hammertoes. The middle phalanx plantar-flexes and the distal phalanx extends.

2. *Double contraction* occurs in 5 per cent of lesser hammertoes conditions, with dorsal dislocation of the head of the proximal phalanx and a dorsal dislocation of the head of the middle phalanx.

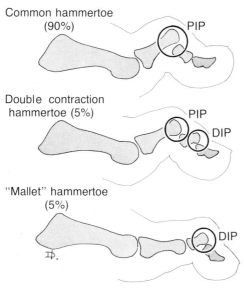

Figure 22–13 Hammertoe pathology. The three types of hammertoes are shown: The most common type, dislocation of proximal joint, occurs in 90 per cent of patients. The double contraction and mallet toe deformities each occur in 5 per cent of patients.

Common hammertoe (90%) — PIP

Double contraction hammertoe (5%) — PIP, DIP

"Mallet" hammertoe (5%) — DIP

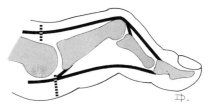

Figure 22–14 Hammertoe correction by tenotomy. Digital arthroplasty is the preferred technique (Fig. 22–3), but an alternate technique for congenital hammertoes is tenotomy, shown here. Extensor and flexor tendons are divided at the locations illustrated. The toe is manipulated dorsally into normal alignment and splinted to the adjacent digit with tape.

3. *Mallet toe* occurs in 5 per cent of the lesser toe deformities. In this condition, the proximal interphalangeal joint is not misaligned, but the distal interphalangeal joint has a dorsal dislocation on the head of the middle phalanx.

4. *Treatment.* Digital arthroplasty is the procedure of choice (Fig. 22–3). Whenever a joint has had both articulating surfaces removed and the raw surfaces come in contact, they eventually will fuse if motion is eliminated. If motion is not eliminated, pain and fibrosis will result. Therefore, at least one surface must be capped or replaced with an artifical surface of the same type of soft tissue in the interspace to maintain the integrity of a functional joint. It is better to preserve at least one surface, leaving the articular surface intact. One preserved surface will permit function of that joint. Nearly all lesser hammertoe surgery can be done effectively by this method.

An alternative method in congenital hammertoe deformity with good functional joints is the tenotomy procedure shown in Figure 22–14.

Overlapping Toes

A condition in which one toe lies on the dorsum of an adjacent toe. Most common is the fifth over the fourth. The second most common type involves the second toe over the first.

Fifth Overlapping Toe

This type is usually due to a congenital deformity or a flaccid type foot, in which there is a short extensor tendon, skin shortening and a contracted dorsal capsule.

Treatment. Conservative treatment consists of teaching the parent or child to tape the toe down or attaching an elastic sling from the toe to the heel. This therapy usually has to be started immediately after birth in order to be effective. Surgical treatment (Fig. 22–15) utilizes a Z-lengthening of the skin, in which the interphalangeal web is incised, followed by a tenotomy and capsulotomy. Suturing is performed in a plantar flexed position.

Second Overlapping Toe

The second toe usually overlaps the first toe as the direct result of hallux valgus. Sometimes the condition may be due to a long second toe. Often there is a partial or complete dislocation at the metatarsophalangeal joint. Short shoes are a contributing factor. Of all the joints in the foot, the second metatarsophalangeal joint exhibits the greatest frequency of dislocation, occurring most commonly with a second hammertoe.

Treatment: When associated with hallux valgus, the hallux valgus must be reduced at the same time. When overlapping is not associated with hallux valgus, a simple tenotomy and capsulotomy will resolve the condition. The procedure should be followed by eight weeks of splinting the toe in a plantar flexed position with a rubber digital prosthesis.

Webbed Toes

A congenital deformity in which the toes are joined together at the web space of the digit. Webbed toes are rarely symptomatic and surgical treatment is performed only for cosmetic reasons.

TRAUMATIC CONDITIONS

Dislocation

Dislocation is a displacement or disruption of the opposing articular surfaces comprising any joint. Subluxation implies a partial or incomplete displacement or disruption of a joint.

Dislocation of some bones and joints of the foot and ankle occur with greater frequency. Some talar bones and proximal phalanges dislocate quite frequently. Specifically, injury to the ankle joint causing an inversion sprain reveals a wide ankle mortice as well as a wide rotation or dislocation.

Treatment of choice consists of either employment of a short leg walking cast or injection therapy followed by a Gibney boot strapping or Unna's paste boot.

Dislocations are common in the proximal phalangeal area and are frequently seen on an outpatient basis. These are usually due to bedroom accidents and there is usually an associated fracture.

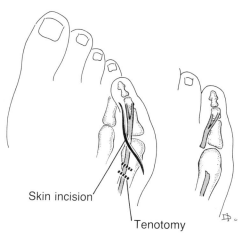

Skin incision

Tenotomy

Figure 22–15 Overlapping toes. Fifth overlapping toe is treated as shown here. A dorsal Z-incision is made. The interphalangeal web is then incised. The extensor tendon is divided and the joint capsule relaxed by a dorsal incision. The toe is sutured in a plantar-flexed position. The operation for uncomplicated second overlapping toe requires only tenotomy and capsulotomy.

Simple taping to the adjacent toe provides sufficient immobilization to insure satisfactory healing of the fracture.

Fractures (See Chapter 11)

Infection

When infections occur in the foot, they are usually devastating, since the foot is difficult to keep clean. Infection poses a constant threat in any injury where the skin has been broken. If the injury has been sustained in an area where there is fertilizer, dirt, rust or fecal bacteria, a full regimen of tetanus therapy must be instituted. The wound must be thoroughly lavaged and cleansed, followed by swabbing with a halogen compound. The wound should be left open to prevent anaerobic bacteria from producing gas gangrene.

When there is no possibility that the skin was exposed to anaerobic bacteria, any broad-spectrum antibiotic may be administered to control impending infection after the wound has been cleansed and the devitalized tissues have been debrided.[24]

Bunnell's solution is an excellent topical treatment for chronic, recalcitrant foot infections. It may be prepared by the pharmacy by mixing. See solution at bottom of this page.

After Bunnell's solution is applied topically, the wound is dressed with sterile gauze and wrapped in polyethylene film such as a plastic "Baggie." The gauze is then moistened and the plastic wrap closed. The principle is to collect body heat, localize the inflammation, and reduce swelling. The dressing should be removed after 48 hours to check for excessive maceration.

Edema

Edema occurs as the result of extravasation of tissue fluids, blood or lymph when trauma has occurred to the tissues.

Whenever bleeding occurs, it is vital to arrest it, but only minimal compression should be employed. If a hematoma develops, aspiration or incision and drainage may be necessary. Simple elevation may permit the lymphatics to drain normally.

Edema in the foot may also be a sign of cardiovascular, hepatic or renal disease. Edema may be the result of obstruction to lymphatic or venous drainage in the leg or abdomen. If no local cause for edema is apparent, consultation with an internist is advisable.

BENIGN SOFT TISSUE TUMORS OF THE FOOT

Lipoma

Lipoma is an abnormal deposit of fatty tissue which may be found in the foot and ankle. It usually occurs as a circumscribed lobulated mass, but may arise where fat does not normally occur. It may appear beneath fascia and periosteum as well as in muscles and joints. A lipoma may also be found in the subcutaneous tissue as a soft, movable mass. Lipomas may be single or multiple. Treatment consists of surgical excision with linear closure.

Ganglion

Ganglionic cysts apparently arise from degeneration in the connective tissue outside of the joints.[11] These lesions are

Benzalkonium chloride	17%	11.8 cc (1:2000)
Acetic acid	36%	56.8 cc
Glycerin		800.0 cc
Distilled	Small qsad 7.0 gallons	
Tint dark pink with 100 mg D + C Red #59 (dissolve D + C Red #30 in Glycerin)		

benign. A ganglion presents as a lobular mass over a joint capsule or tendon sheath, often over a bony prominence, and it contains colorless or strawcolored gelatinous material.[5]

Conservative treatment by aspiration of the cavity gives only temporary relief. The cavity usually refills in a few days. Surgical treatment is the preferred therapy. Complete excision of the mass should be performed.

Morton's Metatarsal Neuroma (Plantar Interdigital Neurofibroma; Perineurofibroma; Morton's Metatarsalgia)

Morton's neuroma is an entrapment of an interdigital nerve. It is most commonly found where the interdigital nerve branches into the contiguous compartments of the digits, most often the third interspace (between the third and fourth toes).

Lasker (1970)[12] observed that the condition was most common in middle-aged women. Neuritic pain radiates from the area of the metatarsal heads into the toes. Pain initially occurs only on weight bearing, but later occurs even at rest. A desire to remove the shoe and massage the foot suggests the diagnosis of neuroma. The major differential diagnosis is metatarsalgia, which causes pain at the plantar aspect of the metatarsal heads. Morton's neuroma causes pain during lateral pressure on the metatarsal heads. If a neuroma is present, it will be compressed against the adjacent metatarsals by pressing against the web space with a pen, thus eliciting pain. Neuroma may also produce numbness or cramping of the contiguous toes.

Treatment. Conservative treatment consists of steroid injections, (1 cc Xylocaine and 1 cc Decadron), for temporary relief of symptoms, and metatarsal pads to redistribute weight bearing.

Surgical treatment is the preferred method. (Fig. 22–16) A 4 cm linear incision is made on the dorsal or plantar aspect of the foot between the metatarsal rays of the third and fourth metatarsals,

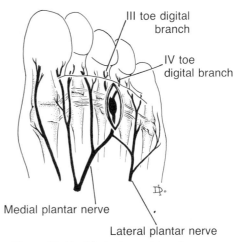

III toe digital branch

IV toe digital branch

Medial plantar nerve

Lateral plantar nerve

Figure 22–16 Morton's metatarsal neuroma. The tender neuroma between metatarsal rays III and IV is excised through a 4 cm incision on dorsal or plantar aspect of the foot.

extending distally between the metatarsal heads. Sharp and blunt dissection is carried down between the metatarsal heads, at which time the tumor becomes visible, bulging into the wound. The neuroma is then grasped with a tenaculum and excised. The proximal nerve trunk is cauterized with 88 per cent phenol. The wound is closed in layers and covered with a nonpressure sterile dressing. Ambulation is begun in a Reese postoperative shoe immediately.

Plantar Warts (Verrucae Plantaris)

Verrucae plantaris are benign lesions of the papillary layer of the skin caused by a filterable virus that is autoinoculable and quite contagious. Infection of several members of a family is not uncommon.

Verrucae vary widely in their clinical course. A single lesion may appear and persist relatively unchanged for many years. However, one single lesion may be followed by the development of satellite verrucae. The mode of spreading may be minor injuries or breaks in the skin of the sole of the foot.

Diagnosis. Verrucae located on the dorsum of the foot present a more spongy consistency, while those on the plantar aspect have a thin layer of callous tissue covering them. They are not necessarily found on weight bearing areas and they occur in both children and adults. The verrucae are exquisitely tender on lateral compression and they bleed profusely when debrided. Verrucae have an affinity for the foot, since it is usually enclosed in a dark, damp shoe. This alkaline, moist environment seems most conducive to growth.

Treatment. There are approximately twenty different treatments for warts, none being entirely satisfactory. Therapeutic modalities vary from suggestion therapy to surgical excision.

Verrucae may respond well to escarotics, e.g., salicylic acid, 88 per cent phenol, sulfuric or nitric acid, or repeated applications of silver nitrate.

Dry ice "snow" (CO_2) and liquid nitrogen have been employed with moderate to good results. Fulguration and desiccation have been used in some cases, but the lesion must then be padded with felt until it has healed.

Our preferred method of treatment for the solitary verruca is enucleation of the diseased tissue under local anesthesia. (Fig. 22–17) The area is anesthetized by block or field anesthesia. The lesion is removed in toto by blunt dissection with a currette-scoop, without traumatizing healthy tissue. This is followed by hyfercation of the base and periphery of the lesion. Aperture padding is employed to take pressure off weight bearing areas.

Complications. The most frequent complication of therapy for verrucae is recurrence. After removal and healing, the patient should be instructed in proper foot hygiene. It is our opinion that verrucae should never be surgically excised by sharp dissection from the plantar aspect of the foot as the resultant scar presents more of a problem than the original lesion.

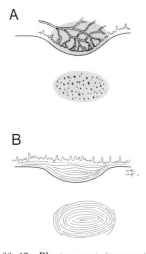

Figure 22–17 Plantar wart (verruca). Plantar wart *(A)* has a thin layer of callus, underneath which is a rich blood supply identified by multiple tiny blood vessel endings which can be seen when callus is removed. A keratoma or plantar callus *(B)* differs from a verruca in having a thick layer of keratin and no abnormal vascularity.

Treatment of a plantar wart is enucleation of the diseased tissue (shaded area) by blunt dissection under local anesthesia. The base and sides of the residual cavity are hyfercated to coagulate the blood vessels.

METABOLIC DISORDERS

Diabetes

The foot is frequently the first place where the objective and subjective signs of diabetes mellitus may be observed.

Diabetics have a well-known propensity toward development of arteriosclerotic peripheral vascular disease, often at a much earlier age than members of the normal population. There are definite subjective and objective pathological changes resulting from insufficient arterial blood supply to the feet and legs. Trophic and ulcerative changes in the lower extremities occur with greater frequency in diabetics because of their tendency to develop peripheral neuritis. A careful examination obviously is important in any patient who presents with neurological findings, or the absence of pain when his feet are injured, such as by a nail protruding from the sole of his shoe. Damage to the skin and subcutaneous tissue may be unnoticed by a diabetic until a trophic ulcer has developed.

Preventive Measures. Proper care of the feet is of the utmost importance to diabetics. Since their condition often reduces the blood supply to the feet, they are more likely than others to develop foot disorders. However, many major foot problems can be avoided. The following instructions should be given to any diabetic patient with foot problems:

Corns and Calluses. Both corns and calluses are caused by the building up of hard skin at points where shoes cause pressure. In general, they should be treated gently with a fine emery board or pumice stone. Consult your physician or podiatrist.

Bathing. Bathe your feet daily in lukewarm (not hot) water, using a mild soap. After thorough rinsing, dry them gently; use a soft towel and a "blotting" technique. Pay special attention to the skin between the toes. If your feet are rough or dry, rub them gently with a moisture restoring cream or lotion. If your feet sweat excessively, rub them gently with alcohol and dust them with foot powder.

Socks. Heavy cotton or wool socks (or stockings) are recommended. They should be of the correct size and need to be free of seams and darns. To ensure cleanliness, it is important to change your socks every day. Loose woolen socks may be worn at night to keep your feet warm.

Exercise. Walking is the best exercise for your feet. Your doctor may advise special exercise.

Shoes. Soft, leather oxford shoes are recommended for daily wear. Shoes should have a leather sole, a flat low heel, and should conform to the shape of your foot. New shoes need to be worn for short periods during the first week of wear (for example, two hours daily). Casual shoes should be worn for short periods. All shoe corrections should be done on the advice of your physician or your podiatrist.

Toenails. Trim or file your toenails straight across so that they are even with the skin on the ends of your toes. A coarse metal file with a blunt tip is a satisfactory instrument to use. (A nail clipper may be used.)

Inspection. Inspect your feet every day. If you notice any redness, swelling, cracks in the skin, or sores, consult your physician or your podiatrist.*

---

*Reprinted from: U. S. Department of Health, Education and Welfare-Public Health Service, Division of Chronic Diseases, Diabetes and Arthritis Program, Washington, D. C. 20201

Ulcers of the Foot in Diabetics

One of the more common findings in diabetics is the formation of ulcers of the foot. The most frequent site is the plantar surface, usually under a metatarsal head. The ulcer is usually of long standing duration and if gently pressed will demonstrate a purulent discharge. The ulcer is always surrounded by a heavy, tough, callus.

Pressure is believed to be an important factor in diabetic ulcers of the feet. The failure to heal properly is probably due to a vascular defect rather than abnormal sugar metabolism.[13]

Treatment. Débridement of necrotic tissue is carried out after aseptic prepping. More complete drainage is established, followed by accomodative padding and topical proteolytic enzyme therapy. A felt pressure pad aperture dressing is used to accommodate the lesion (Fig. 22–18).

Gout

The usual presentation of gouty arthritis is a painful, tender, reddened great toe. There is usually no history of direct trauma and infection is not present. The pain is severe in the morning as well as in the afternoon, in contrast to osteoarthritis, in which pain is worsened by the activities of the day. Diagnosis is made by the finding of elevation in serum uric acid. The disease is differentiated by blood tests from diabetes and rheumatoid arthritis. Blood sugar and serology for rheumatoid factor should therefore also be obtained when patients present with a painful erythematous toe.

We believe that the systemic treatment of gout, diabetes and rheumatoid arthritis is best performed by an internist, and we limit our treatment for these conditions to management of the local problems in the foot.

Treatment of the painful toe consists of relieving pressure on the first metatarsal head by fabrication of an accommodative orthotic inlay which the patient may transfer from shoe to shoe. Wedging of the shoe can be performed if neces-

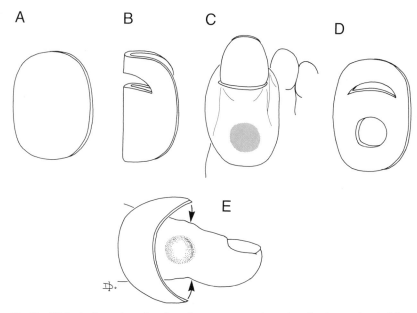

Figure 22-18 Diabetic foot ulcer dressing. A pressure aperture dressing is constructed from felt *(A)* as shown. A slit is made *(B)*, through which the toe is inserted *(C)*. The area of the ulcer, which is usually on the ventral aspect of the metatarsal head, is marked on the pad. The pad is removed and an aperture is cut out *(D)*. The pad is then placed again on the toe.

For lateral ulcers, the same technique is used, except that the pad is rotated 90° and the toe slit is proximal rather than distal *(E)*.

sary, in cases when the patient is not improved sufficiently by the accommodative inlay. Wedging is considerably more expensive, since each pair of shoes must be wedged to be effective.

References

1. Amberry, T. R.: Foot surgery. In Weinstein, F.: Principles and Practice of Podiatry. Philadelphia, Lea and Febiger, 1968.
2. Ashur, M. E.: Onychology. In Weinstein, F.: Principles and Practice of Podiatry. Philadelphia, Lea and Febiger, 1968.
3. Burleson, T.: Glomus tumor. Okla. Podiatry, 4:5, 1964.
4. Davidson, M. R.: A simple method for correcting second, third, and fourth plantar metatarsal head pathology. J. Foot Surg., 8, Nov. 4, 1969.
5. Duvries, H. L. (Ed.): Disorders of synovia and fascia. In Surgery of the Foot. St. Louis, C. V. Mosby Co., 1959. pp. 231–232.
6. Frost, L.: Onychomycosis—treatment by avulsion and onychophytax. J. Amer. Podiat. Assoc., 50:283–287, 1960.
7. Frost, L.: Root resection for incurvated nail. J. Nat. Assoc. Chiropody, 40:19, 1950.
8. Frost, L.: Atraumatic nail avulsion with a novel ungual elevator. J. Amer. Podiat. Assoc., 48:51, 1958.
9. Frost, L.: A treatment for paronychia with concomitant onychocryptosis. J. Amer. Podiat. Assoc., 49:197–201, 1959.
10. Giannestras, N. J.: Foot Disorders; Medical and Surgical Management. Philadelphia, Lea and Febinger, 1967. p. 309.
11. King, E. S. J.: Pathology of ganglion. Austral. and New Z. J. Surg., 1:367–381, 1932.
12. Lasker, A. S.: Intermetatarsal neuroma. Curr. Podiat., 19: March, 1970.
13. Lewis, M. R.: The diabetic foot. In Atlas of Foot Roentgenology. Chicago, Edwards Bros., 1964. p. 43.
14. Macdonald, R. G.: The Stone procedure. Hopedale Medical Complex Podiatry Staff, 4th Annual Surgical Seminar Manual—A Case Report. Hopedale, Ill., 1971.
15. McGlamry, E. D., and Feldman, M. H.: A treatise on the McBride procedure. J. Amer. Podiat. Assoc., 61:170–171, 1971.
16. Ney, G. C.: An operation for ingrown toenails. J.A.M.A., 80:374, 1923.
17. Pillsbury, D. M., Shelley, W. B., and Kligman, A. M.: Dermatology. Philadelphia, W. B. Saunders Co., 1956. pp. 631–635.

18. Podell, R. N.: Issues in the organization of medical care; an illustrative care study-podiatry in the United States. N. Eng. J. Med., *284*:586–589, 1971.

19. Riehl, G. Griseofulvin. Presented at a meeting of the Australia Dermatology Society, Vienna, November 27, 1958.

20. Ross, W. R.: Treatment of ingrown toenails and a new anesthetic method: Surg. Clin. N. Amer., *49*:1499–1504, 1969.

21. Sloan, A. J.: The importance of laboratory examination in a cutaneous disease of the feet. Curr. Podiat., *4*:16, 1955.

22. Steinberg, M. O.: Case report on 24 cases of glomus tumor. J. Podiat., *17*:18–19, 1956.

23. United States Department of Health, Education and Welfare—Public Health Service, Division of Chronic Diseases, Diabetes and Arthritis Program, Washington, D. C. 20201.

24. Weinstein, F. R.: Fractures and dislocations of the foot and ankle. In Weinstein, F. (ed.): Principles and Practice of Podiatry. Philadelphia, Lea and Febiger, 1968.

25. Winograd, A. M.: Modification in technique of operation for ingrown toenail. J.A.M.A. *92*:229, 1929.

23

Pediatric Surgery

By JOHN D. BURRINGTON, M.D.

GENERAL APPROACH

The initial contact between physician and child often determines the magnitude of a surgical procedure which the patient will tolerate as an outpatient.[9,10] If the child is frightened and hurt during the initial examination, much time will be lost in evaluating his problem and the valuable initial rapport may not be achieved. One effective method of contacting the child is through the parent or adult accompanying him to the Emergency Ward. A few words to the parents establishes the exact time and nature of the injury as well as the duration of his symptoms and the status of the child's immunizations. Most important, it indicates to the child that you are a friend who is accepted by the parent. He follows the questions carefully, and once he senses that you are a friend interested in his injury, he will let you examine him. The physician who bursts into the examining room and attempts to overwhelm the child with attention may be greeted by shrieks and complete withdrawal.

Detailed sensory examinations are difficult in an injured child under four or five years of age. However, a very adequate motor examination can be given utilizing the child's natural tendency to reach for shiny or desirable objects and his willingness to play simple games, such as holding a file card between various fingers or wiggling his digits on command. Try it with the normal hand first, and then switch to the injured side.

Immunization

Most children over one year of age brought to an Outpatient Department have had their basic immunization against tetanus. If they have had one or more of their D.P.T. immunizations, a single booster of 0.5 ml of tetanus toxoid should establish adequate immunization.[5] It is superfluous to give an additional injection to a child who has completed his basic immunization and has had a booster shot within three years. If an unimmunized child suffers a burn, a penetrating or crushing injury, or is injured in an area frequented by farm animals, he should receive 1 cc of human hyperimmune globulin. After the lesion has healed, the child must then receive full, active immunization. In all cases where an injection is required, it should be administered after débridement, repair and bandaging are complete. By then the child realizes that you are helping him and often accepts the injection stoically.

Restraint

Whenever possible the nurse who will assist in the outpatient procedure should be introduced to the child and his parents simultaneously. An understanding nurse experienced in working with injured children can be of immeasurable help in getting the child to cooperate. However, virtually all children under eighteen months of age and many children under three years of age require some form of restraint during a surgical procedure or an uncomfortable examination. Wrap-

ping the child with a folded sheet (Fig. 23–1) is usually much more successful than trying to utilize any sort of straps or other standard restraints (Fig. 23–2). While we all abhor physical restraint of a child, I believe it is often misplaced kindness to leave the child unrestrained. His wiggling may prevent complete débridement and cleansing of the wound and compromise the meticulous closure necessary for a good cosmetic result.

For facial lacerations, I prefer to have the extremities immobilized in a folded sheet and then have a nurse complete the immobilization by holding gently but firmly along the sides of his head. The emotional scars from such restraint are far less than those left by an unsightly scar or mismatched vermillion border that can result from inadequate restraint.

Local Anesthesia

A few drops of local anesthetic dripped directly into an open wound renders the margins sufficiently anesthetic so that the remainder of the infiltration can be carried out through the edges of the wound. While it is theoretically undesirable to inject clean tissue through a contaminated area, the degree to which the surrounding skin can be cleansed in the presence of an unanesthetized wound probably renders it not much cleaner than the wound itself. When injecting local anesthetic, it is most important to inject slowly through a 25 gauge needle since rapid injection distends the tissue and causes local pain. In most cases local anesthetic with dilute epinephrine can be used safely in children to aid hemostasis, although it is rarely necessary except in procedures about the face and mouth.

BURNS

The vast majority of thermal burns in children can be treated in the Outpatient

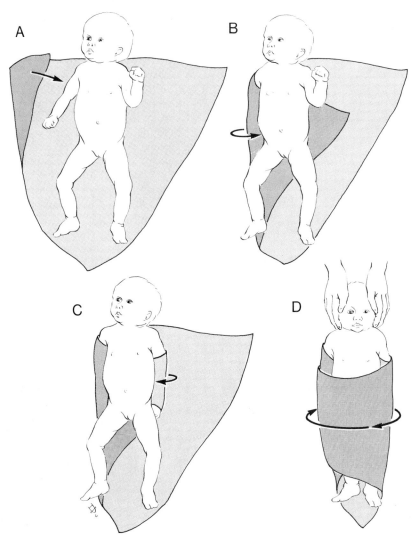

Figure 23–1 Restraint with a folded sheet. *A.* In wrapping the child for restraint it is important to have the sheet or towel large enough to restrain the infant from feet to shoulders. A bed sheet folded as illustrated is preferable. *B.* The first fold goes over the arm, under the body and then, *C,* over the opposite arm and back under the body. *D.* The opposite flap then completely encircles the child and is wrapped snugly to keep him from kicking his feet or legs. A single piece of tape may be necessary to keep the wrapping intact during a prolonged procedure. When working on the face, it is helpful to have an assistant hold the child's head gently as illustrated.

Department.[8] Any burn is a very painful and frightening episode for a child, and if he can be spared the additional experience of a hospital admission, so much the better. Also, the problems with cross infection that are inevitable in any hospital ward are much less likely to occur at home. I have found that most

mothers are capable of doing excellent dressing changes and even local débridement if they are properly instructed and encouraged.

Hot water burns or scalds are the most common burns sustained from infancy through age four or five. Typically, these accidents involve a cup of coffee

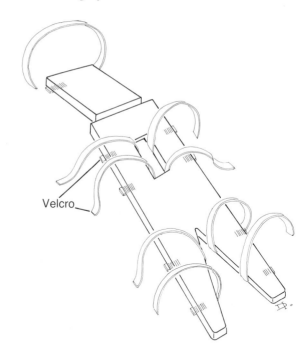

Figure 23–2 Restraint board. This is one of many types of board suitable for restraint. They are excellent for circumcisions or suturing lacerations on the trunk or thighs. They are, however, not suitable for lacerations on the hands, feet or face.

Velcro

or soup being spilled down the child's face, shoulder and arm. This type of burn is usually a second degree and heals very nicely without scarring if kept clean. Initial treatment should consist of a gentle cleansing with a dilute solution of pHisoHex to insure that all food particles, grease and foreign matter are gently removed. Second degree burns on the trunk and extremities are best covered with Vaseline gauze, Furacin gauze or some similar bland dressing. Vaseline gauze should be prepared with a small amount of Vaseline in a coarse-meshed gauze. The interstices of the gauze between the fibers must not be occluded with Vaseline so that if blisters drain, the fluid can seep into the dressing applied over the Vaseline gauze. These dressings must be sufficiently bulky and absorbent to accommodate all serum draining from the burn since an occlusive dressing or a nonabsorbent dressing allows the moist serum to stay in contact with the burn and provides an ideal culture medium for all bacteria, especially Pseudomonas.

Burned portions of the ears, face and neck should be covered with a bland, water-soluble ointment after the initial cleansing has been completed. The extremities and trunk must have a bulky and absorbent dry dressing applied which can be held in place with an Ace bandage or Kerlix dressing. This keeps the burned area clean and also prevents the child from picking at the easily infected areas. For the first 24 hours the diet should be restricted to fluids and bland foods since the fear, pain and crying accompanying the burn lead to aerophagia and resultant anorexia or vomiting.

The initial dressing should be performed by a physician with the parents watching so that they can do subsequent dressing changes at home. The child can then be seen at two to three day intervals or until a dry crust has formed over the burned area. Then only a bulky, dry dressing need be applied to protect the healing area from further trauma. If there appears to be any pus underneath the eschars or crusts, these areas must be debrided and cultured.

Children from ages four to six or

seven are particularly susceptible to flame burns when their pajamas or light clothing ignite. Often these burns are limited to one flank, the axilla, and shoulder. If the areas are quite clearly third degree and constitute less than ten per cent of the surface area, the child is an excellent candidate for admission and for early excision and grafting. If only portions of the burned area appear to be third degree, these can be managed in the Outpatient Department until the granulating bed is ready for skin grafting. The hard eschars of the third degree burn can be debrided at home in the bathtub in a solution of two cups table salt in a full tub of warm water. When the granulating bed is suitably clean, the child can be admitted to the hospital for a short time until grafting is complete.

Electrical burns in childhood are almost exclusively limited to the mouth (Fig. 23–3). Curious toddlers bite into

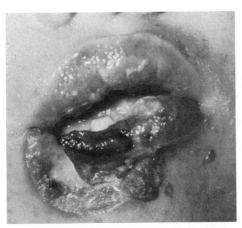

Figure 23–3 Electrical burn of the mouth. This is the appearance of a 13 month old boy who bit into an electrical cord. The current coagulated a large portion of his lower lip and alveolar ridge. The child when first seen may have only a small blister on the lip and a peculiar pallor on the adjacent skin. Electrical burns are always much more extensive than they first appear. Initially, the child may have difficulty with alimentation and drooling from the corner of his mouth. At about 8 to 10 days when the coagulum sloughs, he may bleed from the limbal artery of his lip. All such lesions should be allowed to heal spontaneously and then revised one to two years later if the scar interferes with alimentation.

electrical cords, or careless parents leave the charged male end of an extension cord within the child's reach.[1] Although electrical burns can cause devastating cosmetic problems, they rarely pose any immediate threat to the child's life. The electrical circuit is completed locally in the tissues surrounding the mouth so that the child does not suffer systemic effects from the current. Initial estimation of the tissue destruction can be extremely misleading. Within the first few minutes or hours after the burn is sustained, the child may have only edema and a tiny area of white coagulum on the mucous membranes. Over the next 48 hours the true extent of the tissue destruction becomes apparent, although the devitalized tissue usually does not separate completely until the seventh to tenth day. When this coagulum separates, there may be alarming bleeding from the limbal vessels. A child is often difficult to feed at this stage because his mouth lesion is painful, and the slough from the lower lip may be so great that food and saliva constantly trickle out his mouth. If the parents are reliable and live reasonably close to the hospital. I believe that most of these children can be treated as outpatients for the first five or six days after the burn. Then, however, they must be admitted when the coagulum is about to slough so that bleeding from the raw edges can be controlled by pressure on the limbal vessels or by topical epinephrine solution. During the entire interval between the burn and cicatrization, the child should be kept in a jacket with stiffened sleeves so that he cannot bend his elbow to put his hands or foreign objects into his mouth.

Acid and lye burns are distressingly common, although fortunately most of them do not have serious sequelae. The burns sustained from powdered lye consist of small punctate lesions about the hands and mouth. Flushing with large quantities of water is usually adequate therapy, although many physicians prefer to use vinegar or dilute acetic acid in treating lye burns. This, however, may be painful and extend, rather than curtail, damage to the already injured tissues. Ingestion of powdered lye is not nearly as likely to damage the esophagus as is ingestion of a lye solution. Even the most inquisitive toddler will not put sufficient powdered lye in his mouth to do more than raise some vesicles or areas of white coagulum on the tongue and soft palate. When there is no evidence of injury to the mucous membranes of the pharynx, the child can be sent home as soon as the local hand and oral lesions have been treated. However, if there is reddening or apparent burning of the pharyngeal wall of uvula or if the child was seen to play in a lye solution, he should be admitted immediately and, if possible, induced to swallow a string as a guide for dilators in case later dilations are necessary. If he seems to have excess salivation or appears to be unable or unwilling to swallow, it must be assumed that he has sustained a significant lye burn, and he should be admitted.[11]

Passing a string into the stomach is usually easier than it sounds. Older children can be induced to swallow a string with one or two lead shot attached to the end. Younger children can have the string attached to the end of a nasogastric tube with half a gelatin capsule. After the tip of the tube has been in the stomach for 15 to 20 minutes, the capsule dissolves and the tube can be withdrawn, leaving the weighted string in the stomach.

I have not recently examined any children by esophagoscopy in the acute phase of a lye burn, since the inability of the child to swallow his saliva is adequate indication of an esophageal burn. If the child is esophagoscoped, the scope should never be passed through an area of coagulum or burn. It should be passed only to that level for diagnosis and the child started on steroids and antibiotics.

I personally have never seen a significant burn sustained by ingesting ammonia or any of the standard sodium hypochlorite bleach solutions, and these ingestions require only induced emesis.

LACERATIONS

Lacerations occur predominantly about the toddler's head and face. Because of his large head and unsteady gait, this area absorbs an enormous amount of trauma from the age of about 12 to 36 months. The forehead and lips seem particularly prone to such injuries and are, of course, most likely to develop unsightly scars. Virtually all these can be handled in the Outpatient Department with the toddler wrapped in a sheet and his head gently restrained by an assistant. Since these lacerations are often irregular and have sustained some crushing, the edges must be carefully debrided with iris scissors or a small scalpel blade and closed accurately with 5–0 or 6–0 silk. Rarely is sedation with barbiturates or opiates of much value in treating such lacerations, since doses sufficiently large to render the child somnolent during the procedure induce sedation to such an extent that observation for three or four hours before discharge is usually required. If the facilities are available, a general anesthetic with fluothane is just as quick and often safer than makeshift sedation. Ketalar, given intramuscularly, is also an excellent drug when working around a child's face.

Prepping and draping a child for suture of a facial laceration must be planned so that he does not feel suffocated by the drapes, and, when possible, he should be allowed to look around and see the face of the physician or assistant. Constant verbal reassurance is also very important.

A child's face heals very rapidly if the wounds are properly cleansed and debrided. Early removal of sutures prevents the "cross-hatching" of scars that may ruin an otherwise perfect result.[6] In most instances, one half of the sutures can be removed on the second or third day and the remainder on the fourth or fifth day. If the wound does not appear sufficiently healed to go unsupported, the edges can be reinforced in stages with Steritapes as the sutures are removed. Steritapes are unsatisfactory for preliminary closure of facial lacerations, especially when the child is crying and hot and his skin is moist.

In an older child lacerations tend to occur on the extremities and knees. Whenever possible, the hand or extremity should be examined in the exact position it was in at the time of the injury. This often exposes damaged structures and hidden foreign material not apparent during the initial inspection and cleansing. If there is any question of the laceration involving a tendon, nerve or joint space, the entire repair should be performed in an operating room with the child under general anesthesia or a local block so that the wound can be explored and repaired under optimal conditions. It is often possible to send the child home within several hours after completion of the repair, but a busy Outpatient Department with a wiggling or screaming child is not the place to attempt such delicate procedures.

Many of the childhood injuries involve large areas of abrasions in which gravel or clothing may be deeply imbedded. These wounds can be completely cleansed with sponges moistened with saline or dilute benzalkonium chloride solution. If there still is residual dirt within the wound and the area is not amenable to complete infiltration or a nerve block, it may be necessary to anesthetize the child for complete débridement. Any dirt not removed at this time will become imbedded in the tissues and result in permanant tattooing. Once the débridement is complete, large or deep abrasions should be treated as a second degree burn of equal magnitude.

Intraoral lacerations or lacerations involving the lip and mouth are very common in childhood. The typical intraoral laceration is sustained when the child falls with a ruler, popsicle stick or pencil in his mouth. These lacerations bleed very briskly when they are sustained, although most have stopped by the time they are seen by a physician. Such intraoral lesions usually do not require any suturing and, as with most penetrating injuires, tight closure is con-

traindicated. The exception is the instance when a triangular flap has been raised from the buccal mucosa, tonsillar pillar or mucoperiostium of the palate. These flaps heal as polypoid protrusions of the mucous membrane which are then constantly traumatized by food and chewing. It is usually advisable to tack such a flap down with two or three sutures of chromic catgut. These lacerations should not be closed tightly, and rarely is there any indication to use nonabsorbable suture material.

Tongue lacerations usually result from a fall with the tongue protruding, so that the teeth are driven forcably into it when the mandible strikes the ground. Again, most of these lesions do not require suturing and heal very rapidly on their own. Any flap raised on the top or lateral aspect of the tongue requires closure with buried catgut sutures or complete excision of the flap. When such intraoral lesions are repaired under local anesthesia, the infiltration can be rendered virtually painless by applying a cocaine- or Xylocaine-soaked sponge directly to the surrounding mucosa. The physician who sutures such a laceration without placing a mouth gag or a piece of thick-walled plastic tubing between the molars to prevent the child from biting does so at his own risk. In general, a child under five years of age should have general anesthesia for intraoral surgery.

FOREIGN BODIES

Undoubtedly far more foreign bodies are ingested than ever come to the attention of the parents or physician. Coins are most generally ingested and rarely, if ever, require any therapy. As a general rule, any coin smaller than a quarter passes unimpeded through the gastrointestinal tract of any child old enough to put the object in his mouth. Quarters usually pass without delay in a child two years or over; consequently, I rarely obtain x-rays of such foreign bodies. If the child is eating well, does not have excess salivation indicating esophageal obstruction, and has no evidence of bowel obstruction, the only therapy is to reassure the parents and warn them of the specific symptoms of obstruction.

Sharp objects, including screws, hat-pins, bobby pins and so on, also pass in an astounding number of children without causing any symptoms whatsoever. If there is a fairly clear-cut history of ingestion of a sharp object, I usually obtain a single abdominal x-ray at the time of the first visit. If the foreign body can be seen within the digestive tract, the parents are warned to return immediately should the child develop anorexia, abdominal pain or tenderness, or an unexplained fever. The child is then reexamined every three to four days, and if at the end of a week the object has not passed, I repeat the abdominal x-ray

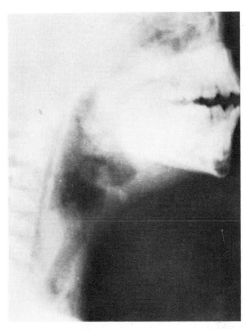

Figure 23–5 Cervical esophagus laceration by goblet fragment. This is a lateral x-ray of the child four hours later. There is considerable free air in the neck and a column of air between the posterior wall of his esophagus and the anterior margin of the spine. He has clinically obvious crepitus in his neck and has sustained a laceration of his cervical esophagus. The glass, however, passed completely unimpeded through the rest of his GI tract.

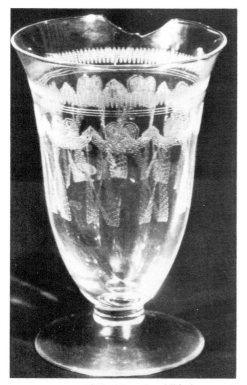

Figure 23–4 Goblet bitten by child. A two year old child bit a large piece of glass from this goblet. He then swallowed the glass fragment intact.

to be sure that the foreign body has moved. Any sharp foreign body remaining in the same position for more than 48 hours usually has impaled the bowel wall and will not progress further. Failure of the pointed foreign object to move, any vomiting, signs of peritonitis, or local irritation are the only indications for surgical removal of a foreign body from a child's digestive tract.

Metallic foreign bodies are often magnetic and can be removed from the stomach by a small round magnet attached to the end of a nasogastric tube. The magnet can be guided to the foreign body under fluroscopic control. With the current trend toward fabricating pins, screws, and other hardware from non-ferrous metal it is helpful if the mother can bring a similar object so that if it proves nonmagnetic, the child can be

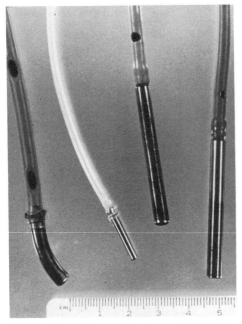

Figure 23–6 Magnets for removal of foreign bodies. These are various magnets available from the V. Mueller Co. (Chicago, Ill.) which have been attached to the ends of nasogastric tubes. They are radiopaque and can be maneuvered under fluoroscopy to remove magnetic foreign bodies from the stomach.

spared the obvious trauma of passing a magnet.

Coins and marbles frequently become lodged in the esophagus, most commonly at the cricopharyngeus, above the aortic arch, or at the cardioesophageal junction. In children with strictures resulting from previous esophageal surgery, peptic esophagitis, or lye ingestion, the foreign body lodges at the level of the stricture.

Marbles are extremely difficult to grasp, but frequently they can be removed with a Fogarty embolectomy catheter. The catheter is passed well beyond the foreign body, the balloon inflated, and then the catheter withdrawn slowly, bringing the marble up into the pharynx where it can be spit out. Coins also can usually be removed by passing a Fogarty or Foley catheter and then inflating the balloon. Under fluoroscopy

it helps to inflate the balloon with contrast material so that it shows up clearly. This is easier and safer than endoscopy and does not require an anesthetic.

Foreign bodies in the tracheobronchial tree are extremely common, and again, they may not come to medical attention until days or weeks after aspiration. The vast majority of nonpointed objects can be recovered by a program of postural drainage and vigorous pulmonary physiotherapy. The child should be admitted to the hospital so that any pointed foreign body can be removed endoscopically.

No foreign body, no matter how benign its appearance, should be left in the tracheobronchial tree for longer than a few days at most, since sepsis distal to the object invariably develops and destroys the pulmonary parenchyma distal to the obstruction.

Aspirated aspirin tablets initiate an especially intense tissue reaction in the tracheobronchial tree. They inevitably fragment as soon as they contact the wet bronchial mucosa so they can rarely be removed intact. All possible fragments should be removed as quickly as possible, and the area should then be washed with copious amounts of sterile 0.9 molar sodium bicarbonate solution. A child often becomes afebrile after aspiration and bronchial lavage and may develop bronchial obstruction secondary to local edema. If this develops, he should be admitted until all atelectasis has resolved. Decadron administered at the time the child is first seen may reduce endobronchial reaction after aspirin aspiration, but this has not been proven.

Around Halloween one is likely to see an epidemic of aspirated beans and split peas coincident with the use of peashooters. Once the dried pea or bean lodges in a bronchus, the bronchial mucosa becomes edematous and entraps the object. It has been stated that dried beans and peas swell in the bronchus, although I have never been impressed by any significant change in the texture of such aspirated beans.

Peanuts and popcorn initiate intense

bronchial reaction, probably in response to salt and vegetable oils covering them, and a child may develop total bronchial obstruction even after the peanut or popcorn has been removed.

If there is an unequivocal history of aspiration and the child is old enough to cooperate, he can usually point to the place where the foreign body is lodged. This is of inestimable help in planning the physiotherapy since it gives a clue as to which bronchus contains the foreign body. Position the child on pillows so that the suspected bronchus is dependent, have him inhale some isoproterenol (a "Medihaler" is very convenient for this), and then have him cough vigorously while his chest wall is percussed rapidly with cupped hands. The isoproterenol reduces the profound bronchoconstriction created by the foreign body in the tracheobronchial tree and aids in clearing the bronchus.

The history of foreign body aspiration can be difficult to document. The child using a pea shooter against his parents' advice or pilfering peanuts from the cupboard may not volunteer this information. In fact, he may not be brought to a physician until he is coughing, wheezing or feverish. Preliminary chest examination may reveal local or generalized wheezing, atelectasis, pneumonia or a combination of all three. Only detailed history and a practice of bronchoscoping all children with localized unresolved pneumonia can lead to a proper diagnosis.

If the child is seen soon after aspiration of a radiolucent foreign object and is too frightened or young to indicate its location, inspiration and expiratory chest x-rays usually aid in locating it. The lung tissue supplied by a partially obstructed bronchus fills more slowly on inspiration and empties more slowly on expiration. On x-ray, then, the obstructed area appears underinflated on inspiration and overinflated on expiration. The mediastinum may shift toward the lesion on inspiration and away from it on expiration.

Beans, dried peas and buttons seem to be favored objects for children to insert in their nose and ears. Most of the foreign objects in the ear can be washed out using a syringe and warm water. Foreign bodies in the nose are best removed under direct vision using topical xylocaine or cocaine to anesthetize the nasal mucosa, although this procedure may require the use of Ketalar or a brief general anesthetic.

I am always amazed at the number of children who step on pins or needles and have the end break off within the foot. If they have been disobeying their parents by going barefoot, they may not reveal the incident until they have a noticeable bump. Removal of such a foreign body is never an emergency and rarely should be attempted under local anesthesia. When a parent or physician calls me about such a child, I arrange to see the child the following morning after he has been fasting for at least five hours. If x-rays confirm the presence of a foreign body, I explore the foot under general anesthesia with x-ray or fluoroscopy available.

The incision should be placed when possible so that the scar will not be on a weight-bearing surface. In the forefoot, the incision is best placed between the metatarsal heads and approximately parallel to the metatarsals.

If I do not find the needle within ten minutes, I insert three No. 25 needles in a circle, all aimed at where I think the needle is. An AP and lateral x-ray will then show the relative position of the foreign body to the three needle tips and facilitate removal.

I do not hesitate to close these wounds with 4-0 silk, but I do drain them with a sterile elastic band if there has been inflammation or sepsis along the needle tract. I check the wound in 48 hours and remove the drain at that time. If there is cellulitis, I remove at least one suture and begin the child on frequent soaks, elevation and reduced activity. Immunization should be the same as for any puncture wound or contaminated laceration.

RECTAL BLEEDING

A child is frequently brought to the Outpatient Department after he has passed some blood mixed with stool or has had blood spotting on his diapers or underclothing. A detailed history and physical examination usually lead to the proper diagnosis, although in some instances the source of bleeding is never discovered.[7]

Anal fissures are quite common in children in the diaper age. The etiology is not clear, but once the fissure has become painful the child develops anal spasm and has difficulty with defecation. He then may get into the vicious circle of spasm, constipation, more pain, and then more spasm. Infants with an acute or chronic fissure usually cry and have obvious discomfort associated with defecation. A tiny amount of blood-streaking appears on the outside of the stool, and a small amount of red blood may stain the diaper after defecation. With the child in the frogleg position, the fissure is readily apparent when the physician firmly separates the buttocks. If the buttocks are held apart for several seconds, the anal sphincter begins to relax, and in most cases the entire anal verge can be viewed directly. Anoscopy, utilizing a tapered centrifuge tube, has been widely described, although I find it of little value. When there is an apparent fissure I apply a small amount of Xylocaine ointment to the painful region and then perform a fairly vigorous anal dilatation. This should be accomplished by slow, gentle pressure in all four directions, and in most cases the sphincter can be felt to relax considerably. Once the dilatation is complete, it is important to insure that the child has soft stools during the time the fissure is healing. If there is a history of constipation, the addition of Metamucil and extra sugar to the formula or extra fruit juice to the diet is usually adequate to keep the stools soft. Local hygiene is also most important. The child's anus should be carefully washed after each defecation, and the perinal area dried carefully with a soft, absorbent towel. The area should then be dusted with cornstarch or talcum powder applied with a cotton fluff or powder puff. If too much starch or talcum powder is applied, it tends to cake and the area remains moist. Only rarely do anal fissures require excision in infancy, and then only when they become chronic or neglected and persist after two weeks of conservative therapy.

A fistula-in-ano may present as bleeding on the diaper, although more often it presents as a perirectal abscess. Fistulas must be treated vigorously, and the principles are exactly the same as for an adult. The tract is identified at anoscopy and laid open. Most of these fistulas are superficial to the sphincter and heal without significant scarring or debility.

Dilated hemorrhoidal veins often appear on routine anoscopy or sigmoidoscopy, but they rarely bleed or thrombose in otherwise normal children. A child with prominent hemorrhoids and bleeding usually has some other underlying pathology, especially portal hypertension. Investigation, management and treatment of the hemorrhoids is again the same as for adults.

Large bowel polyps in children present as bright red rectal bleeding associated with defecation.[3] There may be an occasional blood clot passed with little or no stool present. The amount of blood lost can be significant, and the children often have a mild to moderate iron deficiency anemia associated with chronic, occult bleeding. The blood loss is painless and rarely associated with blood spotting of the underclothes. Since about 90 per cent of these polyps occur within the sigmoid colon or below, many of them can be removed through a sigmoidoscope (Fig. 23–7). In children above the age of about six years, this can be done under sedation with Demerol, 2 mg per kg, given subcutaneously one-half hour before the examination to minimize the cramping pain that

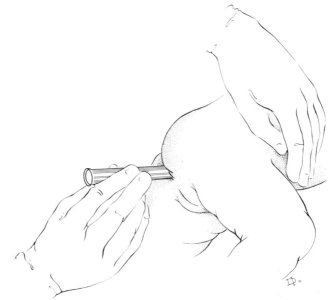

Figure 23–7 Sigmoidoscopy. Sigmoidoscopy in the small child is best performed in the lateral position. With one hand on the abdomen, the tip of the sigmoidoscope can be palpated and loops of colon manipulated onto the end of the sigmoidoscope. This greatly facilitates examination of the sigmoid colon.

often accompanies sigmoidoscopy. Smaller children should be anesthetized or sedated with the mixture of Thorazine, Phenergan, and Demerol used in preparing children for cardiac catheterization (Table 23–1). Ketalar is unsatisfactory anesthesia for sigmoidoscopy or anal procedures because of poor relaxation and frequent laryngeal spasm produced by the anal stretching. Virtually all colon polyps in children are juvenile polyps which are morphologically quite different from the adenomatous polyp of the adult. The juvenile polyp has no potential for malignant degeneration, and in most cases it will pass spontaneously. The only indication for admitting such children for open colotomy is the presence of multiple polyps, a family history of multiple polyposis, or persistent bleeding sufficiently severe to cause symptomatic anemia.

A barium enema is mandatory if no local causes for bleeding can be determined on the basis of examination and sigmoidoscopy. If this shows no obvious source of bleeding, the child should be followed at regular intervals and checked for occult blood and anemia. If he develops episodes of abdominal pain, he should be explored with the presumptive diagnosis of a bleeding Meckel's diverticulum. However, a large number of children never have the bleeding site identified, and it often ceases spontaneously. Some believe that this type of bleeding is from hemangiomas of the bowel, similar to those frequently seen on an infant's skin. These slowly thrombose and probably bleed intermittently during the process.

TABLE 23–1 SEDATIVE MIXTURE FOR OUTPATIENT PROCEDURES IN CHILDREN

The mixture contains 25 mg Demerol, 6.5 mg Thorazine and 6.5 mg Phenergan in each ml of solution. Dosage is 1.0 ml IM per 10 kg, up to a maximum of 1.5 ml.

RECTAL PROLAPSE

Idiopathic rectal prolapse is most common in children aged one to three years and coincides with toilet training. Typically the mother has several other small children, puts the patient on the potty, and leaves him there until he produces. Occasionally there is a history of constipation or difficulty with defecation, although this occurs in surprisingly few patients. Initially, I recommend that the parents abandon toilet training for several months, explaining to them the hazard of leaving the child on the toilet for long periods of time. I have found the usual practices of taping the buttocks or having the child defecate while lying on his side, for instance, are as unsatisfactory as they are impossible. The frequent taping under tension invariably leads to excoriation of the buttocks and another source of irritation and worry.

On initial examination it is important to notice if the prolapse is concentric. When the lumen of the prolapsed bowel is either not visible or is markedly displaced posteriorly, there may be an associated enterocele. Also on initial examination it is most important to be sure that prolapse reduces completely, since occasionally an ileocolic intussusception will present with the intussusceptum prolapsed through the anus. The parents must be taught how to reduce the prolapse promptly whenever it recurs. Once the prolapse has been out several hours, it may become so edematous that replacement is very difficult. Occasionally a child with cystic fibrosis presents with frequent or persistent rectal prolapse, so that a careful family history as well as a history of bowel habits must be obtained. If these are suggestive of cystic fibrosis, the child should have his sweat chlorides measured.

Complicated abdominoperineal prolapse repairs are rarely justified in children. In cases of persistent prolapse or in families where the parents cannot cope, I occasionally use the Lockhart-Mummery procedure, where the retrorectal space is opened just behind the anus and packed with iodoform gauze. This causes dense fibrosis between all layers of the rectum and presacral fascia. This can be done as an outpatient, and

recurrences are infrequent. Only rarely is it necessary to amputate the prolapse from below, although this procedure is usually curative.

Children with severe myelomeningoceles or other causes of paraplegia may be plagued by rectal prolapse. Such children can usually be helped by placing two concentric purse string sutures of monofilament nylon subcutaneously about the anus. Placed much like a Thiersch wire, the sutures are tied just tight enough to make the anus snug about the surgeon's little finger. This can, of course, be done without anesthesia since children with this type of prolapse invariably have an anesthetic perianal region. All the sutures eventually cut out and may have to be replaced. Often, however, there is no recurrence of symptoms after placement of the first pair of sutures. With sutures in place, the child may require intermittent laxatives or enemas to prevent fecal impaction.

CHRONIC ABDOMINAL PAIN

The typical child with chronic abdominal pain is a girl between the ages of eight and ten years who is a perfectly stable and well-adjusted child and who does not appear to use her complaint as a means of getting attention. When having pain, she becomes pale and lethargic, and often her parents can tell at a glance that she is having an "attack." Physical examination at this time shows only a pale, asthenic girl complaining of moderately severe pain throughout her lower abdomen. All physical and laboratory parameters are entirely normal. How much of a work-up is indicated? After the initial physical evaluation I usually examine a clean-catch urine, check the stool for occult blood, ova and parasites, examine a peripheral blood smear, and check the sedimentation rate and sickle cell prep if indicated. If all these are normal, I reassure the child and her parents and encourage them to note the patterns of her pain to see if it can be associated with eating, ingestion of large quantities of fluid, or any particular activities. An intravenous pyelogram or a barium enema may be indicated if there is any suggestion from either the history or from the laboratory that the bowel or urinary tract is involved. Should the family become unduly concerned about these episodes of pain, it may be necessary to perform these x-ray examinations so that the family can be reassured that body systems are radiographically normal. The disease is usually self-limited, although a few children do come to laparotomy and incidental appendectomy. The large percentage of cures resulting from this surgical therapy must be explained on the basis of the art rather than the science, since rarely is any significant pathology discovered. Jackson's membrane kinking the appendix or small ovarian cysts may be noted in these children, but the incidence appears to be the same as in the general population.

When the sedimentation rate is elevated or if there is occult blood in the stool, the clinician must consider the possibility of colitis, enteritis or parasite infestation and proceed with further diagnosis and therapy as indicated.

HERNIAS

Children are often brought to the Outpatient Department because of a lump in the groin. The diagnostic possibilities include a hernia, a hydrocele of the cord, or inguinal lymph nodes. The nodes, of course, are usually distal to the groin crease and can be readily differentiated from hernias, especially if one looks for a contributory lesion somewhere on the extremity. Femoral hernias do occur in children, although they are extremely rare under the age of ten. In older children, when the lump cannot be palpated by the examining physician, he can often produce the hernia by having

the child cough, perform the Valsalva maneuver or jump rope.

One can often elicit the "silk glove sign" when the hernia sac is long. To do this properly, the physician examines the supine child and places gentle traction on the ipsilateral testis. This stretches out the cord structures so that they can be readily palpated just lateral to the pubic tubercle. If there is a significant sac at this level, the cord structures can be felt to slide as the two edges of the sac are rubbed together.

Incarcerated hernias are moderately common in infancy, and statistically the vast majority occur in children under one year of age. Typically, the hernia has not been noticed previously by either the parent or the physician and is first noticed at the time of incarceration. The very large infant hernias containing several loops of bowel almost never incarcerate and even less commonly strangulate. They can, however, cause testicular infarction because of the constant pressure of the viscera on the venous and lymphatic drainage from the testis.

In the small infant with a tender, hard bulge at his external ring, the differential diagnosis between an acute hydrocele of the cord and an incarcerated hernia can be more difficult. In children under one year of age the examining physician can usually palpate the internal inguinal ring with an examining finger in the rectum and the other hand over the region of the cord. If the mass is due to an incarcerated hernia, bowel can be felt entering and exiting through the internal ring. Again, even if the physician is confident that the mass is an acute hydrocele, the testis can infarct if the mass is tense and contained within the rigid walls of the inguinal canal.

While most incarcerated inguinal hernias can be reduced by deep sedation with Nembutal and Demerol, I do not recommend this if facilities and personnel are available for safe emergency surgery, since the level of sedation which must be achieved to reduce the hernia usually borders on general anesthesia.

The children are often so deeply depressed that they must be watched for one to four hours before they can be discharged safely. I personally prefer to repair the hernia at the time of incarceration and discharge the child four to six hours later (Fig. 23–8). Not only have I seen testicles infarcted by prolonged delay in reducing the hernia, but I have seen several testicles ruptured by overzealous attempts to reduce a hernia associated with an ectopic or or undescended testis. If suitable surgical facilities are not available, most hernias can be reduced by sedating the child and elevating his feet.

If for some reason facilities are not available for a safe emergency herniorrhaphy or if the child has some additional medical contraindication to surgery, I believe that once the hernia is reduced the child should be discharged and scheduled for elective herniorrhaphy at least one week later. Rarely do hernias become reincarcerated within this length of time, and the one to two week interval allows all local edema and swelling to subside.

Elective hernia repair can be done on an outpatient basis in most children. I check the urine and hemoglobin at the initial office visit and instruct the parents to bring the child to the hospital on the day of surgery with nothing to eat or drink during the previous four hours. On admission, the child is checked for rashes, upper respiratory illness and cleared for general anesthetia. Two to four hours after surgery, the child is discharged if he is afebrile and taking fluids well.

In general, I explore both groins in female infants, since I have found bilateral hernia sacs in about 70 per cent of the girls explored. In males whom I have operated upon, about 70 per cent of those with a clinical hernia on the left also have a sac or patent processus vaginalis on the right. When the hernia has been on the right, only about 10 per cent of the boys have a sac or patent processus vaginalis on the left. Therefore, in males, I explore the clinically normal side only if the hernia is on the left side. Statistics on the advisability of exploring both sides vary widely and each surgeon must make up his own mind on the subject.

An acute hydrocele of the cord should be treated as an incarcerated hernia unless the physician can be certain of the diagnosis. Acute hydroceles within the scrotum rarely become as hard or as painful as those within the canal, and in most cases they can be dealt with electively.

When there is any tenderness within the testicle associated with the hydrocele, one must be certain that there is no underlying torsion of the testis or torsion of the appendix testis. With torsion of the testis, the cord is usually thickened and foreshortened on the side of the torsion. The testis or cord is also exquisitely tender, and the child usually has anorexia or vomiting and a low-grade fever. The torsion of the appendix testis may be quite subtle at its onset and detectable only as a tender pea-sized nodule immediately adjacent to the testis. The scrotum may become erythematous or edematous soon after a torsion of either the testis or the appendix testis. Transillumination will help differentiate an acute hydrocele from a torsion of the testis. A torsed testis seen soon after the onset can occasionally be reduced by the examining surgeon, but in most cases the swelling in the cord makes it difficult to tell which way the testis should be twisted, and the extreme discomfort experienced by the child makes this maneuver impossible.

A history of trauma to the scrotum often precedes torsion of the testis, but in any instance when the testis remains firm and tender after trauma it must be explored. Every time I have broken this rule I have regretted it.

Umbilical hernias and epigastric hernias rarely incarcerate bowel. They do, however, frequently cause acute pain when a nubbin or properitoneal fat or omentum becomes incarcerated within the sac. If possible these should be re-

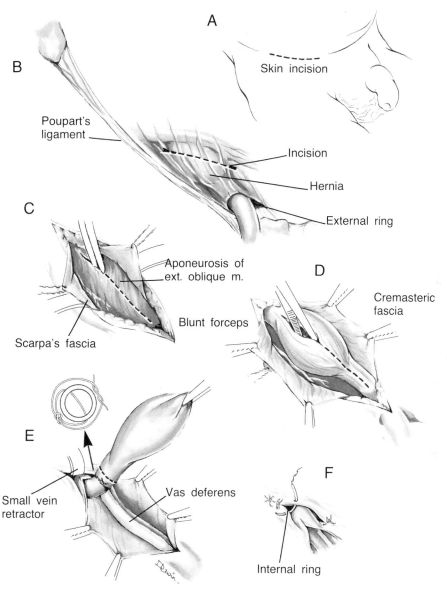

Figure 23–8 Inguinal herniorrhaphy. Infant hernias can be repaired on an outpatient basis. *A*. The skin incision is made in the lowermost abdominal skin crease starting above and slightly lateral to the pubic tubercle. *B*. The external oblique fascia is then exposed down to Poupart's ligament. This reflection is followed inferiorly until the external ring is completely cleared. *C*. The external oblique fascia is then opened in the plane of its fibers down to the external ring. *D*. The cremesteric fascia of the cord is then split in the plane of its fibers and the sac grasped with blunt forceps. *E*. The cord structures are dissected free from the sac, and with a retractor in the internal ring the sac is suture-ligated as high as possible. The excess sac is then trimmed off. *F*. In some cases it is necessary to repair the floor of the canal and internal ring with interrupted sutures. However, in most infants this type of repair is not necessary and only the external oblique fascia need be repaired. The skin is closed with subcuticular catgut in children wearing diapers so that there is little chance of forming stitch abscesses. The child can be discharged from the hospital approximately four hours after completion of his surgery.

duced, but complete reduction may be possible only at operation.

Most umbilical hernias regress spontaneously as the child grows older, although occasionally a small child has a hernia projecting two to three inches and resembling a ram's horn in shape. These have attenuated skin, and I personally have never seen a hernia resolve spontaneously. Taping umbilical hernias serves only to cause excoriation and rarely, if ever, is it beneficial.

INFECTIONS

Although children have excellent circulation and lacerations and abrasions normally heal promptly, their injuries are often heavily contaminated with dirt and debris. All foreign material must be carefully removed from the depths of the wound and all devitalized tissue debrided. Even when these precautions are taken, a small number become infected. However, if the parents are forewarned of the significance of erythema, drainage or increasing pain, they will bring the child back promptly and the infection can be treated simply by removing the sutures and instituting a program of soaks and immobilization. Lacerations about the face and especially the eyebrows seem to be prone to infection in spite of the excellent circulation. This area has the added risk of cavernous sinus thrombosis, and in general, any infection involving the portion of the face draining into the cavernous sinus should be treated by parenteral antibiotics with the child in the hospital. Other infections can usually be treated quite satisfactorily on an outpatient basis, although occasionally the child may have to be seen once or twice daily for antibiotic injections.

The prepatellar bursa and the olecranon bursa also frequently become infected after a trivial laceration, a deep abrasion, or a small puncture wound in the area, even if the bursa was not entered during the initial injury. If the child develops erythema or edema over the region of the bursa, he probably has frank pus within the bursa itself. He also will have rather marked limitation of motion in the involved joint, but no evidence of septic arthritis. With prepatellar bursitis the child limps with his knee slightly flexed. There is no tenderness over the posterior or lateral aspect of the joint, and the child does not keep it flexed as acutely as he would if the joint space were involved. If the erythema does not respond promptly to warm soaks, complete immobilization and parenteral antibiotics, the bursa should be drained.

Joint space infections result primarily from puncture wounds or lacerations which actually enter the joint. At times it may be difficult to differentiate between septic arthritis, hemorrhage into an injured joint, and sympathetic effusion following a direct blow to the joint. If the physician is in doubt, the joint should be aspirated through sterile, undamaged skin, and appropriate therapy initiated. All three conditions are symptomatically improved if as much fluid as possible is aspirated from the joint space.

Children between the ages of about six months and three years frequently present with cervical lymphadenopathy secondary to bacterial tonsilitis. The most common organisms are staphylococci or beta hemolytic streptococci, and if seen early the infection does respond to penicillin. After throat and nasopharyngeal cultures are taken, the child should be started on oral penicillin V, 250 mg four times a day. The parents should be instructed in the technique of warm soaks, which are best applied in this area using a small Turkish towel wrung out in warm water. The towel must be rewarmed frequently and applied for at least ten minutes four times a day. On this regimen many of the cervical lymph nodes regress and require no further therapy.

If they have not shown marked regression after a week to ten days of therapy, I stop all antibiotics and continue only the soaks. Prolonged antibiotic coverage apparently delays markedly the normal process of suppuration, fluctuance and drainage, all of which are inevitable if the adenopathy has not responded to the initial regimen of heat and antibiotics. In no case should cervical lymph nodes be drained until they are unmistakably fluctuant. Premature incision of a hyperplastic lymph node leads to prolonged lymph drainage and it may take months to heal. If the node is truly fluctuant it can be drained through a very small incision carefully placed in a skin crease. The cavity should be loosely packed for 48 to 72 hours, and then the pack can be removed. The drainage site usually heals completely within one week, and I have the parents continue daily soaks during the healing phase. The soaks, if kept warm, stimulate circulation in the skin edges and keep them apart so that the cavity can evacuate completely. The local cleansing keeps the edges free of crusts and debris that harbor bacteria. If the soaks are allowed to cool, they cause vasoconstriction in the skin, thereby defeating the major purpose of the treatment.

Inguinal abscesses can be seen in any age group, although they are most common among children in diapers. Older children may develop inguinal adenopathy in response to infections on their leg or foot, but only a very tiny percentage of these nodes suppurate. The small child who presents with irritability, fever and a palpable mass in the groin may cause difficulty for the physician in differentiating an inguinal abscess from an incarcerated hernia or an acute hydrocele of the cord. The abscesses are, of course, usually below the inguinal ligament and are associated with considerable edema and erythema. To minimize tension in the area of the abscess, the child frequently keeps the hip flexed when he is supine. In contradistinction to the cervical nodes where the temptation is to drain them too early, the groin abscesses usually do not become fluctuant until there is a very large amount of pus present. If the skin over the node is erythematous and has pitting edema, there is usually a significant quantity of pus in or around the lymph node. Children rarely become toxic with inguinal abscess, and most do not require hospitalization.

Small pustular lesions on the hands and feet which do not heal promptly with adequate drainage and soaking usually have a foreign body within the depths. Routine x-rays of such draining areas show a surprising number of fairly large metal objects even though there is no clear-cut history of impalement by a foreign body. Even when x-rays are normal, exploration of any chronic draining sinus in the hand or foot usually produces a splinter or piece of glass.

Ingrown toenails are common in adolescents and usually involve the great toe. By the time these children see a surgeon, there is usually a three or four month history of cellulitis, suppuration and pain. In such cases there is no place for temporizing measures such as wedging pledgets of cotton under the toenail, since the area is so exquisitely tender that the child cannot tolerate a piece of cotton large enough to elevate the nail significantly. If there is surrounding cellulitis, it may be necessary for the child to soak his foot several times a day in warm water for three or four days. He should be instructed to keep off the foot and to keep it elevated. Once the acute cellulitis has regressed, the offending one third of the toenail must be removed completely under a local digital block or a more proximal nerve block. The operation must include complete destruction of the dorsal and ventral components of the nail-forming organ, or else the deformed nail will regrow and the child will have a recurrence of his symptoms within a year or two. If an elastic band is used as a tourniquet about the base of the toe, the incision remains sufficiently dry so that one can inspect the depths and identify the nail-forming organ. This can be removed with a No. 15 scalpel blade or with a small, sharp curette. Any large area of hypertrophic granulation tissue along with lateral edge of the nailbed must also be curetted down to healthy tissue. After the entire area is clean and dry, firm digital pressure should be applied as the tourniquet is released, maintaining pressure for a full five minutes with the foot elevated.

Once the bleeding has stopped, a bulky dressing should be applied to absorb the inevitable drainage and also to protect this very tender toe from further trauma. A small gauze strip liberally covered with neosporin ointment and placed in the raw area keeps the dressing from becoming foul and also minimizes pain and bleeding at the first dressing change. I have found that most children want to stay off the foot and keep it elevated for 24 hours after the excision, and I normally instruct the parents to soak the dressing off in a pan of warm water about 48 hours after excision. After the initial dressing has been removed, I encourage the parents to soak the foot three times a day and keep the open area covered with a Band-aid. In most cases healing is complete in seven to ten days.

Plantar warts are quite common on the weight-bearing surfaces of the feet. Of the numerous treatments available, I find that those using salicylic acid are most likely to succeed, and there is minimal risk of further damage or painful scarring. I instruct the parents to pack 50 per cent to 70 per cent salicylic acid prepared in a vanishing cream base into the small hole in a standard cornplaster and put this carefully over the wart. The dressing is changed every 24 hours and must be continued for at least 10 days after the wart has disappeared. In areas where it is difficult to apply a cornplaster, 50 per cent salicylic acid in Colodion painted onto the wart is effective.

Common warts on the hand respond just as quickly, and in children I prefer this method of destruction to electrodessication or more caustic chemicals.

ANIMAL BITES

Children are frequently bitten by small household pets such as guinea pigs, hamsters, gerbils and other more exotic animals. The bites inflicted by small rodents are rarely very deep, and the jaws are not sufficiently powerful to cause any significant crushing or deep tissue necrosis. If the animal has been raised within the household, there is virtually no possibility that it is rabid, so that cleansing and soaking the extremity in warm water two to three times a day is usually adequate. Such bites become infected less often than human bites, and in general there is no need for local or systemic antibiotics.

The typical dog bite consists mainly of a crushing type of injury to the calf or buttock, with resulting hematoma and superficial skin abrasion. When the clothing has not been torn, the injury requires only adequate local cleansing and soaking. The edges must be debrided and the wound left open if there appears to be a significant component of puncture or laceration.

Dog bites sustained on or near the face are much more likely to be penetrating, and they often produce a jagged flap of skin and raised soft tissue. Such wounds should be carefully debrided, cleansed with a dilute benzalkonium solution, and closed loosely with a 5–0 or 6–0 silk. I have found that only about 3 per cent of the wounds do become infected, and the cosmetic result in the other 97 per cent is far superior if the wounds are closed surgically. It is imperative that the child be followed daily for five days so that sutures can be removed if there is any evidence of cellulitis or sepsis. Every effort should be made to salvage any piece of nose or ear tissue removed and to reapproximate it as a free composite graft. If it is properly cleansed and promptly sutured in place, a surprising number of these grafts will take in small children and save them from a severe cosmetic defect.

Any strange dog or wild animal that

bites should be captured if possible and watched for at least three weeks to see if it develops rabies. In areas where rabies is endemic, any child bitten by a wild skunk, fox, bat, squirrel or mink should be given full active rabies immunization.

The physician working in an Outpatient Department should also familiarize himself with the state laws governing animal bites. In some states they must be reported, while in others antiquated laws require that they be treated with fuming nitric acid and other medieval remedies.

BREAST MASSES

Infants a week or so old are often brought to the Outpatient Department because of an apparent breast mass. This is, of course, the normal button of breast tissue that has hypertrophied under the effects of the maternal hormones. When the mother begins to bathe the infant at home, she notices these for the first time and becomes alarmed. This tissue involutes rapidly and is normally gone within ten days. Staphylococcal abscesses can occur in an infant's breast at this stage and should be considered if there is asymmetry, local erythema or apparent tenderness. These abscesses should be incised and drained through a small circumareolar incision and soaks applied often enough to keep the edges apart while the abscess drains. Such infants should have their daily bath and shampoo with hexachlorophene in an effort to prevent skin colonization with pathogenic staphylococci that were probably picked up in the hospital.

Many adolescent males are troubled with transient breast hypertrophy which may be unilateral or bilateral and which persists for a year or two. The patient most likely seeks medical help because he is extremely sensitive about his feminine bustline and because he suffers as the butt of jokes by his contemporaries.

In all cases the breast enlargement consists of a firm disc of hypertrophied ducts and breast tissue just beneath the areola. The nipple is also usually somewhat conical in shape just as in the normal preadolescent girl. This condition of male gynecomastia is entirely self-limited, although occasionally the emotional and social problems become sufficiently serious to warrant excision. A simple mastectomy through a circumareolar incision can usually be accomplished as an outpatient under general anesthesia.

When a preadolescent girl develops one breast before the other, she may complain of a tender lump in one breast. This appears as a plaque of firm breast tissue placed concentrically beneath a developing nipple, and there is no need for further evaluation. Both the patient and her parents are usually satisfied with an explanation and reassurance.

Obese girls may develop a moderate degree of breast tenderness in association with the onset of their menses. Typically their periods are quite irregular and unpredictable, and the breast tissue has a finely nodular feeling similar to that in an older woman with a mild degree of cystic mastitis. Referred to as adolescent mastitis, this condition is entirely self-limited and usually regresses at about the time that menses become regular. If the discomfort is sufficiently debilitating, it is promptly relieved by a three month course of any one of the combination birth control pills. There is, of course, the slight but significant risk of clotting problems associated with these pills, and the girls may develop ravenous appetites, become even more obese, and thus more miserable than they were with the mastitis.

Solitary nodules in the breast of older girls are usually fibroadenomas. These are particularly common in Negro girls and others with dark skin. Such nodules can be excised completely under local anesthesia in the Outpatient Department. The incidence of carcinoma of the breast in children is so extremely low that there is no indication for an initial surgical procedure more extensive than excisional biopsy.

ABNORMALITIES OF THE NAVEL

Many newborns are left with a small granulating area at the base of the navel when the cord separates. This area should be completely epithelialized by the fourteenth day, although a small polypoid area of chronic granulation tissue may develop deep within the depths of the navel. There is usually little or no drainage, and the child is brought in simply because of the navel's appearance. These polyps regress entirely with several applications of silver nitrate, or they can be removed initially with electrocoagulation. If there is a history suggestive of either bowel contents or urine draining through the navel, the area should be proved with a small blunt probe or sterile catheter. If there appears to be a communication through an omphalovitelline duct or a urachus, the child should be admitted for appropriate surgical correction (Fig. 23–9). X-ray studies may be of help, although the diagnosis can usually be confirmed on the basis of history or by passage of a catheter into the tract.

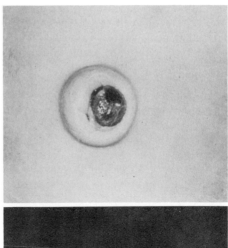
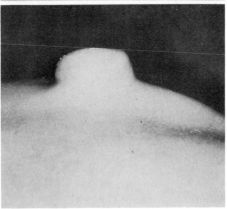

Figure 23–9   Patent omphalovitelline duct. This is the appearance of the navel of a one month old child who had intermittent greenish-brown staining from his navel. On appearance the navel was somewhat more raised than usual and there was a small area of mucosa in the base. A small catheter threaded into the depths of the mucosa passed into the abdominal cavity. Injection of dye outlined terminal ileum and the diagnosis of a patent omphalovitelline duct was confirmed. The child was then hospitalized for surgery.

INTRAORAL LESIONS

Babies are frequently referred for release of tongue-tie because the frenulum appears short and tight owing to feeding problems, or because the parents have noticed the band. At ages three to five the children usually are brought to the physician because of speech impediments. Rarely, if ever, is the degree of tongue-tie sufficient to interfere with normal speech or normal eating. A child who has been swallowing normally must *a priori* have reasonable motion in the tongue, since the swallowing process is initiated by pressing the tip of the tongue against the roof of the mouth. Occasionally a small infant has a frenulum so tight that the tip of the tongue is actually notched and held tightly to the floor of the mouth. It is probably reasonable to release these surgically, but the vast majority of such bands cause no symptoms and require no therapy.

Release of a significant tongue-tie can be done in a minute or two. A Xylocaine- or cocaine-soaked pledget of cotton is applied to the mucosa over the frenulum, and the tongue is then elevated with the heart-shaped end of a grooved director. This instrument has a small cleft in the middle which fits perfectly over the frenulum. When the tongue is elevated, the frenulum is put on the stretch and can be incised with a small pair of iris scissors. One must be careful to avoid injury to the lingual vessels, which are large and quite readily visualized. Any bleeding can be stopped with a few drops of 1:100,000 solution of epinephrine applied with the corner of a sponge.

Inclusion cysts often appear about the lips and intraoral mucosa. These are typically thin-walled and contain thick mucus. While some of these cysts are congenital, some are formed in response to a viral infection. I find that they are most reliably removed by excising the outer portion of the cyst and coagulating the base after the mucous membranes have been suitably anesthetized with topical Xylocaine or cocaine. The coagulum separates in three to five days, leaving a clean new base of mucosa. When the cyst is excised surgically and the incision sutured, there is a reasonably high incidence of recurrence.

Ranulas occur in children of any age, although they appear most often in infants as a rather large inclusion cyst under the base of the tongue. It is soft, cystic and contains thick mucus. Again, I prefer to treat these by excising the transparent anterior wall with electrocautery. I make no effort to remove the deep portion of the cyst, and so far I have seen no recurrences.

INJURIES TO THE EXTERNAL GENITALIA

The commonest injuries to the female external genitalia are labial hematomas and lacerations in the region of the urethra resulting from falls, especially while riding bicycles or tricycles. The major problem is one of urinary retention caused by surrounding edema that is partially blocking the urethra. More often, the child withholds urine because it stings the recently traumatized genitalia. The vast majority of such children can be induced to void if they are allowed to sit in a bathtub filled with warm water and encouraged to void. When left alone for a few minutes and allowed to relax, they are usually able to urinate. Catheterization is necessary only when the bladder is palpable and all other conservative measures have failed. Few of these lacerations require suturing, although when the extent of the laceration is not clear or when the blood appears to be coming from within the introitus, the child must have a complete vaginal examination performed under general anesthesia. If there is a history of any sort of penetrating injury to the vagina or if the injury was inflicted during a sexual attack, the entire vagina must be inspected with the child anesthetized. Upright x-rays of the abdomen should be obtained prior to the anesthesia examination to determine the presence of free air or a foreign body in the abdomen. Either of these findings or a high, deep vaginal laceration necessitates a laparotomy.

Injuries to the male genitalia most often involve direct trauma to the testicles of sufficient magnitude to cause a hematoma within the tunica albuginea or in the spermatic cord (Fig. 23–10). In either case the child should be admitted to the hospital to have the hematoma evacuated surgically; in a surprising number of cases there will be an acute torsion of the testes.

Ruptures of the membranous urethra occur in children much less often than in adults, and I have seen this injury only in association with extensive pelvic fractures.

Paraphimosis results when the foreskin has been retracted for examination or cleansing of the glans and then has not been properly repositioned. This may follow a routine well-baby exam or may result from young parents who have not been sufficiently instructed in cleansing their infant's genitalia. Once the paraphimosis is recognized, it can

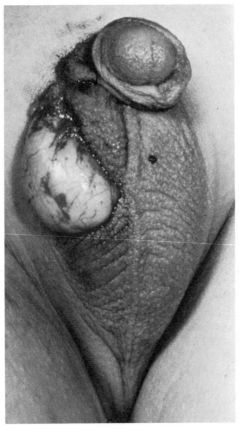

Figure 23–10 Scrotal laceration. This three year old boy lacerated his scrotum on a fence. The testicle was completely exposed at the time of admission. Under general anesthesia the scrotum was debrided and all blood clot and nonviable tissue removed from the testis. It was replaced in the scrotum which was then closed loosely and a small drain led out through the base of the scrotum. The entire injury healed spontaneously and the testis remains normal.

usually be reduced easily in the Emergency Ward, and nothing further is required at that time. If there is sufficient edema or cellulitis to prevent manual reduction, the child must have a dorsal slit of the foreskin. Circumcision should be deferred until all swelling, edema and cellulitis have subsided.

CIRCUMCISION

Since most circumcisions are performed in the newborn nursery for social or religious reasons, the older child presented for circumcision often has a definite indication for operation. Phimosis leading to urinary dribbling or balanitis is the usual preventing symptom. Occasionally a child presents for revision of an inadequate or asymmetrical circumcision performed in infancy.

I personally prefer to do all circumcisions "free hand" under general anesthesia (Fig. 23–11). Starting with dorsal and ventral slits carried down to the reflection of the mucosa and the glans, I then connect the two incisions. All bleeding points are carefully ligated with 5-0 chromic catgut and then the skin and mucosa are approximated with interrupted 4-0 catgut sutures. I dress the glans with Vaseline and several layers of gauze.

At the time of discharge from the recovery room I instruct the mother to apply Vaseline or Obtundia ointment to the glans at each diaper change to prevent irritation and superficial ulcers that will develop if the glans rubs on dry diapers.

The Gomco clamp is widely used, but great care must be taken to excise the foreskin symmetrically and remove excess skin. The clamp must be left engaged at least five minutes, or bleeding will begin when the foreskin is excised.

The new "Plastibell" (Fig. 23–12) seems to work well, although I have treated numerous children with balanitis resulting from this type of circumcision. If the ligation is not tied tightly enough, the foreskin swells and becomes edematous, but will not separate.

In my hands, the free-hand circumcision is easier, less likely to bleed and become infected, and gives the best cosmetic result.

THE BATTERED CHILD

The physician should suspect child abuse whenever he sees a child with an unusual combination of injuries or when there are multiple injuries of different ages and the history does not seem com-

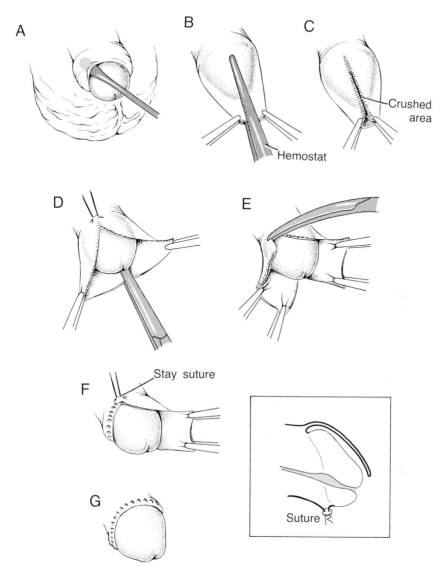

Figure 23–11 "Free hand" circumcision. Circumcision is frequently performed on an outpatient basis. I prefer to use the "free hand" technique of circumcision which is fully described in the text. *A.* The most important preliminary step is to be sure that the foreskin is completely free of the glans. In the newborn there may be some synechiae between the two structures which must be completely broken down. The foreskin can then be retracted completely to allow adequate cleansing and to be sure that the level of circumcision is correct. *B.* The dorsal portion of the foreskin is crushed with a clamp to minimize subsequent bleeding. *C.* An incision along the crushed line. In figure *D,* the dorsal slit has been completed and mosquito clamps are placed on the corners of the incised foreskin. The ventral portion is then crushed in a clamp. *E.* The ventral cut is made well up along the frenulum. There is often a blood vessel in this area which must be suture ligated. *F.* The dorsal and ventral incisions are then connected by an incision that remove the redundant foreskin and mucosa. Interrupted 5–0 chromic catgut sutures are then used to approximate the skin and mucosa and to suture ligate any bleeding points. *G.* The finished circumcision. I instruct the mother to apply Vaseline or Obtundia ointment to the entire glans and sutured area at each diaper change. This minimizes the chance of a meatal ulcer caused by irritation of the diaper on the freshly exposed mucous membrane. Within about ten days the glans become sufficiently toughened to withstand the constant irritation of diapers.

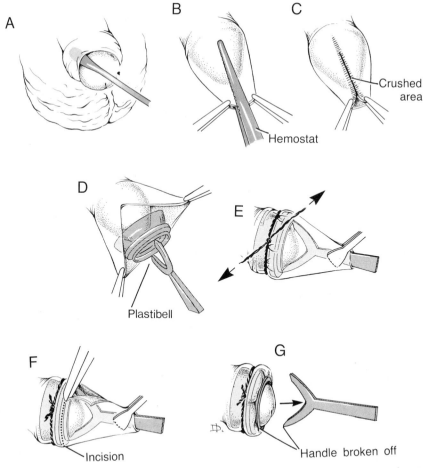

Figure 23-12 "Plastibell" circumcision. Steps *A, B* and *C* are identical to those for the free hand circumcision. *D*. The Plastibell is then inserted over the glans and *E*, the suture tied tightly around the foreskin, holding it against the plastic ring. *F*. The excess foreskin is then removed about 4 or 5 mm beyond the ligature. *G*. The plastic handle is then broken off, leaving the small plastic ring and suture in place. Five to seven days later the foreskin sloughs through the portion crushed by the suture and the entire plastic ring and distal foreskin separate.

patible with these injuries. Lacerations or bruises involving both sides of the head, bruises over the head, shoulders or buttocks, or long, linear bruises indicate that the child has been beaten. Hot water burns in a glove or stocking distribution on an extremity or any deep burn in an unusual place may also indicate maltreatment. Evidence of healing skull fractures, multiple long bone fractures of different ages, and rib fractures are all radiologic signs of the battered child syndrome or "trauma X." Rib fractures especially are rare in children under the age of three and should arouse the physician's suspicion that the child has been beaten.

In most states the physician is obligated to report any suspected battered children to the police, sheriff or state welfare agency (Table 23-2). Separate conversations between the physician and each parent, rather than with both parents together, often reveal the latter's relationships with his child and spouse. It is then usually possible to tell which parent is doing the battering, although it can be both parents or occasionally a babysitter, an older sibling, or another adult who is responsible. In addition to reporting the incident to the appropriate social and law enforcement agencies, the physician should be sure that the family obtains appropriate professional counseling.

ALLEGED SEXUAL ASSAULT (Rape and Molestation)

Any physician who sees a large number of children in an Outpatient Department should be thoroughly familiar with the local laws governing his responsibilities in examining children who have allegedly been sexually molested. In most states he is obligated to report all such cases, and in a few states it is a misdemeanor for him to examine the child before she has been examined by a physician from the office of the Coroner or State Attorney. In recording the history, it is most important to make it quite clear which statements are attributable to the patient, parents or witnesses. After determining the circumstances of the alleged assault, the child should be examined for any signs of physical mistreatment. All clothing, especially her underclothing, should be examined for blood or stains that might be attributable to seminal fluid. The garments must be retained and turned over to local authorities for further laboratory examination.

The child should be examined for evidence of any trauma about the introitus and perineum. The status of the hymen must be carefully noted and recorded. When there is evidence of such trauma, the vagina should be examined using an appropriately sized nasal or vaginal speculum.

Any fluid in the vagina should be examined microscopically for the presence of sperm, with a small aliquot sent to the laboratory for acid phosphatase determination. The presence of either sperm or acid phosphatase presents incontrovertible evidence of recent sexual contact. Rarely are the local injuries sufficiently serious to require hospitalization, although occasionally it is necessary to admit the child temporarily to remove her from the surroundings in which the attack occurred. When the offender is not immediately apprehended for examination, the child should have a two week course of penicillin therapy followed in four to six weeks by a VDRL determination. If there is extensive tearing of the introitus or if there appears to be any blood in the posterior fornices, the child should be observed closely for 24 hours to rule out the possibility that the peritoneal cavity has been entered.

BLEEDING DISORDERS

In any large pediatric population some children will be encountered with known bleeding disorders.[12] For the surgeon the most significant of these are classical hemophilia and Christmas disease. The severity of the defect varies widely, so that it is difficult to formulate general rules for the care of these children. However, in most cases a fracture, laceration or sprain sufficiently severe to bring the child to a physician requires treatment with blood products.

Lacerations large enough to require sutures or those which have not stopped bleeding within 30 minutes require specific replacement with blood products as part of their therapy. In children having documented factor VIII or IX deficiency, treatment of major lacerations without specific clotting factor replacement results in catastrophe. They will continue to bleed into the depths of the wound and return with the wound bulging. Such hematomas inevitably become infected, so the wound must be opened and allowed to granulate. This process may take as long as a month, and the child must be given infusions of specific blood factors daily or every

TABLE 23–2 SUMMARY OF CHILD-ABUSE LEGISLATION*
EXPLANATION

Age: The age of children concerning whom reports are to be made.

Who Reports: For purposes of this paper, only professional health personnel are listed in this column, unless space permits further listings. (H) refers to a provision that hospital administrators are to report when notified by a physician. Some statutes require independent reporting by a hospital. M.D. includes all physicians, surgeons, interns, residents. R.N. refers in most cases to all sorts of nurses, although some statutes include school nurses and visiting nurses and some include nurses only in the absence of a physician. (N) means that reporting a child is nonmandatory.

To Whom Reported: Because of the variations in the levels of authority to whom cases should be reported, this chart uses the letter P to indicate police or sheriff and W to indicate welfare authorities.

Penalty: This indicates if there is any penalty for failure to report. Obviously, the penalties themselves vary from state to state.

State	Age	Who Reports	To Whom	Penalty
Alabama	under 16	M.D., (H) and clinics, teacher, pharmacist, social worker, other person giving aid	P, W	yes
Alaska	under 16	M.D., R.N., teacher, social worker (N)	P, W	. . .
Arizona	under 16	M.D.	P	yes
Arkansas	under 16	M.D., D.O., D.D.S., R.N., (H), any person	P, W	yes
California	minor	M.D., D.D.S., religious practitioner, D.C., school principal	P	yes
Colorado	under 12	M.D., D.O.	P	. . .
Connecticut	under 18	M.D., (H)	P, W	. . .
Delaware	under 18	M.D., (H)	county court	yes
District of Columbia	under 18	M.D.	P	. . .
Florida	under 16	M.D., D.O., (H)	W, P	. . .
Georgia	under 12	M.D., D.O., public health nurse, welfare worker, (H)	W, P	. . .
Hawaii	minor	M.D., D.O., D.D.S., R.N., teacher, (H)	W	. . .
Idaho	child	M.D., (H)	W	. . .
Illinois	under 16	M.D., D.D.S., D.O., D. C., (H)	W, P	. . .
Indiana	under 16	M.D., D.O., D.C.	W, P	. . .
Iowa	under 18	M.D., D.O., D.D.S., D.C., R.N., (H), any person	W, P	. . .
Kansas	under 16	M.D., D.D.S., D.O., D.C., R.N., (H), social worker	juvenile court	yes
Kentucky	under 18	M.D., D.O., (H), other person	W, P	yes
Louisiana	under 17	M.D., D.O.	P	yes
Maine	under 16	M.D., D.O., D.C., (H)	W, county attorney	yes
Maryland	under 16	M.D., D.D.S., R.N., (H) health practitioner, any person	W, P	. . .
Massachusetts	under 16	M.D.	W	. . .

*Adapted from Helfer and Kempe, The Battered Child.

TABLE 23–2 SUMMARY OF CHILD-ABUSE LEGISLATION *(Continued)*

State	Age	Who Reports	To Whom	Penalty
Michigan	under 17	M.D., (H)	W, prosecuting attorney	yes
Minnesota	minor	M.D., R.N., (H), healing practitioner	W, P	yes
Mississippi	under 18	M.D., D.D.S., R.N., (H)	W, juvenile court judge	. . .
Missouri	under 12	M.D., (H), (N)	P	. . .
Montana	under 18	M.D., R.N., (H)	county attorney	. . .
Nebraska	any child	any person	county attorney	. . .
Nevada	under 18	M.D., D.D.S., D.O., R.N., (H), teacher, attorney	P	yes
New Hampshire	under 16	M.D., D.O., (H)	W	yes
New Jersey	under 18	M.D., D.O., (H)	county prosecutor	yes
New Mexico	under 16	health practitioner, R.N., teacher (N)	county attorney	. . .
New York	under 16	M.D., D.D.S., D.O., D.C., R.N., (H)	W	. . .
N. Carolina	under 16	M.D., R.N., school or welfare employees	W	. . .
N. Dakota	under 18	M.D., D.O., D.C., public health nurse	W, juvenile commissioner or state attorney	. . .
Ohio	under 18	M.D., R.N., (H), teacher	P	. . .
Oklahoma	under 17	M.D., D.D.S., D.O., R.N., (H)	W, P	yes
Oregon	under 12	M.D., (H)	appropriate medical investigator	yes
Pennsylvania	under 18	M.D., D.O., (H)	P, juvenile court judge	yes
Rhode Island	under 18	M.D., D.O., (H)	W	. . .
S. Carolina	under 16	M.D., hospital staff	W, P	yes
S. Dakota	under 18	M.D., D.D.S., D.O., D.C., (H), law officer	juvenile court	yes
Tennessee	under 16	any person	juvenile court	yes
Texas	under 18	M.D. (N)	P, juvenile court judge	. . .
Utah	minor	any person, (H)	P, W	yes
Vermont	under 16	M.D., D.O., D.C., (H)	W	yes
Virginia	under 16	licensed healing practitioner, R.N., (H)	P, juvenile court	. . .
Washington	under 18	M.D., D.D.S., D.O., D.C., (H), (N)	P	. . .
W. Virginia	under 18	M.D., doctor of healing arts, R.N., (H)	prosecuting attorney	. . .
Wisconsin	child	M.D., R.N.	W, P	yes
Wyoming	under 19	M.D., D.O., R.N., (H), any person	W	yes
Virgin Islands	under 15	M.D., D.O., (H)	P	yes

other day until the wound is completely epithelialized.

Whenever I see a child with known hemophilia or Christmas disease who has sustained a laceration, I administer sufficient plasma or cryoprecipitate to raise the blood level to about 40 per cent of normal. Then the wound responds as it would in a normal child. The child should return to the Outpatient Department daily or every other day for infusions until all sutures are out and the laceration is completely healed.

A hemophiliac with a significant sprain or with evidence of bleeding into a joint must be hospitalized and given specific replacement therapy; the extremity should be immobilized and as much blood as possible should be aspirated from the joint. Once the bleeding has stopped, he may begin active and passive exercises and may soon resume normal activity, although he must receive factor VIII or factor IX replacement for a minimum of two weeks after such an injury. Occasionally it is possible to keep circulating blood levels of these specific factors in a safe range by administering infusions on alternate days. This must be individualized, however, and carefully documented by determining circulating blood levels.

Hemophiliacs who sustain fractures should be started immediately on specific replacement therapy prior to reduction. In general, they must receive daily infusions until the fragments are stable and callus has begun to form. Premature cessation of replacement therapy may result in late bleeding into the fracture site and in markedly delayed union.

WRINGER INJURIES

In spite of the recent trend toward automatic washing machines, there are still many homes with only the roller type of clothes wringer. The temptation of such a wringer seems irresistible to a small child who either puts his finger directly into the moving rollers or forgets

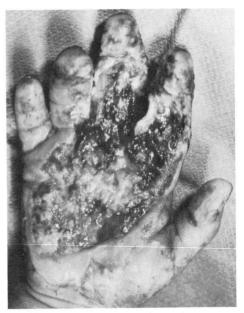

Figure 23–13 Wringer injury. This two year old child put his right hand in a wringer. The hand went in only as far as the palm and the constant rotary motion of the rollers caused extensive tissue destruction. The damage is often more extensive than is initially estimated because of thermal injury caused by the friction of the rubber rollers on the skin. Such injuries should be debrided carefully and dressed daily for several days until the extent of the injury is clear. The child should then have early grafting to preserve as much function as possible in the hand.

to let go of a piece of clothing he introduced. The result is that the arm is drawn in between the rollers up to the wrist, elbow or axilla (Fig. 23–13). Here the rollers continue to turn, creating a tremendous amount of friction with the skin. The result is a combination of crushing injury to the entire extremity as well as a significant thermal burn to the area stuck between the rollers. On initial inspection there may be little to see other than some erythema caused by the turning rollers. Over the next several hours, however, there may be considerable swelling as well as skin necrosis in association with the thermal injury. The acute injuries are rarely associated with fractures and at worst include only an area of third-degree burn. However, because of the crushing nature of the injury, there may be great swelling in the muscle compartments of the forearm that can lead to Volkmann's contracture. Many such tragic late complications have developed when the extent of injury was not initially appreciated.

In the past many hospitals have made it a policy to admit all children with wringer injuries and to treat them with tight wrapping and elevation. This was designed to minimize the chance of late ischemia problems. In recent years I have tended to treat most of these children as outpatients. After initial evaluation to see the extent of the crushing and thermal injuries, I treat the abraded or blistered area just as a second-degree burn and immobilize the arm in a sling. If the injury is acute, I believe that wrapping the extremity in a Turkish towel and then in ice does reduce the edema considerably. If the injury is more than four hours old, the ice seems to have little or no effect. I then arrange to see the child or have the child seen by a responsible physician at 12 hour intervals for at least the first 48 hours. Usually by that time the swelling has subsided remarkably, with the area of tissue necrosis clearly outlined. During the examination in the first two days, I note carefully the capillary filling in the nail beds, the ability to move all fingers, the nature of the radial and ulnar pulses, and the amount of pain in the forearm.

After the initial threat of vascular compromise is passed, the area of thermal injury must be treated like a burn of similar severity. In most wringers only the lower of the two rollers has direct power, and consequently the burned areas are usually on the volar aspect of the wrist, on the medial aspect of the arm, or within the axilla. About one child in ten has sufficient tissue destruction to require eventual skin grafting.

GILL ARCH ANOMALIES

Anomalies involving the development of the first and second gill arches as well as their pouches produce cosmetic problems in childhood. Most common is the first gill cleft remnant which presents as a preauricular sinus. The actual skin dimple may be anywhere in the area anterior to the exterior auditory canal, but it invariably communicates with a sinus or cyst connected to the cartilaginous portion of the external auditory canal. The sinuses and cysts have a strong familial tendency and often three or more generations are involved. Typically, the deeper portions of the sinus become infected, and the child presents with purulent drainage from the skin dimple or a small abscess just anterior to the tragus. When infected, every effort should be made to treat the infection and cellulitis conservatively and then arrange for elective excision of the sinus at a later date. Such excision should always be performed under general anesthesia and in a fully equipped operating room. The dissection is often tedious and involves removing the entire sinus and often some anomalous pieces of cartilage just anterior to the exterior auditory canal. Some of the sinuses come into close approximation to the facial nerve, and local anesthesia is rarely satisfactory since few children are capable of lying still in awkward positions for the required length of time.

First arch remnants appear as small bits of redundant skin or cartilage along a line from the external auditory canal to the angle of the mouth (Fig. 23–14). These may be unilateral or bilateral and often are multiple. These are all very amenable to excision under local anesthesia and rarely have any deep connections.

Branchial cleft sinuses and cysts are remnants of the second gill cleft and appear anywhere along the anterior border of the sternocleidomastoid muscle. Most are associated with a skin dimple, and they usually present as asymptomatic swellings slightly above the area of the dimple. Occasionally the sinus drains a few drops of mucousy material, and of course it may become secondarily infected. These sinuses al-

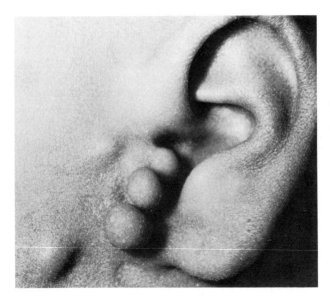

Figure 23–14 Gill arch remnants. This child had a rather unusual accumulation of first gill arch remnants. There may or not be associated sinuses from the first gill cleft that extend down into the middle ear. All such anomalies should be removed under general anesthesia, since the cartilaginous portion is often much more extensive than is apparent.

ways connect with the pharynx in the region of the anterior tonsilar pillar and usually pass through the bifurcation of the carotid artery. Because of the extent of this dissection, it must always be done under general anesthesia. Abscesses and infected cysts must be drained and all cellulitis cleared before the definitive operation is undertaken.

TORTICOLLIS

This relatively common childhood condition is frequently misdiagnosed and often mistreated.[3] Like many chronic diseases of unknown etiology causing no serious debility, it is quite tempting to temporize and defer definitive treatment. In spite of the many theories about the cause of torticollis, none explains the clinical course and microscopic findings.

Typically the child is normal at birth and a firm nodule is noted within the sternocleidomastoid muscle sometime during the first month of life. Since babies at this age have short necks and are often quite chubby, it may not be apparent initially that the nodule arises within the muscle. Many children are

treated for cervical adenopathy, and I have seen drainage attempted in several. There is never any associated skin discoloration and never any microscopic evidence of extravasated blood, so it is doubtful if the nodule results from a hematoma in the sternocleidomastoid muscle.

Whatever the cause, infants at this stage can be treated conservatively. Because of the anatomical arrangement of the sternocleidomastoid muscle, it is stretched to its longest length when the head is turned towards the side of the nodule. I instruct the parents in turning the head through a full range of motion with every diaper change. I then have them position the child's bed so that the window or doorway with the most light is on the side of the nodule when the child is prone. This encourages him to keep the head turned in the proper direction. Some believe that direct massage in the region of the nodule is beneficial, though I have found it of little value. I continue conservative therapy until the child begins to show evidence of facial asymmetry, which begins with a flattening of the malar region and is usually associated with a prominence in the occipital region on the other side. If this deformity develops while the child is undergoing conservative therapy, I then excise the involved area of the sternocleidomastoid as well as a broad sheet of fascia on either side of the nodule. This excision can be performed under general anesthesia as an outpatient, and I normally reinstitute active and passive therapy about one week after surgery. Surgery without adequate postoperative manipulation is doomed to failure. The excision must be extensive, but care taken to preserve the spinal accessory nerve (XI).

In preoperative evaluation it is essential to differentiate between true torticollis with fibrosis of a portion of the sternocleidomastoid and a tight muscle caused by cerebral palsy or some other form of spasticity.

THYROGLOSSAL CYSTS AND SINUSES

As the thyroid descends from the base of the tongue ot its normal position in the neck, there may be remnants of thyroid tissue and occasionally cysts and sinuses left along its track. These are characteristically midline masses just below the hyoid bone. The cyst may become infected and present as an abscess in the anterior portion of the neck. When these abscesses are drained, a chronic fistula may form with intermittent discharge or mucus or pus. When all cellulitis has subsided, the sinus should be excised. Since this always involves a rather extensive dissection with resection of the middle third of the hyoid and removal of the sinus on the base of the tongue, I believe that this should always be done under general anesthesia with the patient hospitalized for at least 48 hours after surgery.

Occasionally a midline neck nodule represents ectopic thyroid and is the only functioning thyroid the child has. This has led some centers to obtain thyroid scans on all children before surgery on thyroglossal duct cysts or sinuses. I rarely obtain a scan, although I do warn the parents preoperatively that the nodule may be the only thyroid tissue present. At operation I explore the region of the normal thyroid digitally. If there is no normal thyroid, I divide the nodule in half, leaving the upper pole vessels intact, and transplant the two portions deep to the sternocleidomastoid muscles. This preserves the child's functioning thyroid tissue and eliminates the rather unsightly bulge in the neck. An alternate treatment involves administering two grains of thyroid a day in an effort to shrink the ectopic thyroid tissue as much as possible.

Acute bacterial thyroiditis is relatively rare, although one still sees an occasional staphylococcal or streptococcal thyroid infection following severe upper respiratory tract infection. The gland will be diffusely tender, and the child will appear quite ill. If the infection does not respond to penicillin therapy, an abscess will form that can be drained like any other abscess. During the phase of acute bacterial infection there may be marked abnormalities in the thyroid function tests, and the uptake will be virtually zero. Yet once infection subsides, function returns to normal.

Thyroid nodules are extremely common in children, especially in adolescent females. Typically the gland is enlarged with one or more firm nodules, and laboratory tests show an increase in thyroglobulin, a decrease in triiodothyromine, and an elevated thyroglobulin antibody. This picture is virtually diagnostic of Hashimoto's thyroiditis, and no biopsy is necessary. If the laboratory findings are not conclusive or if the diagnosis is questioned on clinical ground, I prefer an open biopsy of and palpable nodule, although a needle biopsy will often suffice. Open biopsy can be performed on an outpatient basis and causes little more morbidity than a needle biopsy. The incision need be only two centimeters long and so positioned that it can be extended into a classical thyroid incision if indicated.

I personally believe that all thyroid nodules in children should be treated for at least three months with suppressive doses of thyroid before any thought is given to biopsy. Since the activity of thyroid extract tends to be variable, I prefer the more easily standardized synthetic medication.

There are only about 50 cases of thyroid cancer reported annually in the United States among children 14 years or younger. Of these, about 75 per cent present as palpable nodules outside the thyroid and represent node metastases. Thus, a nodule in a child's thyroid has only a very tiny chance of being malignant when compared to the numbers of children with Hashimoto's thyroiditis or nodular goiter.

DERMOIDS

Dermal inclusion cysts appear very frequently along the lateral aspect of the eyebrow. Initially, they are usually noticed in the first year of life, and they grow slowly as firm, round, movable nodules. There may be an indentation in the skull at the site of the cysts. They may occur at almost any area around the skull, although the vast majority are in the eyebrow region.

Classically, skull x-rays should be obtained before excising any of these cysts so that any underlying cranial defects which might indicate a dumbell-shaped cyst with an intracranial extension will be detected. While this complication does occur, it is extremely uncommon, and in the last seventy patients I have not obtained x-rays. One child had a small tract from the base of the cyst through the calvarium which I tied off. A few months later the child had a very limited craniectomy with removal of the intracranial portion. I believe this is a perfectly suitable way of managing the rare case with intracranial extension.

For cosmetic reasons I prefer an incision within the upper margin of the eyebrow. The cysts are quite circumscribed and shell out without difficulty.

After closing the incision with a subcuticular suture, I apply a pressure dressing to prevent blood from extravasating beneath the skin into the eyelids. This prevents the massive "black eye" which can result from cyst excision. All these cysts can be excised on an outpatient basis.

A much rarer position for dermoids is in the midline between the nasal bones. These are much more formidable lesions and usually communicate with the vomer and occasionally with the meninges at the base of the skull. All these must be performed with the patient in the hospital since they require an extensive dissection with splitting of the nasal bones and tracing the cyst to its origin. Dissection in this location must never be attempted on an outpatient basis.

BIOPSIES

Muscle biopsies are required in children to confirm the diagnosis of muscular dystrophy or in the differential diagnosis of locomotor difficulties. The muscle undergoing biopsy is often dictated by the clinical findings, and when only one muscle or muscle group is involved, this is, of course, the one on which biopsy should be performed. For a generalized disease, however, biopsies around the shoulders and chest should be avoided because of the tendency to develop hypertrophied scars in these areas. A biopsy of the gastroc muscle or the quadriceps femoris is easier to perform and will give suitable results for any disseminated disease. Local field block is usually adequate for anesthesia, and the muscle itself is relatively anesthetic. It is important to avoid any injections of local anesthetic into the tissue being removed for biopsy. In general, I prefer a transverse incision over either the body of the quadriceps femoris or the gastroc. Once the fascia has been divided, a suitable muscle bundle can be isolated by placing suture ligatures of 3-0 or 4-0 silk above the dissection. One or two centimeters of such a nerve is usually adequate for tissue diagnosis. Many surgeons prefer to isolate the sural nerve over the midportion of the gastrocnemius muscle. Here it is usually in the midline and superficial to the investing fascia of the leg. When biopsy is performed on the sural nerve at this level, there is usually no permanent anesthesia over the lateral part of the foot, since there are many interconnections with other sensory nerves in the area. Sural nerve biopsies taken at the level of the lateral malleolus often result in an annoying area of anesthesia over the lateral portion of the foot.

The rectal biopsy in a child with frequent constipation or diarrhea to rule out the possibility of Hirschsprung's disease can be done quite suitably in the Outpatient Department. The pathologist likes to have a full-thickness rectum, but from the surgeon's viewpoint this causes undesirable fibrosis that interferes with the definitive operation. Most pathologists are willing to make the diagnosis of Hirschsprung's disease if ganglion cells are absent in the submucosal Meissner's plexus, especially if there are hypertrophied nerve fibers in that area.

A suitable biopsy can be taken without anesthesia in small infants. A long nasal speculum is passed into the anus with the infant held in the lithotomy position. The biopsy should be taken from the posterior wall greater than 1 centimeter above the pectinate line with a sharp biopsy forceps. If a larger piece is required, a single suture of 3-0 catgut can be placed at the apex of the biopsy site and a long ellipse of tissue removed with scissors. The mucosa and submucosa can then be closed by running the catgut suture along the biopsy site. It is most important to immobilize the biopsy specimen before fixation by tying it to a piece of tongue depressor and noting which end is distal and which is proximal. Then if ganglion cells are absent in one portion, you will know where the area of transition occurs.

References

1. Gross, R. E.: An Atlas of Children's Surgery. Philadelphia, W. B. Saunders Co., 1970.
2. Helfer, R. E., and Kempe, C. H.: The Battered Child. Chicago, University of Chicago Press, 1968.
3. Jones, P. G.: Torticollis in Infancy and Childhood. Springfield, Ill., C. C Thomas, 1968.
4. Jones, P. G.: Clinical Pediatric Surgery. Philadelphia, F. A. Davis Co., 1970.
5. Kempe, C. H.: Current Pediatric Diagnosis and Treatment. Los Altos, Calif., Lange, 1972.
6. McGregor, I. A.: Fundamental Techniques of Plastic Surgery, and Their Surgical Application. Edinburgh, E. & S. Livingstone, 1968.
7. Mustard, W. T., et al., (Ed.): Pediatric Surgery. Chicago, Year Book Medical Publishers, 1969.
8. Polk, H. C., and Stone, H. H., (Eds.): Contemporary Burn Management. Boston, Little, Brown and Co., 1971.
9. Potts, W. J.: The Surgeon and the Child. Philadelphia, W. B. Saunders Co., 1959.
10. Redo, S. F.: Surgery of the Ambulatory Child. New York, Appleton-Century-Crofts, 1961.
11. Swenson, O.: Pediatric Surgery. New York, Appleton-Century-Crofts, 1969.
12. Tarnay, T. J.: Surgery in the Hemophiliac. Springfield, Ill.: C. C Thomas, 1968.

24

Transplantation

By ISRAEL PENN, M.D.

This work was supported by research grants from the Veterans Administration, by grants RR-00051 and RR-00069 from the general clinical research centers program of the Division of Research Resources, National Institutes of Health and grants AI-10176-01, AI-AM-08898, AM-07772, GM-01686, and HE-09110 of the United States Public Health Service.

INTRODUCTION

Many readers have expressed surprise that a chapter on transplantation should be included in a book dealing with outpatient surgery. However, there are currently several thousand organ transplant recipients who are living at home and are being followed periodically in the outpatient clinic. The number of such patients is steadily increasing.

In this chapter we shall discuss the indications for transplantation of various tissues and organs, the pre- and postoperative outpatient care, and complications which may be encountered.

Up to the present time a wide variety of tissues and organs have been transplanted as autografts, homografts or even heterografts. Many transplants have involved relatively simple tissues including blood cells, bone, cartilage, tendon, blood vessels, skin, heart valves, hair, middle ear ossicles and corneas. Transfers of these tissues are well recognized, do not generally require immunosuppressive therapy and will not be discussed further in this chapter, nor will reimplantations of severed limbs. In recent years much experience has been gained with transplantation of complex internal organs and tissues, including the kidney, liver, heart, lung, pancreas, bone marrow, spleen, thymus, larynx and small bowel. As most experience has been gained with transplantation of the kidney, the outpatient management of patients undergoing this procedure will be described in detail. Treatment of recipients of other organs or tissues will be briefly discussed.

Historical Background

The possibility of transplantation of parts of the body from one individual to another or between members of different species has stirred man's imagination since antiquity. Figures in Greek mythology such as the Pegasus and the Satyrs are such examples, as are the Sphinx and Thoth of ancient Egypt. The legend of Daedalus and Icarus concerns an attempt to escape imprisonment on an island with the use of heterologous wings. Unfortunately the beeswax used to attach the wings to the body of Icarus melted in the sun and the escape failed.

Among the earliest known transplants in men was a method of nasal reconstruction using a skin flap that was performed by the Hindu surgeon Sushruta in the sixth century B.C. In the fourth century A.D. the Saints Cosmos and Damian were credited with having transplanted a leg from a cadaver to a faithful churchgoer suffering from gangrene. Apparently no problems with rejection were encountered and the transplant was a success! Today Cosmos and Damian are regarded as the patron saints of transplantation.

In 1597 an Italian surgeon, Gaspar Tagliacozzi, performed elaborate rhinoplasties to reconstruct noses destroyed by syphilis or dueling injuries. In 1804 Baronio first demonstrated the survival of free skin autografts. Crude attempts were made by 18th and 19th century surgeons to perform transplants of various organs and tissues. Among these early efforts were those of the founder of scientific surgery, John Hunter, who was one of the first to use the term "transplanting."

The modern era of transplantation commenced early in the present century when Alexis Carrel and Charles Guthrie perfected techniques of vascular anastomosis, and showed in experimental animals that it was technically possible to transplant kidneys, hearts, lungs, thyroids, ovaries, limbs and heads.

Sporadic attempts to transplant various organs were subsequently made in man but were doomed to failure because of lack of understanding of the immunologic problems involved. During the second World War a major breakthrough came with the work of Medawar and his colleagues, who produced convincing evidence that graft failure was immunologically mediated. Their work opened up avenues for the treatment of rejection and set the stage for successful transplantation of major organs in man.

The work of Willem Kolff from the 1940's onwards established hemodialysis as a method of keeping uremic patients alive for prolonged periods and preparing them for renal transplantation. Although kidney homografts in man were attempted as early as 1902, the significant developments in this field came in the early 1950's in Chicago, France, Boston and Toronto. No immunosuppression was used in these early cases and no long-term function was accomplished except in transplants between monozygotic twins.

Immunosuppression with total body irradiation was introduced in 1958 to prevent rejection in transplants between individuals other than identical twins. The following year this therapy was superseded by the use of 6-mercaptopurine, and in 1961 by the closely related compound, azathioprine (Imuran). In 1963 the use of a combination of azathioprine and prednisone was reported. In addition, splenectomy and thymectomy were added to the immunosuppressive armamentarium. Histocompatibility testing was introduced in 1964 and two years later antilymphocyte globulin (ALG) was used to augment immunosuppression with azathioprine and prednisone. In its evolution kidney transplantation has served as the prototype for the transfer of other major organs. Today it can no longer be looked upon as an experimental procedure but as an accepted method of treatment.

The first liver transplant in man was performed in Denver in 1963, while in the same year the first human lung graft was accomplished in Jackson, Mississippi; in Jackson in the following year a chimpanzee heart was transplanted to a patient. The first transplantation of a human heart was performed in Cape Town, South Africa, toward the end of 1967. Transplantation of the pancreas was performed in Minneapolis in 1966, where the first graft of the small bowel took place in the following year.

KIDNEY TRANSPLANTATION

Much of the management of renal recipients and their living donors can be handled on an outpatient basis.

Selection of Kidney Recipients

In our experience renal transplantation has been performed for uremia caused by subacute or chronic glomerulonephritis in approximately 95 per cent of patients. The others suffered from pyelonephritis, polycystic kidney disease, familial nephritis, Goodpasture's syndrome, medullary cystic disease, lupus nephritis, oxaluria, ethylene glycol nephropathy or postpartum renal failure.

Any patient with irreversible kidney failure is a candidate for renal transplantation provided certain criteria are met:

1. Age. The mortality and morbidity of transplantation is greater in older individuals, whose vascular systems and organs have often suffered the ravages of long-standing hypertension. We seldom perform transplants in patients over 50 years of age. There does not appear to be any lower age limit. Our youngest recipient was three and a half years old but patients as young as nine months have received successful transplants.

2. General physical condition. While renal homograft recipients often have anemia, hypertension and even heart failure, other serious diseases such as pulmonary tuberculosis, angina pectoris or cerebrovascular insufficiency are contraindications to transplantation. We also do not perform the operation in patients with malignant tumors unless these have been previously treated and there is no evidence of recurrent or metastatic lesions.

3. Mental status. Uremia is sometimes complicated by a toxic psychosis. Furthermore, the stress of a serious and potentially fatal illness is often responsible for mental symptoms. These are not contraindications to operation, as they

will often clear up following successful transplantation. However, the existence of a long-standing functional psychosis or severe behavior disorder is a deterrent to operation, as patients with these problems are very difficult to manage postoperatively.

4. Status of the lower urinary tract. Obstruction of the bladder neck or urethra is a contraindication to transplantation unless the underlying lesion is first treated. Although an ileal loop has been substituted for a neurogenic bladder in a few renal transplantations we do not favor this form of treatment, as the risk of complications, especially infection, is very high.

5. Preformed cytotoxic antibodies. These will cause a positive cross match on testing with the lymphocytes of a potential donor. The antibodies are the result of previous exposure to foreign antigens by multiple pregnancies or blood transfusions. In the presence of such antibodies the risk of hyperacute rejection of the homograft is a very serious one, and transplantation should not be performed.

Preoperative Management

Preoperative Preparation of the Recipient

A full history and thorough mental and physical examination are essential. The following studies (Fig. 24–1) are per-

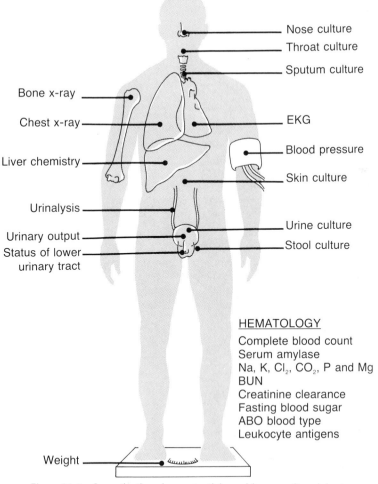

Nose culture
Throat culture
Sputum culture

Bone x-ray

Chest x-ray

EKG

Liver chemistry

Blood pressure

Skin culture

Urinalysis

Urine culture

Urinary output
Status of lower
urinary tract

Stool culture

HEMATOLOGY
Complete blood count
Serum amylase
Na, K, Cl_2, CO_2, P and Mg
BUN
Creatinine clearance
Fasting blood sugar
ABO blood type
Leukocyte antigens

Weight

Figure 24–1 Investigations in a potential renal homograft recipient.

formed: a chest radiograph, full blood count, fasting blood sugar, two hour postprandial blood sugar, electrocardiograph, urinalysis, culture of the urine, blood urea nitrogen, serum creatinine, creatinine clearance, and serum levels of sodium, potassium, chloride, calcium, phosphorus and magnesium.[59] In the course of his illness the patient may have received blood transfusions and been exposed to the risk of hepatitis. Evidence for this is sought by measuring the serum bilirubin, alkaline phosphatase, SGOT, SGPT, serum proteins and prothrombin time and by testing for the Australia antigen.[72] If active hepatitis is suspected, then transplantation should be deferred for several months, owing to the risk of further liver injury by the immunosuppressive drugs.

Immediately before admission to the hospital routine cultures of the throat, sputum, urine, feces and skin are taken.[59]

In cases when the status of the patient's lower urinary tract is doubtful, studies such as voiding cystourethrograms, cystoscopy, retrograde pyelography and cystometrograms may be necessary.

The patient's blood is typed for ABO and RH antigens, and histocompatibility tests are made, using the microcytotoxicity method of Terasaki.[69] A direct cross match between the recipient's serum and the donor's lymphocytes is always performed.[69]

In a few patients the renal failure does not require management with dialysis prior to transplantation. However, the great majority require this treatment to correct fluid and electrolyte imbalance, acidosis, hypertension and pulmonary edema, if present (Fig. 24–2). In most centers such therapy is handled by the renal medicine department and details will not be discussed here. A useful summary of the subject is that of Dunea.[16] In our own center peritoneal dialysis has largely been abandoned because it is only about one fifth as effective as hemodialysis and causes numerous complications.

Arteriovenous Shunts and Fistulas for Hemodialysis

Patients are prepared for hemodialysis by construction of an external arteriovenous shunt or an internal arteriovenous fistula. When a short period of treatment is required the use of an external shunt is adequate. This is usually

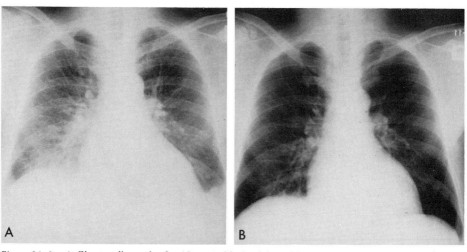

Figure 24–2 *A.* Chest radiograph of a 45 year old physician with chronic renal failure who came to the hospital in pulmonary edema. *B.* Repeat chest radiograph several hours after hemodialysis showing marked improvement in the radiographic appearance.

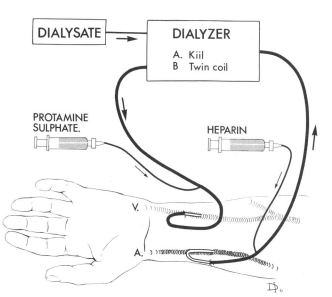

Figure 24–3 Hemodialysis using an arteriovenous shunt.

constructed between a peripheral upper limb artery such as the radial or ulnar and an adjacent vein (Figs. 24–3 and 24–4). The shunt is usually placed on the nondominant extremity to restrict the patient's activities as little as possible. In instances where the distal vessels have previously been used, the same artery is cannulated a centimeter or two more proximally. In those patients requiring repeated shunt revisions, even multiple ligations of one forearm artery have not produced distal vascular insufficiency. In these cases the final shunt in that forearm may lie quite close to the elbow (Fig. 24–4). Because of the small size of the peripheral vessels in children, the initial shunt may have to be placed in the arm between the brachial artery and the cephalic vein.

When vessels in the forearms are unsatisfactory because of thrombosis caused by multiple venipunctures and intravenous infusions, or because of multiple previous shunts, lower extremity shunts may be necessary.[18] Satisfactory types are shown in Figure 24–5 between either the anterior or posterior tibial arteries and the long or short saphenous veins. Occasional patients are seen in whom the distal vessels in the upper and lower limbs have been previously used and have undergone thrombosis. In such instances it may be necessary to anastomose a free graft of the saphenous vein to the superficial femoral artery to provide access to the arterial circulation and to use the proximal divided end of the vein for the venous return (Fig. 24–6).

Shunt devices of the Quinton-Scribner type[54] are supplied as Silastic tubes with separate Teflon tips or as all-Silastic pieces. The standard curved shunt tubes are currently being replaced with straight ones which facilitate removal of blood clots. However, a minor disadvantage of straight tubes is that the site of insertion must be higher in the limb than with conventional shunts because the connecting tube must lie distally rather than proximally. This results in a loss of arterial length and may be important in patients requiring long-term dialysis. A further type of shunt is that described by Thomas,[71] in which each tube has a Dacron skirt at one end for end-to-side anastomosis to artery and vein. Both limbs of the shunt are exteriorized and are connected to one another with a Teflon tube.

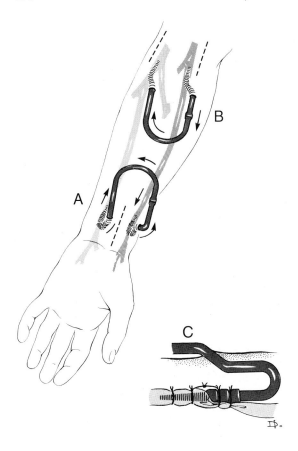

Figure 24-4 *A*. Standard arteriovenous shunt in lower part of forearm. *B*. Shunt near elbow. Direction of tubes is opposite to that in *A* to avoid crossing the antecubital fossa. Dotted lines in *A* and *B* represent incisions used, and arrows indicate direction of blood flow. *C*. Detail showing cannula firmly secured in blood vessel, and buried subcutaneous portion of Silastic tube emerging through the skin.

An advantage of this shunt is that the distal artery is not interrupted as it is with the Scribner shunt. This permits its use in a large artery such as the superficial femoral. The shunt is also said to have a lower incidence of clotting.[20]

The survival rate for external shunts varies considerably from one center to another. With good surgical technique average shunt life is 8 to 17 months for the arterial and 7 to 10 months for the venous limbs.[16] The most common causes of shunt failure are infection and thrombosis.[17] The former can lead to septicemia or bacterial endocarditis. Mild shunt infections, manifested by a small amount of seropurulent drainage with erythema around the cannula sites, may respond to vigorous antibiotic therapy. Otherwise it is necessary, in addition, to remove the shunt completely and

establish a fresh one far removed from the infected area.

Declotting of a thrombosed shunt is often possible by means of syringe suction, an Intracath catheter, a Fogarty balloon catheter, irrigation with heparinized saline or instillation of fibrinolysin to dissolve clot which cannot be mechanically removed. Shunt angiography (Fig. 24-7) is often valuable to establish whether there is a mechanical cause, such as marked angulation of a cannula tip or a stricture in a vessel requiring revision of the affected limb. In the absence of a mechanical fault repeated clotting may be an indication for systemic anticoagulant therapy.

Other problems encountered with shunts are erosion of the skin overlying the buried portion of the tube, hemorrhage around the cannula and false an-

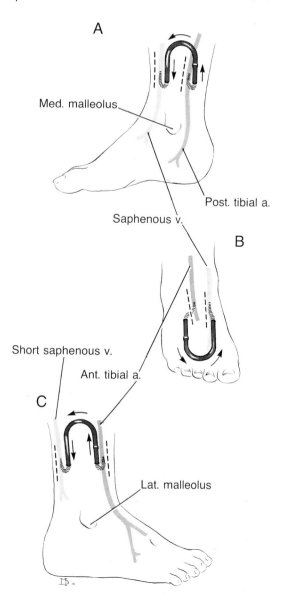

Figure 24–5 A. Shunt between posterior tibial artery and long saphenous vein. *B.* Anterior tibial artery connected to long saphenous vein by the shunt. *C.* Shunt between anterior tibial artery and short saphenous vein. In *A*, *B*, and *C* dotted lines represent incisions used, and arrows indicate direction of blood flow.

eurysm formation at either the arterial or venous ends (Fig. 24–7). The relatively high incidence of complications and the necessity for repeated surgical revisions of the cannulas contribute to the psychological fixations which some patients develop about their shunts.

Internal arteriovenous fistulas are increasingly popular as a means of obtaining access to the patient's circulation for hemodialysis, particularly when a prolonged period of treatment is necessary.[10, 41] A few weeks after creation of such a bypass the veins become arterialized, remain distended and can be easily punctured.

Most fistulas are placed in the distal portion of an upper limb by performing a 5 to 8 mm side-to-side anastomosis between the radial or ulnar artery and an

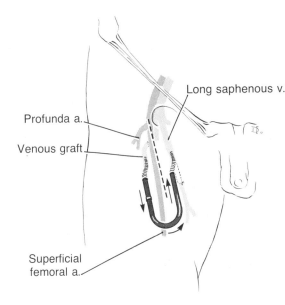

Figure 24–6 Free graft of saphenous vein used for access to the arterial circulation. The proximal divided end of the vein is cannulated for the venous return. Dotted line represents incision used and arrows indicate direction of blood flow.

adjacent vein (Figs. 24–8 and 24–9). Alternatively, an end-to-end or end-of-vein-to-side-of-artery anastomosis can be constructed. An advantage of an end-to-side anastomosis is preservation of continuity of the artery should the vein or fistula become clotted. The artery usually remains patent and the second artery in the same extremity can be used with impunity, if it is needed.[25]

A useful procedure, when there are no suitable veins in the distal forearm, is to place a saphenous vein graft subcutaneously as a straight conduit between the radial or ulnar artery at the wrist and one of the antecubital veins.[25] If the distal vessels are unsatisfactory, a fistula can be made between the lower part of the brachial artery and an adjacent vein, or a segment of long saphenous vein can be placed as a gentle loop in the subcutaneous tissues of the forearm by end-to-side anastomosis with the distal brachial artery and a similar union with the cephalic vein just at or below the elbow. When the upper limb vessels are unsuitable a fistula may be constructed in a lower extremity.[18] (Fig. 24–10). Occasional patients are seen whose peripheral vessels in all extremities have become thrombosed after the repeated use of external shunts. In such cases division of the long saphenous vein in the midthigh and anastomosis of the proximal end to the superficial femoral artery will provide a subcutaneous arteriovenous conduit which can readily be punctured whenever necessary (Fig. 24–11).

Most patients prefer an internal fistula to the external shunt. Complications are less frequent and the patient is freed from having tubes in his arm or leg. Disadvantages are the necessity for two venipunctures for each dialysis, and the fact that blood flow rates are lower than those obtained with shunts. Edema of the extremity distal to the fistula sometimes occurs, and occasional reports have appeared of ischemic changes in the limb, thromboembolic complications, venous aneurysms, cardiac embarrassment, or infection leading to frank septicemia or bacterial endocarditis.[25, 36, 41, 67] Fortunately, these complications are uncommon but they may require excision of the fistula.

The patient with a shunt or fistula may require dialysis two or three times a week for periods of 6 to 12 hours at a time, in preparation for transplantation.

In between dialyses he is maintained on a 2 gm sodium diet containing 30 to

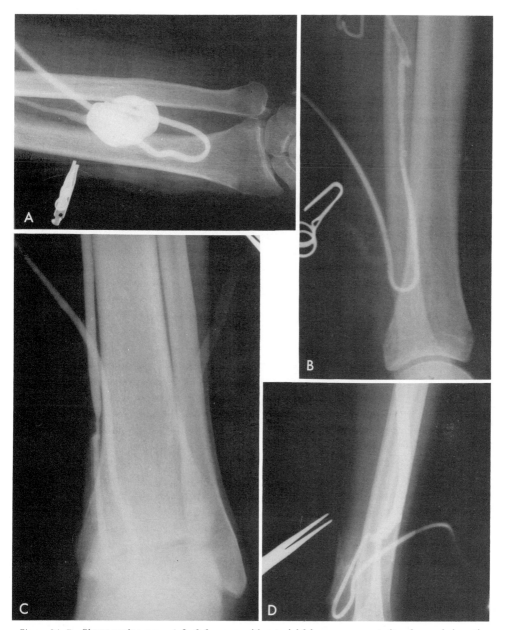

Figure 24-7 Shunt angiograms. *A*. Left forearm with arterial false aneurysm at site of cannula insertion. *B*. Right lower leg with irregular filling defects caused by thrombi in the long saphenous vein. *C*. Right lower leg with stricture of long saphenous vein just above cannula tip. *D*. Left forearm with marked angulation of cannula and stricture of vein.

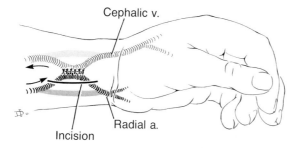

Figure 24–8   Side-to-side arteriovenous fistula. Dotted line shows incision used and arrows indicate direction of blood flow.

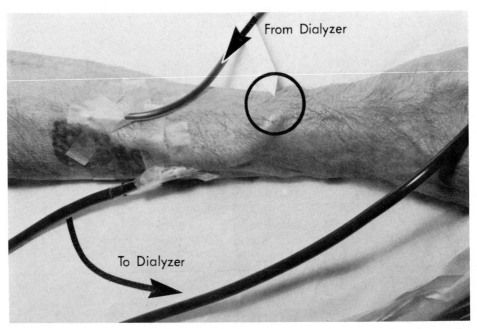

Figure 24–9   Radial artery cephalic vein arteriovenous fistula (indicated by circle). The prominent cephalic vein has been punctured and blood is being returned from the dialyzer through the tube (at the top of the photograph) which is connected to a needle in another forearm vein.

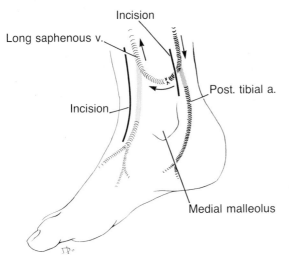

Figure 24–10   End-to-end arteriovenous fistula. Dotted lines represent incisions used and arrows indicate direction of blood flow.

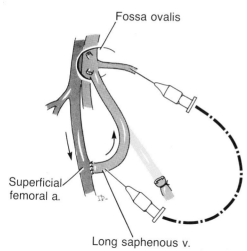

Fossa ovalis

Superficial
femoral a.

Long saphenous v.

Figure 24–11 End-to-side arteriovenous fistula in the proximal thigh. Arrows indicate direction of blood flow. Syringes show sites of venipuncture for obtaining access to the circulation.

50 gm of protein and providing 2000 to 3000 calories. In addition to the water content of the diet the patient is permitted a daily fluid intake of 600 ml plus an allowance equivalent to the previous day's urinary output. Antihypertensive drug therapy may be necessary.

The patient is managed on an outpatient basis until he is ready for transplantation unless he requires admission for a preliminary operative procedure. Depending on circumstances he may require thymectomy for added immunosuppression; a gastric operation to control pre-existing lower urinary tract obstruction; parathyroidectomy for severe secondary hyperparathyroidism; or nephrectomy. This latter operation is performed if renal infection is present, as in pyelonephritis or congenital polycystic disease; for severe hypertension which cannot be controlled by dialysis and drugs; for progressive subacute glomerulonephritis; or for Goodpasture's syndrome. In these cases nephrectomy may precede transplantation by several weeks or months. In the meantime the patient is maintained on regular hemodialysis as an outpatient.

Preoperative Preparation of the Living Donor

In our center approximately 80 per cent of renal transplants are obtained from related living donors. Whenever a patient becomes a candidate for renal transplantation his family is contacted for possible volunteers, all of whom are fully informed about the procedure. Those wishing to proceed are then screened by performing ABO blood grouping and histocompatibility typing for human leukocyte antigens (HL-A).[69] ABO incompatibility between the donor and the recipient automatically eliminates that volunteer.[59] The ideal donor-recipient combinations are identical twins, but these are rarely available. The next best combination is very closely matched siblings (double haplotype identity on lymphocyte typing[26]). Otherwise, HL-A typing has not served as a useful guide to the selection of donors, as many recipients of poorly matched kidneys have done well and conversely, some recipients of well-matched kidneys have had problems with rejection.[26, 63] Further advances in histocompatibility typing will be needed to improve donor-recipient matching.

The best possible donor selected on the basis of blood typing is then thoroughly evaluated as to his general physical and mental condition and renal function.[49] After a full history and physical and mental evaluation, the volunteer undergoes the following tests: chest radiography, electrocardiography, a full blood count, fasting blood sugar, two hour postprandial blood sugar, serum electrolytes, urinalysis, microscopic examinations of the urine, urine cultures, BUN, creatinine, creatinine clearance and intravenous pyelography.[49] Serum is also tested for the Australia antigen to exclude a hepatitis carrier state. Any positive reactors are excused as donors. Only if all the above investigations are satisfactory is the patient subjected to the final test of abdominal aortography. This demonstrates whether single or multiple arteries supply the kidneys, and also whether there is any unsuspected disease involving these vessels. This examination permits the surgeon to choose a kidney which is supplied by a single artery, or—if bilateral double renal arteries are present—the kidney with vessels which will be easiest to anastomose in the recipient. Slight abnormalities, such as an athermatous plaque at the origin of the renal artery, are not a contraindication to donation. The "abnormal" kidney is removed and transplanted to the recipient. Aortography provides protection to the donor, as sometimes serious but unsuspected disorders are present and contraindicate operation in that volunteer.[49] All studies on the donor can be performed on an outpatient basis. He is admitted to the hospital 24 to 48 hours prior to the transplant operation.

Postoperative Management

Postoperative Management of Living Donors

Most donors can be discharged from the hospital 7 to 10 days after the operation. They require little treatment at this stage and their convalescence is usually uneventful. After discharge an occasional patient may need outpatient care for a complication such as a wound infection, persistent wound pain or urinary tract infection.

Immediately following kidney donation renal function is halved. This rapidly improves so that by the end of the first postoperative week the creatinine clearance reaches approximately 70 per cent of preoperative values. Thereafter there is little further change. None of our donors have developed postoperative renal insufficiency.[49]

Postoperative Management of Renal Homograft Recipients

Two aspects are important:
    A. Maintenance therapy with immunosuppressive drugs and other agents.

    B. Prevention and treatment of complications.

A. Maintenance Therapy. The average patient is discharged from the hospital three to five weeks after transplantation. Immunosuppressive therapy in outpatients utilizes four agents: azathioprine (Imuran), prednisone and antilymphocyte globulin (ALG),[60, 61] and cyclophosphamide. At this stage the dose of azathioprine is relatively stable, but the dosage of prednisone and ALG will require reduction in the following weeks.

In our center azathioprine administration is commenced at 5 mgm/kg and is then reduced to daily maintenance levels of 1.5 to 2.5 mgm/kg. Dosage depends on the white blood cell count which is initially done on a daily basis but by the time the patient is discharged from the hospital is performed once or twice a week, and later, less frequently. We are guided more by sudden changes in the count than by the absolute number of cells. A sudden large drop is an indication for reduction in dosage or, if severe, for omission of the drug until the leukocytes have recovered. Daily counts are again performed until the downward trend has been reversed. If the level falls below 2000 cells/cu mm the patient should be admitted to the hospital and placed in reversed isolation because of the risk of serious infection.

During episodes of threatened rejection the dosage of azathioprine should not be increased, as the drug is partially excreted by the kidney and toxic levels may develop rapidly in the presence of impaired renal function. We prefer instead to use larger doses of prednisone.

Another toxic effect of azathioprine is liver injury.[47, 59, 60, 72] Liver chemistries are therefore performed once a month for the first six months and, thereafter, every three months. Evidence of jaundice or serious alteration of liver function is an indication to hospitalize the patient for further investigation to exclude other possible causes, particularly hepatitis. If azathioprine is believed to be responsible dosage is reduced or another immunosuppressive agent such as cyclophosphamide is substituted.[72]

Azathioprine may also have teratogenic effects. While animal studies have shown that it may cause fetal abnormalities[21] the risk in man appears to be small. Thus far our patients have been responsible for 35 pregnancies, of which only two resulted in children with congenital anomalies.[53]

Prednisone dosages vary from time to time. Currently we are using a schedule in which an adult patient initially receives 40 to 60 mgm per day. The daily dose is reduced by 5 to 10 mgm approximately once a month till a final maintenance level of 0.2 to 0.3 mgm/kgm per day or less is reached. Occasionally patients have had their prednisone therapy permanently discontinued.

If threatened rejection occurs, it is managed by an increase in steroid dosage. We have used several different methods of treatment. One technique is to increase dosage to 100 or 200 mgm per day and then to reduce the level progressively, provided of course that the rejection episode is satisfactorily aborted. An alternative method is to give 625 mgm of methyl prednisolone intravenously as soon as rejection is suspected, and to increase the daily maintenance dose of prednisone by 20 to 30 mgm. The intravenous doses can be repeated every second or third day if necessary until the rejection episode is reversed. Thereafter the prednisone dose is gradually reduced toward the original maintenance level. The large intravenous doses cause drastic reductions in the peripheral lymphocyte counts and are very useful in reversing severe rejection episodes.

The corticosteroids have many toxic side effects.[59, 60] In all transplant centers it has been noted that a large percentage of the morbidity following organ transplantation can be attributed to the use of these agents. Obesity is common, mainly because of the tremendously increased appetite engendered by the steroid therapy, and aided by relaxation of the dietary restrictions which the patient may have experienced for many months or years before the transplant operation. Moon

facies, acne, obesity and other manifestations of Cushing's syndrome are a source of considerable distress to some patients, particularly young females. Hypertension is another common problem which requires therapy (see below). Osteoporosis is a frequent complication of prolonged steroid administration and may cause pathologic fractures, while aseptic necrosis of the head of the femur (Figs. 24–12 and 24–13) is another side effect. If this is recognized early and steroid dosage is reduced, obesity treated, and weight bearing avoided, it may be possible to prevent severe degenerative arthritis. Steroid-induced diabetes mellitus is looked for by periodic measurements of the fasting blood sugar and examination of the urine. Treatment includes reduction of prednisone dosage if possible, dietary restriction and administration of oral hypoglycemic agents or insulin if necessary. In many instances we have observed that when steroid therapy is reduced below a critical level the diabetes will completely resolve.

Large doses of prednisone in children may cause stunting of growth (Fig. 24–14). We have attempted to avoid this by administration of the drug on alternate days but, so far, our experience with this mode of therapy is too small to draw any definite conclusions. However, we have repeatedly observed that when steroid dosage is reduced below a critical level normal growth will resume (Fig. 24–14).[39]

Peptic ulcer is a common complication of steroid administration. We have treated patients with known ulcers surgically before the transplant operation to avoid exacerbation of symptoms and complications such as perforation or gastrointestinal bleeding, which we encountered in 8 of 184 (4.3 per cent) of patients who were studied.[46] After transplantation all patients are treated prophylactically with antacids. Initially these are administered every two hours, day and night. As steroid dosage is reduced the frequency of antacid administration is decreased to every four to six hours dur-

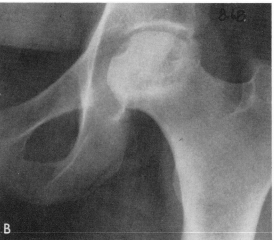

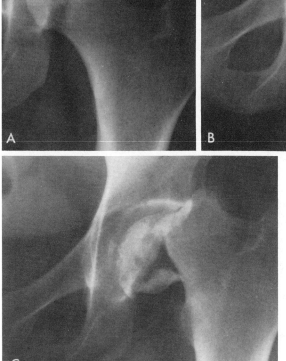

Figure 24–12 Pathologic fracture of head of femur. *A.* Normal appearance of left hip soon after transplantation. Radiograph taken during routine intravenous pyelography. *B.* Sixteen months post-transplantation. Aseptic necrosis of the head of the femur is present. *C.* Fifteen months later a pathologic fracture of the head of the femur is evident.

ing the day, with a double dose before retiring for the night.

Prednisone may also cause fatty infiltration of the liver. This may account for some of the abnormalities in hepatic function which occur postoperatively.[47, 72] Occasionally fat embolism may occur,[30] which may be the cause of aseptic necrosis of the head of the femur.[19]

Psychiatric disorders, particularly depression and lethargy, may result from steroid therapy. In some cases steroids may cause severe toxic psychosis.[50] Symptoms improve with reduction in dosage.

Other complications include pancreatitis and an increased risk of pulmonary tuberculosis. Cataracts are by no means unusual, and any patient who develops visual symptoms should have an ophthalmologic consultation.

In our center ALG therapy consists of intramuscular injections of globulin obtained from antiserum raised in horses and having a leukagglutin titer of 1/4000 to 1/16,000.[60, 61] The usual dose is 4 ml in adults and 2 ml in children. Injections are given daily for the first fourteen days, and on alternate days for a further two weeks. In patients who receive kidneys from related living donors therapy is then continued on a twice weekly basis for three more months and is then discontinued. In cadaveric organ recipients the twice weekly administration is continued indefinitely, provided that there

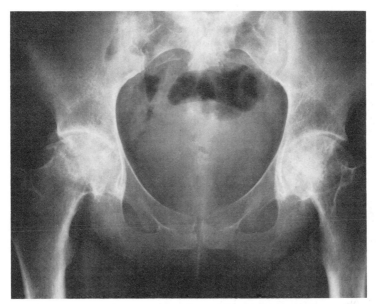

Figure 24–13 Bilateral aseptic necrosis of the femoral heads six years after renal transplantation. The condition had been present for several years at the time the radiographs were taken.

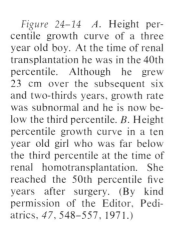

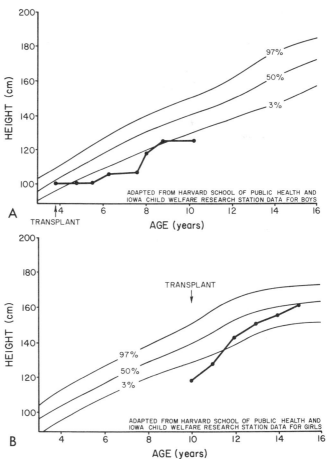

Figure 24–14 A. Height percentile growth curve of a three year old boy. At the time of renal transplantation he was in the 40th percentile. Although he grew 23 cm over the subsequent six and two-thirds years, growth rate was subnormal and he is now below the third percentile. *B.* Height percentile growth curve in a ten year old girl who was far below the third percentile at the time of renal homotransplantation. She reached the 50th percentile five years after surgery. (By kind permission of the Editor, Pediatrics, *47*, 548–557, 1971.)

are no serious reactions. Treatment with ALG has been maintained for periods of almost three years. The most common side effects are pain, tenderness, erythema and swelling at the site of injection.[60, 61] Occasionally the local reaction may simulate cellulitis, but it usually subsides in 24 to 36 hours. Fever is not uncommon after ALG administration and, at times, may cause diagnostic difficulty in patients suspected of harboring an infection. Skin eruptions, usually of urticarial type, occur occasionally. Thrombocytopenia is another occasional complication. It may be severe enough to warrant temporary cessation of ALG therapy and administration of platelet transfusions. Antibodies to ALG develop during the course of treatment. A potential consequence is nephritis due to deposition of antigen-antibody complexes in the microvasculature of the kidney. This has not been a problem in our experience, but may occur following intravenous administration of the globulin.[70]

The major risk of ALG therapy is an anaphylactic reaction.[60, 61] This has caused us to discontinue its administration prematurely in approximately 15 per cent of our patients. The reaction occurs within a few minutes after injection. It manifests itself by a sudden flushing of the face, pain in the lower back, a feeling of constriction in the chest, dyspnea, anxiety and hypotension. Treatment with intravenous hydrocortisone 100 to 400 mgm, Benadryl 50 to 100 mgm, and (if the patient is hypotensive) a liter of saline will usually abort the attack. Occasionally it may be necessary to administer epinephrine as well. We have had two fatalities caused by ALG therapy.

During the past year we have been evaluating cyclophosphamide (Cytoxan) as a substitute for azathioprine in our immunosuppressive regimen.[75, 76] In more than 100 patients treated thus far we have found that cyclophosphamide is as potent and safe as azathioprine when used in low doses in combination with prednisone and ALG. The incidence of side effects, including bone marrow depression, serious infection and gastrointestinal morbidity, is not significantly different with these two agents. Our current practice is to use cyclophosphamide in all new patients for the first three to eight weeks and then switch to azathioprine for chronic therapy. Since these agents have different actions on their target cells, it is hoped that the transition from one agent to the other may promote more effective destruction of immunologically competent cells which are replicating in response to the antigenic stimulus. Whether or not this is true still has to be determined by further clinical observations and controlled laboratory experiments. Patients receiving chronic treatment with azathioprine who manifest evidence of toxicity to the agent, such as hepatic damage, may completely recover after a switch to cyclophosphamide maintenance therapy.

Dosage of cyclophosphamide in our patients is considerably less than that used in cancer chemotherapy, where it has a reputation of being very toxic. Therefore, complications such as gastrointestinal complaints, alopecia and hemorrhagic cystitis either are uncommon or are not observed at all. The dosage of cyclophosphamide per body weight is about 40 per cent of that of azathioprine. When used from the outset, cyclophosphamide is given in a dose of 3 to 5 mgm/kg and is then reduced to daily maintenance levels of 1 mgm/kg or less. Dosage depends on the white blood cell count which is closely followed, as already described for azathioprine therapy. When cyclophosphamide is substituted for azathioprine at some stage in the patient's post-transplantation course, the initial dose is approximately two-thirds of the existing azathioprine level and is then adjusted according to the patient's white blood cell count.

Outpatient visits are initially made twice weekly when the patient is receiving ALG at this frequency. Once this treatment is discontinued the intervals between clinic visits are progressively increased so that patients may be seen once every 6 to 12 months. Recipients who are seen infrequently at our clinic do have periodic checkups performed by their own physicians.

At each clinic visit the patient is questioned regarding any untoward symptoms. His weight, blood pressure, height (if a child) and temperature are recorded. The abdominal incisions and kidney homograft are examined and evidence of peripheral edema is sought. Further examinations are carried out as indicated by the patient's symptoms. A complete blood count, including a platelet count, is performed as a guide to therapy with Imuran and ALG. Adjustments in dosage of immunosuppressive agents and other drugs are made. Other studies include BUN, serum creatinine, creatinine clearance, urinalysis, microscopic examination of the urine, urine culture, and measurement of protein, urea, creatinine, sodium, potassium and chloride in a 24 hour specimen.[59] Liver function tests (bilirubin, SGOT, alkaline phosphatase, prothrombin time and serum protein electrophoresis) and tests for the Australia antigen[47, 72] are performed every one to three months. An intravenous pyelogram is obtained once every 6 to 12 months, or as indicated. Serum calcium, phosphorus, magnesium, amylase, and fasting blood sugar are obtained once a month or more frequently if necessary.

Manifestations of secondary hyperparathyroidism in patients with chronic renal failure usually undergo resolution after successful renal homotransplantation.[1, 29] Despite this, hypercalcemia is frequently noted postoperatively. Among the factors which may contribute to this is the use of phosphate-binding antacids. In many cases we have found that adjustment of the phosphate intake with the use of phosphate-containing compounds such as Phosphaljel (Wyeth) or K-Phos (Beach) will readily control the hypercalcemia.[1] In the last two years we have measured ionized serum calcium levels in all patients with hypercalcemia, and have found persistent hyperparathyroidism much more frequent than we previously believed. We have now performed 25 parathyroidectomies in a series of almost 500 renal homograft recipients.

B. Prevention and Treatment of Complications. The renal homograft recipient is liable to a great variety of complications. The most frequent problems are rejection or infection. The two conditions frequently occur together[63] and one may predispose to the other.

Acute Renal Homograft Rejection

This usually occurs within the first few weeks or months after transplantation. Rejection is usually recognized by evidence of deterioration of renal function or its effects[59]—albuminuria, reduced urinary output, elevated BUN, decreased creatinine clearance, sudden weight gain with peripheral edema, and hypertension. The patient complains of feeling out of sorts and may have fever and leukocytosis. The kidney is often enlarged and tender and there may be edema of the overlying skin. In severe cases the patient requires admission to the hospital for treatment, which can later be continued on an outpatient basis, while the less severe attacks can be treated wholly on an outpatient basis.

Chronic Rejection

Chronic rejection of a renal homograft manifests itself by a slow deterioration of renal function with elevation of the BUN and decline of the creatinine clearance. Albuminuria may become severe with a loss of as much as 20 gm of albumin per day, and hypoproteinemia may ultimately develop. Marked hypertension is often present.

Attempts are being made to prevent this type of rejection with long-term anticoagulation and the administration of platelet deaggregators,[34] but the results are not impressive. Furthermore, there is no effective treatment for the established condition. The patient should continue on immunosuppressive therapy as long as worthwhile renal function can be retained without serious hazard. As renal function fails plans should be made for another renal homograft or for maintenance on permanent hemodialysis.

Infection

Infection represents a serious hazard to the transplant recipient.[59, 63] Immunosuppressive therapy reduces the patient's resistance to a wide variety of bacterial, fungal, viral and protozoal agents. The risk of infection is greatest when immunosuppression is at its height. This is usually at the time of threatened rejection of the organ. In our experience the most common cause of death after renal transplantation is a combination of rejection and infection.[63] Any fever should be treated with the greatest suspicion. A thorough physical examination should be performed, and if no obvious cause is found a chest radiograph should be obtained, as well as cultures of throat, sputum, urine and blood. Mild to moderate fevers can be investigated on an outpatient basis, but if the patient appears obviously ill he should be hospitalized for investigation and treatment.

Common types of infection are herpes labialis and moniliasis involving the mouth and lips. These will usually respond to reduction in immunosuppressive dosage, and topical therapy with deoxyuridine or mycostatin respectively. Occasionally monilial infection may spread to involve the pharynx or larynx or the blood stream. Such cases will require admission for more intensive therapy. Herpes zoster is another common infection. Most cases can be managed as outpatients but occasionally the disease may become disseminated with the risk of a fatal outcome. If there is any suspicion that herpes is spreading the patient should be hospitalized immediately.

Virus warts (verruca vulgaris) occur in about 40 per cent of patients. Most involve the hands but in several patients we have found extensive lesions on the scrotal skin. Large warts may require excision, not only for cosmetic reasons, but also because it may be difficult clinically to distinguish them from carcinoma, which has occurred in three of our patients (Fig. 24–15).

Bacteriuria has been reported in 40 to 80 per cent of patients in several large series during the early post-transplantation period.[62] Most cases respond well to treatment with the appropriate antibacterial agent. Persistent urinary tract infections occur in 6 per cent of cases and may require prolonged treatment, particularly when caused by proteus or pseudomonas organisms. A possible mechanical cause for persistent infection should always be excluded.

Pneumonia is the most common of the more serious infections.[59, 63] A chest radiograph is therefore mandatory in any patient complaining of fever, breathlessness, cough or chest pain. Besides bacterial and viral pneumonias fungal infections are by no means rare, as also is the pneumonia caused by the protozoon *Pneumocystis carinii*. The latter condition frequently manifests itself with breathlessness. Physical examination of the chest is often normal but the diagnosis is suggested by cyanosis, a bilateral infiltrate in the lower lung fields (Fig. 24–16) and evidence of desaturation of the arterial blood. All patients with proven or suspected pneumonia should be hospitalized forthwith.

Infections of the central nervous system, causing meningitis or brain abscess, are not uncommon. Any patient who develops fever and neurologic symptoms must be immediately admitted for investigation.

In our experience wound infections are uncommon and most are superficial. Deep infections usually occur while the patient is still hospitalized and may considerably delay his dismissal. After this occurs the wounds may still require repeated irrigations and dressings, and steroid therapy must be kept as low as possible to permit healing.

Performance of routine liver chemistries has shown that 60 per cent of our patients have evidence of hepatic dysfunction at some stage of their postoperative course.[47, 60, 72] Most disturb-

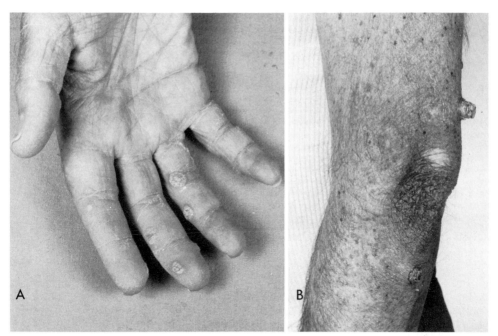

Figure 24–15 *A*. Multiple warts of right hand which appeared approximately one year after renal transplantation. Patient had numerous lesions on both upper extremities and face. *B*. Seventy-four months after transplantation the patient presented with the large lesions near the left elbow. The lower lesion was a squamous cell carcinoma while the upper was a wart. During the following year the patient had multiple lesions excised from the upper limbs and head. The majority were warts but in addition there were multiple squamous cell carcinomas.

ances occur during the early months after transplantation and are usually mild and of short duration. Azathioprine, prednisone or other hepatotoxic drugs may be responsible for some of the changes. Recently we have found that at least half the cases are caused by virus hepatitis, as shown by positive tests for the Australia antigen. Such infections are frequently of low grade but may be

Figure 24–16 Chronic *Pneumocystis carinii* pneumonia in a 15 year old renal homograft recipient. The patient had breathlessness, cough and fever for many weeks. The linear density at the right base is the result of open pulmonary biopsy which was necessary to establish the diagnosis in this case.

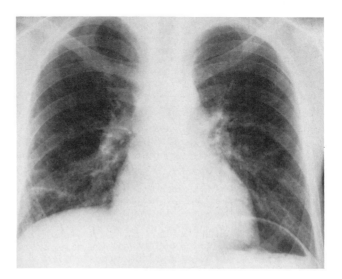

very persistent. The dangers of these infections are twofold. First, they may contribute to the patient's death. Second, they serve as a reservoir for potential spread to other patients and to the medical and nursing staff. Great care must be exercised when drawing blood samples or performing surgical procedures on these individuals.

Other Complications

A great variety of other complications have been seen in renal transplant recipients. Only the more common ones will be mentioned here.

Renal. In transplants between identical twins a high incidence of recurrence of the original disease has been described in patients who required transplantation for glomerulonephritis.[45] This has not been our experience in a small series of cases. Prophylactic penicillin therapy is advisable to prevent this complication. Despite this, recurrent glomerulonephritis has been reported in some cases. Azathioprine is currently being used in some centers in an attempt to prevent this possibly autoimmune complication.

In nontwin transplant recipients we have found a high incidence of glomerulonephritic changes.[63] Definite evidence of this disease was found in 47.6 per cent of 105 patients studied by conventional light microscopy, and another 21.9 per cent had more subtle findings detectable only by ultrastructural or immunofluorescent techniques. In approximately 22 per cent of the cases the pathologic features were suggestive of recurrence of glomerulonephritis, but in the remainder they were probably manifestations of chronic rejection.[63]

Urologic. Urologic complications have occurred in the transplanted kidney or ureter in approximately 10 per cent of our patients.[62] These include persistent urinary tract infections, ureteral stricture, ureteral calculus, hydronephrosis, compression of the ureter by a pelvic lymphocele (Fig. 24–17) and urinary fistulas. Apart from fistulas which occur

early postoperatively while the patients are still hospitalized, the remaining complications are usually recognized by studies performed at routine outpatient follow-up visits. If the complications are mild the patients are followed on an outpatient basis with urine cultures and serial intravenous pyelograms. Recipients with more severe lesions require admission to the hospital for corrective surgery.

Cardiovascular. Hypertension is commonly seen in renal homograft recipients. We have observed this at some stage in at least 50 per cent of our patients. There are several possible causes for this, including acute rejection of the transplant, chronic rejection with thickening of the vascular endothelium and reduced blood flow, high dosage steroid therapy, and persistent hypertension in those patients whose own diseased kidneys have not been removed. The patients are managed with a restricted sodium intake, and the administration of one or more of the following antihypertensive drugs—hydrochlorothiazide, rauwolfia, hydralazine, L-methyl dopa, and guanethidine. If one agent in maximal therapeutic doses is unable to control the blood pressure, other drugs are added as necessary in the order indicated. Other aspects of treatment will vary with the cause of the hypertension. Acute rejection is usually reversed with increased immunosuppressive therapy. Blood pressure often decreases with reduced steroid dosage, but removal of the native kidneys occasionally may be necessary if severe hypertension persists despite drug therapy. Frequently it is possible to reduce or completely eliminate antihypertensive drug therapy as rejection episodes are reversed or steroid therapy is reduced. However, many patients must remain on antihypertensive drug therapy indefinitely.

There is an increased incidence of venous thromboembolism after transplantation. Possible causes include steroid therapy, an increased platelet count following splenectomy, thrombus formation at the renal vein anastomotic line, or

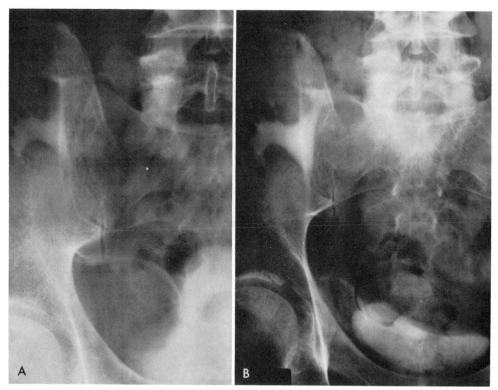

Figure 24–17 A. Marked upward and medial displacement of homograft ureter and compression of the bladder by a large lymphocele. This appeared within a few weeks of transplantation and persisted unchanged for many months without causing hydronephrosis. *B.* Intravenous pyelogram after surgical drainage of lymphocele two and a half years after transplantation showing marked improvement in the course of the ureter and absence of previous filling defect in the bladder outline.

stasis in the stumps of the host renal veins. Any complaint of calf pain or swelling, chest pain, breathlessness or fever requires thorough investigation. Except for cases with mild superficial thrombophlebitis, all suspected cases of thromboembolism should be admitted for treatment. Subsequent to discharge from the hospital the patient is seen regularly as an outpatient to monitor long-term anticoagulant therapy, and to prevent any sequelae of deep vein thrombosis of the legs.

Peripheral arterial thrombosis has been rare in our experience but we have seen progressive intermittent claudication in a young male who had fairly severe arterial disease at the time of transplantation. We have also observed acute coronary artery occlusions in several young patients. Presumably long-standing hypertension and steroid-induced hypercholesterolemia played a role in causing these lesions.

Musculoskeletal. Most of the complications involving this system are the result of steroid therapy. They include osteoporosis with vertebral collapse, pathologic fractures and myopathy. Thirty-eight per cent of a group of our patients who were studied showed other evidence of connective tissue disorders, including avascular bone necrosis, synovitis, arthralgia and diffuse musculoskeletal pain.[9] "Steroid pseudorheumatism" appears to be the underlying cause of many of these problems,[55, 58] but ALG may be responsible for some of the joint and muscle symptoms. Bone and joint sepsis is rare but hand infections or instances of septic arthritis are occasionally seen. Pre-existing uremic neuropathy usually improves after successful transplantation, but recovery may be incomplete even after one year.[7]

Gastrointestinal Complications. These are often the result of steroid therapy. As mentioned earlier we try to prevent peptic ulceration with intensive antacid therapy. Despite this it is sometimes necessary to admit the patient to the hospital because of gastrointestinal bleeding or perforation of a peptic ulcer.[46]

Intestinal obstruction may be caused by adhesions resulting from the previous abdominal surgery and may require admission for treatment.[46]

A form of ulcerative colitis and other colonic lesions have been occasionally observed following transplantation.[48] These often require treatment on an inpatient basis.

Acute pancreatitis or pancreatic pseudocysts are occasionally encountered, usually early in the postoperative period. These lesions may be related to operative trauma during splenectomy and host nephrectomy, high dosage steroid therapy, hyperparathyroidism, azathioprine toxicity, or renal failure.

Despite the young age of most of our patients we have seen acute appendicitis in only 2 of more than 400 renal transplant recipients. For this reason we do not perform prophylactic appendectomy as has been advocated by some workers.[28]

Obstetrical and Gynecologic. A gratifying feature of successful renal transplantation is the restoration of sexual function and the opportunity for parenthood should this be desired. Female patients are advised against pregnancy during the first 18 to 24 months after operation to be certain that kidney function remains stable. Thus far ten of our patients have become pregnant on 13 occasions.[53] Two of the pregnancies were terminated with therapeutic abortions and three more are in progress. The other eight resulted in live births. Frequent outpatient monitoring is necessary, as some deterioration of renal func-

tion occurs during pregnancy in about one-third of the patients. In our experience this returns to its pre-existing state in the postpartum period but other workers have recorded failure of recovery of renal function.[53] There are also increased risks to the infant. Most of these occur early in the neonatal period, but occasional congenital defects may require outpatient management.

Dysplasia of the cervix uteri has been observed in female renal transplant recipients receiving immunosuppressive therapy.[24, 33] In addition, we have collected reports of seven renal homograft recipients who developed carcinoma in situ of the cervix, including three in our own patients.[51, 52, 63] We therefore strongly believe that females should have a pelvic examination and vaginal smear before transplantation and at regular intervals thereafter. If a carcinoma of the cervix is detected, the patient should be admitted for definitive treatment.

The Problem of Malignancy. The use of immunosuppressive agents causes an increased risk of *de novo* malignant disease, and may enhance the growth of pre-existing tumors or of neoplasms inadvertently transplanted with a kidney taken from a cadaver donor who died of cancer.[51, 52, 63] In our own series we have found an approximately 6 per cent risk to the recipient of the development of some form of *de novo* malignancy. We have collected data on 57 tumors which developed in organ transplant recipients treated in centers all over the world. The average period of time after transplantation for development of the lesions is two and a half years. About 60 per cent are of epithelial origin (Fig. 24–15), most commonly carcinomas of the skin, lip or uterine cervix, but highly malignant carcinomas of the internal organs also occur. Of the remaining tumors the majority are varieties of lymphoma, most frequently reticulum cell sarcoma. In transplant recipients this tumor shows a particular predilection for the brain.[56]

It is important to be aware of the danger of malignancy so that any unusual symptoms can be promptly investigated. Most of the patients will require admission to the hospital for appropriate therapy, but tumors of the skin or lip can be widely excised in the conventional manner on an outpatient basis, and uterine cervical carcinoma-in-situ can sometimes be completely removed by performing a wide cone biopsy during a brief stay in the hospital.

Psychiatric Complications. The stress of a potentially fatal illness coupled with a major surgical procedure and prolonged postoperative care is associated with the development of psychiatric symptoms in 32 per cent of patients.[50] Episodes of anxiety and depression are common, particularly when complications mar the postoperative course. An organic psychosis may result from several causes, including large doses of steroids, infectious complications and poor renal function. The antihypertensive drugs may also cause psychological side effects. The patient often has adjustment difficulties, as a successful operation may convert him from a dependent status to one in which he must once again become independent and cope with life's problems. Occasional recipients who are unable to adjust may manifest suicidal tendencies. Those with the more severe psychiatric symptoms should be hospitalized for treatment. The other patients need assurance and guidance and much can be accomplished in the outpatient clinic to help them deal with their problems and resume useful places in the community.

LIVER TRANSPLANTATION

Selection of Liver Recipients

Patients requiring liver transplantation are in the end stages of hepatic disease. Their life expectancy can be measured in days, weeks, or perhaps, a few months. The main indications[60, 64] (Table 24–1) for the operation are as follows: (1) Con-

TABLE 24–1 INDICATIONS FOR ORTHOTOPIC LIVER TRANSPLANTATION*
(University of Colorado Series)

DISEASE	NO. OF PATIENTS
Congenital biliary atresia	20
Hepatoma	12
Cirrhosis	7
Cirrhosis caused by Wilson's disease	3
Chronic active hepatitis	3
Total	45

*Patients aged 11 months to 68 years.

genital biliary atresia in cases in which no reconstructive surgery is possible. (2) End stage cirrhosis of the liver. This represents a large pool of patients, as more than 90 per cent of deaths from liver disease in the U.S. result from this disorder. (3) Hepatoma which is confined to the liver, but is so extensive that it cannot be treated by hepatic lobectomy. (4) Severe chronic active hepatitis. (5) Liver-based metabolic disorders. Hepatic homografts retain their metabolic specificity after transfer to a new host.[60] Theoretically, certain liver-based metabolic disorders might be treatable with hepatic replacement in patients who are severely incapacitated and cannot be adequately treated by more conservative measures. Severe cirrhosis caused by Wilson's disease may be an example of this group of disorders.[64] (6) Acute hepatic failure from fulminating viral hepatitis or ingestion of hepatic poisons. We have not performed any transplants for this indication.

In the selection of patients for transplantation the criteria are similar to those used for renal recipients except, of course, that there is usually no concern about the status of the lower urinary tract. Investigations should be undertaken to exclude other serious disorders, and to rule out metastases in patients with hepatoma. These studies are particularly important in children with biliary atresia in whom other serious congenital anomalies may contraindicate transplantation.

Preoperative Management

Routine liver function studies are necessary to assess the degree of hepatic impairment; ABO blood grouping and lymphocyte typing are performed as a guide to matching with a suitable cadaver donor[69]; and serologic tests are made for the Australia antigen.[72]

Many candidates for liver transplantation are so ill that they cannot be treated as outpatients. Those who can be managed on this basis require supportive therapy until a suitable donor can be found. Treatment includes dietetic control (protein and salt) to prevent hepatic coma and reduce ascites; the latter may also necessitate the administration of diuretics. If the patient is jaundiced and shows a tendency to hypoprothrombinemia, vitamin K is given parenterally. Severe itching may be ameliorated with cholestyramine. Gastrointestinal bleeding, hepatic precoma or serious infections will, of course, necessitate admission to the hospital. All infections, no matter how minor, must be eradicated as quickly as possible so that the patient is in the best possible condition to receive a transplant whenever a donor becomes available.

Postoperative Management

Maintenance Therapy

As a liver transplant operation and the postoperative convalescence are much more complicated than a renal transplantation, the patient is kept in the hospital for six weeks or longer. After being discharged he is maintained on immunosuppression with azathioprine, prednisone and antilymphocyte globulin, as described earlier in connection with cadaver kidney transplantation, except that the daily doses of azathioprine are usually smaller (averaging 1.2 mgm/kg).[60, 64] Sodium dehydrocholate (Decholin) 250 t.i.d. is given to reduce bile viscosity and prevent cholestasis,[6] and antacids are administered. Hyper-

tension is rare after liver transplantation[60] but, if present, it may require drug therapy. Usually there are no fluid or dietary restrictions.

The patient periodically attends the follow-up clinic where he is examined for signs of rejection or other complications. Liver function tests are performed, including serum bilirubin, alkaline phosphatase, SGOT, SGPT, prothrombin time and serum protein electrophoresis. Australia antigen studies are done at regular intervals.[72] When indicated, liver scans are also done, using Technetium-99. Hematologic tests are performed as in renal homograft recipients, as well as urinalysis, BUN and creatinine clearance. Chest radiographs and cultures of the sputum, urine, throat, blood and stool are performed if there is any suspicion of infection.

Prevention and Treatment of Complications

Many of the complications described in renal recipients are seen also in hepatic homograft patients with the exception, of course, of many of the urinary tract complications and hypertension. Again, rejection and infection rank as the major problems.[60, 64]

Rejection

Acute rejection usually occurs in the early weeks after transplantation. Most cases occur while the patient is still hospitalized but occasional instances are seen in the outpatient clinic. The degree of rejection may vary from a mild anicteric episode to a severe rejection crisis. Mild rejection may be detectable only by elevation of the SGOT and SGPT levels and by changes in the liver scan, but in a severe rejection the patient may become severely ill within a few hours.[60, 64] Warning symptoms are anorexia, extreme fatiguability, fever, pain in the back, nausea and vomiting. Evidence of fluid retention may be manifested by weight gain, periorbital and dependent edema. The liver is enlarged and tender and the patient may become frankly icteric. The serum bilirubin and alkaline phosphatase are increased and are often accompanied by elevations of the serum enzymes. Polymorphonuclear leukocytosis may be present. Radioisotope scans usually show enlargement of the homograft. Sometimes the organ may be clinically enlarged, but the scan shows a paradoxically small liver owing to reduced blood flow with consequent poor uptake of the isotope. Irregular filling defects may also be seen in areas of diminished blood flow.

All cases of suspected acute hepatic rejection should be promptly admitted to the hospital for treatment.

Chronic rejection occurs several months after transplantation. The picture resembles obstructive jaundice with elevation of the serum bilirubin and alkaline phosphatase, and dark urine and pale stools.[60, 64] The condition results from gross narrowing of the arteries and arterioles within the liver, causing marked interference with blood flow, necrosis, collapse of lobules, cholestasis and ultimately fibrosis. Serial liver scans show a slow but steady shrinkage of the organ. Deterioration of liver function progresses relentlessly and the eventual clinical picture is of chronic hepatic insufficiency with prominent abdominal wall collaterals, spider angiomata, peripheral edema and ascites. There is currently no way of treating this condition except by replacement of the failing liver with a healthy homograft.[60, 64] One of our patients who was treated in this way lived for a year before he succumbed to liver failure resulting from the same problem affecting the second homograft.

Infection is particularly liable to occur in hepatic transplant recipients as the liver is repeatedly exposed to organisms from the bowel, which reach it either through the portal venous system or via the biliary passages.[60, 64] Infection is especially common during rejection episodes when the poorly functioning organ is unable to deal with the organisms reaching it and septicemia develops.

Frank sepsis may occur in the liver itself in cases with rejection.[60, 64] Ischemic zones in the organ may become colonized by gram negative organisms with resultant areas of gangrene and abscess formation. These can be recognized as filling defects in a radioisotope liver scan. This complication can be prevented by early recognition and vigorous treatment of rejection.

Besides the increased tendency to liver abscesses and septicemia the hepatic homograft recipient is prone to any of the infections mentioned under renal transplantation. Recently we have found that viral hepatitis is common in the long-term survivors after hepatic transplantation. This diagnosis has been facilitated by routine Australia antigen studies.[72] The finding is an important one, as in the past the clinical and biochemical changes would have been interpreted as being caused by rejection, and an increase in immunosuppressive therapy would have resulted. Instead, dosage was maintained or reduced and the patients have made satisfactory recoveries, although they have tended to remain chronic carriers of the antigen.

Recurrence of Malignant Disease. In six of our patients who underwent transplantation for hepatoma and who survived from 2 to 17 months, five developed metastases, and in four instances the recurrences were directly responsible for death.[51, 60, 64] The most common sites of the lesions were the lungs and the homografts themselves and were recognized on serial chest radiographs and liver scans. In addition, serum α-fetoprotein levels remained persistently elevated, suggesting the presence of residual tumor. Only one of our patients, a 4 year old child with intrahepatic biliary atresia and an incidental hepatoma, is alive with no evidence of recurrence 17 months after operation. Occasional successes in the management of hepatoma by liver replacement have also been accomplished by Daloze of Montreal and Calne of Cambridge. At the present time the discouraging results of transplantation for hepatoma lead us to consider this form of treatment only in exceptional cases.

HEART TRANSPLANTATION

Selection of Cardiac Recipients

In the selection of cardiac transplant recipients the cardinal rule is that the patient has terminal heart disease not amenable to any other surgical procedure or medical treatment. Since most heart disease is caused by coronary arteriosclerosis this is the most common reason for cardiac transplantation.[12, 40] Cardiomyopathy is another indication[31] despite the theoretical danger that the immune factors responsible for the original disease could damage the homograft. Rheumatic multivalvular disease, although often correctable by valve replacement, may have caused such severe damage that cardiac transplantation is required. Severe congenital anomalies, not amenable to surgical correction, also warrant excision of the organ and its substitution by a healthy one.

Definite contraindications are infection, carcinoma and severe systemic disorders such as diabetes. Patients with multiple organ disease who are not expected to benefit from improved cardiac function should not undergo cardiac transplantation, and patients of advanced age or questionable emotional status may not be suitable candidates.

Preoperative Management

Most potential recipients are so ill that they require hospitalization. A few can be managed as outpatients with supportive therapy including digitalis, quinidine, diuretics and oxygen. All foci of infection should, of course, be eliminated as expeditiously as possible.

Postoperative Management

Maintenance Therapy

After discharge from the hospital the patient is initially seen twice a week and later at progressively increasing intervals. Immunosuppression is similar to that described under cadaver kidney transplantation and the patients also receive antacid therapy. Besides the hematologic, urinary and liver studies mentioned earlier the cardiac status is evaluated by clinical and laboratory observations. Exercise tolerance is assessed on the history and by tests such as Master's two step test, and if desired, by measurement of the cardiac output before and after exercise.[12] Serial electrocardiographs are a valuable guide to the diagnosis of acute rejection.[40, 65] Ultrasound cardiography permits estimation of total heart size and chamber dimensions, as well as left ventricular wall thickness.[65] Other tests for rejection are serial measurements of the enzymes LDH, CPK and SGOT; and periodic myocardial scintiscanning using Cesium 131 chloride.[32]

Prevention and Treatment of Complications

As with transplantation of other organs the major problems are rejection and infection.[12, 40, 65]

Acute Rejection. Decrease in exercise tolerance is a warning sign of impending rejection. Clinical findings in the early stages are the appearance or accentuation of a previously present pericardial friction rub, and the development of abnormal diastolic heart sounds, usually an early diastolic gallop, although a presystolic gallop has also been noted.

The electrocardiogram serves as the primary index of acute rejection. Characteristic and reversible changes include decreased electrocardiographic voltage, atrial arrhythmias, rightward deviation of the mean electrical axis, and ischemic type ST segment changes.[65] Ultrasound cardiography shows increased total heart and right ventricular chamber size, thickening of the left ventricular wall, and variable decreases in the transverse diameter of the left ventricular cavity.[65] Changes in the levels of the enzymes LDH, CPK and SGOT unfortunately reflect the severity of the rejection process rather than providing an early warning system.[40] Kahn[31] also finds that decreased uptake of Cesium 131 chloride by the myocardium is useful in the diagnosis.

Because there is danger of development of a sudden arrhythmia with potentially lethal consequences, all patients with suspected acute rejection should be immediately hospitalized for treatment.

Chronic Rejection. This results from intimal thickening in the coronary arteries and their branches and has been responsible for many of the late deaths following transplantation.[12] It manifests itself by a progressive reduction in exercise tolerance and the development of cardiac failure. In some centers attempts have been made to prevent this complication with long-term anticoagulant therapy and the use of the platelet deaggregator, dipyridamole.[32] Experience with this form of treatment is still too small to draw any definite conclusions.

As heart failure develops medical treatment for this condition will have to be instituted. Attempts have been made to replace chronically rejecting hearts with further cardiac homografts[12, 31] but no long-term survivals have yet been obtained.

LUNG TRANSPLANTATION

Selection of Pulmonary Recipients

The prime candidates for this procedure are patients who are gravely ill with primary pulmonary hypertension or restrictive lung disease.[15, 74] Unilateral transplantation in patients with chronic obstructive pulmonary disease has failed, largely owing to a serious ventilation-perfusion imbalance between the homograft and the host's residual lung. Attempts are being made to overcome this problem with bilateral lung replacement. Occasional transplants have also

been performed for acute respiratory insufficiency caused by toxic pneumonitis or trauma.[74]

Preoperative Management

Most candidates are so ill that they are already in the hospital. Those few who are outpatients will require work-up to exclude other serious nonpulmonary problems. Supportive pulmonary therapy is essential and foci of sepsis must be eradicated, particularly in the lungs, otherwise there is a grave danger of cross-infection involving the transplanted organ.

Postoperative Management

Little can be said of postoperative care as, thus far, only one patient has survived long enough to be treated on an outpatient basis.[14] Besides immunosuppressive therapy the patient needs careful clinical and radiologic follow-up with periodic studies of arterial blood gases and pulmonary function.

Acute rejection is heralded by general malaise, cough, dyspnea and a fall of arterial pO_2 values.[14] The risk of lung infection is particularly great. It is nearly impossible to distinguish between infection and rejection of the homograft.

PANCREATICO-DUODENAL TRANSPLANTS

Selection of Pancreatico-Duodenal Recipients

Transplantation of the pancreas and duodenum (to provide drainage of the exocrine secretions of the former organ) or of the body and tail of the pancreas alone is indicated in cases of severe juvenile-onset diabetes complicated by marked retinopathy and nephropathy.[37, 38] In most cases which have been treated to date the kidney damage has been so marked as to necessitate renal replacement at the same time as the pancreatic transplantation. As more experience has been gained a trend has developed toward replacing the pancreas before the stage of terminal nephropathy, thus eliminating the need for concomitant renal transplantation.

Preoperative Management

Preoperative care is the same as that already described under renal transplantation, with the additional problem of control of severe diabetes. There are difficulties in treating these patients with dialysis, which has a high morbidity and mortality.[37] The extent of the vascular damage caused by the diabetes needs to be carefully assessed. Particular emphasis is placed on the elimination of septic foci.

Postoperative Management

Maintenance Therapy

After discharge from the hospital the patient's care is much the same as that already described under cadaver renal transplantation. If the pancreatic homograft is functioning satisfactorily the patient does not require insulin, and the fasting blood sugar and glucose tolerance tests are normal.

Additional follow-up studies include periodic measurements of the fasting blood sugar; glucose tolerance; blood insulin, amylase, and lipase levels; and the effects of tolbutamide stimulation.[37, 57, 68]

Prevention and Treatment of Complications

The major problems have been with sepsis and rejection of the kidney transplants, even though in each case they were obtained from the same donors as the pancreases.[37, 38] The pancreatic ho-

mografts have shown very little tendency to undergo rejection. However, the duodenum has suffered rejection on two occasions, and the patients presented with acute abdominal symptoms. Pancreatic rejection should be suspected by recurrence of diabetes or elevation of the serum amylase or lipase levels.[37, 57, 68] Threatened rejection of the kidney, pancreas or duodenum is best handled on an inpatient basis.

Partial pancreatic transplants have not functioned for periods longer than four months. Failure was caused by pancreatitis, infection, autolysis or technical problems associated with the procedure.[37, 38]

BONE MARROW TRANSPLANTATION

Selection of Bone Marrow Recipients

Bone marrow transplants are usually performed in patients who are seriously ill with one of the following disorders[8, 73] which have failed to respond to other forms of treatment: (1) Accidental whole body irradiation. (2) Aplastic anemia. (3) Immune deficiency diseases, including agammaglobulinemia, hypogammaglobulinemia, the Wiscott-Aldrich syndrome and the DiGeorge syndrome. (4) Leukemia. (5) A variety of malignant diseases. The aim of bone marrow transplants in the first three disorders is to repopulate all hemopoietic tissues or to replace a deficiency of only the lymphoid series of cells. In (4) and (5) the object is not only to restore depleted blood elements but to provide immunocompetent cells which, it is hoped, will destroy residual malignant cells which have persisted after other forms of therapy.

Preoperative Management

Preoperative donor work-up should exclude the possibility of transmittable infections or malignant disease. For successful bone marrow transplantation the ideal donor is an identical twin, as there is no need for immunosuppressive therapy in these cases. Otherwise a relative who is carefully matched for the ABO, Rh and HL-A antigens should be used. The "one-way mixed lymphocyte culture test"[4] seems to be particularly useful in selecting well-matched combinations. In the absence of a familial volunteer, an unrelated donor—either living or cadaveric—may be used. However, at the present time the only worthwhile long-term results have been obtained in transplants between ABO and HL-A identical siblings.

Care of the recipient before admission to the hospital for the transplantation is purely supportive and depends on the condition being treated. It may include blood transfusions and antibiotic treatment of infections, which are common in many of the patients. Those with leukemia and other types of cancer usually require treatment with one or more cancer chemotherapeutic agents. Before transplantation immunosuppressive pretreatment is given, using total body irradiation, steroids, azathioprine, cyclophosphamide or antilymphocyte globulin. In some centers pretreatment of the donor with ALG is being investigated.[43]

Postoperative Management

The donor needs no special treatment after discharge from the hospital.

Maintenance Therapy

Except in transplants between identical twins the recipients usually require continuation of immunosuppressive therapy to prevent rejection of the homograft or a graft versus host reaction.

Frequent outpatient hematologic studies are necessary to establish that the grafted bone marrow is functioning and that a state of partial or complete chimerism has been established. The proliferation of the transfused cells is determined by means of erythrocyte or leukocyte antigenic markers, or both. Depending on the patient's condition, transfusion of whole blood or blood constituents such as platelets may still be necessary.

Complications

The most frequent problems are persistence of the original malignant disease, or the development of infection or rejection. Infectious problems are particularly likely to occur because many patients already have impaired immune responses which may be further reduced by the immunosuppressive agents. These complications are frequent indications for hospitalization of the recipients.

Rejection may be of two types.[8] (1) Failure of engraftment is heralded by a disappearance of the initial symptomatic and hematologic improvement. The patient may require admission because of hemorrhage or infection, and further transplantation attempts may be made. (2) Graft versus host disease (G.V.H.D.) is a disorder in which immunologically competent donor cells become established and react to the host's tissues as if they were foreign. The resulting immunologic reaction results in an illness characterized by generalized wasting and malaise, gastrointestinal dysfunction (with anorexia, diarrhea, malabsorption and weight loss), exfoliative dermatitis, destruction of hepatic tissue with abnormal liver function tests and jaundice, fever, and an increased susceptibility to fungal and viral infections.[22] The disorder may occur despite HL-A identity,[22, 44] suggesting that antigenic differences must reside at as yet undetected non HL-A sites. G.V.H.D. occurs in two forms: an acute type which begins within a few days of transplantation and which terminates either in death of the host as early as 14 days later, or by attenuation of reactivity and recovery within 4 to 6 weeks; and a chronic syndrome which occurs more than 30 days after transfusion.

Attempts have been made to prevent

or minimize G.V.H.D. by using grafts of hemopoietic stem cells with as few lymphoid cells as possible.[2] Pretreatment of the recipient with ALG has also been successfully used to prevent G.V.H.D.[43]

LONG-TERM RESULTS OF TRANSPLANTATION

Just over a decade ago the world experience of human organ transplantation consisted of a handful of renal homograft recipients. Apart from transplantation between identical twins the outlook was dismal and survival was for short periods only. During the intervening years the picture has changed dramatically and long-term function has been achieved with kidney, liver, heart, pancreas, lung and bone marrow transplants. In consequence an increasing number of organ recipients are being treated on an outpatient basis.

More than 5826 kidney recipients have been treated throughout the world.[5] With identical twin transplants survival as long as 15 years has been accomplished, with fraternal twins 11 years, with related donors survival of more than 8 years and with nonrelated donors more than 7 years.[63] In our center 236 renal homograft recipients are currently receiving outpatient treatment at postoperative intervals ranging from several weeks to almost 9 years; 49 of these patients have survived 5 years or more.

The world experience with liver transplantation is much less extensive, 139 homografts having been performed. Currently at least 7 patients are alive. Of these, 5 were treated in our center, with survival ranging from several weeks to almost 3 years (the longest survival in the world to date) (Fig. 24–18). In our experience the one-year survival rate after orthotopic liver transplantation is 27 per cent.[64]

Heart transplants have been performed in 168 patients throughout the world. Results have shown that the procedure can rehabilitate very ill patients with secondary effects on the lungs, livers and kidneys, restoring them to satisfactory health for months or even years

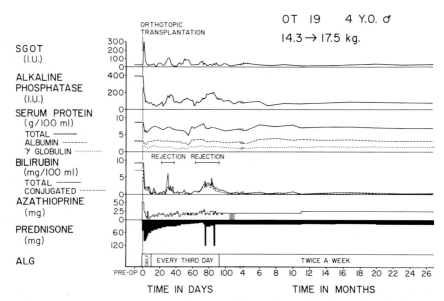

Figure 24–18 Postoperative course of a four year old boy who received an orthotopic liver transplant for congenital biliary atresia. Apart from two mild rejection episodes during early convalescence his liver function has remained excellent. He is now almost three years post-transplantation.

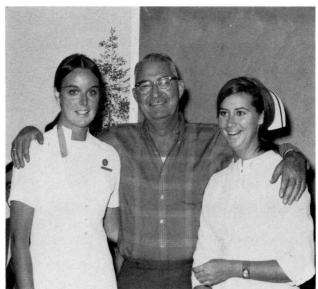

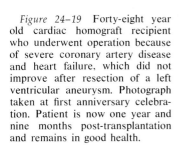

Figure 24–19 Forty-eight year old cardiac homograft recipient who underwent operation because of severe coronary artery disease and heart failure, which did not improve after resection of a left ventricular aneurysm. Photograph taken at first anniversary celebration. Patient is now one year and nine months post-transplantation and remains in good health.

(Fig 24–19). Twenty-five grafts are currently functioning and the longest survivor is 31 months post-transplantation.[5] Shumway's group has reported a one year survival of 34 per cent.[65]

Lung transplants involving the whole lung, a lobe, or both lungs and the heart have been performed in 25 patients.[5, 74] There has been only one long-term survivor; he died ten months after operation of bronchopneumonia and chronic rejection of the transplant.[14]

Pancreatic homografts have been performed in 23 patients and the longest survivor succumbed after 12 months.[37, 38]

Bone marrow transplants have been performed in at least 203 patients.[8] Twenty-two grafts are functioning at present and the longest survival to date has been 31 months.[5]

At least eight patients have received splenic homografts. The chief indication has been terminal carcinoma in patients in whom it was hoped to induce a graft (donor spleen) versus host (recipient's carcinoma) reaction by providing a continuous source of immunocompetent cells which were foreign to the host lymphatic system.[42] The spleen donors had been sensitized with nonviable tumor cells obtained from biopsy of the recipient's malignancy. Other spleen transplants have aimed to replace the suspected enzyme deficiency in Gaucher's disease;[23] to correct the immunologic deficiency in a child with agammaglobulinemia;[42] and to provide Factor VIII in a severe case of hemophilia.[27] The results thus far have been disappointing with no evidence of survival of the transplant for more than a few weeks.

Transplants of fetal thymic tissue have been used in an attempt to restore immunologic competence in various syndromes of congenital immunologic deficiency. Many of these transplants have failed and some patients have developed graft-versus-host disease. However, in two cases of the DiGeorge syndrome (congenital thymic aplasia) immunologic competence has persisted for 16 and 18 months respectively[3, 11] with gratifying clinical improvement; while a child with Swiss type agammaglobulinemia was making good progress almost six months after receiving a cadaver fetal thymus plus a bone marrow transplant from his sister.[13]

Transplantation of the larynx has been performed in one patient who had a total laryngectomy for carcinoma. He died of recurrent cancer 10 months later.[35]

Small bowel replacements have been performed in less than a dozen cases. The longest survival was two and a half months.

The field of organ transplantation is rapidly expanding. In the coming years we can anticipate greater numbers of long-term survivors who will require treatment on an outpatient basis. It is therefore important for the surgeon to be familiar with the handling of these patients.

References

1. Alfrey, A., et al.: Resolution of hyperparathyroidism, renal osteodystrophy and metastatic calcification after renal homotransplantation. New Engl. J. Med., *279*:1349–1356, 1968.
2. Amato, D., et al.: Review of bone marrow transplants at the Ontario Cancer Institute. Transplant. Proc., *3*:397–399, 1971.
3. August, C. S., Levey, R. H., Berkel, A. I., and Rosen, F. S.: Establishment of immunological competence in a child with congenital thymic aplasia by a graft of fetal thymus. Lancet, *1*:1080–1083, 1970.
4. Bach, F. H., and Voynow, N. K.: One way stimulation in mixed leukocyte cultures. Science, *153*:545–547, 1966.
5. Bergan, J. J.: A.C.S.-NIH Organ Transplant Registry, Spring Newsletter, 1971.
6. Bell, P., Homatas, J., MacSween, R., and Brettschneider, L.: Bile secretion following orthotopic transplantation of the liver in dogs. Surg. Forum *20*:295–297, 1969.
7. Bolton, C. F., Baltzan, M. A., and Baltzan, R. B.: Effects of renal transplantation on uremic neuropathy. A clinical and electrophysiologic study. New Engl. J. Med., *284*:1170–1175, 1971.
8. Bortin, M. M.: A compendium of reported human bone marrow transplants. Transplantation, *9*:571–587, 1970.
9. Bravo, J. F., Herman, J. H., and Smyth, C. J.: Musculoskeletal disorders after renal homotransplantation. A clinical and laboratory analysis of 60 cases. Ann. Intern. Med., *66*:87–104, 1967.
10. Brescia, M. J., Cimino, J. E., Appel, K., and Hurwich, B. J.: Chronic hemodialysis using venipuncture and a surgically created arteriovenous fistula. New Engl. J. Med., *275*:1089–1092, 1966.
11. Cleveland, W. W., Fogel, B. J., Brown, W. T., and Kay, H. E. M.: Foetal thymic transplant in a case of DiGeorge's syndrome. Lancet, *2*:1211–1214, 1968.
12. Cooley, D. A., et al.: Cardiac replacement: Current status of cardiac transplants and prostheses. Ann. Int. Med., *73*:677–681, 1970.
13. Dekoning, J., et al.: Transplantation of bone marrow cells and fetal thymus in an infant with lymphopenic immunological deficiency. Lancet, *1*:1223–1227, 1969.
14. Derom, F., et al.: Ten month survival after lung homotransplantation in man. J. Thoracic and Cardiovasc. Surg., *61*:835–846, 1971.
15. Derom, F.: Current state of lung transplantation. Transplant. Proc., *3*:313–317, 1971.
16. Dunea, G.: Peritoneal dialysis and hemodialysis. Med. Clin. N. Amer., *55*:155–175, 1971.
17. Faris, T. D., and Carey, T. A.: Arteriovenous shunts for hemodialysis. Amer. J. Surg., *114*:679–684, 1967.
18. Faris, T. D., Alfrey, A. C., Schorr, W. J. and Ogden, D. A.: Lower extremity shunts for hemodialysis. J.A.M.A., *203*:344–346, 1968.
19. Fisher, D. E., and Bickel, W. H.: Corticosteroid-induced aseptic necrosis. Surg. Forum, *20*:454–455, 1969.
20. Franzone, A. J., et al.: Hemodialysis in children: Experience with arteriovenous shunts. Arch. Surg., *102*:592–593, 1971.
21. Githens, J. H., Rosenkrantz, J. G., and Tunnock, S. M.: Teratogenic effects of azathioprine (Imuran). J. Pediat., *66*:959–961, 1965.
22. Graw, R. G., Jr., et al.: Graft-versus-host reaction complicating HL-A matched bone marrow transplantation. Lancet, *2*:1053, 1970.
23. Groth, C. G., et al.: Splenic transplantation in a case of Gaucher's disease. Lancet, *1*:1260–1264, 1971.
24. Gupta, P. K., Pinn, V. M., and Taft, P. D.: Cervical dysplasia associated with azathioprine (Imuran) therapy. Acta. Cytol., *13*:373–376, 1969.
25. Haimov, M., Singer, A., and Schupak, E.: Access to blood vessels for hemodialysis: Experience with 87 patients on chronic hemodialysis. Surgery, *69*:884–889, 1971.
26. Halgrimson, C. G., et al.: Net histocompatibility ratios (NHR) for clinical transplantation. Transplant. Proc., *3*:140–144, 1971.
27. Hathaway, W. E., et al.: Attempted spleen transplant in classical hemophilia. Transplantation, *7*:73–75, 1969.
28. Hume, D. M.: Progress in clinical renal homotransplantation. In Welch, C. E., Ed.: Advances in Surgery, Vol. 2. Chicago, Year Book Medical Publishers, pp. 419–498, 1966.
29. Johnson, J. J., et al.: Secondary hyperparathyroidism in chronic renal failure: Effects of

renal homotransplantation. J.A.M.A., *215*:478–480, 1971.

30. Jones, J. P., Jr., Engleman, E. P., and Najarian, J. S.: Systemic fat embolism after renal homotransplantation and treatment with corticosteroids. New Engl. J. Med., *273*:1453–1458, 1965.

31. Kahn, D. R., et al.: Human heart transplantation for cardiomyopathy. Surgery, *67*:122–128, 1970.

32. Kahn, D. R., et al.: Effect of anticoagulants on the transplanted heart. J. Thoracic and Cardiovasc. Surg., *60*:616–624, 1970.

33. Kay, S., Frable, W. J., and Hume, D. M.: Cervical dysplasia and cancer developing in women on immunosuppressive therapy for renal homotransplantation. Cancer, *26*:1048–1052, 1970.

34. Kincaid-Smith, P.: Modification of the vascular lesion of rejection in cadaveric renal allografts by dipyridamole and anticoagulants. Lancet, *2*:920–922, 1969.

35. Kluyskens, P., and Ringoir, S.: Follow-up of a human larynx transplantation. Laryngoscope, *80*:1244–1250, 1970.

36. Levi, J., Robson, M., and Rosenfeld, J. B.: Septicemia and pulmonary embolism complicating use of arteriovenous fistula in maintenance hemodialysis. Lancet, *2*:288–290, 1970.

37. Lillehei, R. C., et al.: Pancreatico-duodenal allotransplantation: Experimental and clinical evidence. Ann. Surg., *172*:405–436, 1970.

38. Lillehei, R. C., et al.: Current state of pancreatic allotransplantation. Transplant. Proc., *3*:318–324, 1971.

39. Lilly, J. R., et al.: Renal transplantation in pediatric patients. Pediatrics, *47*:548, 1971.

40. Lower, R. R., et al.: Current state of clinical heart transplantation. Transplant. Proc., *3*:333–336, 1971.

41. Lytton, B., Goffinet, J. A., May, C. J., and Weiss, R. M.: Experience with arteriovenous fistula in chronic hemodialysis. J. Urol., *104*:512–517, 1970.

42. Marchioro, T. L., et al.: Splenic homotransplantation. Ann. N. Y. Acad. Sci., *120*:626–651, 1964.

43. Mathé, G., et al.: Bone marrow graft in man after conditioning by antilymphocytic serum. Transplant. Proc., *3*:325–332, 1971.

44. Meuwissen, H. J., et al.: Graft-versus-host reactions in bone marrow transplantation. Transplant. Proc., *3* 414–417, 1971.

45. Murray, J. E., and Harrison, J. H.: Surgical management of fifty patients with kidney transplants including eighteen pairs of twins. Amer. J. Surg., *105*:205–218, 1963.

46. Penn, I., et al.: Surgically correctable intra-abdominal complications before and after renal homotransplantation. Ann. Surg., *168*:865–870, 1968.

47. Penn, I., et al.: Hepatic disorders in renal homograft recipients. In Zuidema, G. D., and Skinner, D. B., Eds.: Current Topics in Surgical Research, Vol. 1. New York, Academic Press, 1969, pp. 67–76.

48. Penn, I., et al.: Major colonic problems in human homotransplant recipients. Arch. Surg., *100*:61–66, 1970.

49. Penn, I., Halgrimson, C. G., Ogden, D., and Starzl, T. E.: Use of living donors in kidney transplantation in man. Arch. Surg., *101*:226–231, 1970.

50. Penn, I., Bunch, D., Olenik, D., and Abouna, G.: Psychiatric experience with patients receiving renal and hepatic transplants. Seminars in Psychiatry, *3*:133–144, 1971.

51. Penn, I.: Malignant Tumors in Organ Transplant Recipients. New York, Springer-Verlag, 1970.

52. Penn, I., Halgrimson, C. G., and Starzl, T. E.: De novo malignant tumors in organ transplant recipients. Transplant. Proc., *3*:773–778, 1971.

53. Penn, I., et al.: Parenthood in renal homograft recipients. J.A.M.A., *216*:1755–1761, 1971.

54. Quinton, W., Dillard, D., and Scribner, B. H.: Cannulation of blood vessels for prolonged hemodialysis. Trans. Amer. Soc. Artif. Intern. Organs, *6*:104, 1960.

55. Rotstein, J., and Good, R. A.: Steroid pseudorheumatism. Arch. Int. Med., *99*:545, 1957.

56. Schneck, S. A., and Penn, I.: De novo cerebral neoplasms in renal transplant recipients. Lancet, *1*:983–986, 1971.

57. Seddon, J. A., and Howard, J. M.: The exocrine behavior of the homotransplanted pancreas. Surgery, *59*:226, 1966.

58. Slocumb, C. H.: Symposium on certain problems arising from clinical use of cortisone; rheumatic complaints during chronic hypercortisonism and syndromes during withdrawal of cortisone in rheumatic patients. Mayo Clin. Proc., *28*:655, 1953.

59. Starzl, T. E.: *Experience in Renal Transplantation.* Philadelphia, W. B. Saunders Co., 1964.

60. Starzl, T. E.: *Experience in Hepatic Transplantation.* Philadelphia, W. B. Saunders Co., 1969.

61. Starzl, T. E., et al.: A trial with heterologous antilymphocyte globulin in man. Transplant. Proc., *1*:448, 1969.

62. Starzl, T. E., et al.: Urologic complications in 216 human recipients of renal transplants. Ann. Surg., *172*:1–22, 1970.

63. Starzl, T. E., et al.: Long-term survival after renal transplantation in humans (with special reference to histocompatibility matching, thymectomy, homograft glomerulonephritis, heterologous ALG, and recipient malignancy). Ann. Surg., *172*:437–472, 1970.

64. Starzl, T. E., et al.: Indications for orthotopic

liver transplantation: With particular reference to hepatomas, biliary atresia, cirrhosis, Wilson's disease, and serum hepatitis. Transplant. Proc., *3*:308–312, 1971.

65. Stinson, E. B., Griepp, R. B., Dong, E., Jr., and Shumway, N. E.: Results of human heart transplantation at Stanford University. Transplant Proc., *3*:337–342, 1971.

66. Streilin, J. W.: A common pathogenesis for the lesions of graft-versus-host disease. Transplant. Proc., *3*:418–421, 1971.

67. Storey, B. G., et al.: Embolic and ischemic complications after anastomosis of radial artery to cephalic vein. Surgery, *66*:325–327, 1969.

68. Teixeira, E. D., and Bergan, J. J.: Auxiliary pancreas allografting. Arch. Surg., *95*:65, 1967.

69. Terasaki, P. I. in Experience in Hepatic Transplantation. Starzl, T. E., ed. Philadelphia, W. B. Saunders Co., pp. 22–33, 1969.

70. Thiel, G., et al.: Glomerular damage after intravenous administration of antilymphocyte globulin (ALG) in man and Rhesus monkeys. Transplant. Proc., *3*:741–744, 1971.

71. Thomas, G. I.: Large vessel appliqué arteriovenous shunt for hemodialysis. A new concept. Amer. J. Surg., *120*:244–248, 1970.

72. Torisu, M., et al.: Immunosuppression, liver injury and hepatitis in renal, hepatic, and cardiac homograft recipients: With particular reference to the Australia antigen. Ann. Surg. *174*:620–639, 1971.

73. Van Bekkum, D. W.: Bone marrow transplantation. Transplant. Proc., *3*:53–57, 1971.

74. Wildevuur, C. R. H., and Benfield, J. R.: A review of 23 human lung transplantations by 20 surgeons. Ann. Thoracic Surg., *9*:489–515, 1970.

75. Starzl, T. E., et al.: Cyclophosphamide and human organ transplantation. Lancet, *1*:70–74, 1971.

76. Starzl, T. E., et al.: Cyclophosphamide and whole organ transplantation in human beings. Surgery, Gyn. and Obstet., *133*:981–991, 1971.

25

Cancer Chemotherapy

By GEORGE J. HILL, II, M.D.

INTRODUCTION

Cancer chemotherapy is, by the strictest definition, the treatment of cancer with drugs and hormones. However, the use of chemotherapy should not be separated from the total care of the cancer patient.[16] Chemotherapy should not be

907

used as a substitute for potentially curative surgery or radiation therapy. Patients receiving chemotherapy should be considered for reoperation or extended radiation if previously unfavorable tumors become correctible by local eradication.

The cancer chemotherapist must be an oncologist — a student of the biology of neoplasms. The oncologist understands the statistical likelihood of survival as related to type and stage of tumor, and he knows the relative efficacy of therapeutic modalities which are available. He is familiar with the common patterns of tumor growth and metastasis, while always being alert for unusal manifestations of neoplastic growths. He is a clinical pharmacologist, willing to test the effects of some of the most dangerous drugs used in medicine. He observes closely for objective and subjective effects of therapy on the patient and his tumor.[17] He measures dose-related consequences of therapy, and watches for the unexpected, unfavorable idiosyncratic effects of chemotherapy. He is skilled in the age-old techniques of physic: offering comfort, relief of pain, control of anxiety, and — when appropriate — sensible prognostication.[2]

GOALS

The major goals of cancer chemotherapy are (1) palliation, (2) cure and (3) research. These goals are not mutually exclusive.

Palliation. The major effort of cancer chemotherapy at this time is the palliation of patients who have incurable cancer. We define palliation as the prolongation of useful life — life which is relatively free of pain and reasonably full, the patient being returned to his usual occupation or to some other creative activity. Successful palliation is not achieved if the patient requires prolonged hospitalization,[33] or is made sicker by chronic administration of chemotherapy than he would have been if

left untreated. Thus toxic symptoms should be avoided, although mild to moderate toxicity is occasionally required in dosage-seeking during initiation of therapy.

In addition to using antineoplastic drugs, the chemotherapist must be liberal in administration of sedatives, tranquilizers and narcotics. Reassurance is combined with honesty in answers to questions, and the therapist must give sound advice regarding finances, and the use of accumulated time for vacations and sick leave. Other aspects of palliation include dietary instructions, brief hospitalizations for administration of intravenous fluids, laxatives and enemas. Since much of the success in palliation is undoubtedly due to nonspecific aspects of patient care, restoration or preservation of useful life cannot always be related to objective effects of chemotherapy.

Ninety-two percent of 400 consecutive patients treated in Chemotherapy Clinic at Colorado General Hospital received therapy for established incurable tumors — the remainder receiving adjuvant therapy for tumors with a poor prognosis. Of the patients treated for palliation, 70 percent have objectively measurable lesions and 30 percent have known but unmeasurable metastatic or residual cancer.[20]

Approximately 90 to 95 percent of patients treated in Chemotherapy Clinic at Colorado General Hospital at any time are treated as outpatients. Hospitalization is usually reserved for brief courses of intensive chemotherapy, diagnostic evaluation and terminal care.

Approximately 30 percent of patients with a broad spectrum of objectively evaluable solid tumors were found to have tumor regression when treated with chemotherapy using one or more drugs as single agents.[20] Approximately 20 percent of drug courses produced objective responses in these patients.[21]

Prolongation of life per se is not regarded as palliation and heroic efforts to add days or weeks of life are usually not indicated. On the other hand, cancer chemotherapeutic agents should not be used as a form of euthanasia. Therefore, if a life-endangering complication results from chemotherapy, aggressive management is indicated; this may include hospitalization, antibiotics, intravenous fluids, transfusions, and even cardiopulmonary resuscitation in exceptional cases.

Emergency measures may be utilized to treat patients who exhibit sudden, unexpected deterioration. Examples include perforated viscus, tension pneumothorax, hematuria, cardiac tamponade[19] or paraplegia. Hospitalization and surgery should be strongly considered in such cases. Prolongation of life per se may be indicated when the patient needs to attend to specific personal problems, such as religious, family or legal matters. In these cases the physician should consult closely with his colleagues in legal, ministerial and social professions. The presence of nurses and students who are unfamiliar with the entire problem places a special burden on the physician, and he must take the time to explain the rationale of management to them.

Cure. Prolonged survival without evidence of cancer is a goal which is more desirable than palliation of the incurable state. Chemotherapy occasionally has a part in the cure of patients as an adjunct to surgery and radiation. Chemotherapy alone may be a curative modality of treatment in other instances. Unfortunately, at the present time, the majority of tumors are not sufficiently responsive to chemotherapy to be cured by the adjuvant or solo use of therapy. Chemotherapy has, for example, resulted in improvement in the percentage of patients "cured" in acute lymphocytic leukemia of children, Wilms' tumor, choriocarcinoma, Burkitt's lymphoma and carcinoma of the testis. But the common tumors of adults, such as carcinomas of the lung, breast and gastrointestinal tract, have not—in general—been rendered more curable by the addition of adjuvant chemotherapy.

The search for improved methods of adjuvant chemotherapy is a continuing process. Cancer chemotherapeutic drugs are, by and large, also immunosuppressive and carcinogenic. The use of adjuvant chemotherapy, therefore, involves the possibility of harm as well as potential benefit. Prognosis is an important consideration, and adjuvant therapy may be more justifiable if the cure rate is only 10 percent (e.g., melanoma with positive nodes) instead of 85 percent (e.g., Dukes' A carcinoma of the rectum). Adjuvant therapy may also be indicated if average time of survival is short, as in carcinoma of the lung, rather than long, as in follicular carcinoma of the thyroid. Adjuvant therapy might also be warranted if the objective response to therapy in evaluable cases is relatively high, as in carcinoma of the breast. Studies of the adjuvant effect of chemotherapy usually require large institutions or inter-institution cooperative groups. Well controlled, randomized studies are relatively uncommon, because it is difficult to use random findings for all variables which are important—such as age, sex, stage of disease, histology, rate of growth of tumor.

It appears reasonable to offer adjuvant therapy to patients with poor prognosis, for example, in tumors with a cure rate of less than 50 percent. It is obviously important to select doses of drugs which are relatively nontoxic, or the survival may be reduced more by the therapy than by the neoplasm. Individual patients and groups of patients must be observed closely for signs of toxicity, enhancement of tumor growth or new neoplasms.

Chemotherapy Clinic at Colorado General Hospital has utilized poor prognosis as the indication for therapy in approximately 8 percent of patients treated. Virtually all of these patients received weekly low-dose chemotherapy with the most favorable known agent for one year, followed by therapy every two weeks for a second year if no sign of recurrence or metastasis was present.

Research. Each patient should be observed closely for indication of subjective or—preferably—objective signs of improvement. In the absence of objective improvement, the benefit from chemotherapy may be difficult to distinguish from the result of supportive or psychological therapy, or from other forms of palliation such as surgery or radiation therapy. The individual patient is, in this sense, his own control; most patients accept this notion readily, and participate willingly in the measurements, blood tests and x-rays which are required for evaluation.

Evaluation of therapy is important for each chemotherapy clinic. Just as a surgical service must record and criticize its statistics regarding numbers of specific procedures, complications and mortality, so must a chemotherapy clinic study its accession of patients, their length of survival, the objective remission rate and the complications of therapy.

Research begins with establishment of protocols and records. The use of a standard form (Fig. 25–1) for summarization of data has been valuable, both for management of an individual patient and for study of groups of patients. The record is updated on each visit. Sketches and measurements of lesions on the patients and on x-ray are recorded promptly, before they are lost or hidden in files. Graphs and tables of data are prepared frequently as a continuing guide to therapy and for demonstration purposes.

Inevitably, patients read or hear of "new" methods for therapy. The chemotherapist must be conversant with current developments in order to provide answers to questions from patients, relatives and other doctors. Whether or not he is a participant in formal research projects, the cancer chemotherapist will frequently be challenged to attempt unfamiliar or recently developed methods. He must approach this work with caution and objectivity, keeping careful records, obtaining consultation with his colleagues, and written, informed consent from the patients. He must maintain a candid relationship with the patient and his family, and utilize the scientific method in his clinical research.

Experimental drugs supplied by the National Cancer Institute have been administered to approximately 20 percent of patients treated in Chemotherapy Clinic at the University of Colorado Medical Center. (Fig. 25–2) The willingness of patients to cooperate in these studies has been rewarding and challenging. The cancer chemotherapist should anticipate this attitude in his patients and neither be dismayed by it nor accept it as a license to perform irrational or unscientific "experiments" with patients.

THEORY

Several types of therapeutic agents are available, which affect cells in different aspects of metabolism and replication[28, 6] (Fig. 25–3).

Antimetabolites are analogues of normal biochemical molecules which interfere with cellular metabolism and synthesis by competitive inhibition. The most commonly used antimetabolites are analogues of pyrimidines, purines, folic acid and ribose. Pyrimidines and purines are the nitrogenous bases from which the molecules of DNA and RNA are formed. Folic acid is a necessary co-enzyme in reactions which incorporate carbon into DNA and amino acids. Ribose is the 5-carbon sugar contained in DNA.

Examples of antimetabolites in common use are shown in Table 25–1.

Antimetabolites are, in general, "cycle active" drugs and are potentially effective upon all cells which are in the S phase (DNA synthesis) of the cell cycle (Fig. 25–4). On the other hand, cells in other phases of cell life are relatively protected from the effects of antimetabolites. Cells in the resting phase (G_0), or post- and premitotic phases (G_1 and G_2) are relatively insensitive to antimetabolites unless a residual concentration of the drug is present when the cell again enters the S phase. Since antimetabolites may also interfere with RNA synthesis, which occurs in the G phases, antineoplastic effect and drug toxicity are pro-

NAME ______________________
HOSPITAL __________ CHART NO. ______
AGE ____ BIRTH DATE ________ SEX ☐ F ☐ M
WEIGHT ______ LBS ______ KGM HEIGHT ______
RISK STATUS __________ FOOD INTAKE __________
REASON __________ PERFORMANCE STATUS ______

ADDRESSES:
PATIENT ______________
____
PHONE: ______

NEXT OF KIN
NAME ______________
____
PHONE: ______

PRIMARY TUMOR SITE ______________
CELL TYPE ______________
DATE OF TUMOR DIAGNOSIS ______________
ORGAN INVOLVEMENT (Incl. Primary)

LUNGS ☐ CNS ☐
BONE ☐ SKIN ☐
LIVER ☐ OTHER ☐
LYMPH NODES ☐ ______________

RADIATION THERAPY

DOSE	AREA	DATES	RESPONSE	
			OBJ	SUBJ

SUMMARY OF THERAPY:

SURGERY	DATE	RESPONSE	
		OBJ	SUB.

CHEMOTHERAPY
1. ______
2. ______
3. ______
4. ______
5. ______
6. ______

DATE	DRUG	DOSE	WBC	HCT	OTHER LAB	WGT	SIDE EFFECTS	PHYSICAL FINDINGS AND COMMENTS

Figure 25–1 Therapy record. Therapy record for patients in Cancer Chemotherapy Clinic. Stage of disease, types of previous treatment and clinical findings are recorded at initiation of therapy. At each weekly visit, blood count, drug dosage and result are added. (Adapted from form used at University of Wisconsin Hospitals).

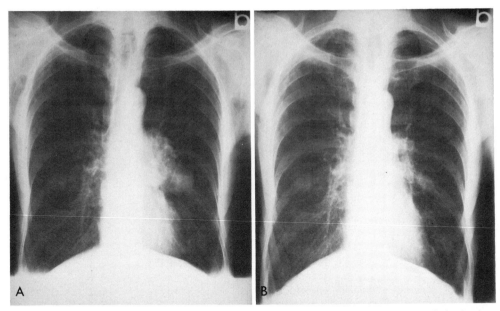

Figure 25–2 Objective tumor regression. Chemotherapy with investigational drug hexamethylmelamine, supplied by National Cancer Institute for treatment of cancer of the lung. To determine objective response, measurable lesion is required, as in this patient, who had an unresectable oat cell cancer. Primary tumor was 8.0 cm in diameter and adjacent metastasis was 2.5 cm in diameter. *(A)* Marked regression apparent in two weeks, *(B)* has persisted for four months. Objective regressions are seen in 30 percent of patients with measureable solid tumors.

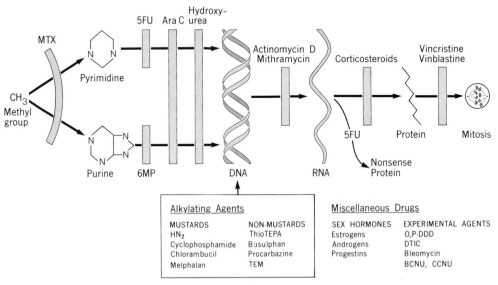

Figure 25–3 Theory of cancer chemotherapy. Theoretical sites of action of drugs in common use. Illustration is schematic and incomplete, since many drugs act at several points in intermediary metabolism.

TABLE 25–1   ANTIMETABOLITES

CHEMICAL OR GENERIC NAME	COMMERCIAL OR OTHER NAME	ABBREVIATION	MECHANISM OF ACTION AND COMMENTS	FORMULATION	DOSE (APPROXIMATE)
5-Fluorouracil	Fluorouracil	5FU	Pyrimidine analogue. Inhibits thymidylate synthetase	500 mg vials	500 mg. IV daily × 5, then once per week
5-Fluorodeoxy-uridine	Floxuridine	5FUDR	Pyrimidine analogue. Inhibits thymidylate synthetase	500 mg vials	0.1–0.6 mg/kg/day intra-arterial
6-Mercaptopurine	Purinethanol	6MP	Purine analogue. Competes with hypoxanthine and inosinic acid in DNA formation	50 mg tablets	50–150 mg PO daily
Methotrexate	Amethopterin. 4-amino-n^{10} methyl pteroylglutamic acid	MTX	Folic acid analogue. Prevents methylation by inhibition of tetrahydrofolate reductase	2.5 mg tablets $\overline{5}$ and 50 mg vials	2.5 mg PO daily $\overline{25}$ mg IV weekly
Cytosine arabinoside	Cytarabine. Cytosar	araC	Ribose analogue. Blocks incorporation of normal purines and pyrimidines into DNA	100 mg and 500 mg vials	1.0–3.0 mg/kg/day for 10–20 days
Hydroxyurea	Hydrea		Blocks DNA synthesis by inhibition of nucleotide reduction	500 mg capsules	20–30 mg/kg/day or 80 mg/kg every third day

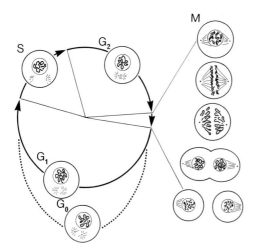

Figure 25–4   Cell cycle. Theoretical diagram of the cell cycle.*

Phase	Usual Duration
G₁–Postmitotic phase (Minimum resting phase) RNA and protein synthesis at normal rate DNA synthesis for repair only Rapid increase in RNA synthesis immediately prior to S phase	hours to days (usually constant for one cell line)
S–DNA synthetic period RNA and protein synthesis at normal rate DNA synthesis for replication	8–30 hours
G₂–Premitotic phase RNA and protein synthesis at normal rate DNA synthesis stops	30–90 hours
M–Mitotic phase RNA and protein synthesis diminish abruptly Segregation of DNA into daughter cells	30–90 minutes
G₀–Nondividing cells Cells which are in resting phase longer than the obligatory minimum period.	indefinite

*Adapted from De Vita, Vincent T. Cell kinetics and the chemotherapy of cancer. Cancer Chemotherapy Reports. Part 3, Vol. 2, No. 1:23–33, 1971.

duced by the presence of residual concentrations of drugs. The emergence of drug-resistant cell populations occurs during prolonged therapy, a phenomenon which is shown in the clinical course of the patient in Fig. 25–5.

In order to avoid the emergence of drug-resistant tumor cell populations, cycle active drugs such as ara-C and 5FU have sometimes been utilized in brief, continuous courses.[22] Other efforts to avoid drug-resistance in tumors have utilized drug combinations, to reduce the populations of drug-resistant cells by simultaneous exposure to drugs with different mechanisms of action.

In practice, the use of antimetabolites is governed more by practical, empirical decisions than by theoretical considerations. Our basic knowledge of the rate of cell turnover, the percentage of resting cells, the percentage of drug-resistant cells, and optimum drug combinations is based mainly on work with transplantable mouse tumors and cultured cell lines. However, human tumors appear to be distressingly variable *in vivo,* and drug toxicity is a greater problem in humans than in mice. Strenuous efforts in the 1950's and 1960's using toxic courses of antimetabolites in solid tumors in humans resulted in a high mortality rate from toxicity and few cures—except in choriocarcinoma. In contrast, a surprisingly high percentage of responses and excellent palliation has been achieved by the use of antimetabolites in long-term, nontoxic therapy on a daily or weekly basis. It seems possible that an unexpectedly high percentage of cells in human tumors may be in resting phase *in vivo.* If this is the case, long-term, low-dosage administration of antimetabolites would provide the best accessibility of drug when DNA synthesis is begun by the resting tumor cells.

Alkylating agents are drugs which add alkyl groups to molecules within the body. In the simplest sense, alkyl groups are methyl groups and straight chain hydrocarbons. Many alkylating agents are complex chemicals which also contain aromatic rings and other atoms in addition to carbon and hydrogen. The most commonly used alkylating agents are shown in Table 25–2. The alkylating agents first used were derivatives of mustard gas (sulfur mustard), a poison manufactured for military purposes. Nitrogen mustard (HN_2), a soluble mus-

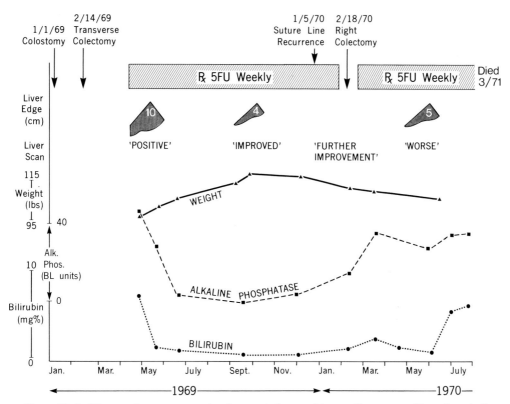

Figure 25–5 Therapeutic response and subsequent drug resistance. Treatment with antimetabolite 5FU produced initial improvement, followed by local tumor recurrence and subsequent deterioration in liver function. Resumption of chemotherapy again produced benefit, but only temporarily.

tard, was first used for cancer chemotherapy in 1946.[10] The symbol used for nitrogen mustard is apparent from its formula:

$$\text{H}_3\text{C}-\text{N}-(\text{CH}_2-\text{CH}_2-\text{Cl})_2$$

Nonmustard alkylating agents which are in common use include a phosphoramide (ThioTEPA), Busulfan (an ester of sulfonic acid), and procarbazine. Alkylating agents are said to be "radiomimetic," because they induce cellular damage similar to that produced by ionizing radiation. The critical mechanism of action of these drugs is believed to be the cross-linking of DNA strands by an alkyl bridge between adjacent nitrogenous bases, leading to fracture or failure of separation of the strands during transcription. Alkylation also occurs with proteins and other reactive molecules, including the glycolipids of the cell membrane.

Alkylating agents exhibit a phenomenon known as "log kill," which refers to the observation in animal tumors that a specific percentage of cells is killed by a given dose of drug, and the same percentage is killed each time the dose is repeated. This phenomenon may produce a cure if successive doses are administered until no living cells are left, unless drug-resistant cells are present, or toxicity precludes administration of drug at sufficiently frequent intervals. Some patients with Burkitt's lymphoma have apparently been cured with cyclophos-

TABLE 25–2   ALKYLATING AGENTS

CHEMICAL OR GENERIC NAME	COMMERCIAL OR OTHER NAME	ABBREVIATION	MECHANISM OF ACTION AND COMMENTS	FORMULATION	DOSE (APPROXIMATE)
Mustards Nitrogen mustard	Mechlorethamine	HN2	Intense local irritant	10 mg vials	Initially: 0.4 mg/kg. (When given IV administer in 4 daily doses of 0.1 mg/kg). Therapy may be repeated at approximately 3–4 wk intervals.
Cyclophosphamide	Cytoxan		Phosphoric acid amide mustard. Inactive until enzymatic activation takes place	50 mg tablets 200 mg and 500 mg vials	50–150 mg/day PO 10–15 mg/kg/wk IV
Chlorambucil	Leukeran		Aminophenylbutyric acid mustard	2 mg tablets	4–6 mg/day PO
Melphalan	Alkeran	PAM	L-phenylalanine mustard	2 mg tablets	2–4 mg/day PO
Ethyleneimines Triethylenethiophosphoramide	ThioTEPA	TSPA	Relatively free of local irritating effects; nausea minimal compared with other alkylating agents	15 mg vials	Initial dose: 30 mg IV or 60 mg intracavitary. Subsequent doses individualized weekly.
Triethylenemelamine		TEM		5 mg tablets	2.5–5.0 mg/wk
Sulfonic Acid Ester Busulfan	Myleran. 1.4-dimethane sulfonoxybutane		Alkylates and dethiolates proteins	2 mg tablets	4–8 mg/day PO
Other Alkylating Agents Procarbazine	Matulane		Alkylates and inhibits transmethylation. Used in "COPP" combination (Table 25–5)	50 mg tablets	50 mg/day PO progressing weekly to 250 mg/day if tolerated

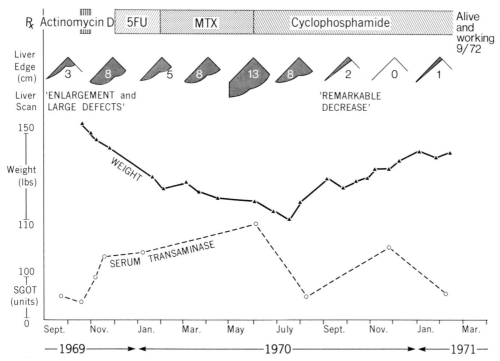

8/66 Rt. Hip Disarticulation
7/67 Lt. Lung Metastasis—Lobectomy
4/68 Rt. Lung Metastasis—Wedge Resection
2/69 Liver Metastasis symptom appeared

Figure 25–6 Selective response to chemotherapy. Therapeutic benefit from cyclophosphamide, a polyfunctional alkylating agent, is seen in this patient with metastatic osteogenic sarcoma. Liver size regressed, liver function tests improved, and patient gained weight. He had not responded to previous therapy with inhibitors of RNA synthesis (actinomycin D) and DNA synthesis (5FU and MTX).

phamide, a derivative of HN_2. The effect of cyclophosphamide in osteogenic sarcoma is illustrated in Fig. 25–6.

Inhibition of RNA Synthesis. The later phases of cell life may be summarized as transcription (formation of RNA), translation (protein synthesis), and cell division. RNA is a single-stranded molecule of nucleic acid formed along a pattern (template) of nuclear DNA. Three types of RNA are known: (1) messenger RNA (mRNA), along which the amino acids are assembled as the "message" of the genetic code is translated; (2) transfer RNA (tRNA), which is the intracellular carrier for individual amino acids; and (3) ribosomal RNA (rRNA), the function of which is still relatively obscure.

DNA-dependent RNA synthesis is blocked in sensitive cells by the antibiotics actinomycin D and mithramycin (Table 25–3), which are derivatives of *Streptomyces* species. Actinomycin D is highly toxic, even in small doses, but has a valuable therapeutic role in chemotherapy because it may eradicate all residual tumor in some instances—particularly in Wilms' tumor, choriocarcinoma, rhabdomyosarcoma and carcinoma of the testis. Kinetics analysis reveals a superficial similarity to the "log kill" action of alkylating agents (Fig. 25–7).

Inhibition of Protein Formation. Adrenal corticosteroids interfere with protein formation and stimulate conversion of amino acids to glucose, a process known as gluconeogenesis. The clinical

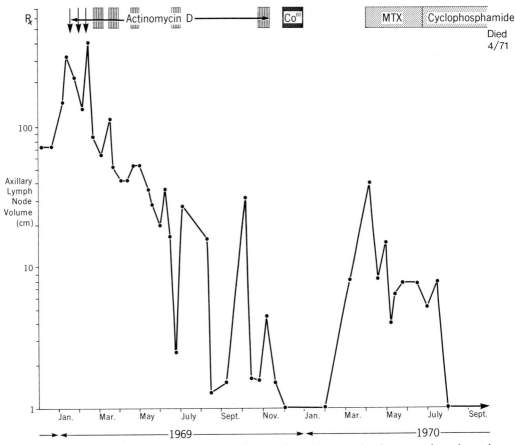

Figure 25–7 "Log kill" of tumor by chemotherapy. Logarithmic scale of tumor volume is used to illustrate percentage of cells killed by single doses and short courses of therapy. In this case, actinomycin D was used to treat metastatic rhabdomyosarcoma. Decrease in tumor volume from either 100 cc to 10 cc or 10 cc to 1 cc represents destruction of 90 per cent of tumor cells present.

picture of protein loss is readily apparent in patients with Cushing's syndrome. The role of corticosteroids in cancer chemotherapy is most prominent in treatment of leukemia and lymphoma (a "lympholytic" effect), and in the treatment of hormone-dependent tumors such as carcinoma of the breast (Table 25–3). The exact mechanism of action of corticosteroids in these cases is not clear.

Various antibiotics and amino acid analogues interfere with translation of the genetic message, blocking assembly of the polypeptides. Examples include the antibiotic puromycin and the ana-logue cycloleucine. None of these drugs are widely used in cancer chemotherapy at the present time.

Mitotic Inhibitors. Cell division is arrested in metaphase by the plant alkaloids vinblastine and vincristine (Table 25–3). These complex molecules were derived from the periwinkle (Vinca rosea *Linn.*), a common garden plant used for ground cover. Like most other chemotherapeutic agents, the vinca alkaloids exhibit toxicity for the marrow and gastrointestinal tract, and also produce neurological toxicity which may be subtle in onset but of permanent consequence.

Sex Hormones. Natural or synthetic androgens, estrogens and progesterones have an important role in cancer therapy (Table 25–3). In general, the selection of a proper agent or procedure can be made on a rational basis. Examples are the use of estrogens in elderly women with carcinoma of the breast and the use of castration and androgens for premenopausal women with breast cancer. Progestational agents are used in treatment of carcinoma of the endometrium. Castration and estrogens are effective in many cases of carcinoma of the prostrate. Occasionally, the mechanism may be debated and the results relatively less predictable, such as in the use of progesterone and androgens for hypernephroma.[3] Frequently, it is necessary simply to embark on a cautious trial of hormones, watching closely for untoward side effects or for acceleration in tumor growth. Dramatic responses may occur in unlikely situations, as in estrogen therapy for elderly men with metastatic carcinoma of the breast.[7]

Miscellaneous Compounds. Many other drugs are currently in use by specialists in experimental chemotherapy (Table 25–3); examples are the chloronitroso ureas: 1,3-bis(2-chloroethyl)-1-nitrosourea (BCNU); 1-(2-chloroethyl)-3-cyclohexyl-1-nitrosourea (CCNU); DTIC—which was mentioned earlier; azacytidine, azaserine, bleomycin, cycloleucine, duanomycin, mitomycin C, and streptonigrin. Many of these drugs are known to be antimetabolites or alkylating agents. The mechanism of action of the others is uncertain at this time. Several of these drugs are currently receiving final scrutiny by the National Cancer Institute and will probably be released for commercial use within the next year.

Another agent in this class is a unique drug used in therapy of adrenal cortical carcinoma: *o, p'*DDD. This drug was developed following the observation that the insecticide DDD caused adrenal cortical necrosis in dogs, particularly in the zona reticularis and zona fasciculata.

METHODS

Methods of Evaluation

Every possible effort should be made to obtain a record of the location and size of tumor prior to starting chemotherapy, and observations should be made at regular intervals during therapy. Palpation, x-rays, photographs and liver function tests are the most common methods used for evaluation. A superficial lesion is more accurately measurable than one which is deep. Lesions of 1.0 to 5.0 cm in size are particularly suitable for measurement. Chest x-ray usually provides more accurately measurable lesions than those which are seen on GI series, bone x-rays, IVP or pneumoencephalogram. However, any of these x-rays may be helpful in following specific lesions. Serum calcium may be a guide to healing of bone lesions or to the control of parathyroid carcinoma or medullary cancer of the thyroid; blood glucose may be a guide in management of retroperitoneal sarcoma or insulin-secreting tumors of the pancreas. Urinary excretion of hormones and their metabolites may be useful in following some tumors, such as trophoblastic tumors of men and women (chorionic gonadotrophin), metastatic carcinoid tumors (5-hydroxyindoleacetic acid), carcinoma of the adrenal gland (17-hydroxycorticosteroids and ketosteroids) and neuroblastoma (vandinyl mandelic acid). Serum α-fetoprotein levels correlate with the mass of hepatoma present in some patients, and serum gastrin levels may be used to monitor the treatment of patients with metastatic Zollinger-Ellison tumors. Serum and urine levels of Bence Jones protein may be followed in some patients with multiple myeloma. Urinary melanin excretion can occasionally be used to monitor response to therapy in melanoma.

Toxicity

Rational management of the patient requires selection of an appropriate drug

TABLE 25-3　Other Cancer Chemotherapeutic Agents

Chemical or Generic Name	Commercial or Other Name	Abbreviation	Mechanism of Action and Comments	Formulation	Dose (Approximate)
Antibiotics					
Actinomycin D	Dactinomycin		Blocks DNA dependent RNA polymerase	0.5 mg vials	15 mcg/kg/day IV for 5 days; course repeated monthly
Mithramycin	Mithricin		Forms complexes with DNA and metallic ions, blocking RNA synthesis and causing hypocalcemia	2500 mcg vials	25 mcg/kg/day IV for 10 days; course repeated monthly
Hormones and Hormonal Antagonists					
Cortisone acetate			Prolonged therapy with all corticosteroids will produce adrenal cortical atrophy. The use of ACTH should be considered when corticosteroid withdrawal is contemplated. Prolonged use at levels greater than physiologic equivalent doses will cause iatrogenic Cushing's syndrome and risk fatal reactions from peptic ulceration, pancreatitis, diabetes, hypertension, infections, fluid retention, hypokalemia and psychosis	5, 10 and 25 mg tablets / 25 mg/cc, vials of 20 cc	25–37.5 mg/day for chronic replacement after adrenalectomy. 50–200 mg/day for leukemia therapy
Hydrocortisone sodium succinate	Solu-Cortef			100, 250, 500, and 1000 mg vials	300 mg IV/24 hr in continuous infusion for Addisonian crisis
Prednisone			Approximately 5 times as potent as cortisone	2.5 mg and 5 mg tablets	15–60 mg/day for responsive tumors, with dose reduced gradually as soon as possible
Prednisolone			Approximately 5 times as potent as cortisone	2.5 and 5 mg tablets	Same as prednisone
Methyl prednisolone	Medrol		Approximately 6 times as potent as cortisone	2, 4 and 16 mg tablets	Same as prednisone

Methyl prednisolone sodium succinate	Solu-Medrol	Approximately 6 times as potent as cortisone (for intravenous use)	40 mg in 1 cc vial; 125 mg in 2 cc vial	Same as prednisone
Methyl prednisolone acetate	Depo-Medrol	Approximately 6 times as potent as cortisone (for intramuscular or intra-articular injection)	40 mg/cc in 1 cc and 5 cc vials 20 mg/cc in 5 cc vials	Same as prednisone
Dexamethasone	Decadron	Approximately 33 times as potent as cortisone	0.25, 0.5, 0.75 and 1.5 mg tablets	0.75 to 3.0 mg PO/day to relieve signs and symptoms of cerebral tumors
Dexamethasone sodium phosphate	Decadron	Approximately 33 times as potent as cortisone (for intravenous use)	1 and 5 cc vials 4 mg/cc	3.0–6.0 mg IV for acute treatment of cerebral tumor signs
Fludrocortisone acetate	Florinef 9-α-fluorohydrocortisone	Potent synthetic mineralocorticoid, used with cortisone in adrenal replacement therapy	0.1 mg tablets	0.1 mg every 1–2 days PO, with 25–37.5 mg cortisone daily, for adrenalectomized patients
Estrogens Diethylstilbesterol	DES	Synthetic estrogenic substance	0.1, 0.25, 0.5, 1.0 and 5 mg tablets	1 mg PO daily for prostate and 5–15 mg PO daily for breast cancer
Diethylstilbestrol phosphate	Stilphostrol	Synthetic injectable estrogenic substance. Used to test responsiveness of tumor to estrogen therapy	0.25 gm ampuls	0.5 gm in 300 ml N/S IV for 3 hrs; increase to 1 gm during next 4 days
Estradiol valerate	Delestrogen	Long-acting intramuscular preparation	10 mg/cc (1 and 5 cc vials) 20 mg/cc (1 and 5 cc syringes) 40 mg/cc (5 cc vials)	20–40 mg IM every 2–3 wks for elderly women with breast cancer
Chlortianisene	Tace	Long-acting oral estrogenic substance	12 and 25 mg tablets	12 or 25 mg per day for prostatic cancer

TABLE 25–3   OTHER CANCER CHEMOTHERAPEUTIC AGENTS (Continued)

CHEMICAL OR GENERIC NAME	COMMERCIAL OR OTHER NAME	ABBREVIATION	MECHANISM OF ACTION AND COMMENTS	FORMULATION	DOSE (APPROXIMATE)
Estrogens, conjugated equine	Premarin		Injectable and oral preparations of natural equine estrogens	20 mg ampul and 1.25, 2.5, 0.625 and 0.3 mg tablets	Available for cautious trial in patients who do not tolerate synthetic estrogens
Androgens					
Testosterone ethanate	Delatestryl		Long-acting injectable androgen	200 mg/cc in 5 cc vials and 1 cc syringes	200 mg/2 weeks, IM for breast cancer in young women
Testosterone cyprionate	Depotestosterone		Long-acting injectable androgen	50 mg/cc (10 cc vials) 100 mg and 200 mg/cc (1 cc and 10 cc vials)	Same as above
Fluoxymesterone	Halotestin Oratestryl		Oral androgen, 5 times as potent as testosterone	2, 5 and 10 mg tablets	15–30 mg/day PO for breast cancer in young women
Testolactone	Teslac Δ'-testololactone		Synthetic derivative of androstadiene; does not masculinize; has been given in doses up to 2000 mg/day PO without side effects	50 mg tablets and 100 mg/cc (5 cc vials)	150 mg/day PO or 100 mg IM 3 times per wk for breast cancer in women

Progestins					
Hydroxy progesterone caproate	Delalutin		Synthetic injectable progestin	125 mg/cc (2 and 10 cc vials) 250 mg/cc (1 and 5 cc vials)	500–1000 mg IM twice a week for endometrial cancer or hypernephroma
Medroxyprogesterone acetate	Provera Depo-Provera		Synthetic progestin in oral and injectable forms	2.5 and 10 mg tablets 50 and 100 mg/cc in 1 cc and 5 cc vials	Doses are titrated by physician for endometrial cancer and hypernephroma. 500–1000 mg/wk is not unusual.
Vinca Alkaloids					
Vincristine	Oncovin	VCR	Mitotic inhibitor. Cell division blocked in metaphase. Neurotoxic	1 and 5 mg vials	0.05–0.15 mg/kg/week IV
Vinblastine	Velban vincaleukoblastine	VLB	Same as above	10 mg vials	0.1–0.3 mg/kg/wk IV
Miscellaneous Compounds					
o, p' DDD	Mitotane, dichloro-dichloro-diphenyl-ethane, Lysodren		Destroys adrenal cortex	500 mg	2–10 gm/day
5 (or 4) dimethyl triazeno imidazole 4 (or 5) carboxamide	NSC45388	DTIC	Investigational drug used for treatment of melanoma	100 and 200 mg vials	4.5 mg/kg/day IV for 10 days, repeated at 4 to 8 wk intervals
Bis-chloronitroso urea		BCNU	Investigational drug for treatment of primary or metastatic brain tumors, lymphomas and melanoma	100 mg vials	0.5 mg/kg/day IV for 5 days, repeated at 6 to 8 wk intervals

and intelligent observation for both therapeutic benefit and toxicity. Most of the drugs used have toxic effects on both normal and neoplastic cells, so the clinician must be keenly aware of the toxic side effects of the drugs. In general, toxicity is greatest in cells of the hematopoietic system and gastrointestinal tract which are undergoing rapid turnover. Hepatic, renal, pulmonary and neurologic complications are commonly observed from chemotherapeutic agents, and many other organs occasionally show toxic manifestations during therapy. Toxicity may be difficult to distinguish from subtle or unusual aspects of progression of cancer, so it is occasionally necessary to discontinue chemotherapy to determine if the patient is toxic or if the tumor is progressing. A common problem, for example, is nausea, which may be due to drug toxicity, cerebral metastases or progression of intra-abdominal tumor.

Route of Administration

Cancer chemotherapeutic agents may be administered by a variety of routes. On an outpatient basis, the preferred methods are: oral, intramuscular or intravenous "push." Less convenient (but often appropriate) methods are: slow intravenous infusion, rapid injection into tubing of intravenous infusion, intracavitary injection (especially intrapleural and intraperitoneal), and chronic intra-arterial infusion. Direct injections into tumor nodules are occasionally performed for symptomatic relief or simultaneously to test the effects of different drugs.

Oral Therapy. Patients who receive drugs by mouth at home will usually reduce the dose when side affects are apparent, and the physician should take this fact into consideration in his instructions to the patients. An informed, intelligent, determined patient will often do an excellent job of regulating his dosage, and will take the maximum safe dosage by careful observation of toxic symptoms and signs. Cyclophosphamide and methotrexate can frequently be administered on a variable, patient-selected schedule, if the therapy is initiated with one tablet every two days, and is increased at weekly intervals until the first symptom appears. The patient must have the side effects described in detail before therapy starts, and a complete blood count should be checked at least every two weeks.

Intramuscular. The intramuscular route is usually reserved for hormone injections or drugs such as ThioTEPA which are relatively free of reactions at the site of injection.

Intravenous. The intravenous (IV) "push" method refers to swift injection of the contents of a syringe. It is commonly used for drugs which have no serious immediate constitutional side effects when rapidly administered, and which do not cause severe local reactions if extravasation occurs. 5FU, cyclophosphamide, methotrexate and the vinca alkaloids may be administered by the "push" method. A 25 ga needle is suitable for use for most patients using veins of the dorsum of the hand. The local side effects of 5FU are limited to mild discoloration and phlebitis of veins during chronic therapy. The volume of solvent is a problem when cyclophosphamide is administered IV, however, since a common weekly dose of cyclophosphamide (600 mg) is dissolved in 30 ml of diluent. On the other hand, the therapeutically equivalent dose of Thio-TEPA (30 mg) may be easily dissolved in only 1.5 ml. Caution should be used in intravenous "push" administration of vinca alkaloids because extravasation may cause troublesome inflammation and necrosis.

Slow intravenous infusion is recommended for large doses of cyclophosphamide (1000 mg or more). Many clinics also utilize slow intravenous infusion for administration of 5FU, following the recommendation of Lemon et al. (1963),[27] since infusion in glucose and water permits larger doses without concomitant increase in toxicity. Patients who exhibit idiosyncratic syncope with "push" therapy often tolerate infusion therapy better.

Rapid injection of the drug into the side-arm or rubber wall of intravenous tubing of a well-running intravenous infusion is the recommended method of administration of any cytotoxic drug with serious local reactions, such as HN_2 and actinomycin D.

Intracavitary. Intracavitary injections of ThioTEPA and 5FU are easily performed in the Outpatient Clinic, and excellent palliation may be achieved with this method. The tolerable dosage of each drug is approximately doubled by using the intracavitary route, and the drug is thereby injected immediately adjacent to the tumor.

Arterial Infusion. Intra-arterial injections or infusions can be performed on an outpatient basis. External carotid or hepatic artery infusions are the most common indications. Intra-arterial infusions are associated with a relatively high incidence of technical and toxic complications, so the method achieves greatest success when an experienced chemotherapist is managing the patient. Various devices may be used to maintain constant pressure. Our preference has been for the Fenwal system, utilizing a plastic bag filled with 1000 ml of glucose and water, plus desired amounts of heparin and the chemotherapeutic agent.[34] The bag containing the antineoplastic agent in solution is surrounded by an outer bag, in which pressure is regulated by a sphygmomanometer bulb and aneroid gauge (Fig. 25–8). The rate of flow is managed by the patient or an attendant, by means of a Hoffman clamp on the infusion tubing. Position of the catheter should be checked by injection of fluorescein or radiopaque dye at regular intervals, usually weekly. An alternative technique is "push" injection of drug once or twice a day, followed by injection of a concentrated solution of heparin (e.g., 10 ml physiological saline containing 5000 units, approximately equal to 50 mg of heparin). The "push" injection of the heparinized saline solution permits temporary discontinuance of the infu-

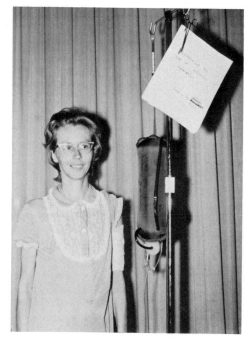

Figure 25–8 Ambulatory arterial infusion chemotherapy. Hepatic arterial infusion of 5FU administered through catheter inserted in brachial artery. Patient regulates flow rate by Hoffman clamp on tubing. She had obstruction of common duct by metastatic adenocarcinoma of colon. She underwent hepaticojejunostomy, followed by 3000 r of Co^{60} to liver, and received 285 mg/kg of 5 FU in a 15 day period. No recurrence of abnormal liver function prior to death 11 months later from ureteral obstruction.

sion, which is also useful if a leak occurs in the plastic bag or pneumatic cuff, or when the patient wishes to have increased mobility from time to time. We have used the Fenwal pack system for administration of 5FU in 315 days of infusion to eleven patients. Objective improvement has been obtained in 80 percent of our evaluable patients who received hepatic arterial infusion for hepatic metastases.

DRUGS

Doses of drugs must be individualized carefully. Previous chemotherapy, especially with alkylating agents, or radiation therapy may limit tolerance to subsequent therapy. Doses should be based on ideal weight (Table 4, Chapter 6) if ideal weight is less than actual weight. Blood counts should be checked frequently when therapy is initiated.

Antimetabolites

5-fluorouracil (5FU, Fluorouracil). 5FU is a broad spectrum *pyrimidine analogue* which is probably the antineoplastic agent most commonly used in treatment of solid tumors at the present time. It has a relatively good therapeutic ratio, in that therapeutic benefit is frequently achieved in the absence of toxicity. It is the least expensive of the fluorinated pyrimidines. 5FU was synthesized in 1957[14] as a derivative of uracil, with which it competes for thymidylate synthetase. It thereby inhibits conversion of uracil into thymidilic acid, a key nucleic acid in DNA. 5FU may also direct formation of "nonsense protein" due to miscoding when it becomes incorporated into RNA.

5FU is the drug of choice for adenocarcinoma of the gastrointestinal tract.[1] It is also effective against adenocarcinoma of the breast and squamous carcinoma of the skin and oral cavity. It is occasionally helpful in management of carcinoma of the lung. Responses have been reported in other tumors, such as sarcomas, brain tumors, carcinoma of the ovary, and hepatoma.

5FU is conjugated by the liver and excreted in part through the kidneys. However, it is remarkably well tolerated in the presence of deteriorating function in these organs, and rarely is the cause of either renal or hepatic dysfunction. The major toxicity of 5FU is on the hematopoietic system (predominantly polymorphonuclear leukocytes) and gastrointestinal tract. It is rare to have a significant degree of thrombocytopenia occur in the absence of leukopenia. Serious gastrointestinal toxicity is usually preceded by nausea, vomiting, loose stools and stomatitis. Therefore, outpatient therapy can be regulated by observing the patient for mild GI toxicity and by maintaining a WBC of 3000 or more.

5FU is relatively inexpensive by comparison with most other antineoplastic agents.

5FU is provided in ampoules of 500 mg. The usual dose is approximately 10 to 12 mg/kg/wk (or, for convenience, 500 mg/wk). The standard method of administration is "push" injection with a 25 ga needle in a small vein of the hand or forearm. Therapy may be begun with five daily doses of 500 mg each in patients with good general health, normal weight and normal bone marrow. Maintenance therapy is then given with 500 to 1000 mg per week. It has recently been suggested that the oral route may be satisfactory or even preferable for patients with metastatic carcinoma of the gastrointestinal tract—especially those with metastases to the liver.[13]

An alternative method for administration of 5FU is the use of monthly "courses" of therapy. The patient should be hospitalized when this method is used. Each course consists of 12 mg/kg/day for four to five days, followed by 6 mg/kg every two days for up to four more doses. The patient must be watched closely for toxicity (diarrhea, stomatitis or leukopenia), since this type of intensive therapy is considerably more hazardous than a loading course of only five days at 500 mg per day.

The advocates of monthly courses of 5FU cite a higher percentage of responses from that method than is observed when weekly doses are used. The advocates of weekly doses point out the increased danger of the intensive courses (up to a 15 percent mortality rate in the hands of inexperienced therapists) and the necessity for hospitalization in initiation of therapy. Since 5FU is not ordinarily expected to "cure" patients with metastatic cancer, our clinic has generally used five daily doses for initiation of treatment and weekly doses for maintenance of therapy.

5FU topical formulations are available for treatment of multiple actinic keratoses. Efudex is prepared in 2 percent and 5 percent cream. Fluoroplex is supplied in 1 percent solution and 1 percent cream. 5FU solutions and creams are not presently recommended for chemotherapy of cancer, although its use in topical chemotherapy is under investigation at the present time.

5-fluoro-2′-deoxyuridine (5-FUDR, Floxuridine). Incorporation of uracil into DNA requires its conversion to thymidilic acid (TMP). As the first step in this conversion, uracil is combined with ribose to form its nucleoside (uridine), followed by reaction with high energy phosphate to form the corresponding nucleotide, uridylic acid (UMP). UMP is then reduced to the deoxy form of ribose (dUMP), which is subsequently 5-methylated to form thymidilic acid. In order to be active as an antimetabolite, 5FU must be converted to its nucleoside (5-FUR), its deoxynucleoside (5-FUDR) and nucleotide (5-FUDRP).

Resistance to 5FU has been observed in tumor cells which are unable to convert 5FU to 5-FUDR and 5-FUDRP. Fluorinated derivatives of 5FU which bypass this mechanism of drug resistance have therefore been prepared for use. 5-FUDR is the only 5-FU derivative currently available for clinical use on a noninvestigational basis. The recommended dose of 5-FUDR is 0.1 to 0.6 mg/kg/day, and it is only authorized for use in arterial infusion therapy. It is supplied in ampoules of 500 mg dry powder, which must be reconstituted before use. Toxicity is essentially the same as that of 5FU.

6-Mercaptopurine (6MP, Purinethanol). This drug is the most effective antineoplastic *purine analogue,* first used in 1952.[8] Of the many sites of action of 6MP, the critical reaction is believed to be competition with hypoxanthine and inosinic acid, which are converted to deoxyadenosine and deoxyguanosine diphosphates in formation of DNA.

6MP and other purine analogues such as azathioprine (Imuran) and 6-thioguanine have potent immunosuppressive activity. For this reason caution is recommended when 6MP is used in chemotherapy, and the patient must be closely observed for acceleration in tumor growth. The most common use of 6MP at present is in the "VAMP" combination drug program for leukemia, which is a combination of *v*incristine, *a*methopterin (MTX), 6-*m*ercaptopurine and *p*rednisone.

6MP is supplied in tablets of 50 mg. The usual dose is 50 to 150 mg/day by mouth, with therapy regulated by observation of white blood count, platelet count and symptomatic side effects, predominantly nausea.

Methotrexate (MTX), amethopterin. MTX is a broad spectrum *folic acid analogue* closely related to the first antimetabolite (aminopterin) used in the chemotherapy of leukemia.

MTX is the only antifolate in common use at the present time. Folic acid analogues interfere with methylation reactions, through competition for the enzyme tetrahydrofolate reductase. A unique feature of MTX is the availability of an antidote, folic acid (in the form of citrovorum factor). When MTX is given by regional infusion, oral citrovorum factor will protect the patient against the generalized effects of MTX toxicity. And in the event of an accidental overdose of MTX, citrovorum factor will eliminate the danger of pancytopenia if it is administered promptly.

MTX has been used with considerable success in chemotherapy of trophoblastic tumors (choriocarcinoma) of women.[15] MTX is also used in the "VAMP" combination for leukemia in children (see 6MP, earlier). In therapy of these diseases, treatment is deliberately initiated with toxic doses on an inpatient basis. MTX is also useful in therapy of squamous carcinoma of the oral cavity, carcinoma of the testis, ovary, breast and lung, and the sarcomas and lymphomas.

MTX *must* be used with caution in outpatient therapy, for it is excreted through the kidneys, and alteration in renal function causes *profound* alteration in MTX toxicity. It is generally advisable to require a normal BUN, creatinine and intravenous pyelogram in patients before prescribing MTX, although very low doses may be used and increased cautiously in the presence of abnormal but stable renal function. The drug *must not be continued* in the presence of deteriorating renal function, whether due to intrinsic renal disease, obstruction, or prerenal azotemia from dehydration (a common manifestation of drug toxicity). MTX also produces chronic hepatic and pulmonary toxicity. Hepatic toxicity is usually seen only in patients treated for more than one year, and may not be fully reversible. Pulmonary fibrosis from MTX is most commonly observed in children on long-term maintenance therapy for leukemia and has usually been reversible when detected in time. In outpatient therapy of solid tumors, the usual toxicity is reflected in the blood count (WBC or platelets) and gastrointestinal toxicity, which may appear as stomatitis, epigastric pain or diarrhea, and progress to fatal septicemia if therapy is continued.

MTX is available in 2.5 mg tablets or 5 and 50 mg vials of the injectable form. Except in urgent situations, the safest initial management is: 2.5 mg by mouth every two days for two weeks, followed by cautious increase in dosage at two week intervals until mild toxicity is observed by the patient or in the blood count. The usual maintenance dose in our clinic is 2.5 mg per day. Because of the rapid renal clearance of MTX, toxicity may be increased by such subtle alterations as taking MTX in two daily doses of 1.25 mg each. On the other hand, a single dose of 50 mg PO or IV may be well tolerated, provided that several days elapse before another dose is given. Fatalities have been reported with as few as one to five consecutive daily doses of 2.5 mg each. The drug is usually well absorbed by mouth, so the oral and intravenous doses are approximately equivalent in effectiveness and toxicity.

Cytosine arabinoside (ara-C, cytarabine, Cytosar). Ara-C is an analogue of the normal cytidine nucleosides in which the 5 carbon sugar arabinose is substituted for ribose. It is a cycle-active drug, blocking DNA formation by inhibition of deoxycytidine synthesis. It also is apparently incorporated into DNA and RNA in small amounts. Ara-C is administered in daily doses of 1.0 to 3.0 mg/kg/day for 10 to 20 days. It is supplied in 100 mg and 500 mg vials.

The optimum method for its use has not been determined. It is frequently administered by a continuous IV drip to inpatients, but for outpatients a single daily IV push dose is most convenient. It has relatively little activity against solid tumors in the doses and intervals tested thus far and is predominantly used in therapy of leukemia. Toxic doses of ara-C cause profound marrow suppression, nausea, vomiting and ulcerative lesions of the gastrointestinal tract.

Hydroxyurea (Hydrea). Hydroxyurea appears to act by blocking DNA synthetase, interfering with reduction of both purine and pyrimidine nucleotides.

Hydroxyurea has had an unimpressive record in clinical chemotherapy, although it has been available for use for many years. It is rapidly absorbed and excreted after oral administration. It causes nausea and a depression in WBC and platelets which is ordinarily promptly reversible when the drug is discontinued.

Hydroxyurea is supplied in capsules of 500 mg. It is usually administered in daily doses of 20 to 30 mg/kg/day (1500 to 2000 mg), or as a single dose of 80 mg/kg every third day.

Alkylating Agents

All alkylating agents may produce permanent leukopenia or impairment of marrow reserve, and this phenomenon should be considered prior to initiation of therapy with these agents. In general, alkylating agents are radiomimetic and are most useful in diseases which would also respond to radiation therapy. The mustards have considerable similarity in the spectrum of their activity, so it is not generally worthwhile to change from one mustard to another in search of a response. On the other hand, nonmustard alkylating agents are frequently useful in treatment of tumors which are not responsive to mustards.

Mustards

Nitrogen Mustard (HN$_2$, Mechlorethamine, "Mustargen"). HN$_2$ is the first synthetic drug used in cancer chemotherapy and is still one of the best, because of its broad spectrum and rapid action. It is particularly useful in management of malignant pleural effusion, where it exhibits specific antineoplastic cytotoxicity and is a sclerosing agent which obliterates the pleural space. It is probably the cytotoxic drug of choice in management of the superior vena cava (SVC) syndrome due to cancer, having been associated with or produced responses in up to 90 percent of patients treated. In the SVC syndrome, it is usually used in conjunction with mediastinal x-irradiation and corticosteroids. In this syndrome, therapy must occasionally be initiated on an emergency basis prior to obtaining a tissue diagnosis. HN$_2$ is highly irritating to tissues and should be used only after the manufacturer's brochure is thoroughly studied for guidelines regarding safety to patient and doctor. It is also unstable in solution and must be used as soon as possible after it has been dissolved.

The usual dose of HN$_2$ is 0.4 mg/kg, given as a single intracavitary dose or in divided doses intravenously on four successive days.

Cyclophosphamide (Cytoxan). Cyclophosphamide is one of many congeners (derivatives) of HN$_2$ which have been produced in the search for an improved therapeutic ratio. Cyclophosphamide is a cyclical phosphoric acid amide derivative of HN$_2$. It is slowly hydrolyzed in aqueous solution but is rapidly converted by liver enzymes to its active form. It is believed that its alkylating activity resides mainly in the chloroethyl fragment, but the phosphoric acid fragment may also be active. The drug is inactive until it has been metabolized, so both the acute toxicity and local side effects are much less than the effects of HN$_2$.

The chronic toxicity of cyclophosphamide is somewhat different from the other mustards, consisting of alopecia and (occasionally) hemorrhagic cystitis in addition to the usual effect of pancytopenia. For this reason, it is believed that the mechanism of action of cyclophosphamide may be more complex than that of HN$_2$. Laboratory studies suggest that cyclophosphamide may be selectively absorbed by tumor cells which are highly sensitive to the drug.[31]

Cyclophosphamide is particularly effective against many of the lymphosarcomas (particularly Burkitt's tumor) and lymphatic leukemia. It is frequently useful in the management of papillary cystadenocarcinoma of the ovary, carcinoma of the breast, multiple myeloma and neuroblastoma. Although responses are not common in sarcomas, occasional dramatic and prolonged responses are observed (Fig. 25-4). It is commonly recommended in the management of lung cancer, but — as with all chemotherapy for this condition — objective responses are uncommon and consist mainly of temporary responses in patients with SVC syndrome, malignant effusions and oat cell cancer.

Cyclophosphamide may be given by mouth in tablet form (one to three tablets of 50 mg each per day) or by injection (approximately 10 to 15 mg/kg/wk). The injectable form is provided in ampoules of 200 mg and 500 mg. It must be dissolved in distilled water prior to use. Patience is required when it is used in a busy clinic, for it dissolves slowly, and a relatively large volume is required for solubilization of the usual weekly dose at the recommended concentration of 20 mg/ml. Cyclophosphamide may also be given in intensive courses or may be injected into body cavities.

Chlorambucil (Leukeran, Aminophenyl-butyric Acid Mustard). The spectrum of action is similar to other alkylating agents, but it has the convenience of smaller doses required to produce similar responses and toxicity — the usual dose is 4 to 6 mg/day, the tablets being 2 mg each. It has been widely recommended for carcinoma of the ovary, and testis and for lymphatic leukemia and the lymphomas.

Melphalan (Alkeran, L-phenylalanine Mustard, L-PAM). (A closely related compound formerly studied was Sarcolysin, which is the racemic mixture, DL-PAM). This mustard was one of many which were prepared to determine if selective incorporation in tumor cells would occur when natural amino acids were linked to alkylating groups. It was originally hoped that this drug would be a specific agent for treatment of melanoma, since phenylalanine is the amino acid precursor of melanin. However, the spectrum of its activity appears similar to that of chlorambucil. The parenteral form remains under investigational use for perfusion of the extremities, and only the oral form is available for regular use on an outpatient basis.

The dose of melphalan is 2 to 4 mg/day, in 2 mg tablets. Leukopenia and thrombocytopenia may occur swiftly from melphalan, preceding nausea, and must be watched for closely — in contrast to cyclophosphamide, which usually produces reversible GI toxicity before serious pancytopenia is observed.

Nonmustard Alkylating Agents

Triethylenethiophosphoramide (Thio-TEPA). ThioTEPA is highly soluble, stable in solution, and causes relatively little systemic toxicity except pancytopenia. The ethyleneimines have a spectrum of therapeutic activity similar to that of the mustards, so it has been particularly useful in chemotherapy of nauseated patients who have tumors which are expected to be sensitive to alkylating agents. It is highly effective in ascites due to papillary cystadenocarcinoma of the ovary, and has a wide range of activity against the lymphomas, carcinoma of the breast and sarcomas. Another advantage of the drug is its relative lack of local irritating side effects, which makes it suitable in most patients for intra-arterial infusion or intramuscular administration.

The first sign of toxicity from Thio-TEPA may be thrombocytopenia, so careful observation of the platelet count is required in patients on maintenance therapy. Persistent mild pancytopenia may follow short courses of ThioTEPA, and may interfere with the use of other cytotoxic drugs later. Therefore, the use of an antimetabolite should be considered *before* use of ThioTEPA in many types of tumors. Although ThioTEPA may be given in short intensive courses, weekly doses are usually preferable in outpatient therapy.

The usual initial dose is 30 mg (intravenous or intramuscular) or 60 mg (intrapleural or intraperitoneal), for patients who have a normal weight and normal blood count. In patients weighing less than 60 kg, the dose should be reduced proportionally. The initial dose and subsequent weekly doses may be given according to the following schedule of blood counts:

WBC	ThioTEPA Dose (weekly, intravenous or intramuscular)
6000 or over	30 mg
5.0–6000	22 mg
4.5–5000	15 mg
4.0–4500	10 mg
3.5–4000	5 mg
3.0–3500	2.5 mg
Less than 3000	Omit Dose

After the therapeutic and toxic results of therapy have been observed for one month, the dosage program can be individualized for the patient.

Triethylene Melamine (TEM). The first ethyleneimine to be studied in detail in cancer chemotherapy, oral TEM appears to have a spectrum of activity similar to other alkylating agents and is therefore not in common usage on an outpatient basis. In parenteral form, TEM is an investigational drug for carotid artery infusion as an adjuvant to surgical therapy of retinoblastomas.

TEM is usually administered in doses of 1.25 to 2.5 mg per day for a total initial course of 20 to 40 mg. Maintenance therapy is given with 2.5 to 5.0 mg/week. Great caution should be used in initiating therapy, since wide individual variance in tolerance to TEM is observed; some patients tolerated only two or three days of therapy in the loading course. Another factor which makes TEM more hazardous than other alkylating agents is the relatively large dose in the individual tablets: TEM is formulated in quarter-scored tablets of 5 mg each. The patient must therefore be cautioned to break the tablets carefully and not to take a whole tablet without specific permission.

Busulfan (Myleran). A sulfonic acid ester, which appears to be particularly effective in therapy of chronic myelogenous leukemia. Pharmacological studies suggest that its action may be alkylation and "dethiolation" of sulfur-containing proteins. The usual dose is 2 mg/day, in 2 mg tablets, and the usual side effects are similar to those of Melphalan.

Procarbazine (Natulan, N-methyl hydrazine). This drug is classed with alkylating agents on theoretical grounds; metabolic studies, however, have shown that it also inhibits transmethylation. It is used in combination chemotherapy of lymphomas, especially Hodgkin's disease, where it is used with Mustargen (HN$_2$), Oncovin (vincristine) and prednisone in the MOPP combination. As a single drug, it is given in doses of 50 to 250 mg/day, and the predominant side effects are pancytopenia and nausea. Depression in blood count may have a delayed onset — up to five weeks after therapy has commenced. Therefore, dosage should not be increased automatically at weekly intervals simply because WBC and platelet count are satisfactory, as is commonly done with other oral alkylating agents.

Antibiotics

Actinomycin D (Dactinomycin). Actinomycin D is believed to act by intercalation of adjacent DNA strands, thereby interfering with DNA-dependent RNA polymerase.

On a molar basis actinomycin D is probably the most potent — and toxic — drug used in cancer chemotherapy. It has an important role in the management of many neoplasms, viz., choriocarcinoma, testicular tumors, sarcomas and Wilms' tumor. It is usually given in short, intensive courses to hospitalized patients, but may be given on an outpatient basis to carefully selected patients who have demonstrated relatively good tolerance to the drug.

The drug is supplied in ampoules containing 0.5 mg of lyophylized powder. It must be mixed with sterile distilled water rather than sterile water containing preservative, for it will not dissolve well in the presence of the preservative. It should be injected into the side of a well-running IV rather than directly into a vein, for local accumulation or extravasation leads to phlebitis or necrosis. In adults, the dose is usually 1.0 mg per week, or courses of 1.0 mg/day for five days repeated at four to six week intervals.[29]

When used with MTX and chlorambucil in "triple therapy" of testicular cancer,[11] it is usually administered on an inpatient basis, and the dose is reduced to 0.5 mg/day for five days. The toxicity usually observed is nausea and vomiting on the day of therapy, followed by pancytopenia, stomatitis, alopecia and (in males) acne, which reaches a peak within two weeks and then subsides slowly.

Actinomycin D has doubled the length and percentage of survival in patients with metastatic Wilms' tumors. However, the intensive use of this drug to pediatric patients in conjunction with surgery and radiation is recommended only for experienced pediatric oncologists.

Mithramycin (Mithricin). This drug binds to DNA and also to metallic cations, inhibiting RNA synthesis and lowering serum calcium in many patients. It has a narrow spectrum of activity in human tumors, as it is effective in metastatic tumors of the testis, but has remarkably little other antitumor activity.[4] It has been used in treatment of hypercalcemia due to benign or malignant disease, the doses being less than the anticancer doses. Initiation of therapy on an outpatient basis is not recommended, for local, systemic and delayed toxicity are frequently severe.

The drug is supplied in vials of 2500 mcg, which are prepared by the addition of 4.9 ml of sterile water. The usual course for testicular tumors is 25 mcg/kg/day for 10 days. The usual course for hypercalcemia is 25 mcg/kg/day for three days.

Severe coagulopathy has been reported in conjunction with the use of mithramycin, in the absence of consistent premonitory laboratory abnormalities, so the patient should be observed carefully for bleeding tendencies during the period of drug administration.

Corticosteroids

Adrenal corticosteroids are commonly used in cancer chemotherapy because of their profound effects on lymphocytes (lympholytic effect), and therapeutic benefit in cancer of the breast (medical "adrenalectomy" by feedback inhibition of endogenous ACTH; also diminishes production of androgens and estrogens by adrenal gland). Corticosteroids are also required for replacement therapy following surgical adrenalectomy (in the form of cortisone and Florinef), and for control of symptoms and signs of primary or metastatic brain tumors (reduction in cerebral edema). Corticosteroids are occasionally used in therapy of other types of cancer, and may produce good results in unexpected situations. Corticosteroids are also used in management of hypercalcemia, the superior vena cava syndrome, lymphangitic tumor spread in the lungs, fever due to necrotic tumor, and Addison's disease due to metastases in the adrenal glands.[18] Considerable palliation is sometimes produced by the euphoric side effect of corticosteroids, though this is generally better sought through the use of tranquilizers and mood elevators. The mechanism is unclear. These hormones may act as enzyme inducers and as either repressors or derepressors of DNA. In long-term therapy corticosteroids produce side effects which may counteract some of the uncommon effects of tumors, such as hypoglycemia from insulinomas or retroperitoneal sarcoma. A dramatic side effect of corticosteroid therapy is an interruption in protein formation, causing negative nitrogen balance and pronounced muscle wasting.

Prednisone, prednisolone and methyl prednisolone are probably the most commonly used corticosteroids in cancer chemotherapy. They have an excellent spectrum of the desired antineoplastic effects, while causing relatively less retention in salt and water than is produced by cortisone or hydrocortisone. Cortisone, hydrocortisone and methyl prednisolone may be given either by mouth or by parenteral injection. In cancer chemotherapy, these agents are usually used for adrenal replacement or suppression. Dexamethasone (Decadron) is used for reduction of cerebral edema, particularly in patients with known or suspected brain tumors. Fludrocortisone acetate (9-αfluorohydrocortisone, Florinef) is used as an adjunct to cortisone in the treatment of adrenal insufficiency, because it produces retention of sodium and chloride.

The dose of an adrenal corticosteroid hormone should always be the minimum dose required to produce the desired effect. Frequently, the initial dose is larger than maintenance dosage in order to determine if an effect will be achieved, or because a therapeutic emergency exists. Since the side effects initially are subtle, the dosage may be inadvertently maintained at an excessively high level. But the chemotherapist must be aware of the devastating, life-endangering complications which result from high doses of corticosteroids. The most common, dangerous complications include activation of peptic ulcer and massive GI bleeding, immunosuppression with septicemia—an especially common phenomenon in patients with lymphomas and lymphatic leukemia—and iatrogenic, drug-induced Addison's disease. Also observed are: diabetes, hypertension, activation of tuberculosis, osteoporosis and psychosis. Diabetic coma, hypertensive stroke, compression fracture or suicide may result from these complications. The equivalent dosage of various corticosteroids may be estimated from the relationship described in the formula:

cortisone	hydrocortisone	prednisone or prednisolone
25 mg	20 mg	5 mg

methyl prednisolone	dexamethasone
4 mg	0.75 mg

For the initial management of the Addisonian patient, intravenous hydrocortisone is begun at a rate of 300 mg/day, or higher, if septicemia is suspected. Cortisone maintenance therapy for the adrenalectomized patient is usually sufficient at 37.5 mg/day, but some patients will require 50 mg and some are managed well with 25 mg/day. Therapy with prednisone (and its 1–2 dehydro analogues, prednisolone and methylprednisolone) is usually initiated with doses of 25 to 100 mg/day, and then tapered as quickly as possible to satisfactory maintenance therapy. We find that 45 mg/day for one week provides a convenient test

of prednisone therapy in most patients (three tablets, three times per day). The dosage may be increased, but substantial benefit in cancer chemotherapy is usually not seen at higher doses if no benefit is seen at the 45 mg daily dose. A convenient tapering routine is 30 mg/day for two weeks followed by 15 mg/day for maintenance therapy. Doses of dexamethasone vary from 0.75 to 6.0 mg per day, depending on the urgency and responsiveness of symptoms and signs of pressure from cerebral tumor. Florinef is administered in doses of 0.1 mg every one to two days.

Vinca Alkaloids

Vincristine (Oncovin). This drug has come into increasing use in adult oncology as one of several drugs used in combination. As a single drug, it has been used predominantly in leukemia and lymphoma chemotherapy. It produces local toxicity, pancytopenia, nausea and vomiting, and insidious progressive neuropathy which may be permanent. The drug may be used in low doses on an outpatient basis if the physician is quick to discontinue therapy at the first sign or symptom of neurotoxicity: absence of patellar reflexes, paresthesias, or abdominal cramps, which may be due to localized areas of diminished peristalsis. The usual dose is 0.05–0.15 mg/kg/wk, and the drug is supplied in ampoules of 1 mg and 5 mg.

Vinblastine (Velban). Velban has a spectrum of action similar to that of vincristine, although it is tolerated in doses which are generally twice as large (0.1 to 0.3 mg/kg/wk), and its neurotoxicity is generally less troublesome than that of vincristine. In adult oncology, it is being used in increasing numbers of patients with miscellaneous solid tumors, in addition to its well-established role in therapy of leukemia and lymphoma. When used as an agent in combined chemotherapy, its effectiveness is difficult to assess precisely.

Sex Hormones

Estrogens. Estrogens are available in several forms. Tablets, injections and intravenous preparations each have specific indications and individual patients may tolerate the side effects of one preparation better than another. Estrogens in cancer therapy are used mainly in metastatic cancers of the prostate and carcinomas of the breast in elderly men and women. The side effects can be troublesome, and patients should be cautioned to reduce or discontinue therapy if they appear. Nausea and vomiting are acute effects which appear from excessive dosage in most patients. Edema and cardiac decompensation are particularly difficult to manage if the patients have serious underlying heart disease. Increased libido or vaginal bleeding may be embarrassing complications in elderly women. Long-term, chronic administration has been associated with the development of hypertensive and arteriosclerotic cardiovascular disease.

Diethylstilbesterol diphosphate (Stilphostrol) is available as a rapid-acting intravenous estrogen preparation. It provides a quick means to determine the responsiveness of a tumor to estrogen therapy. It should be given as a dose of 0.5 gm in 300 ml of saline or glucose solution over a period of one hour on the first day, followed by 1.0 gm on four or more subsequent days. Although nausea may appear, this therapy can be given in the Outpatient Clinic. If the patient develops severe pain in metastases with each infusion, long-term estrogen therapy will probably not be beneficial.

Diethylstilbesterol is a potent oral synthetic estrogen which provides prompt benefit in responsive tumors. It is usually given in doses of 1 mg daily for cancer of the prostate and 5 to 15 mg daily for carcinoma of the breast.

Estradiol valerate (Delestrogen) is a long-acting intramuscular preparation which may be given every two to three weeks. Doses of 20 to 40 mg are usually administered every two to three weeks in metastatic carcinoma of the breast, after careful observation for serious side effects. This preparation is particularly useful in patients with responsive tumors who are not reliable enough to take therapy daily.

Chlortianisene (Tace) is a long-acting synthetic oral estrogen. It is commonly used in therapy of prostatic cancer, in doses of 12 to 25 mg per day.

Androgens. Androgens are used as specific therapeutic agents in premenopausal women with carcinoma of the breast. These hormones also have been reported to produce benefit in some patients with hypernephroma. Protein anabolism is enhanced, and red cell formation is stimulated by androgens. These effects may be undesirable in some patients, but may be exceedingly useful in others. Other side effects commonly observed are nausea and vomiting, fluid retention and hirsutism. Acceleration of tumor growth rate may occur and should be closely watched for when therapy is initiated. Hypercalcemia and cholestatic jaundice are less common but very troublesome complications. Several preparations are available, giving a wide range of options in route, dosage and rapidity of effect. Androgens should not be administered to men with carcinoma of the breast.

Testosterone ethanate (Delatestryl) is a long-acting injectable androgen in sesame oil, in doses of 200 mg per cc. The usual treatment is 200 mg IM every two weeks. Testosterone cyprionate (Depotestosterone) is similar in its effects and is usually used in the same dosage as testosterone ethanate. It is available in dilutions of 50, 100 and 200 mg per cc, which provides greater accuracy when small doses are given to patients who do not require or tolerate large doses.

Fluoxymesterone (Halotestin, Oratestryl). This potent oral androgen exhibits relatively rapid action which allows easy titration of dosage. Because of its short action it should be given in divided doses, and the usual treatment for carcinoma of the breast is 50 to 30 mg per day. Fluoxymesterone is a halogenated methyl testosterone derivative which is said to be five times as potent as the parent compound.

Testolactone (Teslac) is classified with the androgens in this discussion only because of its structural similarity to some androgenic hormones. It is a synthetic derivative of androstadiene, chemically designated Δ'-testololactone. The mechanism of action as an antineoplastic agent is unknown, and it is not androgenic in the usual doses administered for carcinoma of the breast in women. It is available in oral tablets of 50 mg, given in doses of 50 mg three times per day. It is also available in aqueous suspension of 100 mg per cc, given as a dose of 100 mg IM three times per week. Testolactone is the most interesting new single agent recently reported in the treatment of carcinoma of the breast. Doses up to 2000 mg per day have been administered with virtually no side effects attributable to therapy.

Progestins. Progesterone derivatives have been highly effective in some patients with metastatic carcinoma of the endometrium. These drugs have also been useful in some patients with hypernephroma. Natural progesterone cannot be tolerated in doses sufficient to produce significant effects, but the synthetic derivatives cause relatively less edema, nausea and local inflammation at the sites of injection. Thrombophlebitis and pulmonary embolism have also been reported in association with progesterone therapy.

Hydroxyprogesterone caproate (Delalutin) is a long-acting injectable progestin, which is given in doses of 500 to 1000 mg IM twice a week. It is supplied in potencies of 125 and 250 mg/cc.

Medroxyprogesterone acetate is available in a long-acting intramuscular form (Depo-Provera) and an oral form (Provera). The injectable preparation is supplied in concentrations of 50 and 100 mg/cc, and tablets are available at 2.5 and 10 mg. The dosage of medroxyprogesterone must be titrated by the physician for antineoplastic effect. Patients must usually be treated with progressively larger doses until the tolerable limit is reached, if benefit is to be achieved.

Miscellaneous Methods

o,p'-DDD (Mitotane; 1,1-dichloro-2(0-chlorophenyl)-2-(p-chlorophenyl) ethane; Lysodren). This experimental drug has a unique role in the treatment of adrenal cortical carcinoma. It has relieved the Cushingoid side effects of some patients with functioning adrenal tumors, and has been useful in some patients with nonfunctioning adrenal cortical carcinoma. Regressions have been reported in up to 50 percent of patients, persisting for ten months. o,p'-DDD suppresses adrenal cortical activity and produces anorexia, vomiting and diarrhea, plus toxicity in the central nervous system and other organs in some patients. It is supplied in tablets of 500 mg. The usual dose is 9 to 10 gm per day initially, with subsequent therapy adjusted for the desired effect or for toxicity.

DTIC (Dimethyl Triazeno Imidazole Carboxamide, NSC 45388). This analogue of a normal purine precursor was prepared as a random synthetic agent for chemotherapy trial. It had relatively little effect in murine neoplasms, and its major present use in therapy of human tumors is melanoma. The role of DTIC in melanoma chemotherapy was unique and unexpected. It has produced approximately a 25 percent response rate.[25] Many complete responses have been reported, some of which have been maintained for up to three years. No other drug has a similar effectiveness against melanoma, so DTIC is mentioned here even though it is not yet commercially available. Its mechanisms of action remain unclear; the identified products of its metabolism suggest that it may be converted to an alkylating agent *in vivo*: it is also highly carcinogenic in rats, which is an additional clue suggesting that it is active as an alkylating agent.

DTIC is supplied in powdered form in ampoules of 100 and 200 mg. DTIC dissolves rapidly in water, but is unstable in solution and must be used promptly. It is given in doses of 4.5 mg/kg/day for ten days, followed by a four week period of observation, during which pancytopenia may develop at any time.

Immunologic Procedures. The methods reported include (1) specific vaccines prepared from the patient's tumor, other similar tumors or different types of tumors, (2) nonspecific stimulation of resistance by, e.g., BCG, smallpox vaccination, typhoid vaccine, Coley's toxin or etiocholanolone, (3) passive transfer of serum antibody from other patients with similar tumors in remission or cross-immunized patients, and (4) passive transfer of white blood cells from immunized patients. None of these methods has a role in routine clinical management of any type of tumor at the present time. All are under investigational study; they are potentially hazardous, relatively expensive and are apparently rarely effective at present.

TUMORS

The drugs which have been most effective for specific types of tumors at the University of Colorado Medical Center are described in this section. A composite summary of our experience and that of Karnofsky (1968)[23] and Watne (1970)[35] is shown in Table 25–4. We have found the following generalizations useful:

Adenocarcinomas. Adenocarcinomas of gastrointestinal origin are most likely to respond to 5FU. However, adenocarcinomas of the breast may respond as well or better to alkylating agents or MTX, and adenocarcinomas of the lung respond poorly to all forms of therapy.

Squamous Cancers. Squamous cancers are most likely to respond to MTX, although responses to 5FU are

also commonly observed. The toxicity of 5FU is less capricious and usually less dangerous than that of MTX, and failure to respond to 5FU does not preclude later therapy with MTX. Therefore we usually begin chemotherapy of squamous cancers with 5FU. Bronchogenic squamous carcinoma does not respond as well to therapy as tumors which arise in the skin, oropharynx, sinuses or larynx. An experimental agent, bleomycin, is currently being widely distributed for use against squamous cancers. It has been reported to produce responses in cancer of the cervix, penis and esophagus. Bleomycin causes pulmonary rather than hematologic toxicity.

Undifferentiated Cancers. Undifferentiated cancers may respond to any agent, but alkylating agents are usually the best drugs with which to initiate therapy. The reason usually given for this is that most undifferentiated tumors are relatively rapid in their cell turnover and are radiosensitive. Therefore undifferentiated tumors are also sensitive to the type of action achieved by alkylation. Reticulum cell sarcoma may appear as "undifferentiated cancer," especially when the biopsy specimen is small,[26] and reticulum cell sarcoma is also most likely to respond to alkylating agent therapy.

Sarcomas. Sarcomas of "soft tissue" or bone are most likely to respond to alkylating agents or actinomycin D. Embryonal rhabdomyosarcoma is particularly responsive to actinomycin D.

Lymphoid Reticuloendothelial Tumors. Lymphoid reticuloendothelial tumors and the leukemias represent special problems in management, which cannot be summarized in a sentence or two. Combination therapy has become increasingly important, and intensive toxic courses are commonly utilized, followed by outpatient maintenance therapy. Staging and management generally follows the outline of combined radiation therapy and chemotherapy described by Rosenberg and Kaplan (1970).[32] Combination therapy usually utilizes an antimetabolite (MTX or 6MP), an alkylating agent (mustard derivative or procarbazine), a corticosteroid, and one of the vinca alkaloids. The regimen currently in use in our clinic for Stage IV lymphoma is a modified "COPP" program (Table 25–5).

All patients with Stage IIIB and IV lymphosarcomas (lymphocytic, reticulum cell and Hodgkin's) are treated in this fashion. Out of 60 patients, 90 percent of those previously untreated responded, and complete responses occurred in 28 percent of patients previously treated (Kurnick, 1972[24]). Prior performance of splenectomy did not affect the outcome of therapy with the COPP combination at Colorado.

Supportive care with antibiotics and androgens (for anabolism and erythroid stimulation), surgery (especially for staging and splenectomy) and radiation therapy (for palliation or "cure") are important adjuncts to chemotherapy. Experimental agents and new sequences of therapy are in common use by approved investigators. The therapy of most of the tumors of this class should be under the care of a skilled hematologist. However, patients with reticulum cell sarcoma, multiple myeloma, and stage IV lymphosarcoma can be managed effectively by intelligent sequential or combined therapy in a solid tumor chemotherapy clinic.

Melanoma. Therapy is relatively ineffective except when DTIC is utilized, in which case approximately 25 percent of patients show responses. DTIC is presently available on request from the National Cancer Institute, and may soon be marketed commercially.

Testicular Neoplasms. Actinomycin D (with or without chlorambucil and MTX) has been most commonly used, and mithramycin has an important role in embryonal carcinoma. Patients with widespread metastases often show several types of tumor at postmortem; urinary excretion of chorionic gonadotrophin may be present (and is a useful guide to therapy) in any patient with metastatic testicular tumors, regardless of the histologic type of the primary tumor. It is therefore important to treat the patient empirically, measuring results by palpation, x-rays and hormone assays, regardless of the histology of the primary tumor or tumors which have subsequently undergone biopsy.

Breast Cancer. The chemotherapist must integrate the appropriate endocrine manipulations or ablative procedures and bear in mind the fact that a long, indolent course is common—if therapy does not adversely affect the patient's course. Local radiation therapy is useful in up to 70 percent of cases.[30] Chemotherapeutic agents most commonly used are 5FU, cyclophosphamide or Thio-TEPA, and MTX. Premenopausal women should usually undergo oophorectomy when distant metastases are discovered. Responders to oophorectomy would strongly be considered for adrenalectomy when progression again occurs, especially if the recurrent disease is predominantly in skin, axilla or bone. Elderly women are occasionally dramatically benefited by estrogens. Young women may exhibit profound healing of skin or bony metastases from androgen therapy. Testosterone, fluoxymestrone (Halotestin), and testolactone (Teslac) have all been useful in therapy, and masculinizing effects are not essential for useful palliation. Hypophysectomy probably is approximately equal in its effect to that of adrenalectomy, but it has a different type of operative hazard; the preference is, therefore, up to the patient or her physician. Corticosteroids are used to suppress adrenal formation of hormones and in treatment of hypercalcemia. Prednisone is the adrenal steroid most commonly used.

Tumors of Female Genitalia. Carcinoma of the *ovary* is most likely to respond to alkylating agents, and Thio-TEPA, chlorambucil or cyclophosphamide can be used with relatively similar effect. The responses are most frequently observed in papillary cystadenocarcinoma, but may occur in the less common types of ovarian cancers as well. Carcinoma of the *endometrium* is well palliated in many patients by high dose synthetic progestins: Hydroxyprogesterone caproate (Delalutin) or medroxyprogesterone acetate

TABLE 25–4 DRUG SELECTION IN CANCER CHEMOTHERAPY

TYPE OF CANCER	ALKYLATING AGENTS	ANTIMETABOLITES	HORMONES	OTHER DRUGS	COMMENT
Gastrointestinal (colon, rectum, stomach, pancreas, gallbladder, adult hepatoma, and carcinoid) adenocarcinoma		5FU 5FUDR			30–35% respond. Regional arterial infusion may be effective in up to 80% of cases. Responses may persist for many months on maintenance therapy.
Breast, adenocarcinoma	ThioTEPA; cyclophosphamide	5FU MTX	Estrogens (elderly women and men); androgens (young women); adrenal cortical steroids		40–50% improved, some with prolonged complete remissions
Lung, carcinomas	Cyclophosphamide; HN₂	5FU MTX			Oat cell type is most responsive. 20% of patients show temporary benefit, usually with alkylating agents
Sarcomas, soft tissue and bone	Cyclophosphamide			Actinomycin D	20% respond, occasionally for many months
Lymphosarcomas and Hodgkin's disease	Cyclophosphamide,* procarbazine*		Prednisone*	Vincristine*	*Combination therapy with these 4 drugs is COPP program (Table 25–5). Results vary widely with histology and stage of disease. Prolonged remissions in 20–60% of cases
Testis, carcinomas	Chlorambucil*	MTX*		Actinomycin D,* mithramycin	*Combination of these three drugs, or actinomycin D is used alone, except in pure seminoma, which is treated with chlorambucil alone. 30–40% respond, and up to 15% may have long-term complete remissions. Mithramycin has similar results in embryonal carcinoma.

Disease			Results
Ovary, carcinoma	ThioTEPA; chlorambucil	5FU	Up to 50% of cases of papillary cyst-adenocarcinoma respond for several months or longer
Endometrium, carcinoma		Progestins	25% show improvement, which may last for many months
Choriocarcinoma, female	MTX	Actinomycin D	70–80% respond, including many "permanent" regressions
Melanoma		DTIC	25% respond, with complete responses in about 10%
Skin, oral cavity, and upper airway (squamous carcinoma)	MTX 5FU		Up to 30% respond to MTX or 5FU, but mild toxicity is usually needed to maintain response.
Kidney adenocarcinoma (hypernephroma)		Progestins Androgens	20% may show slow improvement, which may be long-lasting
Wilms' tumor		Actinomycin D; vincristine	50% respond, with many prolonged complete remissions; survival time doubled with chemotherapy
Prostate, carcinoma		Estrogens	80% respond, with best results in older men with bony metastases
Neuroblastoma	Cyclophosphamide	Vincristine	50% respond, with some long-term complete remissions
Brain tumors, primary or metastatic		BCNU CCNU	Occasional good results, but usually ineffective
Multiple myeloma	Melphalan; cyclophosphamide	Androgens; adrenal cortical steroids	Difficult to evaluate; pain relief may be excellent and long-lasting for bony disease, but benefit is not common when Bence Jones proteinuria is present
Esophagus, squamous carcinoma			No significant benefit from standard chemotherapeutic drugs
Cervix, squamous carcinoma			

TABLE 25-5 COPP PROGRAM FOR LYMPHOSARCOMAS AT COLORADO

Ten Day Courses	
Cyclophosphamide	10 mg/kg on days 1 and 8 of a 10 day course
Oncovin (vincristine)	0.04 mg/kg on days 1 and 8 of a 10 day course
Procarbazine	2.5 mg/kg on days 1 through 10
Prednisone	1 mg/kg on days 1 through 10, courses 1, 3 and 5 only

For initiation of therapy, five courses are used. The interval without treatment between courses is lengthened successively—two weeks before the second course, three weeks before the third course, four weeks before the fourth course and five weeks before the fifth course. Subsequent courses are given at two month intervals for six months and then three month intervals for one year.

(Provera); both pulmonary and pelvic metastases may respond to this therapy. Carcinoma of the *cervix* has been almost completely resistant to chemotherapy, but some cases may be responsive to the new agent bleomycin, which is available to qualified investigators from the National Cancer Institute. Recurrent and metastatic carcinoma of the *vulva* has occasionally been well palliated with MTX or 5FU. *Choriocarcinoma* has been effectively treated with MTX and actinomycin D, but vigorous, well-informed management in a major medical center is recommended for treatment of choriocarcinoma.

Lung Cancer. These common, highly lethal, rapidly progressive cancers are surprisingly resistant to chemotherapy. Cyclophosphamide is probably the drug of choice for oat cell cancer (small cell undifferentiated cancer). HN_2 has a well-established role in the management of pleural effusions and superior caval syndrome (where it is used in conjunction with local irradiation and high dose therapy with corticosteroids).

Cancers of the Kidney. Wilms' tumor (embryonal carcinoma) is almost exclusively a tumor of childhood. It should be treated by experienced pediatric oncologists, surgeons and radiation therapists, for skilled management can double the cure rate of otherwise unsalvageable cases. The drugs used are actinomycin D and the vinca alkaloids. Adenocarcinoma of the kidney in adults (*hypernephroma*) is almost completely resistant to chemotherapy. Remarkable benefit has been reported in some cases

from the use of androgens and progestins. These results are not commonly seen, although hormone therapy appears to be the best initial therapy at this time.

Prostatic Cancer. Estrogen therapy may be dramatically beneficial, especially in elderly men with slow-growing bony metastases of well-differentiated adenocarcinoma of the prostate. Treatment is relatively less effective in the poorly differentiated cancers of younger men. Chlorotrianisene (Tace) is preferred because of its long-lasting effects; it continues to provide benefit even if the patient forgets to take one or two doses. A trial of therapy may be initiated with intravenous diethylstilbesterol phosphate (Stilphostrol). Diethylstilbestrol (DES) is an alternative and is useful in patients who exhibit nausea, edema or cardiac failure on estrogen therapy, since the side effects subside quickly when DES is reduced or discontinued.

Nervous System. Neuroblastoma, predominantly a tumor of childhood, is effectively treated by a combination of surgery, radiation and chemotherapy, usually with combinations utilizing actinomycin D, vincristine and methotrexate. Prognosis worsens as age increases, and the resources of the chemotherapist are frequently ineffective in neuroblastomas of adolescents. Tumors of children and adolescents present special emotional problems for patients. Their families, their doctors and the chemotherapist should be aware of these challenges.[9, 12] Tumors of the *central nervous system* are generally unresponsive to chemotherapy, although recent reports of the use of the chloronitrosoureas (BCNU, CCNU) for brain tumors are extremely encouraging. BCNU and CCNU are experimental agents which can be obtained from the National Cancer Institute at this time. At the present time, radiation therapy and other chemotherapeutic agents have generally given disappointing results, even when combined with local instillation or infusion.

Other Types of Cancer. The response of other types of neoplasms is unpredictable and generally unsatisfactory. Occasional favorable responses are noted. In general, consultation with a specialist in oncology is indicated to obtain guidance in drug selection and other forms of therapy available for most of the other types of malignant tumors.

SUMMARY

The cancer chemotherapist must be alert to new developments. He must be optimistic but realistic, honest with himself and his patient's family, and willing to measure and record his observations as a guide to further therapy. He must integrate the use of surgery and radiation therapy, palliative drugs and specific chemicals and hormones. Therapy is given by local instillation, infusion, perfusion or by mouth as indicated in specific cases. Consultation and informed consent are important ethical and legal requirements for his work. His goal must always be both the cure of cancer and the relief of suffering.

References

1. Ansfield, F. J.: Chemotherapy of Disseminated Solid Tumors. Springfield, Ill., C. C Thomas, 1966.
2. Bean, W., and Featherman, K.: A time for dying. Curr. Med. Digest, *37*:1039–1042, 1970.
3. Bloom, H. J.: The basis for hormonal therapy. Cancer of the urogenital tract: kidney. J.A.M.A., *204*:605–606, 1968.
4. Brown, J. H., and Kennedy, B. J.: Mithramy-

cin in the treatment of disseminated testicular neoplasms. N. Eng. J. Med., *272*:111–118, 1965.
5. DeVita, V. T.: Cell kinetics and the chemotherapy of cancer. Cancer Chemother. Rep. *2*(3):22–33, 1971.
6. Dowling, M. D., Jr., Krakoff, I. H., and Karnofsky, D. A.: Mechanism of action of anticancer drugs. In Cole, W. H. (Ed.): *Chemotherapy of Cancer.* Philadelphia, Lea and Febiger, 1970.
7. Earley, T. K., et al.: Tumor conference from the University of Colorado Medical Center (carcinoma of the breast). Rocky Mt. Med. J., *68*:43–51, 1970.
8. Elion, G. B., Burgi, E., and Hitchings, G. H.: Studies on condensed pyrimidine systems. IX. The synthesis of some 6-substituted purines. J. Amer. Chem. Soc., *74*:411–414, 1952.
9. Evans, A. E.: If a child must die . . . . N. Eng. J. Med., *278*:138–142, 1968.
10. Gilman, A., and Philips, F. S.: The biological actions and therapeutic applications of the B-chloroethyl amines and sulfides. Science, *103*:409–415, 1946.
11. Goldstein, D. P., and Piro, A. J.: Combination chemotherapy in the treatment of germ cell tumors containing choriocarcinoma in males and females. Surg. Gynecol. Obstet., *134*:61–66, 1972.
12. Gunther, J.: Death Be Not Proud. New York, Harper and Row, 1949.
13. Hall, T. A.: Oral presentation to the American Society of Clinical Oncology. April, 1971.
14. Heidelberger, C., et al.: Fluorinated pyrimidines, a new class of tumour-inhibitory compounds. Nature, *179*:663–666, 1957.
15. Hertz, R., Bergenstal, D. M., Lipsett, M. B., Price, E. B., and Hilbish, T. F.: Chemotherapy of choriocarcinoma and related trophoblastic tumors in women. J.A.M.A., *168*: 845–854, 1958.
16. Hickey, R. C. (Ed.): Palliative Care of the Cancer Patient. Boston, Little, Brown and Co., 1967.
17. Higgins, G. A., and White, G. E.: Cancer chemotherapy and surgery. Surg. Clin. N. Amer., *48*:839–850, 1968.
18. Hill, G. J., II, and Wheeler, H. B.: Adrenal insufficiency due to metastatic carcinoma of the lung: Case report and review of Addison's disease caused by adrenal metastases. Cancer, *18*:1467–1473, 1965.
19. Hill, G. J. II, and Cohen, B. I.: Pleural pericardial window for palliation of cardiac tamponade due to cancer. Cancer, *26*:81–93, 1970.
20. Hill, G. J., II, and Larsen, R. R.: Cancer chemotherapy: I. Methods, agents and overall results in 400 patients. Oncology, *26*:206–222, 1972.
21. Hill, G. J., II, et al.: Cancer chemotherapy: II. Results of 603 courses of therapy in 400 consecutive patients, followed for 18–52 months. Oncology, *27*:137–152, 1973.

22. Hill, G. J., II., Grage, T. B., Wilson, W., and Ansfield, F. J.: 5-Fluorouracil intravenous infusion for 48 hours, repeated every two weeks. J. Surg. Oncol.,*4*:60–70, 1972.

23. Karnofsky, D. A.: Cancer chemotherapeutic agents. Cancer, *18*:72–73, 1968.

24. Kurnick, J. E., and Robinson, W. A.: Combination chemotherapy of advanced lymphomas. Arch. Intern. Med. In press, 1972.

25. Larsen, R. R., and Hill, G. J., II: Improved systemic chemotherapy for malignant melanoma. Amer. J. Surg., *122*:36–41, 1971.

26. Larsen, R. R., Hill, G. J., II, and Ratzer, E. R.: Reticulum cell sarcoma in head and neck surgery. Amer. J. Surg. *123*:338–342, 1972.

27. Lemon, H. M., Modzen, P. J., Mirchandani, R., Farmer, D. A., and Athans, J.: Decreased intoxication by fluorouracil when slowly administered in glucose. J.A.M.A., *185*:1012–1016, 1963.

28. Livingston, R. B., and Carter, S. K.: Single Agents in Cancer Chemotherapy. New York, Plenum Press, 1970.

29. MacKenzie, A. R.: Chemotherapy of metastatic testis cancer: results in 154 patients. Cancer, *19*:1369–1376, 1966.

30. Moore, F. D., Woodrow, S. I., Aliapoulios, M. A., and Wilson, R. E.: Carcinoma of the Breast. Boston, Little, Brown and Co., 1967.

31. Parks, S. D., and Hill, G. J., II: Cyclophosphamide therapy of mouse leukemia: Tumor-induced reduction in drug toxicity. Curr. Top. Surg. Res., *2*:247–256, 1970.

32. Rosenberg, S. A., and Kaplan, H. S.: Hodgkin's disease and other malignant lymphomas. Calif. Med., *113*:23–38, 1970.

33. Solzhenitsyn, A.: Cancer Ward. New York, Farrar, Straus and Giroux, 1969.

34. Wirtanen, G. W., et al.: Hepatic artery and celiac axis infusion for the treatment of upper abdominal malignant lesions. Ann. Surg., *168*:137–141, 1968.

35. Watne, A. L.: Solid tumor chemotherapy, what have we to offer? Amer. J. Surg., *119*:279–287, 1970.

26

The Unconscious Patient

943

By DENNIS BARTON, M.D., *and* GEORGE J. HILL, II, M.D.

INTRODUCTION

A physician's approach to the unconscious patient must be simultaneously diagnostic and therapeutic. This chapter's organization follows this approach. When faced with a completely unknown comatose patient who is nearing respiratory and cardiovascular collapse, one must think clearly and proceed in an orderly fashion.

Life-supporting techniques are outlined in the first portion of the chapter. They are described in the same order as they are applied during resuscitation.

After a measure of respiratory and cardiovascular stability has been achieved, or if it is already present, the physician may proceed with a differential diagnosis that encompasses the common causes of coma. Having arrived at a presumptive diagnosis, he than applies the appropriate treatment. Only those therapeutic measures which have emergency application will be discussed. At this point it will be necessary to utilize laboratory examinations to make or support the diagnosis. A compilation of the more useful laboratory values and their interpretation will be given.

Presuming that the patient is comatose from an obscure cause, a more complex differential diagnosis is required. References will be listed so that the physician can pursue the treatment of these disorders. An exhaustive discussion of the infrequent causes of coma would exceed the purpose of this chapter.

LIFE-SUPPORTING TECHNIQUES — RESPIRATORY SYSTEM

In managing the comatose patient, establishment of adequate ventilation must be the first concern. The physician must train himself to recognize partial and complete airway obstruction. Complete obstruction of the airway may be manifested by a complete lack of air movement, or struggling respirations with suprasternal and supraclavicular retraction. The physician will be unable to inflate the lungs in this situation. Partial obstruction is manifested by air movement with snoring, or by air movement in the presence of excessive secretions, blood or vomitus. The patient may appear to be moving air without obstruction. However, the respiratory rate may be rapid, the volume moved may be insufficient, or the respirations may be arrhythmic: gasps followed by several seconds of apnea or Cheyne-Stokes respiration.

Arterial hypoxemia may result from lung disease or failing circulation, even if the rate and volume of respiration appear to be adequate, and breath sounds are clear to auscultation. Cyanosis is a helpful indicator, if detectable. However, the absence of cyanosis does not guarantee adequate oxygenation. Cyanosis visible to the human eye usually means that at least 5 gm of desaturated hemoglobin per 100 ml blood exist in the arterial blood. Cyanosis can be difficult to detect in anemic or hypovolemic patients, as well as those with darker skin coloration. The physician can be misled by peripheral vasoconstriction secondary to cold. Here peripheral cyanosis exists without arterial desaturation. Arterial hypoxemia can cause anxiety, disorientation, negativism, combativeness, tachycardia, sweating, and somnolence progressing to coma. Retained CO_2, another manifestation of hypoventilation, contributes to this symptom complex.

The immediate goal of airway care in a comatose patient is to deliver 100 per cent O_2 to the alveoli. The percentage of oxygen delivered can be reduced after the patient is stabilized and his condition warrants the reduction. The airway must first be opened and cleared. As demonstrated in Figure 26–1A and B, the patient's neck must be extended and the head tilted backward, a maneuver that lifts the tongue off the posterior pharyngeal wall and opens the airway. One then displaces the mandible down and forward, which further lifts the tongue from the posterior pharyngeal wall and opens the mouth. An open mouth prevents the soft palate from flapping up and closing the nasal passages with expiration. Excessive secretions, blood and vomitus are next suctioned or wiped from the mouth, and the patient is then ventilated. Either mouth-to-mouth resuscitation or bag and mask ventilation can be instituted. Mouth-to-mouth resus-

citation is more effective for immediate delivery of air. Mask fit can sometimes be a real problem, especially in edentulous patients. However, a bag and mask system can quickly supply a high concentration of oxygen and should be utilized if possible. If the airway is still obstructed after these steps have been taken, an oropharyngeal or nasopharyngeal airway will be necessary. The insertion of an oropharyngeal airway is seen in Figure 26–2A. (The application of the breathing mask to the face is shown in Figure 26–2B and C.)

Intubation should be attempted only after the patient has been well oxygenated through a clear airway by a bag and mask system. Dr. Peter Safar has remarked, "Experienced personnel can perform endotracheal intubation more rapidly than tracheotomy. Prolonged attempts at intubation by inexperienced operators, however, have caused asphyxia and cardiac arrest. All hospitals treating seriously ill, or injured patients should have personnel experienced in endotracheal intubation immediately available at all times."[1]

When considering intubation, the physician must choose between cuffed orotracheal or cuffed nasotracheal intubation. The nasotracheal tube can often be inserted by the experienced operator even in the presence of clenched teeth. Furthermore, the tube is more easily tolerated by the semicomatose patient,

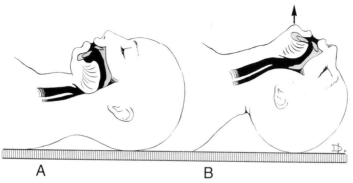

Figure 26–1   A. The tongue often falls onto the pharyngeal wall and occludes the airway. B. By extending the head and lifting the mandible upwards the tongue is pulled off the pharyngeal wall. By opening the mouth the soft palate can no longer act as a flap valve that blocks the nasal passages with expiration.

A

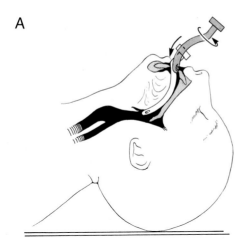

B

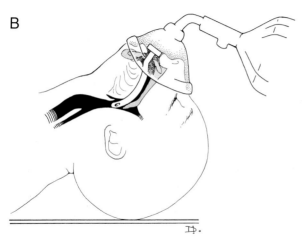

Figure 26–2   A. Insertion of the oropharyngeal airway is accomplished by
placing the airway upside down against
the hard palate. The airway is then
rotated 180° and moved further down
into the mouth. The final position of
the airway is best seen in *B. B.* The
oropharyngeal airway is now in position. It holds the tongue off the
pharyngeal wall and permits an unob-
structive airway. A mask has been
applied to the face so that ventilation
through both oral and nasal passages is
permitted. *C.* The mask is being held
here with the left hand. The thumb and
forefinger press the mask down on the
face. The remaining three fingers of
the hand steady the mandible. The tips
of the fingers rest on the ramus of the
mandible so that pressure is not
exerted on the soft tissue of the neck.
The little finger hooks under the angle
of the mandible and lifts the jaw
forward.

C

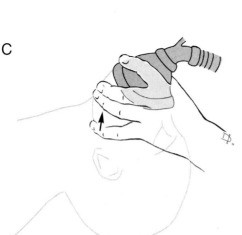

and with proper adjunctive care, the tube can be kept in place for several days, thus avoiding a tracheostomy altogether. The orotracheal tube, however, is more swiftly inserted. A clenched jaw or inadequate visualization of the glottis can frequently be overcome by the injection of succinyldicholine. However, use of muscle relaxants will make aspiration of stomach contents more likely. Before attempting intubation, the operator must have a selection of equipment, best illustrated in Figure 26–3.

The accompanying drawings illustrate the basic differences in the two techniques. Orotracheal intubation is best accomplished with a MacIntosh laryngoscope and endotracheal tube with a well-lubricated stylet (Fig. 26–4). A straight (Miller) laryngoscope blade is

sometimes useful if the patient's mouth can be only slightly opened (Fig. 26–5A and B). If the operator is relatively inexperienced, this blade may inadvertently injure the posterior pharyngeal wall. The patient's head is best supported by a small pillow (Fig. 26–4A). The MacIntosh laryngoscope is held in the operator's left hand and inserted into the right of the patient's mouth. The tongue is followed back (Fig. 26–4B), and pushed to the operator's left until the tip of the laryngoscope falls into the valleculum located at the base of the tongue and the epiglottis. The laryngoscope is then lifted, (not levered) (Fig. 26–4C). This motion moves the mandible, the tongue, and the epiglottis out of the operator's line of sight, and exposes the glottis (Fig. 26–4D).

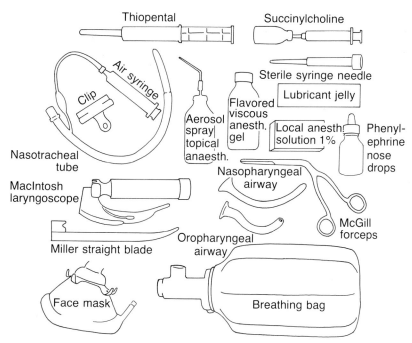

Figure 26–3 A selection of equipment for performing intubation. The components of the tray have been labeled. Airways and a bag and mask system are illustrated to remind the reader that no intubation should be attempted without adequate preoxygenation. Topical anesthesia in the form of viscous gel, liquid or aerosol spray can be used to anesthetize the upper airway if this is deemed necessary. Anesthesia and muscle relaxation can be provided by thiopental and succinylcholine, but great caution is urged when considering these drugs for use in the comatose patient. Phenylephrine nose drops are helpful in shrinking the nasal mucosa and thus facilitating the passage of a nasal tube. A broader description of the pharmacology of the drugs used with intubation is described in the chapter in this book on anesthesia. A cuffed endotracheal tube, two types of blades, and a Magill forceps are also shown. The operator will need a selection of various sizes of endotracheal tubes.

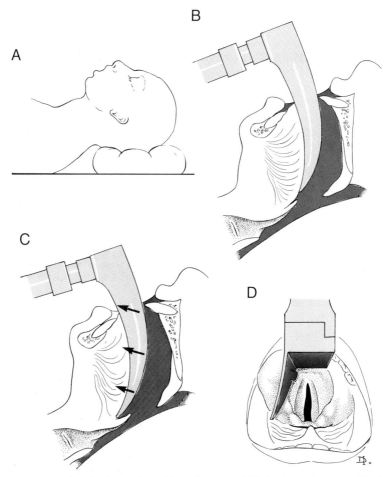

Figure 26–4 *A*. In performing intubation with the MacIntosh blade, the patient's head is placed, slightly flexed, on a small pillow. *B*. The laryngoscope blade follows the tongue back, pushing the tongue to the operator's left. The tip of the blade comes to rest in the valleculum between the epiglottis and the tongue. *C*. The blade is lifted (not levered) in the direction of the arrow. Under no circumstances should the teeth be used as a fulcrum for this maneuver. *D*. Glottic exposure accomplished with the MacIntosh blade. Note how the tongue has been moved to the left. For clarity the size of the tongue has been somewhat exaggerated.

The tube is inserted through the glottis, and the operator is advised to keep it in sight as it passes through the glottis, lest he blindly drop it into the esophagus, which is posterior to the larynx. The tube must not be passed too far, or it will enter the right or occasionally the left main stem bronchus, and deprive the contralateral lung of ventilation. Once the tube is placed, the chest must be inflated with positive pressure. Air will leak around the cuff of the tube. The cuff is then inflated with a volume of air sufficient to stop the leak, and no more. The operator must carefully auscultate the lateral aspects of both lung fields to assure that the breath sounds are equal and that a main stem bronchus has not been intubated. An oropharyngeal airway is inserted so that the patient will not occlude his airway by biting. The operator then cleans the skin of the patient's face, applies tincture of benzoin to the external portion of the endotracheal tube and the skin of the face, and firmly tapes the tube in place. Adhe-

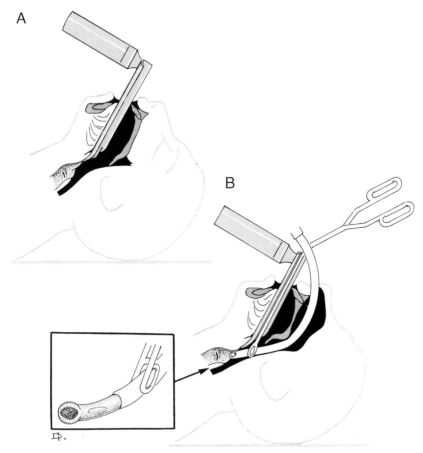

Figure 26–5 A. Here a Miller laryngoscope blade has been used. The blade presses the epiglottis against the tongue, thus permitting exposure of the glottis. Nasotracheal intubation is being accomplished in this drawing. *B*. The nasotracheal tube has been grasped with the McGill forceps and guided toward the glottis. This enlarged view shows the rounded Murphy tip of the nasotracheal tube. The authors have found this type of nasotracheal tube less traumatic to the nasopharyngeal mucosa.

sive tapes are placed across the zygoma and circumferentially around the head. Adequate ventilation may rouse a semicomatose patient enough so that he will pull out the endotracheal tube. Restraints are sometimes required to prevent this unfortunate event.

If nasotracheal intubation is the choice, the nasal passages are best suctioned clean, then sprayed with a vasoconstrictive agent such as $1/4$ per cent neosynephrine. Insertion is also facilitated by anesthetizing the nasal and posterior pharyngeal mucosa with a topical anesthetic spray in order to avoid painful stimuli that will cause struggling in a semicomatose patient. Blind nasotracheal intubation depends on the operator's ability to hear breath sounds through the external portion of the nasotracheal tube. The operator begins by placing the patient's occiput on a small pillow, and cautiously advances the nasotracheal tube. If the trachea is not entered on this attempt, the operator must *flex or extend* the neck of the patient in order to bring the cuffed end of the nasotracheal tube into alignment with the glottis, a matter of some trial and error. However, if a cervical fracture is known, or even suspected, the neck cannot be moved. If visualization of the glottis, or even of the posterior pharyngeal wall is possible with a laryngoscope, the operator can manipulate the cuffed end of the nasotracheal tube with a McGill forcep (see Fig. 26–5*B*) in order to bring the tube into proper alignment with the glottis. Once the tube is through into the trachea proper, cuff location and pressure must be maintained as with an orotracheal tube.

Skill in intubation cannot be gained by reading the description above. The skill must be acquired in the operating room or in the morgue under instruction from someone skilled in intubation.

LIFE-SUPPORTING TECHNIQUES — CARDIOVASCULAR SYSTEM

As soon as the airway is established, hopefully a matter of seconds, the physician's attention is directed to the cardiovascular system. An absence of peripheral pulses and heart sounds immediately requires the institution of closed chest massage. Resuscitation should not be denied any patient until the full status of the patient is known. There are numerous instances of resuscitative efforts being denied "hopeless" trauma patients, only to have these patients "revive" and live on, often with serious neurological deficits. Such patients, with proper resuscitation, could perhaps have resumed full and useful lives.

With the cessation of cardiac activity, physiological events occur which lead inexorably to death. Oxygen stores drop rapidly, leading first to CNS failure of function which results in coma and apnea. Permanent CNS damage is the result of oxygen deprivation for three to five minutes. This time will be less if hypoxia preceded cardiac arrest. As O_2 stores decrease, anaerobic metabolism increases with an increase in hydrogen ion and a fall in pH. Asphyxial death was studied in dogs,[2] where investigators found that PaO_2 of 5–10 torr* (control of 100 torr) or pH_a of 6.5 to 6.45 (control of pH_a 7.40) were both fatal. The effects of hypoxia and acidosis are additive, however, and death in dogs also occurs at a PaO_2 less than 25 torr combined with a pH_a less than 6.8. The rapid arrival of death following O_2 deprivation is illustrated in Figure 26–6.

Acidosis has negative inotropic effects on the myocardium, and if severe, can disrupt intracellular metabolism. An efflux of K+ ions from the liver also occurs with severe hypoxemia. Excessive K+ ions enter the right heart, and increase the possibility of arrhythmia.[3] Disruption of intracellular metabolism eventually stops glycolysis, and blood glucose falls alarmingly. The brain is almost entirely dependent upon glucose for its metabolism,[4] and will begin to die within minutes unless the glucose is replaced, even in the face of adequate oxygenation.

The physician begins resuscitation by a sharp blow to the lower sternum. This maneuver will occasionally start an asystolic heart or ventricle. Some success in cardiac arrest has been achieved by continuous chest pounding. Each sternal blow initiates a myocardial contraction, making closed chest massage unnecessary.[78] Chest thumping has been noted to convert ventricular tachycardia to normal sinus rhythm.[79] If effective cardiac action does not commence, closed chest massage is then begun with direct downward compression of the lower one third of the sternum with the heel of the hand (Fig. 26–7*A*). One hand is placed on the other, so that the strength of both arms can be used (Fig. 26–7*B*). The patient must be lying on a firm surface. Closed chest massage pushes the sternum against the heart and in turn pushes the heart against the vertebral bodies, forcing blood into the systemic and pulmonary circulation (Fig. 26–8).

Resuscitation should be instituted immediately even if only one individual is present. Help is soon required. At least

---

*1 torr equals approximately 1 mm Hg. See ref. 69.

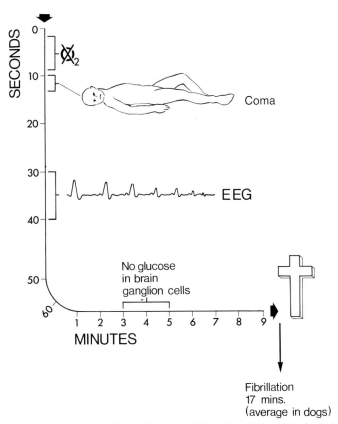

Figure 26–6   Time is of the essence with cardiac arrest. The vulnerability of the brain is quickly demonstrated. Unconsciousness will ensue within seconds, and brain glucose disappears within minutes. The heart can survive longer than the brain. Ventilation with a hypoxic gas mixture will not produce cardiac fibrillation until 17 minutes have passed, but the brain has become functionless long before this (Ref. 2).

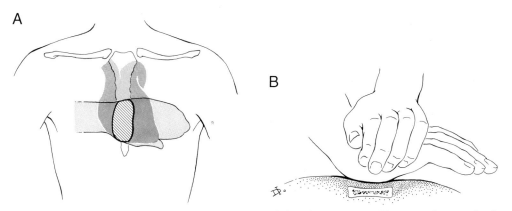

Figure 26–7   *A.* The hands are placed on the lower third of the sternum. *B.* If pressure is exerted only on the lower third of the sternum and not on the ribs, the incidence of rib fracture will be decreased.

A　　　　B

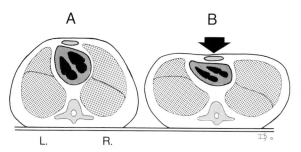

L.　　　R.

Figure 26–8　Closed chest cardiac massage will move blood only if the heart is compressed down onto the vertebral bones by pushing down on the sternum. Adequate time (0.5 sec) is necessary to both empty and then fill the heart. (See text.)

three operators are necessary for efficiency. One should handle the airway and ventilation, another should continue the massage, and the third should connect the monitoring device and administer the proper drugs.

Massage should continue at the rate of 60 times per minute in adults — half a second for the down stroke and half a second for the up stroke. With every five beats there should be a pause for a deep inflation of the lungs with 100 per cent O_2. Oxygen is most efficiently given through an endotracheal tube, but a bag and mask system may be satisfactory.

An intravenous catheter should be inserted and a slow infusion of 5 per cent D/W started as a route for administration of drugs. A greater saphenous vein cutdown at the medial malleolus or a subclavian vein catherization has been the most useful IV route in our hospitals. (See Figs. 3–1, 3–2.) Transcutaneous cardiac puncture for drug administration saves time but often results in unnecessary morbidity (pneumothorax, hemopericardium) and this approach should be used only if an intravenous line is unobtainable.

An electrocardiograph with either an oscilloscope or direct writer print-out is mandatory if resuscitation is unsuccessful in the first minute. A defibrillator should be brought to the scene and used if either diagnosis of defibrillation is established from an ECG tracing, or if the diagnosis is suspect in the absence of a proper ECG trace. Electrode paddle placement follows the precept that the shock is best delivered over the long axis of the heart (Fig. 26–9). One electrode is placed in the region of the right first and

second costal cartilages, while the other is placed just lateral to the left anterior axillary line in the fifth intercostal space[7] (Fig. 26–9). Either direct or alternating current shock can be used for defibrillation, but D.C. defibrillators are preferred.[68]

The effectiveness of massage can be judged from the patient's color and pupil diameter. Fixed dilated pupils are indicative of ineffective circulation while contracted pupils that constrict to light are a good prognostic sign. Brain stem activity in the form of swallowing, reaction to the endotracheal tube or unconscious movements may become evident with improved cerebral circulation. The patient may attempt purposeful movement and become fully aware of what is transpiring. Palpation of pressure waves at various "pulse points" in the body does not indicate blood movement and tissue perfusion, merely pressure change in a column of liquid.[5] The effectiveness of the massage cannot be judged from the palpation of the pulse.

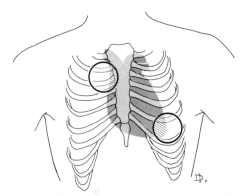

Figure 26–9　This shows the correct paddle placement for defibrillator paddles.

As might be expected, there are many differences between the arrested heart with assisted circulation and the normal heart.[5, 6] With circulatory arrest, venous pressure increases to 20–25 cm H_2O, with resultant cardiac distention. The distention increases the difficulty of defibrillation. Mitral and tricuspid valves become incompetent. This contributes to the observation that closed chest massage produces a cardiac output which is only 30 to 50 per cent of normal. Oxygenation of blood, even with an inspired oxygen concentration of 100 per cent, falls precipitously because of poor pulmonary perfusion. PaO_2 has been measured at less than 100 torr even with PIO_2 of 600 torr. This severe disturbance of the ventilation-perfusion relationship declines gradually after successful resuscitation.

Adjunctive drugs are usually required in cardiopulmonary resuscitation, some more than others. The drugs and their dose limits are listed in Table 26–1.

Sodium Bicarbonate. The rapidly developing acidosis of circulatory collapse cannot be controlled by hyperventilation alone and $NaHCO_3$ is used as a buffer. Acidosis will also greatly reduce the effectiveness of many of the other drugs used in resuscitation. Gilston's formula[8] is often applied to determine the rate of administration of this drug:

$$\frac{\text{Body wt (kg)} \times \text{min cardiac arrest}}{10} = \text{meq } HCO_3 \text{ required}$$

The formula approximates one ampule of 44 meq administered every six minutes to the 70 kg (150 lb.) man. In infants or in patients with congestive heart failure, the continued use of this drug will result in a massive sodium load, which will compound the resuscitation problem.

Epinephrine. This drug usually causes peripheral vasoconstriction by alpha-receptor stimulation. Its usefulness in cardiac resuscitation is probably due to increased myocardial perfusion and improved venous return following its administration.[9] Slow, low voltage fibrillation is often converted to more rapid, higher voltage fibrillation with epinephrine, the latter electrical pattern being more susceptible to defibrillation.[6] The drug is also useful with complete isoelectric cardiac activity. Epinephrine is a double-edged sword: overly enthusiastic use of the drug can lead to arrhythmia, myocardial ischemia and infarction in some patients.

Other Vasopressors. As a general rule these drugs only complicate cardiac resuscitation by increasing the work of the heart. Some success has been claimed with cardiogenic shock by using norepinephrine or metaraminol,[23] but the prognosis is so poor in this condition that it is extremely difficult to judge if any drug offers an advantage.

Calcium Chloride. Calcium, acting directly on the myocardial muscle cell membrane, increases contractility.[10] Calcium chloride is used in states of decreased myocardial contractility when defibrillation has been achieved, but tissue perfusion remains poor. It is especially useful in counteracting the myocardial depressant effects of hyperkalemia. Injudicious use of this drug will be followed by arrhythmia and even ventricular fibrillation. If cardiac resuscitation has been necessitated by digitalis overdose, $CaCl_2$ should be avoided, as the drug potentiates digitalis. Ca gluconate is less irritating to veins and carries less risk of overdosage because of a smaller concentration of Ca^{++} ions. $CaCl_2$ may be preferred in emergency situations, however.

Propranolol (Inderal). This drug blocks beta adrenergic receptors. Propranolol also possesses antiarrhythmic properties unrelated to beta blockade, often referred to as "quinidine-like" activity.[15] It is useful in suppressing arrhythmias secondary to exogenous catecholamines or enhanced endogenous sympathetic nervous system stimulation. The drug has also been used with success in suppressing tachyarrhythmias induced by digitalis overdose.[11] This effect may be due to the quinidine-like activity of the drug. Cardiac arrhythmias which respond to this drug include atrial and ventricular tachycardias, as well as premature ventricular contractions. The drug is not a useful agent for arrhythmias associated with myocardial infarction. Rapid administration of propranolol may precipitate hypotension, and its use may exacerbate congestive heart failure. Its beta-blocking properties *contraindicate its use in asthmatics* and in those patients on insulin or other hypoglycemic drugs.

Lidocaine (Xylocaine). In addition to its well-known local anesthetic action, this drug depresses diastolic depolarization and automaticity in ventricular tissue. It is thus especially useful in ventricular tachyarrhythmias.[70] In the doses recommended, the drug produces no detectable circulatory depression. Procainamide, used clinically in similar situations, can be demonstrated to produce a fall in arterial pressure and a decrease in contractile force of the right ventricle.[12] Lidocaine is best begun as a single intravenous dose of 1–2 mgm/kg. Blood levels of the drug are then maintained by an intravenous drip of 20–50 ug/kg/min which is equivalent to approximately 1.5 to 3.5 mg/min in the 70 kg man. This dose rate avoids the prospect of convulsions, which may occur if an excessive dose of the drug is given.[13] Because of its property of maintaining circulatory stability, the drug is an excellent antiarrhythmic drug in myocardial infarction, in contrast to propranolol.

Diphenylhydantoin (Dilantin). This drug is, like lidocaine, useful in the treatment of ventricular tachyarrhythmia. The drug has few cardiovascular depressant properties in clinical dosages. Because of this fact the drug is probably superior to propranolol for the treatment of digitalis-induced cardiac arrhythmia.[70]

Atropine. Atropine blocks parasympathetic stimulation. This drug may be useful in handling an a-v block which thwarts the efforts of resuscitation. Its effectiveness is probably due to an increased ventricular filling caused by an atropine-induced increase in atrial contraction rate.[14]

Isoproterenol (Isuprel). Isoproterenol is a strong beta receptor stimulator.

Because of this fact, the drug has been recommended in various clinical situations. Both rate and force of myocardial contraction are increased. Additionally, peripheral vasodilation can increase peripheral perfusion by vasodilation and thus decrease the work of the heart. Isoproterenol has been suggested for use in such clinical emergencies as cardiogenic shock and a-v block. Nevertheless, Smith and Corbascio state: "The implications that the seemingly beneficial hemodynamic actions of isoproterenol effectively reverse clinical shock and improve survival is as yet unproven."[9] The authors go on to point out that the inotropic effects of the drug increase oxygen consumption to the heart without increasing coronary blood flow, that the peripheral vasodilation occurs mainly in muscle, where increased flow is not necessary, and that the drug may produce myocardial lesions similar to those seen with hypoxia. The drug is also arrhythmiagenic. Great care should be exercised in its use.

Bretylium Tosylate (Darenthin). Although this drug is not available commercially, it is referred to here because of its apparently unique pharmacological properties. The drug has antifibrillatory effects and has been used with countershock to revert refractory fibrillation. Bretylium also has a marked positive inotropic action, and reduces peripheral resistance by ganglionic blockade.[70]

Glucagon. This hormone has recently received attention in resuscitation because of its positive chronotropic and inotropic effects.[16] It acts directly on the myocardium, and is unaffected by adrenergic blockade. However, the effects of the drug are modest and transient in the hands of most authorities. Injection of glucagon will increase blood sugar and lower serum (K+) levels, and it can therefore be argued that its use is contraindicated if the patient is hypokalemic.

Cardiac Glycosides. Rapid acting preparations of digitalis are invaluable in many resuscitation attempts. There are several preparations which can be given intravenously for rapid effect: ouabain, deslanoside and digoxin. We are more familiar with digoxin, although ouabain has a slightly faster onset of action. The doses of these drugs are listed in Table 26–1. Digitalis' primary effect is a positive inotropic effect—the improvement in cardiac output often results in a slower pulse rate. The digitalis effect on electrical properties of cardiac muscle is much more complicated.[17] The end product of digitalis' electrical effect is to increase atrial-ventricular conduction time, and decrease ventricular rate in atrial dysrhythmias. Other electrical effects, along with changes in autonomic tone, may revert supraventricular dysrhythmias to normal sinus rhythm.

Digitalis may be a hazard in cardiac resuscitation, for the stricken patient may already be taking the drug, and indeed may be in a state of digitalis intoxication. Digitalis intoxication will result in many types of arrhythmias. Ventricular extra systoles culminating in ventricular tachycardia or ventricular fibrillation are some of the more common arrhythmias seen with digitalis overdose. Digitalis toxicity is frequently encountered in hypokalemic patients on digitalis. For this reason serum K+ is always measured. Slow intravenous K+ administration in these patients will often result in abolition of the arrhythmia. Dilantin has been proposed as the most useful drug in combatting digitalis arrhythmia (see earlier) not due to hypokalemia.

Chlorpromazine (Thorazine). The protean actions of this drug include alpha adrenergic blockade. The drug is thus useful in cardiovascular resuscitation, when one wishes to promote a decrease in peripheral vascular resistance. Phentolamine,[24] (Regitine), another alpha receptor antagonist, has also been used for this purpose on an experimental basis. The alpha adrenergic blocker phenoxybenzamine (Dibenzylene) would also be useful, except that it is not commercially available.[72] Decreasing alpha adrenergic tone and causing peripheral vasodilation will unmask hypovolemic states. The central venous pressure must be closely monitored if alpha blockade is performed, and plasma expanders must be judiciously administered.

The outlook for survival after cardiac resuscitation varies with the patient population. Those patients who are closely monitored in hospital intensive care wards or operating rooms have a better prognosis than those who are stricken at home. Unfortunately, a recent in-hospital series reports that only 8.2 per cent of the victims of cardiac arrest live to leave the hospital.[73] Improved survival rates for patients stricken in their homes have been claimed by rushing trained teams in an ambulance equipped with monitors to meet cardiac emergencies.[19] The immediate availability of sophisticated technical equipment such as transvenous pacemakers or various mechanical circulatory assistance devices[84] may also improve prognosis. Occasionally successful electrical complexes are restored on the ECG, but there is no perceptible blood pressure. This is called the state of electromechanical dissociation and carries a very poor prognosis. Fixed dilated pupils for 15 to 30 minutes are clear criteria for abandoning resuscitation.

COMMON CAUSES OF COMA—CARDIOVASCULAR DISORDERS

Cardiogenic Shock

Coma can be caused by poor cerebral perfusion related to failure of the heart to function as a pump. The normal value for cerebral blood flow is around 44 ml/min/100 gm[20] or 750 ml/min for a 70 kg man. Cerebral blood flow is maintained constant when systolic arterial blood pressure is between 60 and 150 torr.[21] When the blood pressure falls below 60 torr, cerebral blood flow decreases and cerebral venous PO_2 is lowered. Unconsciousness is produced[22] by a reduction of flow to roughly one-third of normal (15 ml/min/100 gm brain tissue) or cerebral venous O_2 saturation reduction to 24 per cent. These critical

TABLE 26–1 RESUSCITATIVE DRUGS FOR THE COMATOSE PATIENT

DRUG (TRADE NAME)	SUPPLIED	DOSAGE ROUTE OF ADMINISTRATION	USES
$NaHCO_3$	Amps 44.6 meq/amp	See text p. 953	Correction of metabolic acidosis, including the acidosis of cardiac arrest. Correction of respiratory acidosis if ventilation is adequate.
Epinephrine (Adrenalin)	Amps 1:1000 concentration	1 amp IV or rarely intracardiac	Cardiac arrest – see text
$CaCl_2$	Amps 100 mgm/cc. 1 gm	3–5 cc. IV slowly	Cardiac arrest – see text. Counteracts hyperkalemia
Ca Gluconate	Same	Same	
Isoproterenol (Isuprel, Isoprenaline)	Amps of 1 mgm/5 cc. 0.2 mgm/cc	IV drip: 1–4 ug/min or rarely 0.02–0.04 mgm intracardiac	Bradycardia secondary to heart block. Powerful myocardial stimulant (see text) with peripheral vasodilating properties
Propranolol (Inderal)	Amps 1 mgm/cc 1 cc/amp	1–3 mgm/min – no faster than 1 mgm/min. Total dose limit: 0.1 mgm/kg body weight	Arrhythmias of sympathetic stimulation, possible digitalis overdose (see text)

Drug	Preparation	Dose	Comments
Diphenylhydantoin (Dilantin)	Amps 250 mgm crystals with diluent	100 mgm q 5 min. Total dose limit: 1000 mgm in adult	Arrhythmias of digitalis overdose (see text)
Lidocaine (Xylocaine, Lignocaine)	Vials 1.0–2% (without preservative)	q 1–2 mgm/kg, then IV drip 20–50 ug/min	Arrhythmias, especially those of myocardial infarction (see text)
Bretylium (Darenthin)	Unavailable commercially	3–5 mgm/kg IM or IV	Ventricular fibrillation, and so forth (Ref. 70)
Atropine	Vials various concentrations	0.4–1.0 mgm IV	A-V block
Glucagon	Amps 10 mgm in powder with diluent	3–5 mgm bolus IV adult	Transient inotropic action in cardiac arrest
Digitalis Preparations: Ouabain	Amps 0.25 or 0.5 mgm/ml	0.25–0.5 mgm IV	3–10 minute onset of action; regresses after 8–12 hours
Deslanoside (Cedilanid-D)	Amps 2–4 ml of 0.2 mgm/ml	1.2–1.6 mgm IV	10–30 minute onset of action; regresses after 16–36 hours
Digoxin	Amps 0.25 mgm/cc	0.5–1.0 mgm IV	5–30 minute onset of action; regresses after 8–10 hours
Chlorpromazine (Thorazine, Largactil)	Amps or vials 25 mgm/cc	5 mgm IV, repeat dose q 5 min to effect	For vasodilation, see text for alternative drugs

levels are rapidly approached—with cardiogenic shock—in the hypertensive patient, or in the patient with arteriosclerotic cerebral vascular disease.

Patients with cardiogenic shock are most often the victims of severe myocardial infarction, although myocarditis, cardiac tamponade or massive pulmonary emboli may also present in this fashion. As the cardiac output begins to fall in these patients, adrenergic impulses cause increased peripheral vasoconstriction, which will maintain flow to critical parts of the body. As the cardiac output continues to fall, the patient is left hypotensive, with cold, wet, cyanotic extremities. The patient will then lapse into coma and cardiorespiratory collapse.

Treatment of coma due to pump failure is frustrating.[83] The patient's CVP and arterial pressure must be closely monitored. Because of peripheral vasoconstriction, arterial pressure is best monitored directly with an intra-arterial cannula and strain gauge. Controlled ventilation and administration of oxygen is usually mandatory. The real difficulties come when one attempts to support the cardiovascular system. Some measure of success has been claimed using norepinephrine and metaraminol, which have both beta adrenergic cardiac stimulating and alpha adrenergic vasoconstrictive properties.[23] These drugs can be administered as a slow intravenous infusion, with continuous monitoring. A recent review of the problem of cardiogenic shock concluded that there is as yet no satisfactory means for treating this disorder.[9] The mortality for cardiogenic shock remains distressingly high.

Malignant Hypertension

Hypertension can lead to cerebral events which are the cause of coma. It is sometimes difficult to determine if the coma is due to a cerebral hypertensive event, or due to uremia related to a kidney disorder. If the coma is due to a cerebral hypertensive event, the bulk of these will be focal in nature: focal brain ischemia, cerebral or subarachnoid hemorrhages (see below). Some patients may be comatose from these causes alone. Other patients may have convulsions related to these cerebral events. The syndrome of hypertensive encephalopathy is rare.[25] Hypertensive encephalopathy is an acute *generalized* cerebral episode manifested by increasing blood pressure, headache, drowsiness, vomiting, visual impairment, convulsions and focal neurological signs without focal brain lesions.

The patient with malignant hypertension may present with a variety of neurological findings, including coma. Unfortunately, intracranial mass lesions with increased intracranial pressure can also present in this fashion. If the patient has an intracranial mass and secondary hypertension, lowering the blood pressure will reduce cerebral blood flow, often to fatal levels. The physician should support the airway and ventilation, and, if the neurologic lesion is due to malignant hypertension, he should attempt to lower the blood pressure.

The objective of this therapy is to lower the diastolic pressure to 100 mm Hg without excessive risk from cerebrovascular ischemia, myocardial ischemia or renal shutdown.[26] Trimethaphan camphorsulfonate (Arfonad) used as a drip has an immediate hypotensive action, and has the advantage that its action is rapidly terminated when the drip is stopped. Tachyphylaxis to Arfonad can develop in some patients, however. The drug is made up as 1 mg/cc solution in D5W and the flow rate adjusted so that the desired blood pressure is obtained. Apresoline (Hydrolazine HCl) 10–20 mgm IV can also be used, but this drug has cardiac stimulating properties and is not recommended for patients with coronary artery disease—a condition often present in hypertensive patients.

Hypovolemic Shock

As with cardiogenic shock, coma is produced because cerebral blood flow falls below critical levels. Replacement of lost fluids is the goal of resuscitation. The mental status of the patient gives a clue to the volume of blood lost. An acute decrease of 20 to 25 per cent of the circulating blood volume produces anxiety, 30 to 35 per cent volume loss produces restlessness, and 35 to 40 per cent volume loss produces obtundation.[27] Loss of half the circulating volume will produce coma in patients with hypertension, cardiac impairment or cerebrovascular disease. Other symptoms of shock are pallor, intense peripheral vasoconstriction and sweating—all related to the sympathetic discharge that is the body's defense in hypovolemic shock.

The diagnosis of massive blood loss is easy if there is obvious external trauma. Shock can also occur from blood loss associated with internal bleeding from a fractured femur, from occult gastrointestinal hemorrhage, and from blunt trauma to the chest or abdomen. Such patients can present in coma with few clues to the diagnosis.

There is no ideal substitute for human blood. Treatment of massive blood loss must inevitably utilize blood replacement. Unfortunately, patients may present with severe hypovolemia due not only to blood loss, but also to loss or sequestration of plasma or electrolytes. Severe burns, prolonged vomiting or diarrhea may play a variable part in bringing these patients to collapse. The physician must judge what combination of fluids he will infuse. The judgment is based on his diagnosis. His judgment is subject to revision during continuous monitoring of arterial and venous blood pressure, heart rate, EKG, urinary output, ventilation and pulmonary compliance. The last named value is important in the early detection of pulmonary edema caused by fluid overload. Controlled ventilation in the comatose or anesthetized shock patient allows the physician to gauge when increasing pressure is required to maintain a constant minute volume. (The decreased compliance evidenced here may be due not only to fluid overload, but also to tension pneumothorax or an obstruction in the endotracheal tube.) CVP monitoring is a helpful guide during fluid replacement, although this measurement can be misleading. Volume-depleted patients may exhibit an abnormally high CVP during infusion of blood. This phenomenon is transitory, and the intense peripheral resistance recedes as volume is restored. If a high CVP (over 15 cm saline) persists, one should look for the cause: misplaced or blocked CVP line, occult tension pneumothorax, overtransfusion, congestive heart failure and so on. In the rush to restore blood volume, it is far too easy to resort to the infusion of balanced salt solutions such as Ringer's lactate. Such action is pardonable only when blood or plasma cannot be obtained. It should be remembered that with every liter of Ringer's lactate infused, only 250 cc remains in the intravascular space.[35]

The transfusion of blood can be hazardous to the patient if several rudimentary precautions are not taken. Blood which has been crossmatched with that of the patient is, of course, preferable. However, type specific, or even O− or O+ blood may be necessary for the rapidly dying patient. Administration of incompatible blood is disastrous, but can easily occur in mass casualty situations where comatose patients are known only by numbers or fictitious names. Blood should be warmed. A thermostatically controlled water bath or a thermostatically controlled infrared oven are both quite suitable, but even a pan of warm water with extra coils of tubing on the blood line will do well in an emergency. If the blood is not warmed, the transfused patient may inadvertently be rendered hypothermic to the point of ventricular fibrillation.

Banked blood is acidic. Massive transfusion usually requires buffering with $NaHCO_3$. We give 1 ampule 44.6 meq $NaHCO_3$ with every three to five units of blood on an empirical basis. If blood gas analysis is available, frequent checks of the patient's pH and acid base balance are advisable. Banked blood is hyperkalemic, the potassium content rising with the age of the blood. Electrocardiographic monitoring may allow the early detection of hyperkalemia: increasing height of the waves leading to standstill and ventricular fibrillation.

Banked blood is buffered with citrate. Replacement with several units of transfused blood does not appear to significantly lower serum calcium. However, the massively transfused patient may exhibit a widened P-R interval on the electrocardioscope, or may exhibit Chvostek's sign (the latter is sometimes encountered after hyperventilation also). In these instances the slow infusion of 100 to 500 mgm IV $CaCl_2$ is advisable,

Banked blood has an altered oxyhemoglobin dissociation curve. The curve is shifted to the left with hypothermia. Furthermore, the hemoglobin of stored red cells shows an increased O_2 affinity secondary to reduced 2,3 DPG levels.[74] Both these effects prevent oxygen from reaching body tissue. The effects can be diminished by infusing warmed blood that is as fresh as possible.

Ventilation must be supported in the patient who is comatose from hemorrhagic shock. Pulmonary blood flow decreases, and the resultant poor perfusion of alveoli will drop the PaO_2. Intubation and ventilation with 100 per cent O_2 will be required to overcome this problem.

Severe Pulmonary Disease

Coma can result from severe cerebral hypoxia, severe hypercarbia or combinations of these two. All these states can be the result of severe pulmonary disease. Hypoxia is far more dangerous than hypercarbia, although hypercarbia and attendant acidosis certainly potentiate the deleterious effects of hypoxia. Neurologic signs that may precede coma include a symptom complex of headache, papilledema, drowsiness, confusion, tremor and arrhythmic twitching reminiscent of hepatic coma.[28] Coma occurs from hypoxia when the normal O_2 consumption of the brain of 3.3 ml O_2/100 gm tissue/min falls to 2.0 ml O_2/100 gm tissue/min.[29] Hypercarbia, if severe, can cause convulsions and deep anesthesia, but the changes are reversible.[30] Hypoxia can result from exposure to high altitudes, impairment of O_2 diffusing capacity, and hypoventilation based on central or peripheral neurological problems, diaphragmatic impairment or obesity, However, most paients with coma induced by respiratory failure are the victims of intrinsic lung disease. Asthmatic or emphysematous patients will become comatose when their disease is exacerbated by pulmonary infection or severe bronchospasm. We have encountered ambulatory patients of PaO_2's of less than 50 torr. How thin a margin of pulmonary reserve these patients have! It is easy to see that a minor exacerbation of the patient's pulmonary disease can become a fatal illness. Small doses of sedative drugs to control "restlessness" from hypoxia can prove calamitous.

Diagnosis of coma caused by respiratory failure can be difficult, as outlined in the resuscitation portion of this chapter. Arterial blood gas analysis is essential in diagnosing and following the course of illness, and the reader is referred to two excellent books that cover this topic in more detail.[31, 32] The basis of treatment is the institution of artificial ventilation through a cuffed endotracheal tube. Immediate tracheostomy is not advisable as the goal of therapy in *short term* ventilatory support, since it carries an unnecessary morbidity and mortality for such short term support.

Two important warnings should be recalled when ventilation of these patients is undertaken: severely hypercarbic patients may be dependent on hypoxic drive to maintain ventilation. Exposing such patients to an oxygen-enriched atmosphere may result in hypoventilation. Such patients must have ventilatory support. On the other hand, abrupt change in pH by assisted ventilation (or intravenous buffering) may cause cardiac arrhythmia. This phenomenon can be explained by alkalosis in the presence of hypoxia, activation of catecholamines or hypokalemia. Rapid reversal of respiratory acidosis can also cause cerebral problems, manifested by convulsions, coma and sometimes death. The etiology of this complication appears to be in part related to changes of cerebral spinal fluid pH that accompanies sudden alkalosis.[85] Diamox (carbonic anhydrase inhibitor) has been used experimentally to combat central depression during correction of severe respiratory acidosis.

Once the cuffed endotracheal tube is in place, ventilation is instituted with one of a variety of breathing bags. Most of these bags will not produce an output of 100 per cent O_2.[34] The use of these bags should be considered an intermediate step to the use of a mechanical ventilator.

Frequent checking of blood gases, minute volume, inspired O_2 concentration and so on are necessary when these machines are used. The reader is again referred to the excellent book listed in the bibliography[31] for a further understanding of respiratory intensive care.

ENDOCRINE DISORDERS—GLUCOSE METABOLISM

Hypoglycemia is a common cause of coma. The brain is almost solely dependent on glucose for metabolism and will not survive long without an adequate blood glucose level. Patients can adapt to relatively low levels of blood glucose, so that the rate of the fall of blood glucose is also important.[4] It is thus difficult to cite a blood glucose level at which a particular patient will become comatose.

The most common cause of hypoglycemic coma is insulin overdose in diabetics. The patient may have taken too much insulin, may have not eaten his meals, or may have engaged in excessive physical exercise. Oral hypoglycemic agents are capable of precipitating comas which can be prolonged and difficult to treat.[36] Alcoholism can precipitate hypoglycemia. Alcohol can act independently of insulin and inhibit hepatic glu-

coneogenesis.[37] Severe liver disease will also cause hypoglycemia by the same mechanism.

Hypoglycemia precipitated by an overnight fast is usually caused by pancreatic islet beta cell tumors. Extra pancreatic tumors that produce hypoglycemic coma are infrequently encountered.[38]

The neurologic manifestations of hypoglycemia include: (1) a spectrum of delerium from confusion to mania, (2) epileptic seizures with postictal coma, (3) coma associated with hypothermia and hypotension with pupils which react to light, and (4) a strokelike illness.[39] A history of diabetes and insulin use is often obtained.

The diagnosis is easily made with Dextrostix analysis of the patient's blood. This procedure takes about one minute and should be done in any coma of unknown etiology. Treatment is equally simple. After a blood sugar sample is taken, the patient is given 25 gm glucose IV. This is useful even in nonhypoglycemic coma because, as has been mentioned before, the brain utilizes glucose for all its metabolic needs.

Hyperglycemia, with its associated metabolic disorders, can also be the cause of coma. Diabetic ketoacidosis frequently causes coma, and demands prompt recognition and treatment. Diabetic ketoacidosis is found in untreated diabetics, in diabetics who do not take their insulin or who overeat, in diabetics who have severe infections, and in diabetics with alcohol overdose. The hyperglycemia results in osmotic diuresis leading to dehydration and electrolyte depletion. Lack of insulin also results in increased lipolysis with increased ketogenesis. The acidosis of this disorder results from both HCO_3 ion loss in the osmotic diuresis and an increase in the H+ ion from the ketogenesis. The exact cause of the coma is still not clear. Acute acidosis with cerebrospinal fluid pH below 7.23 will cause coma,[86] but the cerebrospinal fluid pH has been found above this level in diabetic coma.[87, 88]

The patient presents with dehydration and often is febrile. There may be a detectable odor of acetone on the breath. Excess acetone is produced as the result of increased ketogenesis. The patient may initially hyperventilate as a result of acidosis, but if the coma has deepened, respirations may be depressed. A history of thirst and copious urinary output, as well as abdominal pain, may be obtained. (Diagnosis is quickly made from blood glucose Dextrostix determinations, as well as urinary and serum acetone.) Treatment of this disorder must begin with determining baseline measurements of the deranged aspects of the body's metabolism. Insulin therapy and correction of electrolyte imbalance follows. Basic laboratory determinations are blood glucose, electrolytes ($Na+$, $K+$, Cl^-, and HCO_3^-), blood gases (especially pH and base deficit determinations), and serum acetone. As there is often renal, pancreatic and cardiac disease associated with this disorder, BUN and amylase determinations as well as an EKG should be obtained. Urine output, urine glucose and urine acetone should be followed. The patient may require urethral catheterization. If the patient is comatose, aspiration of vomitus should be prevented with a cuffed endotracheal tube. Oxygen supplementation, or even ventilatory assistance may be necessary, depending on the ventilatory status of the patient.

Insulin therapy should begin with 100–200 u of regular insulin subcutaneously. Intravenous insulin is used in the presence of circulatory collapse. Insulin doses of 50–200 u are required hourly or even more frequently, depending on the status of the patient. Electrolyte imbalance is best corrected with hypotonic bicarbonate solutions. Potassium supplementation is usually required as the acidosis is corrected. The reader is referred to an excellent source for further discussion of the treatment of diabetic ketoacidosis.[40]

Hyperglycemia without ketoacidosis is a feature of two other forms of coma in diabetics. Tissue hypoxia in the diabetic may result in coma with severe lactic acidosis. In other patients the blood sugar may rise to astronomical levels (1000 mg/100 ml or more). Seizures may result. Treatment of this group of patients depends on rehydration rather than on insulin therapy.[41]

HEPATIC COMA

There is still uncertainty as to why hepatic disease should cause coma. The most likely explanation is that blood ammonia rises to a point that causes the patient to become comatose. With liver failure, there is no control over ammonia liberated into the portal circulation by colonic micro-organisms. The ammonia level rises especially with GI hemorrhage or high protein intake in the diet. Three groups of patients may develop hepatic coma: those with chronic liver disease and progressive loss of hepatic function, those with acute liver failure secondary to infections, hepatotoxins or autoimmune reactions, and finally, those patients with hepatic encephalopathy due to shunting from portal circulation directly into the vena cava. Significant hepatic encephalopathy developed in 8 of 21 patients submitted to portacaval anastomosis procedures.[42] Short chain fatty acids,[81] certain amino acids,[82] and false neurotransmitters[90] have also been implicated as a cause of hepatic coma.

The presentation of the patient has been epitomized as a "generalized disorder of movement coupled with a lack of external stimuli proceeding into coma."[43] The bulk of these patients will have cirrhosis, mainly of the alcoholic variety. Increasing drug abuse in our society has increased the number of patients with infectious hepatitis. Liver failure from this disease will also cause coma. Signs of severe liver disease may be quite evident in the patient: jaundice, ascites, spider angiomata, hepatomegaly and splenomegaly. However, all clinical signs of liver disease may be absent, and in this case, one must depend on laboratory diagnosis. An elevated blood ammonia (normal 40 to 70 ug per cent) or BSP retention of greater than 5 per cent in one hour may be the only clues to the diagnosis of a deep coma.[45]

A list of the less common causes of coma due to systemic disease is found at the end of this chapter. The following section deals with coma associated with systemic toxicity of exogenous origin.

BARBITURATE OVERDOSE

Barbiturate coma may be preceded by nystagmus, ataxia and dysarthria. When coma appears, pupillary light reflexes are preserved and neurological signs are symmetrical, providing some clue in the differential diagnosis. The coma is accompanied by respiratory depression and later, or deeper, by circulatory depression. Death will occur unless respiration and circulation are supported.

Treatment begins with airway care, and the steps leading to intubation are performed as outlined earlier in this chapter. Cardiovascular instability must be treated with vasopressors. Gastric lavage is performed only in the presence of an endotracheal tube. An attempt should be made to identify the poison by the presence of empty pill boxes or by a history from friends and relatives. Laboratory analysis of blood or gastric juice should be done to identify the type of depressant drug.

Supportive hospital treatment with close monitoring of physiological functions produces an excellent survival rate. Cerebral stimulant drugs are no longer recommended by any authority. There is controversy as to the effectiveness of diuresis or peritoneal dialysis as an adjunct in therapy. One recent series[46] found that supportive treatment offered less morbidity than diuresis or dialysis. These last two methods did not decrease the length of coma in the series. It must be remembered, however, that other investigators[47] advocate osmotic diuresis,

and that phenobarbital coma can be shortened with alkalinization of the urine.

OTHER SEDATIVE INGESTIONS

Doriden (Glutethimide) produces an appearance of dilated or midposition pupils that may be unequal or fixed to light.[39, 80] The patient can sometimes be roused to movement by vigorous stimulation, only to lapse into immobility with cessation of stimulation. Supportive treatment is complicated by the fact that glutethimide coma exhibits a prolonged and unpredictable course. The cyclic nature of glutethimide coma has been attributed to enterohepatic circulation of the drug, but this postulate has been disputed.[77]

Miltown (Meprobamate, Equanil)

Miltown can be fatal with the ingestion of 30 gm. Coma is seen with blood levels of 6 to 12 mgm per cent. Coma is characterized by hypotension, hypoventilation and hypothermia.[48]

Imipramine Type Antidepressants (Elavil, Tofranil, Aventyl)

These have a variable fatal dose — possibly 10 to 30 times the daily dose. These patients are notoriously difficult to manage. Coma is accompanied by cardiovascular depression, cardiac arrhythmia, hypoventilation, and disturbances of temperature regulation. The picture may resemble that of atropine overdose.

Over-the-Counter Sedatives

Scopolamine is the most troublesome ingredient is these compounds. Fortunately this compound can be counteracted with intravenous physostigmine in a dose of 1 to 2 mgm for every 0.5 to 1.0 mgm scopolamine.[49]

Alcohol (Ethanol)

Coma produced by ethanol ingestion alone is uncommon except among those who vaingloriously swallow an entire fifth at once. Ethanol in combination with other drugs or disease states figures prominently in any tabulation of comatose patients brought to the Emergency Room. Levels of ethanol above 110 mgm/100 ml blood produce staggering, mental confusion and perhaps euphoria. At 310 mgm/100 ml blood the patient is comatose or arousable only with vigorous stimulation. Assessment of coma due to ethanol is difficult, since ethanol is an analgesic. Ethanol also acts as a peripheral vasodilator, and the resultant heat loss may result in hypothermia. As blood ethanol rises, the patient becomes more liable to death by respiratory obstruction, vomiting with aspiration, and eventually respiratory arrest. Supportive airway care is mandatory. Alcohol disappears at the rate of 50 to 200 mgm/kg/hr. If the drunken patient cannot be aroused within a few hours after cessation of drinking, other causes for his coma should be sought.

Alcoholism can be complicated by the simultaneous ingestion of other drugs. Barbiturates and other hypnotics are additive in their depressant effect. Phenothiazines, reserpine, meprobamate, amitryptylene, morphine and heroin are hyperadditive.[50] Alcohol derelicts have been known to ingest methyl alcohol,[51] isopropyl alcohol (rubbing alcohol),[52] and ethylene glycol (antifreeze)[53] as a substitute for alcohol.

Chronic alcoholism can lead to a number of disease states that can, in turn, lead to coma.[54] Liver disease, either acute (as in acute fatty degeneration of the liver), or chronic (as in cirrhosis) can result. This in turn leads to coagulopathies. Thrombocytopenia, independent of portal cirrhosis and hypersplenism, can also occur. The coagulopathies make the patient quite susceptible to intracranial bleeding, for the alcoholic frequently falls and injures his head. Portal cirrhosis also leads to varices, which

in turn lead to massive hemorrhage, shock and coma. Alcohol ingestion also can result in hypoglycemia, and this state can be complicated by liver disease.

Rarely one encounters alcoholics who are comatose from vitamin deficient states or thiamine deficient (Wernicke's) encephalopathy, or in cardiogenic shock from alcoholic cardiomyopathy. This latter state is unresponsive to thiamine in the majority of cases and appears different from beriberi heart disease.[55] Alcohol withdrawal is also associated with coma. The patient may be comatose from a postictal state following withdrawal seizures, or further on in the course of withdrawal he may be moribund from delerium tremens.

NARCOTIC OVERDOSE

Coma can be caused by opium, heroin, morphine, paregoric, demerol and even methadon, a drug used in the treatment of heroin addiction.[89]

The first type of coma encountered in narcotic overdose can be expected from the pharmacology of narcotics. The patient has very slow, deep respiration and "pinpoint" pupils. The coma can be reversed with levellorphan (Lorfan), nalorphine (Nalline) or naloxone (Narcan). The injection of the antagonist may lead to an acute narcotic withdrawal syndrome characterized by hallucinations, fever, pain, perspiration and combative behavior. A second type of narcotic-induced coma is associated with pulmonary congestion and pneumonitis but does not respond to narcotic antagonists.[56] These patients need cardiovascular and ventilatory support.

SALICYLISM

Aspirin overdose is extremely common in children. Adults with aspirin overdose are less frequently encountered, but all age groups can present real problems in management. The comatose patient presents with hyperventilation and flushed, often cyanotic skin. The picture is reminiscent of diabetic ketoacidosis. High concentrations of salicylate stimulate respiration centrally and result in an initial respiratory alkalosis. This phase is followed by a metabolic acidosis due to an accumulation of keto and hydroxy acids. Late manifestations of salicylate overdose are hyperthermia — from salicylate-induced uncoupling of oxidative phosphorylation — and gastrointestinal hemorrhage. The presence of salicylate will cause development of a purple color when 5 ml of urine is tested with 1 ml of 10 per cent $FeCl_3$ solution. Serum salicylate levels above 30 mgm/100 ml blood confirm the diagnosis. However, there is a poor correlation of salicylate level in serum with clinical signs.[57]

Most patients will respond to intubation, gastric lavage (although the salicylates are rapidly absorbed), and osmotic diuresis (although kidney function must be intact). Metabolic acidosis can be combatted with $NaHCO_3$. As a rule of thumb: Wt in kg $\times$ 0.3 $\times$ base deficit meq/L = amt (meq) $NaHCO_3$ administered. It is imperative to keep checking the progress of therapy with frequent analyses of the blood for acid base status and salicylate levels.[75] Prognosis for adult patients with salicylate levels of 70 mgm/100 ml is not good, and these patients may be candidates for hemodialysis.[58]

INTRACRANIAL PATHOLOGY

The discussion now turns to another major cause of coma — intracranial pathology. As a general rule, supratentorial mass lesions alone rarely cause coma unless these lesions are both quite widespread and destructive. It is only when the lesion is infratentorial, or when it is of such a size that the brain stem is compressed from above that coma is usually produced.

Diagnosis

The progression of brain herniation with a supratentorial lesion can be quite orderly and can often be followed by successive physical signs. Every physician who handles comatose patients must recognize these signs and act upon his knowledge of them. Of prime importance to the physician are those lesions in which immediate operative intervention can be lifesaving.

Every comatose patient must be evaluated for the presence of a head injury. Examination of the head may reveal obvious lacerations, hematomas or blood in the external auditory canal — a sign of a basilar skull fracture. Less obvious signs are blood behind the tympanic membrane, a bruise or hematoma over the mastoid area, spinal fluid rhinorrhea, or even minor lacerations that the unwary physician may tend to dismiss as insignificant.

Eye signs are of great importance. They often indicate increasing intracranial pressure, and resultant temporal uncus herniation with compression of the vulnerable ipsilateral oculomotor nerve (Fig. 26–10). Oculomotor nerve injury may demonstrate the following sequence as the compression of the nerve progresses (Fig. 26–11 *A, B, C, D*) (1) pupillary miosis appears sec-

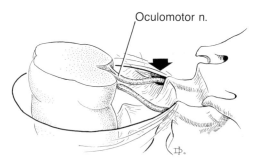

Figure 26–10 Downward pressure on the tentorium causes pressure on the oculomotor nerve. Damage to this nerve produces the dilated pupil of increased intracranial pressure.

ondary to parasympathetic stimulation. This sign may be absent or fleeting in its appearance. (2) (Fig. 26–11 *B*). Further compression leads to parasympathetic paralysis which results in isolated sympathetic stimulation. This leads to the ominous dilated pupil of head injury. Consensual response to light in the contralateral pupil will not be lost if the dilated pupil is the result of oculomotor injury. Ophthalmic nerve damage will also cause a dilated pupil, but there will be no consensual light reflex. With complete pupillary dilation, (Fig. 26–11 *C*) oculomotor ophthalmoplegia occurs, and the eye assumes the characteristic outward and downward gaze of third nerve palsy.

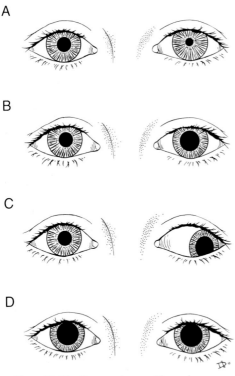

Figure 26–11 Progressive pupillary changes as might be seen with a progressive increase of intracranial pressure: *A.* Pupillary constriction secondary to irritation of the nerve is a transient sign, and is often absent. *B.* Isolated sympathetic stimulation of the pupil leads to dilation. *C.* Motor paralysis results in an outward, downward gaze to the affected eye. *D.* Bilateral dilated pupils, frequently, but not always, connoting death.

The lesion may be difficult to localize by physical examination. For example, the dilated pupil is not always on the same side as the lesion. The dilated pupil may be contralateral to the actual mass lesion which is causing the temporal uncus herniation, especially if the patient has suffered a chronic increase in intracranial pressure. In addition, there may be bilateral mass lesions which complicate the diagnosis. Anisocoria, unrelated to head injury, may have been present in the patient before the onset of his coma.

Bilateral dilated pupils (Fig. 26–11 *D*) are a grave sign and quite frequently indicate cerebral death or severe cerebral hypoxia. Rarely the cardiovascular system may appear to be intact and the bilateral pupillary dilation will be the result of bilateral optic nerve lesions with frontal lobe trauma. We have seen this sign only with obvious external signs of trauma.

The presence of an oculocephalic response ("doll's eyes") is helpful in assessing head injury in coma. The physician turns the head to the left or right. If the eyes move so that they stare in the same direction despite the head being turned (Fig. 26–12), the reflex is intact. If the eyes remain centered, midbrain function is lost. Deep comas of systemic disease, poisoning or massive brain stem injury do not exhibit this sign. Light systemic coma and supratentorial mass lesions that have not sufficiently damaged the brain stem will exhibit this sign. Presence of the oculocephalic response in coma is thus a more favourable sign than its absence. Likewise the disappearance of the sign with the course of time indicates deepening coma or further brain stem injury. If oculomotor ophthalmoplegia is present (see the paragraphs above), the oculocephalic response will be lost in the affected eye. If brain herniation has proceeded so far as to produce ophthalmoplegia, the brain stem may be so compromised that the oculocephalic response disappears altogether.

A wide variety of neurological signs indicative of upper motor neuron damage can sometimes be found. Vigorous

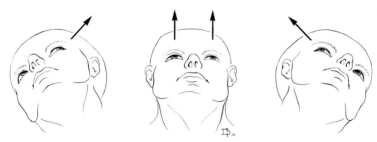

Figure 26–12 The oculocephalic response ("doll's eyes"). The eyes stare straight up, despite the head being turned. The presence of the reflex indicates that at least some brain stem activity has been preserved.

stimulation may cause the comatose patient to move one side and demonstrate an occult hemiplegia. Unfortunately, these signs do not satisfactorily localize all mass lesions, and emergency diagnostic procedures should be undertaken if the physician feels that the patient is stable enough to permit them. Echoencephalography is useful in detecting shifts of the brain midline which are indicative of a supratentorial mass lesion.[76] Skull x-rays are mandatory and films taken with difficulty from a struggling, semicomatose patient are of more use than no films at all. The physician must check for shift of a calcified pineal gland (again indicative of a midline shift), and for fractures. The Waters' view is necessary for visualization of many basilar fractures, but the hyperextension required for x-ray should be avoided until the patient has been evaluated for the presence of cervical fractures or dislocation. Even a trained radiologist finds fractures difficult to locate at times. Cerebral angiography and even pneumoencephalography are considered if the patient is stable and the diagnosis is unclear. In a patient who is rapidly deteriorating, neurosurgery is often begun on the basis of conclusions drawn only from the neurological examination and, perhaps, skull films. It is, therefore, important that the physician constantly observe and record neurological signs at frequent intervals when treating a comatose patient suspected of head injury. Deterioration may be sudden and unexpected. Operative intervention is then forced to proceed with few, if any, concrete guidelines.

Treatment

Monitoring of the patient cannot be confined to the neurological exams. These patients all need intubation, and many need hyperventilation (see later discussion). With increased intracranial pressure most patients manifest an increased sympathetic discharge by an elevated blood pressure and a slow pulse rate — caused reflexively or by direct cephalic hypoxia and vagotonia. These patients may exhibit cardiac arrhythmias and even pulmonary edema.[59, 60] Frequent checks of blood pressure and heart rate must be done.

Even before surgery can begin, intracranial pressure should be decreased. Reduction of CO_2 by hyperventilation reduces cerebral blood flow and the size of intracranial vascular compartment. A $PaCO_2$ of 25 torr is felt to be a safe level for this purpose,[61] and represents an approximate 25 per cent reduction in cerebral blood flow. Authorities all agree that hyperventilation does reduce intracranial pressure over the short term, but the extension of this technique for several days is still experimental. Other means of reducing intracranial pressure are often employed to gain time before surgical treatment. Hypertonic mannitol or urea infusion, hypothermia and dexamethasone (dose: 4 to 8 mgm IV) can be employed for this purpose. A recent critical review of these methods[62] concludes that hypothermia per se may not be effective, and that cooling brain patients is merely prophylactic against the hyperthermia that may accompany brain injury.

Major Causes

There is a wide variety of intracranial mass lesions that cause coma. Only the major varieties will be considered here.

Epidural Hematoma. The most common cause of this lesion is laceration of the middle meningeal artery or its branches. The lesion is frequently associated with skull fracture. The enlarging mass of extravasated blood produces a rapidly progressive syndrome of increased intracranial pressure, temporal uncus herniation, brain stem compression, and death. Early homolateral pupillary dilation can be seen, and as herniation progresses, the contralateral eye also becomes affected.[63] Bilateral fixed and dilated pupils are a poor prognostic sign. Immediate operative intervention is mandatory (see section on Neurosurgery).

Subdural Hematoma. Acute and subacute hematomas are often found in conjunction with brain damage. The brain damage contributes to the high mortality of the disease. Skull fracture is less common here than with epidural hematoma, and may be opposite to the hematoma. Rapid enlargement of the hematoma makes the lesions clinically indistinguishable from acute epidural hematoma.

Chronic subdural hematoma can be notoriously difficult to diagnose correctly. The clinical picture may make the physician suspect brain tumor, various forms of cerebral vascular disease, senile dementia, encephalitis or psychosis.

The chronic subdural hematoma evolves with a definite lining or membrane. The interior is filled with decomposing blood and protein rich fluid. Fresh blood can leak from the vessels in the containing membrane, and the hematoma enlarges further. As the hematoma enlarges, headache, progressive neurological signs and obtundation ensue. The symptoms may fluctuate, and the patient may appear to move in and out of a syndrome of brain stem compression.[39]

As with other mass lesions, unconsciousness will result from central or uncal herniation. Coma is a late and grave sign of subdural hematoma. Pupillary signs are often homolateral with respect to the lesions, but the physician cannot depend on it.

When the diagnosis of chronic subdural hematoma is suspected in a comatose patient, immediate steps must be taken to save the patient's life. Hyperventilation with oxygen through a cuffed endotracheal tube is instituted to reduce the brain size and to increase oxygen to the brain. Other methods to reduce intracranial pressure must also be undertaken. Surgical intervention must occur soon after the diagnosis, perhaps even before cerebral angiography can be done.

Chronic and occasional acute subdural hematomas can be successfully aspirated in infants. Emergency aspiration through the open fontanelle is indicated when the lesion is suspected.

Other Supratentorial Vascular Lesions. Coma associated with supratentorial hemorrhage is due to brainstem compression, the irritative effects of blood in the subarachnoid space, or large intraventricular hemorrhage. The last named catastrophe appears to affect the brainstem via pressure changes in the ventricular system.[39] Coma with supratentorial hemorrhage can be found with: (1) a rupture of an intracerebral blood vessel, sometimes associated with subarachnoid hemorrhage; (2) leakage or rupture of an arterial aneurysm at the base of the brain, with resultant hemorrhage; or (3) leakage or rupture of vascular malformations. Blood in the subarachnoid space appears to produce vascular spasm of blood vessels at the base of the brain with resultant vascular spasm and diffuse cerebral ischemia.[91] Chemical meningitis may also occur from blood. Blood in the subarachnoid space can thus cause diffuse neurological symptoms and even coma without brainstem herniation.

Patients with supratentorial vascular lesions are often hypertensive. If coma occurs, the onset is usually rapid, although preceded by headache and localizing signs. If there is no history of symptoms preceding the coma, the patient has suffered either infratentorial hemorrhage with direct damage to the brainstem, or intraventricular hemorrhage. If coma ensues with supratentorial vascular hemorrhage, the prognosis is poor. Surgical intervention for bleeding aneurysm can be successful. The surest way to complicate an already desperate situation is to fail in supporting ventilation. All comatose patients require endotracheal intubation. Hyperventilation and other adjunctive measures to decrease intracranial pressure should be considered. There is some evidence that hyperventilation will also reduce the area of cerebral infarction following vascular occlusion or hemorrhage,[64] but this approach must be considered experimental in man.

Subtentorial Vascular Lesions. Sudden coma is seen in the case of a brainstem hemorrhage, whereas coma preceded by occipital headache is strongly suggestive of cerebellar hemorrhage. If the patient survives, the coma presents with varying discrete and localizing neurological signs. Coma associated with systemic disease or intoxication will produce no such discrete and localizing signs, but rather overall dysfunction of the brainstem. It is difficult to separate cerebral herniation-brainstem compression comas from comas caused by direct brainstem injury. As a rule, brainstem compression proceeds as an orderly erasure of brainstem function while direct brainstem injury has a spotty and variable presentation of loss of neurological function.[39] Brainstem vascular lesions are the result of occlusions of the basilar artery or its branches, pontine hemorrhage, or rupture of a vertebrobasilar artery aneurysm. Cerebellar hemorrhage is also a subtentorial event, and here coma is caused by compression or involvement of the brainstem. Aggressive neurosurgical intervention may salvage some patients if this entity is recognized quickly.[65] Likewise basilar artery aneurysm has become more amenable to surgical correction.[67] Prognosis for most patients with coma and subtentorial hemorrhage is poor.

Seizures

The physician will frequently encounter seizures in known epileptics, in alcoholics in the early stages of alcohol withdrawal, in patients with craniocerebral trauma, in patients with brain damage secondary to cardiac arrest or brain hemorrhage, and in patients with brain tumors or abscesses. Fortunately for the puzzled diagnostician, the ensuing postictal coma rarely lasts for more than an hour. Often the patient is a known epileptic, or there have been witnesses to the seizures. The airway should be secured in the postictal patient.

The physician is sometimes confronted with a patient having uncontrollable seizures. Again the airway should be secured and the patient given oxygen to increase the supply of oxygen to the brain. The patient can be given medication to control the seizure. Dilantin 500 mgm IV,[43] Valium 5–10 mgm IV, or phenobarbital in 100–200 mgm IV doses have proven effective in the adult. Seizures can sometimes injure a patient. The onset can be sudden, resulting in a fall with fractures and head trauma, or the muscular activity can become so violent as to result in dislocation, ligamentous strains or fractures. A trained anesthesiologist can administer a short-acting muscle relaxant such as succinylcholine in order to control muscular activity. Here endotracheal intubation and a means of positive pressure ventilation with oxygen are required. This therapy is limited to seizures that cannot be easily controlled with sedation, or in those instances when the seizures are the result of overdose with local anesthetic drugs.[66] In the latter case the seizures are limited in time, and oxygen and prophylactic muscle relaxants are all that are required.

SUMMARY

The preceding sections survey the common causes of coma as they present in the Emergency Room. Various emergency diagnostic and therapeutic measures to identify and alleviate the coma are reviewed. They are summarized in Figure 26–13. The following section (Tables 26–2, 26–3, 26–4, and 26–5) will list laboratory blood examinations that are helpful in differentiating the causes of coma. The final section will present references to causes of coma not covered by this chapter.

The authors gratefully acknowledge the assistance of Dr. Peter Cohen, Dr. Ernst Fuchs and Dr. Ralph Lehman in preparation of this chapter.

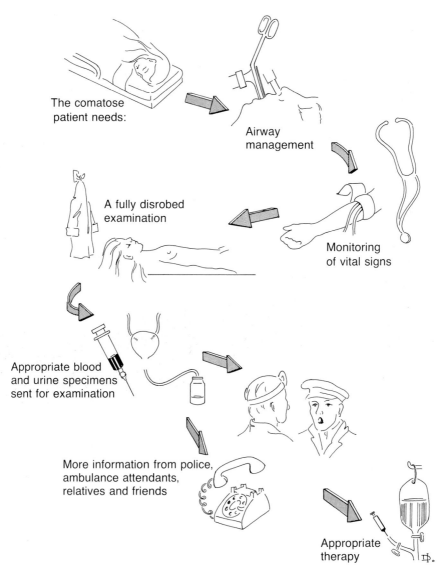

The comatose patient needs:

Airway management

Monitoring of vital signs

A fully disrobed examination

Appropriate blood and urine specimens sent for examination

More information from police, ambulance attendants, relatives and friends

Appropriate therapy

Figure 26–13   This figure summarizes the chapter.

TABLE 26-2   ELECTROLYTE DETERMINATIONS (NORMALS)

Ca — 9.0–10.6 mgm/100 ml	Very high or very low values result in coma.
Mg — 1.8–3.0 mgm/100 ml	Very high levels may result in cardiac arrest. Very low levels are associated with nutritional deficiency.
P — 3.0–4.5 mg/100 ml	
Na — 136–142 meq/L	Extremely high or low values can accompany coma.
Cl — 95–103 meq/L	If the value is abnormally low, excessive HCO_3 may be the cause. Excessive high values usually reflect Na overload. It is usually not necessary to measure Cl on an emergency basis.
K — 3.5–4.5 meq/L	Extremely high or low values can be lethal.

TABLE 26-3   ACID BASE VALUES 37°C

	Arterial	Venous
pH	7.37–7.44	7.35–7.45
pCO_2	34–45 torr	36–50 torr
Base	−2.4–+2.3 meq/L	0–+5.0 meq/L
Oxygen		
Sea Level	80–95 torr	
	96–97 per cent sat.	
Denver	67–76 torr	25–40 torr
	92–94 per cent sat.	40–70 per cent sat.

TABLE 26-4   OTHER IMPORTANT VALUES (ENDOGENOUS)

AMMONIA	Collect with heparin, analyze immediately — 40–70 ug/100 ml
ACETONE	Serum — normal negative on qualitative exam with acetest tablet
GLUCOSE	Collect with heparin-flouride — 65–100 mgm/100 ml
LACTIC ACID	Draw without stasis — 5–20 mgm/100 ml normal
UREA NITROGEN	8–20 mgm/100 ml — abnormally high values are often associated with coma

TABLE 26-5   EXOGENOUS TOXIC SUBSTANCES

ALCOHOL   Whole blood. Collect without cleansing skin with alcohol.
10–50 mgm/100 ml — no influence
50–250 mgm/ml — increasing drunkenness
250–300 mgm/100 ml — "falling down" drunkeness
300– and up/100 ml — coma
100/100 ml prima facie evidence of alcoholic intoxication (A.M.A.)

METHYL ALCOHOL   Whole blood. Fatal ingestion with 30–100 gm

BARBITURATES   Whole blood, or stomach contents. With 3–9 mgm/100 ml blood, coma is observed.

BROMIDE   Whole blood. 100–200 mgm/100 ml serum — toxic manifestations (level variable)

DILANTIN   If dilantin is present, it may interfere with barbiturate determinations, and should be noted as suspect on blood request slip.

GLUTETHEMIDE   3.0 mgm/100 ml produces coma.

METALS
Pb urine — 0.01–0.15 mgm/day normal
Blood — 0.01–0.08 mgm/100 ml normal
As urine — 0.1 mgm/24 hr indicative of As poisoning
Fe blood — hemolysis should be avoided. 50–150 ug/100 ml serum

OPIATES   Not detectable in blood. Urine must be used.

AMPHETAMINES   Detectable in urine. Difficult to detect in blood.

LSD   No test available.

SALICYLATE   30 mgm/100 ml — toxicity

References

1. Safar, P.: Recognition and management of airway obstruction. J.A.M.A., *208*:1008–1011, 1969.

2. Kristoffersen, M. B., Rattenborg, C. C., and Holaday, D. A.: Asphyxial death: The roles of acute anoxia, hypercarbia, and acidosis. Anesthesiology, *28*:488–497, 1967.

3. Lund, I., and Lind, B. (eds.): Aspects of resuscitation. Proceedings of the second international symposium on emergency resuscitation. Acta Anesthesial. Scand., Suppl. 29, 1968.

4. Etheridge, J. E.: Hypoglycemia and the central nervous system. Ped. Clin. N. Amer., *14*:865–880, 1967.

5. Harley, H. R. S.: Reflections on cardiopulmonary resuscitation. Lancet, *2*:1–4, 1966.

6. Grossman, J. I., and Rubin, I. L.: Cardiopulmonary resuscitation. Parts I and II. Amer. Heart J., *78*:569–572; 709–714, 1969.

7. Jude, J. R., and Elam, J. O.: Defibrillation. In Fundamentals of Cardiopulmonary Resuscitation. Philadelphia, F. A. Davis Co., 1965.

8. Gilston, A.: Clinical and biochemical aspects of cardiac resuscitation. Lancet, *2*:1039–1043, 1965.

9. Smith, N. T., and Corbascio, A. N.: The use and misuse of pressor agents. Anesthesiology, *33*:58–101, 1970.

10. Leonard, E., and Hajdu, S.: Action of electrolytes and drugs on the contractile mechanism of the cardiac muscle cell. In Handbook of Physiology, Circulation I. p. 165–170, 1962.

11. Theilen, E. O., and Wilson, W. R.: Beta-adrenergic-receptor-blocking drugs in the treatment of cardiac arrhythmias. Med. Clin. N. Amer., *52*:1017–1029, 1968.

12. Harrison, D. C., Sprouse, J. H., and Morrow, A. G.: The antiarrhythmic properties of lidocaine and procaine amide. Circulation, *28*:486–491, 1963.

13. Gianelly, R., von der Groeben, J. O., Spivack, A. P., and Harrison, D. C.: Effect of lidocaine on ventricular arrhythmias in patients with coronary heart disease. N. Eng. J. Med., *277*:1215–1219, 1967.

14. Eger, E. I.: Atropine, scopolamine and related compounds. Anesthesiology, *23*:365–383, 1962.

15. Dollery, C. T., Paterson, J. W., and Conolly, M. E.: Clinical pharmacology of beta-receptor-blocking drugs. Clin. Pharmacol. Ther., *10*:765–799, 1969.

16. Williams, J. F., Jr.: Glucagon and the cardiovascular system. Ann. Intern. Med., *71*:419–423, 1969.

17. Koch-Weser, J.: Current concept: Mechanism of digitalis action on the heart. N. Eng. J. Med., *277*:417–419; 469–471, 1967.

18. Dietzman, R. H., and Lillehei, R. C.: The treatment of cardiogenic shock. IV. The use of phenoxybenzamine and chlorpromazine. Amer. Heart J., *75*:136–138, 1968.

19. Pantridge, J. F., and Geddes, J. S.: A mobile intensive-care unit in the management of myocardial infarction. Lancet, *2*:271–273, 1967.

20. Lassen, N. A., and Lane, M. H.: Validity of internal jugular blood for study of cerebral blood flow and metabolism. J. Appl. Physiol., *16*:313–320, 1961.

21. Lassen, N. A.: Autoregulation of cerebral blood flow. Circ. Res., *15* (Suppl. 1): 201–204, 1964.

22. Lennox, W. G., Gibbs, F. A., and Gibbs, E. L.: Relationship of unconsciousness to cerebral blood flow and to anoxemia. Arch. Neurol. Psychiat., *34*:1001–1013, 1935.

23. Leavitt, M. A., and Polansky, B. J.: Cardiogenic aspects of shock and coma. Surg. Clin. N. Amer., *48*:273–285, 1968.

24. Shubin, H., and Weil, M. H.: Treatment of shock complicating acute myocardial infarction. Prog. Cardiovasc. Dis., *10*:30–54, 1967.

25. Clarke, E., and Murphy, E. A.: Neurological manifestations of malignant hypertension. Br. Med. J., *2*:1319–1326, 1956.

26. Treatment of hypertensive crisis. Med. Lett. Drugs Ther., *12*:31–32, 1970.

27. Williams, L. F.: Hemorrhagic shock as a source of unconsciousness. Surg. Clin. N. Amer., *48*:263–272, 1968.

28. Austen, F. K., Carmichael, M. W., and Adams, R. D.: Neurologic manifestations of chronic pulmonary insufficiency. N. Eng. J. Med., *257*:579–590, 1957.

29. Posner, J. B., and Plum, F.: Toxic effects of carbon dioxide and acetazolamide in hepatic encephalopathy. J. Clin. Invest., *39*:1246–1258, 1960.

30. Ferguson, A., and Gaensler, E. A.: Respiratory failure and unconsciousness. Surg. Clin. N. Amer., *48*:293–310, 1968.

31. Bendixen, H. H., Egbert, L. D., Hedley-Whyte, J., Laver, M. B., and Pontoppidan, H. (eds.): Respiratory Care. St. Louis, C. V. Mosby Co., 1965.

32. Whipple, H. E. (ed.): Respiratory failure. Ann. N.Y. Acad. Sci., *121*:651–958, 1965.

33. Ayres, S. M., and Grace, W. J.: Inappropriate ventilation and hypoxemia as causes of cardiac arrhythmias. The control of arrhythmias without antiarrhythmic drugs. Amer. J. Med., *46*:495–505, 1969.

34. Carden, E., and Bernstein, M.: Investigation of the nine most commonly used resuscitator bags J.A.M.A., *212*:589–592, 1970.

35. Albert, S. N., Shibuya, J., Economopoulos, B., Radice, A., Cuevo, N., Varrone, E. V., and Albert, C. A.: Simultaneous measurement of erythrocyte, plasma and extracellular fluid volumes with radioactive tracers. Anesthesiology, *29*:908–916, 1968.

36. Cushman, P., Jr., Dubois, J. J., Dwyer, E., and Izzo, J. L.: Protracted tolbutamide hypoglycemia. Amer. J. Med., *35*:196–204, 1963.

37. Arky, R. A.: State of unconsciousness associated with alcohol. Surg. Clin. N. Amer., *48*:403–413, 1968.

38. Hurwitz, D.: Hypoglycemic and hyperglycemic coma. Surg. Clin. N. Amer., *48*:361–370, 1968.

39. Plum, F., and Posner, J. B.: The Diagnosis of Stupor and Coma. Philadelphia, F. A. Davis Co., 1966.

40. Marble, A. (ed.): Joslin's Diabetes Mellitus. Philadelphia, Lea and Febiger, 1971.

41. Hyperosmolar nonketotic diabetic coma. Ed-

itorial. Can. Med. Assoc. J., *99*:1099–1100, 1968.

42. Read, A. E., Laidlaw, J., and Sherlock, S.: Neuropsychiatric complications of portacaval anastomosis. Lancet, *1*:961–963, 1961.

43. Wallis, W., Kutt, H., and McDowell, F.: Intravenous diphenylhydantoin in treatment of acute repetitive seizures. Neurology, *18*:513–525, 1968.

44. Adams, R. D., and Foley, J. M.: The neurological disorders associated with liver disease. Assoc. Res. Nerv. Ment. Dis. Proc., *32*:198–237, 1953.

45. McDermott, W. V., Jr.: Liver disease in the differential diagnosis of coma. Surg. Clin. N. Amer., *48*:327–333, 1968.

46. Hadden, J., Johnson, K., Smith, S., Price, L., and Giardina, E.: Acute barbiturate intoxication. J.A.M.A., *209*:893–900, 1969.

47. Shapiro, F. L., and Smith, H. T.: The treatment of barbiturate intoxication. Mod. Med., *37*, Part 2:104–110, April 21, 1969.

48. Davis. J. M., Bartlett, E., and Termini, B. A.: Overdosage of psychotropic drugs: A Review. Part I. Major and minor tranquilizers. II. Antidepressants and other psychotropic agents. Dis. Nerv. Sys., *29*:157–164; 246–256, 1968.

49. Duvoisin, R. C., and Katz, R.: Reversal of central anticholinergic syndrome in man by physostigmine. J.A.M.A., *206*:1963–1965, 1968.

50. Forney, R. B., and Harger, R. N.: Toxicology of ethanol. Ann. Rev. Pharmacol., *9*:379–392, 1969.

51. Doe, R. P.: Metabolic acidosis nondiabetic. Arch. Intern. Med., *116*:717–728, 1965.

52. Juncos, L., and Taguchi, J. T.: Isopropyl alcohol intoxication. J.A.M.A., *204*:732–734, 1968.

53. Fuller, E. W., Jr.: Ethylene glycol: A review. Medicoleg. Bull., *198*:1–8, 1969.

54. Carson, D. J. L.: Pathologic findings following alcohol. Anesth. Analg., *48*:670–675, 1969.

55. Brigden, W., and Robinson, J.: Alcoholic heart disease. Brit. Med. J., *2*:1283–1289, 1964.

56. Cherubin, C. E.: The medical sequelae of narcotic addiction. Ann. Intern. Med., *67*:23–33, 1967.

57. Done, A. K.: Salicylate intoxication. Significance of measurements of salicylate in blood in cases of acute ingestion. Pediatrics, *26*:800–807, 1960.

58. Beveridge, G. W., Forshall, W., Munro, J. F., Owen, J. A., and Weston, I. A. G.: Acute salicylate poisoning in adults. Lancet, *1*:1406–1409, 1964.

59. Simmons, R. L., Martin, A. M., Heisterkamp, C. A., and Ducker, T. B.: Respiratory insufficiency in combat casualties. II. Pulmonary edema following head injury. Ann. Surg., *170*:39–44, 1969.

60. Webb, W. R.: Pulmonary complications of nonthoracic trauma: Summary of the national research council conference. J. Trauma, *9*:700–711, 1969.

61. Alexander, S. C., and Lassen, N. A.: Cerebral circulatory response to acute brain disease: Implications for anesthetic practice. Anesthesiology, *32*:60–68, 1970.

62. Shenkin, H. A., and Bouzarth, W. F.: Clinical methods of reducing intracranial pressure. N. Eng. J. Med., *282*:1465–1471, 1970.

63. Sunderland, S., and Bradley, K. C.: Disturbances of oculomotor function accompanying extradural hemorrhage. J. Neurol. Neurolsurg. Psychiat., *16*:35–46, 1953.

64. Soloway, M., Nadel, W., Albin, M. S., and White, R. J.: The effect of hyperventilation on subsequent cerebral infarction. Anesthesiology, *29*:975–980, 1968.

65. McKissock, W., Richardson, A., and Walsh, L.: Spontaneous cerebellar hemorrhage: A study of 34 consecutive cases treated surgically. Brain, *83*:1–9, 1960.

66. Moore, D. C., and Bridenbaugh, L. D.: Oxygen: The antidote for systemic toxic reactions from local anesthetic drugs. J.A.M.A., *174*:842–847, 1960.

67. Drake, C. G.: Further experience with surgical treatment of aneurysms of the basilar artery. J. Neurosurg., *29*:372–392, 1968.

68. Lown, B., Neuman, J., Amarasingham, R., and Berkovits, B.: Comparison of alternating current with direct current electroshock across the closed chest. Amer. J. Cardiol., *10*:223–233, 1962.

69. Smith, T. C.: Editorial. Toward Better Measurement. Anesthesiology, *30*:125–126, 1969.

70. Lieberman, N. A., Harris, R. S., Katz, R. I., Lipschutz, H. M., Dolgin, M., and Fisher, V. J.: The effects of lidocaine on the electrical and mechanical activity of the heart. Amer. J. Cardiol., *22*:375–380, 1968.

71. Hitchcock, P., and Keown, K. K.: The management of cardiac arrhythmias during cardiac surgery. South. Med. J., *52*:702–706, 1959.

72. Dietzman, R. H., and Lillehei, R. C.: The treatment of cardiogenic shock. IV. The use of phenoxybenzamine and chlorpromazine. Amer. Heart J., *75*:136–138, 1968.

73. Hollingsworth, J.H.: The results of cardiopulmonary resuscitation. A 3-year university hospital experience. Ann. Intern. Med., *71*:459–466, 1969.

74. Bunn, H. F., and Jandl, J. H.: Control of hemoglobin function within the red cell. N. Eng. J. Med., *282*:1414–1421, 1970.

75. Siggaard-Andersen, O.: Therapeutic aspects of acid-base disorders. In Evans, F. T., and Gray, T. C. (eds.): Modern Trends in Anaesthesia. New York, Appleton-Century-Crofts, 1967.

76. Grossman, C. C.: The use of diagnostic ultrasound in brain disorders. Springfield, C. C Thomas Co., 1966.

77. Charytan, C.: The enterohepatic circulation in glutethimide intoxication. Clin. Pharmacol. Ther., *11*:816–820, 1970.

78. Wild, J. B., and Grover, J. D.: The fist as an external cardiac pacemaker. Lancet, *2*:436–437, 1970.

79. Pennington, J. E., Taylor, J., and Lown, B.: Chest thump for reverting ventricular tachycardia. N. Eng. J. Med., *283*:1192–1195, 1970.

80. Wright, N., and Roscoe, P.: Acute glutethimide poisoning. Conservative management of 31 patients. J.A.M.A., *214*:1704–1706, 1970.

81. Walker, C. O., McCandless, D. W., McGarry, J. D., and Schenker, S.: Cerebral energy metabolism in short-chain fatty acid-induced coma. J. Lab. Clin. Med., *76*:569–583, 1970.

82. Steigmann, F., Condon, R. E., Silverman, D. A., Bombeck, C. T., Alavi, I., and Dubin, A.: Hepatic coma: Newer pathogenetic and therapeutic factors. Amer. J. Gastroenterol., *54*:355–362, 1970.

83. Mueller, H., Ayres, S. M., Gregory, J. J., Gianelli, S., and Grace, W. J.: Hemodynamics, coronary blood flow, and myocardial metabolism in coronary shock: response to 1-norepinephrine and isoproterenol. J. Clin. Invest., *49*:1885–1902, 1970.

84. Sanders, C. A., Buckley, M. J., and Austen, W. G.: Mechanical circulatory assistance: Current status. N. Eng. J. Med., *285*:348–350, 1971.

85. Cotev, S., and Severinghaus, J. W.: Role of cerebrospinal fluid pH in management of respiratory problems. Anesth. Analg., *48*:42–47, 1969.

86. Posner, J. B., and Plum, F.: Spinal-fluid pH and neurologic symptoms in systemic acidosis. N. Eng. J. Med., *277*:605–613, 1967.

87. Ohman, J. L., Marliss, E. B., Aoki, T. T., Munichoodappa, C. S., Khanna, V. V., and Kozak, G. P.: The cerebrospinal fluid in diabetic ketoacidosis. N. Eng. J. Med., *284*:283–290, 1971.

88. Ketones and coma. Editorial. N. Eng. J. Med., *284*:328–329, 1971.

89. Sopira, J. D., and McDonald, R. H., Jr.: Drug abuse – 1970. Disease-A-Month. November, 1970.

90. Fischer, J. F., and James, J. H.: Treatment of hepatic coma and hepatorenal syndrome. Amer. J. Surg., *123*:222–230, 1972.

91. Echlin, F.: Experimental vasospasm, acute and chronic, due to blood in the subarachnoid space. J. Neurosurg., *35*:646–656, 1971.

Supplementary Reading List: Coma

This list is arbitrarily divided by organ systems. Systemic diseases, such as myasthenia gravis, will be found under the organ primarily effected, i.e., the lung.

Adrenal

Egdahl, R. H.: Shock and the adrenal. Surg. Clin. N. Amer., *48*:287–291, 1968.

Blood

Symposium on malaria. Bull. N.Y. Acad. Med., *45*:997–1101, 1969.

Baird, R. L., Weiss, D. L., Ferguson, A. D., French, J. N., and Scott, R. B.: Studies in sickle cell anemia. XXI. Clinicopathological aspects of neurological manifestations. Pediatrics, *34*:92–100, 1964.

DesForges, J. F., and Wang, M. Y. F. W.: Sickle cell anemia. Med. Clin. N. Amer., *50*:1519–1532, 1966.

Bodansky, O.: Methemoglobinemia and methemoglobin-producing compounds. Pharmacol. Rev., *3*:144–196, 1951.

Brain

O'Higgins, J. W.: Fat embolism. Brit. J. Anesth., *42*:163–168, 1970.

Resnick, M. E., and Patterson, C.: Coma and convulsions due to compulsive water drinking. Neurology, *19*:1125–1126, 1969.

Miller, R. B.: Central nervous system manifestations of fluid and electrolyte disturbances. Surg. Clin. N. Amer., *48*:381–393, 1968.

Gitelman, H. J., and Welt, L. G.: Magnesium deficiency. Ann. Rev. Med., *20*:233–242, 1969.

Plum, F., and Posner, J. B. (eds.): Vitamin deficiency: Cofactor deficiency. In The Diagnosis of Stupor and Coma. Phiadelphia, F. A. Davis Co., 1966.

Oxbury J. M., and Whitty, C. W. M.: Causes and consequences of status epilepticus in adults. Brain, *94*:733–744, 1971.

Ingvor, D. H., and Sourander, P.: Destruction of the reticular core of the brain stem. Arch. Neurol., *23*:1–8, 1970.

Heart and Cardiovascular System

Blair, E., Wise, A., and MacKay, A. G.: Gram-negative bacteremic shock: Mechanisms and management. J.A.M.A., *207*:333–336, 1969.

Weil, M. H., and Shubin, H.: Diagnosis and Treatment of Shock. Baltimore, Williams and Wilkins Co., 1967.

Wayne, H. H.: Syncope. Physiological considerations and an analysis of the clinical characteristics in 510 patients. Amer. J. Med., *30*:418–438, 1961.

Hutchinson, E. C., and Stock, J. P. P.: The carotid-sinus syndrome. Lancet, *2*:445–449, 1960.

Kidney

Earley, L. E.: Effects of uremia on the cardiovascular and central nervous system. Surg. Clin. N. Amer., *48*:371–380, 1968.

Liver

De Matteis, F.: Disturbances of liver porphyrin metabolism caused by drugs. Pharmacol. Rev., *19*:523–557, 1967.

Eales, L.: The porphyrins and the porphyrias. Ann. Rev. Med., *12*:251–270, 1961.

Lung

Bigelow, D. B., Petty, T. L., Ashbaugh, D. G., Levine, B. E., Nett, L. M., and Tyler, S. W.: Acute respiratory failure. Med. Clin. N. Amer., *51*:323–340, 1967.

Grant, J. L., and Arnold, W.: Idiopathic hypoventilation. J.A.M.A., *194*:119–122, 1965.

Osserman, K. E. (Chairman): Myasthenia gravis. Conference. N. Y. Acad. Sci., *135*:1–680, 1966.

Kott, H. S.: Crisis in myasthenia gravis. Med. Clin. N. Amer., *53*:285–291, 1969.

Jenkins, M. T., and Luhn, N. R.: Active management of tetanus. Based on experiences of an anesthesiology department. Anesthesiology, *23*:690–709, 1962.

Sankaran, S., and Wilson, R. F.: Factors affecting prognosis in patients with flail chest. J. Thorac. Cardiovasc. Surg., *60*:402–409, 1970.

Abrahamsen, A. M., and Nitter-Hauge, S.: Extreme obesity with respiratory failure, necessitating artificial ventilation. Acta. Med. Scand., *180*:113–136, 1966.

Pruitt, B. A., Flemma, R. J., DiVincenti, F. C., Foley, F. D., and Mason, A. D.: Pulmonary complications in burn patients. A comparative study of 697 patients. J. Thorac. Cardiovasc. Surg., *59*:7–18, 1970.

Pancreas

Toffler, A. H., and Spiro, H. M.: Shock or coma as the predominant manifestation of painless acute pancreatitis. Ann. Intern. Med., *57*:655–659, 1962.

Parathyroid

Kreisler, B., Dinbar, A., and Tulcinsky, D. B.: Postoperative atetanic hypocalcemic coma: Report of a case. Surgery, *65*:916–918, 1969.

Wilson, R. E., Bernhard, W. F., Polet, H., and Moore, F. D.: Hyperparathyroidism: The problem of acute parathyroid intoxication. Ann. Surg., *159*:79–93, 1964.

Pituitary

Blau, J. N., and Hinton, J. M.: Hypopituitary coma and psychosis. Lancet, *1*:408–409, 1960.

Thyroid

Rosenberg, I. N.: Hypothyroidism and coma. Surg. Clin. N. Amer., *48*:353–360, 1968.

Ingbar, S. H.: Management of emergencies. IX. Thyrotoxic storm. N. Eng. J. Med., *274*:1252–1254, 1966.

Coma: Secondary Exogenous Factors

This list is divided into several arbirtrary headings.

Poisons — General

Arena, J.: Treatment of poisoning. Clin. Sympos., *18*:3–31, 1966.

Gleason, M. N., Gosselin, R. E., and Hodge, H. C.: Clinical Toxicology of Commercial Products. Baltimore, Williams and Wilkins Co., 1969.

Schreiner, G. E.: Dialysis of poisons and drugs — Annual review. Trans. Amer. Soc. Artif. Intern. Organs, *16*:544–568, 1970.

Dreisback, R. H.: Handbook of Poisoning: Diagnosis and Treatment. Los Altos, Calif., Lange Med. Publications, 1971.

Poisons — Food

Lamanna, C., and Carr, C. J.: The botulinal, tetanal and enterostaphyloccal toxins: A review. Clin. Pharmacol. Ther., *8*:286–332, 1967.

Tyler, V. E.: Poisonous mushrooms. Prog. Chem. Toxic., *1*:339–384, 1963.

Coma: Secondary to Prescription Drugs

Westlin, W. F.: Desferal (Deferoxamine) in the treatment of acute iron intoxication. Clin. Pediat., *5*:531–535, 1966.

Adams, P., and Waite, C.: Isoniazid induced encephalopathy. Lancet, *1*:680–682, 1970.

McBay, A. J., and Algeri, E. J.: Ataraxics and non-barbiturate sedatives. Progr. Chem. Toxic, 157–190, 1963.

Xanthaky, G., Freireich, A. W., Matusiak, W., and Lukash, L.: Hemodialysis in methyprylon poisoning. J.A.M.A., *198*:1212–1213, 1966.

Teehan, B. P., Maher, J. F., Carey, J. J. H., Flynn, P. D., and Schreiner, G. E.: Acute ethchlorvynol (Placidyl) intoxication. Ann. Intern. Med., *72*:875–882, 1970.

Finkelstein, R., and Jacobi, M.: Fatal iodine poisoning: A cliniopathologic and experimental study. Ann. Intern. Med., *10*:1283–1296, 1937.

Wooster, A. G., Dunlop, M., and Joske, R. A.: Use of oral diuretic (Doburil) in treatment of bromide intoxication. Amer. J. Med. Sci., *253*:23–26, 1967.

Kerr, F., Kenoyer, G., and Bilitch, M.: Quinidine overdosage. Brit. Heart J., *33*:629–631, 1971.

Coma: Secondary to Illicit Drugs and Psychotropic Agents

Swissman, N., and Jacoby, J.: Strychnine poisoning and its treatment. Clin. Pharmacol. Ther., *5*:136–140, 1964.

Espelin, D. E., and Done, A K.: Amphetamine poisoning. Effectiveness of chlorpromazine. N. Eng. J. Med., *278*:1361–1365, 1968.

Ginsberg, M., Hertzman, M., and Schmidt-Nowara, W. W.: Amphetamine intoxication with coagulopathy, hyperthermia and reversible renal failure: a syndrome resembling heatstroke. Ann. Intern. Med., *73*:81–85, 1970.

King, A. B., and Cowen, D. L.: Effect of intravenous injection of marijuana. J.A.M.A., *210*:724–725, 1969.

Cole, J. O., and Wittenborn, J. R., (eds.): Drug Abuse: Social and Psychopharmacological Aspects. Springfield, C. C Thomas, 1969.

Taylor, R. L., Maurer, J. I., and Tinklenberg, J. R., Management of "bad trips" in an evolving drug scene. J.A.M.A., *213*:422–425, 1970.

Cohen, S.: Psychotomimetic agents. Ann. Rev. Pharmacol., *7*:301–318, 1967.

Freedman, D. X.: The psychopharmacology of hallucinogenic agents. Ann. Rev. Med., *20*: 409–418, 1969.

Taylor, G. J., and Harris, W. S.: Cardiac toxicity of aerosol propellants. J.A.M.A., *214*:81–85, 1970.

Bass, M. Sudden sniffing death. J.A.M.A., *212*:2075–2079, 1970.

Poisoning: Secondary to Industrial Products and By-Products

Jenkins, R. B.: Inorganic arsenic and the nervous system. Brain, *89*:479–498, 1966.

Noe, F. E.: Mercury as a potential hazard in medical laboratories. N. Eng. J. Med., *261*:1002–1006, 1959.

Chisolm, J. J., and Kaplan, E.: Lead poisoning in childhood: comprehensive management and prevention. J. Pediatrics, *73*:942–950, 1968.

Bour, H., and Ledingham, I. (eds.): Carbon monoxide poisoning. Progr. Brain Res., *24*:1967.

Quinby, G. E., Loomis, T. A., and Brown, H. W.: Oral occupational parathion poisoning treated with 2-PAM iodine (2-pyridine aldoxime methiodide). N. Eng. J. Med., *268*:639–643, 1963.

Heyndrickx, A.: Toxicology of insecticides, rodenticides, herbicides, and phytopharmaceutical compounds. Progr. Chem. Toxic, *4*:179–256, 1969.

DePalma, A. E., Kwalick, D. S., and Zuckerberg, N.: Pesticide poisoning in children. J.A.M.A., *211*:1979–1981, 1970.

Frazer, A. C.: Pesticides. Ann. Rev. Pharmacol., *7*:319–342, 1967.

Maehly, A. C.: Volatile toxic compounds. Progr. Chem. Toxic, *3*:63–98, 1967.

Coma From Hostile Environmental Factors

Menon, N. D.: High-altitude pulmonary edema: A clinical study. N. Eng. J. Med., *273*:66–73, 1965.

Singh, I., Khanna, P. K., Srivastava, M. C., Lal, M., Rey, S. B., and Subramanyam, C. S. V.: Acute mountain sickness. N. Eng. J. Med., *280*:175–184, 1969.

Andrews, I. C., and Orkin, L. R.: Environmental cold and man. Anesthesiology, *25*:549–559, 1964.

Lapp, N. L., and Jurgens, J. L.: Frostbite. Mayo Clin. Proc., *40*:932–948, 1965.

Wakim, K. G.: Bodily reactions to high temperature. Anesthesiology, *25*:532–548, 1964.

Levine, J. A.: Heat stroke in the aged. Amer. J. Med., *47*:251–258, 1969.

Cahill, J. M.: Drowning: The problem of nonfatal submersion and the unconscious patient. Surg. Clin. N. Amer., *48*:423–430, 1968.

Webster, D. P.: Skin and scuba diving fatalities in the United States. Public Health Rep., *81*:703–711, 1966.

Williams, L. F.: Dysbarism as a source of unconsciousness. Surg. Clin. N. Amer., *48*:453–459, 1968.

Lee, W. R.: The nature and management of electric shock. Brit. J. Anesth., *36*:572–580, 1964.

Jiménez-Porras, J. M.: Pharmacology of peptides and proteins in snake venoms. Ann. Rev. Pharmacol., *8*:299–318, 1968.

Russell, F. E.: Clinical aspects of snake venom poisoning in North America. Toxicon, *7*:33–37, 1969.

Barnard, J. H.: Severe hidden delayed reactions from insect stings. New York J. Med., *66*:1206–1210, 1966.

27

Excruciating Pain

By GEORGE J. HILL, II, M.D.

Pain is always a baleful gift, which reduces the subject of it, and makes him more ill than he would be without it.

(Leriche, R., *The Surgery of Pain* 1939. p. 24)

Severe or excruciating pain is a dramatic challenge to the physician or surgeon, but few guidelines are available for diagnosis and management of this type of crisis. It is a topic which is generally neglected in medical schools, and the student or intern usually must learn to grapple with the problem on his own.

Other emergencies are discussed in detail in classrooms, textbooks and small groups. The student learns to deal with hemorrhage, asphyxia, open fractures and dislocations. He is taught to manage thermal burn, accidental electrocution, poisoning, trauma, and cardiac or respiratory arrest. Acute psychosis, advanced labor, perforated viscus and uncon-

sciousness are traditional subjects for detailed classroom presentation. Several of these problems are of particular interest to surgeons, and their management is described elsewhere in this book. Excruciating pain may be an antecedent or concomitant problem with each of these emergencies, and with a host of other acute illnesses or symptoms. And in many cases it is *pain* which is the greatest *immediate* challenge for the physician.

Excruciating pain is similar in many respects to the problem of the unconscious patient (Chapter 26). The diagnosis is often obscure, the urgency is apparent, the danger is unknown, and the

977

outcome frequently depends on intelligent, rapid assessment of the patient and institution of correct therapy.

This chapter will discuss many of the common pain syndromes which are seen by surgeons in outpatient clinic and emergency rooms. The historical aspects, psychology and physiology of pain will be presented to provide a general perspective for the problem. The discussion of pain syndromes will be organized anatomically, since this is the way the patient presents them in his plea for help. Although many of the syndromes do not require surgical treatment, they are all problems which have presented themselves to the author or to other surgeons for diagnosis or therapy.

Throughout all of his work, the surgeon should endeavor to relieve pain as soon as it is feasible and safe. Pain itself complicates the management of many illnesses, by provoking prolonged stimulation of the sympathetic nervous system and by reducing the patient's ability to cooperate in treatment. The surgeon who shows sincere concern and awareness of his patient's pain will be able to make a diagnosis in many cases in which it would otherwise be impossible. And when the lesion is believed to be surgically correctible, the humane physician will administer appropriate sedative or narcotic drugs to permit the patient to rest until operation is performed. Knowledge of the benefits and side effects of mood-altering drugs must therefore be a part of every surgeon's experience. When all reasonable avenues for pain relief have been explored, neurosurgical control of pain may still be possible, and should be sought before the patient is a hopeless drug addict or psychologically unbalanced by prolonged, unbearable pain.

HISTORY

> Pleasure is oft a visitant; but pain
> Clings cruelly to us.
> Keats, *Endymion*, 1818 Bk. 1, line 906

In preparation for dealing with the problem of severe pain, the physician should familiarize himself with the historical and philosophical aspects of pain.

The legendary figure of Job in the Old Testament is a classic example of the sorely tested man who must occasionally endure great distress for reasons which are obscure.

> My bone cleaveth to my skin and to my flesh, and I am escaped with the skin of my teeth. Have pity upon me God . . . why do ye persecute me . . . ? (Job, Ch. 19:20–22)

Every surgeon can appreciate the suffering described by the ancient author: "My bowels boiled, and rested not . . ." (Job 30:27). Although modern scientific thought rejects the notion of illness or suffering as occurring either by God's whim or as a heavenly punishment, the primitive wail of Job is still repeated by our patients. How many times have we all heard, "What did I do to deserve this?" Quiet reassurance is necessary to remind the patient that physical pain is not an earthly retribution for his misdeeds.

Ancient and primitive societies have in common an almost universal belief that illness is caused by demoniac influence, and a belief that illness must be conjured out of the afflicted patient. In each society a system of taboos and fetishes is closely involved with the prevention, diagnosis and treatment of disease. The fascination with witchcraft and its relationship to pain is apparent even in the so-called civilized countries, where the "Witches' Mark" is considered by the superstitious a sure sign that the bearer is in the service of the Devil. The Witches' Mark is traditionally described as a small spot, usually blue or brown, on the surface of the body, which is entirely insensible to pain, and when pricked with a needle does not bleed.[18] The witchcraft delusion was at its height in Europe and America in the 17th and 18th centuries, but a strong undercurrent of belief persists in modern times.[12] The Catholic ritual "Exorcising the Possessed"[18] is said to have been used even in the present century. The enormous literature on witchcraft and disease was reviewed by Lea (pp. 1464–1485), describing many cases of "sharp pains," "spasms of hands and feet," "pain around the heart," "paroxysms" as if "burned with red-hot iron" and so forth. We can only speculate on the many diseases such as biliary colic, arterial occlusive disease, angina pectoris and tic douloureux which such patients may have had. We sadly note the accusations and tortures which they must have suffered as the result of superstition.

Primitive societies have long used a variety of drugs and beverages to relieve pain, and modern medicine is indebted to these early discoveries.

Alcoholic fermentation is believed to be one of the first technical processes carried out by man, for what appears to be the preparation of mead from honey is depicted in prehistoric drawings on the walls of caves in Europe. Ingestion of ethyl alcohol has subsequently become a widespread, insidiously addictive and frequently abused method for analgesia used by laymen and physicians alike. The most precise use of alcohol for pain relief is the destruction of sensory nerves and nerve roots by local injection of absolute alcohol.[20] This technique can be performed in the outpatient clinic for relief of unbearable pain, such as that due to incurable cancer, although subarachnoid injection of phenol in glycerin has supplanted the use of alcohol in many clinics.[21]

The effects of cannabis preparations (including marihuana and hashish) and the opiates were discovered in Asia. These drugs were probably introduced into Europe by returning Crusaders (1096–1270), by adventuresome traders such as the Polo family from Venice, whose expeditions to the East spanned the period 1255–1295, and by physician-travelers, the most famous of whom was Paracelsus (1493–1541).

General anesthesia began with analgesia obtained from Sir Humphry Davy's nitrous oxide (1800). Surgery was still performed without anesthesia, however, and excruciating pain was commonplace during the next four decades. It was in this period that John Keats, as a young sensitive graduate surgeon from Guy's Hospital penned the lines from *Endymion*, which are shown above.[1] Effective inhalation anesthesia for major surgery was later discovered independently by the dentists Crawford W. Long of Georgia (1842, published 1849) and William T. G. Morton of Boston. Morton's use of ether (1846) with Henry Bigelow and John Collins Warren was followed one year later (1847) by the introduction of chloroform as a general anesthetic agent in England. The anesthetic effects of chloroform were discovered by the distinguished archaeologist Sir James Young Simpson, who was also an eminent gynecologist and midwife to Queen Victoria. The original citations for the literature in the field of anesthesia are summarized in Morton (1970).[16]

Topical and local anesthesia from cocoa leaves had long been known in some primitive societies, but the medical applications of this form of pain relief were first recognized by Carl Koller (1884)—who used cocaine topically—and by William Stewart Halsted (1885)—who introduced local infiltration with cocaine. Halsted accidentally developed a nearly fatal addiction to the drug, but after patient rehabilitation he subsequently became the first Professor of Surgery at the Johns Hopkins University, and the leading American surgeon of the early 20th century.

The psychiatric implications of pain are particularly important in selecting patients as candidates for operations to relieve pain. The subject was reviewed by Dr. Stanley Cobb in White and Sweet[20] in which the problems of psychoneurosis and malingering are discussed in detail and illustrated by case histories. In addition, a case report of the rare congenital anomaly of absence of the sense of pain is presented. The mechanism of this anomaly is unknown, although it is believed not to be due to an absence of pain terminals in the skin, but rather to a defect at the thalamic or cerebral level. Most important for our consideration is the excellent adaptation which such individuals make to the absence of pain. In contrast to this rare condition is the common, desperate situation of the patient with terminal cancer, causalgia, thalamic pain and many other excruciating pain syndromes, who know that frequently

Pain issues a warning with kindly intent,

but also

Pain may stay. Transformed into a torturer,
it clings and claws to no good purpose.
(Wilder Penfield in White and Sweet, 1969,
p. vii)

Difficulty in quantitating pain has long been a stumbling block to the application of the scientific method in this field of research. A major contribution came from Hardy, Wolff, and Goddell, who developed a reliable quantitative technique to elicit pain, using thermal stimulus from an electric light bulb placed near skin which was blackened to provide uniform absorption of heat. These investigators also measured the intensity of pain and provided the first satisfactory index of this subjective sensation: they described the standard unit of pain as the "dol," defined in multiples of a smaller unit known as the "jnd" (just noticeable difference). Maximum (unbearable) pain was defined as 10 dols. Since 21 steps of jnd were recognized by most experimental subjects between no pain (0 dols) and unbearable pain, each dol was defined as 2 jnd's. The intensity of stimulus was recorded quantitatively in mc/sec/cm^2 (millicalories per second per square centimeter). The scale of pain intensity versus stimulus intensity was logarithmic through much of the range of values. An increasing intensity of heat was required to produce a "just noticeable difference" at the higher levels of pain stimulation. This team of investigators noticed that the threshold for pain was 45° C, which was the temperature at which protein denaturation begins. They postulated that pain was produced by destruction of tissue, particularly proteins, a theory which has been developed further in the last few years.[11]

Individual tolerance to discomfort or pain is highly variable, as illustrated in the classic fairy tale of the princess and the pea. It is difficult for us to understand the ability of primitive men to walk on red hot coals, and the remarkable feats of mystics and fakirs of the Indian subcontinent. Differences in tolerance to pain between various ethnic and racial groups and of great tolerance to pain in the past have been repeatedly reported in anecdotal instances.[20] Tolerance to pain is clinically conditioned by excitement—which raises tolerance—and by anxiety—which decreases it. But tolerance is difficult to quantitate, and the phenomenon of tolerance could not be demonstrated in the initial studies by Hardy et al. Subsequently, a model of thermal stimulation by immersion in hot water was designed by A. G. M. Weddell and his colleagues of Oxford University. Weddell reported that transient pain was observed at temperatures lower than the 45° C threshold of Hardy's group. Hardy and Stolwijk (1966)[10] confirmed Weddell's observation. They found that transient or "phasic" pain occurred within 1 to 5 seconds after immersion in water at 37–41° C, adapting in 2 to 6 seconds—a phenomenon which we all notice when we enter a bath which is warmer than we desire. The important observation made by Hardy and Stolwijk was that tolerance to pain could be demonstrated on a reproducible, quantitative basis, and that the characteristics of the data were consistent with a second-order kinetic system. Alternative mechanisms were considered to be subcutaneous thermal gradients, vasomotor reactions and thermochemical changes in the nerve membrane.

The history of our knowledge of the anatomy of the nervous system regarding pain and its mechanisms was thoroughly reviewed by White and Sweet (1955).[20] One of the most important early contributions was S. Weir Mitchell's summary of his experience as a neurologist in the American Civil War, and his vivid description of causalgia in 1872. The role of the sympathetic nervous system in transmitting visceral afferent stimuli dates to the turn of the twentieth century with the work of François-Franck and Jannesco. At about the same time, René Leriche demonstrated the role of vasoconstriction due to sympathetic stimulation in producing pain. This discovery was followed by his use of periarterial sympathectomy to relieve pain in ischemic extremities. The first neurotomy for tic douloureux is said to have been performed in the seventeenth century, but accurate neurosurgery for this condition was not performed until the present century. Harvey Cushing was the first to completely excise the Gasserian ganglion, in 1920.

Charles Brown-Sequard had noticed in 1851 that lesions of the spinal cord caused ipsilateral paralysis and contralateral anesthesia. Knowledge of the spinal tracts was advanced enough to permit the first successful cordotomy to be performed in 1912, and the spinal dermatomes were mapped by 1933. Pain fibers are known to ascend to the thalamus, where awareness of pain takes place. The diffuse thalamic projection system was identified in the cat and macaque monkey by Thomas Starzl and his co-workers in 1951. Impulses are relayed from the thalamus to the sensory cortex (postcentral convolution), where localization and quantitation of pain are accomplished.[6] Concern, anxiety and personality are functions of the frontal lobes. Only one year after the discovery that monkeys could be relieved of frustration by excision of the frontal lobes, Moniz performed (1936) the Nobel prize-winning operation of frontal leukotomy to relieve psychotic anxiety. Even though a complete understanding of pain is still elusive, many modalities for its control are now available. Specific operations, drugs and injections may be used to combat the primary illness. Physical therapy and psychological care can be supportive, reinforcing the effects of primary care. And for intractable, excruciating pain, surgical or chemical destruction of neural pathways can usually be achieved to relieve the patient of pain "which serves no useful purpose . . . and . . . so often becomes his chief tormentor."[20]

A brief comment is in order regarding acupuncture. This ancient oriental form of medical practice has recently been brought to the attention of the Western medical world by scientist-authors such as E. G. Dimond (1971).[5] It now appears that skilled practitioners of acupuncture are able to reduce or eliminate the pain usually associated with major surgery. Acupuncture anesthesia utilizes percutaneous placement of solid needles in sites distant from the site of surgery. Examples cited are: needle placement in the forearm producing anesthesia for thyroidectomy; needles in the pinna of the ear for analgesia during subtotal gastrectomy; manipulating of a needle in the forearm supplemented by 10 mg of morphine producing anesthesia for thoracotomy.

The mechanism of reduction in pain is unknown, although hypnotism and posthypnotic suggestion have previously been considered possible mechanisms for success in acupuncture. It is now suggested that neural pathways may be involved. Acupuncture sites are said to be highly specific in the areas to which anesthesia is referred, and the distant anesthetic effects have been blocked by infiltration of local anesthesia around the acupuncture needles.

It is logical to assume that if acupuncture anesthesia can be verified and reproduced by Western medical researchers, our ability to understand and control pain of many types will be enormously enhanced.

ANATOMY AND PHYSIOLOGY

All pain fibers enter the spinal cord through the dorsal roots, their nuclei being contained in the dorsal root ganglions. The fibers enter the posterior horns, where they synapse with neurones of the lateral spinothalamic tract. The spinothalamic neurones ascend for one or two segments, then cross the midline to the opposite side and continue upwards through the brainstem to the posterolateral and posteromedial nuclei of the thalamus. Impulses are then transmitted to the sensory cortex (postcentral convolution) and hypothalamus.

Classification of Pain

Pain is classified according to depth, modality and speed of perception. The anatomical regions for pain perception are classified on the basis of depth from the skin, being "superficial," "deep" and "visceral" in location. The modalities of discomfort are pain, deep pressure, heat and cold. Pain is usually described as either "quick" or "slow."

Cutaneous Pain

Superficial nerve endings are located in the skin; they transmit impulses which are perceived as pain, touch, heat or cold. It is still debated whether the intensity or type of stimulus is responsible for the quality (modality) of the perception, and whether or not different stimuli are received at different end organs. Traditional teaching is strongly in favor of modality-specific sensory endings,[6] in spite of the difficulty which investigators have in confirming this hypothesis. The traditional anatomic receptors in the epidermis are: bare nerve endings for pain (although White and Sweet believe that other nerve endings also subserve pain); Pacinian and Meissner's corpuscles and Merkel's discs for touch; Ruffini's organ for warmth and heat; and Krause's end-bulb for cold.

Deep Pain

Deep pain and pressure are perceived in receptors in the dermis by Ruffini's endings and the Golgi-Mazzoni endings. Other deep pain receptors are located in muscles, tendons, joints, adipose tissue and fascia.

Visceral Pain

Visceral pain is more complex and has been studied less completely than somatic pain. Painful stimuli in the deep viscera apparently travel with the sympathetic nervous system, except for the pelvic viscera, which are served by the parasympathetic system. Pain from viscera is described as (a) true visceral pain, (b) referred pain, and (c) pain due to secondary skeletal muscular contraction. Each visceral afferent nerve passes through the sympathetic ganglion for its segment, then through its white ramus communicans, its spinal nerve and its posterior root where the nucleus is located in the dorsal root ganglion. It then enters the posterior grey matter of the spinal cord. The visceral afferent dendrite synapses with a visceral efferent sympathetic fiber in the posterior horn of the spinal cord. Most authors state that there is no synapse in the cord between the visceral afferent and a secondary spinothalamic neurone, so the means by which visceral pain is perceived can only be surmised on theoretical grounds. It has been proposed that the visceral sympathetic relay in the posterior horn triggers an afferent response in the adjacent spinothalamic neurone; other authors propose a separate, synapsing visceral afferent pathway with short neurones in the spinothalamic tract. The mechanism of referred pain is also unknown; in this situation visceral pain is perceived erroneously in the skin or other surface area. Theories are based on dissections in man and lower animals, and on complex analogies. Among the hypotheses are: dual innervation of skin and deep viscera by branched afferent neurones; or a discharge taking place by a "short circuit" or "reverberation" in the synapse between the somatic afferent and spinothalamic neurone when transmission occurs in the adjacent synapse between visceral afferent and visceral efferent fibers.

Whatever the mechanism of pain transmission from viscera, the most important clinical aspect is the fact that interruption of sympathetic innervation of viscera will stop visceral pain. But if peritoneum and muscles are involved, the posterior spinal roots or lateral spinothalamic tract must be divided to control pain.

A *Fibers and* C *Fibers*

Painful stimuli are transmitted by rapid-conducting (myelinated) and slow-conducting (unmyelinated) nerves. *A* fibers are the largest and most heavily myelinated of the peripheral nerves. They are $2-20\mu$ in diameter and have a conduction velocity of 15–40 m./sec. "Quick" pain is transmitted by the delta group of the *A* fibers, which are $2-5\mu$ in diameter. *B* fibers are of medium size, and have a conduction velocity which is midway between the *A* and *C* fibers. *C* fibers are the smallest nerves and have little or no myelin, and the slowest transmission velocity. They are 2μ or less in diameter, and have a conduction time of 0.6–2.0 m./sec. "Slow" or "delayed" pain is transmitted over *C* fibers, which also have a threshold for stimulation approximately five times greater than the delta group of *A* fibers.

Dermatomes, Myotomes and Sclerotomes

Dermatomes, myotomes and sclerotomes are the regions of skin, muscle and bone, respectively, which correspond to the embryonic segmental anatomy.[7] The segmental distribution of each spinal nerve has been mapped in detail. Variations due to biological variability, method of testing, and (apparently) to artistic license are illustrated in White and Sweet.[20] The dermatomes are usually depicted from the anterior and posterior views; a useful lateral view is given by Finneson.[6] There is general agreement on the following guidelines for dermatome innervation:

C2 — angle of the mandible

C4 — acromioclavicular region (shoulder)
C6 — thumb
T2 — medial humerus (arm)
T4 — nipples
T10 — umbilicus
L2 — knee
L5 — great toe
Sl — lateral foot
S4 — perineum

Sensory Pathways in the Spinal Cord and Brain

The posterior roots fan out widely as they enter the spinal cord, as was beautifully shown by the 1906 Nobel Prize winner, Ramon y Cajal. The large myelinated fibers which subserve proprioception pass medially into the dorsal columns and ascend directly to the fasciculi gracilis and cuneatus. The other sensory modalities are carried in the spinothalamic tract of the opposite side of the spinal cord. The spinothalamic-sensory nerve synapse for pain is just deep to the gelatinous substance of Rolando in the outer aspect of the posterior horn. The fibers for the other sensory modalities synapse with the spinothalamic fibers deeper in the posterior horn. The lateral spinothalamic tract mainly carries fibers for pain and temperature, whereas the fibers for light touch are predominantly grouped in the ventral spinothalamic tract. The higher (thoracic) fibers travel in the medial (deep) portion of the spinothalamic tract, and the lower (sacral) fibers are arranged laterally (superficially). Cordotomy is the operation in which the entire spinothalamic tract is cut to relieve pain in the lower part of the body. In order to relieve all pain the operation is usually performed at the cervical level, with an incision anterior to the dentate ligament, penetrating to a depth of 4.5 mm. The anterior horn is occasionally injured by this procedure, producing some degree of ipsilateral paresis (see diagram in Finneson, p. 13)[6]

The fibers for pain are gathered and regrouped in the thalamus, which is located adjacent to the third and lateral ventricles. Other afferents in the thalamus include auditory and visual sensation. Thalamic efferents are relayed to the ipsilateral cerebral cortex. Thalamic destruction by sterotaxic instruments has been widely employed but has not been particularly satisfactory. Occasionally severe pain develops from surgery as a result of injury to the thalamus or vascular lesions. This type of "central" pain is particularly distressing if it occurs as the result of an attempt to treat some other form of pain by a surgical procedure on the thalamus. The "thalamic syndrome" of Déjerine and Roussy is caused by thrombosis of the thalamogeniculate artery. The syndrome is characterized by excruciating pain which occurs with minimal stimuli, following a stroke in which transient hemialgesia has occurred. The pain of this syndrome is usually poorly localized and may eventually become protracted or permanent. Central pain may occur from any lesion of the central nervous system,[4] but apparently it is most commonly the result of damage to the thalamus.

The role of the cerebral cortex in pain perception is poorly understood. The somatic cortex has been identified as the postcentral convolution of the parietal lobe, and it is here that the corticothalamic tracts terminate. However, anatomical localization of pain is not served by specific areas of the cortex to the degree that is seen in the motor cortex. Likewise, surgery on the somatic cortex has revealed puzzling results, with relatively little pain produced from direct stimulation, and with relatively poor pain relief achieved by resection of this portion of the brain.

Biochemistry

The thermal threshold for sustained cutaneous pain is approximately 45° C, which is approximately the temperature at which tissue injury begins to occur. It has been postulated that tissue injury effects release of bradykinin, which thereby becomes a major endogenous cause of pain.[14] According to this theory, the lysosomal enzymes released from damaged cells initiate the process of conversion of bradykinin from its precursor, kininogen. The proposed sequence begins when the pre-kallekrein is converted to kallekrein by the action of Factor XII (Hageman Factor) in tissues. Kallekrein is a peptidase which splits bradykinin from kininogen, an $\alpha 2$ globulin. Bradykinin is a nonapeptide which causes intense pain when it is injected in amounts as small as 10 nanomatars beneath the skin. It is rapidly inactivated by kininases in blood and tissues, such as carboxypeptidase B, which removes its terminal amino acid, arginine.

The chemical theory of the origin of pain states that bradykinin and other chemicals such as histamine, acetylcholine and 5-hydroxytryptamine (serotonin) stimulate chemoreceptors in axons of the afferent nerves. Variation in intensity of pain could be due to differences in concentrations of chemicals which are released in the damaged tissues, and to differences in the rate of transmission of the afferent impulses.

The chemical theory of pain is an attractive proposition to explain pain in which there is gross or microscopic evidence of tissue injury. It appears to offer little help for the problem of central pain, such as that which develops following cordotomy and in the Déjerine-Roussy syndrome. It is also doubtful that the chemical mechanism can be invoked successfully as the cause of severe, chronic pain due to metastatic cancer. Indeed, the review of pain produced by chemicals by Keele and Armstrong (1969)[11] relates the chemical theory to clinical conditions only when necrosis, inflammation, vasodilatation or constriction is present. These authors discuss pain due to endogenous chemicals such as histamine, acetylcholine, kinins and serotonin, and exogenous chemicals such as canthardin and other vesicants. They clearly distinguish two types of pain — pain from physical and pain from chemical stimuli. But the subjects of cancer and central pain are not discussed by Keele and Armstrong. Apparently the chemists, neurologists and psychiatrists are still unable to formulate a unified hypothesis which even begins to explain all of the aspects of pain.

PRESENTATION OF THE PATIENT

Pain is almost invariably localized to one or more specific regions of the body, and classification of the problem may begin with anatomical areas. In each region, three types of problems are generally encountered: surgical, medical and psychiatric. A complete discussion of many of the diseases mentioned here is presented elsewhere in this book. In other conditions, a full discussion in a surgical textbook would obviously be inappropriate.

Head

Pain in the head or face may be localized in either a general area or at a specific point. The pain may be referred to a spot which is some distance away from the pathology. A typical example is pain in the external auditory canal due to carcinoma of the nasopharynx. Likewise, severe toothache may be a manifestation of angina pectoris. The wise physician therefore does not limit his examination to the area of pain or tenderness.

Tic douloureux is severe and usually intermittent pain which occurs in the face—the distribution of the trigeminal nerve. Other causes of severe facial, oral or ear pain are cancer, alveolar (tooth) caries or abscess, bony fracture, stomatitis from bacteria (streptococcus, diphtheria, Ludwig's or Vincent's angina, and so on), parotitis (mumps, salivary calculus or idiopathic), mastoiditis, otitis media (bacterial or serous, including "air otitis" following an airplane trip), angina pectoris with pain referred to face or jaw, foreign body, and herpes zoster ("shin-gles," with pain preceding the rash by 24–72 hours).

Pain which is located in the general region of the calvarium may be localized or diffuse. Of the many causes which are sometimes seen, several are relatively more common. These include brain tumor, brain abscess, metastases to the skull, skull fracture, acute hypertensive crisis, cerebral hemorrhage (from hypertension, aneurysm, tumor,) migraine headache (usually preceded by a typical "aura"), and sinusitis. Acute sudden pain in the eye may be due to glaucoma, hemorrhage, infection, iritis, a foreign body or corneal scratch, and other conditions described in Chapter 9.

It is remarkable how often the patient is unaware of the antecedent history which would seem to make many of these conditions simple to diagnose. Occasionally the trauma occurred while the patient was drunk or under the influence of drugs. Sometimes he is embarrassed to relate the key point in the history, especially in the presence of his friends or family. And sometimes either a language barrier or a physician's failure to ask the proper question is the reason for confusion in diagnosis.

Neck

Many causes of pain in head or face also produce simultaneous or referred pain to the neck. "Tension" headache may produce a severe crisis in an anxious patient who has an intolerable family situation—although the doctor may correctly be concerned with the possibility of meningitis or subarachnoid hemorrhage. Causes of pain in the neck which are especially frequent in outpatient and emergency clinics are whiplash injuries (some of which cause pain that increases over a period of several days or weeks), cervical arthritis and herniated cervical intervertebral discs. Less common are various types of cancer, including cancer of the thorax with pain referred to the neck, such as a Pancoast (superior sulcus) tumor. Deep-seated infections of the neck may be puzzling, though the pain of a sore throat is usually sufficiently well-localized to guide the physician to the proper examination. The possibility of carcinoma of the upper airway, pharynx, or esophagus should be considered in every patient over the age of forty with a sore throat. These patients should not be simply sent home with a handful of antibiotic capsules — re-examination is always indicated in 7 to 14 days. A practical and well-illustrated guide to cervical pain has been prepared by Caillet (1964).[3]

Chest

Pleurisy (inflammation of the pleura) is frequently the cause of a crisis, especially when it occurs in previously healthy persons. Most of these patients are "breathless" because of splinting. Spontaneous pneumothorax is a common cause of pleurisy in young people, or in elderly patients with emphysematous blebs. Although patients with pleurisy will usually have normal blood gases, they will frequently describe difficulty in "getting breath." Relief of anxiety and administration of nasal oxygen is more important in most of these patients than an endotracheal tube or immediate insertion of a chest tube. If the patient with a small pneumothorax strains owing to anxiety, a tension pneumothorax may develop. On the other hand, if the air is temporarily evacuated with a needle connected to an intravenous tube, the end of which is placed underwater, the pneumothorax can be removed and the patient immediately made comfortable.

Many other causes of pleurisy are occasionally discovered in the course of the work-up: tuberculosis, viral pneumonia, pulmonary embolus, carcinoma of the lung, mesothelioma. Severe chest pain also always raises the question of a myocardial infarction, especially if the pain is located anteriorly or on the left. Dissecting aneurysm is also considered seriously, especially if the pain is posterior, and radiates to the neck, arm or abdomen. Pericarditis may be extremely

painful, and the pain may begin as acutely as a myocardial infarction. The patient with acute idiopathic costal chondritis (Tietze's syndrome) may be extremely concerned, although these patients usually can be reassured when they are found not to have myocardial ischemia. Incarcerated paraesophageal diaphragmatic hernia may cause acute, severe pain, and the situation may require immediate surgery to avoid infarction of the entrapped viscera. Asthmatic patients may develop painful mediastinal emphysema. Subcutaneous emphysema in the neck in these patients may cause great alarm, since ruptured bronchus or esophagus also causes this physical finding. Post-thoracotomy pain may be severe, though usually the diagnosis is clear, since the nerve involved is located above the course of the incision. Compression fracture of the spine may cause local pain and an obvious gibbous deformity. The diagnosis may be missed initially, however, if the patient's complaint is pain in the distribution of the intercostal nerves which were crushed with collapse of vertebra. Rib fractures may be a puzzling cause of chest pain, for it may occur in patients who are unaware of the severe cough or trauma which caused it. This problem is most common in older patients, who have partially decalcified ribs. A nondisplaced fracture may not be fully apparent until a callus has appeared some weeks later. If the fracture occurred when the patient was inebriated, he may have been unaware of the trauma, or he may wish to suppress the incident. Pathologic fracture of a rib during minor trauma or a cough may be the first sign of the presence of a primary or metastatic tumor in the rib.

Abdomen

The differential diagnosis of the acute abdomen is discussed in Chapter 18. In this portion of the text we wish to focus on those problems which frequently present with severe pain.

Ruptured viscus generally produces excruciating pain, if the perforation occurs into the free peritoneal cavity. Perforated duodenal ulcer and a perforated colon are the two most common causes of the "boardlike" abdomen in which free air is found on x-ray in the subdiaphragmatic spaces. Every portion of the gastrointestinal tract is subject to rupture, of course. Free air may also escape from the esophagus, stomach or small bowel if the rupture is into the peritoneal cavity. Gastric perforation may, however, occur into the lesser sac, and although great pain is present, free air may be difficult to identify on x-ray. Likewise, retroperitoneal colonic perforation may be very painful but difficult to identify on x-ray. Rupture of the common bile duct or gallbladder is usually due to erosion by calculi, and the acute bile peritonitis which develops usually causes intense pain. Rupture of the rectum usually raises the question of sadomasochism or other aberrant sexual behavior. Rupture of the uterus usually is a complication of pregnancy or direct trauma. Rupture of the urinary tract (kidney, ureter, bladder or urethra) usually is accompanied by severe trauma or is associated with significant localizing antecedent history. Rupture of any of these organs may cause pain from either the escape of irritating contents, or because of the sudden traction placed on the serosa or the mesentery of the abdominal viscera. The appropriate studies for the patient with a suspected ruptured viscus include x-rays (AP, upright or lateral decubitus), in which a careful search is made for air shadows in the retroperitoneum, subhepatic and subphrenic areas. Contrast medium must frequently be instilled in order to localize the lesion. Water-soluble material is preferred (e.g., Gastrografin for intestinal examination and Hypaque for the bladder and urethra). But if other causes of abdominal pain can reasonably be excluded, it is frequently necessary to operate for identification and correction of the problem.

Intraperitoneal bleeding is frequently associated with severe pain. The mechanism is not clear, since slow instillation of blood in the abdomen is commonly said not to cause pain. The pain from ruptured aneurysm or ectopic pregnancy may be due to tension and pressure on the mesentery or serosa. In any case, the distinction between "apoplexy" (intraperitoneal hemorrhage) and ruptured viscus can usually be made preoperatively, since the patient with a ruptured viscus does not ordinarily go into shock immediately. Shock from peritonitis occurs slowly, as intravascular volume is lost in the form of plasma.

Severe ischemia or infarction of viscera usually produces intense pain. Mesenteric infarction from thrombosis or embolus may cause intense pain, and volvulus of the stomach, small bowel, cecum or sigmoid may also cause similar pain. An internal hernia may produce the same type of pain as infarction incurs. In a patient with severe constant abdominal pain, the management should be in the direction of surgery, since a small abdominal incision is usually less dangerous than prolonged deliberation in an attempt to make a definitive diagnosis prior to surgery.

Gynecological causes of severe pain include a variety of conditions including normal pregnancy (labor or false labor), ectopic pregnancy, acute pelvic inflammatory disease (gonococcal, bacteroides, pneumococcal, for instance), cancer (especially from pelvic wall invasion in cervical cancer) or even Mittelschmerz and endometriosis, which ordinarily do not cause severe pain but may be acute and confusing to the physician who sees the patient for the first time when she is having an episode of pain. The pain which follows instillation of air for hysterosalpingogram may mimic the pain of a perforated ulcer, and free air is also present!

Urologic causes of severe pain are usually localized to the diseased organ, or can be identified because of the area to which pain is referred (e.g., ureter referring pain to testicle and kidney referring pain to the costovertebral angle). Urologic lesions causing severe pain include calculi, bleeding, infection, trauma and tumor. Noteworthy is the severe pain from acute infection: pyelonephritis, cystitis, perinephric abscess, prostatitis and urethritis. Waves of acute pain followed by relatively pain-free intervals are characteristic of calculi, and when the pain subsides it is usually because the calculus has finally passed into the bladder or out of the urethra. Bleeding into the renal pelvis may cause acute pain which mimics the colic produced by renal calculi. A distended bladder causes great pain. When relieved by passage of a catheter or by percutaneous aspiration, the gratitude of the patient is unbounded. Frequently, a drug-induced postoperative urinary retention will be self-limited after only one catheterization.

The pancreas is the site of pain for a variety of reasons. Acute pancreatitis may cause severe pain in the back or generalized peritoneal pain and tenderness. Chronic pancreatitis may cause equally severe episodes of abdominal or back pain, but the patient usually does not develop fever, hypotension and tachycardia. Carcinoma of the pancreas rarely causes acute pain, though the pain, if present, may truly be excruciating. Pain from end-stage carcinoma of the pancreas may not respond well to the largest doses of narcotics. Pseudocyst of the pancreas and the pain after ingestion of alcohol in patients with Hodgkin's disease are rare and confusing causes of severe pain in this area.

Colic may be as common and frustrating as the problem of colicky babies. Or it may occur as biliary colic, colic due to calculi in the gallbladder or bile ducts; or as intestinal colic, from obstruction (gallstones, tumor, stricture) or inflammation, as in staphylococcal food poisoning or "traveler's diarrhea." Colic from ureteral obstruction was mentioned above. All forms of colic have in common the severe, intermittent nature of the pain, and they may be difficult to distinguish from each other. When pain is intermittent, it rarely requires immediate surgery, and it is therefore usually possible to take time to localize the lesion and determine if medical or surgical treat-

ment is needed. Intussusception in children is a cause of colicky pain which cannot be passed off as physiologic, since bowel infarction may be occurring even though the baby is not crying constantly. So continued observation and repeated examinations are needed in patients with colic, along with a generous amount of suspicion that surgery *may* indeed be necessary.

Penetrating trauma should be mentioned as a cause of pain, only to emphasize the role of surgery. When a major penetration has occurred, or when the penetrating instrument is still protruding from the patient, it is especially important to take the patient immediately to the operating room. Until the site of perforation has been identified, and the vessels in the area are secured, a sudden, irretrievable change may occur in the patient's condition. It is usually best not to remove the knife or protruding foreign body until the patient is in the operating room. The final preparations for surgery may be somewhat more leisurely than the trip to the operating room, which should be swift. Extra IV lines can be placed if desired and the trachea can be intubated *after* the patient has been placed on the operating table and a team gathered for instant action in case of sudden deterioration.

Hepatic pain may occur from hepatitis, and sometimes this pain may be acute and severe. However, severe hepatic pain is more commonly due to a sudden event, as in hemorrhage into a primary or metastatic tumor, rupture of an abscess or some other acute lesion. Elevation of intrahepatic pressure from biliary tract obstruction may cause considerable discomfort, but rarely is it the cause of excruciating pain.

Acute intra-abdominal infections may cause severe pain and may be confused with such problems as bowel obstruction or infarction, or perforated viscus. The most common infection is appendicitis. The problem in diagnosis usually arises in cases in which the diagnosis is obscured by an atypical history. Usually the pain of appendicitis begins in the midabdomen, associated with mild nausea. The pain usually increases gradually as it shifts and localizes in the right lower quadrant. But in retrocecal appendicitis, or in obese, elderly or chronically ill patients, the disease may evolve in different ways. It may occasionally bring the patient to the doctor only when severe, excruciating pain is finally present. The next most common abdominal infections are cholecystitis, diverticulitis and pelvic inflammatory disease. Each may produce severe abdominal pain, usually most intense in the organ involved. Although infection can occur in all of the other abdominal viscera, the main differential diagnosis must be with several types of disease which mimic infection and intra-abdominal surgical crises. The nonsurgical conditions include lead poisoning, Henoch-Schönlein purpura, sickle cell disease, acute intermittent porphyria, acute gastroenteritis, peptic ulcer, pancreatitis, hepatitis, familial Mediterranean fever and other forms of acute polyserositis such as lupus, rheumatic fever and rheumatoid arthritis. Unfortunately, some of these so-called "medical" conditions also may require surgery. For example, the patient with Henoch-Schönlein purpura may develop intussusception; the patient with serositis may develop cholecystitis, and sickle cell crisis may lead to splenic or renal infarct.

Foreign bodies in the gastrointestinal tract may cause great discomfort and may be a challenge to locate if the foreign body was ingested some time previously. The acute impaction of food in a hiatal hernia is much easier to suspect than perforation of the colon by a poultry bone or toothpick. Sedation and relief of anxiety in the patient with obstruction of a hiatal hernia is especially important, to avoid perforation of the esophagus by uncontrolled attempted emesis.

Thrombosed or acutely inflamed hemorrhoid is the most common cause of sudden, severe perianal pain. The diagnosis can usually be made over the telephone but the patient must be examined in person in order to determine if the hemorrhoid can be evacuated surgically or if local astringents are indicated (Chapter 21).

Acute, severe pain in the groin may be due to incarcerated (or strangulated) inguinal or femoral hernia. In my experience it is more common for severe groin pain to be caused by acutely inflamed lymph nodes than by an incarcerated hernia. In any case, the best course usually is to explore the area surgically, unless a very definite history of infection and lymphadenitis is obtained.

Constipation, on the other hand, may cause a tremendous problem with pain, especially in overly anxious patients and in young people with overly anxious parents. It is difficult but sometimes necessary in these patients to make the diagnosis of constipation and to treat with a laxative or an enema. It is especially difficult when the patient complains of *severe* pain, and the parents are perspiring and agitated. But an x-ray may help by revealing a large volume of feces in the colon and a careful history, taken in private, may uncover the background of the problem and its presentation.

Back Pain

Acute lumbosacral back strain may cause a severe, incapacitating episode of pain. The patient obviously must be thoroughly evaluated for pathological fracture, abdominal aortic aneurysm and malingering, but if these conditions can be ruled out it may be gratifying to institute the proper measures of bed rest, sedation, heat and muscular relaxants (Chapter 12).

Extremities

An orderly examination of the extremities will usually uncover the cause of acute pain in this area. An understanding of some of the more common causes of severe pain may direct the examiner to a speedier solution.

Ischemia—acute or chronic—may cause severe pain. Chronic arterial insufficiency may cause claudication and rest pain. Acute arterial insufficiency may be the cause of pain from thrombosis or embolus. In all of these cases a careful inspection of the vascular system (pulses, bruit, color, temperature) will usually give the clues to diagnosis. If the pain from ischemia is continuous and severe, emergency arteriography and surgery is usually indicated, since infarction is always suspected in such cases. If muscular contraction is present, a "cramp" or "charley horse" must be ruled out, however, since it would be embarrassing to operate for ischemia and find that muscular rigor was not due to impaired vascularity!

Rupture or tear of muscles and their sheaths may occur with trauma or great effort; the pain may be severe. The most common sites are the plantaris and palmaris muscles and the pronators of the forearm. Other forms of trauma may be identified by their location: cartilaginous injury, ligamentous strain or tear, sprained ankle or fracture. Some of these problems may be difficult to diagnose, and the treatment may be diametrically opposed (e.g., rupture of the plantaris muscle vs. deep thrombophlebitis). Pain due to rupture of the Achilles tendon is usually severe, and physical examination combined with history will provide the diagnosis. In each condition, the treatment is relatively straightforward (see Chapters 11, 12 and 13). But diagnosis is the challenge; a dislocation may be difficult to recognize on x-ray, and the patient's agony may interfere with the examination—he may not even give an adequate history. So the physician must let his mind range over the *types* of problems which can afflict the area in which pain is located. Pain also may be referred in an exasperating pattern, as with pain in the knee from disease in the hip. (Watch for a pathologic fracture of the hip in a patient with previous history of carcinoma who develops severe pain in the knee), or pain in the arm as the predominant symptom in angina pectoris. Specific syndromes are discussed in greater detail by Tarsey (1953),[19] Fin-

neson (1969)[6] and Hale (1971).[7] The section on thoracic outlet syndrome by Whelan (pp. 45–56) in Hale's monograph is particularly useful.

Gout may affect any part of the extremities, though usually the patient will have a problem of tenderness and pain in the great toe at some time in his history. Elevation in serum uric acid level will confirm the suspicion. Neurological syndromes are occasionally seen, including amputation stump neuroma, Sudek's atrophy and causalgia.

"Minor" lesions may produce a lot of pain when the patient is bearing all of his weight on them: e.g., stress fracture of a metatarsal in a hiker or gymnast, blisters in a hiker (especially in sandy country), a large plantar wart on the metatarsal heads, or an infected ingrown toenail.[15] All of these may cause such severe pain that the physician is called out of his bed to give relief to the suffering patient. Sometimes it takes patience to deal with these problems. But the doctor has only to think how he would feel if the situation were reversed, and he will give the care that is needed to send a happy patient on his way.

Skin

Severe pain in the skin raises the question of serious deep visceral pain with referral to the integument. Localized pain in the skin may occur due to herpes zoster ("shingles") which may actually cause psychic derangement because of severe discomfort. These patients are sometimes seen by surgeons because the dermatome involved overlies an area of surgical interest, such as the right lower abdomen. Every surgeon will eventually mistake "shingles" for appendicitis or cholecystitis, just as the internist will occasionally mistake the pain for myocardial infarction. The pain and tenderness of herpes zoster may precede the appearance of the first vesicles by as much as 24–72 hours.

First and second degree burns also cause severe pain. If the burn is extensive, generous use of narcotics may be required. Loss of the epidermis by abrasion—rope burns, mat burns (wrestlers), floor burns (basketball players), and blisters—are all problems of the integument which are not life-endangering, but require prompt attention for relief of pain. Cold water usually provides a safe method of alleviating the pain. If topical analgesics are used, the danger of sensitization should be remembered. Johnson and Johnson's "First Aid Cream" appears to be an innocuous and relatively effective topical analgesic cream for these abrasions.

Cancer of the skin will occasionally present severe problems in pain control. The lesion may be a neglected or recurrent basal or squamous cell carcinoma. Rare and very painful lesions such as glomus tumors and Kaposi's sarcoma are occasionally encountered. If the cancer has recurred and is no longer amenable to radiation therapy or resection, the pain may be difficult to control perfectly. This sort of patient will probably live long enough to become resistant to relief from most of the narcotics. Metastases may also appear in the skin from almost every type of cancer. We have seen cutaneous spread of tumors as diverse as carcinomas of the lung, stomach, colon, breast, larynx, oral cavity, bladder, vulva, melanoma, sarcomas and bone tumors. We have seen local recurrence of glioblastoma multiforme in a scalp incision. Local radiation therapy may be very helpful in controlling the growth of these tumors. But when the tumor recurs in a previously irradiated area, the pain may be an unbearable combination of radiation dermatitis and cancer, treatable only with cordotomy.

Genitalia

Pain in the external genitalia may occur from local lesions such as infection, insect bites, trauma from sadomasochism or accident, or cancer. Pain may also be referred from deep seated lesions, such as ureteral calculi, gonorrheal urethritis or vaginitis, and perirectal abscess. Gonococcal infections are especially troublesome because they may be atypical and—if unsuspected—may be transmitted to the examining physician. Patients with gonorrhea are often somewhat uncooperative as well as being tender to palpation. The surgeon should always avoid getting vaginal or urethral discharge in his eyes, and should be scrupulous in his own hygiene after each examination of a patient's genitalia. Accidental infection with gonorrhea during a physical examination led to conjunctivitis and unilateral blindness, and was nearly fatal for America's first female physician, Elizabeth Blackwell.

Drug-Induced Problems

The most common problem in this category is narcotic withdrawal, in which the patient may present a well thought out history of disease in order to trick the unwary physician into giving him a dose of morphine (e.g., colicky pain with hematuria, boardlike abdomen with a history of previous ulcer disease, and so on.) It is necessary to study every previously unknown patient for signs of needle marks, excessive agitation, perspiration and the consistency of history. Occasionally, mistakes will be made, since drug addicts can develop surgical lesions, and patients who appear to be unreliable may have significant problems other than drug addiction. Pain due to withdrawal reaction is not the only type of problem produced by drug abuse, for LSD or mescaline intoxication may produce severe abdominal pain.

Generalized Pain

Widespread, severe pain is a puzzling and—fortunately—uncommon situation. The patient's appearance will usually give a clue to drug addiction, if it is a withdrawal reaction. The prodromal pain of myalgia, arthralgia and headache which precedes the localized signs of adeno- or enteroviral infection would rarely be considered excruciating. However, tetanus, rabies, malaria and dengue may all be associated with severe generalized pain. Acute polyserositis may involve many of the areas of the body and may appear generalized; this syndrome may occur as an acute or delayed manifestation of drug toxicity, serum sickness or streptococcal illness. The bizarre pain of Déjerine-Roussy syndrome was discussed earlier. Generally speaking, diffuse, poorly localized pain is usually not a surgical problem; it is either medical or psychiatric, or both.

TREATMENT

Treatment should ideally be given only *after* the etiology has been determined. However, it may be necessary to compromise with the ideal. As mentioned above, when operation has been decided upon, it is reasonable to give sufficient premedication to be humane, although the patient must not be given so much morphine that his respiration ceases or blood pressure falls. Likewise, it is sometimes necessary to make a presumptive diagnosis of myocardial infarction and give morphine to allay anxiety and prevent progression of the infarct. Morphine will also relieve some of the muscular spasm which accompanies fracture of a bone and will prevent secondary destruction or hemorrhage in soft tissue. Morphine may be given subcutaneously, IM, or intravenously, and the action is progressively more rapid in each of these routes (see Chapter 2).

Specific aspects of treatment of several of the painful lesions were discussed in previous chapters. An amazing amount of relief is often obtained simply by the presence and attention of a physician or nurse. Likewise, hospitalization for one or two days may be a great help in management of many puzzling or essentially incurable pain problems. In this way, a proper program of medication can be worked out, and the patient is given the opportunity to see that it will be successful, at least for the time being.

Pain from recurrent cancer can be relieved in up to 70 per cent of patients by treatment with supervoltage irradiation therapy. Some forms of cancer, such as lymphoma and carcinoma of the breast, are more responsive to radiation than others, such as carcinoma of the colon and melanoma. But radiation may succeed even in unexpected cases.

Pain from infection should usually be treated by both antibiotics and surgical drainage. As mentioned in Chapter 4, the indications for antibiotics and drainage must be individualized, based on the type and location of the infection, and the status of the individual patient. When the pain is severe, it is usually necessary to perform drainage, and in such patients the likelihood of need for antibiotics is also highest.

Interruption of the sensory nerves may be needed in some cases of severe, intractable pain. Causalgia (from trauma or amputation of the extremities) and recurrent cancer are the most common indications for nerve interruption. Causalgia may be relieved by sympathectomy. However, causalgia and recurrent cancer may require subarachnoid instillation of alcohol or phenol, or rhizotomy, cordotomy or frontal leukotomy. Cold saline irrigations of the subarachnoid space recently received a flurry of interest. This technique has not been universally acclaimed, but it has fewer complications and fewer permanent side affects than the nerve interruption procedures.[2] Local injections with short or long-acting local anesthetics also may be helpful. If relief is obtained with local injection of lidocaine, an injection of dibucaine in oil or bupivacaine may be tried. Sympathetic block with local anesthetic has been reported to be successful for pain caused by carcinoma of the pancreas; we have never found it useful, however, presumably because the retroperitoneum has been invaded by tumor.

The local effects of counterirritants such as oil of wintergreen, Bengay or Mentholatum are remarkably helpful in relief of musculoskeletal strains and trauma. In treating athletic injuries, the surgeon will profit from a study of the methods used by osteopathic physicians and athletic trainers.

CONCLUSION

Successful management of the crisis of excruciating pain begins with a physician who is able to be calm, compassionate and alert in the presence of an agitated patient and distraught bystanders. Each physician must learn to control himself by practice and self-discipline. No one has described this goal better than Sir William Osler (1905):[17]

I…have urged you to educate your nerve centres so that not the slightest dilator or contractor influence shall pass to the vessels of your face under any professional trial.

…an inscrutable face may prove a fortune. In a true and perfect form, imperturbability is indissolubly associated with wide experience and an intimate knowledge of the varied aspects of disease.

From its very nature this precious quality is liable to be misinterpreted, and the general accusation of hardness, so often brought against the profession, has here its foundation. Now a certain measure of insensibility is not only an advantage, but a positive necessity in the exercise of a calm judgment, and in carrying out delicate operations. Keen sensibility is doubtless a virtue of high order, when it does not interfere with steadiness of hand or coolness of nerve; but for the practitioner in his working-day world, a callousness which thinks only of the good to be effected, and goes ahead regardless of smaller considerations, is the preferable quality.

Cultivate, then, gentlemen, such a judicious measure of obtuseness as will enable you to meet the exigencies of practice with firmness and courage, without, at the same time, hardening "the human heart by which we live."

References

1. Bate, W. J.: John Keats. Cambridge, Harvard University Press, 1963.
2. Battista, A. F.: Subarachnoid cold saline wash for pain relief. Arch. Surg., *103*:672–675, 1971.
3. Cailliet, R.: Neck and Arm Pain. Philadelphia, F. A. Davis Co., 1964.
4. Cassinari, V., and Pagni, C. A.: Central Pain; A Neurosurgical Survey. Cambridge, Harvard University Press, 1969.
5. Dimond, E. G.: Acupuncture anesthesia. Western medicine and Chinese traditional medicine. J.A.M.A., *218*:1558–1563, 1971.
6. Finneson, B. E.: Diagnosis and Management of Pain Syndromes, 2nd Ed. Philadelphia, W. B. Saunders Co., 1969.
7. Hale, M. S.: A Practical Approach to Arm Pain. Springfield, Ill., Charles C Thomas, 1971.
8. Hannington-Kiff, J. G.: Treatment of intractable pain by bupivacaine nerve-block. Lancet, *1*:1392–1394, 1971.
9. Hardy, J. D., Wolff, H. G., and Goodell, H.: Pain Sensations and Reactions. Baltimore, Williams and Wilkins Co., 1952.
10. Hardy, J. D., and Stolwijk, J. A. J.: Tissue temperature and thermal pain. In Reuck, A. V. S., and Knight, J. (eds.): Ciba Foundation Symposium: Touch, Heat and Pain. Boston, Little, Brown and Co., 1966.
11. Keele, C. A., and Armstrong, D.: Substances Producing Pain and Itch. London, Edward Arnold Ltd., 1964.
12. Lea, H. C.: Materials Toward a History of Witchcraft. Howland, A. C. (ed.), 3 Vol. New York, Thomas Yoseloff, 1957.
13. Leriche, R.: The Surgery of Pain. [Trans. by Archibald Young] Baltimore, Williams and Wilkins Co., 1939.
14. Lim, R. K. S.: A revised concept of the mechanism of analgesia and pain. In Knighton, R. S., and Dumke, P. R. (eds.): Pain. Boston, Little, Brown and Co., 1966.
15. Mennell, J. M.: Foot Pain. Boston, Little, Brown and Co., 1969.
16. Morton, L. T.: Garrison and Morton's Medical Bibliography. London, British Book Centre, 1970.
17. Osler, W.: *Aequanimitas,* with other addresses to medical students, nurses and practitioners of medicine. Philadelphia, P. Blakiston's Son and Co., 1905.
18. Summers, M.: The History of Witchcraft and Demonology. New York, University Books, Inc., 1956.
19. Tarsey, J. M.: Pain Syndromes and Their Treatment with Special Reference to Shoulder-Arm Pain. Springfield, Ill., Charles C Thomas, 1953.
20. White, J. C., and Sweet, W. H.: Pain: Its Mechanisms and Neurosurgical Control. Springfield, Ill., Charles C Thomas, 1955.
21. White, J. C., and Sweet, W. H.: Pain and the Neurosurgeon: A Forty-Year Experience. Springfield, Ill., Charles C Thomas, 1969.

28

Outpatient Surgery in Developing Countries

By ROBERT R. LARSEN, M.D.

INTRODUCTION

Half of the world's population live in developing countries. Most of these people are hungry, undernourished and have little access to even basic medical care. The United States has one doctor for every 750 people, whereas India has only one doctor for every 5000 people and northern Nigeria has only one doctor for every 140,000 people. Complicating this picture, developing countries are burdened with high unemployment rates, high birth rates, low per capita income, a large rural population, and little foreign exchange for importing medical supplies and equipment. Although this picture is rapidly changing, doctors from medically advanced countries will be needed for several generations to share their skills. Gradually medical organizations in well-doctored, medically advanced countries are realizing their responsibility to the other half of the world.

Traditionally the experience of serving overseas in a developing country was limited to only a few career medical missionaries, but today there are increasing numbers of opportunities for short periods of overseas service. Besides the various Christian mission societies, agencies such as the American Peace Corps, A.I.D., Ford Foundation, HOPE Foundation, and the British Ministry of Overseas Development are seeking doctors for varying periods of medical service. Many group medical practices allow their members regular periods of sabbatical leave for such service. At the same time military programs place more and more physicians in developing countries at some time during their tenure of military practice.

In most developing countries, top medical administrative positions are filled by national doctors, and the role of the foreign practitioner is usually that of teacher, organizer, supervisor and consultant in the local medical institution. The foreign physician is seldom the administrative authority in the hospital, and he must be prepared to work under the national administrator. It is essential that the foreign physician be aware of this changing role before he arrives at his destination for practice. The physician should also be prepared to adapt his methods of medical care to provide the best care for the largest number of persons with the least expenditure of resources. This can be the most difficult task for a physician from a medically advanced country. But to simply export foreign ideas and approaches to medical care to the culture of a developing nation is not satisfactory. I strongly recommend that any physician who is to practice medicine in a developing country should first read the book *Medical Care in Developing Countries,* edited by Maurice King and published by the Oxford University Press.[15]

ANESTHESIA

In developing countries there are two factors which restrict anesthesia: the lack of trained personnel and the limited availability of equipment and materials. In most hospitals anesthesia is the responsibility of the operating surgeon. The surgeon must, therefore, promptly become familiar with the use and limitations of a few simple, safe, inexpensive agents and techniques. A book such as *Regional Block* by D. C. Moore[18] will be of more value than an expensive gas anesthesia machine.

For setting fractures or for procedures of less than half an hour on the extremities, intravenous local anesthesia (the Bier block) is safe and simple. This procedure and several other commonly used regional blocks are adequately described in Chapter 2. Because the Bier block with intravenous local anesthesia utilizes a blood pressure cuff tourniquet, this technique should not be used in areas of the world where sickle cell disease is prevalent (see following discussion).

Regional block is ideal for outpatient operative procedures, but unfortunately few American-trained surgeons have sufficient experience with the technique to obtain good results. Familiarity with axillary, digital, pudendal, pericervical, ulnar, radial, median and sciatic nerve blocks is extremely valuable (see Chapter 2). Don't expect success right away, but persist in your efforts to master one technique for each block. Use 0.05 per cent solutions for infiltration of peripheral nerve blocks so that larger volumes will be possible without the risk of reactions. It is seldom necessary to use solutions with epinephrine, and the complications produced by improper use of epinephrine are serious. It is advisable to keep anesthetic solutions containing epinephrine well apart from the usual anesthetic solutions.

Systemic toxic reactions to anesthetic solutions must be treated immediately and properly to avoid death. If the reaction appears to be an allergic response manifested by angioneurotic edema, asthma or other histamine-type symptoms, give 50 mg of diphenhydramine (Benedryl) intravenously (IV) and 0.3 cc of epinephrine 1:1000 intramuscularly (IM). If, however, an anaphylactic allergic reaction or a reaction from high blood levels of the agent occur, much more aggressive therapy is indicated.

1. Maintain ventilation by giving oxygen through an endotracheal tube
2. Start an IV
3. Maintain the blood pressure with IV vasopressors
4. Monitor the cardiac action by ECG
5. Stop convulsions with frequent 50 mg doses of thiopental in or with 40 mg of succinyl choline, and assist ventilation.

Single dose spinal (subarachnoid) anesthesia is suitable for outpatient use under some circumstances. It is convenient for hernia repairs, lower extremity operations, and perianal or genital procedures. These procedures are seldom considered outpatient procedures in the United States, but are commonly done as outpatient procedures in countries with limited inpatient beds, so the technique will be reviewed here:

1. Start an IV.
2. Have the assistant hold the patient on his side with his knees drawn up to his face, or sitting upright with the back arched towards the anesthetist and the head held down on the assistant's chest.
3. Aseptically prepare the skin of the entire back with an iodine solution.
4. Locate the L3–L4 interspace just cephalad to an imaginary line connecting the two iliac crests.
5. Make a wheal in the skin overlying the interspace and infiltrate the underlying interspinous ligament with 1 per cent procaine solution.
6. A 24 or 25 gauge spinal needle is then inserted through the interspace into the subarachnoid space by aiming at the umbilicus. It will pass through the interspinous liga-

ment and ligamentum flavum with moderate resistance, then less resistance will be felt when it reaches the epidural space, and finally the "pop" will be felt as it pierces the dura.

7. At this point the stylet is withdrawn and the needle checked for spinal fluid return, with frequent rotations of the needle. If fluid does not return, slowly advance the needle another 5 mm and check again.

8. A syringe containing 0.2 cc epinephrine 1:1000 solution, plus 1.0 cc (10 mg) of tetracaine (Pontocaine), plus 1.2 cc of 10 per cent dextrose solution is attached to the spinal needle. Spinal fluid is aspirated until the syringe contains a total of 3.0 cc, and then slowly injected over a period of three minutes. Before removing the needle a small amount of spinal fluid is again aspirated and reinjected, to be sure the anesthetic solution was injected in the subarachnoid space.

9. The patient is put in the supine position with the head and shoulders on a pillow, adjusting the table to achieve the proper level of anesthesia. (The anesthetic solution is hyperbaric, and will therefore flow downhill.) *Do not* put the patient in Trendelenburg position.

10. Every 30 seconds for 15 minutes monitor the patient's blood pressure, and test the level of anesthesia with a pin prick. After 15 minutes the solution is "fixed."

11. Once the level is fixed a nurse can safely be trusted to monitor the patient's vital signs and responses every 15 minutes during the operative procedure.

The spinal anesthetic agents which are least expensive and most readily available are tetracaine and procaine. 100 mg of procaine crystals dissolved in 2.0 cc of distilled water or normal saline produce a hyperbaric solution with a shorter du-

ration of anesthesia. When using prepared solutions be sure to check whether they are hyperbaric or hypobaric before starting the procedure. Hypotensive complications are more common with the longer-acting agents and in patients with a low circulating blood volume, because of the vasodilatory effect of this form of anesthesia. This hypotension will nearly always respond rapidly to methedrine, neosynephrine or other mild vasopressors.

General anesthetics have very limited usefulness in outpatient surgery, but a few words of advice are in order. In developing countries personnel are rarely available who are capable of handling general anesthetic agents and equipment. It is therefore essential that very simple techniques be used, and that the operating surgeon constantly be aware of the patient's level of anesthesia. He must observe respiratory motions, and frequently ask the nurse anesthetist about the patient's status. The narrow margin of safety of the intravenous barbiturates limits their use as a sole agent to those who are very experienced with this technique. In many countries chloroform is still used, but again, its margin of safety is much less than that of ether. Chloroform provides more rapid induction and avoids the hyperexcitability of ether during induction, but it should be used with extreme caution and replaced by ether after induction. Ether evaporates readily in the tropics. Its use can quickly be taught to a nurse anesthetist, but the surgeon must still be constantly aware of the patient's level of anesthesia. The open drop technique seems somewhat crude to the refined surgeon and is difficult to use for induction, but it is safe in inexperienced hands with a little guidance.

Many hospitals in developing countries use the EMO (Epstein, Macintosh, Oxford) inhaler with the Oxford inflating bellows (Fig. 28–1). This machine is very simple, quite safe and has the convenience of use with either a mask or endotracheal tube (Fig. 28–2). The volume of ether vapor is controllable, and of a

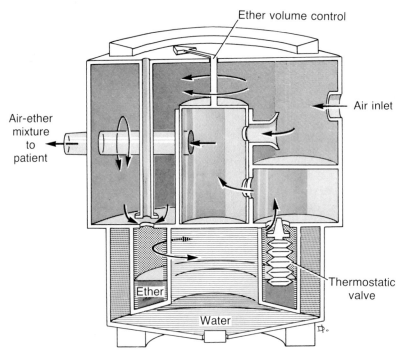

Figure 28–1　Cutaway view of the EMO anesthesia machine.

concentration independent of the air temperature. The surgeon must be thoroughly familiar with the machine, for death can occur with its use in endotracheal anesthesia by not allowing for blow-off of CO_2 during expiration. The Oxford inflating bellows are particularly useful, for they afford the surgeon a constant visual indicator of the patient's respiratory volumes.

Before leaving the subject of anesthesia a few comments concerning sickle cell disease are in order. Although this is primarily a disease of patients of African descent, it is wise for the surgeon to keep it constantly in his mind. Hemoglobin S is an inherited defect in the globin portion of the hemoglobin molecule where one glutamic acid group is replaced by a valine group. In the heterozygous patient with sickle cell trait, up to 40 per cent of the hemoglobin will be hemoglobin S, but this is insufficient to produce clinical symptoms. Whenever the capillary pO_2

of the patient with sickle cell disease falls below 45, the erythrocytes become distorted to the sickle shape. These cells then tend to tangle and clump, and along with fibrin formation, block the capillaries, resulting in tissue infarction. The following anesthetic conditions may lead to a local or general fall in tissue pO_2, and are therefore potentially lethal to the patient with sickle cell disease or trait: (1) hypoxia, (2) acidosis, (3) hypothermia, (4) hypotension, (5) use of tourniquets. Even minor surgery should not be done on a patient of African descent until the hematocrit has been checked. If the hematocrit is less than 30 per cent, sickle cell disease must be ruled out prior to surgery. To prepare for emergency surgery in patients with sickle cell disease, exchange about 70 per cent of the patient's blood with nonsickling blood; in addition, use sodium bicarbonate to prevent acidosis and avoid the conditions listed above during the procedure.

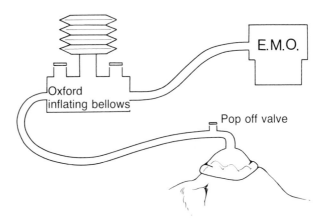

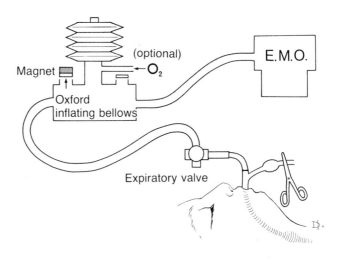

Figure 28–2 The EMO machine with the Oxford inflating bellows. *A*, with expiratory valve and mask; *B*, with an endotracheal tube.

KELOIDS, SCARS AND SKIN GRAFTING

When working with dark-skinned patients, the surgeon must constantly keep in mind the principles of wound healing and scar formation. Unsightly hypertrophic scars and keloids can develop even after minor procedures. To prevent troublesome keloids, a few basic facts must be remembered.

1. The presternal and upper back skin is particularly susceptible to keloid formation.
2. The incision must extend to the fatty subcutaneous layer for a keloid to form. Keloids do not form in the scrotum or penis where the skin contains no fat.
3. Always make the skin incision parallel to the lines of skin tension. To demonstrate these lines, pinch the skin in two perpendicular directions and observe the natural crease.
4. The wound must be absolutely free of tension when closed. *Use subcutaneous sutures.*
5. Avoid "cross hatching" marker scratches, and when possible avoid skin sutures by careful closure of the subcutaneous layer. When possible use tapes for sutureless skin closures.
6. Trauma to the skin edges, wound

hematoma and infection must be avoided.

For cosmetic removal of a keloid, extra care is necessary or the patient will develop an even larger keloid. First be certain you are dealing with a keloid and not a hypertrophic scar. In time (up to three years) a hypertrophic scar will gradually shrink to a normal-appearing scar. Histologically keloids and hypertrophic scars are indistinguishable but there are a few clinical features to help in the differential diagnosis. The hypertrophic scar:

1. Is confined to the area of the original scar.
2. Appears earlier (within weeks of the injury).
3. Is frequently associated with burn scars.
4. Is the more common type.
5. Usually has associated signs and symptoms of irritation.

Radiotherapy or local injection of hydrocortisone will suppress hypertrophic scars and may help prevent recurrence following surgical excision of a keloid. Neither radiation nor hydrocortisone is adequate treatment for a mature keloid. Complete surgical excision is possible, but the recurrence rate is high since the new wound must be larger than the initial wound. Total excision requires undermining the skin edges to relieve all tension on the new wound, but trauma to skin edges must be kept to a very minimum. Better results are reported by partial excision and grafting. With this technique, most of the keloid is excised but the subcutaneous fatty layer is not entered. The defect in the dermis is closed with a split thickness skin graft from the keloid itself or from the anterior thigh. No sutures are used to hold this graft in place. Do not be trapped into treating presternal keloids, for in this location all forms of treatment result in a larger keloid than before.

Although skin grafting is usually an inpatient operative procedure, small defects can be grafted in the outpatient operating room. These can be taken free hand by the skilled surgeon, but a useful tool is the safety razor dermatome (Fig. 28–3). The central strut supporting the skin guard must be filed off on one side of an ordinary household safety razor. Shims are made from old blades, by placing the blade in a vise with only the beveled cutting edge exposed, and then tapping off this edge with a screwdriver and hammer. The thickness of the graft to be taken can be varied by adding shims below the cutting blade. One shim under the blade will cut the skin 0.010 inch thick and each additional shim will increase the thickness by 0.004 inch. The split thickness skin is removed by keeping the donor site under tension and holding the razor dermatome at a 60° angle to the skin. Then pressing gently, rapid side-to-side oscillations of about one-half inch are made. The whole process can be made even easier by utilizing the vibrating safety razor, but this is a much more expensive tool.

ABSCESSES AND INFECTIONS

In tropical countries the maxim of early incision and drainage (I and D) of subcutaneous abscesses does not always apply. For example, I and D is not the treatment of choice in parasitic abscesses caused by Onchocerca, Dracunculus, or *Diphyllobothrium latum*. These infections not only are confused with bacterial abscesses, but are often mistaken for inguinal or femoral hernias.

Onchocerca larvae migrate from the site of the host black fly bite to bony prominences around the iliac spines, greater trochanter or the sacrococcygeal area. Here the adults and their microfilaria soon produce a 2–3 cm irregular nodule or adenolymphocele. Needle aspiration and smear will reveal the microfilaria. These nodules are best treated by excision, not incision. Surgical treatment should be combined with the administration of diethylcarbamazine (Hetrazan).

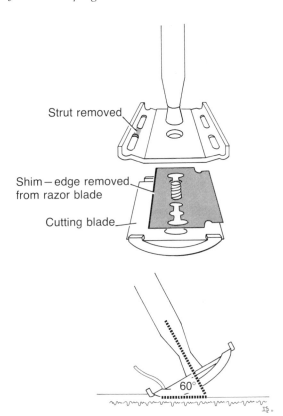

Figure 28–3 The safety razor dermatome.

Guinea worms (Dracunculus) gain entrance to the systemic circulation following ingestion, and then spend the next few months burrowing subcutaneously. Some adult worms eventually die and disintegrate, but most come to the skin surface. Here they produce local cellulitis and emerge, or form a 2–10 cm cyst or abscess. The emerging worm should be "helped out" by winding on a matchstick after killing it with large doses of diethylcarbamazine. Persistent cysts or abscesses should be excised.

Similar to the Guinea worm in the tropics is the abscess of *D. latum* (sparginosis) seen in East Asia. The ingested larvae invade the subcutaneous tissue, where they form localized abscesses or nodular pustules. While incising one of these abscesses the operator may be greeted by the moving tapeworm, and frequently the patient describes the feeling of something moving in the lump. Incision and removal of the worm or excision of the nodule is the preferred treatment.

Tuberculous cervical lymphadenitis (Fig. 28–4) is still commonly seen in developing countries, especially in children. Tuberculosis must be kept in mind whenever the surgeon is about to incise and drain a fluctuant neck mass. Since it is common to find associated tuberculous lesions elsewhere in the body, antibiotics are the treatment of choice. In some cases radical excision of involved lymph nodes may shorten the length of treatment. Always do an acid-fast stain of any cervical ulcer or draining sinus before planning surgical treatment.

A tropical condition of the head and neck which simulates abscess is Burkitt's lymphoma. Burkitt's lymphoma is the most common cause of tumor in the jaws of children in tropical Africa. The maxilla is more often involved than the mandible, and the child frequently presents with the complaint of loose

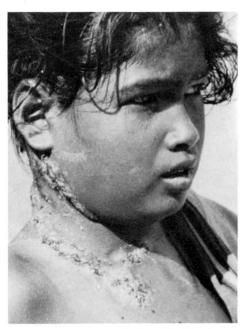

Figure 28–4 A young Indian girl with tuberculous cervical lymphadenitis.

molars or premolars. The orbit is involved early in the course of the disease, making Burkitt's lymphoma also the commonest cause of exophthalmos in African children. The tumors are often bilateral and usually multiple. Peripheral lymph node involvement is rare. Associated features may be abdominal tumors and paraplegia. As with any lymphoma of the head and neck, it is important to distinguish these tumors from osteomyelitis, Ewing's tumor, or other primarily surgical conditions. The primary treatment for Burkitt's lymphoma is chemotherapy, the present drugs of choice being methotrexate and cyclophosphamide (Cytoxan).

Ulceration of the skin and soft tissues in the region of the ankle and calf are so common in the tropics that this condition is often considered a separate disease entity, "tropical ulcer." Factors contributing to these ulcers are malnutrition and vitamin deficiency, lack of shoes or protective clothing, lack of pure water for cleansing minor wounds, and contamination of wounds with fusiform bacilli. Other causes of ulceration and infection of the skin and soft tissues in the lower extremity include foreign bodies, leprosy, guinea worm, *Schistosoma hematobium,* rhinoscleroma, tuberculosis, ameba, syphilis and other treponemes, leishmania, spider bites, other insect bites and carcinoma. One very common type of ulceration seen on the ankles and feet contains mixed fusiform bacilli and Vincent's spirochetes. It may be either acute or chronic, and not uncommonly proceeds to involve bone as well as soft tissue. The early lesions will respond dramatically to penicillin. Large or chronic ulcers require thorough excision followed by split thickness or rotational flap graft.

Abscesses in large muscle masses are so common they have earned the label "tropical pyomyositis." These abscesses are most common in the muscles of the posterior or lateral abdomen, and muscles of the thigh. They may be confused with abscesses of perforated appendicitis or diverticulitis, but lack the signs and symptoms of peritonitis. Localized psoas spasm and tenderness are helpful signs. Frequently they contain large volumes of pus (up to several liters) which will culture coagulase positive *Staphylococcus aureus.*

A mixed bacterial infection frequently occurs in the mouth, from a combination of malnutrition, anemia, vitamin deficiency and debilitating general illness. In this condition, invasive fusiform bacilli, spirochetes and secondary bacteria produce necrosis in periodontal tissues. *Cancrum oris* is the extension of this acute ulcerative gingivitis to surrounding tissues. Soon varying amounts of lips, cheek and nose tissue slough away and are gradually replaced by disfiguring scar. Trismus is a common late complication of the scar formation. In the early acute phase, medical treatment will usually control the infection. Therapy should include antibiotics and treatment of the associated debilitating disease, as well as supplemental iron, protein and vitamins. Unfortunately, the patient seldom consults a physician in the early phase. Surgery is usually reserved for the reconstructive phase, which presents challenging problems. The aims of this reconstructive surgery are to release the trismus and replace both the lost mucosal and skin tissue. The magnitude of the problem of reconstructing the face with flaps and pedicle grafts usually dictates inpatient management.

Since footwear is seldom used in developing countries, a high incidence of foot infections is not surprising. Mycetoma pedis (Madura foot) is the result of inoculation with either the fungus *Maduromycetes* or the related bacteria *Actinomycetes* when the patient, usually a male, steps on either a piece of thorn bamboo or acacia shrub. Slowly there develops swelling of the foot, multiple draining sinuses and a discharge containing black, yellow or red granules (Fig. 28–5). The process may extend over a period of several years. Gradually it progresses to involve bones and joints. Pain is seldom a prominent feature.

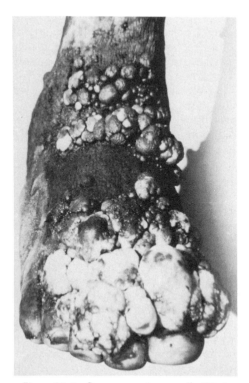

Figure 28–5 Severe mycetoma pedis (Madura foot).

Roentgenograms show cystic cavitation, osteoporosis and bone erosion. Any new bone formation is totally disorganized, usually at right angles to the cortex. Medical treatment is generally discouraging. *Nocardia brasiliensis,* one of the yellow granule producers, is susceptible to prolonged streptomycin or sulfone treatment. Other organisms have shown no consistent *in vivo* susceptibility to agents presently available. Prior to amputation, a course with one of the systemic antifungals such as amphotericin B is advisable. Surgical excision is satisfactory for the early lesion confined to soft tissues, but the lesion is seldom seen early. The newcomer may confuse the early stages of mycetoma with the superficial fungus and bacterial infections of the skin so commonly seen during the monsoon season (Fig. 28–6). This more superficial infection will respond to systemic and local treatment with combined antibacterials and antifungals.

Ainhum is another foot problem seen throughout both Africa and Asia. Although fungus infection is often blamed for this disease, there is no good evidence to support this theory. All cases which I have seen occurred in barefoot patients and many of them remembered relatives who had experienced the same disease. Just distal to the plantar digital fold, a groove forms and spreads towards the dorsum of the toe (Fig. 28–7). Slowly the groove widens and deepens, and it may later ulcerate. By this time it has the appearance of an encircling constriction of the soft tissue around the toe. Most commonly the fourth or fifth toe is involved, but it has been reported on the fingers as well. Eventually bone becomes involved in the groove, resulting in slow autoamputation. In the late stages, pain may be a prominent feature, and often the patients come at this stage requesting the surgeon to complete the amputation for pain relief. It is possible simply to complete the amputation at the level of the groove, but the preferred treatment is amputation at the metatarsal-phalangeal joint under local anesthesia. In addition

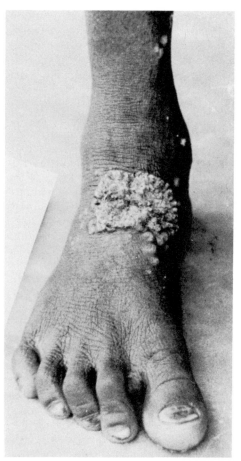

Figure 28–6   Chronic combined fungal and bacterial infection of the foot. This type of infection is commonly seen during the monsoon season, and is not to be confused with early mycetoma.

to attention to aseptic technique, a course of tetanus toxoid before surgery is advisable. If the disease is seen before ulceration or bone involvement has occurred, the toe can be saved by performing two or three Z-plasties on the constricting groove.

It is customary in most tropical countries for people to create various holes, scars or wounds for cosmetic or therapeutic purposes. Ear piercing is universal, and the jewelry may consist of large pieces of bamboo or ivory, which necessitate very large holes. Tattoos are often used for permanent cosmetics. Incisions made in intricate designs on the face or abdomen are used for tribal markings in

Africa. Indian women often perforate the nasal alae for jewelry. Lip perforations for insertion of ivory pegs are seen in both Africa and Asia. Constricting bands are applied as bracelets or necklaces in Indochina. In most developing countries the most common method of treatment for pain used by the local medicine men is burn escharification. It is frequently possible to make a diagnosis by simply observing the locations of these scars. It is amazing how rarely these various wounds become infected, in spite of the septic conditions under which most of them are produced. Tetanus, however, can be a complication of these wounds and they should not be considered totally harmless. Occasionally with educational achievement people find these tribal marks or facial cosmetics distasteful and come requesting their removal.

LEPROSY

Leprosy is not limited to developing countries, but does have a high incidence in Africa and Asia. The clinical picture of infection with *Mycobacterium leprae* is usually divided into two patterns, but most cases are a mixture of the two with one form predominating. The tuberculoid form is characterized by a vigorous defense reaction against the bacilli, manifested by a tuberculoid follicle consisting of giant cells surrounded by epithelioid cells. This reaction affects skin appendages and melanocytes, resulting in patches of skin devoid of hair, sweat and pigment. The lepromatous type has minimal host reaction and is characterized by nodules of granulation tissue and bacilli located in the peripheral nerves.

The diagnosis is usually made by the clinical picture, but to confirm this suspicion and to follow the response to therapy the laboratory is essential. Smears of the serum from the papillary dermis bordering an active lesion, or from the mucosa of the nasal septum are used for this test. A positive test may be difficult to

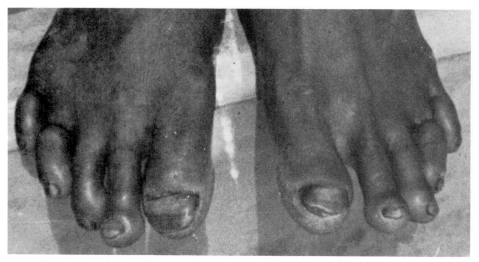

Figure 28–7 Ainhum. The constricting bands of ainhum on the fourth and fifth digits.

obtain in the tuberculoid form. In those cases the lepromin test or surgical biopsy of a lesion may be helpful for diagnosis. To make a smear, prepare the skin with alcohol and then squeeze a skin fold between the left thumb and index finger. Then make a 5 mm incision into, but not through, the papillary dermis. Scrape the sides of the incision with the blade for the clear juice and pulp and smear this onto a glass slide and stain with Ziehl-Neelsen* stain. Since the nasal mucosa is the last area to become negative on therapy, a smear from this area is best for following the response to therapy. After removing any nasal mucus, scrape the hyperemic mucosa or a nodule with a blunt scraper. (A portion of a bicycle spoke hammered to a fusiform flat end

makes a good nasal scraper.) Then smear it on the slide and stain as above. If blood is obtained, repeat the procedure, for this will make it difficult to interpret the smear.

Although the primary treatment of leprosy is medical (diaminodiphenyl sulphone [DDS]) the surgeon should be thoroughly familiar with the disease and its management in order to avoid the mistakes commonly made when a physician is asked to enter into the patient's management. Many talented young surgeons have seen their technically beautiful surgical procedures totally wasted because the extremity was treated instead of the patient. Before the surgeon operates, he must consider certain principles:

---

*Technique of the Ziehl-Neelsen stain:

1. Fix the film on the glass slide by passing it once or twice through a flame.

2. Cover the slide with strong carbol fuchsin and heat gently for 5 minutes (letting the stain steam but not boil).

3. Wash in running water and drain.

4. Cover slide with 0.5 per cent acid alcohol for three to five minutes (use 3 per cent acid alcohol for TB preparations).

5. Wash rapidly and drain.

6. Counterstain momentarily with malachite green or 2 per cent picric acid.

7. Wash and rapidly dry.

1. Be sure everything possible to prevent deformity is being done. Time spent in prevention of deformity will reap more fruit than time spent in correction of deformity.

2. Freedom from ulceration is more important to a patient than fine dexterity.

3. Physical and occupational therapy programs must be planned and started long before and continued long after any surgical procedures are performed.

4. In many cultures the stigmata of leprosy prevent a patient from returning to his village even after arrest of the disease. Amputation of a deformed foot may therefore do more for a patient than an intricate tendon transfer.
5. Lost sensation is never restored by surgery.
6. The patient's motivation is more important than the surgeon's motivation.

When there is definite indication for surgical intervention in leprosy, many of the procedures can be done in the outpatient operating room with little or no anesthesia. The complications of leprosy most frequently requiring surgical treatment are ulcers, cosmetic repair of deformities, acute neuritis, acute reaction in the eye or hand, and paralytic conditions of the hand or foot.

The primary treatment of ulcers is prevention. Constant education will make the patient aware of the three principles of preventing ulcers:

1. Care to avoid trauma.
2. Inspection of hands and feet daily.
3. Protective footwear.

Chronic ulcers are best treated conservatively with frequent cleansing, dressings and antibiotics. As a last resort, conservative amputation may be necessary for severe multiple nonhealing ulcers.

Cosmetic repair need not be elaborate, but is based upon correcting those factors considered as stigmata of the disease by the community. Simple procedures such as full thickness graft of hair-bearing skin to replace lost eyebrows, or correction of gynecomastia may be all that is needed.

Pain is the primary reason for treating acute neuritis. Conservative measures include plaster casts to put the extremity at rest, systemic steroids, and injection of the involved nerve with anesthetic agents and hydrocortisone. When paralysis is complete and severe pain persists, the nerve sheath may be incised along the entire length of the enlarged nerve. While doing this, abscesslike cavities may be noted and should be evaluated. But do not confuse these with bacterial abscesses, for they are sterile. The wound should be closed primarily without drainage.

Acute iridocyclitis should be recognized and treated early to prevent blindness. Treatment consists of bed rest, eye patches, twice daily instillation of atropine, systemic steroids, and daily injection of 0.1 or 0.2 mg of cortisone subconjunctivally. Acute reactions in the hands are treated by plaster splints and systemic steroids.

Most paretic and paralytic conditions will respond to conservative nonoperative care, including splints, massage, wax baths and Faradic stimulation of weak muscles. Interphalangeal arthrodesis can be done with a very small incision and no anesthesia, holding the bone surfaces together by means of Kirschner wires. This will not only remove some of the dreaded stigmata, but will provide useful grasp and pinch. Tendon transfers, such as the sublimis tendon transfer to provide opponens-abductor action of the thumb, are reserved for highly motivated patients, or those with skilled jobs requiring these functions.

BITES AND STINGS

Snakebite is a common problem wherever people walk barefoot, spend most of their time in the fields, and where the climate is warm and moist. There are at least 300,000 bites by poisonous snakes in the world each year. Estimated annual deaths from snakebite are 25,000 for Southeast Asia and 1000 for Africa. During childhood, most local residents learn to differentiate poisonous from harmless snakes, so that the history of a bite by a poisonous snake should be considered reliable. Unfortunately many victims are very young children or patients bitten while walking at night without a lantern or torch. The physician must then make a guess as to the nature of the biting animal.

Description and Classification of Snakes

Of the 3500 species of snakes in the world, about 200 are poisonous. These are generally classified by physical characteristics (Table 28–1). Subclassification by type of venom action is difficult, for no venom has a single mode of action. It is nevertheless possible to classify venoms by their primary mode of action. Most local residents classify snakes as either "highly toxic" or "not so toxic," and this may actually be the best classification.

Cobra venom is responsible for more deaths than any other venom. It is reported to be 10,000 times more toxic than botulinum toxin A. The primary action of the cobra, krait and mamba venom is neurotoxic. Russell's viper, phoorsa and adder venom is cytotoxic or hematoxic. Pit viper venom may be neurotoxic or cytotoxic, or mixed, in which case no action may be called primary. All poisonous snakes have proteolytic toxins which produce local destruction and swelling of tissues, but the viperine group produce the most intense local reactions. The wise physician will early acquaint himself with appearance and venom of the poisonous snakes in his area.

Not all bites from poisonous species of snakes are dangerous. Generally bites in children are more dangerous than in adults, because of the greater relative concentration of toxin. A snake which bites after a recent kill may have little or no stored venom. Other factors which determine the toxic effect include depth of the bite, weather conditions, site of the bite, and even the mood of the snake. As with rabies, head and trunk bites are more serious.

Treatment

Because of rapid-acting toxins, the treatment of cobra, krait, Russell's viper and mamba bites must be prompt and vigorous. Immediate application of a tourniquet above the bite is helpful, with suction applied to remove as much of the uncirculated venom as possible. With these species, death may come in minutes to hours, with an average of eight hours from bite to death. Polyvalent antivenom vaccine is always indicated, but does not insure saving the patient's life. Large doses (30 to 200 ml) should be given intravenously or intra-arterially as soon as possible in either adults or children. Anaphylactic reactions to horse serum are a danger, but can usually be controlled with epinephrine and hydrocortisone. Unfortunately, the conventional preparations of antivenom have a short half-life of potency, and must be discarded about six months after preparation. Many countries now have

TABLE 28–1   A Simple Classification of Common Poisonous Snakes

Group Name	Identification	Primary Toxic Effect	Common Examples		
			Asia	Africa	Americas
Colubrine	Back fang	Hematoxic		Boomslang	
Elapine	Fixed front fang	Neurotoxic	Cobra Krait	Mamba Cobra	Coral snake
Viperine	Hinged front fang	Hematoxic Marked local reaction	Russell's viper Phoorsa	Puff adder	
Crotaline (pit viper)	A pit between the eye and nostril	Mixed hematoxic or neurotoxic	Malay pit viper Habu		Bushmaster Rattlesnake

available a new freeze-dried antivenom, which has a two to three year duration of potency. If respiratory paralysis occurs in spite of these measures, respiratory assist is indicated, for the heart beat will persist long after respiratory arrest has occurred.

Other snake bites have a slower response and a longer time available for therapy. Morbidity or mortality is the result of bleeding, fluid loss from swelling, and necrosis of local tissues. Although hemolysis frequently occurs, hemorrhage is a more common problem. The venom initiates abnormal coagulation which exhausts fibrin and fibrinogen, leading to a bleeding diathesis. Alertness to this problem will prompt early study and correction of the coagulation factors with fresh blood. It appears that heparin or epsilon aminocaproic acid (Amicar) may reverse this coagulopathy. Following viper and adder bites, swelling of an extremity can be considerable. In the early phase, the patient may become oligemic from the loss of serum and blood into the extremity. This must be corrected with intravenous colloid solutions or plasma expanders to prevent shock. At the same time, frequent evaluation of the perfusion of the swollen extremity must be done, and fasciotomy performed whenever there is evidence that the swelling is obstructing arterial flow. Tissue necrosis may be extensive as a direct effect of the venom, but necrosis is not life-endangering unless it leads to sepsis. Tissue slough should be treated like a third degree burn.

Recent work with rattlesnake bites in the United States indicates that one gram of hydrocortisone IV every six hours for 72 hours, combined with immediate fasciotomy from the joint above to the joint below the bite, prevented tissue loss from necrosis and made antivenom unnecessary. This should be kept in mind in handling other pit viper bites.

Scorpion stings are seldom fatal, but are always extremely painful. Management with rest, analgesics and local injection of an anesthetic solution about the area of the bite will control symptoms. Tissue necrosis does not occur. With some rare varieties, systemic symptoms of a neurotoxin may be seen. These include salivation, nausea and vomiting, increased respiratory rate, slow pulse, shock, convulsions, and signs and symptoms of an acute abdomen. Abdominal pain is due to the effect of toxin on the pancreas. Ergotamine and atropine injections should be used to control these systemic symptoms.

The most common toxic response to spider bites is local necrosis surrounding the bite, but hemolytic and neurotoxic effects can occasionally be severe, such as those due to the black widow spider. Corticosteroids and subcutaneous epinephrine will usually prevent collapse. In the United States there is a commercial antivenom available for the black widow spider, but this is not available in developing countries. The usual necrotic ulcer following the brown spider bite is very slow to heal. The period of morbidity can be shortened by thorough débridement as soon as the area of necrosis is demarcated. Usually the subcutaneous tissues and fat are also necrotic, and débridement must include these layers as well as the skin. It may be possible to undermine the edges and pull the defect of a small ulcer together when the base is clean. More often a split thickness skin graft is required. Antibiotic coverage is essential to control the secondary invaders.

Venomous marine life is a problem in all coastal areas of the world, not just in developing or tropical countries. Sea urchins and spiny starfish have brittle spines which will cause severe local pain for up to 48 hours after contact. Local anesthetic injection and removal of any of the visible spines is the only treatment. The toxic effects of jelly fish and the Portuguese man-o-war are more severe and can be fatal. Immediate cramps and muscle spasms may render a swimmer totally helpless. For stings of these anemones, intravenous hydrocortisone and calcium gluconate is the recommended treatment. The venom of the sting ray and scorpion fish is thermolabile, so that the immediate application of hot compresses to the site of the wound, or immersion of the wound into water of 110–115° for 30 minutes will considerably minimize the toxic effects. The venom from the stings of these fish produces unusually severe local pain. Shock secondary to the pain is not uncommon. The local pain can be relieved by local anesthetic infiltration and 30 mg of pentazocaine lactate intravenously. If shock still persists, IV hydrocortisone and vasopressors are indicated.

Wounds produced by wild animals are best treated like open human bites, with special emphasis on prevention of sepsis, especially gas gangrene and other anaerobic infections. Generally speaking, delayed closure of these wounds following extensive débridement is advisable. Crocodiles seize their victims by an extremity and try to pull them into the water. The result is either a stripping injury or avulsive amputation or disarticulation. It is amazing how well most of these injuries heal, but they should be left open. Monkey bites are deep puncture wounds or lacerations. These wounds are always heavily infected and should be debrided thoroughly and left open. Monkey bites may transmit viral encephalomyelitis with symptoms ensuing several days after the bite. Elephants and water buffalo produce crushing and goring wounds. Damage to thoracic or abdominal viscera frequently require exploration. Since hippopotami are herbivorous, delayed primary closure is satisfactory for their enormous bites.

Rabies

Rabies is the dreaded outcome of bites by jackals, monkeys, bats and especially of stray dogs. Unprovoked attack by any of these animals should alert the physician to the possibility of the animal being rabid. Symptoms of rabies infection in an animal include snapping, drooling, vocal cord paralysis, and unusual purposeless movements. Seldom is a biting animal impounded in developing countries, so the physician must make a decision based upon the patient's impressions and descriptions. In most developing countries rabies is endemic, and rabies vaccine is used more liberally than in the United States. Nevertheless, remember that both the sheep brain vaccine and the duck embryo vaccine may produce lethal anaphylactic reactions, and this risk must be weighed before committing the patient to treatment. The management recommended by the World Health Organization for treatment of exposure to rabies is outlined in Table 28–2. Do not overlook the local treatment. Antirabies serum is not available in all countries, but is indicated in cases of severe exposure.

Once symptoms of rabies occur in the patient, supportive measures are indicated, but the mortality rate is essentially 100 per cent. Only one recovery has ever been reported following the onset of symptoms.

UNUSUAL WOUNDS, FOREIGN BODIES, AND TETANUS

The variety of wounds and foreign bodies seen by the surgeon in developing countries is unlimited.

The wounds of bamboo, particularly thorn bamboo, have already been discussed in relation to the feet. Thorn bamboo is commonly used for fencing material, and is therefore a common cause of hand wounds as well. Thorn bamboo wounds are slow to heal and tend to form chronic draining sinuses. Such drainage usually indicates that a piece of the bamboo is still buried and will have to be removed before healing can occur. Frequently these thorns will visualize by radiograph using a soft tissue technique.

Fishhooks imbedded in the finger or foot are a common problem everywhere in the world. The classical method of removal is to rotate the hook, advancing the point until it emerges from the skin,

TABLE 28–2 WHO GUIDE FOR TREATMENT OF EXPOSURE TO RABIES

A. LOCAL TREATMENT OF WOUNDS INVOLVING POSSIBLE EXPOSURE TO RABIES

(1) Recommended in all exposures

(a) *First-aid treatment*

Immediate washing and flushing with soap and water, detergent or water alone (recommended procedure in all bite wounds including those unrelated to possible exposure to rabies).

(b) *Treatment by or under direction of a physician*
   (i) Adequate cleansing of the wound.
   (ii) Thorough treatment with 20% soap solution and/or the application of a quaternary ammonium compound or other substance of proven lethal effect on the rabies virus.[1]
   (iii) Topical application of antirabies or its liquid or powdered globulin preparation (optional).
   (iv) Administration, where indicated, of antitetanus procedures and of antibiotics and drugs to control infections other than rabies.
   (v) Suturing of wound not advised.

(2) Additional local treatment for severe exposures only.
(a) Topical application of antirabies serum or its liquid or powdered globulin preparation.
(b) Infiltration of antirabies serum around the wound.

---

[1] Where soap has been used to clean wounds, all traces of it should be removed before the application of quaternary ammonium compounds because soap neutralizes the activity of such compounds.

B. SPECIFIC SYSTEMIC TREATMENT

| Nature of Exposure | Status of Biting Animal (Irrespective of Whether Vaccinated or Not) | | Recommended Treatment |
	At Time of Exposure	During Observation Period of Ten Days	
I. No lesions; indirect contact	Rabid	—	None
II. Licks: (1) unabraded skin	Rabid	—	None
(2) abraded skin, scratches and un-abraded or abraded mucosa	(a) healthy	Clinical signs of rabies or proven rabid (laboratory)	Start vaccine[1] at first signs of rabies in the biting animal
	(b) signs suggestive of rabies	Healthy	Start vaccine[1] immediately; stop treatment if animal is normal on fifth day after exposure
	(c) rabid, escaped, killed or unknown	—	Start vaccine[1] immediately
III. Bites: (1) mild exposure	(a) healthy	Clinical signs of rabies or proven rabid (laboratory)	Start vaccine[1,2] at first signs of rabies in the biting animal
	(b) signs suggestive of rabies	Healthy	Start vaccine[1] immediately; stop treatment if animal is normal on fifth day after exposure
	(c) rabid, escaped, killed or unknown	—	Start vaccine[1,2] immediately
	(d) wild (wolf, jackal, fox, bat, etc.)	—	Serum[2] immediately, followed by a course of vaccine[1]
(2) severe exposure (multiple, or face, head, finger or neck bites)	(a) healthy	Clinical signs of rabies or proven rabid (laboratory)	Serum[2] immediately; start vaccine[1] at first sign of rabies in the biting animal

TABLE 28–2   WHO Guide for Treatment of Exposure to Rabies (*Continued*)

B. Specific Systemic Treatment

| Nature of Exposure | Status of Biting Animal (Irrespective of Whether Vaccinated or Not) | | Recommended Treatment |
	At Time of Exposure	During Observation Period of Ten Days	
	(b) signs suggestive of rabies	Healthy	Serum[2] immediately, followed by vaccine; vaccine may be stopped if animal is normal on fifth day after exposure
	(c) rabid, escaped, killed or unknown		
	(d) wild (wolf, jackal, pariah dog, fox, bat, etc.)	–	Serum[2] immediately, followed by vaccine[1]

[1] Practice varies concerning the volume of vaccine per dose and the number of doses recommended in a given situation. In general, the equivalent of at least 2 ml of a 5% tissue emulsion should be given subcutaneously daily for 14 consecutive days. Many laboratories use 20 to 30 doses in severe exposures. To ensure the production and maintenance of high levels of serum-neutralizing antibodies, booster doses should be given at 10 days and at 20 or more days following the last daily dose of vaccine in *all* cases. This is especially important if antirabies serum has been used, in order to overcome the interference effect.

[2] In all severe exposures and in all cases of unprovoked wild animal bites, antirabies serum or its globulin fractions together with vaccine should be employed. This is considered by the Committee as the *best* specific treatment available for the post-exposure prophylaxis of rabies in man. Although experience indicates that vaccine alone is sufficient for mild exposures, there is no doubt that here also the combined serum-vaccine treatment will give the best protection. However, both the serum and the vaccine can cause deleterious reactions. Moreover, the combined therapy is more expensive; its use in mild exposures is therefore considered optional. As with vaccine alone, it is important to start combined serum and vaccine treatment as early as possible after exposure, but serum should still be used no matter what the time interval. Serum should be given in a single dose (40 IU per kg of body weight) and the first dose of vaccine inoculated at the same time. Sensitivity to the serum must be determined before its administration.

and then cut the shaft of the hook and pull the hook out by the point. This technique requires local anesthesia (usually digital block) and increases the trauma to the digit. An alternative method first reported by Dr. Theo Cooke is painless and requires no anesthesia, but does require courage to attempt the first time (Fig. 28–8). The technique described by Dr. Cooke is as follows: "The person who is to remove the hook makes a loop of ordinary string and winds the end securely around his right index finger. The loop, about 18 inches long, is slipped over the shank of the hook. The finger (or foot) which the hook has entered is placed on a firm surface with the eye of the hook pointing to the left of the manipulator, who then takes the eye and shank between the thumb and index finger of his left hand. Holding the shank rigidly, he depresses it, painlessly disengaging the barb unless the hook is moved sideways. He slowly straightens the loop of the string horizontally in the plane of the long axis of the shank. This is a test maneuver to make sure the loop will not become tangled on coat buttons, and to bring the center of the loop gently against the curve of the hook. The tip of the operator's left third finger then holds the center of the loop against the finger (or foot) at the point where the hook enters. The operator brings his right hand back to the hook and suddenly jerks it away in the same direction as in the test maneuver, with full follow-through. The hook is spun back out of the finger without enlarging the track or the hole of entry."

In parts of Egypt, Sudan and Nigeria, unusual wounds include ritual circumcision of the female. This disappearing tribal ritual varies from trimming the labia minor and tip of the clitoris to radical procedures which may damage the urethra and include infibulation (attempt to produce vulvar stenosis by encourag-

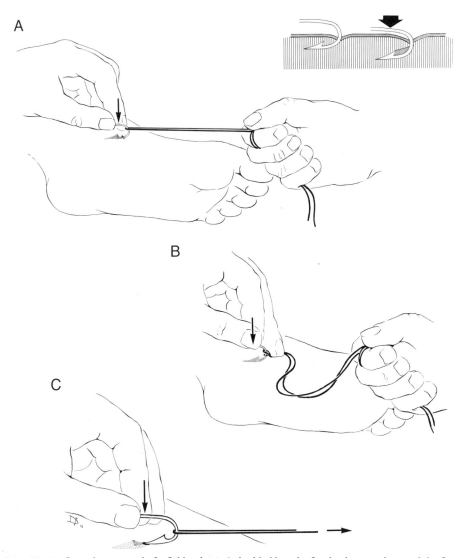

Figure 28–8 Stepwise removal of a fishhook. *A.* A doubled length of string is wound around the finger of the person who is removing the fishhook, and looped over the shank of the hook. *B.* The shank is depressed with the thumb of the left hand, disengaging the hook from the tissues (see inset). The middle finger of the left hand is used to secure the loop of string in the middle of the curve of the hook, at the point of entry into the skin. *C.* After a slow test maneuver to insure that unobstructed motion of the right hand is possible, the hook is removed by a sudden jerk on the string, with a full follow-through of the right hand.

ing raw edges of the labia to adhere across the midline). In many parts of the world, caustics are commonly inserted into the vagina to treat gonnorrhea. The management of most of these wounds is not an outpatient procedure, and must be done meticulously to avoid damage to the urethra.

Tetanus

As long as it is common practice to treat wounds with cow dung, mud or other excrement, tetanus will be a problem. Compounding these habits is the lack of pediatric immunization. The sanitary disposal of human excrement is unusual, so that all soil should be considered contaminated with the *Clostridium tetani* organisms. Puncture wounds into bare feet are a daily occurrence. In fact, the high incidence of tetanus is not surprising; indeed, it is surprising there is not more.

After an average incubation period of six to ten days, the prodromal symptoms begin: stiffness in the jaw, restlessness, yawning and headache. These symptoms last for about 24 hours. If there is no treatment, the neurotoxin causes progressive trismus, tonic contracture of skeletal muscles, abdominal pain, convulsions, and finally death. The exact cause of death is not known, but certainly hypoxia from the sustained convulsions is a major factor.

Seldom do patients come to the hospital with puncture wounds. But there are other wounds with dead or dying tissue and a low local tissue pO_2 which are prone to tetanus. These include burn wounds, gunshot wounds, open fractures, gorings, wounds from arrows or spears, and neglected lacerations. The prophylactic management of these patients is as follows:

1. If the patient has had tetanus immunization in the past six years, give 0.5 cc of tetanus toxoid booster.
2. If the patient was immunized more than six years ago, do the same unless there is an overwhelming possibility that tetanus will develop, in which case also give 250 units of human tetanus immune globulin and penicillin.
3. If the patient has never been immunized and the wound is clean and unlikely to grow tetanus, begin immunization with 0.5 cc of tetanus toxoid.
4. For other wounds in nonimmunized patients, begin immunization with 0.5 cc of tetanus toxoid, and give 250–500 units of human tetanus immune globulin plus penicillin.
5. Human tetanus immune globulin is

unavailable in many countries. The only choice in this situation is horse serum antitoxin.

Test for horse serum sensitivity with 0.1–0.2 ml intradermally and question the patient before giving the therapeutic dose. If there is no sensitivity give at least 3000 units. If there is sensitivity begin immunization with toxoid and give penicillin, but do not give any antitoxin.

Emergency Treatment of Tetanus

The management of the patient with prodromal or active symptoms is not an outpatient procedure, but since the program of treatment is usually started or outlined in the Emergency Room, the measures are included herein:

1. *Maintenance of an adequate airway.* This means early tracheostomy in all except the very mild forms which present with a long incubation period prior to the onset of symptoms.
2. *Wound care.* Through débridement without closure of the primary wound.
3. *Neutralization of the toxin.* If human tetanus immune globulin is available give 1000 to 1500 units in multiple IM injections, particularly in the suspected area of the infection. If this is unavailable, give 50,000 to 100,000 units of equine tetanus antitoxin IV and an additional 50,000 units injected into and around the wound following débridement. Since recent evidence questions the value of this measure, it is not advisable to give any equine antitoxin if the patient is sensitive to horse serum.
4. *Control tetanospasms.* Paraldehyde up to 12 cc IM every four hours or diazepam (Valium) 5–20 mg and chlorpromazine 25–50 mg IM every four hours combined with meperidine (Demerol) and barbiturates as necessary.
5. *Antibiotics.* These have no effect on the neurotoxin producing the symptoms, but it is advisable to give penicillin prophylactically, 10 million units per day IV, and kanamycin 0.5 mg IM every eight hours.
6. *Maintenance of respiration.* In the

severe fulminating form with a two to four day incubation period it is usually necessary to perform a tracheostomy. The patient is then curarized and ventilated by means of a respirator. These patients should be monitored by frequent arterial blood gases.

About 10 per cent of the patients with tetanus have a mild form following a long incubation period of 10–14 days. These patients develop rigidity of the face and neck muscles, but have no convulsions. They can be managed adequately with ordinary nursing care and supportive measures as indicated.

Tetanus in Septic Abortion

It has been my experience that tetanus complicating attempted abortion is unusually severe and fulminant, with a high mortality rate. The plentiful culture medium and rich blood supply for rapid transport of the neurotoxin may be responsible for this. One or two hours after administration of the human tetanus immune globulin of the antitoxin, the uterus should be removed, preferably by vaginal hysterectomy. This should be followed by the same measures outlined for severe tetanus.

Tetanus is a reversible disease. The patient will recover with no physiologic or anatomic sequelae if careful attention is paid to the six measures of management outlined above.

Neonatal Tetanus

The same basic principles of treatment apply to neonatal tetanus. This disease usually begins between the fifth and tenth day of life. The mother first notices a poor suck, and within 36 hours the typical spasms are manifest. Again, paraldehyde is an excellent agent for sedation and control of the spasms (0.2 cc/kg every four to six hours IM). Aspiration is more likely to occur in the infant. Since feeding via a nasogastric tube is

unwise, nutrition must be maintained by using 10 per cent dextrose solutions, or preferably with a parenteral hyperalimentation formula. Neither adult nor neonatal tetanus should have a mortality of greater than 40 per cent in any hospital.

MISCELLANEOUS

Family Planning

No concerned surgeon can practice in a developing country without becoming involved in family planning programs. In countries where the literacy rate is low, the birth rate per thousand is two or three times greater than in countries with a high rate of literacy. All progress in developing countries is hindered by a high birth rate and exploding rate of population growth. Rare are the hospitals today that do not have Family Planning Clinics, mobile clinics, or conduct family planning camps. Taking their example from Japan, many countries are liberalizing abortion laws in attempts to lower the birth rates. Vasectomies, D and C's and even tubectomies are being done as outpatient procedures. See Chapters 17 (Gynecology) and 18 (Urology) for procedural techniques.

Postmortem Examinations

In many countries it is impossible to obtain permission for postmortem examination of a body. One solution to this problem is the percutaneous biopsy needle. With a little practice, tumor masses as well as all major organs of the body can be sampled postmortem by a percutaneous needle biopsy. Few hospitals in developing countries stock these needles and they are seldom purchasable. It is therefore advisable to become familiar with a nondisposable variety and take one with you.

SUMMARY

Many procedures considered to be inpatient procedures in medically developed countries will be done as outpatient procedures in developing countries. There are three reasons for this:

Financial—costs must be kept to an absolute minimum.

Patient—many patients will refuse surgery because of their fear of staying in a hospital, while for others it may be a considerable inconvenience.

Beds—Inpatient beds are always in short supply.

Some of the surgical procedures that can be done in the outpatient operating room will include:

vasectomy
tubectomy
D and C
skin grafts
hernia repair
hydrocelectomy
scar revisions
pedicle graft advancement
abscess drainage
breast biopsy
skin or lymph node biopsy

Precautions must be taken, including close follow-up to prevent infections. The advantages to the patient and to the hospital outweigh the risks of complications. These operations are suitable for local or regional anesthesia, and this, too, will reduce the time of postoperative observation.

It has not been the purpose of this chapter to discuss all the potential surgical procedures to be done in the outpatient operating room of a hospital in a developing country. Most of the cases presenting to the surgeon in a developing country involve principles of therapy discussed in other chapters of the text. Instead, this has been an attempt to discuss those conditions peculiar to tropical or developing countries.

References

1. Rob, C.: Clinical Surgery. (Vol. 8, A. K. Basu). Washington, Butterworths, 1965.
2. Bowesman, C.: Surgery and Clinical Pathology in the Tropics. Edinburgh, E and S Livingstone Ltd., 1960.
3. Chatterji, K. K.: Tropical Surgery and Surgical Pathology. London, John Bale, Sons and Danielsson, Ltd., 1927.
4. Christensen, N. A., and Thurber, D. L.: Current treatment of clinical tetanus. Mod. Treat., *5*:729–757, 1968.
5. Christy, N. P.: Poisoning by venomous animals. Amer. J. Med., *42*:107–128, 1967.
6. Cole, L., and Youngman, H.: Treatment of tetanus. Lancet, *1*:1017–1019, 1969.
7. Cooke, T.: How to remove fish-hooks with a bit of string. Med. J. Aust., *1*:815–816, 1961.
8. Davey, W. W.: Companion to Surgery in Africa. Edinburgh, E and S Livingstone Ltd., 1968.
9. Furste, W., Skudder, P. A., and Hampton, O. P., Jr.: The evolution of prophylaxis against tetanus from the civil war to the present. Bull. Amer. Coll. Surg., *52*:(5), 227 passim, 1967.
10. Glass, T. G., Jr.: Cortisone and immediate fasciotomy in the treatment of severe rattlesnake bite. Tex. Med., *65*:40–47, 1969.
11. Green, W. O., and Adams, T. E.: Mycetoma in the United States. A review and report of seven additional cases. Amer. J. Clin. Path., *42*:75–91, 1964.
12. Hershey, F. B., and Aulenbacher, C. E.: Surgical treatment of brown spider bites. Ann. Surg., *170*:300–308, 1969.
13. Hunter, G. W., Frye, W. W., and Schwartzwelder, J. D.: A Manual of Tropical Medicine. Philadelphia, W. B. Saunders Co., 1966.
14. Kerr, W. F.: Surgery. London, Oxford University Press, 1957.
15. King, M.: Medical Care in Developing Countries. London, Oxford University Press, 1966.
16. Linaweaver, P. G.: Toxic marine life. Mil. Med., *132*:437–442, 1967.
17. McNair, T. J. (ed.): Hamilton Bailey's Emergency Surgery. Baltimore, Williams and Wilkins Co., 1967.
18. Moore, D. C.: Regional Block: A Handbook for Use in the Clinical Practice of Medicine and Surgery. 4th Ed. Springfield, Ill., C. C Thomas, 1971.
19. Shoul, M. I.: Skin grafting under local anesthesia using a new safety razor dermatome. Amer. J. Surg., *112*:959–963, 1966.
20. World Health Organization. Technical Report Series. 321. Expert Committee on Rabies, 5th Report.

29

Surgery and Medicine in the Field

By BRUCE C. PATON, M.R.C.P. (Ed.), F.R.C.S. (Ed.)
and BEN EISEMAN, M.D.

INTRODUCTION

The average physician is poorly prepared to play an effective role in assisting in the rescue of a patient hurt or seriously ill in a remote area. Increase in the number of people seeking solitude and recreation in remote areas provides a concomitant increase in the frequency with which a physician lacking any prior

training may be asked to perform in this unaccustomed milieu.

It is not possible to estimate how many people in the United States walk, climb or camp in the mountains, but more than two million visitors came to the Rocky Mountain National Park, Colorado in 1968. A distressing majority are neither trained for preventing injury nor prepared for the unexpected event

TABLE 29–1   Mountain Rescue
Association, 1967

Active membership (approx.)	600
Number of rescues	236
Man hours spent on rescues	36,877
Number of victims killed	73
Number of victims injured	290

which so often precedes an accident. The American Alpine Club annually records and analyzes fatal accidents that occur in the mountains of the United States and Canada. Between 1951 and 1966 there was an average of 14 deaths per year. It was found that 421 of the 936 recorded accidents occurred to people without appreciable previous mountaineering experience. Inexperience compounds dangers that already exist.

The Mountain Rescue Association, a group of dedicated volunteers organized on a regular basis, records and analyzes their own experience annually. Table 29–1 summarizes their statistics for 1967.

Although most people probably go to the mountains or seashore, the deserts, canyonlands and rivers all attract large numbers of vacationers. The types of accidents and the possible complications depend upon all aspects of the environment including terrain, temperature, season and remoteness from and availability of help.

CALL FOR HELP AND EARLY ORGANIZATION

If disaster is to strike, two principles minimize delay in rescue: (1) All parties should leave a detailed climbing or camping plan with a responsible agency (Forest Service) or friend. (2) No one should make solitary expeditions or climb alone.

These principles are, however, often overlooked. Unnecessary delays occur because it is not recognized when a party is overdue, or the location of a possible accident is only vaguely known.

Time is of the essence in evacuating a casualty. Exposure to wind, rain, cold, and high altitude may enormously complicate even a relatively simple injury. Indeed, cold injury may be fatal to a poorly equipped person immobilized by a simple extremity injury. It must be remembered that cold injury is the product of temperature plus time plus the chill factor (Table 8–1) of wind and humidity. One cold, wet night in the wind at high altitudes may be uncomfortable to a casualty. A second may be lethal. If the accident occurs during winter, these factors are readily obvious to everyone. But even in the summer, temperatures at night at high altitudes may drop to dangerously low levels, especially when combined with strong winds.

The physician should seldom organize the search and rescue operation. This is a job for professionals, who should be called at once. The best trained, equipped, and manned group in the United States is the Mountain Rescue Association which has branches adjacent to most recreation areas. The Forest Service and police usually know how to reach these groups, who maintain a 24-hour, 365-day-a-year watch.

Successful location, care and retrieval of a casualty in a remote area is largely a matter of organization, logistics and discipline. The following brief outline gives the physician an idea of the organization in which he will be involved. By its demands, a search closely resembles a military operation. One person is the Director of the search and rescue. He establishes a base of operations at which he gathers his trained personnel and equipment, and from which he has good communication both with the outside and with the searchers on the site of the accident.

Locating a missing person in a remote area is a fascinating science and art, but is not germane to this discussion, since the physician will probably play no important role in its activation. Details of search and rescue vary as to terrain, weather and available rescue equipment.

Once the injured party is located, a well-equipped and strongly manned contact party is sent to the scene. Unless the physician is himself very fit (and a strong climber), he had best not try to keep up with this initial group, which is apt to keep a quick pace.

Although the purpose of the initial contact group is primarily to assess the injury and the locale of the accident, its members should have splints, bandages and other basic first-aid equipment, as well as sleeping bags, food and warm clothing. Their primary aim is to report back by radio or messenger an accurate assessment of the situation. One or two of its members will then stay with the casualty.

The physician should be close to the Director at the base camp. He should spend his time assuring himself that his equipment is in order and that all means have been prepared for casualty evacuation (by helicopter, sled, litter, horse and so on) and hospitalization.

As soon as the physician is notified of the exact status and location of the casualty, he should set off, taking with him not only the necessary medical equipment, but also his own warm clothes, gloves, parka and sleeping bag, for he may have to spend at least one night with the casualty in an exposed area.

Although it is the Director's responsibility to see that sufficient manpower is sent with the physician to accomplish the task of evacuation, it is well for the physician himself to remember that 10 to 18 men may be required to evacuate each casualty.

HELICOPTER EVACUATION

In the absence of more highly trained personnel, the physician may have to select and prepare a helicopter casualty evacuation site. The following principles should be kept in mind:

(1) Do not risk the life of helicopter personnel by choosing a risky site, if a safe site can be reached by carrying the casualty farther. Unwarranted alarm may overtake the uninitiated under the conditions of a rescue, and unnecessary risks are often urged. Speed of evacuation is not always essential once the condition of the patient is stable.

(2) Ability of a helicopter to land and lift off may be limited at altitudes over 10,000 feet. Factors to be considered are power of the machine available, load and temperature. There is less lift in warm air than in cold.

(3) Size of landing zone. Although a straight vertical ascent requires a clearing no greater than 100 feet on a side, risks increase directly with the surrounding clearing. In general, no area cleared less than 100 yards square should be considered. Low trees or bushes can compromise this minimum, but each encroachment increases the risk, particularly in windy exposed landing zones.

(4) Ground cover. Stumps, boulders, brush and even high grass can interfere or exclude a landing zone. The pilot himself will usually weigh the factors previously mentioned, but the ground party must confirm the safety of the terrain for him.

(5) Recovery while hovering is extremely difficult and should be avoided, especially in windy areas, if the pilot is inexperienced in such a tricky procedure, or when the helicopter is underpowered.

(6) Marking the zone. In wooded terrain, it may be difficult for the pilot to locate the landing zone. Brightly colored parkas are adequate substitutes for the panels used in military medical evacuation operations. Radio communication between ground and air is ideal but not always available in civilian life.

PRINCIPLES OF FIRST-AID

A general scheme for organizing a medical evacuation is given in Figure 29–1.

Forewarned is forearmed. Since re-

TRANSPORTATION   SITE   ACTION

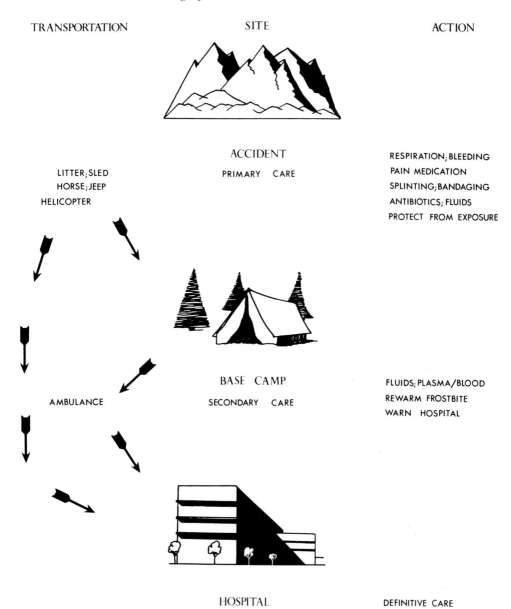

ACCIDENT

PRIMARY   CARE

LITTER;SLED
HORSE;JEEP
HELICOPTER

RESPIRATION; BLEEDING
PAIN MEDICATION
SPLINTING; BANDAGING
ANTIBIOTICS; FLUIDS
PROTECT FROM EXPOSURE

BASE   CAMP

SECONDARY   CARE

AMBULANCE

FLUIDS; PLASMA/BLOOD
REWARM FROSTBITE
WARN HOSPITAL

HOSPITAL   DEFINITIVE CARE

Figure 29-1   Scheme for action to be taken at various sites during evacuation of victim from mountain accident.

ports of accidents are often vague and even erroneous, as accurate a description of the emergency as possible should be obtained before the rescue party starts off from the base. Don't carry splints to a case of appendicitis, and make suitable arrangements for the treatment of the injured after they are brought off the mountain.

The most important principle in handling all problems, both medical and surgical is: "Do the minimum necessary to make the patient safe and comfortable for transportation." If this principle is followed, unnecessary time will not be spent undertaking measures better done at a lower level or under more advantageous circumstances. Do not neglect to make as full an examination as time and circumstances permit. Do not neglect the first-aid of a serious injury because of failure to make an examination. Vital signs should be recorded when the patient is first seen and regularly thereafter, depending upon the injury or illness. A label detailing all medications given and the time of administration should be attached to the patient, especially if the doctor cannot accompany the patient to the hospital.

ENVIRONMENTAL HAZARDS

Injuries and illness in the field usually are a combination of a disease or injury plus the complicating factor of exposure to the elements. The physician obviously must consider both, but for simplicity, hazards of the environment can be identified and means of treatment indicated.

High Altitude Sickness

Campers, climbers and hunters often become ill or injured in high mountains, a complication not often considered by the hospital-based surgeon.

Altitude is unlikely to be of serious consequence below 7000 feet, unless the patient has a pre-existing cardiac or pulmonary lesion. Partial pressure of oxygen in dry air at 5000 feet is about 130 mmHg. Arterial oxygen tension at 5000 feet is 55–75 mmHg. Only above 9000 feet is there a serious threat of hypoxia from altitude per se complicating the problems of the injured.

High altitude sickness itself is a fascinating syndrome which may variously occur at any height above 9000 feet.[1] Although the critical altitude varies in different parts of the world (U.S.A. above 8500 feet; Himalayas and Andes, 11,000 to 12,000 feet), the factors involved are altitude, exercise, conditioning and duration of exposure. During the Chinese invasion into India in 1966 more than 2000 cases occurred in unacclimatized Indian troops rushed from lowlands to the Himalayas.

The manifestations of acute mountain sickness may be primarily respiratory and cardiovascular (dyspnea, cough and pulmonary edema), gastrointestinal (anorexia, nausea, vomiting, abdominal pain), cerebral (headache, giddiness), psychosomatic (insomnia and restlessness), or general (tiredness and weakness). Individual patients may present primarily with one of these groups of symptoms or with a combination of types.

Nausea, anorexia, headache, insomnia and confusion have been recognized for many years by mountain climbers as part of the intrinsic hazards and discomforts of climbing at high altitudes. But it is only in recent years that pulmonary and cardiovascular problems—especially pulmonary edema—have been clearly defined as secondary effects of altitude hypoxia.

Pulmonary edema develops either in those who normally reside at high altitudes, go to lower levels for two or three weeks, then return to the original altitude; or in those who have never previously been at high altitudes and are rapidly transported to high country. In either case, pulmonary edema usually develops within about three days of exposure or re-exposure to altitude. The onset may be acute and explosive with the patient rapidly becoming moribund, or it may be insidious. The patient usually has associated symptoms of mountain sickness, with headache, anorexia, and sometimes oliguria. For two or three nights before the development of severe symptoms, he may experience shortness of breath and coughing and have to sit up in order to regain his breath.

The amount of exertion during the first few days at high altitude does not necessarily determine who will develop symptoms. Some people develop pulmonary edema although sedentary, while others are able to exert themselves without symptoms. Occasional individuals develop edema on repeated occasions.

Circulatory responses vary. Blood

pressure may be higher or lower than normal. The pulse rate may be faster or slower than normal. Total blood volume does not change, but pulmonary blood volume increases as much as 80 per cent, and peripheral blood volume decreases. Pulmonary artery pressure is high, secondary to an increase in precapillary arteriolar resistance, but pulmonary wedge pressures and left atrial pressures are normal.

The treatment of high altitude sickness and high altitude pulmonary edema is based upon three principles: (1) Increase arterial pO_2 by giving oxygen; (2) Decrease pulmonary blood volume by giving diuretics; and (3) Reduce overall activity by rest.

Arterial pO_2 can be increased either by administration of oxygen by face mask or by evacuation of the patient to an altitude lower than 9000 feet. Two to three liters of oxygen per minute may be sufficient to relieve symptoms.

Diuretics have been strongly advocated both for cure of established sickness and prophylactically during the first few days of exposure to high altitude. Furosemide 80 mg twice daily for two to three days on arrival at high altitude may reduce the incidence of severe symptoms. Furosemide may induce a rapid diuresis and relieve symptoms during acute pulmonary edema.

Morphine sulfate 15 mg given intravenously with a diuretic has been found very effective. Morphine and furosemide together may induce a greater diuresis than furosemide by itself. No danger of respiratory depression has been encountered by the use of IV morphine under these circumstances.

If cerebral symptoms are severe and cerebral edema is thought to be present, betamethasone should be given in conjunction with a diuretic. There is no evidence that pulmonary symptoms are helped by steroids.

Activity should be reduced to a minimum. Reduction in bodily activity and evacuation to a lower altitude may, by themselves, result in marked improvement in many patients.

Effect of High Altitude on Fluid and Caloric Requirements

Climbing at high altitudes requires the expenditure of much energy and results in dehydration. Estimates of this dehydration should be taken into account when rehydration with intravenous fluids is attempted. Mountain explorers have found that a fluid intake of 3–4 liters per day is necessary to maintain a urine output of 1500 cc per day. At moderate altitudes of 10,000 to 15,000 feet, caloric requirements for an active climber may be as high as 4500 cc per day. For the victim of an accident, however, the caloric requirements are of secondary importance. Most victims of mountain accidents are healthy and young, and with appropriate indications, can be given 500 to 1000 cc lactated Ringer's intravenously in 60 minutes without fear of overloading the circulation. If the patient has pulmonary edema or a primary cardiac condition, this volume of fluid would be contraindicated.

Avalanche Victims

Occasionally a physician skier will be drafted to join an avalanche rescue team. Usually he is unfamiliar with the problem that he must face. The following precepts are helpful:

Speed in reaching the victim is the essence of success because death is due to suffocation, freezing and blunt injuries. Of victims located within 15 minutes, 85 per cent survive; within 35 minutes, 75 per cent live; and within one hour 55 per cent are saved. This is the golden period and all efforts and even reasonable risks should be taken to reach the victim within one hour. It is well to hurry to the scene, but not to risk the lives of the rescuers two hours after an avalanche.

Density of new snow may be as little as 5 per cent that of water and is thus mostly air.[2] Avalanche snow is usually much more dense, but is reasonably permeable to air. Depending on the type of snow in the slide, the victim may obtain some air for exchange if not too deeply buried.

While the search team looks and probes for the victim, the physician should set up an aid station near the base of the slide area. Once a slide has occurred, there is no immediate danger of another avalanche in the same slide path.

First-aid supplies should include endotracheal tube, an ambu bag or other means of ventilation, splints, warm clothes and intravenous resuscitative solutions. Once set up, the physician and the search Director should locate and prepare a helicopter evacuation area if such is appropriate.

Frostbite[3]

Immediate treatment is influenced by those factors which seriously influence ultimate injury and accentuate tissue damage. Remove wet clothing and socks and replace them with dry clothes from the rescuers' packs. Shelter the victim, because of the additional cooling factor of wind. The chilling effect of wind is related to several factors including the air temperature, wind velocity, the insulating properties of clothing, the activity of the man and the amount of exposed skin. In order, therefore, to reduce the effects of wind, the patient should be sheltered, well-insulated, and completely covered. Contact between the exposed part and wetness or metal greatly accelerates heat loss and increases the likelihood of loss of tissue.

Reflex vasodilatation induced by warming the rest of the body is a good method for restoring circulation in a frozen limb. While the victim is being removed from the scene of the accident, keep the rest of his body as warm as possible. Alcohol induces vasodilatation, but increases heat loss: avoid its use (until the end of the rescue mission)!

The best definitive treatment of frostbite is rapid rewarming in water no hotter than 42°C (107.6°F) after the patient has been brought to a care center or base camp beyond which good transportation is assured. Do not attempt rewarming of a frozen foot in exposed conditions when continued warmth of the part is not assured. Under extreme circumstances, it is possible to walk on a frozen foot. Walking on a thawed-out painful foot, too swollen for a boot, is an impossibility.

Generalized Body Hypothermia

In addition to frostbite, a localized condition, accident victims often develop generalized body hypothermia. General body hypothermia may be lethal. If body temperature falls below 27°C cardiac arrhythmias and, ultimately, ventricular fibrillation ensue. Atrial fibrillation is the commonest arrhythmia to develop first, followed by conduction disturbances, ventricular arrhythmias, and ventricular fibrillation.

There have been several well-recorded cases of patients who survived body temperatures below 25°C. Why ventricular fibrillation did not develop in these individuals is not known.

The treatment of hypothermia is rewarming. Blankets, hot water bottles, heating pads or warm water tubs are all suitable agents. Cold tissues are, paradoxically, more easily burned than normothermic tissues. Therefore, great care should be taken to ensure that the temperature differential between the patient and the rewarming modality is not more than 10°C, and the maximum temperature for the rewarming medium should be 40°C (104°F). When cold tissues are rewarmed, a metabolic acidosis may develop as acidic metabolic end products re-enter the circulation. Obviously, acidosis cannot be detected in the field, although it may be suspected. In the hospital, appropriate measurements should be made of blood gases and other acid-base parameters and the acidosis treated with sodium bicarbonate.

Cardiac arrhythmias usually disappear upon rewarming and do not require specific treatment. If atrial fibrillation should persist at a rapid rate, digitalis would be indicated.

Lightning[4]

Approximately 160 people die each year in the United States after being struck by lightning. Most are either golfers or mountain climbers. The former usually either take refuge under a tree or are caught in the open after refusing to quit when a lightning storm approached. Mountaineers are usually caught on an exposed ridge where their bodies act as a lightning rod. Approaching lightning danger is often predicted by Saint Elmo's Fire — audible and visible discharge of electricity from hair or metal equipment. Given such warning, the mountaineer or sportsman must quickly minimize his exposure. Mountaineers must familiarize themselves with such techniques. Wherever the threat occurs, a group must disperse so one bolt cannot immobilize potential assistance.

Lightning kills immediately by cardiac arrest and injures by burning. It consists of an enormous electrical discharge (millions of volts and up to 20,000 amps) through the atmosphere into the victim's body. If the victim is standing near a tree which is struck the electrical charge may jump from the tree to the victim. The repulsive charge thus built up may throw the victim many feet.

Immediate therapy consists of external cardiac massage and artificial ventilation. Cardiac rhythm should be determined electrocardiographically as soon as possible and the patient defibrillated if indicated. Because many victims are young and without underlying vascular disease, the possibilities of resuscitation are good and attempts to restore a normal cardiac action should be continued for at least one hour.

Associated injuries include temporary deafness, often with a perforated ear drum, confusion or even coma, arterial spasm of major vessels in the legs where the discharge travelled up the legs, burns, and late appearance of cataracts.

The arterial spasm will usually disappear spontaneously, but we have used both heparin and sympathetic blocks on occasion. Seldom is either necessary.

Lightning victims with cardiac arrhythmias should be hospitalized and monitored for several days, as would be routine after an acute myocardial infarction.

Heat Stroke

Unacclimatized, unfit or obese persons working or exercising in a warm, humid atmosphere are liable to heat stroke or heat injury. Such patients lose salt and water, become unable to maintain a normal temperature and develop hyperthermia. Presenting symptoms may be confusion, headache, dizziness and hyperthermia. Occasionally, if seriously hypotensive, the skin may be cool, but usually the victim is flushed.

The physiologic defect is counteracted by rest, placement in a cool environment, removal of warm clothing, and cold sponging to reduce body temperature. An intravenous infusion of physiologic saline solution or one-sixth molar lactate solution should be started immediately through two large-gauge needles, one in each arm. One to two liters administered to an otherwise healthy adult within 30–45 minutes will usually restore adequate intravascular sodium and water, overcome hypotension and restore urine output. In severe cases, there may be oliguria or even renal shutdown.

Following initial resuscitation, heat stroke victims may complain of headache and should be hospitalized or otherwise closely observed to confirm that a good urine output is maintained.

Drowning

The problem of treating a person drowned in either fresh or salt water is one of clearing the airway and establishing artificial ventilation. As with suffocation beneath an avalanche, duration of hypoxia must be minimized. Although victims of fresh water drowning absorb water from their alveoli and develop detectable hemolysis, anoxia — not hemolytic anemia — is the prime cause of death.

The physician should be ready to administer artificial respiration by mouth-to-mouth or mechanical means (ambu bag) using 100 per cent oxygen if available. Endotracheal intubation is ideal to allow better delivery of positive pressure ventilation, to avoid gastric distention from air forced into the mouth and to improve endotracheal suction. Ideally, some means of suction should be available to remove airway secretions.

A blanket or warm clothes should be available, since most victims of drowning feel very cold after resuscitation.

Snake Bite

Any camping group or expedition passing through snake-infested country should be familiar with the types of snake likely to be encountered.

Space is insufficient to detail all the many types of snake likely to be encountered throughout the world, or even in North America. Certain principles, however, can be stated briefly and should be kept in mind when treating snake bite.[5]

Specific antivenin should always be used whenever toxic symptoms are of sufficient severity to endanger life or limb. Because antivenin is made from horse serum and carries a risk of allergic reactions, if symptoms are not severe, judgment must be used in deciding whether the risks of using horse serum are justified. But in severe cases of envenomation specific antivenin must be used, and other subsidiary forms of treatment such as tourniquets, incision and suction are inadequate substitutes.

The use of cold has been widely advocated as treatment for rattlesnake bite but ill-advised and prolonged immersion of bitten limbs in ice water may result in greater tissue loss than from the snake bite alone. Ice packs, immersion in ice water or similar treatment should be used only as a temporary expedient until adequate treatment with antivenin is available. Incision, suction and tourniquets are of limited use and may be either inadequate or dangerous, depending upon the care, knowledge and energy with which they are applied.

Most venoms are absorbed via the lymphatics; lymphatic flow rates are increased by motion and therefore immobilization of the bitten limb reduces the rate of absorption of venom.

In the United States, polyvalent crotalid antivenin (Wyeth) is suitable for treating the bites of rattlesnakes, moccasins, and copperheads. It will keep for many years at room temperature.

The dose of antivenin depends upon the severity of symptoms and the response to treatment. About three to five 20 cc vials are necessary for treating an average bite in an adult. Intramuscular administration is best, but the intravenous route may be used in a severe emergency with the additional administration of hydrocortisone 100 mg to diminish chances of an allergic reaction.

SURGICAL AND MEDICAL EMERGENCIES

Nontraumatic surgical emergencies, such as appendicitis and ruptured peptic ulcer, may occasionally occur in the field. Immediate evacuation to a hospital is mandatory. Nasogastric intubation and the administration of intravenous fluids are within the realm of first-aid management, especially if the patient has been vomiting, is dehydrated, and faces a litter trip of several hours duration.

First-Aid Care of Injuries

Shock

The clinical manifestations of shock are the same, even at moderately high altitudes, as at sea level. Resting pulse rates are higher at altitudes and the response of the pulse rate to work is greater at altitude than at sea level. Therefore, in a resting man at a high altitude a rapid pulse may not have the same significance as in a patient seen in the Emergency Room. Low blood pressure, very rapid pulse, pallor, clammy sweating, and vasoconstriction have, however, their usual significance.

Above 10,000 feet the resting respiratory rate may be increased by 2–4 breaths per min. Hyperventilation and dyspnea should, therefore, be regarded as important signs of respiratory difficulty.

Soft Tissue Injuries

Do not attempt to debride or repair soft tissue injuries. Gross contamination by wood, grass or rock fragments can be dealt with immediately, provided that no more than a few minutes are taken for this task. Stop hemorrhage by pressure, or rarely, by the application of a hemostat and ligature. Leave ligature ends long for subsequent identification of the bleeding point. A dry, sterile dressing should be applied and copiously bandaged in position. If hemorrhage is likely during the evacuation, try to arrange the patient in such a way that bandages can be examined for blood with minimum disturbance.

Fractures

Limbs. All limb fractures should be splinted using available materials, inflatable or cardboard splints. Do not set fractures except to obtain roughly correct alignment of the limb. Check circulation in the distal part of the limb before and after applying the splint. If compromise of the circulation is a possibility (i.e., with a supracondylar fracture of the humerus or injuries around the knee), keep the distal part of the limb available for frequent inspection. Overinflated inflatable splints may diminish circulation, especially if it is already decreased for other reasons. Fractures of the major bones, such as the femur, may be associated with blood loss of 2 to 3 liters into the soft tissues of the limb. Blood loss of this magnitude should be recognized in making calculations for fluid replacement and may be as great a cause for shock as exposure or exhaustion. If a patient has both a skull laceration and a fractured femur, don't forget that more blood may be lost into the thigh than through the more obvious scalp wound.

Skull. A careful evaluation should be made of:

1. State of consciousness, including a history of lucid periods, deepening or lightening of coma.
2. Obvious neurological defects, such as hemiplegia, speech difficulties, gross sensory and motor loss.
3. Scalp and oropharyngeal lacerations. Do they communicate with intracranial contents? Is the airway compromised now or likely to be compromised by subsequent swelling?
4. Bleeding or escape of CSF from ears or nose.

Lacerations of the scalp may bleed profusely. Bleeding can be controlled by finger pressure around the bleeding area, compressing the scalp against the cranium.

Closed skull fractures require no special management and may not be amenable to superficial clinical diagnosis. Compound fractures should not be explored, but should be copiously dressed. The circular "doughnut" hematoma that sometimes develops after a blow on the head may be mistaken for a depressed fracture. Resist the temptation to elevate the "depressed" fragment.

Mannitol or urea to diminish cerebral swelling is not indicated. Decadron (dexamethasone sodium phosphate) 4 mg, IM or IV, may be valuable for the reduction of edema in severe cerebral injury.

Unconscious or semiconscious victims should be transported in the semi-prone position, with constant attention to maintenance of the airway, and with vigilance for the possibility of vomiting. During transportation the head should be kept uphill to reduce intracranial pressure and diminish bleeding from scalp lacerations.

Spinal Column. Notice areas of local pain and make a careful examination for motor and sensory deficits. Because of the obvious danger of neurologic complications, actual or suspected victims of vertebral column injuries must be moved with maximum care. Keep the patient as straight as possible. No advantage is gained by adopting positions of flexion or extension. Movement must be avoided during transportation. A fixation collar is valuable in suspected cervical injuries. If the patient is already paraplegic and a prolonged evacuation of several hours is anticipated, a urethral catheter should be passed and attached to any convenient drainage system, or clamped and released every two hours. An inflatable splint makes a convenient urine container.

Chest Injuries

Simple chest injuries such as fractures of one or two ribs require only support of the patient in the litter and medication for pain.

Pneumothorax is treated by needle aspiration, which can be repeated as necessary. Open sucking wounds of the chest should be plugged by a large, bulky dressing made as airtight as possible.

In all cases of serious thoracic injury, additional oxygen may not only be valuable, but life-saving, especially if ventilation is impaired and the accident has occurred at high altitude.

Abdominal Injuries

Little can be done for closed abdominal injuries. Fluids and volume expanders must be given intravenously if the patient is in shock because of a ruptured viscus or blood loss. Give only the minimal doses of narcotics needed to make transportation comfortable.

Penetrating abdominal injuries should be covered by a sterile dressing. Cover bowel that is visible in the wound with Vaseline gauze or a saline-soaked sponge. Intact, healthy unperforated bowel should be washed with sterile saline and replaced in the abdominal cavity. The wound should be covered securely by a large dressing to prevent repeated evisceration. Bowel left protruding from a small wound can become strangulated by the abdominal wall. Give large doses of antibiotics. If the bowel is gangrenous or has ruptured, do not replace it within the peritoneum. Keep it exteriorized and covered adequately by dressings.

Vascular Injuries

Hemorrhage must be stopped by pressure. Clamping or ligation is advisable only if a large bleeder is clearly seen. Even large vessels, such as the brachial artery, may stop bleeding if completely torn across. It is, however, unsafe to transport someone with the proximal end of a large artery unsecured even if no bleeding is occurring from it. The vessel should be ligated and the ends of the ligature left long for future identification.

Speed is essential in the evacuation of patients with major vascular injuries. Much can be done surgically to restore blood flow, but time is important and the sooner definitive care is given the better are the chances of recovery.

CARDIAC EMERGENCIES

Angina or frank myocardial infarct will frequently first occur in the middle-aged, overweight, unconditioned, enthusiastic, occasional outdoorsman when in a remote area. The relief of pain and hypoxia is a prime consideration. Oxygen should be administered, especially at altitudes above 5000 feet, and narcotics should be used to relieve pain. It is safer to use small frequent doses of narcotics rather than large doses which may depress respiration.

Occasional patients develop cardiac arrhythmias in response to exertion and hypoxia. If atrial fibrillation develops with a rapid ventricular response the patient should be digitalized and evacuated by means other than walking. If the patient has anginal pain and an arrhythmia suspected of being ventricular in origin, Xylocaine (lidocaine) 50–100 mg, IV, followed by 0.5–1.0 mg per min. in an IV drip may be life-saving by averting ventricular tachycardia.

In all patients with cardiac symptoms exertion should be reduced to an essential minimum.

DRUGS AND SUPPLIES

The list of drugs in Table 29–2 is based upon the most likely requirements, both medical and surgical. Table 29–3 lists essential supplies. Because the doctor will almost certainly have to carry his own supplies, nothing is gained by too elaborate a kit. All drugs should be clearly labeled with name and dose so that a nonmedical rescue worker could administer them if necessary.

Drugs

Narcotics. Morphine or Demerol. Morphine is the better analgesic, but may induce vomiting, undesirable in a patient already nauseated from altitude. Small doses intravenously at frequent intervals are preferable to larger doses intramuscularly or subcutaneously, especially in cold, shocked patients. The recommended dose of morphine sulfate is 5 mg IV or 10 mg IM, and for Demerol, 80 to 100 mg IM. The doses for children are morphine sulfate 1 mgm/10 kg and Demerol 1 mgm/1 kg, both IM.

Antibiotics. Wide-spectrum antibiotics capable of being given intramuscularly. Alternatives should be carried, because of frequent allergies to penicillin.

Tranquilizers, Antiemetic. Nausea and vomiting are common at high altitudes and after injury. Chlorpromazine (25–50 mg IM) is effective in reducing nausea and as a general tranquilizer. Given intravenously, chlorpromazine induces vasodilatation and hypotension

TABLE 29–2   DRUGS AND MEDICATIONS

Morphine, Demerol	Digitalis, aminophylline
Chlorpromazine	Isuprel, nitroglycerine
Barbiturate,	Adrenaline,
chloralhydrate	antihistamine
Dilantin, dexamethasone	Aspirin, Darvon
Penicillin, tetracycline	50 per cent glucose
Lactated Ringer's,	pHisohex
dextran 70	Diuretic, Furosemide
Lomotil	Water purifying tablets
Xylocaine	Furacin gauze
Sunburn ointment	

TABLE 29–3   BASIC SUPPLIES

Ace bandages	Bandaids
Sterile dressings	Adhesive tape
Safety pins	Triangular bandages
Hemostats	Scissors
Note pad and pencil	Oral thermometer
Stethoscope	Clinical thermometer
	Sphygmomanometer

Razor blades or sterile scalpel blades
IV fluid administration sets
Disposable syringes, needles
Instant soups, bouillon
Small mountain stove, fuel, pan, matches, flashlight

and should not be given to patients in shock unless adequate intravenous fluid replacement is available.

Cardiac Drugs. Digoxin acts within 30 to 45 minutes after intravenous administration. The total digitalizing dose for a previously undigitalized patient is 0.75 mg to 1.25 mg IV. An initial dose of 0.5 mgm IV can safely be given to adults and repeated within four hours.

Diuretics may be of value in a patient with pulmonary edema, especially if several hours are likely to elapse before evacuation to a lower altitude. Furosemide 80 mg IV has been shown to be of value.

Nitroglycerine is indicated for ischemic myocardial pain.

Xylocaine (lidocaine) may occasionally be of great value in treating ventricular arrhythmias (see Cardiac Emergencies earlier).

Anticonvulsant. Convulsions may occur after head injuries. The development of convulsions during a difficult evacuation might obviously be hazardous to patient and rescuer alike. Dilantin is the most effective anticonvulsant and does not depress respiration. The dose is 150 mg to 250 mg IV at a rate not greater than 50 mg per min.

Fluids. Fluids are heavy to carry, but may be life-saving. The most useful fluid for intravenous use is lactated Ringer's solution. Its use presents neither problems of sensitivity nor bleeding complications. It is a safe temporary blood volume expander and simultaneously

TABLE 29–4 Items for Physician-
Climber's Pack on Major
Mountain Expedition

pHisohex in small container
Dexedrine, 12 pills
Blistex, 1 tube
Nevafil ointment, 1 tube
Bandaids, 25
Dial soap, 1 bar
Moleskin for blisters, 12 × 12
Adhesive tape, one 2″ roll
Darvon compound (65 mgm), 15
Zinc oxide, 1 tube
Lasix (Furosemide), 1 amp, w/ 5 cc syringe and
 20g needle
4 × 4 bandage, 2 packages of 2
Lomotil, 30
Neosporin, ophthalmic ointment, 1 tube
Gelusil, 10 tablets
Vibramycin, 7 tablets
Pen V-K, 250 mgm #28
Ornade, #20 decongestant
Humatin (puromomycin), 16 tablets
Barbiturate (Seconal, gr 1½), 12
Chloralhydrate (500 mgm), 12 (or other sleeping
 pill as per individual choice)

restores extravascular deficits in dehydrated patients.

Dextran 70 is a better plasma volume
expander than Ringer's solution, but as
an "all purpose" fluid, the latter is preferable. None of the physiologic intravenous solutions is of high enough concentration to inhibit freezing at
temperatures likely to be encountered
during a winter rescue mission. If the
fluid freezes, it can be thawed by putting
it inside the clothing of a rescuer.

Basic Supplies

Bandages, dressings, tape, etc., considered necessary are listed in Table 29–
4. Numbers, quantities and doses are not
given because these may vary with individual requirements. The list should
serve as a checklist for anyone preparing
a first-aid supply kit.

MAJOR EXPEDITIONS

Medical logistic support for a major
expedition requires the thought, planning
and presence of an expert climber and
physician. Surprisingly little is written on
the subject. Lessons learned in support
of such expeditions involving dozens of
men, isolated for many weeks, can be
applied to planning for less pretentious
outings. Medical needs of an expedition
are analogous to those embarking on
space travel, both as to scope and weight
restriction.

Individual packets should be bound in
rugged plastic bags, small enough to fit
into each man's pack. Packaging should
be color coded and each item should be
available without destroying the packaging of the remaining items. Brief indications and dosage should be included with
each drug. Resupply should be from the
expedition's major medical source. All
antibiotics can be kept in one bottle with
color code directions on the outside.

The items suggested for the climber's
pack are listed in Table 29–4. Much of
this equipment is dispensed, en route, to
porters and local population.

Table 29–5 lists the presterilized and
double-packed surgical equipment packs
necessary for a major expedition.

References

1. Singh, I., Khanna, P. K., Srivastava, M. C., Lal,
 M., Roy S. B., and Subramanyam, C. S. V.:
 Acute mountain sickness. N. Eng. J. Med.,
 280:175–184, 1969.
2. Snow Avalanches. Handbook of Forecasting
 and Control Measures. U.S. Department of
 Agriculture Handbook No. 194. Washington,
 D.C., U.S. Government Printing Office,
 1968.
3. Washburn, B.: Frostbite: What it is—How to
 prevent it—Emergency treatment. N. Eng. J.
 Med., *266*:974–989, 1962.
4. Taussig, H. B.: "Death" from lightning and the
 possibility of living again. Amer. Sci.,
 57:306–316, 1969.
5. Paton B. C.: Treatment of snake-bite In Kyle,
 J. (ed.): Pye's Surgical Handicraft. Bristol,
 John Wright and Sons, 1969.
6. Wilkerson J. A. (ed.): Medicine for Mountaineering. Seattle, Washington, The Mountaineers, 1967.

TABLE 29–5 SURGICAL PACKS FOR A MAJOR EXPEDITION

Small Instruments × 3
Size 8 gloves, 3 pairs
Eye drape, 1
Small curved clamp, 2
Suture pack, 4/0 silk, 2
Suture pack, 2/0 chromic gut, 2
4/0 silk on curved cutting needle, 6
Suture scissors, 1
Adson pickups, 1
Pickups with teeth, 1
Knife handle, disposable, 3
Bard-Parker #15 blades, 3
Bard-Parker #11 blades, 3
Needle holder, 1

Chest Tube Tray
5 cc syringe, 1
Size 8 gloves, 2 pairs
Trochar, 1
Curved Kelly, 2
Small eye drape, 1
Chest tube with Heimlich valve
Suture scissors, 1
Needle holder, 1
4/0 silk on cutting needle, 1
Vaseline gauze, 2 strips
4 × 4 gauze, 4 packages
50 cc plastic syringe with threeway stopcock
Disposable scalpel handle with blades

Tracheostomy Set
Eye drape, 1
#34 Portex cuffed tube, 1
#36 Portex cuffed tube, 1
Bard-Parker #15 blade with appropriate handle, 1
Curved mosquito clamp, 2
Curved Kelly clamp, 1
Trachea hook, 1 (or towel clip)
Army-Navy retractor, 2
Trachea spreader, 1
Allis forceps, 1
4/0 silk on a curved cutting needle, 2
4/0 silk suture pack, 1
#14 red French catheter, 1
4 × 4 flats, 8
5 cc syringe with #20 1½ inch needle, 1

Neurosurgical Pack
Plastic disposable razor with blade, 1
#10 Bard-Parker blade with appropriate handle, 1
Eye drape
Hemostats, small and curved, 2
Straights, 3/0 silk suture pack, 1
4/0 silk on a curved Kelly needle, 2
3/0 chromic on tapered needle
Duroclips, 2
Silver nitrate cautery sticks, 4
Trephine (not drill), hard type, 1

Emergency Laparotomy Set
Disposable paper drape set, 1
Vidrape, 1
Abdominal lap pads, 12
Brush, detergent-impregnated scrubbing, 1

Sponges, 4 × 4, 24
Knife handle, Bard-Parker #3, 2
Knife blades, Bard-Parker #10, 2
Knife blades, Bard-Parker #11, 2
Knife blades, Bard Parker #15, 2
Clamps, towel clips, 4
Clamps, hemostat, Crile, 6
Clamps, curved Kelly, 4
Clamps, Mayo-Robson, GI, 10 inch, 2
Clamps, Babcock, 2
Needle holders, Mayo Hegar, 8 inches, 1
Needle holders, Crile-Wood, light, 6 inches, 1
Retractors, Deaver, medium, 2
Retractors, Harrington, 1
Pickup forceps, without teeth, medium, 1
Pickup forceps, without teeth, long, 1
Pickup forceps, two teeth, Adson, 1
Scissors, suture, 1
Scissors, tissue, 1
Scissors, Metzenbaum, 1
Sutures, silk, 3/0, precut, 6
Sutures, silk, 4/0, tapered needle, 3
Sutures, silk, 5/0, tapered needle, 3
Sutures, silk, 1/0, tapered needle, 3
Sutures, chromic gut, 2/0, dispensing reel, 3
Sutures, chromic gut, 3/0, dispensing reel, 3
Sutures, chromic gut, 2/0, tapered needle, 4
Needles, assorted pack, 1

Anesthesia Set
Syringes, 2 cc, 2
Syringes, 5 cc, 2
Syringes, 10 cc, 2
Spinal needles, 22 g, 2
Needles, 25 g, 2
10% dextrose, 30 cc
Pontocaine 1%
Xylocaine 1%
Procaine 1%
Epinephrine, 1:1000
Towels, 18″ × 27″, − 4

Urinary Catheterization Tray
Foley catheters, three sizes, 5 cc bag
Lubricant
Towels, 18″ × 27″, 2
Syringe, 5 cc, 1
Clamp, catheter, 1

General Supplies
Syringes, re-usable, glass
Needles, re-usable, all metal
Towels, drapes
Gloves, sterile, 7½ and 8
Solution for skin preparation
Solution for cold sterilization of instruments
Pan for boiling instruments
Presterilized commercially available packed kits
    for urinary catheterization, spinal tap, etc. May
    be preferable to above listed items, but these
    cannot be resterilized.
Dental instruments — syringes, local anesthetic and
    extraction forceps

Index

Note: Numbers in *italics* indicate pages containing illustrations; numbers in **bold-face** indicate pages containing tables. Inclusive page numbers are given for chapters only.